ENCYCLOPEDIA
OF
BIOSTATISTICS

ENCYCLOPEDIA
OF
BIOSTATISTICS

Volume 3
H–MEA

Editors-in-Chief

PETER ARMITAGE

University of Oxford, UK

THEODORE COLTON

Boston University, USA

John Wiley & Sons
Chichester • New York • Weinheim • Brisbane • Singapore • Toronto

Copyright © 1998 John Wiley & Sons Ltd,
        Baffins Lane, Chichester,
        West Sussex PO19 IUD, England

    National   01243 779777
    International (+44) 1243 779777
    e-mail (for orders and customer service enquiries): cs-books@wiley.co.uk
    Visit our Home Page on http://www.wiley.co.uk
            or http://www.wiley.com

A website containing full descriptive details of the *Encyclopedia of Biostatistics*
can be accessed on the following URL–http://www.wiley.co.uk/eob/

Reprinted with corrections April 1999

Other Wiley Editorial Offices

John Wiley & Sons, Inc., 605 Third Avenue,
New York, NY 10158-0012, USA

WILEY-VCH Verlag GmbH, Pappelallee 3,
D-69469 Weinheim, Germany

Jacaranda Wiley Ltd, 33 Park Road, Milton,
Queensland 4064, Australia

John Wiley & Sons (Canada) Ltd, 22 Worcester Road,
Rexdale, Ontario M9W 1L1, Canada

John Wiley & Sons (Asia) Pte Ltd, 2 Clementi Loop #02-01,
Jin Xing Distripark, Singapore 129809

Library of Congress Cataloging-in-Publication Data

Encyclopedia of biostatistics/editors-in-chief, Peter Armitage,
    Theodore Colton.
        p. cm.
    Includes bibliographical references and index.
    Contents: v. 1. AAL–Cox − v. 2. Cra–G − v. 3. H–Mea − v. 4. Med
-Pre − v. 5. Pri–Sph − v.6. Spi–Z.
    ISBN 0-471-97576-1 (set)
    1. Medical statistics−Encyclopedias. 2. Biometry−Encyclopedias.
I. Armitage, Peter, 1924− . II. Colton, Theodore.
RA409.E53 1998
610′.2′1−dc21   98-10160
                                                                   CIP

British Library Cataloguing in Publication Data

A catalogue record for this book is available from the British Library

ISBN 0 471 975761

Typeset in $9\frac{1}{2}/11\frac{1}{2}$ pt Times by Laser Words, Madras, India
Printed and bound from PostScript files in Great Britain by Bookcraft (Bath) Ltd
This book is printed on acid-free paper responsibly manufactured from sustainable forestry,
in which at least two trees are planted for each one used for paper production.

Editorial Board

Editors-in-Chief

Peter Armitage
2 Reading Road
Wallingford
Oxon
OX10 9DP
UK

Theodore Colton
Department of Epidemiology and
Biostatistics
Boston University School of Public Health
715 Albany Street
Boston, MA 02118-2394
USA

Editors

CATEGORICAL DATA ANALYSIS

Alan Agresti
Statistics Department
University of Florida
204 Griffin-Floyd Hall
Gainsville, FL 32611-8545
USA

INSTITUTIONAL AND HISTORICAL

Douglas G. Altman
ICRF Medical Statistics Group
Centre for Statistics in Medicine
Institute of Health Sciences
PO Box 777, Headington
Oxford OX3 7LF
UK

SURVIVAL ANALYSIS

Per Kragh Andersen
Department of Biostatistics
University of Copenhagen
Blegdamsvej 3
Copenhagen N
DK-2200
Denmark

MULTIVARIATE ANALYSIS

Ralph B. D'Agostino, Sr
Department of Mathematics
Boston University
111 Cummington Street
Boston, MA 02215
USA

HEALTH SERVICES RESEARCH

Paula Diehr
Department of Biostatistics
University of Washington
F-670 Health Sciences Building
Box 357232
Seattle, WA 98195-7232
USA

HUMAN GENETICS

Robert C. Elston
Department of Epidemiology and
Biostatistics
Case Western Reserve University
MetroHealth Medical Center
2500 MetroHealth Drive, R-258
Cleveland, OH 44109
USA

Preface

The first duty of the Editors-in-Chief of a work as ambitious as the *Encyclopedia of Biostatistics* is to define its scope and to explain its purpose. What is it about, and why is it needed?

The scope is easily defined. We use the term "Biostatistics" to denote statistical methods in medicine and the health sciences. This usage is standard in many, if not most, parts of the world, but of course it is etymologically curious: we make no attempt to cover systematically the more general use of statistics in biology, for which the term "Biometry" is perhaps now more widely used. Our scope might have been defined as "Medical Statistics", a term which we avoided as it is sometimes taken to imply a more restricted field than that represented here. The field of biostatistics is indeed wide. We have needed to cover applications in clinical medicine, public health, epidemiology, health services research, demography, genetics, and laboratory studies. We have attempted to provide a very broad coverage of general statistical theory and methodology, which has developed enormously during the last half-century, building on the foundations laid down during the interwar period. Some branches of statistics have been especially stimulated by their applications in medical research, notably the analysis of survival data, which receives especially full treatment in these pages.

Many of the 1208 articles concern topics that might be relevant in investigations in almost any branch of medicine: the design of experiments and observational studies, the problems associated with data collection, the technical aspects of statistical inference, and so on. We have also included many articles concerning specific fields of medicine, such as Communicable Diseases, Neurology, and Ophthalmology. Many articles describe institutions of particular interest to biostatisticians, such as research organizations, professional societies, and journals. Finally, we include biographical memoirs of many statisticians and others, now deceased, who have contributed notably to the theory and practice of biostatistics.

Why, then, is all this information needed? During the last few decades, the use of statistical methods in medical research has grown more rapidly than in any other field of application. Parallel growth has naturally taken place in the numbers of practitioners, in medical schools, hospitals and medical centers, research establishments, government agencies, pharmaceutical firms, and elsewhere. The technical literature also has grown, so that medical applications assume a prominent role in general statistics journals, specialist journals have been founded, and statistical methods are commonly described in research articles in the medical literature. Books have appeared in large numbers, but these necessarily deal broadly with the simpler aspects of the subject, or narrowly with only a part of it. The publishers of this *Encyclopedia*, and the editorial team, took the view that a comprehensive work was overdue, and that it would fulfill a widely recognized need.

There are, of course, other relevant large-scale reference works, notably the *Encyclopedia of Statistical Sciences*, edited by S. Kotz & N.L. Johnson (Executive Editor C.B. Read), published in 9 Volumes by John Wiley & Sons (1982–1988, with a Supplement Volume in 1989 and Update Volumes currently in the course of publication). This highly important work has served as an inspiration to us, and we have followed many of the design features adopted by its publisher and editors. However, the present *Encyclopedia* is not intended as in any way a competitor to its forerunner, but should rather be regarded as complementary to it. The *Encyclopedia of Statistical Sciences (EoSS)* provides coverage in considerable depth for virtually the whole theory of statistics and probability, with much detail concerning the methodology of statistical analysis. The *Encyclopedia of Biostatistics (EoB)* also aims at a wide coverage of general statistical theory, but usually in less depth than the *EoSS*, and with some emphasis on topics of practical application. Secondly, the *EoSS* covers applications in virtually every direction, in the physical, biological, and social sciences, so that medical applications form merely one category amongst many. In the *EoB* we concentrate on the technical and practical aspects of biostatistics in what we believe is a comprehensive way. Thus, the two works overlap in their coverage, but each contains material extending far beyond the scope of the other. For instance, readers of the present work who wish to learn more about some of the more theoretical topics are likely to find the *EoSS* particularly helpful.

An earlier predecessor is the *International Encyclopedia of Statistics* (1978, W.H. Kruskal & J. Tanur, eds, Free Press, New York) based on the *International Encyclopedia of the Social Sciences* (1968, D.L. Sill, ed., Macmillan and Free Press, New York). We have made use of various other biographical and lexicographic works, and have found the *Cambridge Dictionary of Statistics in the Medical Sciences* (1995, B.S. Everitt, Cambridge University Press, Cambridge) and the *Dictionary of Scientific Biography* (1981, C.C. Gillispie, Scribner New York) particularly useful.

When we were approached by the publishers in 1995 we realized that a work of the magnitude that we believed to be required must necessarily be a highly cooperative enterprise. We defined 17 (later increased to 18) sections of the subject, and sought the appointment of one or more Section Editor for each section. The titles of the sections, and the names of the Section Editors, are listed under Editorial Board (pp. *v–vii*). The sections covered broad types of biostatistical work (clinical trials, epidemiologic studies, clinical epidemiology, vital and health statistics, health services research, laboratory studies, biological models, health surveys and biomedical experiments); medical specialties with statistical applications; human genetics (a discipline with an important role in medicine and a long history of statistical input); particular branches of statistical methodology of special biostatistical interest (statistical models, longitudinal data analysis, multivariate analysis, survival analysis); statistical computing (an essential feature of modern statistical analysis); the general range of statistical theory and methodology, including probability theory; and the institutional and historical topics referred to earlier.

We have ourselves commissioned a number of articles on topics that were not easily assigned to a particular section. These include articles from leaders in the field, giving an overview, invariably from a personal perspective, of a broad range of scholarly work, such as "Biostatistics, Overview" (B.W. Brown, Jr), "Frontiers of Biostatistics" (L.E. Moses & F. Mosteller), and "Statistics, Overview" (D.R. Cox). Likewise, among the articles commissioned by the Section Editors, there are a number that provide a broad perspective of a particular field, many of them being designated with the word "Overview" in the title. Most of these articles contain cross-references to more specialized articles on related topics, and thus may serve the reader as a guide and introduction to the overall coverage of the *Encyclopedia*. A list of these review articles appears on pp. *xv–xvi*.

The Section Editors were responsible for drafting the list of entries, subject of course to later amendment, for the recruitment of contributors, and for the editing and (with others) proofreading of the contributions. Articles were graded according to intended length and level of mathematical detail, again subject to revision as time went on. Whatever success the *Encyclopedia* has is largely due to the sustained efforts and enthusiasm of the Section Editors. In addition to the listed Section Editors, initial planning for the section on Vital and Health Statistics, with recruitment of contributors, was undertaken by K.H. Dunnell, M.P. Coleman and A.J. Fox, of the Office of National Statistics, London, UK; and initial planning of the section on Statistical Models was done by Annette J. Dobson, of the University of Newcastle, New South Wales. We are grateful for their help.

The sections referred to above are ignored in the final presentation of the articles, which is strictly alphabetic. The variety of length and style is obvious. Some of the more theoretical and specialized topics are directed towards the practicing biostatistician, interested in extending his or her command of statistical theory. Other articles deal more directly with practical issues, and have little or no mathematical content. We have aimed to interfere as little as possible with a contributor's individual style, although articles have been reviewed by editors, and occasionally by external referees. Contributors have been encouraged, even in the more mathematical articles, to introduce their topic verbally so that the less mathematical reader can gain some general understanding of it. A few short, unsigned articles have been written by the Editors-in-Chief.

Most of the articles include a list of citations to the scientific literature. Occasionally the contributors have added also a Bibliography of books or articles not directly cited in the text of the article, but useful for additional reading.

We have used various forms of cross-reference. Terms leading directly to other articles appear in bold type on their first occurrence in an article; however, very common terms such as "mean" are not always emboldened in this way. Frequently, the wording in the current article may be slightly different from the title of the article referred to, but the intention will normally be quite clear. Thus, "... a **crossover trial**..." will refer to the article entitled "Crossover Designs". When a direct reference of this sort is not possible, we refer explicitly in parentheses to the intended article; e.g. "... a changeover design (*see* **Crossover Designs**)". Sometimes the first word of emboldened terms in the text will not lead directly to the article's location, but this will be indicated clearly by subsequent terms; for example, "... a **nested case-control study**..." refers to the article entitled "Case-Control Study, Nested". Occasionally, useful additional sources of information, in articles not conveniently referenced in the text, are listed at the end of an article, as "(*See also*...)".

Additionally, and importantly, we include in the alphabetic list of entries 1477 terms, cross-referenced to specific articles.

No work of this sort can be wholly error-free. We and our production colleagues have tried to eliminate as many errors as possible. We should greatly appreciate notification of any remaining errors – technical, factual, or typographic – which we may be able to remove in future versions of this project.

Our predominant impression, on coming to the end of this collaborative effort, is of the unfailing enthusiasm and good nature of everyone involved. We have mentioned our debt to the Section Editors. Contributors also have responded to our cajoling with good humor, and have been willing, when asked, to modify their original intentions to comply with the overall plan. The project was initiated by Helen Ramsey, of John Wiley & Sons, and that she has been able to see her vision made manifest within a little over three years is in very large measure due to her assiduity, tact, and clear sense of direction. We are grateful to her, and to many of her colleagues at Chichester, notably Juliet Booker and Sharon Clutton, for helping to guide our progress throughout the various stages of the project, and tactfully keeping us up to schedule. We should like to acknowledge the generous support from John Wiley & Sons throughout our work on this project. From the outset, our publishers have supported technical computer and communication activities, and clerical administrative needs, and have also provided funding for several of our meetings as Editors-in-Chief as well as our meetings with the Section Editors.

Our thanks are given to Suzanne Thompson, of Boston University, who assisted most ably with file-management throughout the project. We thank also David Gagnon, of Boston University, who was extremely helpful in developing the computerization of entries, which proved invaluable in the management of the project and in providing a basis for the system of cross-referencing. John and Celia Hall joined the project as Managing Editors and have played a major part also in distributing, correcting, and collating proofs. The Section Editors received valuable help from many individuals; in particular they would like to thank Diane Ames, LeiLane D'Agostino, Leslie Powers, Heidy Kwan Russell, Denise Tanner, and Liza Thong.

For our part, we have greatly enjoyed our role in this remarkable enterprise. We have learnt much from the articles that we have read and edited, and our knowledge of the field has greatly increased over these past three years. Clearly, the amount of material we have read is far beyond our powers of retention, so we can make no claim to have achieved an encyclopedic knowledge of biostatistics. We have, however, obtained a good grasp of where to find information on virtually any aspect of our field in the *Encyclopedia of Biostatistics*. We hope that readers who become familiar with these volumes will similarly attain this ability. That we have been able to devote so much time to the *Encyclopedia* is a tribute most of all to the patience and understanding cooperation of our wives, Phyllis Armitage and Carolyn Colton, and, indirectly, that of our families. To them, as to our technical colleagues, we offer our deep thanks.

Peter Armitage
Wallingford, UK

Theodore Colton
Boston, USA

Editors-in-Chief

1997

Review Articles

Several articles in the *Encyclopedia of Biostatistics* provide broad reviews of important branches of the subject or areas of application. We give here a selected list of such review articles, some of which are designed by the term "Overview". The selection is admittedly arbitrary, and the reader may well encounter other articles of this type that are not included in the list. Most of these articles contain cross-references to more specialized articles dealing with specific topics, as well as references to the scientific literature. The list will, we hope, serve as a rapid index to review articles on the main components of biostatistics, and should provide the reader with an immediate impression of the extensive coverage of the *Encyclopedia*.

CATEGORICAL DATA ANALYSIS
  Categorical Data Analysis
  Contingency Table
  Mantel–Haenszel Methods
  Polytomous Data
  Quantal Response Models

CLINICAL EPIDEMIOLOGY
  Administrative Databases
  Clinical Epidemiology
  Pharmacoepidemiology, Overview
  Screening, Overview

CLINICAL TRIALS
  Clinical Trials, Overview
  Data and Safety Monitoring
  History of Clinical Trials
  Meta-Analysis of Clinical Trials

COMPUTATION
  Computer-Intensive Methods
  Graphical Displays
  Software, Biostatistical

DESIGN OF EXPERIMENTS AND SAMPLE SURVEYS
  Experimental Design
  Missing Data
  Sample Surveys

DISEASE MODELING
  Epidemic Models, Deterministic
  Epidemic Models, Stochastic
  Image Analysis and Tomography
  Mathematical Biology, Overview
  Pharmacokinetics and Pharmacodynamics
  Stochastic Processes
  Tumor Incidence Experiments

EPIDEMIOLOGY
  Case–Control Study
  Causation
  Clustering
  Cohort Study
  Confounding
  Environmental Epidemiology
  Geographical Analysis

Acronyms and Abbreviations

AAAS	American Association for the Advancement of Science
AAF	Ascertainment assumption-free method
AC	Available-case analysis
ACF	Autocorrelation function
ACME	Automated Classification of Medical Entities
A&E	Accident and emergency
AES	American Epidemiological Society
AHCPR	Agency for Health Care Policy and Research
AHEAD	Asset and Health Dynamics Among the Oldest-Old
AHP	Analytic hierarchy process
AHSR	Association of Health Services Research
AI	Artificial intelligence
AIC	Akaike Information Criterion
AIDS	Acquired immune deficiency syndrome
AJE	*American Journal of Epidemiology*
ALGOL	Algorithmic language
ALL	Acute lymphocytic leukemia
ALLHAT	Antihypertensive and Lipid-Lowering Treatment to Prevent Heart Attack Trial
ALR	Alternating logistic regression
AMA	American Medical Association
ANCOVA	Analysis of covariance
ANLL	Acute nonlymphocytic leukemia
ANOVA	Analysis of variance
ANP	Analytic network process
ANSI	American National Standards Institute
APC	Annual Patient Census
APDF	Approximate degrees of freedom
APHA	American Public Health Association
APM	Affected-pedigree-member
AQCESS	Automated Quality of Care Evaluation Support System
AR	Attributable risk
ARE	Asymptotic relative efficiency
ARF	Area Resource File
ARFS	Area Resource File System
ARIMA	Autoregressive integrated moving average
ARL	Approximate likelihood ratio
ARMA	Autoregressive moving average

ARS	Adaptive rejection sampling
ART	Anturane Reinfarction Trial
ASA	American Statistical Association
ASH	Averaged shifted histogram
ASN	Average sample number
ASPO	American Society for Preventive Oncology
ASTPM	American Society of Teachers Preventive Medicine
ATBC	Alpha-Tocopherol, Beta Carotene Cancer Prevention Trial
BAN	Best asymptotic normal
BBM	Branching Brownian motion
BBS	Basic stratified samples
BBT	Basal body temperature
BCDDP	Breast Cancer Detection Demonstration Project
BED	Biologically effective dose
BFGS	Broydon–Fletcher–Goldfarb–Shanno algorithm
BHAT	β-Blocker Heart Attack Trial
BIBD	Balanced incomplete block design
BIPF	Bayesian version of IPF
BJP	*British Journal of Psychiatry*
BL	Bilinear models
BLAS	Basic linear algebra subroutines
BLS	Bureau of Labor Statistics
BLUE	Best Linear Unbiased Estimate
BM	Brownian motion
BMDP	Biomedical Data Processing Program
BMI	Body mass index
BMJ	*British Medical Journal*
BPH	Benign prostate hyperplasia
BRFSS	Behavioral Risk Factor Surveillance System
BRR	Balanced Repeated Replication
BSAC	British Society of Antimicrobial Chemotherapy
BSE	Bovine spongiform encephalopathy
BSM	Basic structural model
CABG	Coronary artery bypass graft
CAC	Computer-Assisted Coding
CADI	Computer-Assisted Data Input
CAHRV	Chronome alterations of heart rate variability
CAI	Computer-assisted interviewing
CAPI	Computer-Assisted Personal Interviewing
CAPM	Capital asset pricing model
CAPS	Cardiac Arrhythmia Pilot Study
CARET	Beta-Carotene and Retinol Efficacy Trial
CART	Classification and Regression Trees
CASI	Computer-Assisted Self-Interviewing

CASRO	Council of American Survey Research Organization
CASS	Coronary Artery Surgery Study
CAST	Cardiac Arrhythmia Suppression Trial
CATCH	Child and Adolescent Trial for Cardiovascular Health
CATI	Computer-assisted telephone interviewing
CBA	Cost-benefit analysis
CBER	Center for Biologics Evaluation and Research
CC	Complete-case
CCA	Canonical correlation analysis
CCD	Central Composite Design
CCF	Cross-correlation function
CCNSC	Cancer Chemotherapy National Service Center
CCOP	Community Clinical Oncology Program
CDC	Centers for Disease Control
CDER	Center for Drug Evaluation and Research
CDF	Cumulative distribution function
CDP	Coronary Drug Project
CDR	Communicable Disease Report
CDRH	Center for Devices and Radiological Health
CFSAN	Center for Food Safety and Nutrition
CGF	Child Growth Foundation
CGOP	Cooperative Group Outreach Program
CHAT	Circadian hyper-amplitude tension
CHD	Coronary heart disease
CHF	Congestive heart failure
CHI	Community Health Index
CHW	Castle–Hardy–Weinberg's law
CIOMS	Council of International Organizations of Medical Sciences
CISC	Complex instruction-set computers
CJD	Creutzfeldt–Jakob Disease
CLT	Central limit theorem
CMF	Comparative mortality figure
CMIB	Continuous Mortality Investigation Bureau
CMRR	Capture–mark–release–recapture
COMMIT	Community Intervention Trial for Smoking Cessation
COPSS	Committee of Presidents of Statistical Societies
corr	Correlation
cov	Covariance
CPF	Corner-point feasible
CPMP	Committee of Proprietary Medical Products
CPS	Current Population Survey
CQI	Continuous quality improvement
CRA	Clinical research associate
CRF	Case report form
CRL	Coefficient of racial likeness
CRLB	Cramér–Rao lower bound

CRO	Contract Research Organization
CSF	Cancer slope factor
CSR	Complete spatial randomness
CT	Computed tomography
CTFS	Corneal Transplant Follow-up Study
CTRW	Continuous-time random walk
CTS	Community Tracking Survey
CUSUM	Cumulative sum
CVD	Cardiovascular disease
CVM	Center for Veterinary Medicine
DAWN	Drug Abuse Warning Network
DBCG	Danish Breast Cancer Cooperative Group
DBMS	Database management system
DEERS	Defense Enrollment Eligibility Reporting System
DEF	Double exponential family
DES	Diethylstilbesterol
DESI	Drug Efficacy Study Implementation project
df	Degrees of freedom
DFT	Discrete Fourier transform
DHFS	Diet Heart Feasibility Study
DHHS	Department of Health and Human Services
DHR	Decreasing hazard rate
DHRA	Decreasing hazard rate on the average
DIG	Digitalis Investigation Group
DLT	Dose-limiting toxicity
DMIS	Defense Medical Information System
DMPLE	Discrete maximum penalized likelihood estimator
DNA	Deoxyribonucleic acid
DPCP	Detectable preclinical phase
DRAM	Dynamic RAM
DRG	Diagnosis related group
DSMB	Data and Safety Monitoring Board
DSMC	Data and Safety Monitoring Committee
DSP	Disease Surveillance Point
DVA	Department of Veterans Affairs
E	Expectation
EB	Empirical Bayes
EC/IC	Extracranial/Intracranial Bypass Trial
ECG/EKG	Electrocardiogram
ECMO	Extracorporeal membrane oxygenation therapy
ECOC	Essential Care of Obstetric Complications
ECST	European Carotid Surgery Trial
ECT	Electro-convulsive therapy
EDF	Empirical distribution function

EDF	Equivalent degrees of freedom
EE	Estimating equation
EEC	European Economic Community
EEG	Electroencephalogram
EF	Estimating function
EFSPI	European Federation of Statisticians in the Pharmaceutical Industry
EGG	Electrogastrogram
EM	Expectation-maximization algorithm
EMCOC	Emergency Care of Obstetric Complications
EMEA	European Medicines Evaluation Agency
EMG	Electromyogram
EMODS	Econometric Model of the Dental Sector
ENAR	Eastern North American Region
ENT	Ears, nose, and throat
EOC	Emergency obstetric care
EORTC	European Organization for Research and Treatment of Cancer
EPA	Environmental Protection Agency
EPTRV	Expert Panel on the Theory of Reference Values
ERB	Ethics review board
ERP	Event-related potential
ESRF	End-stage renal failure
ETS	Educational Testing Service
EWE	Experiment-wise error rate
EWMA	Exponentially weighted moving average
FACT	Functional Assessment of Cancer Therapy
FDA	Food and Drug Administration
FDASA	FDA Statistical Association
FEV	Forced expiratory volume
FFQ	Food frequency questionnaire
FFT	Fast Fourier transform
FKPP	Fisher, Kolmogorov, Petrovskii and Piskunov equation
FLM	Fraction of labeled mitosis
fMRI	Functional magnetic resonance imaging
FNF	False negative fraction
FOBT	Fecal Occult Blood Test
FOCE	First-order conditional estimation
FPE	Final Prediction Error criterion
FPF	False positive fraction
FSR	Feedback shift register
FTC	Federal Trade Commission
FVC	Forced vital capacity
FWE	Familywise error rate
GAM	Generalized Additive Model
GBD	Generalized birth-and-death process

GCV	Generalized cross validation
GDP	Gross domestic product
GEE	Generalized estimating equation
GFSR	Generalized feedback shift register
GIS	Geographic information system
GISSIM	Gruppo Italiano per lo Studio della Streptochinasi/Sopravvivenza hell'infarto Miocardio
GLM	Generalized linear model
GLMM	Generalized linear mixed model
GLS	Generalized least squares
GLSE	Generalized least squares estimator
GMC	General Medical Council
GOF	Goodness of fit
GRP	Good review practice
GUSTO	Global Utilization of Streptokinase and Tissue Plasminogen Activator for Occluded Coronary Arteries trial
HAAS	Honolulu Asia Aging Study
HAD	Hospital anxiety and depression
HARE	Hazard regression
HCC	Hepatocellular carcinoma
HCFA	Health Care Financing Administration
HCT	Historical control trial
HCUP-3	Healthcare Cost and Utilization Project
HDFP	Hypertension Detection and Follow-up Program
HEAST	Health Effects Assessment Summary Tables
HH	Hansen–Hurwitz estimator
HI	Hospital Insurance claims
HIP	Health Insurance Plan
HIV	Human immunodeficiency virus
HLA	Human leukocyte antigen gene complex
HMA	Hospital market area
HMM	Hidden Markov model
HMO	Health Maintenance Organization
HNBUE	Harmonic new better than used in expectation
HNWUE	Harmonic new worse than used in expectation
HRSA	Health Resources and Service Administration
HRT	Hormone replacement therapy
HRV	Heart rate variability
HT	Horvitz–Thompson estimator
HUI	Health Utilities Index
HWE	Hardy–Weinberg Equilibrium
HYE	Healthy years equivalent
I MUST	International Marrow Unrelated Search and Transplant Study
IADL	Instrumental Activities of Daily Living
IARC	International Agency for Research against Cancer

IBD	Identity-by-descent
IBS	International Biometric Society
ICC	Intraclass Correlation Coefficient
ICD	International Classification of Diseases
ICH	International Conference on Harmonization
ICIDH	International Classification of Impairments, Disabilities, and Handicaps
ICM	Iterated conditional modes algorithm
ICPM	International Classification of Procedures in Medicine
ICRDB	International Data Bank
IDDM	Insulin-dependent (type I) diabetes mellitus
ID/MS	Isotope dilution/mass spectrometry
IEA	International Epidemiological Association
IEEE	Institute of Electrical and Electronics Engineers
IEF	Industrial Epidemiology Forum
IFCC	International Federation of Clinical Chemistry
IGF-1	Insulin growth factor-1
IHD	Ischemic heart disease
IHR	Increasing hazard rate
IHRA	Increasing hazard rate on the average
IID	Independent and identically distributed random variables
ILCR	Incremental lifetime cancer risk
IMS	Institute of Mathematical Statistics
IMSE	Integrated mean square error
INCLEN	International Clinical Epidemiology Network
IND	Investigational New Drug
IOM	Institute of Medicine
IPA	Independent Practice Association
IPCW	Inverse probability of censoring weighted
IPF	Inverse production functions
IPF	Iterative proportional fitting
IPS	Interpenetrating sampling
IRB	Institutional review board
IRF	Item response function
IRIS	Integrated Risk Information System
IRLS	Iterative reweighted least squares
IRMA	Immunoradiometric assay
IRT	Item response theory
ISC	International Statistical Congress
ISCB	International Society for Clinical Biostatistics
ISI	Indian Statistical Institute
ISI	International Statistical Institute
ISIS	International Studies of Infarct Survival
ISO	International Organization for Standardization
ISPE	International Society for Pharmacoepidemiology
ITT	Intention to treat
IUD	Intrauterine device

IVF	*In vitro* fertilization
IWM	Independence working model
JAMA	*Journal of the American Medical Association*
JASA	*Journal of the American Statistical Association*
JBS	*Journal of Biopharmaceutical Statistics*
JCD	*Journal of Chronic Diseases*
JEM	Job-exposure matrices
JNCI	*Journal of the National Cancer Institute*
JRR	Jackknife Repeated Replication
JRSS	*Journal of the Royal Statistical Society*
LCG	Linear congruential generator
LLN	Laws of large numbers
LMP	Locally most powerful tests
LMS	Least Mean Squares
LOS	Length of stay
LRS	Linear risk score
LRTS	Likelihood ratio test statistic
LS	Least squares
LSD	Latin square design
LSD	Least significant difference
LSHTM	London School of Hygiene and Tropical Medicine
LST	Large-sample theory
MA	Moving average
MAC	*Mycobacterium avium* complex disease
MAD	Mean absolute deviation
MAD	Median absolute deviation
MAE	Mean absolute error
MANOVA	Multiple analysis of variance
MANOVA	Multivariate analysis of variance
MAR	Missing at random
MARS	Multivariate adaptive regression splines
MCA	Medicines Control Agency
MCAR	Missing completely at random
MCBS	Medicare Current Beneficiary Survey
MCEM	Monte Carlo EM
MCF	Mean cumulative function
MCG	Matrix congruential generator
MCG	Multiplicative congruential generator
MCMC	Markov chain Monte Carlo
MCP	Multiple comparison procedure
MDC	Major diagnostic category
MDI	Mutation–deletion–insertion model
MDPIT	Multicenter Diltiazem Post-infarction Trial
MED	Median effective dose

MED	Minimum effective dose
MEPS	Medical Expenditure Panel Survey
MEU	Maximizing expected utility
MFI	Master Facility Inventory
mgf	Moment generating function
MGS	Modified Gram–Schmidt QR algorithm
MI	Multiple imputation
MIC	Minimum inhibitory concentration
MICAR	Medical Information, Classification, and Retrieval
MILIS	Multicenter Investigation of Limitation of Infarct Size
MINQUE	Minimum norm quadratic unbiased estimation
MLCG	Multiplicative linear congruential generator
MLE	Maximum likelihood estimate/estimator
MLP	Multilayer perceptron
MLP	Multilocus probe
MOLS	Mutually orthogonal Latin square
MONICA	Monitoring of trends and determinants in cardiovascular disease
MOR	Mortality odds ratio
MP	Most powerful (test)
MPLE	Maximum penalized likelihood estimator
MPN	Most probable number
MPS	Medical Provider Survey
MRC	Medical Research Council
MRE	Minimum risk equivariant
MRF	Markov random field model
MRFIT	Multiple Risk Factor Intervention Trial
MRG	Multiple recursive generator
MRI	Magnetic resonance imaging
MRL	Mean residual life
MRLF	Monthly Report on the Labor Force
MSE	Mean square error
MSEP	Mean square error of prediction
MSIS	Medicaid Statistical Information System
MSO	Management Service Organization
MSS	Medicare Statistical System
MSSP	Most stringent and somewhere most powerful
MTD	Maximum tolerable dose
MTED	Minimum therapeutically effective dose
MVD	Measure-valued diffusion
MVU	Minimum variance unbiased estimation
NAMCS	National Ambulatory Medical Care Survey
NAS	National Academy of Sciences
NCHS	National Center for Health Statistics
NCI	National Cancer Institute
NCTR	National Center for Toxicological Research

NDI	National Death Index
NED	Normal equivalent deviate
NEHIS	National Employer Health Insurance Survey
NEJM	*New England Journal of Medicine*
NFIP	National Foundation for Infantile Paralysis
NFOC	Necessary first-order condition
NFP	Natural family planning
NHAMCS	National Hospital Ambulatory Medical Care Survey
NHANES	National Health and Nutrition Examination Survey
NHCS	National Health Care Survey
NHDS	National Hospital Discharge Survey
NHI	National Heart Institute
NHIS	National Health Interview Survey
NHLBI	National Heart, Lung, and Blood Institute
NHLI	National Heart and Lung Institute
NHP	Nottingham Health Profile
NHPI	National Health Provider Inventory
NHS	National Halothane Study
NHS	National Health Service
NHSCR	National Health Service Central Register
NHSDA	National Household Survey on Drug Abuse
NIA	National Institute on Aging
NICU	Neonatal intensive care unit
NIH	National Institutes of Health
NINDS	National Institute of Neurological Disorders and Stroke
NIS	Nationwide Inpatient Sample
NK	Newman–Keuls method
NLMA	Nonlinear moving average model
NLMS	National Longitudinal Mortality Study
NLSY	National Labor Survey of Youth
NLTCS	National Long Term Care Surveys
NMAR	Not missing at random
NMES	National Medical Expenditure Survey
NMFI	National Master Facility Inventory
NMIHS	National Maternal and Infant Health Survey
NND	Nearest neighbor distance
NNHES	National Nursing Home Expenditure Survey
NNHS	National Nursing Home Survey
NNIS	National nosocomial infections study
NNT	Number needed to treat
NORC	National Opinion Research Center
NPMLE	Nonparametric maximum likelihood estimate
NSAID	Nonsteroidal anti-inflammatory drug
NSAS	National Survey of Ambulatory Surgery
NTA	Neyman's type A distribution
NTD	Neural tube defect

NTP	National Toxicology Program
nvCJD	New variant CJD
OC	Operating Characteristics
ODE	Ordinary differential equation
OEB	Office of Epidemiology and Biostatistics
OECD	Organization for Economic Cooperation and Development
OLS	Ordinary least squares
OMB	Office of Management and Budget
OME	Otitis media with effusion
ONS	Office for National Statistics
OPC	Out Patient Care
OPRR	Office for Protection from Research Risks
OR	Operations Research
ORL	Otorhinolaryngology
OSEM	Ordered subsets EM algorithm
OTCOM	Office of Training and Communication
OUP	Ornstein–Uhlenbeck process
PACF	Partial autocorrelation function
PAI	Patient Assessment Instrument
PBIBD	Partially balanced incomplete block designs
PCA	Principal components analysis
PCE	Per-comparison error rate
PCP	Pneumocystis carinii pneumonia
PCR	Polymerase chain reaction
PCR	Principal component regression
pdf	Probability density function
PDR	Pharmacoepidemiologic dose–response
PE	Pharmacoepidemiology
PEFR	Peak expiratory flow rate
PET	Positron emission tomography
PF	Preventable fraction
PF	Production function
pgf	Probability generating function
PHLS	Public Health Laboratory Service
PHM	Proportional hazards model
PHO	Physician Hospital Organization
PI	Prognostic index
PIC	Polymorphism information content
PIR	Proportional incidence ratio
PK/PD	Pharmacokinetic and pharmacodynamic model
PKU	Phenylketonuria
PL	Product-limit estimator
PLCO	Prostate, Lung, Colorectal, and Ovarian Cancer Screening Trial
PLSR	Partial least square regression

PMLE   Partial maximum likelihood estimate/estimator
PMOR   Proportional mortality odds ratio
PMR   Proportional mortality ratio
PMTED   Population MTED
Post-CABG   Post-Coronary Artery Bypass Graft study
PPK   Population pharmacokinetic modeling
PPS   Probability proportional to size
PQL   Penalized quasi-likelihood
PRE   Proportional reduction in error
PRNG   Pseudo-random number generator
PSA   Prostate specific antigen
PSI   Statisticians in the Pharmaceutical Industry
PSU   Primary sampling unit
PTF   Patient Treatment File
PYLL   Person-years of life lost

QALY   Quality-adjusted life year
QAS   Quality-adjusted survival
QI   Quasi-independence model
QL   Quasi-likelihood
QMR   Quantitative Methods and Research
QOL   Quality of life
Q–Q   Quantile–quantile plot
QSAR   Quantitative structure–activity relationships
Q-TWiST   Quality-adjusted TWiST
QWB   Quality of well-being

RAC   Random coefficient autoregressive model
RCBD   Randomized complete block design
RCGP   Royal College of General Practitioners
RCT   Randomized (controlled) clinical trial
RCT   Residual cancer tissue
RDD   Random digit dialing
RECS   Research in Epidemiology and Communication Science
REML   Restricted maximum likelihood estimation
RfD   Reference dose
RFLP   Restriction fragment length polymorphism
RIA   Radioimmunoassay
RIGLS   Restricted iterative generalized least square
RISC   Reduced instruction-set computer
RLA   Radioligand assay
RM   Rasch model
RMNE   Random man is not excluded
RNA   Ribonucleic acid
ROC   Receiver operating characteristic
RPSNFTM   Rank-preserving structural nested failure time model

RR	Randomized response
RR	Relative risk
RRF	Relative risk function
RSC	Code of statistical conduct
RSCL	Rotterdam Symptom Checklist
RSMS	Relative SMR
RSS	Royal Statistical Society
RST	Repeated significance testing
RTM	Regression to the mean
SA	Simpson Angus scale
SA	Surface area
SAR	Secondary attack rate
SBP	Systolic blood pressure
SCC	Sufficient-component cause model
SCMD	Smallest clinically meaningful difference
SCRV	Scandinavian Committee on Reference Values
sd	Standard deviation
SDS	Standard deviation score
se	Standard error
SEER	Surveillance, Epidemiology, and End Results Program
SEM	Standard errors of measurement
SEM	Structural equation model
SEQ	Second linear combinations
SER	Society for Epidemiologic Research
SG	Standard Gamble
SH	Sitting height
SID	State Inpatient Database
SIDS	Sudden infant death syndrome
SIMEX	Simulation extrapolation
SIP	Sickness Impact Profile
SIR	Standardized incidence ratio
SIS	Susceptible–infective–susceptible model
SLE	Significance level to enter
SLL	Subischial leg length
SLLN	Strong law of large numbers
SLP	Single layer perceptron
SLP	Single locus probe
SMI	Supplementary Medical Insurance
SMR	Standardized mortality ratio
SNFTM	Structural nested failure time model
SOLVD	Studies of Left Ventricular Dysfunction
SOP	Standard Operation Procedures
SPDE	Stochastic partial differential equation
SPECT	Single photon emission (computed) tomography
SPMR	Standardized proportional mortality ratio

SPRT	Sequential probability ratio test
SQL	Structured Query Language
SRAM	Synchronous static random access memory
SRG	Shift register generator
SROC	Summary ROC curve
SRP	Stationary renewal process
SRR	Standardized rate ratio
SRS	Simple random sampling
SRSWOR	Simple random sampling without replacement
SSPS	Sum symmetric power series distribution
SSU	Secondary Sampling Unit
STD	Sexually transmitted disease
STR	Short tandem repeat system
SUTSE	Seemingly unrelated time series equations model
SVD	Singular value decomposition
SWB	Subtract-with-borrow generator

TAR	Threshold autoregressive models
TCI	Treatment–covariate interaction
TENS	Transcutaneous electrical nerve stimulation
TLSE	Trimmed least squares estimator
TMJPDS	Temporomandibular joint pain dysfunction syndrome
TPF	True positive fraction
TQM	Total quality management
TSS	Toxic shock syndrome
TTT	Total time on test
TWiST	Time without symptoms and toxicity

UGDP	University Group Diabetes Program
UICC	Union Internationale Contre le Cancer
UMPU	Uniformly most powerful among unbiased test
UMV	Uniformly minimum variance
UMVUE	Uniformly minimum variance unbiased estimate
UNICEF	United Nations International Children's Emergency Fund
USDA	United States Department of Agriculture

VA	Visual acuity
VAR	Vector autoregression
var	Variance
VARMA	Vector ARMA
VAS	Visual analog scale
VIF	Variance inflation factor
VNTR	Variable number of tandem repeat
VPS	Variable probability sampling

WAIFW	Who Acquires Infection From Whom
WCP	Weak conditional principle
WHI	Women's health initiative
WHO	World Health Organization
WHOQOL	World Health Organization Quality of Life
WLS	Weighted least squares
WLSE	Weighted least squares estimation
WNAR	Western North American Region
WOSCOPS	West of Scotland Coronary Prevention Study
WPRC	Weighted pairwise rank correlation
WSP	Weak sufficiency principle
WTP	Willingness to pay
WWW	World Wide Web

Contents

xlvi   Contents

Contributors

Aalen, O.O. *University of Oslo, Norway*
Abrahamowicz, M. *McGill University, Canada*
Aday, L.A. *University of Texas, USA*
Agresti, A. *University of Florida, USA*
Ahsanullah, M. *Rider College Lawrenceville, USA*
Aitken, C.G.G. *University of Edinburgh, UK*
Aitkin, M.A. *University of Newcastle, UK*
Alberman, E. *London, UK*
Alemi, F. *Cleveland State University, USA*
Alexander, K.S. *University of Southern California, USA*
Algina, J. *University of Florida, USA*
Altan, S. *RW Johnson Pharmaceutical Research Institute, New Jersey, USA*
Altham, P. *University of Cambridge, UK*
Altman, D.G. *ICRF Medical Statistics Group, Oxford, UK*
Andersen, E. *University of Copenhagen, Denmark*
Andersen, P.K. *University of Copenhagen, Denmark*
Andersen, R.M. *UCLA School of Public Health, USA*
Anderson, D.R. *Colorado State University, USA*
Anderson, R.J. *University of Illinois at Chicago, USA*
Anderson, R.L. *ClinTrials Research Inc., Lexington, USA*
Andrews, D.F. *University of Toronto, Canada*
Anello, C. *Rockville, USA*
Arjas, E. *University of Oulu, Finland*
Armitage, P. *University of Oxford, UK*
Arnett, R.H. *Agency for Health Care Policy and Research, Rockville, USA*
Ash, A. *Boston University School of Medicine, USA*

Ashley, J. *NHS Centre for Coding and Classification, Loughborough, UK*
Asmar, L. *University of Texas, USA*
Atkinson, A.C. *London School of Economics and Political Science, UK*
Austoker, J. *University of Oxford, UK*
Axelson, O. *Linkoping University, Sweden*

Babb, J. *Fox Chase Cancer Center, Philadelphia, USA*
Bacchetti, P. *University of California, San Francisco, USA*
Bailar, B. *National Opinion Research Center, Chicago, USA*
Bailey, B.J.R. *University of Southampton, UK*
Bailey, N.T.J. *Fang, Switzerland*
Balakrishnan, N. *McMaster University, Hamilton, Canada*
Ball, F. *University of Nottingham, UK*
Balzi, D. *Centre for the Study and Prevention of Cancer, Florence, Italy*
Barker, D. *MRC Environmental Unit, Southampton, UK*
Barlow, W. *Group Health Cooperative, Seattle, USA*
Barnard, Jr, J. *Harvard University, USA*
Barnett, V. *University of Nottingham, UK*
Baron, J. *Dartmouth Medical School, Hanover, USA*
Barry, S.C. *Australian National University, Canberra, Australia*
Basu, A.P. *University of Missouri, USA*
Baur, M.P. *University of Bonn, Germany*
Beach, M. *Dartmouth Medical School, Hanover, USA*
Beacon, H.J. *Harvard School of Public Health, USA*
Becker, M. *University of Michigan, USA*
Becker, N. *La Trobe University, Victoria, Australia*

Beckett, L.A. *Oak Park, IL, USA*
Bedrick, E. *University of New Mexico, USA*
Begg, C. *Memorial Sloan Kettering Cancer Center, New York, USA*
Begg, M. *Columbia University, New York, USA*
Behrens, R.H. *London Hospital for Tropical Diseases, UK*
Bellhouse, D. *University of Western Ontario, Canada*
Bemis, K.G. *Indianapolis, USA*
Benichou, J. *Unité de Biostatistiqué, Rouen, France*
Bennett, S. *Australian Institute of Health and Welfare, Canberra, Australia*
Bentler, S.E. *University of Iowa, USA*
Berman, M. *CSIRO Mathematical and Information Services, North Ryde, Australia*
Berry, D.A. *Duke University, Durham, USA*
Berry, G. *University of New South Wales, Australia*
Best, N. *Imperial College of Science, Technology and Medicine, London, UK*
Bethel, J. *Westat Inc., Rockville, USA*
Bhapkar, V. *University of Kentucky, Lexington, USA*
Bienias, J.L. *Rush Institute for Healthy Aging, Chicago, IL, USA*
Bigby, M.E. *Massachusetts General Hospital, Charlestown, USA*
Biggeri, A. *University of Florence, Italy*
Billard, L. *University of Georgia, USA*
Bingham, S. *MRC Dunn Nutrition Unit, Cambridge, UK*
Birkes, D.S. *Oregon State University, USA*
Bithell, J. *University of Oxford, UK*
Blackwelder, W.C. *Bethesda, USA*
Blackwell, P. *University of Sheffield, UK*
Blangero, J. *SW Foundation for Medical Research, San Antonio, USA*
Blesch, K. *New Jersey, USA*
Blettner, M. *German Cancer Research Centre, Heidelberg, Germany*
Blot, W. *International Epidemiology Institute, Rockville, USA*
Bollen, K. *University of North Carolina, USA*
Bonney, G. *Fox Chase Cancer Center, Cheltenham, USA*

Boos, D. *North Carolina State University, Raleigh, USA*
Borgan, O. *University of Oslo, Norway*
Bowman, A. *University of Glasgow, UK*
Bowman, K.O. *Oak Ridge National Laboratory USA*
Box, J.F. *Madison, USA*
Boyle, P. *European Institute of Epidemiology, Milan, Italy*
Bradley, R. *University of Georgia, USA*
Braun, H.I. *Education Testing Service, Princeton, USA*
Breslow, N. *University of Washington, USA*
Brinkley, E. *Belconnen, Australia*
Brock, D. *Office of Epidemiology, Demography and Biometry, Bethesda, USA*
Brogan, D. *Emory University School of Public Health, Atlanta, USA*
Brookmeyer, R. *Johns Hopkins University, Baltimore, USA*
Brown Jr, B.W. *Stanford University, USA*
Brown, K.S. *University of Waterloo, Ontario, Canada*
Brown, L.D. *University of Pennsylvania, USA*
Brown, P.J. *University of Kent at Canterbury, UK*
Brown, S. *University of Waterloo, Canada*
Browne, M.W. *Ohio State University, USA*
Bryant, J.L. *NSABP, Pittsburgh, USA*
Buckland, S. *University of St Andrews, Edinburgh, UK*
Buiatti, E. *Centre for the Study and Prevention of Cancer, Florence, Italy*
Buonaccorsi, J.P. *University of Massachusetts, USA*
Burmaster, D.E. *Alceon Corporation, Cambridge, USA*
Burnham, K.P. *Colorado State University, USA*
Byers, R.H. *Atlanta, USA*

Cabilio, P. *Acadia University, Wolfville, Canada*
Cairns, A. *Heriot-Watt University, Edinburgh, UK*
Caliński, T. *University of Poznan, Poland*
Campbell, M. *Northern General Hospital, Sheffield, UK*

Caporaso, N. *National Cancer Institute, Rockville, USA*

Carlson, B.L. *Mathematical Policy Research, Princeton, USA*

Carr, D.B. *George Mason University, Burke, USA*

Carriquiry, A. *Iowa State University, USA*

Carroll, J.D. *Rutgers University, Piscataway, USA*

Carroll, R.J. *Texas A & M University, USA*

Casady, B. *US Department of Labor, Washington, USA*

Casella, G. *Cornell University, Ithaca, USA*

Chakraborti, S. *University of Alabama, USA*

Chakraborty, R. *University of Texas, USA*

Chakravarti, A. *Case Western Reserve University, Cleveland, USA*

Chalmers, I. *UK Cochrane Centre, Oxford, UK*

Chandler, R. *University College London, UK*

Chang, I-S. *National Central University, Taiwan, ROC*

Chao, A. *National Tsing Hua University, Taiwan, ROC*

Chatfield, C. *University of Bath, UK*

Chen, C.W. *US EPA, Washington, USA*

Chen, H.J. *University of Georgia, USA*

Cheng, B. *University of Kent at Canterbury UK*

Chernoff, H. *Harvard University, USA*

Chiang, C.L. *University of California, Berkeley, USA*

Childs, A. *McMaster University, Hamilton, Canada*

Chinchilli, V.M. *Penn State University, Harrisburg, USA*

Choi, B.C.K. *Health Canada, Ottawa, Canada*

Chow, S-C. *Bristol-Myers-Squibb, Plainsboro, USA*

Chow, W-H. *Affiliation Unknown*

Churchill, G. *Cornell University, Ithaca, USA*

Ciampi, A. *McGill University, Montreal, Canada*

Clapp, R. *Boston University, USA*

Cnaan, A. *University of Pennsylvania, USA*

Cohen, S. *Division of Statistics, DHSS, Rockville, USA*

Cole, T.J. *MRC Dunn Nutrition Unit, Cambridge, UK*

Coleman, M. *Office of Population Censuses and Surveys, London, UK*

Collett, D. *University of Reading, UK*

Collins, J.F. *V.A. Medical Center, Perry Point, USA*

Colton, T. *Boston University, USA*

Conaway, M. *Duke University, Durham, USA*

Conrad, D.A. *University of Washington, USA*

Cook, N.R. *Brigham and Women's Hospital, Boston, USA*

Cook, R.J. *University of Waterloo, Canada*

Corey, L.A. *Virginia Institute, USA*

Cornelissen, G. *University of Minnesota, USA*

Coster, D.C. *Utah State University, USA*

Costigan, T. *Ross Laboratories, Cleveland, USA*

Couturier, A. *McGill University, Quebec, Canada*

Cox, C. *University of Rochester Medical Center, USA*

Cox, D.F. *Statistical Laboratory, Ames, USA*

Cox, D.R. *University of Oxford, UK*

Crichton, N. *Royal College of Nursing, London, UK*

Cronin, W.M. *NSABP, Pittsburgh, USA*

Crowder, M.J. *University of Surrey, Guildford, UK*

Crowley, J.J. *Fred Hutchinson Cancer Research Center, Seattle, USA*

Cui, J. *La Trobe University, Victoria, Australia*

Cumberland, W.G. *UCLA School of Public Health, USA*

Currall, J. *University of Glasgow, UK*

Cutler, D.R. *Utah State University, USA*

Cuzick, J. *ICRF, London, UK*

Czaja, R. *North Carolina State University, USA*

D'Agostino, R.B. *Boston University, USA*

D'Agostino, Jr, R. *Waker Forest University, Winston-Salem, USA*

Dabrowska, D.M. *UCLA School of Public Health, USA*
Dalal, S. *Bellcore, New Jersey, USA*
Darby, S. *ICRF Radcliffe Infirmary, Oxford, UK*
Darlington, G.A. *Cancer Care Ontario, Canada*
Das, S. *Indian Statistical Institute, India*
Das Gupta, S. *Indian Statistical Institute, India*
DasGupta, A. *Purdue University, West Lafayette, USA*
Datta, G.S. *University of Georgia, USA*
Davey-Smith, G. *University of Bristol, UK*
David, H.A. *Iowa State University, USA*
Davies, N. *Nottingham Trent University, UK*
Davis, C.E. *University of North Carolina, USA*
Davis, C.S. *University of Iowa, USA*
Davis, J. *Maryland, USA*
Davis, P. *University of Auckland, New Zealand*
Davis, T. *Addenbrookes Hospital, Cambridge, UK*
Davison, A.C. *Ecole Polytechnique Federale de Lausanne, Switzerland*
Dawson, D.V. *Case Western Reserve University, Cleveland, USA*
Dawson, R. *Affiliation Unknown*
Day, S.J. *Leo Pharmaceuticals, Princes Risborough, UK*
De Angelis, D. *University of Cambridge, UK*
de Bock, T. *Leiden University, The Netherlands*
de Bruin, A. *Statistics Netherlands, Voorsburg, The Netherlands*
de Gruttola, V. *Harvard School of Public Health, Boston, USA*
De Soete, G. *University of Ghent, Belgium*
de Vet, H. *University of Limburg, The Netherlands*
Dean, C. *Simon Fraser University, Burnaby, Canada*
DeMets, D.L. *University of Wisconsin, USA*
Demidenko, E. *Dartmouth Medical School, Hanover, USA*
Dempster, A.P. *Harvard University, USA*
Deng, L-Y. *University of Memphis, USA*

Dengler, H.J. *Medizinische Klinik der Universität Bonn, Germany,*
Denniston, C. *University of Wisconsin, USA*
Derr, J.A. *Pennsylvania State University, USA*
Desmond, A.F. *University of Guelph, Canada*
Dewanji, A. *Indian Statistical Institute, India*
Dewey, M. *Trent Institute for Health, Nottingham, UK*
Dey, A. *Indian Statistical Institute, India*
Diamond, I. *University of Southampton, UK*
Dickey, J.M. *University of Minnesota, USA*
Diehr P. *University of Washington, USA*
Dietz, E.J. *North Carolina State University, USA*
Dietz, K. *Institut für Medizinische Biometrie, Tubingen, Germany*
Diggle, P. *University of Lancaster, UK*
Dillman, D. *Washington State University, USA*
Dinse, G. *NIEHS, North Carolina, USA*
Dixon, D.O. *Coordinating Centers Branch, Bethesda, USA*
Doksum, K. *University of California, Berkeley, USA*
Doll, R. *Radcliffe Infirmary, Oxford, UK*
Dong, J. *Michigan Technical University, USA*
Dorfman, A.H. *US Bureau of Labor, Washington, USA*
Dorling, D. *University of Bristol, UK*
Dorsaz, F. *Swiss Federal Institute of Technology, Lausanne, Switzerland*
Doyon, F. *Institut Gustave-Roussy, Villejuif Cedex, France*
Draper, D. *University of Bath, UK*
Drum, M. *University of Illinois at Chicago, USA*
Dubey, S. *FDA, Rockville, USA*
Duffy, S.W. *MRC Biostatistical Unit, Cambridge, UK*
Dukes, K.A. *Stoneham, USA*
Dunn, G. *University of Manchester, UK*
Dunnell, K. *Office of Population Censuses and Surveys, London, UK*
Dunnett, C. *McMaster University, Hamilton, Canada*
Dykstra, R.L. *University of Iowa, USA*

Ederer, F. *The EMMES Corporation and University of Minnesota, USA*

Edwards, A.W.F. *University of Cambridge, UK*

Elbourne, D. *ICRF Radcliffe Infirmary, Oxford, UK*

Ellenberg, J. *Westat, Rockville, USA*

Elliott, P. *Imperial College School of Medicine, London, UK*

Elston, R.C. *Case Western Reserve University, Cleveland, USA*

Elwood, J.H. *Affiliation Unknown*

Elwood, P. *MRC Epidemiology Unit, Penarth, UK*

Endrenyi L. *University of Toronto, Canada*

Evans, S. *Medicines Control Agency, London, UK*

Everitt, B. *Institute of Psychiatry, London, UK*

Ewens, W. *University of Pennsylvania, USA*

Fahrmeir, L. *Universität München, Germany*

Farewell, V.T. *University College London, UK*

Fargot-Largeault, A. *Centre National de la Recherche Scientifique, Paris, France*

Farley, T.M. *World Health Organization, Switzerland*

Farrington, C.P. *PHLS Communicable Disease Surveillance Centre, London, UK*

Fearn, T. *University College London, UK*

Feinleib, M. *Georgetown University, Washington, USA*

Feinstein, A.R. *Yale University, New Haven, CT, USA*

Felson, D.T. *Boston University, MA, USA*

Fergusson, P. *University of Manitoba, Canada*

Fetter, R.B. *Florida, USA*

Fienberg, S. *Carnegie-Mellon University, Pittsburgh, USA*

Finch, S. *State University of New York at Stonybrook, USA*

Finlay, E. *Affiliation Unknown*

Fisher, L.D. *University of Washington, USA*

Fisher, N.I. *CSIRO, North Ryde, Australia*

Fitzmaurice, G. *University of Oxford, UK*

Flagle, C. *Johns Hopkins University, Baltimore, USA*

Fleming, T.R. *University of Washington, USA*

Folks, J.L. *Oklahoma State University, USA*

Foulkes, M. *SmithKline & Beecham, Rixenart, Belgium*

Fox, J. *Office of Population Censuses and Surveys, London, UK*

Frankel, M. *City University of New York, USA*

Franklin, L. *Indianna State University, USA*

Freels, S. *University of Illinois at Chicago, USA*

Freeman, D. *University of Texas, USA*

Friedman, L.M. *Rockledge Center, Bethesda, USA*

Frydman, H. *New York University, USA*

Furner, S. *University of Illinois at Chicago, USA*

Gafni, A. *McMaster University, Hamilton, Canada*

Gail, M.H. *National Cancer Institute, Bethesda, USA*

Gaines Das, R.E. *National Institute for Biological Standards, Potters Bar, UK*

Galbraith, R.F. *University College London, UK*

Gange, S. *Johns Hopkins University, Baltimore, USA*

Gani, J. *Australian National University, Canberra, Australia*

Gastwirth, J. *George Washington University, USA*

Gatsonis, C. *Brown University, Providence, USA*

Gauvreau, K. *Harvard School of Public Health, USA*

Gaylor, D.W. *National Center for Toxicological Research, Jefferson, USA*

Gehan, D. *Quintiles, Inc, Austin, TX, USA*

Gehan, E.A. *Georgetown University Medical Center, USA*

Geller, N.L. *Office of Biostatistics Research, Bethesda, USA*

George, E.O. *Memphis State University, USA*

George, S. *Duke University Medical Center, Durham, USA*

Germolec, D. *National Institute of Environmental Health Sciences, Research Triangle Park, USA*

Ghosh, J.K. *Indian Statistical Institute, India*
Ghosh, P.K. *Brentwood, USA*
Ghosh, S. *University of California, Riverside, USA*
Gilbert, E. *ICRF, Radcliffe Infirmary, Oxford, UK*
Gilks, W. *Institute of Public Health, Cambridge, UK*
Gill, R. *University of Utrecht, The Netherlands*
Giltinan, D. *Genentech Inc., San Francisco, USA*
Gilula, Z. *Hebrew University, Jerusalem, Israel*
Gittins, J.C. *University of Oxford, UK*
Gladman, D.D. *Toronto Hospital, Canada*
Glasbey, C. *University of Edinbugh, UK*
Glasziou, P. *University of Queensland Medical School, Australia*
Glimm, E. *Affiliation Unknown*
Glynn, R. *Harvard Medical School, USA*
Godambe, V. *University of Waterloo, Canada*
Godley, M.J. *Zeneca Pharmaceuticals, Macclesfield, UK*
Goldsmith, C. *McMaster University, Hamilton, Canada*
Goldstein, H. *Institute of Education, London, UK*
Goldstein, R. *Brighton, USA*
Goodman, S. *Johns Hopkins University, Baltimore, USA*
Gordon, T. *Biostatistics Center, Rockville, USA*
Gore, S. *MRC Biostatistics Unit, Cambridge, UK*
Gower, J.C. *St Albans, UK*
Graf, E. *Albert-Ludwigs-Universität Freiburg, Germany*
Grambsch, P.M. *Affiliation Unknown*
Green, S.B. *National Cancer Institute, Bethesda, USA*
Greenhalgh, D. *University of Strathclyde, UK*
Greenhouse, J. *Carnegie-Mellon University, Pittsburgh, USA*
Greenhouse, S. *George Washington University, USA*
Greenland, S. *Topanga, USA*

Grembowski, D.E. *University of Washington, USA*
Griffith, J. *Boston, USA*
Gross, A.J. *Medical University of Southern California, USA*
Grummer-Strawn, L. *Centers for Disease Control and Prevention, Atlanta, GA, USA*
Grzebyk, M. *Institut National de Recherche et de Sécurité, France*
Guess, H. *Chapel Hill, USA*
Guo, S-W. *School of Public Health, Minneapolis, USA*
Gupta, S. *Northern Illinois University, USA*
Gusev, Y. *Johns Hopkins University, Baltimore, USA*
Guyatt, G.H. *McMaster University, Hamilton, Canada*

Haber, M. *Emory University, Atlanta, USA*
Haberman, S. *Northwestern University, USA*
Haberman, S. *City University, London, UK*
Hakulinen, T. *Finnish Cancer Registry, Helsinki, Finland*
Halberg, F. *University of Minneapolis, USA*
Hall, P. *Australian National University, Canberra, Australia*
Halloran, E. *Emory University, Atlanta, USA*
Hampel, F. *University of Zurich, Switzerland*
Hand, D.J. *Open University, Milton Keynes, UK*
Hanley, J. *McGill University, Montreal, Canada*
Hapsara, H. *World Health Organization, Switzerland*
Harrell, F. *University of Virginia, USA*
Harrington, D.P. *Dana Farber Cancer Institute, Boston, USA*
Harris, E.K. *Madison, USA*
Hartford, R.B. *Cedar Crest, New Mexico, USA*
Hartge, P. *National Cancer Institute, Rockville, MD, USA*
Harvey, A. *University of Cambridge, UK*
Haseman, J.K. *NEIHS, Research Triangle Park, USA*

Hastie, T.J. *Stanford University, USA*

Hatzinger, R. *Vienna University of Economics, Austria*

Hawkins, D.M. *University of Minneapolis, USA*

Hazelton, M.L. *University College London, UK*

Healy, M. *Harpenden, UK*

Heesterbeek, J.A.P. *Centre for Biometry, Wageningen, The Netherlands*

Heitjan, D.F. *Columbia University School of Public Health, USA*

Helfenstein, U. *Zurich University, Switzerland*

Hettmansperger, T.P. *Penn State University, USA*

Heyse, J. *Merck and Co. Inc., West Point, USA*

Hill, B. *Ann Arbor, USA*

Hill, C. *Institut Gustav Roussy, Villejuif Cedex, France*

Hill, H.A. *Emory University, Atlanta, USA*

Hills, M. *London, UK*

Hilton, J.F. *University of California, San Francisco, USA*

Hirotsu, C. *University of Tokyo, Japan*

Hoaglin, D.C. *Abt Associates, Cambridge, USA*

Hochberg, Y. *University of Tel Aviv, Israel*

Hodge, S.E. *New York State Psychiatric Institute, USA*

Hoem, J. *Stockholm University, Sweden*

Holford, T. *Yale University School of Medicine, USA*

Holland, W.W. *London School of Economics and Political Science, UK*

Hoppe, F.M. *McMaster University, Hamilton, Canada*

Hopper, J.I. *University of Melbourne, Australia*

Hosmer, Jr, D.W. *University of Massachusetts, USA*

Hougaard, P. *Novo Nordisk, Bagsvaerd, Denmark*

Hsiung, C.A. *Academia Sinica, Taiwan, ROC*

Hsu, H. *FDA, Rockville, USA*

Hu, B. *Brigham and Women's Hospital, Harvard University, USA*

Huang, W. *Boston University School of Public Health, Boston, MA, USA*

Hudson, H.M. *Macquarie University, New South Wales, Australia*

Hughes, C. *University of Wales, Cardiff, UK*

Hughes, M.D. *London School of Hygiene and Tropical Medicine, UK*

Hunt, N. *University of Coventry, UK*

Hutton, J. *University of Newcastle, UK*

Iglewicz, B. *Temple University, Philadelphia, USA*

Imrey, P.B. *University of Illinois, USA*

Inskip, H. *University of Southampton, UK*

Irwig, L. *University of Sydney, Australia*

Israel, R.A. *Bowie, USA*

Jackson, J.E. *Rochester, USA*

Jacobs JR, D.R. *University of Minnesota, USA*

Jadad, A. *McMaster University, Hamilton, Canada*

Jagers, P. *Chalmers University of Technology, Göteborg, Sweden*

James, I. *Murdoch University, Australia*

Janacek, G.J. *University of East Anglia, Norwich, UK*

Janssen, P. *Limburgs Universitair, Diepenbeek, Belgium*

Jensen, D.R. *Virginia Polytechnic Institute and State University, USA*

Johnson, A. *Institute of Public Health, Cambridge, UK*

Johnson, T.P. *University of Illinois at Chicago, USA*

Jolliffe, I.T. *University of Aberdeen, UK*

Jones, B. *De Montfort University, Leicester, UK*

Jones, D.R. *University of Leicester, UK*

Jovanovich, B. *University of Illinois at Chicago, USA*

Juniper, E. *McMaster University, Canada*

Kalbfleisch, J.D. *University of Waterloo, Canada*

Kass, R.E. *Carnegie-Mellon University, Pittsburgh, USA*

Katz, J. *Cambridge, USA*

Keen, K.J. *University of Manitoba, Canada*

Keiding, N. *University of Copenhagen, Denmark*

Kelly, P.J. *University of Teeside, UK*

Kemp, A.W. *University of St Andrews, Scotland, UK*

Kemp, D. *University of St Andrews, Scotland, UK*

Kendall, W.S. *University of Warwick, UK*

Kendrick, S. *Scottish Health Service, Edinburgh, UK*

Kennessy, Z. *Director, ISI, The Netherlands*

Kenward, M.G. *University of Kent at Canterbury, UK*

Khamis, H.J. *Wright State University, Dayton, USA*

Kiernan, K. *London School of Economics and Political Science, UK*

Kilpatrick, K. *University of North Carolina, USA*

King, B. *Boca Raton, USA*

Kingman, J.F.C. *University of Bristol, UK*

Klein, J.P. *Medical College of Wisconsin, USA*

Kleinbaum, D. *Emory University, Atlanta, USA*

Knatterud, G. *Maryland Medical Research Institute, USA*

Koch, G. *University of North Carolina, USA*

Kocherlakota, S. *University of Manitoba, Canada*

Koehler, K.J. *Iowa State University, USA*

Koepsell, T. *University of Washington, USA*

Kokic, P. *University of Southampton, UK*

Kolkiewicz, A. *University of Waterloo, Canada*

Kolonel, L.N. *University of Hawaii, USA*

Konrad, T.R. *University of North Carolina, USA*

Koopman, S.J. *London School of Economics, UK*

Kostyu, D.D. *Duke University Medical Center, Durham, USA*

Kraemer, H.C. *Stanford University, USA*

Kravitz, H. *Rush Medical College, Chicago, USA*

Kreiner, S. *University of Copenhagen, Denmark*

Krieger, A.M. *University of Pennsylvania, USA*

Krótki, K.P. *ESSI, Washington, USA*

Krutchkoff, R. *Virginia Polytechnic Institute, USA*

Krzanowski, W. *University of Exeter, UK*

Kuha, J. *Nuffield College, Oxford, UK*

Kunst, A.E. *Erasmus University, The Netherlands*

Kupper, L. *University of North Carolina, USA*

Kuritz, S.J. *Health Information Solutions, USA*

Kviz, F. *University of Illinois at Chicago, USA*

Laake, J. *National Marine Fisheries, Seattle, USA*

Laan, M. *University of California, Berkeley, USA*

Lachenbruch, P.A. *FDA, Rockville, USA*

Lachin, J.M. *George Washington University, USA*

Lai, T.L. *Stanford University, CA, USA*

Laird, N. *Harvard School of Public Health, USA*

Lakatos, E. *Forest Laboratories, New York, USA*

Lancaster, H.O. *Spit Junction, Australia*

Landis, J.R. *Penn State University College of Medicine, USA*

Lang, J.M. *Boston University, USA*

Lange, N. *McLean Hospital, Belmont, USA*

Langholz, B. *University of Southern California, USA*

Laupacis, A. *Loeb Institute of the Ottowa Civic Hopsitals, Canada*

Läuter, J. *Editor, Biometrical Journal*

Lave, J.R. *University of Pittsburgh, USA*

Lavori, P.W. *Stanford University, USA*

Lawless, J. *University of Waterloo, Canada*

Lawrance, A.J. *University of Birmingham, UK*

Lawrence, C.J. *University of Exeter, UK*

Lawson, A.B. *University of Abertay, UK*

Le Cam, L.M. *University of California, Berkeley, USA*

Le Marchland, L. *University of Hawaii, USA*

Lee, A.F.S. *Boston University, USA*

Lee, J.J. *Texas Medical Center, USA*

Lee, J. *Belle Mead, NJ, USA*

Lee, M-L.T. *Channing Laboratory, Boston, USA.*

Lee, Y.J. *National Institute of Child Health and Human Development, USA*

Lehoczky, J. *Carnegie-Mellon University, Pittsburgh, USA*

Lei, T. *USA, affiliation unknown*

Lemeshow, S. *University of Massachusetts, USA*

Lepowski, J.M. *University of Michegan, Ann Arbor, MI, USA*

Leufkens, H.G. *Utrecht University, The Netherlands*

Levin, D.L. *Division of Cancer Prevention and Control, Bethesda, USA*

Levy, P.S. *University of Illinois at Chicago, USA*

Lew, R. *Lexington, USA*

Lewis, R.J. *UCLA Medical Center, USA*

Liang, K-Y. *Johns Hopkins University, Baltimore, USA*

Liao, Q. *Harvard School of Public Health, USA*

Lin, D. *University of Washington, USA*

Lindley, D.V. *Minehead, UK*

Lindsay, B. *Penn State University, USA*

Lindsey, J. *Limburgs Universitair Centrum, Belgium*

Lindstrom, M. *University of Wisconsin, USA*

Link, W.A. *Patuxent Wildlife Research Center, Laurel, USA*

Lipsitz, S. *Harvard School of Public Health, USA*

Little, J. *University of Aberdeen, UK*

Little, R. *University of Michigan, USA*

Liu, I-M. *National Chung Hsing University, Taiwan, ROC*

Liu, J-P. *National Cheng-Kung University, Taiwan, ROC*

Lo, S-H. *Columbia University, USA*

Lohr, K.N. *Research Triangle Institute, Research Triangle Park, USA*

Longini, I. *Emory University, Atlanta, USA*

Looney, S.W. *University of Louisville, USA*

Lopez, A.D. *World Health Organization, Switzerland*

Loynes, R.M. *University of Sheffield, UK*

Lyles, C.A. *Johns Hopkins University, Baltimore, USA*

Lynge, E. *Danish Cancer Society, Copenhagen, Denmark*

Lyu, M.R. *AT & T Research, Murray Hill, USA*

Macauley, D. *Belfast, UK*

Macfarlane, A. *Radcliffe Infirmary, Oxford, UK*

Machin, D. *MRC Clinical Trials and Research Unit, Singapore*

Magnello, M.E. *Wellcome Institute, London, UK*

Maindonald, J. *University of Newcastle, Australia*

Majumder, P.P. *Indian Statistical Institute, India*

Malec, D. *National Center for Health Statistics, Hyattsville, USA*

Mallows, C.L. *AT & T Research, Murray Hill, USA*

Mandel, J. *National Institute of Standards Technology, Gaithersburg, USA*

Manton, K. *Duke University, Durham, USA*

Marler, J. *National Institutes of Health, Bethesda, USA*

Marriott, F.H.C. *University of Oxford, UK*

Marron, J.S. *University of North Carolina, USA*

Marsh, M.J. *Johns Hopkins University, Baltimore, USA*

Marshall, G. *Pontificia Universidad Católicade Chile, Chile*

Martin, M. *Australian National University, Canberra, Australia*

Martin, R.J. *University of Sheffield, UK*

Massaro, J. *Quintiles Inc., Cambridge, USA*

Matthews, D. *University of Waterloo, Canada*

Matthews, J.N.S. *University of Newcastle, UK*

Matthews, J.R. *Williamsburg, USA*

Matthysse, S. *McLean Hospital / Harvard Medical School, USA*

McColl, J.H. *University of Glasgow, UK*

McCullagh, P. *University of Chicago, USA*

McDonald, J.W. *University of Southampton, UK*

McFadden, E. *ECOG Coordinating Center, Brookline, USA*

McGee, D. *Loyola University, Maywood, USA*

McGilchrist, C.A. *Australian National University, Canberra, Australia*

McKnight, B. *University of Washington, USA*

McLaughlin, J.K. *Johns Hopkins University, Baltimore, USA*

McLean, Jr, D.C. *Medical University of South Columbia, USA*

Meenan, R. *Boston University School of Public Health, USA*

Mehta, C. *Cytel Software Company, Cambridge, USA*

Meier, P. *Columbia University, USA*

Meinert, C. *Johns Hopkins School of Hygiene and Public Health, Baltimore, USA*

Mendell, N.R. *State University of New York at Stonybrook, USA*

Mick, R. *University of Pennsylvania, USA*

Milne, R.K. *University of Western Australia, Nedlands, Australia*

Milner, P. *University of Bath, UK*

Milton, R. *EMMES Corporation, Potomac, USA*

Mode, C.J. *Drexel University, Philadelphia, USA*

Moolgavkar, S. *Fred Hutchinson Cancer Center, Seattle, USA*

Morgan, B.J. *University of Kent at Canterbury, UK*

Morgan, D.D.V. *Hoechst Marion Roussel, UK*

Morgenstern, H. *UCLA School of Public Health, USA*

Morrison, D.F. *University of Pennsylvania, USA*

Moses, L.E. *Stanford University, USA*

Mosteller, F. *Harvard University, USA*

Muller, H-G. *University of California, Davis, USA*

Muller, K.E. *University of North Carolina, USA*

Murphy, J.R. *Denver, USA*

Murray, G.D. *University of Edinburgh, UK*

Murray, L. *New Mexico State University, USA*

Nadarajah, S. *University of Plymouth, UK*

Nassim, J. *Washington, USA*

Neale, M.C. *Virginia Commonwealth University, USA*

Nelson, W. *Stat Consulting, Schenectady, USA*

Neuburger, H.L. *Office for National Statistics, London, UK*

Neuhaus, J. *University of California, San Francisco, USA*

Nevill, A.M. *Liverpool John Moores University, UK*

Newcombe, R.G. *University of Wales, Cardiff, UK*

Newell, D.J. *University of Sydney, Australia*

Nielsen, S.F. *University of Copenhagen, Denmark*

Nolan, D. *University of California, Berkeley, USA*

O'Brien, B. *McMaster University, Hamilton, Canada*

O'Brien, C.M. *Ministry of Agriculture Fisheries and Food, Lowestoft, UK*

O'Brien, P.C. *Mayo Clinic, Rochester, USA*

O'Fallon, M.W. *Health Science Research, USA*

O'Neill, R. *Silver Spring, MD, USA*

O'Neill, R.T. *FDA, Rockville, USA*

O'Neill, T.J. *Australian National University, Canberra, Australia*

O'Quigley, J. *University of California, San Diego, USA*

Oakes, D. *University of Rochester, USA*

Obeyesekere, M. *UT MD Anderson Cancer Center, Holcombe, USA*

Olkin, I. *Stanford University, USA*

Olshen, R.A. *Stanford University, USA*

Olson, J.M. *Case Western Reserve University, Cleveland, USA*

Olschewski, M. *Albert-Ludwigs-Universität Freiburg, Germany*

Owen, M. *Royal Statistical Society, London, UK*

Pak, A.W.P. *Brock University, USA*

Palmer, S. *Public Health Laboratories, Cardiff, UK*

Palmgren, J. *Rolf Nevanlinna Institute, Finland*

Parmigiani, G. *Duke University, Durham, USA*

Parsons, V. *Office of Research and Methodology, Hyattsville, USA*

Patel, N.R. *Cytel Software Corporation, Cambridge, USA*

Patil, G.P. *Penn State University, USA*

Patrick, D.L. *University of Washington, USA*

Pawitan, Y. *University College Dublin, Ireland*

Peace, K. *Journal of Biopharmaceutics, USA*

Pearl, D.K. *Ohio State University, USA*

Peele, P.B. *University of Pittsburgh, USA*

Pelias, M.Z. *Louisiana State University, USA*

Peña, E.A. *Bowling Green State University, USA*

Pendergast, J. *University of Florida, USA*

Pereira, B. de B. *Universidade Federal do Rio De Janeiro, Brasil*

Perrin, E.B. *University of Washington, USA*

Peters, T.J. *University of Bristol, UK*

Pettitt, A. *Queensland University, Australia*

Piantadosi, S. *Johns Hopkins University, Baltimore, USA*

Picavet, H.S.J. *RIVM/CCM, Bilthoven, The Netherlands*

Pickles, A. *Institute of Psychiatry, London, UK*

Piegorsch, W.W. *University of South Carolina, USA*

Pierce, D.A. *Radiation Effects Research Foundation, Hiroshima, Japan*

Plackett, R.L. *Newcastle upon Tyne, UK*

Podgor, M. *National Eye Institute, Bethesda, USA*

Pollack, E. *Center to Protect Workers' Rights, Washington, USA*

Portier, C. *NIEHS-BRAP, Research Triangle Park, USA*

Potthoff, R.F. *Greensboro, USA*

Poullier, J.P. *Organization for Economic Cooperation and Development, Paris Cedex, France*

Prentice, R.L. *Fred Hutchinson Cancer Center, Seattle, USA*

Prescott, P. *University of Southampton, UK*

Press, S.J. *University of California, USA*

Preston, D. *Radiation Effects Research Foundation, Hiroshima, Japan*

Pringle Smith, R. *Brown University, Providence, USA*

Prokhorskas, R. *World Health Organization, Copenhagen, Denmark*

Prorock, P.C. *National Institute of Health, Bethesda, USA*

Quasney, A.O. *US Bureau of the Census, Washington, USA*

Rabe-Hesketh, S. *Institute of Psychiatry, London, UK*

Raboud, J.M. *Canadian HIV Trials Network, Vancouver, Canada*

Raghavaro, D. *Temple University, Philadelphia, USA*

Ramakrishnan, V. *University of Illinois at Chicago, USA*

Rao, D.C. *Washington University Medical School, USA*

Rao, P.S.R. *University of Rochester, USA*

Rao, S.B. *Affiliation Unknown*

Rathouz, P.J. *University of Chicago, IL, USA*

Ratnaparkhi, M. *Wright State University, Dayton, USA*

Raz, J. *University of Michigan, USA*

Razzaghi, M. *Bloomsburg University, USA*

Rebbeck, T. *Fox Chase Cancer Center, Philadelphia, USA*

Redmond, C.K. *Medical University of South Carolina, USA*

Reid, N. *University of Toronto, Canada*

Reisner, E. *Duke University Medical Center, Durham, USA*

Renshaw, E. *University of Strathclyde, UK*

Reynolds, G. *Center for Disease Control, Atlanta, USA*

Rice, T. *University of Washington, USA*

Ridout, M. *Horticulture Research International, East Malling, UK*

Ripley, B. *University of Oxford, UK*

Roberts, M.G. *Wallaceville Animal Research Centre, Upper Hutt, NZ*

Roberts, R. *Henderson Hospital, Hamilton, Canada*

Robins, J.M. *Harvard School of Public Health, USA*

Robinson, G. *CSIRO, Clayton, Australia*

Rocke, D.M. *Graduate School of Management, Davis, USA*

Rogatko, A. *Fox Chase Cancer Center, Philadelphia, USA*

Rogers, C. *Cardiothoracic Transplant Audit, Bristol, UK*

Rohatgi, V.K. *Bowling Green State University, USA*

Rolin, J-M. *Institut de Statistique, Louvain-la-Neuve, Belgium*

Romano, P. *University of California, Davis, USA*

Roos, L. *University of Manitoba, Canada*

Rosalsky, A. *University of Florida, USA*

Rosenbaum, P. *Wharton School, Philadelphia, USA*

Rosenberg, L. *Boston University, USA*

Rosenberg, P.S. *National Cancer Institute, Bethesda, MD, USA*

Rosner, B. *Channing Laboratories, Boston, USA*

Rothman, K. *Newton Executive Park, Newton Lower Falls, USA*

Rotnitzky, A.G. *Harvard School of Public Health, USA*

Routledge, R. *Simon Fraser University, Burnaby, USA*

Royston, P. *Royal Postgraduate Medical School, London, UK*

Rubin, D.B. *Harvard University, Cambridge, MA, USA*

Rubinstein, L.V. *National Institute of Health, Bethesda, USA*

Russell, H. *Muro Pharmaceutical Inc., Tewksbury, USA*

Rust, P. *Medical University of South Carolina, USA*

Ryan, L.M. *Harvard School of Public Health, USA*

Saaty, T.L. *University of Pittsburgh, USA*

Sackett, D.L. *University of Oxford, UK*

Salsburg, D.S. *New London, USA*

Samet, J. *Johns Hopkins University, Baltimore, USA*

Sasieni, P.D. *ICRF, London, UK*

Satten, G. *Centers for Disease Control and Prevention, Atlanta, USA*

Sauerbrei, W. *Universität Freiburg, Germany*

Schaible, W. *Silver Spring, USA*

Schaid, D.J. *Mayo Clinic, Rochester, USA*

Scheaffer, R.L. *University of Florida, USA*

Schechter, S. *National Center for Health Statistics, Hyattsville, USA*

Schenker, N. *UCLA School of Public Health, USA*

Schieve, L. *Norcross, USA*

Schilder, A.G.M. *University Hospital, Utrecht, The Netherlands*

Schluchter, M.D. *The Cleveland Clinic Foundation, USA*

Schmid, C.H. *Tufts University, Boston, USA*

Schneiderman, M. *Deceased April 1997*

Schork, M.A. *Ann Arbor, USA*

Schork, N. *Case Western Reserve University Metro Health, Cleveland, USA*

Schucany, W.R. *Southern Methodist University, Dallas USA*

Schwartz, D. *INSERM, France*

Scott, A. *University of Auckland, New Zealand*

Scott, D. *Rice University, Houston, USA*

Searle, S.R. *Ithaca, USA*

Seber, G. *University of Auckland, NZ*

Seeber, G.U.H. *Universität Innsbruck, Austria*

Seidenfeld, T. *Carnegie-Mellon University, Pittsburgh, USA*

Seldrup, J. *Quintiles Inc., Tanneries Cedex, France*

Selvin, S. *University of California, Berkeley, USA*

Sen, P.K. *University of North Carolina, USA*

Seneta, E. *University of Sydney, Australia*

Senn, S. *University College London, UK*

Shafer, G. *Rutgers University, Piscataway, USA*

Shah, B.V. *Research Triangle Institute, Research Triangle Park, USA*

Sham, P. *Institute of Psychiatry, London, UK*

Shannon, H.S. *McMaster University, Hamilton, Canada*

Shapiro, S. *Boston University, USA*
Sharp, T.J. *University of North Carolina, NC, USA*
Shenton, L. *Athens, USA*
Sherman, C.D. *NIEHS, Research Triangle Park, USA*
Shiboski, S. *University of California, San Francisco, USA*
Shimuzu, I. *National Center for Health Statistics, Laurel, USA*
Shoukri, M. *University of Guelph, Canada*
Shuster, J. *University of Florida, USA*
Siemiatycki, J. *University of Quebec, Canada*
Silagy, C. *Flinders University of South Australia, Australia*
Simon, R. *National Institutes of Health, Bethesda, USA*
Simonoff, J.S. *University of New York, USA*
Simpson, J. *University of Sydney, Australia*
Sireci, S.G. *University of Massachusetts, USA*
Sirken, M. *National Center for Health Statistics, Hyattsville, USA*
Skinner, C. *University of Southampton, UK*
Slud, E.V. *University of Maryland, USA*
Smalls, M. *Scottish Health Service, Edinburgh, UK*
Smith, C. *Zeneca Pharmaceuticals, Macclesfield, UK*
Smith, L. *Australian National University, Canberra, Australia*
Smith, R. *British Medical Journal, London, UK*
Smith, R.P. *New York Presbyterian Hospital, NY, USA*
Smith, W. *West Tisbury, USA*
Smyth, G.K. *University of Queensland, Australia*
Sobel, E. *Stanford University School of Medicine, USA*
Soper, K.A. *Merck and Co., Inc., USA*
Sowan, B.J. *Executive Editor, Biometrika, UK*
Sox Jr, H.C. *Dartmouth-Hitchcock Medical Center, Lebanon, USA*
Speed, T. *University of California, Berkeley, USA*
Spence, M.A. *UC Irvine Medical Center, Orange, USA*

Spiegelhalter, D.J. *MRC Biostatistics Unit, Cambridge, UK*
Spiegelman, D. *Harvard School of Public Health, USA*
Sprent, P. *Newport-on-Tay, UK*
Sprott, D.A. *University of Waterloo, Canada*
Steele, J.M. *University of Pennsylvania, USA*
Steinwachs, D.M. *Johns Hopkins University, Baltimore, USA*
Stevenson, C. *The Australian National University, Canberra, Australia*
Stewart, F. *SmithKline and Beecham, King of Prussia, USA*
Stinnett, S. *Duke Clinical Research Institute, Durham, USA*
Stone, M. *University College London, UK*
Storer, B.E. *University of Wisconsin, USA*
Storm, H. *Danish Cancer Registry, Copenhagen, Denmark*
Straatman, H. *University of Nijmegen, The Netherlands*
Strachan, D. *University of London, UK*
Strawderman, H. *Rutgers University, Piscataway, USA*
Street, A.P. *University of Queensland, Australia*
Street, D.J. *University of Technology at Sydney, Australia*
Strom, B. *University of Pennyslvania, USA*
Suarez, B.K. *University of Washington, USA*
Subba-Rao, T. *UMIST, Manchester, UK*
Sudman, S. *University of Illinois at Urbana-Champaign, USA*
Suhov, Y. *Statistical Laboratory, University of Cambridge, UK*
Suissa, S. *McGill University, Montreal, Canada*
Sullivan, L. *Stoneham, USA*
Sullivan, S.D. *University of Washington, USA*
Sun, J. *Harvard School of Public Health, USA*
Sun, J-Y. *University of Missouri, USA*
Sutherland, I. *Cambridge, UK*
Swerdlow, A.J. *London School of Hygiene and Tropical Medicine, UK*

Sylvester, R. *Therapeutics in Cancer (EORTC) Data Center, Brussels, Belgium*

Taillon, S. *CIHI, Ottowa, Canada*

Tamblyn, R. *McGill University, Montreal, Canada*

Tan, W-Y. *Germantown, USA*

Taqqu, M. *University of Boston, USA*

Ten Have, T. *Penn State University, USA*

Terwilliger, J. *University of Columbia, USA*

Thall, P.F. *Anderson Cancer Center, Houston, TX, USA*

Therneau, T.M. *Mayo Foundation, Rochester, USA*

Thisted, R. *University of Chicago, USA*

Thode, H.C. *State University of New York at Stonybrook, USA*

Thomas, D. *University of Southern California, USA*

Thompson, E.A. *University of Washington, USA*

Thompson, S.G. *Royal Postgraduate Medical School, London, UK*

Tibshirani, R. *University of Toronto, Canada*

Tilley, B. *Henry for Health Systems, Detroit, USA*

Timæus, I. *Centre for Population Studies, London, UK*

Titterington, D.M. *University of Glasgow, UK*

Todorov, A.A. *University of Washington, USA*

Tonascia, S. *Johns Hopkins University, Baltimore, USA*

Tong, H. *University of Kent at Canterbury, UK*

Tong, Y.L. *Georgia Institute of Technology, USA*

Torrance, G. *McMaster University, Hamilton, Canada*

Tosteson, A. *Dartmouth Hitchcock Medical Centre, Lebanon, USA*

Tosteson, T.D. *Dartmouth Medical School, Lyme, NH, USA*

Travis, C. *Informatics International, Knoxville, USA*

Tritchler, D.E. *Ontario Cancer Institute, Canada*

Tsiatis, A. *University of North Carolina, USA*

Turetsky, B. *University of Pennsylvania, USA*

Tutz, G. *Technische Universität Berlin, Germany*

Ungerleider, R. *Affiliation unknown*

Upton, G. *University of Essex, Colchester, UK*

Vach, W. *Universität Freiburg, Germany*

Væth, M. *Institute for Biostatistik, Arhus, Denmark*

Valliant, R. *US Department of Labor, Washington, USA*

Van der Laan, M. *University of California, Berkeley, CA, USA*

Van Houwelingen, J.C. *Leiden University, The Netherlands*

Van Oortmarssen, G.J. *Department of Public Health, Rotterdam, The Netherlands*

Vangel, M.G. *National Institute of Standards and Technology, Gaithersburg, USA*

Venables, W.N. *University of Adelaide, Australia*

Vieland, V. *University of Iowa, USA*

Wacholder, S. *National Cancer Institute, Rockville, USA*

Wadsworth, J. *Deceased July 1997*

Wadsworth, M.E.J. *MRC National Survey of Health and Development, London, UK*

Wainer, H. *Educational Testing Service, Princeton, USA*

Waksberg, J. *Westat, Rockville, USA*

Walker, N. *University of Cambridge, UK*

Wallenstein, S. *Teaneck, USA*

Walter, S.D. *McMaster University, Hamilton, Canada*

Wang, C.Y. *Fred Hutchinson Cancer Center, Seattle, USA*

Wang, J. *De Montford University, Leicester, UK*

Wang, J-L. *University of California, Davis, USA*

Wang, M-C. *Johns Hopkins University, Baltimore, USA*

Ware, J. *Harvard School of Public Health, USA*

Warnecke, R. *University of Illinois at Chicago, USA*

Wasserman, S. *University of Illinois at Chicago, USA*

Watanabe, K. *Tulane University, New Orleans, USA*

Wei, L.J. *Harvard School of Public Health, USA*

Weinberg, C. *National Institute of Environmental Health, USA*

Weiner, M.G. *University of Pennsylvania, USA*

Weir, B. *University of North Carolina, USA*

Weller, S. *University of Texas Medical Branch, Galveston, USA*

Welsh, A.H. *Australian National University, Canberra, Australia*

Wensing, F. *Affiliation Unknown*

Wermuth, N. *Universität Mainz, Germany*

Whaley, F. *Pharmacia and Upjohn, Kalamazoo, USA*

Whitaker, L. *Imperial College of Science and Technology, UK*

White, C. *Yale University, USA*

White, R.A. *UT MD Anderson Center, Houston, USA*

Wieand, H.S. *University of Pittsburgh, USA*

Wijsman, E.M. *University of Washington, USA*

Wilcox, R.R. *University of Southern California, USA*

Wild, P. *Institut National de Recherche et de Securité, Vandoeuvre Cedex, France*

Wiley, J. *University of California, Berkeley, USA*

Wilkens, L.R. *Cancer Research Center of HI, Honolulu, USA*

Wilkinson, L. *The Wellcome Institute for the History of Medicine, UK*

Williams, D. *University of Bath, UK*

Williams, P. *Harvard School of Public Health, USA*

Williams, S. *University of Pennsylvania, USA*

Williams, S. *San Diego State University, USA*

Willson, J.C. *Kleinfelder Inc., Lakewood, USA*

Wilson, S.R. *Australian National University, Canberra, Australia*

Witte, J.S. *Case Western Reserve University, Cleveland, USA*

Wittes, J. *Statistics Collaborative, Washington, USA*

Wolfe, D.A. *Ohio State University, USA*

Wolff, R.C.L. *University of Queensland, Australia*

Woolson, R.F. *University of Iowa, USA*

Wright, D. *University of Bristol, UK*

Wright, E. *New England Research Institute, Watertown, USA*

Wypij, D. *Harvard School of Public Health, USA*

Xia, Z. *Mayo Clinic, Rochester, USA*

Xie, X. *Fred Hutchinson Cancer Research Center, Seattle, USA*

Xu, R. *University of California, USA*

Young, G.A. *University of Cambridge, UK*

Young, P.J. *University of York, UK*

Young, S.G. *University of Glasgow, UK*

Zabell, S. *Northwestern University, Evanston, USA*

Zacks, S. *Binghamton University, Binghamton, USA*

Zar, J.H. *Northern Illinois University, USA*

Zaslavsky, A. *Harvard Medical School, USA*

Zeger, S. *Johns Hopkins University, Baltimore, USA*

Zelen, M. *Harvard School of Public Health, USA*

Zelterman, D. *Yale University, USA*

Zhang, H. *Yale University School of Medicine, New Haven, CT, USA*

Zhang, M-J. *Medical College of Wisconsin, USA*

Zielhuis, G.A. *University of Nijmegen, The Netherlands*

Zucker, D. *Hebrew University, Jerusalem, Israel*

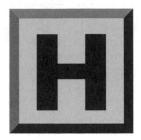

H–H **Plot** *see* Cox Regression Model

Hadamard Matrix *see* Response Surface Methodology

Haldane's Map Function *see* Genetic Map Functions

Half-Normal Distribution

The half-normal distribution will arise in sampling from a standard normal population when the signs of the negative observations are lost or not relevant. The half-normal distribution was introduced by Daniel [2] in connection with the **analysis of variance** of **factorial experiments**. An example of the use of the half-normal in biostatistics is given by Berlin et al. [1], where the outcome of interest was the difference in treatment effects between two treatments in a number of **clinical trials**. The treatment effects (and hence their differences) were assumed normally distributed, but there was no reason to assign either treatment as the first of the pair, so the sign of the difference was made to be positive.

Formally, if z is normally distributed with mean equal to zero and variance equal to one, then the half-normal distribution is the distribution of $\sigma|z|$. The probability density function (pdf) is given by

$$f(x) = \frac{1}{\sigma}\sqrt{\frac{2}{\pi}}\left\{\exp\left[-\left(\frac{x}{\sigma}\right)^2\Big/2\right]\right\}, \quad x \ge 0. \tag{1}$$

The first four central **moments** of the half-normal are given by Elandt [3]:

$$m_1 = \sigma\sqrt{\frac{2}{\pi}}, \tag{2}$$

$$m_2 = \left(1 - \frac{2}{\pi}\right)\sigma^2, \tag{3}$$

$$m_3 = \sqrt{\frac{2}{\pi}}\left(\frac{4-\pi}{\pi}\right)\sigma^3, \tag{4}$$

$$m_4 = \left(\frac{3\pi^2 - 4\pi - 12}{\pi^2}\right)\sigma^4. \tag{5}$$

The standardized third and fourth moments (**skewness** and **kurtosis**, respectively) are

$$\sqrt{\beta_1} = \frac{(4-\pi)\sqrt{2}}{(\pi-2)^{3/2}} = 0.995272 \tag{6}$$

and

$$\beta_2 = \frac{3\pi^2 - 4\pi - 12}{(\pi-2)^2} = 3.86918. \tag{7}$$

The parameter σ can be estimated by equating the noncentral theoretical and sample moments:

$$\hat{\sigma}^2 = \sum_{i=1}^{n} x_i^2/n, \tag{8}$$

where n is the sample size. According to Johnson [4], this is also the **maximum likelihood** estimator.

The half-normal distribution is a special case of the folded normal distribution, where the point of folding is at zero. The folded normal was investigated by Leone et al. [5], Elandt [3], and Johnson [4].

References

[1]   Berlin, J.A., Begg, C.B. & Louis, T.A. (1989). An assessment of publication bias using a sample of published clinical trials, *Journal of the American Statistical Association* **84**, 381–392.

[2]   Daniel, C. (1959). Use of half-normal plots in interpreting factorial two-level experiments, *Technometrics* **1**, 311–341.

[3]   Elandt, R. (1961). The folded normal distribution: two methods of estimating parameters from moments, *Technometrics* **3**, 551–562.

[4]   Johnson, N.L. (1962). The folded normal distribution: accuracy of estimation by maximum likelihood, *Technometrics* **4**, 249–256.

[5]   Leone, F.C., Nelson, L.S. & Nottingham, R.B. (1961). The folded normal distribution, *Technometrics* **4**, 543–550.

R.H. BYERS

Halley, Edmond

Born: November 8, 1656, in Haggerton, UK.
Died: January 14, 1742, in Greenwich, UK.

Edmond Halley was a major English astronomer, mathematician, and physicist, who was also interested in **demography**, insurance mathematics (*see* **Actuarial Methods**), geology, oceanography, geography, and navigation. Moreover, he was considered an engineer and a social statistician whose life was filled with the thrill of discovery. In 1705, he reasoned that the periodic comet – now known as Halley's comet – that appeared in 1456, 1531, 1607, and 1682, was the same comet that appears every 76 years, and accurately predicted that it would appear again in December 1758. His most notable achievements were his discoveries of the motion of stars, which were then considered fixed, and a scheme for computing the motion of comets and establishing their periodicity in elliptical orbits.

Edmond Halley, whose name was also spelled Edmund, was the eldest son of a prosperous landowner, soapmaker, and salter in London. He was tutored at home before attending St Paul's School, where he learned Latin, Greek, and mathematics, including geometry, algebra, the art of navigation, and the science of astronomy. In 1673, at the age of 17, he entered Queen's College, Oxford, and was introduced to John Flamsteed, who was appointed Astronomer Royal in 1676.

In November 1676, Edmond Halley sailed to the island of St Helena, where he cataloged the stars of the southern hemisphere, and incidentally discovered a star cluster in Centaurus, a constellation in the Southern Hemisphere. In 1677, he timed a transit of Mercury and of Venus across the sun and made rough calculations of the mean distance between Earth and the sun. In 1678, he published his results in Catalogus Stellarum Australium, was elected a fellow of The Royal Society, and received the M.A. degree from Oxford University. He married Mary Tooke in 1682, and they had three children – two daughters and one son. He established a home and small observatory center at Islington, and saw the comet of 1682.

Halley encouraged Newton to expand his studies on celestial mechanisms and contributed important editorial aid and financial support to the publication of Newton's major work, *Philosophiae Naturalis Principia Mathematica*, in 1686. From 1685 to 1696 he was assistant of the secretaries of the Royal Society, and from 1685 to 1693 he edited the *Philosophical Transactions of the Royal Society*. In 1698 he was the frequent guest of Peter the Great, who was studying British shipbuilding in England. He was the technical adviser to Queen Anne in the War of Spanish Succession, and in 1702 and 1703 she sent him on diplomatic missions to Europe to advise on the fortification of seaports.

Between 1687 and 1720 Halley published papers on mathematics, ranging from geometry to the computation of logarithms and trigonometric functions. He also published papers on the computation of the focal length of thick lenses and on the calculation of trajectories in gunnery. In 1684 he studied tidal phenomena, and in 1686 he wrote an important paper in geophysics about the trade winds and monsoons. From 1683 to 1692 he published two important papers in geophysics about terrestrial magnetism and made a chart of the variation of the compass. In 1716 he suggested that the aurora was governed by the terrestrial magnetic field.

Halley was a man of great curiosity who combined his astronomical knowledge to help in the dating of historical events. In 1691 he published a paper on the date and place of Julius Caesar's first landing in Britain, and in 1695 he published a paper on the ancient Syrian city of Palmyra. In 1695 he began an intensive study of the movement of the comets, using the hypothesis that cometary paths are nearly parabolic. In 1696 he became deputy controller of the mint at Chester. Between 1698 and 1700, Halley was appointed as a naval captain. He charted magnetic variations while crossing the Atlantic, and was the first to adopt isogonic lines to connect points of equal magnetic variation. In 1704 he was appointed Savilian Professor of Geometry at Oxford and was granted the degree of Doctor of Civil Law. In 1705 he published his cometary views in *Philosophical Transactions,* and *A Synopsis of the Astronomy of Comets.* In 1706 and 1710 he translated and published *Conics,* and *Sectio Rationis of Apollonius.* In 1712 Halley and Newton published *Historia Coelestis,* an edition of Flamsteed's observations, using material deposited at the Royal Society, and infuriated Flamsteed.

Although the major scientific interest of his life was astronomy, Halley wrote a seminal paper on **life tables**. Since the end of the sixteenth century, registers of births and deaths by sex and age had been well kept in Breslau, Silesia. Caspar Neumann, a prominent evangelical pastor and scientist, used the data to combat some popular superstitions about the influence on health of the phases of the moon and certain ages (those divisible by seven and nine). Neumann sent his results to Leibniz, who in 1689 brought them to the attention of the Royal Society. Since the work of **Graunt** and **Petty**, members of the Royal Society were waiting to receive observations suitable for construction of a life table and sent the data to Halley for analysis. In 1693 Halley wrote the paper "An estimate of the degrees of the mortality of mankind, drawn from curious tables of the births and funerals at the City of Breslaw, with an attempt to ascertain the price of annuities upon lives." Halley assumed a constant number of births per year, mortality by age constant in time, and no migration. He did not present the data in detail, but he calculated a life table based on the number of survivors by year, including the first empirical distribution of deaths according to age. He used the life table to calculate the number of men able to bear arms from age 18 to 56, the **median** remaining lifetime for an individual of age x (*see*

Life Expectancy), the total population size, and certain calculations relating to annuities. He found that the value of an annuity is the sum of the expectation of the payments made to the living, a concept later pursued by **Abraham de Moivre**. His expectation became the fundamental quantity in life insurance, today called the pure endowment. Having written an important paper on life tables, Halley never returned to the topic, which was far from his main interests.

In 1715 Halley published a paper on novae, and nebulae, and recorded ideas and experiences of living underwater. In 1720 Halley succeeded John Flamsteed in his appointment as Astronomer Royal. In 1729 he was elected a Foreign Member of the Academie des Sciences at Paris. By 1731 he had published a method of using lunar observations for determining longitude at sea. He also studied the question of the size of the universe and the number of stars it contained.

At his death, Edmond Halley was 86 years old and widely mourned. He was a famous and a friendly man of rare intelligence who was always ready to support young astronomers. As Joseph Laland said about Halley, he was "the greatest of English astronomers ... ranking next to Newton among the scientific Englishmen of his time".

For more complete information about Halley's life, see the following references.

References

[1]   Abbott, D. (1984). *The Biographical Dictionary of Scientists: Astronomers.* Peter Bedrick Books, New York.

[2]   Armitage, A. (1966). *Edmond Halley.* Nelson, London.

[3]   Gillipsie, C.C. (1972). *Dictionary of Scientific Biography,* Vol. VI. Charles Scribner's Sons, New York.

[4]   Hald, A. (1987). On the early history of life insurance mathematics, *Scandinavian Actuarial Journal* **4**, 18.

[5]   Hald, A. (1990). *A History of Probability and Statistics and Their Applications Before 1750.* Wiley, New York.

[6]   Muirden, J. (1968). *The Amateur Astronomer's Handbook: A Guide to Exploring the Heavens.* Thomas Y. Crowell, New York.

[7]   Ronan, C. (1969). *Astronomers Royal.* Doubleday, New York.

[8]   Safra, J.E., chairman. (1997). *The New Encyclopedia Britanica,* Vol. 5. Encyclopedia Britanica, Chicago.

[9]   Stephen, L. & Lee, S., eds (1968). *Dictionary of National Biography,* Vol. 8. Oxford University Press, Oxford.

LINA ASMAR

Halperin, Max

Born: November 5, 1917, in Omaha, Nebraska.
Died: February 1, 1988, in Fairfax, Virginia.

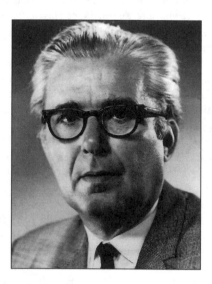

Max Halperin was a leading statistician in biostatistics for over 40 years both at the **National Institutes of Health** and at the Biostatistics Center at the George Washington University. At the time of his death he was Research Professor of Statistics and Director of the Biostatistics Center of the George Washington University.

Halperin graduated from the University of Omaha in 1940 with a B.S. degree and from the University of Iowa in 1941 with an M.S. degree, both in mathematics. He earned his Ph.D. in mathematical statistics from the University of North Carolina in 1950. From 1941 to 1946, Halperin served in the Armed Forces primarily with the US Air Force in the China–Burma–India theater of operations.

A brief review of his career begins with the year 1948–1949 when he was a research mathematician at the RAND Corporation where he worked with Alex Mood. He then spent the years 1950–1955 in the Biometrics Department of the US Air Force School of Aviation Medicine at Randolph Field, Texas. He first came to the National Institutes of Health (NIH) in 1951, joining Felix Moore in the Biometrics Research Branch of the National Heart Institute (NHLBI). From 1955 to 1958 he was Chief of the Biometrics

Office of the Division of Biologic Standards, NIH. For the next eight years he held positions as statistician in private industry with the General Electric Company and with the Sperry-Rand Corporation. He returned to the NIH in 1966 as Assistant Chief and Chief of the Biometrics Research Branch, NHLBI. After retirement from the NIH in 1977, he spent the remaining years of his career as Research Professor of Statistics and Director of the Biostatistics Center of the Department of Statistics at the George Washington University.

Max Halperin entered the Statistics Department at the University of North Carolina shortly after **Harold Hotelling** became chairman of the Department. His first attempt at a dissertation had to be scrapped since a paper was published on the same topic. In 1948 he met Alex Mood who suggested that he write on the estimation of parameters in truncated samples. He successfully completed his dissertation on this theme, publishing one of the first papers on this subject in the *Annals of Mathematical Statistics* [3].

Max Halperin was widely respected and recognized for his contributions to theoretical and applied statistics and biostatistics. He took great joy in working on theoretical problems, particularly those initiated by his consultations with investigators engaged in scientific research. His theoretical work reflected his strength in **multivariate analysis** and his adeptness in deriving **large sample**, asymptotic distributions. His interests in both theoretical and applied research ranged over a broad spectrum of subjects. He contributed significantly to (i) various topics in **regression** such as inverse estimation [16], **errors in variables** [7, 13], interval estimation in **nonlinear regression** [9, 12]; (ii) interval estimation (*see* **Estimation, Interval**) of parametric nonlinear functions [11, 14, 21]; and (iii) distribution-free tests (*see* **Nonparametric Methods**) [4, 23, 25, 30]. In addition, he wrote on applied probability [5, 19], on reliability [10, 18], and on other problems in general statistical methodology [6, 8, 15, 20]. Halperin collaborated with **Cornfield** and others to write on an alternative solution for the **multiple comparison** problem [24] which turned out to be a powerful method to detect **outliers**, and to write on an adaptive procedure for sequential clinical trials (*see* **Sequential Analysis**) [1].

Halperin and his colleagues in the Biometrics Research Branch of the NHLBI were to a large extent responsible for developing the statistical foundations of the **multicenter clinical trial**. During this period, as Chief of the Biometrics Branch in the NHLBI and later as Director of the Biostatistics Center, his interests were primarily directed to the **clinical trial**. The more he became involved in the conduct of clinical trials the more he realized that the clinical trial was much more complicated than a simple extension of a laboratory experiment into the community. He was led to consider special aspects of design [17, 31] and problems in **data and safety monitoring** [27]. His greatest effort at this time was devoted to two major topics: stochastic curtailment [28, 32] and early stopping of a clinical trial [2, 22]. His ideas and writings in these areas had a great impact on the planning and direction of clinical trials (*see* **Clinical Trials Protocols**). In addition to his personal research related to clinical trials, Max Halperin greatly influenced the design and conduct of clinical trials through his service on steering, policy advisory, or **data and safety monitoring boards** of many major clinical trials sponsored by the NHLBI.

Towards the end of his career, he was responsible for another novel idea related to multiple comparisons. Conventionally, statisticians looked for protection against making no errors – in an experiment, or family of experiments, etc. Halperin, however, relaxed the requirement by seeking protection against making at most one error, or at most two errors, etc. [29].

Halperin was a member of the Board of Directors of the **American Statistical Association** (1975–77) and served as an Associate Editor of the *Journal of the American Statistical Association* (1971–74) and of the *American Statistician* (1976–80). He was a member of a committee on standards for statistical symbols and notation together with H.O. Hartley and P.G. Hoel and was the senior author of the Committee's report [26]. He was Chairman of the Biometrics Section of the American Statistical Association in 1974.

Max Halperin received many honors. He was a Fellow of the American Statistical Association, the Institute of Mathematical Statistics, the American Association for the Advancement of Science, and an elected member of the **International Statistical Institute**. He received a Superior Service Award from the Department of Health, Education and Welfare (1973) and the Statistics Section Award from the **American Public Health Association** in 1985.

Max not only worked on statistical problems – he also loved to talk about statistics, especially to point out the difficulties he was running into on a specific problem. Many of these discussions would occur at lunch, which for his associates became special occasions. The problems on which he worked were primarily those motivated by his work. The sole criterion: Was it real and interesting?

Max married Mary Ann Thomas whom he met while both were working at the National Heart Institute. They have a daughter, Martha.

References

[1]   Cornfield, J., Halperin, M. & Greenhouse, S.W. (1969). An adaptive procedure for sequential clinical trials, *Journal of the American Statistical Association* **64**, 759–770.

[2]   DeMets, D. & Halperin, M. (1982). Early stopping in the two-sample problem for bounded random variables, *Controlled Clinical Trials* **3**, 1–12.

[3]   Halperin, M. (1952). Maximum likelihood estimation in truncated samples, *Annals of Mathematical Statistics* **23**, 226–238.

[4]   Halperin, M. (1960). Extension of the Wilcoxon–Mann–Whitney test to samples censored at the same fixed point, *Journal of the American Statistical Association* **55**, 125–138.

[5]   Halperin, M. (1960). Some asymptotic results for a coverage problem, *Annals of Mathematical Statistics* **31**, 1063–1076.

[6]   Halperin, M. (1961). Almost linearly-optimum combination of unbiased estimates, *Journal of the American Statistical Association* **56**, 36–43.

[7]   Halperin, M. (1961). Fitting of straight lines and prediction when both variables are subject to error, *Journal of the American Statistical Association* **56**, 657–669.

[8]   Halperin, M. (1963). Approximations to the non-central "t", with applications, *Technometrics* **5**, 295–305.

[9]   Halperin, M. (1963). Confidence interval estimation of non-linear regression, *Journal of the Royal Statistical Society, Series B* **25**, 330–333.

[10]   Halperin, M. (1964). Some waiting time distributions for redundant systems with repair, *Technometrics* **6**, 27–40.

[11]   Halperin, M. (1964). Interval estimation of non-linear parametric functions II. *Journal of the American Statistical Association* **59**, 168–181.

[12]   Halperin, M. (1964). Note on interval estimation in non-linear regression when responses are correlated, *Journal of the Royal Statistical Society, Series B* **26**, 267–269.

[13]   Halperin, M. (1964). Interval estimation in linear regression when both variables are subject to error, *Journal of the American Statistical Association* **59**, 1112–1120.

[14] Halperin, M. (1965). Interval estimation of non-linear parametric functions III. *Journal of the American Statistical Association* **60**, 1191–1199.

[15] Halperin, M. (1967). An inequality on a bivariate Student's "*t*" distribution, *Journal of the American Statistical Association* **62**, 603–606.

[16] Halperin, M. (1970). On inverse estimation in linear regression, *Technometrics* **12**, 727–734.

[17] Halperin, M. (in the MRFIT Group Report) (1977). Statistical design considerations in the NHLBI multiple risk factor trial, *Journal of Chronic Diseases* **30**, 261–275.

[18] Halperin, M. & Burrows, G.L. (1960). The effect of sequential batching for acceptance–rejection sampling upon sample assurance of total product quality, *Technometrics* **2**, 19–26.

[19] Halperin, M. & Burrows, G.L. (1961). An asymptotic distribution for an occupancy problem with statistical applications, *Technometrics* **3**, 79–89.

[20] Halperin, M. & Lan, K.K.G. (1987). A two sample ordered alternative test for means and variances, *Communications in Statistics - Theory and Methods* **16**, 1297–1313.

[21] Halperin, M. & Mantel, N. (1963). Interval estimation of non-linear parametric functions, *Journal of the American Statistical Association* **58**, 611–627.

[22] Halperin, M. & Ware, J.H. (1974). Early decision in a censored Wilcoxon two-sample test for accumulating survival data, *Journal of the American Statistical Association* **69**, 414–422.

[23] Halperin, M., Gilbert, P.R. & Lachin, J.M. (1987). Distribution free confidence intervals for $\Pr\{X(1) < X(2)\}$, *Biometrics* **43**, 71–80.

[24] Halperin, M., Greenhouse, S.W., Cornfield, J. & Zalokar, J. (1955). Tables of percentage points for the Studentized maximum absolute deviate in normal samples, *Journal of the American Statistical Association* **50**, 185–195.

[25] Halperin, M., Hamdy, M. & Thall, P.F. (1989). Distribution-free confidence intervals for a parameter of Wilcoxon–Mann–Whitney type for ordered categories and progressive censoring, *Biometrics* **45**, 509–521.

[26] Halperin, M., Hartley, H.O. & Hoel, P.G. (1965). Recommended standards for statistical symbols and notation, *American Statistician* **19**, 12–14.

[27] Halperin, M., Lan, K.K.G., Ware, J.H., Johnson, N.J. & DeMets, D.L. (1982). An aid to data monitoring of long term clinical trials, *Controlled Clinical Trials* **3**, 311–323.

[28] Halperin, M., Lan, K.K.G., Wright, E.C. & Foulkes, M.A. (1987). Stochastic curtailing for comparison of slopes in longitudinal studies, *Controlled Clinical Trials* **8**, 315–326.

[29] Halperin, M., Lan, K.K.G. & Hamdy, M. (1988). Some implications of an alternative definition of the multiple comparison problem, *Biometrika* **75**, 773–778.

[30] Halperin, M., Ware, J.H. & Wu, M. (1980). Conditional distribution-free tests for the two-sample problem in the presence of right censoring, *Journal of the American Statistical Association* **75**, 638–645.

[31] Lan, K.K.G., DeMets, D. & Halperin, M. (1984). More flexible sequential and non-sequential designs in long-term clinical trials, *Communications in Statistics - Theory and Methods* **13**, 2339–2353.

[32] Lan, K.K.G., Simon, R. & Halperin, M. (1982). Stochastically curtailed testing in long-term clinical trials, *Communications in Statistics - Theory and Methods* **1**, 207–219.

Samuel W. Greenhouse

Hanes Plot *see* Michaelis–Menten Equation

Hansen–Hurwitz Estimator *see* Horvitz–Thompson Estimator

Haplotype Analysis

Haplotype analysis examines and attempts to specify the genetic information descending through a pedigree, thus providing a useful visualization of the gene flow. Specifically, a haplotype for a given individual and set of loci is defined as the set of alleles inherited, one per locus, from the same parent (*see* **Gene**). Thus, for each person there are two haplotypes, one of maternal origin and the other paternal. Usually, the loci under consideration are syntenic, i.e. the haplotype consists of alleles all on a single chromosome. Traditional haplotype analysis, also known as haplotype reconstruction or simply haplotyping, is the process of obtaining a "best" estimate for each of the two haplotypes for each person in a pedigree. This set of haplotypes is the inferred haplotype vector for that pedigree. For example, Figure 1 shows for a small fully typed pedigree the most likely of the 262 144 haplotype vectors consistent with the data [11, 15].

In addition to traditional haplotyping that simply specifies from which parent each child's allele is descended, there is a more complete form of haplotyping that specifies from which parental *allele* each child's allele is descended, i.e. specifies grandparental

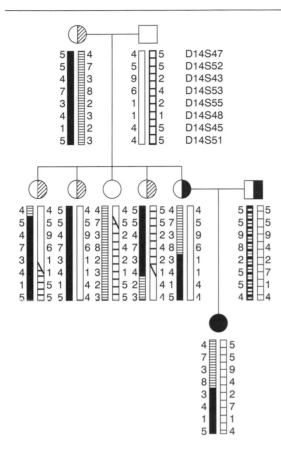

Figure 1 Example of a haplotyped pedigree in which each founder haplotype has been uniquely hatched. This is the most likely of the 262 144 haplotypes consistent with the fully typed pedigree [15]. This pedigree comes from a study of Krabbe disease: the full-black symbol indicates an affected person; half-black indicates obligate carriers; half-hatched indicates carriers identified by an enzyme assay [11] (*see* **Genetic Counseling**). Reproduced from Sobell et al. [15] by permission of Springer-Verlag

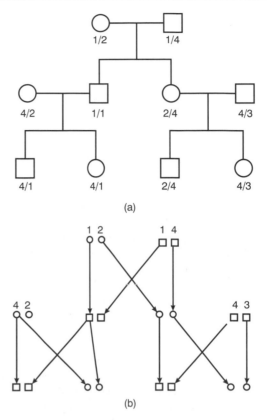

Figure 2 (a) Pedigree data set with one locus in which ordered genotypes have been inferred for each person. (Ordered genotypes are shown as maternal-allele/paternal-allele.) The grandparental origin of the "1" allele cannot be determined; (b) one of the four gene flow representations consistent with the data in (a). Reproduced from Sobel & Lange [14] by permission of the University of Chicago Press

source information. This more complete haplotype analysis includes sufficient information to describe completely gene flow through a pedigree. For example, consider Figure 2(a), which demonstrates a traditional haplotyping solution at a single locus, i.e. everyone has been assigned an ordered **genotype**. (Here, an ordered genotype is listed with the maternal allele on the left, paternal allele on the right.) However, notice that the gene flow is not completely specified, in that the grandparental source of the "1" allele in the grandchildren cannot be determined. Grandparental source information can be displayed by using a gene flow representation. Figure 2(b) shows one of

the four gene flow representations consistent with the data in Figure 2(a). Here, each individual is represented by two nodes at each locus: one for the allele of maternal origin and one for the paternal allele. The founders' nodes have specific alleles assigned to them and then arcs are drawn connecting each child node with the parental node from which it descended. This more complete form of haplotyping can be defined as the task of reproducing the complete gene flow information for a pedigree at the loci under consideration.

Applications of Haplotype Analysis

Haplotype analysis has several common applications. An early goal of haplotyping was to make the genetic data used in **linkage analysis** more informative. A locus is defined to be informative at a mating, i.e. for two parents and their child, if the observed typing information at that locus allows one to infer from which parental allele each allele in the child is inherited (*see* **Polymorphism Information Content**). To illustrate this, consider a locus at which the parents are typed as **heterozygotes** with no alleles in common, e.g. a/b and c/d, then one is assured an informative mating. Conversely, consider the mating in Figure 3(a) in which all three loci are individually uninformative. To increase informativeness, one may construct a single, highly polymorphic "mega-locus" from a number of less polymorphic, but closely linked, loci. (Indeed, some researchers still use the term haplotyping to refer only to this application or to the related problem of finding the population frequencies of the newly defined "mega-alleles".) The creation of a mega-locus is advantageous because each locus alone may be uninformative for many matings in the pedigree, while the combined mega-locus will often be informative at nearly all matings. For example, the mating in Figure 3(a) is uninformative at all three loci. However, if one can create haplotypes for these three loci using the rest of the pedigree (not shown), then the newly defined mega-alleles may make the mega-locus informative. Such an informative mega-locus is seen in Figure 3(b). By treating the combined loci as a single point in the genome, the results of standard linkage analysis will often be improved. Clearly, this approach is best suited for closely linked loci, usually with no recombination between the loci.

Haplotyping is also used to identify genotyping or data-entry errors. Even relatively few mistyping errors can have a significant effect on the determination of genetic maps and gene localization [1, 8]. Haplotyping, by exhibiting the gene flow within a pedigree, permits a visual check of the data to find likely mistypings. Mistyping that results in non-Mendelian inheritance is easy to detect, e.g. a 1/3 child from two 1/2 parents. (Of course, if these data stand up to retyping, then nonpaternity or nonmaternity must be considered.) However, mistyping a true 2/2 child as a 1/2, when both parents are 1/2, is difficult to detect. Haplotyping across this locus may highlight the possibility that the child's typing was in error. For example, in Figure 4 haplotyping reveals a double recombination, one on either side of the questionable allele. If the distance between

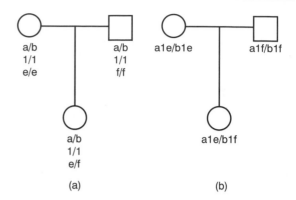

Figure 3 (a) Unordered genotypes at three loci. Each locus is uninformative in this mating; (b) shows the three loci haplotyped and combined into one "mega-locus" that is informative

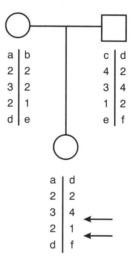

Figure 4 Haplotyping results that suggest that the child's typing may be in error at the "1" allele. The arrows indicate flanking recombination events

these flanking markers is small, then the "1" allele in the child would be a definite candidate for retyping. Several papers have discussed statistical tests (usually **likelihood ratio tests** or their approximation) that indicate which typings are most likely to be in error [1, 8].

Finally, haplotype analysis may provide a more precise localization of a putative trait locus than standard linkage analysis. The introduction of a rare trait in an isolated population, by new mutation or immigration, probably occurred in only a few ancient individuals. Many of the living affected persons will have inherited the trait from a common founder, even though it is not apparent that they are related. Haplotyping of these affected persons, over loci linked to the trait, may reveal a conserved haplotype inherited through many generations from a common founder. The conserved haplotypes will be flanked by alleles not part of the inferred ancient haplotype. These nonconserved alleles are evidence of recombination events that may have occurred in any generation since the introduction of the trait into the population. The interval contained within all such flanking recombination points is most likely to contain the trait locus. This localization technique, using conserved affected haplotypes in isolated populations, employs recombinations from the entire history of the trait's segregation within the population. Classical linkage analysis can only work with the recombination events manifested within the pedigrees observable today. Thus, it is not surprising that this use of haplotype analysis in an isolated population can often localize a trait to a smaller interval than can classical linkage analysis alone.

As an example of this use of haplotype analysis, consider the localization of the autosomal recessive disorder ataxia-telangiectasia (A-T). In early 1995, classical linkage analysis on an international consortium of 176 pedigrees generated an approximately 500 kb (kilobase) support interval for an A-T gene located on the short arm of chromosome 11 [7]. This support interval roughly spanned the region from S1819 to S1294, which contains the markers S384 and S535 (*see* **Genetic Markers**), as shown in Figure 5. No recombination events were seen in the 176 pedigrees between the A-T locus and either S384 or S535. Figure 6 shows an ancestral haplotype analysis of Costa Rican A-T affected persons and demonstrates that 20 out of the 27 seemingly unrelated affected individuals (and 34 out of the 54 haplotypes) contain a region from an identical ancestral haplotype [19]. Moreover, the boundaries of the conserved haplotypes (see individuals 26–3, 35–3,

and 13–3) indicate that the trait locus must be distal to S384. (Here, distal is the direction away from the centromere and proximal is the reverse.) A similar haplotype analysis of a subpopulation of British A-T affected persons concluded that the locus must be proximal to S535 [16]. Haplotype analysis thus localized the A-T gene to the approximately 200 kb interval between S384 and S535; the approximately 100 kb A-T gene, now called ATM, was subsequently found within this interval [12].

Origins of Computational Complexity

Haplotyping is not conceptually difficult – it is simply determining the parental (and grandparental) origin of the children's alleles. What makes haplotyping exceedingly difficult in practice is the amount of missing information usually encountered in a pedigree data set. With even moderate amounts of missing data, the number of haplotype vectors that are consistent with the observed data can grow to astronomical levels. Thus, the search for the "best" haplotype vector is often a nontrivial combinatorial optimization problem.

For typical haplotyping problems the missing data come in the following three forms: (i) Unknown typing is seen in real pedigrees because there are often some people who are simply unavailable for reliable typing at all the loci under consideration. These people may be too remote for sampling; they may decline to participate; or they may simply be deceased. (ii) Phase information for a locus at a typed individual specifies which allele is maternally inherited and which paternally. Modern genetic data, usually marker genotypes and trait phenotypes, do not specify phase. Marker loci are missing phase information because almost all are codominant loci that yield unordered genotypes. In the case of trait phenotypes, even the underlying alleles may be obscured, e.g. a dominant allele will hide the value of the other allele. (iii) Grandparental source information is also

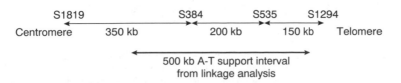

Figure 5 Map of four loci on chromosome 11 that are closely linked to the A-T gene. The 500 kb support interval is indicated for the A-T locus found using linkage analysis

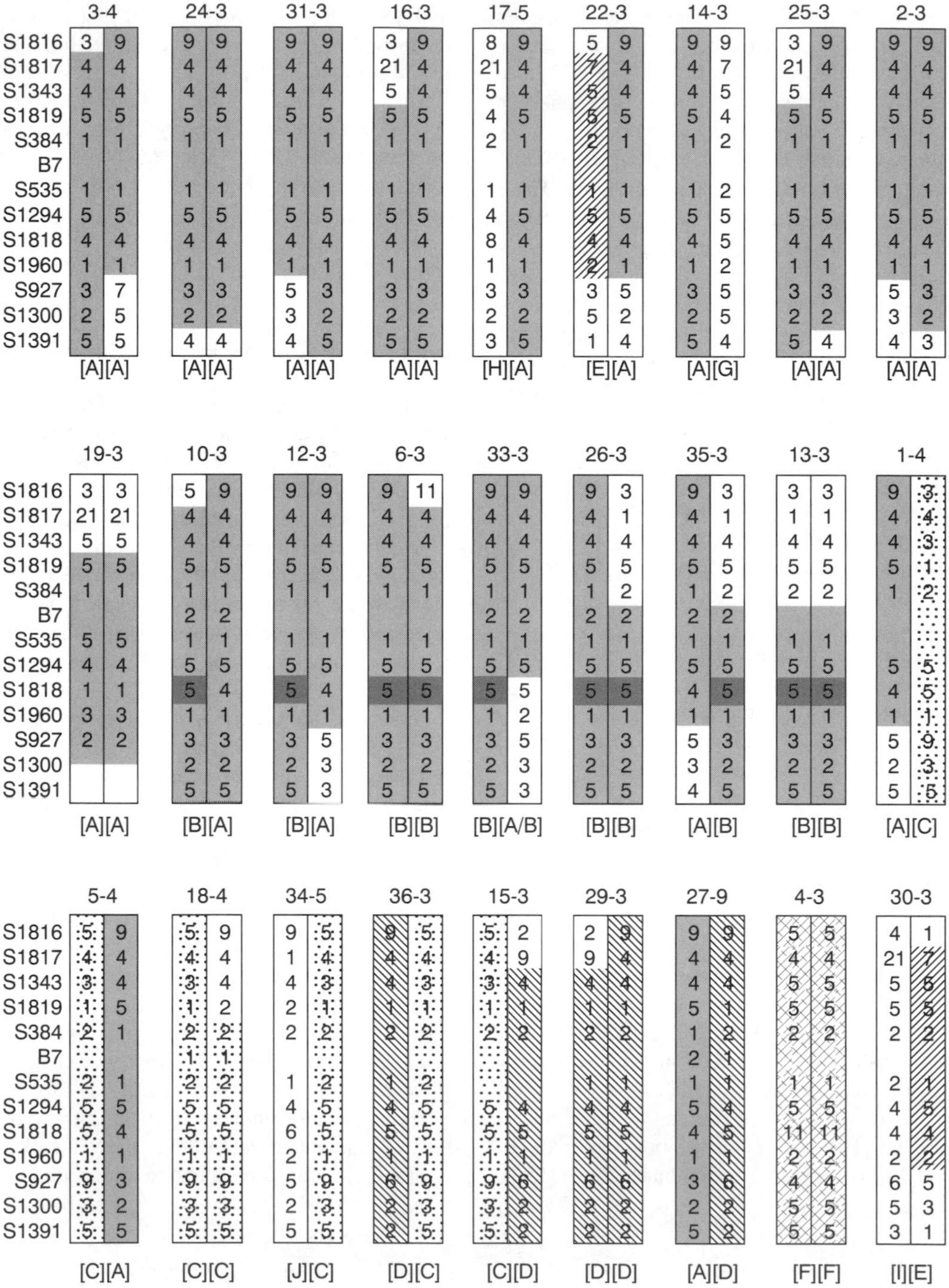

Figure 6 Haplotyping results of 27 living Costa Rican A-T affected persons. The individuals are labeled above the haplotypes; the haplotypes are labeled by bracketed capital letters. The haplotypes of common ancestral origin are similarly hatched. Unique haplotypes (G, H, I, and J) are not hatched. Reproduced from Uhrhammer et al. [19] by permission of the University of Chicago Press

required to be assured of complete knowledge of the gene flow through a pedigree (see Figure 2). However, no source information is specifically included in conventional pedigree data, although occasionally some can be directly inferred.

Much missing data of any type will result in a large number of possible haplotype vectors, each consistent with the data. For example, without phase information even a fully-typed pedigree can have an abundance of consistent haplotype vectors. Specifically, with p people fully typed over l loci there can be as many as 2^{pl} haplotype vectors consistent with the data [15]. For real fully typed pedigrees this value is usually significantly smaller, lowered by homozygosity in the founders and informativeness in the matings. The inheritance patterns in the vicinity of the people with missing data can help one infer the missing values, but the trend towards highly **polymorphic** marker loci increases the number of possible haplotypes the missing data imply. Considering the extent to which each of the three types of data is usually absent, it is not surprising that searching for the best haplotype vector is often computationally complex.

To demonstrate the size of the space that one must search to choose a best haplotype vector for a pedigree, consider the 36 person pedigree structure shown in Figure 7. This pedigree is from a study of dopa-responsive dystonia [10]. We simulated

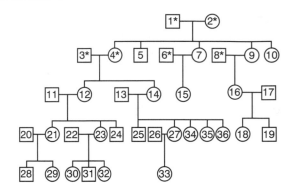

Figure 7 This 36-person pedigree structure is part of the data set used to generate Table 1. The individuals marked with an asterisk have no typing information assigned to them. Everyone else is typed at 14 polymorphic linked loci. Reproduced from Sobel et al. [15] by permission of Springer-Verlag

randomly complete gene flow data on the 14 linked polymorphic markers used in the linkage study. We considered then only the resulting unordered typing information for each individual, except for the six people unavailable for typing in the actual study, for whom no typing information was included. Table 1 lists for each person the number of haplotype pairs consistent with the simulated data. The number of haplotype vectors for the pedigree would be somewhat less than the product, over all people, of these

Table 1 The number of possible haplotype pairs for each individual in the pedigree in Figure 7. Reproduced from Sobel et al. [15] by permission of Springer-Verlag

Person	Haplotype pairs	Person	Haplotype pairs
1	29,421,583,551,360	19	1
2	29,421,583,551,360	20	2048
3	85,944,603,802,337,280	21	2
4	46,558,955,520,000	22	2048
5	75,776	23	2
6	1,024,479,830,005,632	24	2
7	2048	25	8
8	987,891,264,648,288	26	256
9	256	27	2
10	7168	28	2
11	2048	29	1
12	2048	30	2
13	256	31	8
14	2048	32	1
15	4	33	1
16	4	34	16
17	2048	35	8
18	2	36	1

numbers of haplotype pairs. Thus, an exhaustive search of the possible haplotype vectors is well beyond practical computability. (This analysis was previously reported by Sobel et al. [15].)

Algorithms for Haplotype Analysis

The algorithms that have been devised to overcome the computational complexities of haplotyping have evolved considerably with changes in technology. The trend has been away from heuristic and rule-based approaches toward more **likelihood**-based methods, while using sophisticated techniques to avoid as much as possible the computational bottleneck of calculating likelihoods for pedigrees with significant missing data. Manual haplotyping, the first method used, and still used by some, is likely not to consider all the possibilities, even for moderate-sized pedigrees. Indeed, the majority of published haplotype vectors we have examined can be improved; for examples, see Sobel et al. [15]. Another problem with manual haplotyping is that it is difficult to prove that one has performed sufficient analysis to enable others to have confidence in the results. Clearly, the tedious and error-prone nature of haplotyping lends itself to computer-based approaches.

The first class of widely-used computer **algorithms** specifically designed for haplotype analysis were rule-based: PATCH by Wijsman [24] and CHROMLOOK by Haines [4]. By using logical rules to transform the available typing information into inferred underlying haplotypes these programs avoided all likelihood calculations. This approach was developed because at that time the major likelihood calculation programs were fairly limited, by computer memory and time constraints, in the size and complexity of the pedigrees they could handle. Thus, these nonnumeric rule-based algorithms are faster than any other approach. However, rule-based algorithms are by their nature somewhat *ad hoc*. Particularly in the presence of nontyping or uninformative matings, these approaches may leave portions of the haplotypes undetermined. Also, by not considering the recombination fractions between loci, which can be quite varied, these methods may miss a more likely solution.

In contrast to the qualitative rule-based methods, several quantitative algorithms have been devised.

All are based on searching for the haplotype vector that maximizes a likelihood calculation. The most straightforward is the exhaustive enumeration technique. For small pedigrees with few untyped people, one can consider systematically every possible haplotype vector and rank them by exact likelihood. This brute-force approach has become feasible with the speed of modern computers and likelihood calculation programs [21]. This algorithm is guaranteed to find the **maximum likelihood** solution, but is only practical for small pedigrees.

To handle larger pedigrees it is necessary to invoke some scheme to reduce the number of possible haplotype vectors that are considered or to reduce the number of calculations required for each vector. One such strategy is not to compute exact likelihoods over the untyped and uninformative loci, which is where the calculations become complex because the number of possible configurations becomes large. This is the strategy used by the CHROMPIC option of the CRI-MAP program developed by Green et al. [2]. Again, however, nontyping may lead to significant uncertainty or even leave portions of the haplotypes undetermined.

Another implemented strategy reduces the number of configurations that need be considered by using a sequential conditional probability algorithm. Here, the haplotype pairs are assigned to people in the pedigree in a sequential fashion. Once the first $i - 1$ haplotype pairs have been assigned, individual i is assigned the most probable haplotype pair given the observed data and the previously assigned haplotypes. This is the method used in the program HAPLO developed by Weeks et al. [15, 21]. This method can accommodate pedigrees with a modicum of missing data, in which case the order in which the haplotypes are assigned can affect significantly the amount of computation required.

The next strategy for surveying the space of possible haplotype vectors in reasonable time employs the combinatorial optimization technique known as simulated annealing. This technique has been shown to work on many previously intractable optimization problems in many fields [20]. However, the stochastic nature of simulated annealing implies that one is assured only of reaching a near-optimal solution and repeated applications are normally suggested for confidence. SIMCROSS, developed by Weeks et al. [15, 21], includes a particularly fast implementation of simulated annealing for haplotyping. The speed is attained by using an easily calculated **pseudo-likelihood** for the haplotypes. Specifically, for each locus interval i with recombination fraction θ_i, let $\rho_i = \theta_i$ if interval i contains a crossover, and $1 - \theta_i$, otherwise; SIMCROSS uses the pseudo-likelihood $\prod_i \rho_i$. Missing data and large pedigrees can be accommodated by simulated annealing, because it visits only a small fraction of the possible configurations and can escape local maxima of the search space.

Yet another strategy for efficiently searching the space of haplotype vectors uses the gene flow representation of pedigrees as modeled in Figure 2(b). If one ignores the actual alleles assigned to the founder nodes in such a complete gene flow representation, then one is left with only the graph of inheritance paths. Two facts are notable about the space of all such graphs that are consistent with the observed typing. First, the number of these graphs is smaller than the number of possible haplotype vectors – much smaller if there is nontyping in the pedigree. Secondly, given a graph it is straightforward to find the set of founder alleles such that the complete gene flow representation (that is, the combination of the graph and the founder alleles) has maximum likelihood [14]. Thus, one can search the relatively small space of graphs and rank each graph by the maximum likelihood of all haplotype vectors consistent with the graph. Moreover, by conducting this search of the space of graphs, one is, in effect, searching the space of all possible haplotype vectors.

Two haplotyping programs use inheritance graphs, although with different techniques for searching the graph space. For pedigrees in which $2n - f \leq 16$, where n is the number of nonfounders and f the number of founders, GENEHUNTER, by Kruglyak et al. [5], uses the Viterbi algorithm over hidden **Markov chains** to search the graph space comprehensively in reasonable time. Thus, as with the exhaustive enumeration technique, GENEHUNTER is guaranteed to find the maximum likelihood solution and yet is practical for pedigrees of small to modest size, including those with missing data.

However, for large complex pedigrees even the space of inheritance graphs can become too large for deterministic analysis. Similar to SIMCROSS, SIMWALK2, by Sobel & Lange [14], also uses simulated annealing, but to survey the graph space and thus obtain an estimate of the most likely graph. The simulated annealing is performed on a **Markov process** that moves between graphs using the Metropolis criterion [9], i.e. in proportion to the ratio of their exact likelihoods. Although SIMWALK2 may be somewhat slower than the above programs for simple pedigrees (except for the exhaustive enumeration approach, which is, of course, the slowest), it can provide in reasonable time a good estimate of the best haplotype vector for even the most complex pedigree data set.

Conclusions

Haplotype analysis has evolved considerably, driven by the rapid change in genetic and computer technology. This evolution has moved from an *ad hoc* qualitative methodology to quantitative estimations based on maximum likelihood considerations. Despite this progress, haplotype reconstruction can still fail to recover the true haplotype vector for a pedigree, particularly in the presence of large intervals between loci and significant amounts of nontyping. It may simply be that the true state is not the most likely state consistent with the observed data [15]. However, the process of haplotyping may well reveal those specific regions in which more information is needed to pinpoint the true underlying haplotype vector [5].

It is interesting to note that the most recent advances in haplotyping involve techniques that are also proving useful in other branches of pedigree analysis. For example, many areas of pedigree analysis have profited from the use of the gene flow representation of genetic data (see Sobel & Lange [13] and Thompson [18] for reviews). Clearly, haplotyping to the level of complete gene flow information is equivalent to specifying all the identity by descent (IBD) characteristics in the pedigree (*see* **Identity Coefficients**). Thus, it is not surprising that the directed inheritance graphs and the Markov process techniques mentioned above have also been proposed for use in robust nonparametric IBD-based linkage statistics [3, 5, 14, 22, 23] and for **Markov chain Monte Carlo** (MCMC) **multipoint linkage analysis** [5, 6, 13, 14, 17]. These multiple applications demonstrate the importance and flexibility of the gene flow representation and the Markov process methods employed. Moreover, it shows that haplotype analysis can play a central role in the confluence of statistics and genetics that exists in the field of pedigree analysis.

References

[1]   Ehm, M.G., Kimmel, M. & Cottingham, R.W., Jr (1996). Error detection for genetic data, using likelihood methods, *American Journal of Human Genetics* **58**, 225–234.

[2]   Green, P., Falls, K. & Crooks, S. (1990). Documentation for CRI-MAP 2.4. (Unpublished software documentation.)

[3]   Guo, S.-W. (1995). Proportion of genome shared identical by descent by relatives: concept, computation, and applications, *American Journal of Human Genetics* **56**, 1468–1476.

[4]   Haines, J.L. (1992). CHROMLOOK: An interactive program for error detection and mapping in reference linkage data, *Genomics* **14**, 517–519.

[5]   Kruglyak, L., Daly, M.J., Reeve-Daly, M.P. & Lander, E.S. (1996). Parametric and nonparametric linkage analysis: a unified approach, *American Journal of Human Genetics* **58**, 1347–1363.

[6]   Lander, E. & Green, P. (1987). Construction of multilocus genetic linkage maps in humans, *Proceedings of the National Academy of Sciences of the United States of America* **84**, 2363–2367.

[7]   Lange, E., Borresen, A.-L., Chen, X., Chessa, L., Chiplunkar, S., Concannon, P., Dandekar, S., Gerken, S., Lange, K., Liang, T., McConville, C., Polakow, J., Porras, O., Rotman, G., Sanal, O., Sheikhavandi, S., Shiloh, Y., Sobel, E., Taylor, M., Telatar, M., Teraoka, S., Tolun, A., Udar, N., Uhrhammer, N., Vanagaite, L., Wang, Z., Wapelhorst, B., Yang, H.-M. Yang, L., Ziv, Y. & Gatti, R.A. (1995). Localization of an ataxia-telangiectasia gene to an ~500-kb interval on chromosome 11q23.1: linkage analysis of 176 families by an international consortium, *American Journal of Human Genetics* **57**, 112–119.

[8]   Lincoln, S.E. & Lander, E.S. (1992). Systematic detection of errors in genetic linkage data, *Genomics* **14**, 604–610.

[9]   Metropolis, N., Rosenbluth, A., Rosenbluth, M., Teller, A. & Teller, E. (1953). Equations of state calculations by fast computing machines, *Journal of Chemical Physics* **21**, 1087–1092.

[10] Nygaard, T.G., Wilhelmsen, K.C., Risch, N.J., Brown, D.L., Trugman, J.M., Gilliam, T.C., Fahn, S. & Weeks, D.E. (1993). Linkage mapping of dopa-responsive dystonia (DRD) to chromosome 14q, *Nature Genetics* **5**, 386–391.

[11] Oehlmann, R., Zlotogora, J., Wenger, D.A. & Knowlton, R.G. (1993). Localization of the Krabbe disease gene (GALC) on chromosome 14 by multipoint linkage analysis, *American Journal of Human Genetics* **53**, 1250–1255.

[12] Savitsky, K., Bar-Shira, A., Gilad, S., Rotman, G., Ziv, Y., Vanagaite, L., Tagle, D.A., Smith, S., Uziel, T., Sfez, S., Ashkenazi, M., Pecker, I., Frydman, M., Harnik, R., Patanjali, S.R., Simmons, A., Clines, G.A., Sartiel, A., Gatti, R.A., Chessa, L., Sanal, O., Lavin, M.F., Jaspers, N.G.J., Taylor, A.M.R., Arlett, C.F., Miki, T., Weissman, S.M., Lovett, M., Collins, F.S. & Shiloh, Y. (1995). A single ataxia-telangiectasia gene with a product similar to PI-3 kinase, *Science* **268**, 1749–1753.

[13] Sobel, E. & Lange, K. (1993). Metropolis sampling in pedigree analysis, *Statistical Methods in Medical Research* **2**, 263–282.

[14] Sobel, E. & Lange, K. (1996). Descent graphs in pedigree analysis: applications to haplotyping, location scores, and marker-sharing statistics, *American Journal of Human Genetics* **58**, 1323–1337.

[15] Sobel, E., Lange, K., O'Connell, J.R. & Weeks, D.E. (1996). Haplotyping algorithms, in *Genetic Mapping and DNA Sequencing, IMA Volume 81 in Mathematics and its Applications*, T.P. Speed & M.S. Waterman, eds. Springer-Verlag, New York, pp. 89–110.

[16] Taylor, A.M.R., McConville, C.M., Rotman, G., Shiloh, Y. & Byrd, P.J. (1994). A haplotype common to intermediate radiosensitivity variants of ataxia-telangiectasia in the UK, *International Journal of Radiation Biology* **66**, S35–S41.

[17] Thompson, E.A. (1994). Monte Carlo likelihood in genetic mapping, *Statistical Science* **9**, 355–366.

[18] Thompson, E.A. (1996). Likelihood and linkage: from Fisher to the future, *Annals of Statistics* **24**, 449–465.

[19] Uhrhammer, N., Lange, E., Parras, O., Naiem, A., Chen, X., Sheikhavandi, S., Chiplunkar, S., Yang, L., Dandekar, S., Liang, T., Patel, N., Teraoka, S., Udar, N., Calvo, N., Concannon, P., Lange, K. & Gatti, R.A. (1995). Sublocalization of an ataxia-telangiectasia gene distal to D11S384 by ancestral haplotyping in Costa Rican families, *American Journal of Human Genetics* **57**, 103–111.

[20] van Laarhoven, P.J.M. & Aarts, E.H.L. (1987). *Simulated Annealing: Theory and Applications*. Reidel, Dordrecht.

[21] Weeks, D.E., Sobel, E., O'Connell, J.R. & Lange, K. (1995). Computer programs for multilocus haplotyping of general pedigrees, *American Journal of Human Genetics* **56**, 1506–1507.

[22] Whittemore, A.S. & Halpern, J. (1994). Probability of gene identity by descent: computation and applications, *Biometrics* **50**, 109–117.

[23] Whittemore, A.S. & Halpern, J. (1994). A class of tests for linkage using affected pedigree members, *Biometrics* **50**, 118–127.

[24] Wijsman, E.M. (1987). A deductive method of haplotype analysis in pedigrees, *American Journal of Human Genetics* **41**, 356–373.

E. SOBEL & D.E. WEEKS

Haplotype-Based Haplotype Relative Risk (HHRR) *see* Disease–Marker Association

Hardware *see* Computer Architecture

Hardy–Weinberg Equilibrium

The Hardy–Weinberg Equilibrium (HWE) principle, the most fundamental rule of **population genetics**, prescribes the **genotype** frequencies at a locus in terms of its allele frequencies in a population. In the most general form, it states that in the absence of mutation, selection, migration, and random genetic drift (*see* **Population Genetics**), and with random mating in a population, the genotype frequencies at an autosomal locus in a large population will reach equilibrium in a single generation and will continue to be in proportions given by the expansion of $(p_1 A_1 + p_2 A_2 + \cdots + p_k A_k)^2$, where p_i, $i = 1, 2, \ldots, k$, are the frequencies of k alleles $A_1, A_2, \ldots, A_k$ at the locus in the population. In other words, the frequency of a homozygote $A_i A_i$ becomes p_i^2 and that of a **heterozygote** $A_i A_j$ becomes $2 p_i p_j$, the rule that was independently discovered by the British mathematician G.H. Hardy [8] and the German physician Weinberg [20]. Of course, before them, Yule [22], Pearson [15], and Castle [1] noted that this rule works for the special cases of allele frequencies at a biallelic locus (see [12] and [17] for historical notes on the discovery of HWE).

Several authors attempted to pay tribute to Castle's [1] work by renaming this rule as Castle–Hardy–Weinberg's (CHW) law (see, for example, [13]). HWE, as a predictive equation for genotype frequencies in a large population in terms of the allele frequencies at a locus, has played a pivotal role for many other population genetic principles. For example, since the equilibrium is reached in a single generation, it implies that if mating is at random, then to understand the genotypic composition of a population it is not necessary to investigate the past

history of the population. Also, the rule implies that random mating (with regard to the locus under study) is equivalent to random union of gametes. Furthermore, under this rule, the frequency of a rare recessive gene is about one-half of its heterozygote carrier frequency, and, for rare dominant diseases, the frequency of affected individuals in a large population is approximately twice the allele frequency.

Since the conditions (i.e. no preferential mating, no viability and/or fertility differential of alleles, no immigration or emigration, no mutation, and infinite population size) under which HWE is strictly valid are quite severe, and perhaps no real population satisfies most of these conditions, the applicability of HWE in predicting genotype frequencies is still being questioned in current work (see, for example, [11]). The early optimism of the robustness of HWE, however, has turned out to be justified, since for most loci for which the allelic effects are not physiologically meaningful (e.g. **blood groups**, enzyme-proteins, DNA markers), the rule provides a good approximation to reality. This is so, because, in nonexperimental populations, the extent of deviation from HWE is generally so small that the statistical **power** of its detection is "notoriously" small [5, 19].

While HWE can be extended to X-linked loci, to polyploid genetic systems, and even to genotype frequencies at linked loci, the critical difference is that the approach to equilibrium under these systems is gradual, instead of being reached in a single generation (see [7] for discussions on these systems). Deviations from HWE, in the presence of "nondetectable" alleles, and/or mixture of subpopulations that do not completely interbreed, are also well studied (see, for example, [2], [3], [6], [16], [18], and [21]), indicating that unless subpopulations are genetically well differentiated, or the nondetectable alleles are at high frequency in the population, the approximation of HWE is accurate relative to the usual sampling error of genotype frequency evaluation. Both of these factors cause the expected frequencies of homozygotes to be increased, with corresponding deficiencies of heterozygotes in relation to the predictions of HWE, although the deviations are small and are not generally detectable [4, 14]. In contrast, the finite size of a population is expected to cause a reduction of homozygote frequency, with heterozygote frequencies correspondingly increased by a factor of the order of the inverse of twice the breeding size of a population [7, 9, 10].

References

[1]   Castle, W.E. (1903). The laws of heredity of Galton and Mendel, and some laws governing race improvement by selection, *Proceedings of the American Academy of Arts and Sciences* **39**, 223–242.

[2]   Chakraborty, R. & Danker-Hopfe, H. (1991). Analysis of population structure: a comparative analysis of different estimators of Wright's fixation index, in *Handbook of Statistics*, Vol. 8, C.R. Rao & R. Chakraborty, eds. Elsevier, Amsterdam, pp. 203–254.

[3]   Chakraborty, R. & Jin, L. (1992). Heterozygote deficiency, population substructure and their implications in DNA fingerprinting, *Human Genetics* **88**, 267–272.

[4]   Chakraborty, R. & Kidd, K.K. (1991). The utility of DNA typing in forensic work, *Science* **254**, 1735–1739.

[5]   Chakraborty, R. & Rao, D.C. (1972). Detection of the inbreeding coefficient from ABO blood-group data, *American Journal of Human Genetics* **24**, 352–354.

[6]   Chakraborty, R., Zhong, Y., Jin, L. & Budowle, B. (1994). Non-detectability of restriction fragments and independence of DNA-fragment sizes within and between loci in RFLP typing of DNA, *American Journal of Human Genetics* **55**, 391–401.

[7]   Crow, J.F. & Kimura, M. (1970). *An Introduction to Population Genetics Theory*. Harper & Row, New York.

[8]   Hardy, G.H. (1908). Mendelian proportions in a mixed population, *Science* **28**, 49–50.

[9]   Hogben, L. (1946). *An Introduction to Mathematical Genetics*. Norton, New York.

[10]   Levene, H. (1949). On a matching problem arising in genetics, *Annals of Mathematical Statistics* **20**, 91–94.

[11]   Lewontin, R.C. & Hartl, D.L. (1991). Population genetics in forensic DNA typing, *Science* **254**, 1745–1750.

[12]   Li, C.C. (1967). Castle's early work on selection and equilibrium, *American Journal of Human Genetics* **19**, 70–74.

[13]   Li, C.C. (1976). *First Course in Population Genetics*. Pacific Grove, California.

[14]   NRC (1996). *Evaluation of Forensic DNA Evidence*. National Research Council, Washington.

[15]   Pearson, K. (1904). On a generalized theory of alternative inheritance, with special reference to Mendel's laws, *Philosophical Transactions of the Royal Society of London, Series A* **203**, 53–86.

[16]   Smith, C.A.B. (1970). A note on testing the Hardy–Weinberg law, *Annals of Human Genetics* **33**, 377–383.

[17]   Stern, C. (1943). The Hardy–Weinberg law, *Science* **97**, 137–138.

[18]   Wahlund, S. (1928). Zusammensetzung von Populationen und Korrelationserscheinungen von Standpunkt der Vererbungslehre aus betrachtet, *Hereditas* **11**, 65–106.

[19]   Ward, R.H. & Sing, C.F. (1970). A consideration of the power of the χ^2 test to detect inbreeding effects in natural populations, *American Naturalist* **104**, 355–365.

[20]   Weinberg, W. (1908). Uber den Nachweis der Vererbung beim Menschen, *Jahreshefte des Vereins für Vaterändische Naturkunde in Württemberg* **64**, 368–382.

[21]   Weir, B.S. & Cockerham, C.C. (1984). Estimating *F*-statistics for the analysis of population structure, *Evolution* **38**, 1358–1370.

[22]   Yule, G.U. (1902). Mendel's laws and their probable relations to intra-racial heredity, *New Phytologist* **1**, 193–207 and 222–237.

RANAJIT CHAKRABORTY

Harmonic Analysis *see* Spectral Analysis

Harmonic Mean *see* Mean

Harrington–Fleming Test *see* Linear Rank Tests in Survival Analysis

Harris–Kaiser Rotation *see* Orthoblique Rotation

Hat Matrix *see* Diagnostics

Hawkins, Francis Bisset

Born: 1796
Died: 1894

Bisset Hawkins is most widely remembered as the author of the first book on medical statistics in the English language [2]. He was the first Professor of Materia Medica at King's College, London, and was a prolific author in the fields of industrial medicine and public health. He was a founder member in 1834 of the Statistical Society of London (later the **Royal Statistical Society**), although he does not appear to have played a very active part in its later proceedings, and his death at an advanced age went unrecorded in the Society's *Journal* (*see* ***Journal of the Royal Statistical Society***).

According to **Greenwood** [1], Hawkins "was instrumental in obtaining the insertion in the first Registration Act of a column containing the names of the diseases or causes by which death was occasioned", initially on a voluntary basis. That may prove to be a more lasting claim to fame than the celebrated book.

Unfortunately, *Elements of Medical Statistics* now has only curiosity value. Hawkins adopts a purely descriptive approach, relying heavily on crude death rates, but with some appreciation of the effects of the age structure of a population on demographic measures such as the **average age at death**. His detailed comments often show a remarkable lack of critical awareness. The book contains many complimentary remarks about Manchester, which he apparently thought to have a remarkably low death rate (1 in 74, as compared with 1 in 43 for Birmingham and 1 in 40 for London). Unfortunately, he had made an arithmetic slip, and in a copy of the book owned by the Royal Statistical Society all the complimentary references to Manchester are scored out, apparently in his own hand. Again, he seems to have accepted anecdotes from classical antiquity with a degree of naivety. He refers uncritically to reports of individuals living to ages greater than 150 years; and he uses a fatality rate from acute fevers quoted by Hippocrates as a control for more favorable figures recorded in 1825.

As Greenwood remarks, Hawkins "had been diligent and brought together numerical data from all parts of the world and was certainly one of the first physicians to advocate a serious study of hospital records". The work of pioneers often shows traces of fallibility, but they deserve to be remembered for their achievements rather than their weaknesses. Hawkins lacked the mathematical abilities of the younger physicians **W.A. Guy** in England and **Jules Gavarret** in France, but he helped to ensure that medical applications played a significant part in the enormous growth of statistical activity during the first half of the nineteenth century.

References

[1]   Greenwood, M. (1948). *Medical Statistics from Graunt to Farr*. Cambridge University Press, Cambridge.
[2]   Hawkins, F.B. (1829). *Elements of Medical Statistics*. Longman, Rees, Orme, Brown & Green, London.

P. ARMITAGE

Hawthorne Effect

The Hawthorne effect is an effect on study participants that results from their knowing that they are being studied. For example, in a study of methods to promote smoking cessation, it might be necessary to contact study participants each year to determine smoking status. The Hawthorne effect could distort study results if this repeated annual contact affected smoking behavior or the reporting of smoking behavior.

M.H. GAIL

Haybittle–Peto Boundaries *see* Data and Safety Monitoring

Hazard Identification; Hazard Index (HI); Hazard Quotient *see* Risk Assessment for Environmental Chemicals

Hazard Plotting

Hazard plotting and nonparametric statistical inference for **hazard rate** (intensity) models have been vigorously studied in the mathematical framework of counting processes, as illustrated by such articles as **Counting Process Methods in Survival Analysis**, **Nelson–Aalen Estimator, Kaplan–Meier Estimator, Aalen–Johansen Estimator, Repeated Events, Duration Dependence,** and **Goodness of Fit in Survival Analysis**. Common to these versions of the simple techniques for analysis of hazard rate models are some specific model assumptions which were not made by W. Nelson when he originally proposed what is here termed the *Nelson–Aalen estimator* of an integrated hazard.

Nelson's approach is described in the article **Hazard Plotting: The Nelson Approach**, and his generalization to repeated events in the article

Hazard Plotting and Nonparametric Repeated-Events Analysis: the Nelson approach. Some of these generalizations are also natural and obvious in the counting process approach, as evidenced in some of the above-mentioned articles.

To help the reader appreciate the particular characteristics of the two approaches, we provide here a brief introduction to Nelson's derivation of the estimator and its properties in the repeated events situation, referring to the entries mentioned above for the counting process approach. See [1] for further discussion and generalization.

Let the "total cost (or number) of recurrences" or "cumulative cost histories" $X_1, \ldots, X_n$ be independent, identically distributed (iid) nondecreasing, nonnegative, random functions of $t \geq 0$; $X_i(0) = 0$. Let $J_1, \ldots, J_n$ be independent of $X_1, \ldots, X_n$; 0–1 valued and nonincreasing. $X_i(t)$ is the counterfactual cumulative number of events (or more generally, cumulative cost) on unit i, up to time t, when there is no **censoring**. $J_i(t)$ is the indicator that unit i is still uncensored at time t. Note that, as emphasized by Nelson in his entries, no assumptions are made concerning a mechanism generating the functions X; the iid property suffices for the theory. This is in contrast to the counting process approach, in which $X_i(t)$ is a sample function from a stochastic (counting) process.

We *observe* $\tilde{X}_i(t) = \int_0^t J_i(s)\mathrm{d}X_i(s)$ and $J_i(t)$, $t \geq 0$.

Let $X(t)$ denote a generic $X_i(t)$. We assume the "population mean cumulative function" at age t, $x(t) = \mathrm{E}X(t) < \infty$ and we *estimate* it by

$$\hat{x}(t) = \int_0^t \frac{\sum_{i=1}^n \mathrm{d}\tilde{X}_i(s)}{\sum_{j=1}^n J_j(s)} = \sum_{i=1}^n \int_0^t \frac{J_i(s)}{\sum_{j=1}^n J_j(s)} \mathrm{d}X_i(s),$$

where the second expression is the formula used for calculation, while the third is better suited for theoretic developments. Here $\sum_j J_j(t)$ is the number "at risk at age t".

Since we assume that $(J_1, \ldots, J_n)$ is independent of $(X_1, \ldots, X_n)$, and $X_1, \ldots, X_n$ are iid we may condition on $J_1, \ldots, J_n$. We leave $\hat{x}(t)$ undefined for t such that $\sum_1^n J_j(t) = 0$. We see that (conditional on $J_1, \ldots, J_n$), and for t such that $\sum_1^n J_i(t) > 0$, $\hat{x}(t)$ is a sum of n independent contributions.

Using nonnegativity, by Fubini we have (always conditioning on $J_1, \ldots, J_n$)

$$\mathrm{E}\hat{x}(t) = \sum_{i=1}^n \int_0^t \frac{J_i(s)}{\sum_{j=1}^n J_j(s)} \mathrm{d}\mathrm{E}X_i(s)$$

$$= \sum_{i=1}^n \int_0^t \frac{J_i(s)}{\sum_{j=1}^n J_j(s)} \mathrm{d}x(s)$$

$$= \int_0^t \left(\sum_i \left(J_i(s) \bigg/ \sum_{j=1}^n J_j(s) \right) \right) \mathrm{d}x(s)$$

$$= x(t),$$

where we have used that $\sum_1^n J_i(t) > 0 \Rightarrow \sum_1^n J_i(s) > 0$ for all $s \leq t$, and

$$\sum_1^n \frac{J_i(s)}{\sum_j J_j(s)} \equiv 1.$$

Since $\hat{x}(t)$ is a sum of independent contributions, its variance is a sum of variances of each term. We can compute the variance of one term, the ith, as expectation of its square minus the square of its expectation. For the expectation of its square we have, writing $j(s) = j_i(s) = J_i(s)/\sum_j J_j(s)$, $X(s) = X_i(s)$,

$$\mathrm{E}\left(\int_0^t j(s)\mathrm{d}X(s) \right)^2$$

$$= \int_{u=0}^t \int_{v=0}^t j(u)j(v)\mathrm{E}(\mathrm{d}X(u)\mathrm{d}X(v)).$$

Assuming that $\mathrm{E}X(t)^2 < \infty$ this is finite, and by Fubini unbiasedly estimated by substituting, for $u \leq v$,

$$\mathrm{E}(\mathrm{d}X(u)\mathrm{d}X(v))$$

by

$$\sum_{i=1}^n \frac{\mathrm{d}\tilde{X}_i(u)\mathrm{d}\tilde{X}_i(v)}{\sum_{i=1}^n J_i(v)}$$

$$= \sum_{i=1}^n \left(J_i(v) \bigg/ \sum_{j=1}^n J_j(v) \right) \mathrm{d}X_i(u)\mathrm{d}X_i(v).$$

A natural variance estimator is therefore

$$\sum_{i=1}^{n} \left(\iint_{0<u<v\leq t} 2j_i(u)j_i(v) \sum_{j=1}^{n} j_j(v) \mathrm{d}\tilde{X}_j(u) \mathrm{d}\tilde{X}_j(v) \right.$$
$$\left. + \sum_{u=0}^{t} j_i(v)^2 \sum_{j=1}^{n} j_j(u) \Delta\tilde{X}_j(u)^2 - \left(\int_0^t j_i(s) \mathrm{d}\hat{x}(s) \right)^2 \right).$$

Reference

[1] Lawless, J.F. & Nadean, C. (1995). Some simple robust methods for the analysis of recurrent events. *Technometrics* **37**, 158–168.

RICHARD D. GILL & NIELS KEIDING

Hazard Plotting and Nonparametric Repeated-Events Analysis

Recurrent event data arise in many applications where individuals are observed over time and undergo repeated recurrences of events of interest (*see* **Repeated Events**). For example, reliability work on repairable systems yields data on the age of systems when repaired and the cost of repairs. Similarly, medical data on recurrent disease episodes consist of the patients' dates of episodes and costs of treatment. Recurrence data also arise in sociology, criminology, factory simulation, and many other applications.

This article presents a simple hazard-like nonparametric estimate for analyzing recurrence data on the numbers or costs of repeated recurrences of events in a random sample of individuals. It appears similar to the **Nelson–Aalen** estimate of the cumulative hazard function of a life distribution, but differs from that. When plotted, this estimate of the mean cumulative function (defined below) is most informative. It can be used to

1. evaluate whether the population recurrence (or cost) rate increases or decreases with age; this can yield insight on the nature of the recurrences; for example, for repair data, rate information is

useful for system retirement and burn-in decisions;

2. compare two samples; in system repair work, samples come from different designs, production periods, maintenance policies, environments, operating conditions, etc.; in medical work, samples come from different treatments, hospitals, etc.;

3. predict future numbers and costs of recurrences; and

4. reveal unexpected information and insight – an important advantage of plots.

Recurrence Data

This section describes typical recurrence data on a sample of individuals.

Bladder Data

Table 1 displays typical recurrence data from Byar [3] on 38 patients on a new treatment in a clinical study of recurrent bladder tumors. Information sought from the data include (i) the nature of the recurrence rate over time and (ii) how this compares with the rate for patients under a standard treatment. For each patient, the data consist of the number of months (i) in the study at each recurrence and (ii) that the patient was observed. For example, the data on patient 66 are a recurrence at 6 months and the months observed 27+, indicated with +. Nelson [6–8] gives repair data on blood analyzers, residential heat pumps, window air conditioners, power supplies, turbines, and other applications.

Censoring

An individual's current (latest) age under observation is called the "**censoring** age", because the individual's recurrence history beyond that age is censored (unknown) at the time of the data analysis. Usually individual censoring ages differ. The different censoring ages complicate the data analysis and require the methods given here. An individual may have no recurrences; then the data are just the censoring age. Other individuals may have one, two, three, or more recurrences to date. End of a history (say, death of a patient or retirement of a system from service) is

Table 1 Tumor recurrence data for new treatment (+ denotes months observed)

Patient	Months at recurrence
49	1+
50	1+
51	5 5+
52	9+
53	10+
54	13+
55	3 14+
56	1 3 5 7 10 17+
57	18+
58	17 18+
59	2 19+
60	17 19 21+
61	22+
62	25+
63	25+
64	25+
65	6 12 13 26+
66	6 27+
67	2 29+
68	26 35 36+
69	38+
70	22 23 27 32 39+
71	4 16 23 27 33 36 37 39+
72	24 26 29 40 40+
73	41+
74	41+
75	1 27 43+
76	44+
77	2 20 23 27 38 44+
78	45+
79	2 46+
80	46+
81	49+
82	50+
83	4 24 47 50+
84	54+
85	38 54+
86	59+

a complication not discussed here and is a form of informative censoring. Here censoring is assumed to be random (noninformative).

Age

Here "age" (or "time") means any useful measure of usage or exposure, for example days since diagnosis or months under treatment, number of treatment administrations, etc. For repairable products, usage includes mileage, days, cycles, months, etc.

The Population Model and its Mean Cumulative Function

Model

The required information on the recurrence behavior of a population of individuals is given by the population mean cumulative function (MCF) vs. age t. This function, which is defined below, is a feature of the following uncensored model for a population. At a particular age t, each population individual has accumulated a total cost (or number) of recurrences. These cumulative individual totals usually differ. Figure 1 depicts such cumulative cost histories as smooth curves for easier viewing. In reality, the histories are staircase functions, where the rise of each step is the cost or number of recurrences at that age. However, staircase functions are difficult to view in such a plot. Consequently, there is a population distribution of the cumulative cost (or number) of recurrences at age t. It appears in Figure 1 as a continuous density. Suppose this distribution at age t has a population mean, $M(t)$. $M(t)$ is plotted vs. t as a heavy line in Figure 1. $M(t)$ is called the "population mean cumulative function" (MCF) for the cost (or number) of recurrences. As shown below, it provides most information sought from repair data. In **stochastic process** theory for a counting process, $M(t)$ is called the mean value function (*see* **Counting Process Methods in Survival Analysis**).

Repair Rate

When $M(t)$ is the cumulative number of recurrences, the derivative

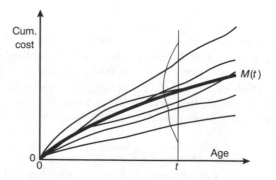

Figure 1 Population cumulative cost histories and MCF $M(t)$

$$m(t) = dM(t)/dt$$

is assumed to exist and is called the population "instantaneous recurrence rate" or the "intensity function". It is expressed in recurrences per unit time per individual, e.g. tumor recurrences per patient per month. For repairable systems, $m(t)$ is called the "repair rate"; some mistakenly call $m(t)$ the "failure rate", which causes confusion with the quite different failure rate (hazard function or **hazard rate**) of a life distribution for nonrepaired units (usually components). The failure rate for a life distribution has an entirely different definition, meaning, and use.

Estimate and Plot of the MCF

Steps

The following steps yield an unbiased nonparametric estimate, $M^*(t)$, of the population MCF, $M(t)$, for the number of repairs from a random sample of N individuals. Superficially the following calculation of $M^*(t)$ for recurrence data appears like the Nelson–Aalen estimate $H^*(t)$ from life data of a population cumulative hazard function $H(t)$ of a life distribution. However, the underlying meaning, properties, and use of the population models for $M(t)$ and $H(t)$ and their estimates differ in important ways.

1. List all recurrence and censoring ages in order from the smallest to the largest, as in column (1) of Table 2, which contains the tumor data. Denote each censoring age with a +. If a recurrence age of an individual equals its censoring age, then put the recurrence age first. If two or more individuals have a common age, then list them in a suitable order, possibly random.
2. For each sample age, write the number R of individuals that have reached that age ("at risk at that age") in column (2) as follows. If the earliest age is a censoring age, then write $R = N - 1$; otherwise, write $R = N$. Proceed down column (2) writing the same R value for each successive recurrence age. At each censoring age reduce the R value by 1. For the last age, $R = 0$.
3. For each recurrence, calculate its observed mean number of recurrences at that age as $1/R$. For example, for the recurrence at 10 months, $1/34 = 0.029$, which appears in column (3). For a censoring age, the observed mean number is zero,

Table 2   MCF Calculations

Months, t (1)	Number at risk, R (2)	Mean number, $1/R$ (3)	Sample MCF, $M^*(t)$ (4)
1	38	0.026	0.026
1	38	0.026	0.052
1+	37		
1+	36		
2	36	0.028	0.080
2	36	0.028	0.108
2	36	0.028	0.136
2	36	0.028	0.164
3	36	0.028	0.192
3	36	0.028	0.220
4	36	0.028	0.248
4	36	0.028	0.276
5	36	0.028	0.304
5	36	0.028	0.332
5+	35		
6	35	0.029	0.361
6	35	0.029	0.390
7	35	0.029	0.419
9+	34		
10	34	0.029	0.448
10+	33		
12	33	0.030	0.478
13	33	0.030	0.508
13+	32		
14+	31		
16	31	0.032	0.540
17	31	0.032	0.572
17	31	0.032	0.604
17+	30		
18+	29		
18+	28		
19	28	0.036	0.640
19+	27		
20	27	0.037	0.677
21+	26		
22	26	0.038	0.715
22+	25		
23	25	0.040	0.755
23	25	0.040	0.795
23	25	0.040	0.835
24	25	0.040	0.875
24	25	0.040	0.915
25+	24		
25+	23		
25+	22		
26	22	0.045	0.960
26	22	0.045	1.005
26+	21		
27	21	0.048	1.053
27	21	0.048	1.101

(continued overleaf)

Table 2 (*continued*)

Months, t (1)	Number at risk, R (2)	Mean number, $1/R$ (3)	Sample MCF, $M^*(t)$ (4)
27	21	0.048	1.149
27	21	0.048	1.197
27+	20		
29	20	0.050	1.247
29+	19		
32	19	0.053	1.300
33	19	0.053	1.353
35	19	0.053	1.406
36	19	0.053	1.459
36+	18		
37	18	0.056	1.515
38	18	0.056	1.571
38	18	0.056	1.627
38+	17		
39+	16		
39+	15		
40	15	0.067	1.694
40+	14		
41+	13		
41+	12		
43+	11		
44+	10		
44+	9		
45+	8		
46+	7		
46+	6		
47	6	0.167	1.861
49+	5		
50+	4		
50+	3		
54+	2		
54+	1		
59+	0		

corresponding to a blank in column (3). However, the censoring ages determine the R values of the recurrences and thus are properly taken into account.

4. In column (4), calculate the sample mean cumulative function, $M^*(t)$, for each recurrence as follows. For the earliest recurrence age, this is its mean number of recurrences, namely 0.026 in Table 2. For each successive recurrence age, this is its corresponding mean number of recurrences [column (3)] plus the previous mean cumulative number [column (4)]. For example, at 10 months, this is $0.029 + 0.419 = 0.448$. Censoring ages have no mean cumulative number.

5. For each recurrence, plot on graph paper its mean cumulative number [column (4)] against its age [column (1)] as in Figure 2. This plot displays the nonparametric estimate $M^*(t)$, the sample MCF. Censoring times are not plotted.

Figure 2 was plotted by Nelson & Doganaksoy's [9] program MCFLIM, which does the calculations above.

Confidence Limits

MCFLIM also calculates pointwise nonparametric approximate 95% **confidence limits** for $M(t)$, shown in Figure 2 above and below each data point by −. Nelson's [8] complex calculations of these limits requires a computer program to calculate Nelson's unbiased estimate of the true variance, var[$M^*(t)$]. The square root of his variance estimate is the **standard error** for $M^*(t)$, and 95% confidence limits for $M(t)$ based on a large-sample normal approximation to the sampling distribution of $M^*(t)$ are $M^*(t)$ plus or minus two standard errors. MCFLIM is available from Wayne Nelson at 739 Huntingdon Drive, Schenectady, NY 12309, USA. The SAS Institute [10] does these calculations in the new RELIABILITY PROCEDURE in the SAS QC Software, available from Dr Gordon Johnston of SAS Institute (*see* **Software, Biostatistical**).

How to Interpret and Use a Plot

The Estimate

The plot displays the nonparametric estimate $M^*(t)$ of $M(t)$. That is, the estimate involves no assumptions about the form of $M(t)$ or a process generating the individual histories. Thus, the estimate is a staircase function that is flat between repair ages, but the flat portions need not be plotted. The MCF of a large population is usually regarded as a smooth curve, and one usually imagines a smooth curve through the plotted points. Interpretations of such plots appear below. See Nelson [6–8] for more details.

Mean Cumulative Number

An estimate of the population mean cumulative number of recurrences by a specified age is read directly from such a curve through the plot. For example, from Figure 2 the graphic estimate of this by

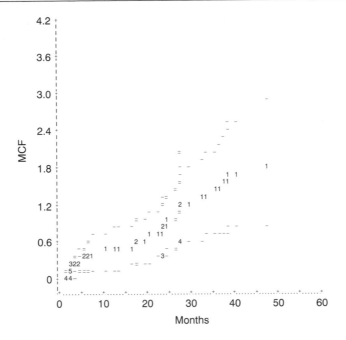

Figure 2   Sample MCF and 95% limits for new treatment

12 months is 0.5 recurrences per patient (on average) – an answer to a common question. This estimate can also be read from Table 2 and is 0.478 recurrences at 12 months. Corresponding 95% confidence limits are 0.16 and 0.79.

Recurrence Rate

The derivative of such a smooth MCF curve (imagined or fitted) estimates the population recurrence rate, $m(t)$. If the derivative increases with age, then the population recurrence rate increases with age. If the derivative decreases, then the population recurrence rate decreases with age. In reliability work, the behavior of the rate is used to determine burn-in, overhaul, and retirement policies. In Figure 2 the tumor recurrence rate (derivative) is constant as the population ages, thus answering a basic question. A **Poisson process** has a constant recurrence rate, but it is not suitable for the tumor recurrences, which do not have independent increments – a key property of the Poisson process.

Burn-In

In a factory burn-in, systems typically are run and repaired until the instantaneous (population) repair

rate decreases to a desired value, m'. An estimate of the suitable length, t', of burn-in is obtained from the sample MCF, as shown in Figure 3. A straight line segment with slope m' is moved until it is tangent to the MCF. The corresponding age t' at the tangent point is suitable, as shown in Figure 3.

Other Information

Nelson [6–8] provides other applications and information on

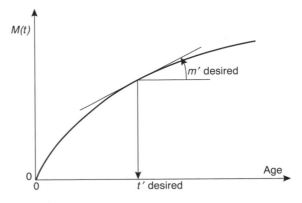

Figure 3   Method to estimate desired time, t', of burn-in

1. predicting future numbers or costs of recurrences for a population;
2. analyzing recurrence cost data (or other noninteger data);
3. analyzing data with more complex censoring where individual histories have gaps with missing recurrence data;
4. analyzing data with a mix of types of recurrences, and the minimal assumptions on which the nonparametric estimate $M^*(t)$ and confidence limits depend; and
5. analyzing continuous history functions, for example on up-time for system availability data, which includes downtime for repair.

Literature

In reliability work most models and data analysis methods for repair data are parametric and involve further assumptions, which often are unrealistic. For example, Englehardt [4] and Ascher & Feingold [2] present such parametric models, analyses, and assumptions for a single individual, not for a sample from a population. The simplest such parametric model is the Poisson process. In biomedical work most models and data analysis methods for recurrence data are nonparametric. For example, Fleming & Harrington [5] and Andersen et al. [1] present such results.

Comparison of Two Samples

This section shows how to compare two statistically independent samples of recurrence data. The comparison is illustrated using the Byar [3] tumor data.

Standard Treatment

Figure 4 displays the estimate of the MCF from 48 patients given a standard treatment for bladder tumor recurrences. The purpose of the study was to compare the standard and new treatments. This sample MCF also has a constant derivative, and this MCF is above that for the new treatment. Over most of the time range the pointwise 95% confidence limits for one treatment overlap the estimate for the other, suggesting that the observed difference is not statistically significant. A better comparison follows.

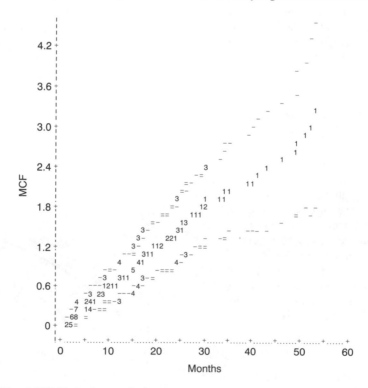

Figure 4   Sample MCF and 95% limits for standard treatment

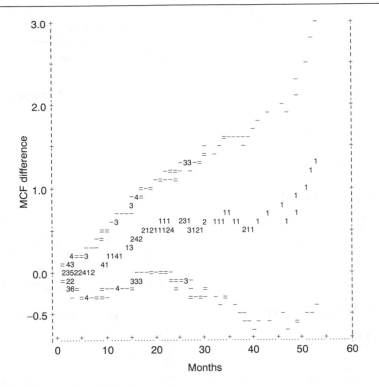

Figure 5   Plot of MCF difference (standard minus new)

Difference

Figure 5 displays the difference $M_1^*(t) - M_2^*(t)$ of the two sample MCF functions (standard minus new). The figure also includes pointwise approximate 95% limits for this difference. These limits all enclose zero, indicating that the two treatments do not differ statistically significantly in this pointwise sense. Limits based on incorrectly assuming that the population has independent increments are too narrow and falsely suggest a significant difference. A treatment population appears better modeled as a mixture of Poisson processes with a different recurrence rate for each patient; such a mixture does not have independent increments.

Limits

The limits for the difference employ the variance $\text{var}[M_1^*(t) - M_2^*(t)] = \text{var}[M_1^*(t)] + \text{var}[M_2^*(t)]$. The square root of its estimate is the standard error of the difference, and the pointwise approximate 95% confidence limits for the difference are the difference plus or minus two such standard errors. Nelson

& Doganaksoy [9] provide a computer program, MCFDIFF, that calculates and plots the sample MCF difference and the approximate 95% limits, as does the SAS Institute [10].

References

[1]   Andersen, K., Borgan, O., Gill, R.D. & Keiding, N. (1993). *Statistical Models Based on Counting Processes.* Springer-Verlag, New York.

[2]   Ascher, H. & Feingold, H. (1984). *Repairable Systems Reliability.* Marcel Dekker, New York.

[3]   Byar, D.P. (1980). The Veterans' Administration study of chemoprophylaxis for recurrent stage I bladder tumors, in *Bladder Tumors and Other Topics in Urological Oncology*, M. Pavone-Macaluso, P.H. Smith & F. Edsmyn, eds. Plenum, New York.

[4]   Englehardt, M. (1995). Models and analyses for the reliability of a single repairable system, in *Recent Advances in Life-Testing and Reliability*, N. Balakrishnan, ed. CRC Press, Boca Raton, pp. 79–106.

[5]   Fleming, T.R. & Harrington, D.P. (1991). *Counting Processes and Survival Analysis.* Wiley, New York.

[6]   Nelson, W. (1988). Graphical analysis of system repair data, *Journal of Quality Technology* **20**, 24–35.

[7]   Nelson, W. (1990). Hazard plotting of left truncated life data, *Journal of Quality Technology* **22**, 230–238.

[8]   Nelson, W. (1995). Confidence limits for recurrence data - applied to cost or number of repairs, *Technometrics* **37**, 147–157.

[9]   Nelson, W. and Doganaksoy, N. (1994). Documentation for MCFLIM and MCFDIFF - Programs for Recurrence Data Analysis, available from Wayne Nelson, 739 Huntingdon Drive, Schenectady, NY 12309, USA.

[10] SAS Institute (1997). *The RELIABILITY PROCEDURE*. Document available from Dr Gordon Johnston, SAS Institute, SAS Campus Drive, Cary, NC, USA.

(*See also* **Hazard Plotting; Hazard Plotting: The Nelson Approach**)

WAYNE NELSON

Hazard Plotting: The Nelson Approach

This article surveys **hazard plotting**, which provides a nonparametric estimate of a cumulative life distribution from multiply right-**censored** and other types of data. Such right-censored data consist of intermixed failure and nonfailure (censoring) times, which are known exactly. Also called the Nelson or **Nelson–Aalen estimate**, it is an alternative to probability plotting of the **Kaplan–Meier** [6], Herd [4], and Johnson [5] median rank, and other estimates. Hazard plotting involves simple calculations and directly provides a parametric or nonparametric estimate of the population **hazard rate** (instantaneous failure rate), as well as an estimate of its cumulative distribution function (*see* **Survival Distributions and Their Characteristics**). A hazard plot also allows one to assess how well a parametric distribution fits the data (*see* **Parametric Models in Survival Analysis**). Terminology here is a mix from biomedical and manufacturing reliability applications.

The hazard plotting method is illustrated with life data in Table 1 from Nelson [11, p. 174] on a new design of a snubber, which is a toaster component. For each of 52 toasters, the corresponding snubber age is its number of cycles on test. An age with a + denotes a snubber ran that number of cycles without failure (a censored life); otherwise, the snubber failed at the age shown. The test purpose was to predict the percentage of new snubbers failing on warranty (typically 500 cycles) and their median life (*see* **Median Survival Time**).

Concepts and Distributions

The hazard estimate and plot employ the cumulative hazard function of a life distribution. Its properties are presented here and provide theory for hazard plotting papers (Figures 1 and 2).

Concepts

We assume that time t to failure has a continuous cumulative distribution function (cdf) $F(t)$ for the population fraction failed by age t. Then the "survival (reliability) function" is $R(t) \equiv 1 - F(t)$. The probability density $f(t) \equiv dF(t)/dt$ is assumed to exist. The "hazard function" (or rate) $h(t) \equiv f(t)/R(t)$ is a measure of population proneness to failure as a function of population age t. $h(t)$ is also called the *force of mortality* and the *instantaneous failure rate*. Useful in various ways, $h(t)$ plays a key role in life data analysis. The "cumulative hazard function" is

$$H(t) \equiv \int_0^t h(t)dt = -\ln[1 - F(t)] = -\ln[R(t)].$$
(1)

Its derivative is $h(t)$, a fact used to interpret hazard plots.

Hazard Paper

As shown below, the time and cumulative hazard scales on hazard paper (Figures 1 and 2) for a parametric theoretical distribution are constructed so that any such $H(t)$ plots as a straight line on the corresponding paper. Eq. (1) can be written

$$F(t) = 1 - \exp[-H(t)].$$
(2)

This "basic relationship" is used to calculate the probability scale on hazard paper for a parametric distribution; also, that probability scale is exactly the same as the one on probability paper for that distribution. The cumulative hazard scale is merely a convenience for plotting sample failure times. Available from TEAM [16] are hazard plotting papers for the **exponential, Weibull** (two papers), **lognormal, normal**, and **extreme value distributions**.

Exponential

The exponential cdf is $F(t) = 1 - \exp(-t/\theta), t \geq 0$, where $\theta > 0$ is the mean time to failure and the 63.2th percentile (*see* **Quantiles**). Its hazard function is $h(t) = 1/\theta$, which is constant over time $t \geq 0$. $H(t) = t/\theta, t \geq 0$, is a linear function of time t. Thus, exponential hazard paper is square grid paper, as in Figure 1. On such paper, the probability scale for the population cumulative percentage failed is given by (2).

Weibull

The Weibull cdf is $F(t) = 1 - \exp[-(t/\alpha)^\beta], t > 0$; here $\beta > 0$ is the shape parameter, and $\alpha > 0$ is the scale parameter (called the characteristic life) and 63.2th percentile. The Weibull hazard function is $h(t) = t^{\beta-1}(\beta/\alpha^\beta), t > 0$. $h(t)$ increases with time t for $\beta > 1$ and decreases for $\beta < 1$; for $\beta = 1$, $h(t)$ is constant and the Weibull distribution is exponential. Thus, the β value determines the failure-rate behavior. $H(t) = (t/\alpha)^\beta, t > 0$, which is a power function of time and is a straight line on log–log paper. Thus, Weibull hazard paper is log–log paper, as in Figure 2. On the paper, the cumulative probability scale is given by (2) and is exactly the same as that on Weibull probability paper. The slope of the straight line equals β, a fact used to estimate β from a plot, as shown below.

Hazard Plot

This section shows how to make and interpret a hazard plot.

How to Plot

Make a hazard plot of multiply right-censored data as follows.

1. Order the n times (failures are unmarked and nonfailures are marked +) from smallest to largest, as in column (1) of Table 1. Label the times with reverse ranks (the number r at risk) as in column (2) of Table 1. That is, label the first (smallest) time with rank n, the second with $n - 1$, etc. and the nth with 1. There are $n = 52$ snubbers in the data set.

Table 1 Hazard calculations for snubber data

Age (1)	Reverse rank, r (2)	Hazard, $100/r$ (3)	Cum. hazard (4)	Cum. prob. (%) (5)
90	52	1.9	1.9	1.9
90	51	2.0	3.9	3.8
90+	50			
190+	49			
218+	48			
218+	47			
241+	46			
268	45	2.2	6.1	5.9
349+	44			
378+	43			
378+	42			
410	41	2.4	8.5	8.1
410	40	2.5	11.0	10.4
410+	39			
485	38	2.6	13.6	12.7
508	37	2.7	16.3	15.0
600+	36			
600+	35			
600+	34			
600+	33			
631	32	3.1	19.4	17.6
631	31	3.2	22.6	20.2
631	30	3.3	25.9	22.8
635	29	3.4	29.3	25.4
658+	28			
658	27	3.7	33.0	28.1
731	26	3.8	36.8	30.8
739	25	4.0	40.8	33.5
739+	24			
739+	23			
739+	22			
739+	21			
790	20	5.0	45.8	36.7
790+	19			
790+	18			
790+	17			
790+	16			
790+	15			
790+	14			
790+	13			
790+	12			
790+	11			
790+	10			
790+	9			
855	8	12.5	58.3	44.2
980	7	14.3	72.6	51.6
980	6	16.7	89.3	59.1
980+	5			
980+	4			
980+	3			
980+	2			
980+	1			

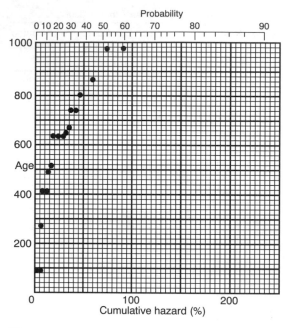

Figure 1 Plot of snubber data on exponential hazard paper

2. Calculate a hazard value for each failure time as $100/r$, where r is its reverse rank (number at risk that passed through that age), as shown in column (3) of Table 1. For example, for the failure at 268 cycles, the hazard value is $100/45 = 2.2\%$.

3. Calculate the cumulative hazard value for each failure as the sum of its hazard value and the cumulative hazard value of the preceding failure, as in column (4) of Table 1. For example, for the failure at 268 cycles, its hazard value 2.2 plus the preceding cumulative hazard value 3.9 is its cumulative hazard value 6.1. Steps 2 and 3 are easy to carry out on a pocket calculator. Nonfailures do not have hazard or cumulative hazard values. Cumulative values have no physical meaning beyond Eqs. (1) and (2) and may exceed 100%.

4. Choose a hazard paper, available from TEAM [16]. The choice is usually based on experience with such data. Label the time-scale to enclose the data and times of interest, as in Figures 1 and 2.

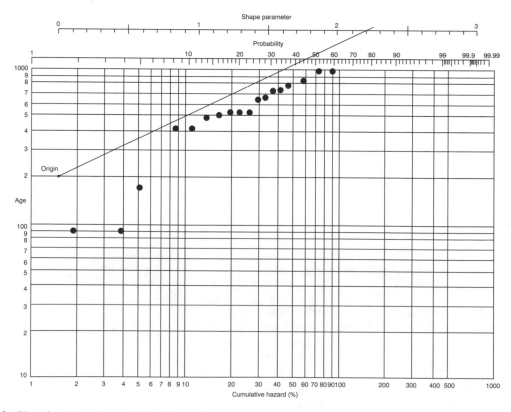

Figure 2 Plot of snubber data on Weibull hazard paper

5. On the paper, plot each cumulative hazard value against its failure time, as shown in Figures 1 and 2. Nonfailure times are not plotted. However, the reverse ranks of nonfailures determine the proper plotting positions of failures.

6. If the plot of failure times is straight enough, then the paper's theoretical distribution adequately fits the data. By eye (or least squares) fit a straight line through the data as a graphic parametric estimate of the population cdf. Also, one can use just the plotted points or a smooth curve through them as a nonparametric cdf estimate.

Motivation

The following informally motivates hazard plotting positions. Formal theory is surveyed later. For a sample failure time t_i with reverse rank r_i, the observed failure (hazard) rate among the r_i units that passed through that age is one out of r_i, i.e., the hazard value $1/r_i$, which is expressed as a percentage above for convenience. This observed hazard rate approximates the population hazard rate at age t_i. Similarly, the sum of the sample hazard values of the failures up through age t_i smooths the data and approximates the integral $H(t_i)$ of the hazard function up to age t_i.

Probability Plot

Such data can be plotted on probability paper. Convert the cumulative hazard percentages to fractions and use them in (2) to calculate the corresponding fractions failed [shown as percentages in column (5) of Table 1]. These fractions (or percentages) failed are used as plotting positions in a probability plot.

How to Use

Once the points are on a hazard plot, it is used like a probability plot (*see* **Graphical Displays**). The cumulative hazard calculations and scale are just convenient means for properly plotting the failure times. Some uses are given below. Nelson [8-11] and Meeker & Escobar [7] give further uses and examples.

1. Using straightness of a plot, one can subjectively assess whether the paper's theoretical distribution adequately fits the data. The exponential plot (Figure 1) is curved, so that distribution is not adequate; the increasing derivative of the plot indicates an increasing failure (or hazard) rate. The Weibull plot (Figure 2) is straight enough, so a Weibull distribution adequately describes the data. Note that the exponential plot compresses the data in the lower tail and spreads out the data in the upper tail. The Weibull plot spreads out and better displays life data in the lower tail, which is usually of greatest interest, especially in product reliability work.

2. The plot yields an estimate of the population percentage failed by an age of interest as follows. Go from that age on the time-scale to the fitted line (or curve) and then to the probability scale to read the percentage. In Figure 2, the percentage failed by age 500 cycles (typical use on a one-year warranty) is 15%; this is too high, so another snubber design was needed.

3. The plot yields estimates of percentiles as follows. Go from the percentage of interest on the probability scale to the fitted line (or curve) and then to the time-scale to read the percentile. In Figure 2, the 50th percentile (snubber median life), interpolating linearly between plotted points, is 940 cycles, just under two years with typical usage of 500 cycles per year. This result also indicated that the design was unsatisfactory.

4. The plot yields estimates of the theoretical distribution's parameters. For example, the estimate of the Weibull scale parameter, α, is the estimate of the 63.2th percentile, 1100 cycles (slightly off scale) from Figure 2. The Weibull shape scale yields an estimate of the shape parameter, β, as follows. Through the paper's "origin", draw a line parallel to the line through the data. Where that line intersects the shape scale is the estimate of the shape parameter. It is 2.2 from Figure 2. This shape value above 1 indicates that the snubber population has an increasing failure rate.

Theory and Extensions

Censoring

The following theory for hazard plotting and for virtually all other analyses of censored data assumes that censoring is random (noninformative). Loosely speaking, censored sample units must have failure times that are independent of their censoring times. This assumption often is not satisfied in practice; then any estimate is biased. For example, patients lost from a survival study often have a shorter remaining life than those who remain in the study and thus are not randomly censored. Treating patient lifetimes as censored when lost will yield a life distribution estimate that is biased toward longer life. Similarly, products removed unfailed from service because they seem likely to fail soon are not randomly censored. Another example arises if a sample comes from a population with strata each with a different life distribution and different censoring. Then the pooled sample is not randomly censored, and any estimate of the life distribution from the pooled data is biased. This is so because the strata with short censoring times do not contribute to the cdf estimate at longer times. This situation may arise with products made in different production periods with different life distributions and times in service.

History

The following briefly surveys the history of the hazard estimate and plotting. In 1967, an engineer brought to Wayne Nelson a set of multiply right-censored life data for which the engineer had calculated cumulative hazard values and had incorrectly plotted them on probability paper. Nelson [8; 11, Chapter 4] published the hazard calculation and various hazard plotting papers he developed for this engineer. A later discovery showed that Leadbetter had previously described hazard calculations and had plotted data on simple log–log paper to make a Weibull-type plot. Nelson [9; 11, pp. 173–187] extended the hazard calculations and plotting to data with a mix of independent competing failure modes (*see* **Competing Risks**). Nelson [10] extended the estimate to data multiply censored on the left, and on both the right and left. For a multiple failure (type II) censored sample, which is rare in practice, Nelson [10] formally justified the cumulative hazard value $H^*(T_i)$ of the ith ordered failure time T_i by showing that value is the expectation of $H(T_i)$ for that sample's censoring pattern; he also gave the variance of $H(T_i)$ and its covariance with $H(T_j)$. Aalen [1] derived the asymptotic properties

of $H^*(t)$ for multiply time (type I) censored samples, which are common in practice; such properties appear in Fleming & Harrington [3] and Andersen et al. [2]. Nelson [13] extended hazard plotting to left **truncated** data; here the sample consists of several groups of individuals where failures in each group were unobserved before some common truncation age for the group; one observes failure and censoring times of a group only after its common truncation age (*see* **Delayed Entry**). Also, hazard plotting is widely used to assess the fit of the **Cox regression model** to life data; one makes hazard plots of data from selected population strata on log–log paper; if the plots are parallel, then the corresponding strata have **proportional hazards**.

Recurrence Data

Nelson [12] extended hazard-type estimates and plotting to recurrence data (stochastic counting and continuous processes) (*see* **Repeated Events**); the estimates extend to cost or other recurring quantities over time (*see* **Hazard Plotting and Nonparametric Repeated-Events Analysis**). Nelson [14] provided approximate **confidence limits** for recurrence data. The recurrence data estimate, plot, and confidence limits are available in [15] (*see* **Software, Biostatistical**).

Interval Data

Strictly speaking, hazard plotting applies only to multiply censored data where all failure times are exact and distinct since the cdf is continuous, and censoring times are exact. Suppose now that the failure and censoring times are grouped into a common set of intervals (say, by month), which need not have equal length (*see* **Interval Censoring**). Then the hazard values must be modified as follows. Suppose interval i is $(t_{(i-1)}, t_{(i)}]$, $i = 1, 2, \ldots, I$, where $t(0) = 0$ or the lower limit of the distribution. Suppose that the number entering interval i is $n_i (n_1 = n)$, the number failing in the interval is f_i, and the number censored "randomly" in the interval is c_i. Then the "average" number at risk in interval i is $r_i = n_i - c_i/2$, and the corresponding hazard value for interval i is $h_i = f_i/r_i$. The upper endpoint, $t_{(i)}$, of interval i is plotted against the cumulative hazard value $H_{(i)} = h_1 + h_2 + \ldots + h_i = H_{(i-1)} + h_i$.

References

[1]   Aalen, O.O. (1978). Nonparametric inference for a family of counting processes, *Annals of Statistics* **6**, 701–726.

[2]   Andersen, K., Borgan, Ø., Gill, R.D. & Keiding, N. (1993). *Statistical Models Based on Counting Processes*. Springer-Verlag, New York.

[3]   Fleming, T.R. & Harrington, D.P. (1991). *Counting Processes and Survival Analysis*. Wiley, New York.

[4]   Herd, G.R. (1960). Estimation of reliability from incomplete data, in *Proceedings of the Sixth National Symposium on Reliability and Quality Control*. IEEE, New York, pp. 202–217.

[5]   Johnson, L.G. (1964). *The Statistical Treatment of Fatigue Experiments*. Elsevier, New York.

[6]   Kaplan, E.L. & Meier, P. (1958). Nonparametric estimation from incomplete observations, *Journal of the American Statistical Association* **53**, 457–481.

[7]   Meeker, W.Q. & Escobar, L.A. (1998). *Statistical Methods for Reliability Data*. Wiley, New York.

[8]   Nelson, W. (1969). Hazard plotting for incomplete failure data, *Journal of Quality Technology* **1**, 27–52.

[9]   Nelson, W. (1970). Hazard plotting methods for analysis of life data with different failure modes, *Journal of Quality Technology* **2**, 126–149.

[10]   Nelson, W. (1972). Theory and applications of hazard plotting for censored failure data, *Technometrics* **14**, 945–966.

[11]   Nelson, W. (1982). *Applied Life Data Analysis*. Wiley, New York.

[12]   Nelson, W. (1988). Graphical analysis of system repair data, *Journal of Quality Technology* **20**, 24–35.

[13]   Nelson, W. (1990). Hazard plotting of left truncated data, *Journal of Quality Technology* **22**, 230–238.

[14]   Nelson, W. (1995). Confidence limits for recurrence data – applied to cost or number of product repairs, *Technometrics* **37**, 147–157.

[15]   SAS Institute (1997). *The RELIABILITY PROCEDURE*. Document available from Dr Gordon Johnston, SAS Institute, SAS Campus Drive, Cary, MC, USA.

[16]   TEAM (1997). Catalog of Graph Papers, Box 25, Tamworth, NH 03886, USA.

WAYNE NELSON

Hazard Rate

The hazard rate at time t of an event is the limit $\lambda(t) = \text{limit}_{\Delta \downarrow 0} \Delta^{-1} \Pr(t \preceq T \prec t + \Delta | t \preceq T)$, where T is the exact time to the event. Special cases and synonyms of hazard rate, depending on the event in question, include force of mortality (where the event is

death), instantaneous incidence rate, **incidence rate**, and **incidence density** (where the event is disease occurrence).

For events that can only occur once, such as death or first occurrence of an illness, the probability that the event occurs in the interval $[0, t)$ is given by $1 - \exp(-\int_0^t \lambda(u)du)$ (*see* **Survival Analysis, Overview; Survival Distributions and Their Characteristics**). The quantity $\int_0^t \lambda(u)du$ is known as the **cumulative hazard**.

Often, the theoretical hazard rate $\lambda(u)$ is estimated by dividing the number of events that arise in a population in a short time interval by the corresponding **person-years at risk**. The various terms, hazard rate, force of mortality, incidence density, person–years incidence rate, and incidence rate are often used to denote estimates of the corresponding theoretical hazard rate.

M.H. GAIL

Hazard Ratio Estimator

In **survival analysis**, statistical models are frequently specified via the **hazard** function $\alpha(t)$. A simple model for the relation between the hazard functions in two groups (e.g. a treatment group 1 and a control group 0) is the **proportional hazards model** where

$$\alpha_1(t) = \theta\alpha_0(t), \qquad (1)$$

with θ being the treatment effect. For a parametrically specified baseline hazard, $\alpha_0(t)$, both the treatment effect and the parameters in the baseline hazard are usually estimated using **maximum likelihood**. In a semiparametric model where the baseline hazard is left unspecified, several estimators for θ are available: the maximum **partial likelihood** ("Cox") estimator, cf. [5] (*see* **Cox Regression Model**), a class of **rank** estimators, and some *ad hoc* estimators.

Assume that the available data are

$$(X_{ij}, D_{ij}; i = 1, \ldots, n_j, j = 0, 1),$$

where the X_{ij} are the times of observation: a failure time if the corresponding indicator D_{ij} is 1, a right-censoring time if D_{ij} is 0. The Cox estimator, $\hat{\theta}$, is then the solution to the following equation:

$$O_1 = E_1(\theta), \qquad (2)$$

where, for $j = 0, 1, O_j = \sum_i D_{ij}$ and

$$E_1(\theta) = \sum_{ij} \frac{Y_1(X_{ij})\theta}{Y_0(X_{ij}) + Y_1(X_{ij})\theta} D_{ij}.$$

Here, $Y_j(t) = \sum_i I(X_{ij} \geq t)$ is the number at risk at time $t-$ in group j, $j = 0, 1$. Notice that (2) expresses that for $\theta = \hat{\theta}$, the observed number, O_1, of failures in group 1 should be equal to a corresponding "expected" number, $E_1(\theta)$ under the proportional hazards assumption. The Cox estimator $\hat{\theta}$ is **consistent** and asymptotically normal under mild regularity conditions when n_0 and n_1 tend to infinity (*see* **Large-Sample Theory**).

A class of explicit "rank" estimators originally introduced by Crowley et al. [6] and further discussed by Andersen [1] is for a given *weight process* $L(t)$ given by

$$\hat{\theta}_L = \frac{\sum_{i=1}^{n_1} L(X_{i1})(D_{i1}/Y_1(X_{i1}))}{\sum_{i=1}^{n_0} L(X_{i0})(D_{i0}/Y_0(X_{i0}))}. \qquad (3)$$

For $L(t) = I(t \leq t^*)$, $\hat{\theta}_L$ is simply the ratio between the **Nelson–Aalen estimators** for the cumulative hazards in groups 1 and 0 evaluated at t^*. Under the same kind of regularity conditions as for $\hat{\theta}$, the rank estimators given by (3) are also consistent and asymptotically normal if the weight process is well behaved in large samples. It was shown in the above-mentioned papers that the Cox estimator $\hat{\theta}$ given by (2) is always less dispersed than any $\hat{\theta}_L$ given by (3). However, for the particular choice

$$L(t) = \frac{Y_0(t)Y_1(t)}{Y_0(t) + Y_1(t)}, \qquad (4)$$

$\hat{\theta}_L$ is nearly fully **efficient** when θ is close to 1. Furthermore, a fully efficient estimator is the two-step estimator of Begun & Reid [3] that is obtained with

$$L(t) = \frac{Y_0(t)Y_1(t)/\theta^*}{Y_0(t) + Y_1(t)\theta^*},$$

where θ^* is some preliminary, consistent estimator, e.g. $\widehat{\theta_{L=1}}$.

Using an estimator $\hat{\theta}_L$ and its estimated variance (see, for example, Andersen et al. [2, Section V.3.1]) the hypothesis $\theta = 1$ of no treatment effect may be tested. This gives all the standard linear nonparametric two-sample tests for survival data (*see* **Linear Rank Tests in Survival Analysis**) and, in particular, the weight process given by (4) gives the **logrank test**.

Another explicit *ad hoc* estimator, discussed by Breslow [4], is given by

$$\tilde{\theta} = \frac{O_1/E_1(1)}{O_0/E_0(1)},$$

with

$$E_0(\theta) = \sum_{ij} \frac{Y_0(X_{ij})}{Y_0(X_{ij}) + Y_1(X_{ij})\theta} D_{ij}.$$

The estimator $\tilde{\theta}$ is generally inconsistent when $\theta \neq 1$ but it has gained some popularity due to its simplicity and close connection to the logrank test, which is also based on the observed, O_0 and O_1, and expected, $E_0(1)$ and $E_1(1)$, numbers of failures.

Tests for the proportional hazards assumption (1) based on $\hat{\theta}_L$ were studied by Gill & Schumacher [7] and further developed by Lin [9]; see, for example, Andersen et al. [2, Example VII.3.5].

The estimators discussed above only make sense under the proportional hazards model (1). However, Kalbfleisch & Prentice [8] defined, for a given survival function, S, the *average hazard ratio* by $\theta_1(S)/\theta_0(S)$ where, for $j = 0, 1$,

$$\theta_j(S) = -\int_0^\infty \frac{\alpha_j(t)}{\alpha_0(t) + \alpha_1(t)} dS(t). \qquad (5)$$

Under the model (1) the average hazard ratio reduces to θ. Particular emphasis was paid to survival functions of the form $S(t) = (S_0(t)S_1(t))^\gamma$ where, for $j = 0, 1, S_j(t)$ is the survival function corresponding to the hazard function $\alpha_j(t)$. In this case (5) reduces to the following quantity:

$$-\int_0^\infty S_0(t)^\gamma dS_1(t)^\gamma,$$

which, for a given value of γ, is easily estimated by replacing the survival function $S_j(t)$ by its **Kaplan–Meier estimator**.

References

[1]   Andersen, P.K. (1983). Comparing survival distributions via hazard ratio estimates, *Scandinavian Journal of Statistics* **10**, 77–85.
[2]   Andersen, P.K., Borgan, Ø., Gill, R.D. & Keiding, N. (1993). *Statistical Models Based on Counting Processes.* Springer-Verlag, New York:
[3]   Begun, J.M. & Reid, N. (1983). Estimating the relative risk with censored data, *Journal of the American Statistical Association* **78**, 337–341.
[4]   Breslow, N.E. (1975). Analysis of survival data under the proportional hazards model, *International Statistical Review* **43**, 45–58.
[5]   Cox, D.R. (1972). Regression models and life-tables (with discussion), *Journal of the Royal Statistical Society, Series B* **34**, 187–220.
[6]   Crowley, J.J., Liu, P.Y. & Voelkel, J.G. (1982). Estimation of the ratio of hazard functions, in *Lecture Notes – Monograph Series* 2, *Survival Analysis*, J.J. Crowley & R.A. Johnson, eds. Institute of Mathematical Statistics, Hayward, pp. 56–73.
[7]   Gill, R.D. & Schumacher, M. (1987). A simple test of the proportional hazards assumption, *Biometrika* **74**, 289–300.
[8]   Kalbfleisch, J.D. & Prentice, R.L. (1981). Estimation of the average hazard ratio, *Biometrika* **68**, 105–112.
[9]   Lin, D.Y. (1991). Goodness-of-fit analysis for the Cox regression model based on a class of parameter estimators, *Journal of the American Statistical Association* **86**, 725–728.

(*See also* **Survival Distributions and Their Characteristics**)

PER KRAGH ANDERSEN

Hazard Regression (HARE) *see* Drug Utilization Patterns

Health Belief Model *see* Health Care Utilization and Behavior, Models of

Health Care Financing

The methods used to finance personal health care service play a major role in shaping a country's

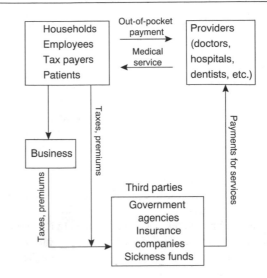

Figure 1 Health care financing. Source: adapted from [10]

health care system. Personal health care services are those services such as hospital care, physician care, dental services, and drugs that are provided directly to individuals. The financing methods influence the terms under which people access the health care delivery system, the types of health care provided, and the mechanisms used to allocate health care services. They also influence how the costs of health care services are distributed over the population by income and by health status.

Two aspects of health care financing are the focus of this article: the sources of funds for health care services and the mechanisms used to pay individuals and institutions who provide health care services. Figure 1 presents a diagrammatic representation of these two aspects of health care financing and provides a framework for the discussion that follows.

Sources of Payments for Health Care

Overview

Individuals may simply use their own incomes to purchase health care services from health care providers (physicians, hospitals, clinics, laboratories, and other firms/individuals). In most other markets this is the way goods and services are purchased. However, the market for health care services has evolved quite differently. In this market, other mechanisms such as private insurance plans, sickness funds, and national health insurance systems have been developed to pay for a significant proportion of personal health care services.

Nevertheless, as indicated in Figure 1, all health care is eventually paid for by individuals. It is individuals who ultimately pay the premiums to insurance companies and the taxes to governments which in turn pay for health care services. Furthermore, even though business may be a source for collecting premiums and/or taxes, the amounts paid by businesses are passed back to individuals and households through lower wages, higher prices, or lower returns on invested capital.

The total payments made for health care are sometimes referred to as the *cost* of personal health care. The way that the funds are raised to pay for health care services affects the distribution of the cost of health care within a country. Two types of distributions of the cost of health care are frequently considered: the distribution by health status (across the healthy and the sick), and the distribution by income. Analysts classify funding sources with respect to income as progressive, regressive, or proportional. In a progressive funding system the fraction of a person's income paid in taxes (or premiums) rises as their income rises; in a regressive funding system the fraction of a person's income paid in taxes (or premiums) declines as their income rises; while under a proportion funding system, this fraction is constant regardless of a person's income. This section will discuss the sources of funds in some detail and comment on the distribution of the cost of health care.

Payments by Third Parties

A basic characteristic of health care systems in all developed countries is that the majority of payments for medical services flows through third parties. A third party is an entity, usually an insurance company or government agency, that pays for medical services but does not receive or provide health care services. This payer is the third party, while the patient and the health care provider are the first two parties. This distinction between the third party and the providers is becoming blurred, particularly in the US. In the US, groups of health care providers may assume some financial risk (thus acting as insurers) by contracting with governments, businesses, and/or individuals to provide medical care at a fixed rate per person covered.

In general, third-party financing arose for two reasons: individuals wanted to insure against the large and uncertain financial costs associated with illness, and governments wanted to ensure that the population at large or certain vulnerable portions of the population had access to needed health care.

As indicated in Figure 1, there are three basic sources of third-party funds: general taxes, payroll taxes, and insurance premiums. General taxes include income taxes, value added or consumption taxes, and other specific taxes. Payroll taxes are employment-related taxes which are normally set as a percentage of payroll or wages. (Payroll taxes may apply to all wages, or to wages up to a certain amount.) Insurance premiums are the amount paid for an insurance policy – premiums vary according to the type and amount of insurance purchased as well as the characteristics of the individuals covered under the policy.

Premiums are the price paid for an insurance policy. (An individual's policy may cover the individual, or the individual and other persons dependent on that individual.) Payments made by the insurance company for covered medical services used by individuals enrolled in the insurance plan are funded by the premiums. If premiums are the sole funding source for the plan, then premiums must reflect the expected cost of health care services used by the individuals covered under that plan. There are two different approaches to setting the health insurance premiums: community rating and experience rating. Community rating systems use the average, expected cost of medical care for all individuals in a community and assign this premium to each individual in the community. An experience rating system groups individuals by some common characteristic (i.e. place of employment, age, whether or not they smoke) and assigns individuals of like characteristics the same premium which is based on the average, expected cost of medical care for individuals with those characteristics (*see* **Actuarial Methods**).

Major Sources of Third Party Funds in Selected Countries.   Payroll taxes are the major source of third-party funds in France and Germany. In both of these countries, employees and employers pay a certain percentage of their wages into sickness funds. In Germany there are several sickness funds, and employees often have a wide choice of sickness funds in a region. Once an employee selects a fund, the fund has the right to collect its premiums (which vary from fund to fund) as a percent of the employee's gross wages – half the premium is paid by the employer and half by the employee. There is a limit on the amount of wages subject to premiums. In France there is one large sickness fund (which covers about 80% of the population) and several small funds. The contributions paid by employers and employees are set by the Central Government: the employer pays about 12.6% of total wage bill and the employee pays about 6.8% of wages. In both of these countries, systems have been developed to cover individuals who are unemployed and those who are retired.

General taxes are the major source of third-party funds in the UK and Canada. The British National Health Service is a national program. The Canadian Medicare program is a decentralized program and the cost of the program is shared between the federal and provincial governments. Each Canadian province administers its own program and exercises some discretion regarding which medical services are covered.

Third-party financing in the US is fundamentally different from that in all other developed countries because of the large mix of funding methods used. Multiple types of third parties exist, including government programs such as Medicare and Medicaid, nonprofit insurance companies such as Blue Cross/Blue Shield, and numerous private insurance plans vended to employers, unions, and individuals. This variety of third-party payers results in a mix of sources of third-party funds, including premiums by individuals and businesses, general taxes, and payroll taxes.

In the US, the majority of employed people and their dependants obtain health insurance through their employment. However, the provision of health insurance by employers is strictly voluntary (other than the State of Hawaii which mandates that employers provide health insurance). The fact that many employers voluntarily offer health insurance reflects the strong incentives in the current tax system for employers to provide health insurance. Under current tax codes, employer-paid premiums are considered a cost of doing business and are treated as a business expense. (Large companies frequently self-insure and hire administrators to manage their health benefits. Thus, these companies do not strictly pay premiums. Nevertheless, conceptually, one can think of expected, average health care costs as the premium.) Furthermore, these employer-paid premiums are not considered income for employees and are

exempt from individuals' income taxes. Wide differences exist across firms with respect to the proportion of the premium paid by the employer, and employers generally pay a higher proportion of the total premium for their employees than for their employees' dependants who might also be included in the insurance coverage. Employers sometimes offer employees a choice among health insurance plans.

Active competition exists among insurance companies in the employment-offered health insurance market, and premiums are set competitively. Premiums tend to be experience rated rather than community rated, and businesses with healthy employees have lower premiums than businesses with generally sicker employees.

In the US, health insurance is also available to individuals and groups, independent of employment. Premiums are experience rated and reflect the average, expected cost of illness for individuals within the defined group covered by a particular policy. The sicker the pool of individuals covered by an insurance policy, the higher the premiums. A number of states have passed legislation which set limits on the range of premia.

Although the US lacks universal health insurance, it provides public health insurance for the poor, the disabled, and the elderly through two publicly funded programs, Medicaid and Medicare. Medicaid, which is jointly funded by the Federal and State governments, provides medical services to low-income individuals who meet specific eligibility criteria. Eligibility criteria may vary slightly across states. In general, the Medicaid enrollees are medically disabled and poor. Medicaid contains specific benefits for low-income women and their children, and the majority of those covered by Medicaid are women and children. (The majority of payments, however, go for the disabled and the elderly to pay for long-term care services not covered under the Medicare program.) The federally funded Medicare program insures most people aged 65 and over as well as a small subset of the general population who are medically disabled. The Medicare program is funded through a combination of payroll taxes, general tax revenues, beneficiary premiums, and direct beneficiary payments.

It should be pointed out that health insurance markets have developed in many countries to supplement government health insurance programs. For example, people in the UK may purchase private health insurance as an additional source of third-party funding which facilitates access to specialists and allows individuals to jump queues and to use private facilities not covered by government programs. Canadians may purchase supplemental health insurance policies to pay for medical services not covered under the provincial Medicare programs and to pay for nonessential amenities such as private rooms. Likewise, American Medicare beneficiaries may purchase supplemental insurance (called Medigap insurance) to cover expenses not included in the Medicare program, such as outpatient prescription drugs and extended nursing home care, as well as Medicare cost-sharing liabilities.

Direct Payments by Individuals

Individuals may also pay health care providers directly for services rendered. Direct payments to providers are often referred to as *out-of-pocket payments*. People may pay directly for health care services for several reasons: they are uninsured, or a particular service is not covered by their health insurance plan, or the health insurance coverage is not complete. For example, many insured individuals routinely make some out-of-pocket payments because their health insurance policies (including the national health insurance programs discussed above) contain explicit *cost-sharing* provisions mandating some amount of direct payment by the individual. Cost-sharing provisions take several different forms including: deductibles (a fixed amount that must be paid by the insured before any third party payment will be made); co-payments such as a specific payment that the insured must pay for each service (e.g. $6.00 for each prescription filled or $5.00 for each visit to a physician); or a specific percentage of the bill (such as the 20% co-payment Medicare beneficiaries must pay for physician services).

Wide variations exist across countries with respect to the level of out-of-pocket payments for health care. For example, in both Canada and the UK there are no out-of-pocket payments for basic services covered under the respective national health insurance systems. In Germany, out-of-pocket payments are very limited, whereas France has substantial cost-sharing (i.e. 20%–30%) for many health care services.

In general, out-of-pocket payments in the US are high relative to those in other developed countries for a number of reasons: a significant number of people are uninsured (no third-party payer), and private health insurance plans are not standardized with respect to the types of services covered or the level of cost-sharing provisions on covered services. Note that although the Medicare program does contain significant cost-sharing requirements, few Medicare beneficiaries actually pay out of pocket. Indigent Medicare beneficiaries have their cost-sharing covered under the Medicaid program, while the majority of other Medicare beneficiaries purchase private Medigap policies.

Uninsured Individuals

Among the developed countries, only the US has a large number of people without insurance because it is the only country without a universal health insurance program. Approximately 17% of the US nonelderly population was uninsured in 1994 [2]. However, the uninsured do use health care services. Theoretically, the uninsured would purchase medical care with out-of-pocket payments, but in practice a large portion of the cost of medical care for the uninsured comes from publicly funded clinics, specifically designated charity funds, and "cost-shifting". Cost-shifting occurs when a provider charges some groups of patients higher than normal fees in order to cover the cost of services provided to other groups of patients for whom the provider receives no or inadequate payments.

Implication of Funding Sources on the Burden of Illness

In general, health insurance programs funded predominately by income taxes are the most progressive with respect to income. Individuals with the most income pay proportionately more than individuals with the lowest incomes, regardless of their use of medical services. Health insurance programs funded by premiums are the most regressive with respect to income. Payroll taxes tend to be moderately regressive because the percentage of a person's income from wages tends to decline as total income rises. Value-added or consumption taxes are also regressive with respect to income because low-income individuals tend to spend a higher proportion of their income on consumption goods than do upper-income individuals. However, the regressive nature of health insurance programs financed by consumption taxes can be reduced by excluding specific items (such as food) from taxation.

The broader and more inclusive the funding base for health insurance programs, the more the financial cost of illness is shifted from the sick to the healthy. The more out-of-pocket payments serve as the source of funds for health care, the more the burden of the financial cost of illness is borne by the sick. The more experience rating is used to set premiums, the more the relatively sick have to pay for health care. Thus, under national health insurance systems such as those in the UK, Germany, and Canada, the *financial* cost of illness is borne socially and distributed broadly across the population. Actual expenditures (in out-of-pocket payments and premiums) made by the sick are much less than the total cost of their medical care. This is in contrast to the US where a higher proportion of costs are paid out of pocket and a large number of insurance plans are experience rated.

Third-Party Payments and Consumer Demand

Health insurance affects the price that a person pays for medical service, but the effect can be complicated. For example, a person who has complete insurance coverage pays a price of zero for each medical service used. A person with an insurance plan specifying a $500 deductible, 20% cost-sharing, and a $3000 limit on out-of-pocket payments, pays out of pocket for the first $500 of medical services used and then pays 20% of charges for additional medical services until a total of $13 000 in medical services has been used. At that point the person will have spent $3000 in total out-of-pocket expenses and the insurance policy will cover all additional costs. Thus, individuals covered under the former plan may choose to use medical services differently than those covered under the second plan since they face very different prices for the same unit of medical care.

Not surprisingly, there is considerable interest in how the structure of cost-sharing influences the number of health care services used, i.e. in determining how responsive consumers are to out-of-pocket payments for medical services. Since the US is the only country in which direct patient payments are a significant source of funds, most research on this issue has been done in the US using that country's data.

Several different analytical structures have been employed to examine the use of services (*see* **Health Care Utilization, Data**) by individuals who pay different prices for the same service including the examination of natural experiments (e.g. some exogenous event changes the price that an individual pays for health care), analyses of self-reported utilization data

from large-scale surveys such as the National Medical Care Expenditure Survey, and analyses of claims data from different health insurance plans [7]. The need to control for nonprice factors that influence the use of health care services, as well as **selection bias**, complicates this research. (Selection bias arises when people who need more services choose plans with more extensive coverage, and vice versa.) The best study examining these issues uses data from the Health Insurance Experiment, a randomized clinical trial (*see* **Clinical Trials, Overview**) conducted by the RAND corporation [5]. This experiment, conducted in the 1970s, randomized people from six different locations (both urban and rural) in the US into one of 14 insurance plans which differed by the amount of the deductible, consumer cost-sharing, and maximum out-of-pocket expenses.

The research revealed that consumers generally respond to the price of health care services, and the extent to which they respond varies by the type of medical service. For example, the price of emergency services produces very little response, while people are more highly responsive to the price for elective services. The demand for mental health care services is more price responsive than that for physical health care services (*see* **Health Services Organization in the US**).

As argued above, the presence of health insurance affects an individual's behavior, relative to what it would be if he or she were not insured. This effect is sometimes referred to as *moral hazard*.

Moral hazard is said to occur when insured individuals change their behavior because they have insurance. The term was first applied in the life and fire insurance markets. For instance, moral hazard is said to exist if a person burns down the house in order to collect fire insurance, or fakes death with the intent of collecting the life insurance payments. The use of the term in the life and fire insurance markets implies some immoral behavior on the part of the insured.

In the health insurance market, *moral hazard* refers to insured individuals engaging in riskier (in terms of their health) behavior because of the presence of health insurance or otherwise changing their health-related behavior, such as using more health care services or failing to seek out low-cost providers. However, most commonly the term *moral hazard* simply reflects the basic law of demand: as the out-of-pocket price of medical services decreases, people use more medical services. In this sense, moral hazard

Table 1   Source of payment for personal healthcare: 1994. Total: $831.7 billion (US: 1994).
Source: Levit et al. [6]

Type of service	Total	Patient direct	Private health insurance	Other private	Federal[a]	State and local[b]
Hospital care	100.0%	2.9	34.2	4.0	49.1	10.9
Physician care	100.0%	18.9	47.3	1.6	25.7	6.5
Dentist services[c]	100.0%	52.7	43.4	0	2.2	1.8
Drugs and other[c]	100.0%	69.9	15.1	0	7.9	7.1
Nursing homes	100.0%	37.2	3.0	1.9	37.3	20.6
Total	100.0%	21.0	32.1	3.4	33.7	9.8

[a]Includes Medicare, Federal Share of Medicaid, and Veterans Administration.
[b]Includes state share of Medicaid and subsidies to health care providers.
[c]Data from 1993.

and price responsiveness (known as price elasticity of demand) are intimately related. Thus, there is nothing immoral about this type of moral hazard; it is simply a manifestation of rational human choice.

Funding Sources in the US

As indicated above, the financing of health care services in the US is more complex than in other countries. Table 1 presents information on the sources of funds for personal health care services in the US, both total and by type of service. In 1994, expenditures on personal health care services were $831.7 billion, of which 21% was paid by direct patient payments (out-of-pocket payments) and 79% by third parties. However, the proportion of expenditures covered by third parties ranges from 97% for hospital care to 30% for drugs and other services.

Data Sources

Information on health care expenditures is reported by the government agencies for each country. For example, the *Health Care Financing Review* annually publishes detailed information on health care expenditures in the US. The Department of National Health and Welfare in Canada publishes data on Canadian health expenditures. The Organization for Economic Cooperation and Development (OECD) maintains an ongoing data collection and analyzes effort aimed at producing timely, consistent data for 24 nations in Asia, Europe, and North America. The journal

Health Affairs periodically publishes data on the performance of health systems in OECD countries.

Paying Health Care Providers

A number of methods exist for paying health care providers (physicians, hospitals, clinics, labs, and other individuals/firms supplying health care services) for medical care services rendered to individuals. This section presents an overview of the most important of these payments methods.

Paying for Physician Services

Physicians are generally paid using one of three general methods of payment: fee-for-service, capitation, or salary. In some cases, physicians receive payments under more than one of these payment methods. The use of multiple payment methods occurs when either a given payer uses a combination of methods, or, as occurs in the US, a physician receives payments from more than one third-party payer, each of which uses a different payment method.

Fee-for-Service.   Under the fee-for-service method of payment, physicians receive a fee for each service provided. The medical service rendered is the *unit of payment*, and there is a certain degree of discretion regarding how a service is defined. A service unit can be very distinct (e.g. a urinalysis) or relatively comprehensive (e.g. an appendectomy where the physician payment covers all care associated with the procedure, including the preoperative visit, the surgical procedure itself, and some follow-up care). Thus, the service on which the unit of payment is based can actually be some bundle of separate, discrete services.

Payments to physicians for medical services may be based on the fees that physicians set for their services or on a specific fee schedule. A fee schedule defines the amount or relative amount of fees for each physician service. In general, only third-party payers use fee schedules. Individuals without insurance for physicians' services are usually billed according to charges set by the physician.

In the US, third-party payers using the fee-for-service method may pay physicians an amount based on the physician's charges, prenegotiated rates, or a fee schedule. Because different third-party payers may use different rates or schedules, physicians can receive different payment amounts for the same type of service depending upon the third-party payer involved. By contrast, in most other countries using the fee-for-service method, physicians receive payment based on a single negotiated fee schedule or on regional negotiated fee schedules.

The best known fee schedule in the US is the *Medicare fee schedule*, the fee schedule used by the Medicare program to pay physicians for services rendered to Medicare beneficiaries. The Medicare fee schedule assigns each defined unit of service a relative value quantifying the resources (such as physician time, skill, and use of support services) needed to produce the service. The Medicare fee schedule employs a conversion factor to translate the value of the resources used into a specific payment amount. In addition to the Medicare program, some of the other third-party payers in the US have adopted the Medicare fee schedule for use with their own resource conversion factors to set payments for physician services.

Capitation. The capitation method of payment provides physicians with a defined, periodic, per patient payment (usually monthly), regardless of the number or type of covered services the physician provides to a patient. Most commonly used to pay primary care physicians, the periodic payment reflects the expected cost of providing the covered services. The covered services and terms of the care provided under capitation vary with the actual capitation agreement. When used to pay primary care physicians,

some subspecialty services provided to patients by other physicians may be charged to the primary care physician for payment out of the primary care physician's capitated fee. Likewise, some specified services provided by the primary care physician may not be included in the capitated fee and instead may be paid for on a fee-for-service basis. Again, these arrangements vary by the actual capitation agreement.

The capitation fee may be adjusted to reflect patient characteristics such as age in order to compensate physicians for variations in the expected use of services by groups of patients with similar characteristics. In the US, managed care plans use the capitation method widely to pay primary care physicians, as does the British National Health Service.

Salary. The salary method of payment provides physicians with a fixed monthly or annual salary that does not vary with the number of patients treated or services provided. However, not all physicians are paid the same salary, which is based on such factors as specialty, hours worked, special duties (such as administrative tasks), and years of experience. In many European countries, hospital-based physicians are paid using the salary method, while physicians working in the outpatient setting receive payment under other methods. In the US, physicians working for government agencies, some Health Maintenance Organizations, or large group practices often receive payment by the salary method.

It should be noted that a physician can receive payment under a single payment method, while third-party payers make payments for the physician's services using several different payment methods. For example, a physician belonging to a large group practice may receive a salary even though insurance plans pay for services rendered by physicians in the group via a capitation method.

Paying Other Professionals. For other health care professionals (physical therapists, dieticians, social workers, home care nurses, etc.) the fee-for-service and salary methods are widespread, while capitation is rarely used.

Paying Hospitals

Numerous methods are used to pay for hospital services, such as payment based on established charges, retrospective costs, per diem rates, per case rates, capitated payments, or budgets. Because there are many different third-party payers in the US, hospitals located there frequently receive payments under a host of different methods. In contrast, hospitals in other countries tend to be paid according to a single payment method.

Charge-Based Payments Method.   Prevalent only in the US, the charge-based method requires hospitals to define a price or "charge" for each service the hospital provides. This hospital-established charge for each service is then paid either directly by the patient or by the patient's health insurance company. If the insurance policy requires copayments, then the hospital's charge is split between the patient and the health insurance company according to the conditions of the insurance contract. The charge-based method allows the hospital to determine the price of hospital services. This method is not used by government payers.

Retrospective-Cost-Based Payment Method.   The retrospective-cost-based payment method pays hospitals on the basis of the actual costs of providing hospital services as opposed to a hospital set charge (which may not be linked to the cost of providing services). Under this method a set of accounting rules allocates hospital costs to a group of patients. Although relatively common in the US from 1966 to 1983 because it was used by the Medicare program, most state Medicaid programs, and several Blue Cross plans, this method has lost importance since the mid-1980s when Medicare introduced the Prospective Payment System. When this method is used, hospital payments are typically subject to limitations – either limits on the extent to which reimbursable costs can rise from year to year and/or limits on the maximum allowable costs. Limitations on the maximum allowable costs are normally set relative to costs reported by other, similar hospitals.

Per Diem Payment Method.   The per diem payment method pays hospitals a set amount for each day that a patient spends in the hospital. In general, the per diem rate is independent of patient characteristics, (e.g. the same per diem rate is paid for patients undergoing heart surgery as for maternity cases). However, the per diem rate may vary by hospital. The rate is generally set via negotiations between the third-party payers and the hospital. The per diem method is relatively common in Europe. In Canada, provincial

governments use the per diem method to pay hospitals located outside the province for hospital care rendered to residents of the province. These transfer payments represent only a small proportion of hospitals' budgets.

Per Case Payment Method.   The per case method pays a hospital a set amount for each patient discharged from the hospital. In the most extreme form of the per case method, hospitals receive a defined amount per discharge irrespective of the patient's condition. More commonly, patients are classified into groups on the basis of the expected costs for necessary care (known as case mix formulations). Using a cost weight established for each group, the hospital receives a payment related to the patient's group classification. A number of patient classification systems exist, but the most frequently used systems are based on the **diagnosis related groups (DRGs)** developed at Yale University [3]. (See Hornbrook [4, 5] for an overview of case-mix classification issues.)

The *Medicare Prospective Payment System* is the best known of the case-mix-based per case payment systems. This system classifies patients into one of approximately 492 DRGs. A cost weight assigned to each group reflects the expected relative cost of treating patients within that group. For each patient discharged, the hospital receives a set payment which varies by the DRG assigned to the patient. This particular per case payment system also contains provisions for additional payments for patients whose treatment cost are exceptionally high (referred to as outlier payments).

Capitation Payment Method.   The capitation payment method pays hospitals a fixed, periodic fee per patient for a defined group of patients, often referred to as a panel of patients. The capitation payment does not vary with the actual use of services. Thus, even if no hospital services are used by any patient in the hospital's panel of patients in a given period, the hospital still receives payment. Unexpectedly high use of hospital services by the patients in the panel can result in net hospital losses for the period. This payment method shifts financial risk from the third-party payer to the hospital itself and its use is relatively rare.

Budget Payment Method.   The budget payment method provides hospitals with a global budget designed to cover all services provided by the hospital over the course of the year. The global budget may be unilaterally set by some government agency; it may be established according to some generally accepted formulas which account for inflation and changes in the size of the inpatient population; or it may be negotiated between the payer and the hospital. In some countries, global budgets involve the use of case-mix information. For example, in the Canadian provinces of Ontario and Alberta, the provincial governments use case-mix information to identify hospitals with global budgets which may be over or under-funded relative to other hospitals serving similar patients.

Like a capitation system, a global budget system shifts financial risk from the third party to the hospital system. However, it differs from the capitation system because it is not so closely related to the number of covered lives.

Paying Other Institutional Providers.   The same methods that have been developed to pay for hospitals are used to pay other institutional providers.

Data Sources

Government agencies publish reports that include the detailed specifications of their health care payments. For example, the rules for both the Medicare Hospital Prospective Payment System and the Medicare Physician Payment system are published annually in the *Federal Register*. The former includes a listing of all DRGs, the associated costs, the relative cost weights, and other information needed to transform DRG relative costs into payment rates. The latter includes a list of physician services, associated codes, associated relative values, and the conversion factor. The Ontario Ministry of Health publishes the *Schedule of Benefits* for physician services under the Health Insurance Act. This includes the listing of services, the associated codes, and the payment amounts.

Incentives Embedded in the Payment Methods

Theoretical Effects of Provider Payment Mechanisms

The effects of these different methods of paying providers have been the focus of a large body of

research. The basic approach to assessing providers' response to methods of payment is to identify those actions which either increase the providers' profits or decrease their losses. This can be done through formal theoretical modeling (see, for example, Ellis & McGuire [1]) as well as through a thoughtful consideration of the issues.

In general, analysts believe that the fee-for-service payment method creates incentives for providers to increase the number of services provided. Furthermore, the fee-for-service payment method lacks incentives for physicians to combine services in a way that minimizes the total cost of treating a patient to obtain a specific outcome. This effect, combined with a physician's desire to deliver thorough and comprehensive care, can result in too many services being provided.

The capitation payment method eliminates the incentive in the fee-for-service method to increase the number of services rendered. Instead, the capitation method creates strong incentives for physicians to manage a patient's care efficiently – at least with respect to the services covered under the capitation fee. However, the capitated payment method may result in under-treatment of patients when physicians are not involved in the long-term planning of patient care. Furthermore, there may be some incentives for physicians actively to seek out or recruit relatively healthy (i.e. less costly) patients and to discourage relatively sick (i.e. more costly) patients from joining or remaining in the physician's panel of patients. This is possible because physicians can influence the nature of the interaction that they have with patients.

The salary payment method removes all physician incentives to provide either too many or too few services. However, this method lacks any incentives for physicians to manage patient care efficiently. Furthermore, while the salary payment method removes the incentive for excessive use of medical services, physicians may respond by decreasing their work output. Thus, this method may necessitate productivity enhancement and monitoring measures to ensure an adequate level of work effort on the part of physicians.

Analysts examine the same factors when they consider the incentive effects embedded in the different methods used to pay hospitals. Under a charge-based payment system or a retrospective-cost-based payment system (when most of the payments are made by third parties), there are few financial incentives for hospital administrators to decrease costs or to develop systems that encourage physicians to manage care efficiently. Under a per diem payment method, financial incentives exist to manage the daily costs of hospital care but not the number of days. Therefore, as long as the per diem payment rate is higher than the marginal daily costs, incentives exist to increase the length of the hospital stay.

The per case payment method creates strong incentives to manage the use of inpatient services efficiently but also creates incentives to shorten hospital stays. Hospitals may achieve shorter stays by transferring patients to other facilities. The per case payment method also contains financial incentives for hospital decision-makers to under-treat patients, to discriminate against relatively sick patients, and to encourage actively the admission of relatively healthy patients.

Empirical Research on Supply Response

Research on the supply response to payment methods has been concentrated in the US because of the variety of payment schemes in effect there, the extensive changes in the level and structure of payments that have been made by third parties, and the accessibility of electronic data bases (*see* **Administrative Databases**) suitable for testing hypotheses about supply response.

Different analytical approaches analyzing provider response to employer changes have been used. Two approaches are commonly used: before–after studies comparing the outcomes for a common set of providers before and after some specific change in payment method and **fixed effect** models analyzing the effect of payment method using categorical variables to characterize the payment method. Analysts also use a difference in the differences approach in which they analyze the relative differences across two panels of medical providers (or patients) over time where one panel has experienced a change in payment methods and the other panel has not. In general, empirical results are consistent with the incentive effects as discussed above (see [9] for a review of physician supply response).

Data Bases

As noted, research on supplier response has been facilitated by the existence of large, electronically available data bases. For example, the Medicare program's administrative records include detailed information on all payments made under the traditional Medicare program. In the Medicare system, an electronic claim record is created for each service provided to a Medicare beneficiary by a physician or other individual medical care provider. A comprehensive electronic claim record is also created for each hospital admission for a Medicare beneficiary. Each provider of medical services (including hospitals and clinics) and each Medicare beneficiary has a unique identifier. Therefore, it is possible to develop records of episodes of care for beneficiaries and to assess the effect of payment changes for hospital care on length of stay, hospital transfers, the characteristics of hospital patients, and the use of nonhospital services. Detailed data linking providers and recipients (*see* **Record Linkage**) are also available for some state Medicaid programs. Additionally, some states require hospitals to report detailed diagnostic and charge information on all their discharges or mandate the collection of limited clinical data on all patients. These data are available from the relevant state agencies. Finally, the American Hospital Association surveys all hospitals in the US about the number of beds, the number of admissions, and costs. The results are reported in the *AHA Annual Guide to the Health Care Industry* as well as electronically.

Macroeconomic Concerns: A Comment

In all countries the health care system is shaped by the general regulatory environment within which consumers make decisions about accessing the health care system, and providers make decisions about the types of treatments to provide or recommend. There are significant differences across countries with respect to the extent of centralized controls over the number and location of hospital beds, the number and specialties of physicians in training, physician licensing, practice location and mobility, and the ability of hospitals or groups of providers to establish clinics or purchase advanced technology. In addition, all health plans (government and private) define the types of services they will cover, the relative frequency with which some services (e.g. preventive services) will be paid for, and the conditions under which patients can seek specialty care. Under some plans patients are allowed to self-refer to specialists; in others they must obtain permission from a primary care physician to visit a specialist.

In addition to the regulatory controls, the level of control that government authorities have over aggregate health care budgets varies. In general, the more a health care system is directly budgeted, the more governmental control there is over the size of the health care system (subject of course to the give and play of the political environment). In those cases where governments or regulatory authorities control the prices of care (per service, per day, or per case), providers can influence the outcomes by altering the mix of services or the volume of care. However, it is possible to impose budgetary control in a system where prices are directly controlled. For example, the US has imposed physician expenditure targets called Volume Performance Standards for physicians under the Medicare program. The conversion factor applied to determine the Medicare fee schedule is a function of how well physicians in the aggregate meet the volume performance standard. In the province of Ontario, the government sets income limits for individual physicians. As payments to individual physicians reach the limit, the proportion of the fee paid decreases. In general, there is much less aggregate control over the health care delivery system in the US than there is in other countries.

The financing methods and the type of aggregate controls imposed on a country do not appear to have a major independent effect on the size of the health care sector relative to the aggregate economy. Health care expenditures per capita are highly correlated with gross domestic product per capita. In fact, a study of health care costs in countries that were members of the Organization for Economic Cooperation and Development (OECD) found that R^2 (*see* **Correlation**) was 0.93 for a simple model in which log of a country's per capita expenditures on health care was regressed against the log of the country's per capita domestic product [7].

References

[1] Ellis, R.P. & McGuire T.G. (1986). Provider behavior under prospective reimbursement: cost sharing and supply, *Journal of Health Economics* **5**, 107–193.

[2] Employee Benefit Research Institute (EBRI). *Sources of Health Insurance and Characteristics of the Uninsured, Analysis of the March 1995 Current Population Survey.* EBRI Issue Brief 170.

[3] Health Systems Management Group (1982). *The New ICD-9-CM Diagnosis-Related Group Classification Scheme*, Final Report. Yale School of Organization and Management.

[4] Hornbrook, M.C. (1982). Hospital case mix: its definition, measurement, and use: Part I. The conceptual framework, *Medical Care Review* **39**, 1–43.

[5] Hornbrook, M.C. (1982). Hospital case mix: its definition, measurement, and use: Part II. Review of alternative measures, *Medical Care Review* **39**, 75–123.

[6] Levit, K.R., Lazenby, H.C., Sirarajan, L., Stewart, M.W., Braden, B.R., Cowan, C.A., Donhgam, C.S., Long, A.M., McDonnell, P.A., Sensing, A.L., Stiller, J.M. & Won, D.K. (1996). Health expenditures, 1994, *Health Care Financing Review* **17**, 205–242.

[7] Newhouse, J.P. (1993). *Free for All? Lessons from the RAND Health Insurance Experiment*. Harvard University Press, Cambridge, Mass.

[8] Phelps, C.E. (1992). *Health Economics*. Harper Collins, New York.

[9] Phelps, C.E. & Newhouse, J.P. (1974). Effects of coinsurance: the price of time and the demand for medical service, *Review of Economics and Statistics* **56**, 334–342.

[10] Reinhardt, U.E. (1993). An "all-American" health reform proposal, *Journal of American Health Policy* **13**, 11–17.

[11] Rice, T. (1996). Recent changes in physician payment policies: impacts and implications, in *Annual Review of Public Health*, J.E. Fielding, L.B. Lave & B. Starfield, eds. Annual Reviews Inc., Palo Alto.

JUDITH R. LAVE & PAMELA B. PEELE

Health Care Personnel *see* Health Services Organization in the US

Health Care Utilization and Behavior, Models of

Models of health care utilization behavior provide guidance for defining variables, specifying the relationships between them, and evaluating programs and policies concerned with access to and utilization of health care services (*see* **Health Care Utilization, Data; Health Care Utilization, Data Analysis**). Diagrams (as in Figure 1) are used to categorize the relevant variables and their interrelationships.

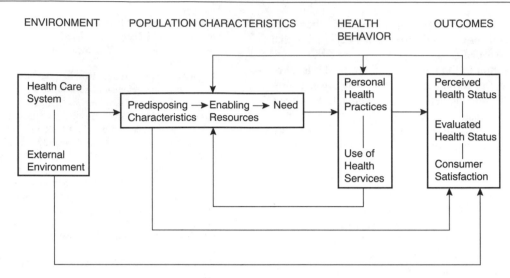

Figure 1   An emerging model – phase 4. Reprinted from [3] by permission of the publisher

Models may be used to guide the conduct of descriptive, analytic, or evaluative studies of the operation and performance of the health services delivery system. Descriptive studies focus on profiling the variables in the model (represented by boxes in Figure 1) for a population or subgroup. Analytical designs speculate on the hypothesized relationships between the implied predictors (independent variables) and outcomes of interest (dependent variables) (displayed by arrows). **Experimental designs** or **quasi-experimental designs** test the impact of a specific program or intervention on desired outcomes (the end-points in Figure 1).

Four major types of conceptual models have been developed and applied in specifying the interrelationships of the array of possible predictors of health care utilization behavior, and in guiding the conduct of analytic and evaluative research in this area [2]. These include (i) models of patient decision making, grounded in sociological theory and research (particularly those developed by Suchman, Kosa and Robertson, and Mechanic); (ii) the health belief model, based in social psychological theory (developed by Becker); (iii) economic models of the demand for medical care (as amplified by Grossman); and (iv) the behavioral model of health services utilization (developed by Andersen and his colleagues, displayed in Figure 1) that has guided the conduct of much **health services research** on access to and utilization of health care services [1, 5]. The first three types of models will be reviewed next and the behavioral

model discussed in more detail in the section that follows.

Models of Patient Decision Making

Suchman

Suchman's framework for stages of decision making about seeking medical care is focused on episodes of illness. In Suchman's paradigm, the sequence of seeking medical care for illness is divided into five stages: (i) experience of the symptom; (ii) assumption of the sick role; (iii) medical care contact; (iv) dependent patient role; and (v) recovery or rehabilitation. A group with more parochial or traditional, in contrast to more cosmopolitan, affiliations and a popular, rather than more scientific, orientation toward medical care would, he suggests, be more likely to delay in recognizing symptoms, linger longer in the stage of using home remedies, be suspicious of medical providers and perhaps shop around more, fail to adhere to prescribed therapies, and relinquish the sick role as soon as possible.

Kosa and Robertson

Whereas Suchman's model tended to offer more sociological or structural explanations for why individuals might respond differently at different stages of an illness episode, a model developed by Kosa and Robertson focused more on psychological explanations. Behavior is motivated by the individual's psychological need to reduce the anxiety aroused by the threat of illness. The Kosa and Robertson model also assumes stages of individual decision making in response to illness: (i) an assessment of a disturbance in usual functioning; (ii) anxiety arousal based on the perception of the symptoms; (iii) the application of one's medical knowledge to address the problem; and (iv) the performance of activities to alleviate the anxiety. Activities may be of two kinds: therapeutic interventions directed at the removal of the specific health problem, or interventions aimed at relieving the anxiety of satisfying other needs (e.g. fear) without addressing the health problem directly.

Each stage of decision making is influenced by these psychological dynamics as well as the culture and social groups (e.g. family) of which they are a part or with whom they come in contact (e.g. professional medical providers).

Mechanic

Mechanic's model catalogues an array of social and psychological factors that might influence the likely impact of symptoms on individuals care-seeking. These include: (i) perception of symptoms (e.g. salience, seriousness, disruptiveness, frequency); (ii) characteristics of individuals (e.g. tolerance of discomfort, knowledge of illness, competing needs); and (iii) accessibility of care causing disruption in the treatment process (e.g. inconvenient location or hours of service, out-of-pocket costs). However, the need for care from the point of view of the patient (self-defined illness) may not always agree with the need for care as defined by the provider (other-defined illness), which may have significant consequences for patient compliance and continuity [1].

Health Belief Model

The health belief model was originally conceived to understand preventive health care (health behavior) but has subsequently been applied to explaining care-seeking in response to illness (illness behavior) and those activities required for recovery from illness (sick role behaviors). The major components of this social–psychologically oriented model are as follows: (i) an individual's subjective state of readiness to take action, based on the individual's perceived likelihood of susceptibility to the illness, as well as its

seriousness; (ii) an individual's assessment of engaging in a given health care-seeking behavior, based on weighing the benefits (reducing susceptibility or seriousness) relative to the likely costs (physical, financial, etc.); (iii) the presence of cues to action to trigger the appropriate action, coming from either internal (e.g. symptoms) or external (e.g. interpersonal interactions, mass media) sources; and (iv) the role of other modifying factors, such as demographic, socio-psychological, and structural. These factors all influence the perceived threat of the disease and the subsequent likelihood of taking action [1].

Models of Consumers' Demand for Medical Care

Economic models of consumer choice stress means (e.g. health insurance or income) through which people can attain services or translate their perceived need into economic demand for medical care. An important contribution to the demand models was made by Grossman, who argued that what consumers really demand when they purchase medical care is health [5]. A number of hypotheses might be generated by this model of joint demand for health and care including: (i) as people age and their stock of health declines they will increase their consumption of medical care to offset the decline; (ii) as people's income increases, their consumption of medical care will increase because they will place increased value on healthy days; and (iii) as people's education increases, their demand for medical care will decline because they will be more efficient in producing health [4]. The best known application of the demand for medical care model is the RAND Health Insurance Study which employed randomized trials (*see* **Clinical Trials, Overview; Health Care Financing**) to estimate the effects of changes in health insurance benefits on people's use of medical care and their health status [6].

Behavioral Model of Health Services Utilization

The behavioral model of health services utilization is arguably the most comprehensive and widely applied model in health services research focusing on access to and use of health care services [2, 3]. The most current adaptation of the model is displayed in Figure 1.

The original version of the model developed in the 1960s suggested that people's use of services is a function of their predisposition to use services (predisposing variables), factors which enable or impede use (enabling variables), and their need for care (need variables). Predisposing variables include demographic and social structure factors (e.g. employment, social class, occupation, race) and health beliefs. The enabling component encompasses both resources specific to individuals (e.g. income, insurance coverage, regular source of care) and attributes of the community in which they live (e.g. physician and hospital bed supply). The need for care may be based on perceptions of the individuals themselves or diagnostic assessments by providers.

The model provides an empirical approach to assessing the equity of health services utilization. Andersen and Aday (originators of the model) assume that in an equitable system, need (rather than predisposing and enabling) components will be the primary basis for accounting for subgroup variations in use. They also distinguish those components which are more mutable (alterable by the health care system) – enabling factors – vs. those that are not – demographic or social structural characteristics.

In later versions of the model (1970s) the health care system was explicitly included in the model in recognition of the important impact of organizational and financial factors on the distribution and delivery of services. The dimensions of health services use measures (type, site, purpose, and time interval for care) were elaborated, and satisfaction added as another important (subjective) indicator of individuals experience of care-seeking.

More recently (during the 1980s and 1990s) the model allowed for the growing recognition of the importance of considering the impact of health care utilization in the context of other likely predictors of health outcomes. Revisions acknowledged that the external environment (physical, political, and economic) and personal health practices (such as diet, exercise, and self-care) influence formal health services utilization and (ultimately) health outcomes. The revised model added people's perception of their health status and clinical (evaluated) measures of health status as well as patient satisfaction with service as outcomes. Finally, it incorporated feedback loops showing that health outcomes, in turn, affect subsequent predisposing factors, perceived need for services, and health behavior.

Limitations of Dominant Models and New Directions

A number of criticisms have been offered of the original and expanded behavioral model of health services utilization, which may be seen as establishing the grounding for new substantive and methodological research based on the model [2, 7]. These criticisms relate principally to the specification of the independent and dependent variables in the model, the causal pathways between and among them, and the generalizability and policy relevance of research based on the model.

Independent Variables

The criticisms of the major predictors of utilization relate primarily to the validity or accuracy of the operational definitions used to measure major study concepts; the fact that most studies in which the model is used do not fully encompass all components of the model; the need to add other dimensions to capture adequately the relevant predictors for selected types of utilization or populations; and the likelihood of significant **interactions** between subcomponents of the model.

Dependent Variables

Important extensions of the model in terms of the utilization variables themselves would be to explore more systematically the interrelationships (or trade-offs) between different types of service use (e.g. ambulatory vs. inpatient), as well as the relationship of utilization to both patient satisfaction and health outcomes.

Relationships between Variables

Full tests of the interrelationships between and among variables entail the use of stronger analytic and evaluative research designs and the application of more sophisticated modeling techniques in empirically examining these interrelationships.

Generalizability

Major criticisms of the model have focused on the fact that most studies in which it has been utilized explain only a small amount of the variation in health services utilization. Also, the program and policy relevance of the model would be enhanced by the design of studies and analyses to relate more directly the impact of utilization on patient satisfaction, health outcomes, and costs.

Summary

In summary, various factors may account for those who ultimately seek health care. Substantial progress has been made in specifying and measuring the relationships among these factors. The conceptual models reviewed here provide integrative frameworks for considering many of these factors and their interrelationships. However, health services research can provide continued guidance in refining these models, designing and implementing empirical studies to test and evaluate them, and shaping the formulation and interpretation of the policy relevance of research guided by such models.

References

[1]   Aday, L.A. (1993). Indicators and predictors of health services utilization, in *Introduction to Health Services*, S.J. Williams & P.R. Torrens, eds. 4th Ed. Delmar, Albany, pp. 47–70.

[2]   Aday, L.A. & Awe, W.C. (1997). Health services utilization models, in *Handbook of Health Behavior Research*, Vol. I *Determinants of Health Behavior: Personal and Social*, D.S. Gochman, ed. Plenum, New York, pp. 153–172.

[3]   Andersen, R.M. (1995). Revisiting the behavioral model and access to medical care: does it matter?, *Journal of Health and Social Behavior* **36**, 1–10.

[4]   Feldstein, P.J. (1979). *Health Care Economics*. Wiley, New York, pp. 78–79.

[5]   Grossman, M. (1972). *The Demand for Health: A Theoretical and Empirical Investigation*, Occasional Paper 117. National Bureau of Economic Research, New York.

[6]   Newhouse, J. & the Insurance Experiment Group (1993). *True for All? Lessons Learned from the RAND Health Insurance Experiment*. Harvard University Press, Cambridge, Mass.

[7]   Pescosolido, B.A. & Kronenfeld, J.J. (1995). Health, illness, and healing in an uncertain era: challenges from and for medical sociology, *Journal of Health and Social Behavior* **Extra issue**, 5–33.

Lu Ann Aday & Ronald M. Andersen

Health Care Utilization, Data

Many important questions about the fairness, efficacy, or efficiency of health care delivery systems require examining utilization data. Ideally, we would have information on the nature, timing, cost, and setting of each person's utilization, and the ability to link that information with personal demographics, health status characteristics, and health outcomes.

Health services research works best when there is a complete list of persons whose care is tracked and longitudinal records of the medical problems addressed, all care given, and health outcomes. In the US, records maintained by the Health Care Financing Administration (HCFA) for its Medicare program (which covers over 30 million people, including almost all US citizens over the age of 65) are a unique resource for health services research. HCFA works actively to create **confidentiality**-protected, research-quality, longitudinally-linked, person-level records which track virtually all elderly people from their 65th birthday onwards, through geographical moves and changes in providers, until death.

However, even the Medicare data have limitations. One such limitation is that care not covered by Medicare is not recorded in the data: most notably, long-term care services and prescription pharmaceuticals. There is extensive information on the patient's diagnosis for hospitalizations (Part A data), but less for outpatient services (Part B data). Also, unfortunately, as more Medicare beneficiaries come to receive their care from managed care organizations (*see* **Health Services Organization in the US**) which receive a lump-sum, "capitated" payment for each person they enroll, HCFA's data, as a record of what services were offered to an entire national age cohort, will deteriorate. The problem of loss of information about what care is actually delivered is of growing concern to the research and policy community within all health care databases, not just for Medicare.

In sharp contrast to the relative completeness and continuity of Medicare data is the fragmented information available in the US for low-income persons with Medicaid health coverage. Each state administers its own Medicaid program, eligibility requirements frequently change, people move on and off the system as their incomes and other circumstances which affect eligibility change, and the same person will sometimes appear under different identification numbers.

Data from privately insured populations in the US have intermediate-level quality, with most people remaining enrolled through the same employer year after year, although they may switch health plans during annual, open-enrollment periods. Other problems arise because coverage is usually offered to "families" of employees; thus, marriage, divorce, alternate coverage that becomes available (or is lost) to a spouse or child, job loss and geographical movement can all disrupt the continuity of the data. Typically, employer-based coverage systems do not record why someone disenrolls; they may not even have an explicit record ("positive enrollment") of each person entitled to receive care in their "family" contracts. There is often less **covariate** information available about the characteristics of insured dependents than about the contract holder.

Only some health records are computer accessible and even fewer can be reliably tracked at the patient level. This limits the questions that a **population-based study** can address. For example, many state-wide databases capture in a uniform format and make available for research a file with one record for each inpatient admission. Available variables include the age, sex, and zip-code of residence of the patient, the principal problem which caused the admission and other medical problems present (using the **International Classification of Diseases** diagnostic coding system), major procedures (such as surgeries) received, dates of admission and discharge, discharge disposition (e.g. in-hospital death, transfer to another facility, discharge home), days of stay in special care units (e.g. intensive care units), and hospital billing information, including "payor". These data capture very much the same information that Medicare requires for hospitalizations, in very much the same format [1]. However, despite the richness of these data a great deal of important medical information is missing, some of which can (with time and effort) be captured by retrospectively abstracting information that is usually recorded in patients' medical charts [1].

Another way to improve the completeness of available information is through prospective data collection, which ensures that desired elements will be present by collecting them while care is being administered. In certain health care systems, various additional computerized information, such as laboratory findings as well as tests ordered, drugs prescribed, and amounts dispensed, can round out the picture of what medical problems were being seen and resources used.

Patient **surveys** can capture "outside" or "out-of-pocket" utilization, such as purchases of nonprescription drugs and use of alternative or uncovered services, like chiropractic or acupuncture, and provide insight into patients' views of their own health or the care they receive. Although self-report is not an ideal way to capture health care utilization, it may be necessary when more reliable information is not available. For example, many of the large managed care organizations in the US have agreed to use a survey instrument called the "P_{ra}" with their elderly enrollees, to capture numbers of hospitalizations and doctor visits during the past year. The P_{ra}, which estimates the probability of repeated hospital admission, is used as a screening tool to identify frail elders in need of specialized management. It records a variety of medical problems that may require attention and could become an important source of uniform data on elderly populations [1].

Measures of Utilization

Utilization studies may focus on a particular kind of use, or on a summary measure of total utilization or cost. Kinds of use include hospital admissions, specific surgeries, such as hysterectomies and tonsillectomies, ambulatory care (such as doctor's office visits and outpatient surgeries), readmissions to hospital (within, say, two weeks of an earlier discharge), diagnostic tests, referrals for specialist care, and intensive care unit stays.

Average annual costs per person is a natural summary measure of health care expenses. In the case of a purchaser of medical care, such as the Medicare program administered by the HCFA, "cost" is most commonly defined as the sum of all dollars that it pays for covered services; "cost" can also include overheads (the administrative costs associated with running a program). "Total" health care costs are larger than this, however, including at least the "out-of-pocket" expenses of health care consumers for covered services (copayments and deductibles) and consumers' expenditures for noncovered goods and services, such as over-the-counter medicines and devices, dental, psychiatric or long-term care, and visits to nonorthodox practitioners such as acupuncturists or chiropractors. Some calculations attempt also to capture costs ancillary to the receipt of care, such as the price of transportation to providers or the value of time lost in care-seeking, as well as costs ancillary to being sick (lost productivity). However, these last costs are less relevant to a study of "utilization".

Most health care providers do not know the cost of particular instances of care-giving. First is the question of whether average or marginal costs are sought. If average costs, then the accounting system used to allocate fixed overhead expenses to particular cases matters, as does the universe of cases over which the average is computed (e.g. all admissions at the same hospital, admissions to the same administrative unit, pneumonia cases, admissions paid for from a single source).

The "charges" which appear on many billing records often bear little relationship to either what payors actually pay or what expenses were actually incurred. Charge comparisons are suspect, especially when pooling or comparing cases from institutions with different accounting systems. Health services researchers sometimes use the method of "cost-to-charge ratios" to convert charges to a more credible estimate of costs.

Another way to summarize utilization is by "pricing" and counting each unit of care; a "synthetic" total cost is calculated by summing the imputed costs associated with the care given. The price of a service may be generated internally (e.g. as the average charge associated with it in the data) or externally, as a "book rate". The technique is credible so long as most relevant services are likely to be captured in the data and the relative prices, at least, form a believable weighting system. Any summary cost figure is essentially a weighted sum of inputs.

When comparing utilization across different delivery systems, it is important to recognize that some data systems are substantially more complete than others. As a rule, records are most complete and accurate when payments are linked to individual services through bills; "what was done" is often less easy to track when capitated and "lump-sum" payment systems are used.

Extensive discussion about billing records and coding conventions can be found in [2].

References

[1]   Boult, C., Pacala, J.T. & Boult, L.B. (1995). Targeting elders for geriatric evaluation and management: reliability, validity, and practicality of a questionnaire, *Aging: Clinical Experimental Research* **7**, 159–164.

[2]   Iezzoni, L.I., ed. (1994). *Risk Adjustment for Measuring Health Care Outcomes*. Health Administration Press, Ann Arbor, Chapter 3.

ARLENE ASH

Health Care Utilization, Data Analysis

Data on the use of health services can be used to answer many important questions concerning what health care is provided for whom, and can shed light on why the care was provided and with what outcome, in the large segment of economic life that "delivers" health care services to populations. We discuss several kinds of studies and some of the analytic issues that commonly arise.

Important concerns when studying utilization are (i) identifying all instances of use, (ii) identifying the at-risk population, (iii) accounting for differential risk of individuals, and (iv) distinguishing real differences from random noise. These issues are explored in more detail in this article, and in the articles on **Health Care Utilization, Data** and **Risk Adjustment**.

Types of Studies

An influential class of **small area variation** studies has established that people in different parts of a country and in different communities within the same region receive very different care. For example, population-based rates for tonsillectomy, hysterectomy, or hospitalization vary greatly by geographic region. Research has been undertaken to explain these differences; for example, by asking if areas with high hospitalization rates also have high rates of inappropriate hospital admission. Geographic variation in patterns of use may reflect lack of agreement within the medical community about treatment options and may help identify opportunities for improving care through standardization to better treatment protocols.

Variations in treatment by patient race, or sex may reflect societal discrimination in the allocation of expensive resources. Variations by payor class, such as Medicaid vs. private insurance, or by payment method, such as fee-for-service vs. capitation, may point to inequities or inefficiencies related to financing (*see* **Health Care Financing; Health Services Organization in the US**).

Other studies seek to estimate the effect of various factors on utilization during an instance of care-giving, such as a hospital admission. Potential predictors of utilization include patient characteristics (socio-demographic, medical), characteristics of doctors or other medical providers (socio-demographic, training, and experience), and characteristics of the conditions of practice (the particular site or its features, or the organizational/financial structures under which the care is given). Predictor variables can be heavily confounded (*see* **Confounding**); for example, most patients seen at high-volume hospitals may be city dwellers, and patients of public hospitals tend to have low income, making it difficult to sort out the separate effects. **Hierarchical models** are needed to explore the influence of facility-specific factors.

Another goal of utilization analysis is to describe differences in **case-mix**, as a guide to why providers may differ in the care they give and the outcomes achieved. Case-mix differences may serve as the basis for redistributing money among providers, so that those who treat the sickest patients receive the highest per-patient reimbursements.

Yet another goal is to provide reports on the quality of health care provided (*see* **Quality of Care**), which can guide patients and health care purchasers, assessing what health care providers do and what they achieve with the people they serve. An important initiative in the US in the 1990s has been developing a protocol for comparing managed health care plans (HEDIS), using measures such as what fraction of a plan's women of a certain age receive annual mammograms. However, HEDIS measures are generally not risk-adjusted and few HEDIS measures assess the quality of care given to the very sick, largely because this is so difficult to do.

Cost effectiveness studies seek to relate the cost of the health care inputs used to the value of an achieved outcome. They require data on utilization and a plausible methodology for "pricing" this, as well as a numerical measure of the outcome, such as quality-adjusted life years (QALYs) (*see* **Quality of Life and Health Status**). Health care strategies with the highest QALY yield per dollar might be the first to be implemented (or the last to be eliminated) in a health care system with constrained dollars.

Provider profiling is used to identify individual doctors, hospitals, or health care systems with exemplary or problematic practices (*see* **Profiling Providers of Medical Care**). Unfortunately, when providers are compared in public releases of analyzed data, much harm can be done if providers are "flagged" as problematic either because of random variation (small numbers) or because they care for an unusually difficult mix of patients. Clearly, appreciation of the "small numbers" problem and the importance of risk adjustment is critical to provider profiling.

Special Features of Utilization Data that Require Analytic Attention

Skewness and Heteroscedasticity

Health care utilization variables often have a mode at zero and a distribution with a long, heavy, right tail. Although the data are often counts, they tend to have a **lognormal distribution** rather than a **Poisson distribution**. This is true for variables such as numbers of office visits or hospitalizations per year, days of stay in a hospital for hip fractures, and costs of care for individual hospitalizations or in fixed periods of time. For example, in a working insured population during a one-year period, upward of 50% of people eligible to receive health care may incur no costs, many more have low-level, nonhospital expenses, and the 5% with the most intense use may account for around 50% of all expenses; the magnitude of the **standard deviation** for expenditures is generally similar to the **mean**, and in a system where average costs range between $2000 and $4000 per year, the very most expensive cases can run as high as $250 000 to over a million dollars. A few large **outliers** can substantially distort analyses even in data sets that contain tens of thousands of cases, and decisions about whether to truncate or remove these extreme cases can affect study findings.

One technique for addressing the concentration of zero values (*see* **Structural and Sampling Zeros**) is to use a two-part model [2], in which the first equation predicts the probability of having any use and a second equation is used to predict the level of use (on the log scale) among the users only. The expected level of use for an individual is then calculated by multiplying these two estimates together. This framework has been extended to a four-part model in which the probability of hospital use is estimated for users, and then the costs for users without hospitalization and for those hospitalized are separately estimated [2].

To address **skewness**, many authors transform the utilization variable, for example, by analyzing the logarithm of dollars (*see* **Transformations**). This can help in identifying factors which affect use because it makes findings about the significance of individual predictors more credible, but may be problematic when the goal is to predict use, since the modeling predicts log dollars rather than dollars. When retransforming into the original scale, a smearing estimate [2] can be used to address bias. Retransformed estimates often fit the data less well than models constructed from the untransformed data. **General linear modeling** provides an attractive framework for simultaneously addressing the problems of skewness and nonconstant **variance** of the outcome variable, while predicting it in its original, untransformed scale. For example, the function which "links" costs to predictors can be specified as the log function and variances can be specified as proportional to means.

Lack of Independence

When studying hospital admissions, multiple hospitalizations for the same patient cannot usually be identified. Thus, the data may not be able to answer questions such as: Now that patients are being discharged from hospitals earlier, have readmission rates increased? Furthermore, random variation is greater when rehospitalizations are common than when single hospitalizations are the norm. When clustered data (*see* **Clustering**) are analyzed as if independent, chance variability can be misinterpreted as evidence of systematic differences [1].

When examining the role of a site-specific characteristic such as "do hospitals which see more **AIDS** cases provide them better care?" or "do major teaching hospitals see sicker patients?", the analysis needs to account for the fact that patients are nested within hospitals which are in turn nested within hospital type. Otherwise, effects attributed to hospital "characteristics" can easily be dominated by the experience of a few large facilities.

The Effect of Death

Patients who die shortly after entering hospital often use the least resources, while those who remain alive a few days but eventually die are among the most expensive. Some authors propose treating utilization (a nonnegative variable) as the time variable in a **survival analysis**, with death as the censoring variable (*see* **Censored Data**). The resources that a patient would have used had he or she not died are then estimated, which may or may not be a useful concept. In addition, death is an "informative" reason for censoring, which may muddle the interpretation of findings. In general, it is unclear how and whether to use information about death in predicting utilization.

The Study Population

It is not always easy to identify the population of interest. For studies involving Health Maintenance Organizations (HMOs) or all people covered by a particular insurance plan, the population is clear. If the population is all people who receive care from public facilities, then the result is less clear, because many are eligible but few would ever use that facility. Defining a study population based on use of services, such as "all people who have used services in the last year" provides a biased, higher-using group of patients for study, as compared with the set who would attend for care if it were needed. The estimate of the proportion of people in the "population" who receive services will probably be too high. If the population is those people who reside in a particular geographic catchment area (*see* **Hospital Market Area**), then findings may be unclear if people travel outside their area for care.

To learn how medical problems are treated and what outcomes are achieved requires problem-defined study **cohorts**, such as people with diabetes, with hypertension, or with low back pain. Eligibility criteria affect the type of patient seen. For example, if the data from health plan A identify all people who are even mildly diabetic, while health plan B data identify only hospitalized diabetics, then there will tend to be lower rates of diabetes, but more intensive treatment and worse outcomes per diabetic patient in health plan B.

Breadth of Use Within Relevant Populations

Gross measures of use (such as number of hospital admissions per thousand person-years of experience) are important to payors, but administrators need to understand where inefficiencies occur. Thus, for example, numbers of hospitalizations for respiratory problems for patients with asthma, and the prevalence of blood sugar tests and eye examinations for diabetics provide more focused views of how a health care delivery system works. One difficulty in conducting such studies is that few systems maintain **disease registers** which would specifically allow the utilization patterns of persons with a disease to be tracked.

Individual payors are principally interested in monitoring the utilization for which they pay, but the larger community has an interest in tracking the outcomes associated with all the care that individuals receive.

Utilization in a Population vs. During a Period of Treatment

Some services, such as hysterectomy, are delivered at most once to any one person. However, many services can be delivered more or less often and with variable intensity. Thus, each of the following questions may be of interest about inpatient hospital care for a population: What fraction was ever hospitalized during a given year? How many hospitalizations occurred per person-year of exposure? How many days of hospital care were incurred per person-year? How many days of intensive care unit stay were used per person-year?

Examples of relevant measures when the hospital admission is the **unit of analysis** are: total length of stay, presence of any special care unit stays, number of days in special care units, number of X-rays ordered, and total cost of diagnostic testing. Comparisons are meaningful only among relatively similar cases; little can be gained by pooling information for patients admitted for heart attacks with those admitted for hernias.

The appropriate measure of utilization depends upon the purpose for which the study is conducted. For example, when utilization is examined for quality-monitoring purposes, the most relevant measure may be whether an appropriate medication or service was delivered, rather than how often; for hospice programs which provide supportive care for people thought to be near death, per-person utilization, rather than services per month of enrollment, may be most relevant.

The Unit of Analysis

When summing total hospital costs over a group of admissions, it does not matter whether an expense relates to a single admission, to several admissions for the same individual, or to one admission for each of several people. (The variance of the sum will, of course, depend upon such factors.) Such distinctions are important, however, to explore whether low costs per admission are due to frequent readmission for people discharged "early". "Unbundling" and "cost-shifting" may also produce apparent shifts in utilization that are not real. For example, hospital costs may appear lower simply because of separate billing for procedures that might have been subsumed in a global hospital bill, or because some services have been shifted to the outpatient setting.

Episodes of Care and Calendar-Based Time Frames

Utilization per episode of care, ranging from first problem identification through active treatment and follow-up can be used to compare the efficiencies with which providers handle a defined medical problem, such as "stomach pain due to an ulcer". Episodes can be studied only when care offered to the same person in different settings can be linked. Other potential difficulties arise in defining when one episode ends and a second one begins; the concept may not be helpful for studies of chronic conditions. Also, when the same person has more than one medical problem, it is not obvious which services should be assigned to which episode. No **algorithm** for defining episodes has widespread acceptance.

When a medical event has a readily identifiable starting point, but no clear endpoint, it often makes sense to examine utilization within a fixed window of observation which is long enough for most follow-up care to have occurred. For example, we may seek to capture all stress tests that occur within 30 days following a hospital admission for heart attack, whether or not they are done in the hospital;

or, all respiratory-related tests and services offered within the first six months after a breathing problem is identified.

Even costs per "episode" may not capture efficiencies associated with preventive care, since the number and/or severity of episodes may be affected by the presence and quality of preventive services. A yet more global way to examine utilization is through the lens of total use per **person-year** of coverage.

References

[1]   Diehr, P., Cain, K., Connell, F. & Volinn, E. (1990). What is too much variation? The null hypothesis in small area analysis, *Health Services Reports* **24**, 741-771.

[2]   Duan, N., Manning, W.G., Morris, C.N. & Newhouse, J.P. (1983). A comparison of alternative models for the demand for medical care, *Journal of Business and Economic Statistics* **1**, 115-126.

ARLENE ASH

Health Economics

The principal foundations of health economics are based in microeconomic theory and welfare economics [16]. Essentially, this field of specialization within the discipline of economics addresses the allocation of resources directed to health improvement and the organization, delivery, and financing of health services. Under this broad purview, practitioners in the field of health economics have tackled such questions as:

1. How does the uncertainty of health outcomes influence the optimal forms of organizing and paying for medical care [1]?
2. What mix of cost-sharing between patients, health plans (insurers), and health care providers (e.g. hospitals and physicians) will produce optimal outcomes in terms of the most improved health for the least incremental cost [8, 9]?
3. Under what conditions would increased competition among providers of health services be likely to produce improvements in health status and efficiency relative to existing market arrangements for health care [27]?
4. What are the economic costs to society of prevailing patterns of illness [31, 32]?
5. How does one measure the cost and benefit of programs directed toward the improvement of health [20, 25]?
6. What are the aggregate results of health care, when measured as increased **life expectancy** for given levels of health care expenditure [3]?
7. What are the differences in performance (e.g. in the quality and efficiency of services) between not-for-profit and for-profit organizations in health care [13]?

These questions illustrate, but of course do not fully characterize, the range of issues subsumed in health economics. A common theme cutting across theory and empirical work in health economics is to discover which forms of market structure, industrial organization, and individual behavior lead to efficient and equitable outcomes. Potential market structures range from the one extreme of "perfect competition", in which large numbers of consumers and providers interact in an environment of perfect information, to monopoly, with one large firm controling the market. Virtually no health care services are provided in a market structure that is close to the perfectly competitive or monopoly model.

Indeed, health care is distinguished from other economic markets by specialized information, principal–agent relationships, a relatively small number of providers in any given local area (an "oligopoly"), an inherently intimate and highly personalized service, and the dominance of third-party insurance. Arrow [1] highlights the special nature of health care from the perspective of the economist as uncertain medical consequences resulting in demand for treatments determined by physicians with payment emanating from third-party insurance carriers. Thus, the consumer is unable to predict the illness, not responsible for selecting the services he will receive, and will not – for the most part – pay the bill. This peculiarity of medical care markets challenges the traditional theoretic paradigms.

Accordingly, health economists have approached market structure from a different tack: What kinds of economic incentives and countervailing power would induce consumers and concentrated provider oligopolies, characterized by few, large firms producing highly differentiated services for a wide array of consumers, to behave efficiently and to achieve equitable outcomes?

In attempting to answer such questions, the economist's attention inevitably turns to the related issue of how health care providers are organized; in terms of "vertical" integration among the suppliers of inputs (e.g. pharmaceutical manufacturers) and the "output" providers (e.g. hospitals and medical groups), and the "horizontal" integration in local markets of providers of similar services (e.g. hospital mergers and consolidations of medical groups) (*see* **Health Services Organization in the US**). Moreover, while market structure and industrial organization exert a strong influence on health services outcomes, the factors governing the individual behavior of consumers and providers are equally pivotal in the study of health economics (*see* **Health Care Utilization and Behavior, Models of**). Seminal studies of the role of coinsurance and deductibles (patient "cost-sharing") in encouraging the efficient use of services [28] have contributed greatly to our understanding of health care, as has the theoretic and empirical research on different modes of provider payment [15, 16] (*see* **Health Care Financing**).

Defining "Efficiency"

In defining efficiency, the economist has in mind two distinct and quite specific types:

1. Technical efficiency refers to the production of a given amount of services ("output") for the least amount of resources ("cost"). This can be imagined as minimizing average cost per unit of output, or – equivalently – minimizing the total cost of producing a predetermined level of output.
2. Economic, or "allocative", efficiency examines "tradeoffs" in the allocation of resources. An arrangement is allocatively efficient when the incremental benefits of services provided are equal to the incremental costs of those services. Thus, allocative efficiency is measured "at the margin": Is the change in total cost (marginal cost) of services matched by an equal change in patient health benefit (marginal benefit) from those services?

Following these definitions then, the search for efficient arrangements follows the so-called Pareto

criterion: social welfare is optimized when no arrangement can be devised under which some individual(s) could be made better off without others being made worse off. This criterion effectively requires both technical and allocative efficiency. Either failure to produce at least cost or failure to deliver the correct output (aligning marginal benefit with marginal cost) would violate the Pareto principle.

Kaldor [19] and Hicks [14] refined the Pareto rule into a potential compensation criterion. Assuming that the gains to the "winner(s)" under some new arrangement could be measured, a situation was optimal if and only if no change could be effected that would leave winners with sufficient gains to compensate fully the losers. The use of a standard of "potential", rather than actual compensation, reflects the existence of real world costs of information and exchange (so-called "transaction costs") that impede actual exchange of compensation.

In recognition of the centrality of efficiency within economics, a set of methodologies for economic evaluation has been developed. Those methods can be broadly categorized as follows:

1. cost–benefit analysis;
2. cost–effectiveness analysis;
3. cost–utility analysis.

Over the past 20 years or so, a substantial literature has developed in the applied area of health economic evaluation [7]. Each of these techniques is grounded in economic theory, and their application to health services problems is illustrated in what follows.

Cost–Benefit Analysis

Cost–benefit analysis translates all costs and benefits into monetary units. The opportunity cost concept underlies the logic and implementation of all three economic evaluation methodologies. Opportunity cost is defined as the value of the resources used up in a given activity, measured as the value that those resources would have produced in their next best alternate use. Hence the value of opportunities foregone constitutes the opportunity cost of a given employment of resources. Even if no money changes hands – for example, in the case of time and assets donated for a particular activity – the resources do have this opportunity cost, which includes both direct, observable monetary costs and implicit opportunities forgone.

The time value of resources, captured in normal financial dealings through the rate of interest, is another crucial element in cost–benefit analysis. Looking forward from today, a cost incurred a year from now is somewhat less onerous than the same monetary cost incurred today. Similarly, a benefit realized one year from now is perceived as less valuable than a benefit of equivalent magnitude delivered today.

This rate of time preference is reflected in the practice of "discounting" costs and benefits through the use of a discount rate – analogous to the interest rate or rate of return required in financial transactions. The use of a discount rate in valuing costs and benefits implies that those consequences are long-lived, or spread over a period of time. Thus the discounting approach is appropriate for health programs that take the form of investments, which involve commitment of resources over time in return for future benefits.

Whereas persons considering *financial* investments generally accept the logic of requiring *interest* (some additional amount above what they invested originally) as compensation for having to wait to receive returns in the future, a thought experiment may be useful for the reader seeking to convince himself or herself that this approach can be applied appropriately to investments the direct payoffs of which are in terms of *health*, not dollars. Suppose that investing in a new positron emission tomography (PET) scanner costs $1.2 million today, and is expected to produce health benefits starting three months from now and lasting for the useful life of the scanner (estimated to be 10 years, for example). Furthermore, assume that those health benefits are expressed as earlier detection of, and more rapid recovery from, a variety of acute health problems. For purposes of the hypothetical, let the incremental (specific) costs of caring for those health problems *if not* detected earlier by PET scanning, be valued cumulatively at $200 000 per year (say, 20 cases per year at $10 000 costs saved per case).

The use of costs of caring avoided as the value of the scanner's *health benefit* simplifies the illustration that benefits can be converted into monetary equivalents. Then, to complete the reasoning, if one assumes that health investments "compete" with financial investments for scarce resources, it makes sense that the expected rate of return on the

next best alternate financial investment of comparable risk should become the rate of return required for a given health investment. Thus, a discount rate equal to the foregone financial return should be used to convert the future stream of benefits into its (time zero) present value equivalents.

Now let the required return on investments of comparable risk be 20%. In this case, if the initial costs of the scanner were subtracted from the discounted present value of the future health benefits (in a technique described in the next section), using 20% as the discount rate, one would calculate the scanner's net benefit valued as of now to be a negative $361 506. The reason is that, given that the benefits accrue over the future 10 years, they are not sufficiently large to offset the time costs of waiting (the 20% rate of return foregone) to recover the initial investment cost of $1.2 million.

Inflation would not affect these comparisons, because the health benefit values and the discount rate both would simply be increased by the same proportionate amount to reflect the rising cost of living. Thus, one can think of these examples as valuing costs and benefits in "real terms" (i.e. having abstracted from inflation).

Not only does the discount rate capture the time value of resources, but also the risk involved in the costs and payoffs from different programs. In reality, since health programs often do not adopt the language of owners, investors, and return on investment, the notions of business risk, financial risk, and systematic risk – so central to mainstream economic analysis of investments – have only infrequently been applied in health program applications of cost–benefit analysis. Nonetheless, to the extent that the benefits and costs of health programs are stochastic, not deterministic, it is appropriate to increase the discount rate from the level appropriate for a "riskless" investment, to compensate for the riskiness of the project.

To convince oneself of the appropriateness of building a positive "risk premium" into the discount rate for health investments, let us revisit the earlier thought experiment of the PET scanner. Suppose in that case that the benefits of the scanner were risky, in the sense that the estimated savings in cost of caring were dependent on alternate treatments available and environmental conditions affecting personal and public health for the kinds of health problems detected by the scanner. Then it seems reasonable that to a risk-averse decision maker the health benefits per year would be worth something less than the stated amount of $200 000. Put differently, the decision maker would accept a "certainty equivalent" amount of something less than $200 000 per year *for sure* in exchange for the current risky "claim" to an *expected* value of $200 000 per year.

Modern finance theory allows one to calculate the size of the premium to be built into the discount rate (or to value the certainty equivalent amount per year) for a given level of riskiness. The risk premium to be added to the discount rate might, for example, be calculated from the capital asset pricing model (CAPM) developed by William Sharpe, Jan Mossin, and John Lintner [5]. The CAPM model assumes that: (i) the capital market is perfectly competitive; (ii) transaction costs are zero; (iii) investors have homogeneous beliefs about the risk and return on assets in the economy; and (iv) investors hold well-diversified portfolios (assumptions that, while not strictly true, seem to generate patterns of asset returns generally consistent with empirical experience in the security markets, although the CAPM's specific validity has come under recent challenge [10]. If these assumptions hold true, the required return on a particular investment – "health" or "financial" – is given by the following equation: $r_i = r_F + \beta_i(r_M - r_F)$, where r_i is the expected (required) return on a risky investment i, r_F is the return on a riskless investment (say, in 10 year Treasury bonds), r_M is the expected return on the "market portfolio" of economy-wide assets, and β_i is the systematic, or "market", risk of investment i. This systematic risk, or "beta", is measured by the **regression** coefficient (**covariance** of returns on i with returns on M, divided by the **variance** of the market portfolio's returns), and represents the notion that only such systematic risk will be "priced" in required returns. Non-systematic risk, the unique variability associated with each asset's returns, will be averaged out ("diversified away", in the finance lexicon) by holding a large number of assets not perfectly correlated with each other in one's portfolio. Or one might find, equivalently under the CAPM, that all the risk in the payoffs from the scanner investment had been diversified away by the decision maker's holding of a well-diversified portfolio of health *and* financial investments. That is, suppose the risk was all "diversifiable"; in other words, the returns on the scanner

investment had zero covariance with broader activity in the market. In this case, no "risk premium" would be built into the discount rate. For the purposes of the preceding example, assume that this "risk premium" accounts for, say, 10%, or half of the 20% required return. That implies that, if the health benefits were known with certainty, the appropriate discount rate would be a smaller amount, 10%. Then the net benefit in present value would change to +$28 913, and the scanner investment would be worth undertaking, on balance. The trick in factoring risk into health investments is to determine this risk premium, which in theory should reflect the extent to which the health payoffs (and costs) covary with returns on assets reflecting the larger economy (the "market portfolio"). In practice, this is extremely difficult to do, and analysts instead generally perform **sensitivity analyses** of the impact of different discount rate assumptions on estimated net benefits.

The analyst's perspective is crucial in implementing a specific cost–benefit analysis. Alternative points of view include the following:

1. society's – for example, in the case of public programs, in which the costs and benefits are broadly diffused among a large population (a publicly funded mobile coronary care unit for emergencies represents such an investment);
2. third-party payers' – for example, if a private health plan were structuring a new covered benefit (say, bone marrow transplantation), and wished to evaluate whether the long-term benefits in terms of market share (additional premium revenues) would offset the expected costs of the additional coverage;
3. health care providers' – for example, if a hospital or medical group were implementing a new information system and wished to compare the capital and operating costs of the investment with the future benefits of improved patient care and enhanced clinical efficiency over the long run; and
4. patients' – for example, in the case of a consumer cooperative organized for the health care of its members, the decision to develop a specialized home care unit (say, for persons with chronic obstructive pulmonary disease), with the costs to be fully funded through a surcharge to member premiums and with caregiver support to be provided by member volunteers.

Each one of these points of view suggests a potentially different perspective on costs and benefits. For example, the nature of the publicly funded mobile coronary care unit implies that a social opportunity cost viewpoint be used to assess that program. A full accounting of the direct monetary costs and implicit opportunity costs of the investment would be appropriate, as would a broad conception of population benefit. In contrast, the third-party payer might not incorporate the value of volunteer resources (e.g. donated time) in its calculation of program cost and would likely value benefit more narrowly in terms of gains in premium earned net of health care costs incurred for subscribers only. Similarly, providers and patients will view costs and benefits in narrower terms, based on the inflows and outflows of resources internalized by them.

Another important consideration in cost–benefit analysis is the methodology used to measure program benefits. Two basic approaches exist: (i) the human capital approach [31, 40], which measures program benefits as the sum of direct treatment costs (for illness) saved plus the value of increased production (in the work-for-pay labor force) attributable to the program; and (ii) "**willingness to pay** (WTP)", which values program benefits according to what prospective program "beneficiaries" would be willing to pay in return for receiving those benefits. The WTP technique has certain conceptual advantages relative to the human capital methodology, in that it includes the perceived value of leisure and nonmarket production as well as the **quality of life** and other indirect benefits of health program investments [17, 33].

These advantages come at a practical price, however. Measures of willingness to pay generally require either that careful population-based **surveys** be performed to collect sample estimates of benefit, or that intended beneficiaries' preferences be inferred by examining their choices in real-life situations in which health and money are "traded off". The "revealed preference" approach is exemplified in surveys of airline passengers, regarding their willingness to pay for improved airline travel safety [18] and for improved air quality [38]. Examples of the "revealed preference" approach include the classic work by Viscusi [37], which inferred the implicit value of human life by comparing the wage premium demanded for jobs at different levels of occupational health risk. Similar safety choices that have been analyzed include the use of automobile safety belts [4]

and the decision to purchase new cars with improved safety features [2].

The Cost–Benefit Analysis Algorithm: A Geometrical and Numerical Example

The logic of cost–benefit analysis is displayed graphically in Figure 1. Consider the case of a small local health plan deciding whether to contract with an independent information systems company for its information technology support of its patient care arrangements with hospitals and physicians. The contract is for one year, and the present (year 0) value of the plan's total assets is $2 million. The plan expects additional net revenues (revenues minus costs) next year of $1 080 000 from the additional transaction processing efficiencies estimated from this one-year contract.

The curve BDE, labeled "project opportunity set", depicts the set of all projects available to the plan for investment. The "capital market line", drawn as CDF, reflects the tradeoffs for borrowing and lending (rates of return and interest rates) available for investing in comparably risky projects. The revenues and costs are quite risky for this project, in light of the control given up by "outsourcing" this traditional insurance function, so the plan assigns a 20% discount rate to the contract.

The project will require $400 000 in initial investment (represented as a movement from point B to point A, drawing down plan assets from $2 million to $1.6 million), to cover the costs of canceling existing contracts for this information systems support function and the incremental costs of hiring staff to monitor the new arrangement. As shown in Figure 1, this proposed project would add an

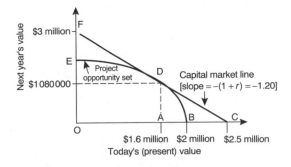

Figure 1 The logic of cost–benefit analysis

estimated $500 000 to the net value of the health plan's assets. This is represented by the horizontal distance between the plan's original position (point B, pre-investment) of $2 million and the ending position (point C) of $2.5 million. This amount equals the net present value (NPV) of benefits less costs. Put another way, based on the plan's estimates, the company's next year value would be $3 million, or $600 000 more in year one terms than would have been the case if the plan's assets were simply invested in the capital markets for a 20% rate of return [$3 million − 1.2($2 million) = $0.6 million]. This $600 000 in increased "future (year 1) value" is equivalent to receiving $500 000 ($600 000/1.2) in increased value today (year 0).

Next, consider the example of a local community not-for-profit hospital deciding whether or not to acquire 49% ownership interest in a large multispecialty medical group that is preeminent in its service area (*see* **Hospital Market Area**). The hospital's total assets are presently worth $400 million. Acquisition of the group practice would not compromise the hospital's not-for-profit status, but would require an investment of $60 million cash by the hospital and lease arrangements with the medical group for use of imaging and laboratory technology. The hospital estimates that the proposed lease contract represents a subsidy to the medical group (hospital costs greater than revenues recouped by the hospital) of $20 million, for a total net investment of $80 million in present value. The expected rate of return to the hospital on comparably risky investments is 15%, which the hospital's chief financial officer chooses as the discount rate for the costs and benefits of the hospital's investment in the medical group.

The hospital takes the "provider's" perspective in this cost–benefit analysis. The future revenues (benefits) are estimated at $20 million per year for 25 years (the expected "economic life" of this investment), and annual costs to the hospital of supporting the medical group (e.g. with information systems, health plan contracting support, billing services) are estimated as $5 million. Thus, the "net benefit" of this project, measured as total benefits minus total costs discounted to their present value, is represented as

net present value benefit

$$= \sum_{t=0,1,\ldots,n} (\text{benefits in year } t \text{ minus costs}$$

in year t)/[1/(1 + annual discount rate)^t],

summed over years $t = 0$ (now), $1, 2, \ldots, n$, where n is the terminal year of the project.(1)

In this case the estimated net present value (NPV) is

NPV (in $millions)

$$= \left\{\sum t = 1, \ldots, 25(20 - 5)/[1.15^t]\right\}$$
$$- 80(\text{the time "0" net investment})$$
$$= 15(6.4641) - 80 = \$16 962 236. \qquad (2)$$

Thus, based on this cost–benefit analysis, the investment should be undertaken because the present value of the net benefits of the project is positive. The figure of 6.4641 is termed the "annuity factor", and it represents the value today (time zero) of $1 paid in each of n years (= 25 years in this case) invested at a rate of return r (= 0.15 in this case). The formula for calculating this factor is $\{(1/r)[1 - (1/(1 + r)^n)]\}$.

In the case of publicly funded programs with widely dispersed beneficiaries and many implicit (rather than direct monetary) costs, it is likely to be more difficult to isolate the annual stream of costs, benefits, risk, correct discount rate, and the "economic life" of the program, but the principles remain the same.

Cost–Effectiveness Analysis

Cost–effectiveness analysis compares the incremental medical costs and health outcomes of alternate health care programs. In contrast to cost–benefit analysis, the denominator of the cost–effectiveness ratio represents health effects expressed in natural units (e.g. life-years gained (*see* **Person-Years of Life Lost**), days free of symptoms, cases avoided) rather than monetary units. Valuation of outcome using monetary units favors those with greater income, to the extent that health outcomes are a "normal good", the value of which increases with income [26]. The cost–effectiveness approach to economic evaluation avoids the somewhat controversial monetary valuation of improved health outcomes such as lives saved. However, it should be noted that – in effect – even cost–effectiveness analysis requires an *implicit* monetary value of health outcomes; otherwise, the decision maker would not know at what level to set the cost–effectiveness threshold for minimally acceptable projects. Under most conditions, results from cost–benefit and cost–effectiveness methods lead to similar conclusions [30]. The interest in the cost–effectiveness model currently stems from its broader acceptance within the health care field and, perhaps, from a working assumption that health decision makers generally operate under externally imposed budget constraints that effectively *fix* the threshold for minimally acceptable projects [22].

A maximization hypothesis underlies the method of cost–effectiveness analysis. Health outcomes are maximized for a given level of medical resource input [11]. The analytic perspective for cost–effectiveness analysis should be that of the health care decision maker, as it is the decision maker who seeks to maximize aggregate health benefits given a budget constraint. This perspective, however, has been criticized as inconsistent with the theoretic axioms of welfare economics, and not in the interest of society [12, 17]. Whereas cost–benefit analysis is strictly based upon a compensation test such as Kaldor–Hicks, cost–effectiveness analyses do not always result in a desirable reallocation from gainers to losers, unless the threshold for minimally acceptable investments is set according to the net benefit maximization rule [11].

The types of questions appropriate for cost–effectiveness analysis include the following:

1. Which of two drug products is most cost-effective for the treatment of major depression [34]?
2. Is heart transplantation a cost-effective strategy [36]?
3. Are work-site intervention programs for hypertension cost-effective [23]?

At the heart of the cost–effectiveness method is the determination of the average and marginal ratios of costs and effectiveness [39]. The average cost–effectiveness ratio is the net cost of each program divided by its measure of effectiveness, resulting in an estimate of the cost of the intervention per unit of outcome gained (e.g. cost per case avoided, or cost per life-year gained). The marginal cost–effectiveness ratio shows the costs and effectiveness of one program in relation to the alternate program.

Specifically, the marginal cost–effectiveness ratio is defined as the difference in medical care costs (net costs) over the difference in program effectiveness (net effectiveness) when comparing at least two alternatives. The marginal cost–effectiveness ratio can be expressed as

$$(TC_a - TC_b)/(O_a - O_b),$$

where TC is the total direct medical care costs associated with the intervention, O is the health outcome associated with the intervention, a is program a (new), and b is program b (existing level of care).

Cost–effectiveness analysis is most useful when there are multiple health programs with a common measure of effectiveness, thus allowing direct comparison between alternative programs. This is not always possible, for most medical interventions lack a common outcome measure. For example, medical interventions for hypertension involve an outcome measured in blood pressure units, while antibiotic treatments are assessed in terms of cases resolved.

Selection of the comparator is important, as the marginal cost–effectiveness ratio reflects a direct comparison of the new intervention compared to a base case. The cost–effectiveness ratio can vary dramatically depending upon the characteristics (cost and effectiveness) of the base case comparator.

The analytic horizon of a cost–effectiveness study should correspond to the expected period over which program costs and outcomes will be realized. For acute conditions such as treatment for infection, a less than one-year horizon is appropriate. However, programs for treatment of chronic disease (e.g. hypertension, diabetes, or asthma) and strategies for primary prevention (e.g. vaccination or disease screening) require a longer time frame. In those instances in which costs and outcomes extend beyond one year, discounting to adjust for time preference of the cost stream as a consequence of the program is recommended. Discounting nonmonetary clinical benefits is less widely accepted. Current recommendations for the selection of discount rates for economic evaluations of health care interventions range from 3% to 5% in the US and Canada [21].

Discounting health care costs and benefits has intended and unintended consequences. Time preference adjustment, also known as net present value calculation, of cost streams from comparator programs that accrue at different rates and at different time periods allows for a standardized valuation of the numerator of the cost–effectiveness ratio. One potential down side to discounting is that public health prevention programs (e.g. immunization or health promotion interventions) often have relatively high up-front costs. Monetary savings that offset these costs may not be realized until much later. Thus, some programs may be judged as not cost-effective simply because of the discount factor.

For resource allocation purposes, the cost–effectiveness ratio can suggest that a new program: (i) improves allocative efficiency (same or better outcome at lower costs); (ii) reduces allocative efficiency (same or worse outcome at higher costs); or (iii) is potentially cost-effective (better outcome at higher cost) relative to the comparator. The latter result requires some interpretation by the decision maker as to the amount of additional resources that they are willing to allocate from other sources in order to realize the incremental gain in health outcome [6].

Cost–Utility Analysis

Cost–utility analysis is a special form of the cost–effectiveness model in which the lack of a common outcome measure is overcome by estimation of some composite metric such as the quality-adjusted life year (QALY) (*see* **Quality of Life and Health Status**). This single outcome measure incorporates the effect of the program or treatment on the quality and quantity of life and allows for comparison of a wide array of interventions [35]. The quality adjustment is derived from preference weights or health utility scores. Several direct and indirect approaches have been developed to measure health utilities or preferences for various outcomes (*see* **Health Status Instruments, Measurement Properties of; Outcomes Research**).

The QALY is not the only outcome measure used for cost–utility analysis. The healthy-year equivalent (HYE) has been proposed as an alternative to the QALY, in part because of the restrictive assumptions about preference measurement [24]. The acceptance of the HYE for cost–utility analysis remains controversial.

The primary application of cost–utility analysis is in cases in which programs or treatments generally impact the health status of individuals rather than improve survival or some other clinical outcome measure. Most importantly, cost–utility ratios can be used to compare programs and treatments across different disease states.

A Cost–Utility Analysis Example

Suppose that three different medical options are available for the treatment of inoperable stage 3 to 4 nonsmall cell lung cancer. Option 1 is supportive care without the use of chemotherapy agents. Option 2 is a chemotherapy regimen that consists of two concurrently administered agents. Option 3 is a chemotherapy regimen that consists of three concurrently administered agents. Patient survival, preference weights (utility scores), and cost data are depicted in Table 1. These data show that option 2 is more effective than either option 1 or option 3 from the standpoint of **median** survival. However, best supportive care without chemotherapy (option 1) provides better quality of life for patients. Options 2 and 3 are more expensive, owing in part to the additional cost of the chemotherapy agents, than option 1.

When comparing option 2 to a baseline of option 1, the incremental cost–utility ratio is $[(9985 - 4639/214 - 112) \times 365]$, or $19 130 per QALY gained. Option 3 compared to option 1 yields an incremental cost–utility ratio of $[(6606 - 4639/165 - 112) \times 365]$, $13 546 per QALY gained.

Table 1 A cost–utility example

| | Treatment options | | |
Parameter	Option 1, best supportive care	Option 2, two-drug regimen	Option 3, three-drug regimen
Median survival (days)	112	214	165
Preference weight	0.61(±0.22)	0.34(±0.30)	0.34(±0.30)
QALY	0.187	0.199	0.154
Cost ($)	4639	9985	6606

The Use of Cost–Effectiveness and Cost–Utility Studies by Decision Makers

How are cost–effectiveness and cost–utility analyses used to augment resource allocation decisions? The possible outcomes of a cost–effectiveness or cost–utility study comparing program or treatment A to program or treatment B are illustrated in Table 2. When the overall cost of A is less than B and the health outcomes associated with A are greater than for B, then A is considered to be "dominant", and should be adopted by providers and purchasers as they improve efficiency in the delivery of care. On the other hand, if A is more costly and provides reduced health benefits when compared to B, the new technology should be rejected. Most new programs or treatments are not consistent with the previous two examples. The third row of Table 2 shows the cost–outcome relationship of most new medical technology or programs. Health benefits are improved at some incremental cost for program A compared to program B. Clinicians, patients, and payors must decide whether the improvement in health outcome is "worth" the additional costs. Tradeoffs or substitutions must be made in order to finance and make available treatment A. The final possible result of a cost–effectiveness study is one in which A is less costly when compared to B and also is less effective. Again, if a health system or insurance plan were to adopt such a treatment (e.g. some population **screening** strategies), then tradeoffs would have to be made in terms of foregone benefit.

How attractive does a new treatment have to be to warrant adoption and reimbursement? At what level of cost per health outcome gained would decision makers choose to accept and use new medical innovations? Currently, a cutoff point for cost–effectiveness determination remains uncertain. The value of $100 000 per QALY has been discussed by policy makers as the level below which a new

program would be described as cost-effective and, therefore, worth the investment.

Summary

Health economics is a field of specialization within the discipline of economics that addresses the allocation of resources directed to health improvement and the organization (*see* **Health Services Organization in the US**), delivery, and financing of health services (*see* **Health Care Financing**). In recognition of the centrality of efficiency within economics, a set of methodologies for economic evaluation of health care programs and interventions has been developed. These methods include cost–benefit, cost–effectiveness, and cost–utility analysis. The application of these tools to health economic problems, and particularly to resource allocation decisions, is an area of intense interest. For analysts considering the use of these methods, a complete understanding of the role and limitations of each is necessary.

References

[1] Arrow, K. (1963). Uncertainty and the welfare economics of medical care, *American Economic Review* **53**, 941-973.

[2] Atkinson, S.E. & Halvorsen, R. (1990). The valuation of risks to life: evidence from the market for automobiles, *Review of Economics and Statistics* **72**, 133-136.

[3] Auster, R.D., Leveson, I. & Sarachek, D. (1969). The production of health: an exploratory study, *Journal of Human Resources* **4**, 411-436.

[4] Blomquist, G. (1979). Value of life saving: implications of consumption activity, *Journal of Political Economy* **87**, 540-558.

[5] Brealey, R.A. & Myers, S.C. (1986). *Principles of Corporate Finance*, 3rd Ed. McGraw-Hill, New York.

[6] Detsky, A.S. & Nagalie, G. (1990). A clinician's guide to cost-effectiveness analysis, *Annals of Internal Medicine* **113**, 147-154.

[7] Elixhauser, A., ed. (1993). Health care cost-benefit and cost-effectiveness analysis (CBA/CEA) from 1979 to 1990: a bibliography, *Medical Care* **31**, 1-141.

[8] Ellis, R.P. & McGuire, T.G. (1986). Provider behavior under prospective reimbursement: cost-sharing and supply, *Journal of Health Economics* **5**, 129-152.

[9] Ellis, R.P. & McGuire, T.G. (1990). Optimal payment systems for health services, *Journal of Health Economics* **9**, 375-396.

Table 2 Results of cost–effectiveness and cost–utility analyses for resource allocation decisions

Cost difference	Outcome difference	Implication
Cost (A) < Cost(B)	O(A) > O(B)	Accept A
Cost (A) > Cost(B)	O(A) < O(B)	Reject A
Cost (A) > Cost(B)	O(A) > O(B)	Tradeoff
Cost (A) < Cost(B)	O(A) < O(B)	Tradeoff

[10] Fama, E.F. & French, K.R. (1993). Common risk factors in the returns on stocks and bonds, *Journal of Financial Economics* **33**, 3–56.

[11] Garber, A.M. & Phelps, C.E. (1997). Economic foundations of cost–effectiveness analysis, *Journal of Health Economics* **16**, 1–31.

[12] Gold, M.R., Siegel, J.E., Russell, L.B. & Weinstein, M.C., eds (1996). *Cost–Effectiveness Analysis in Health and Medicine*. Oxford University Press, Oxford.

[13] Gray, B.H., ed. (1986). *For-Profit Enterprise in Health Care. An Institute of Medicine Report*. National Academy Press, Washington.

[14] Hicks, J.R. (1939). *Value and Capital, Part 1*. Oxford University Press, Oxford.

[15] Hillman, A.L., Pauly, M.V. & Kerstein, J.J. (1989). How do financial incentives affect physicians' clinical decisions and the financial performance of health maintenance organizations?, *New England Journal of Medicine* **321**, 86–92.

[16] Hornbrook, M. & Rafferty, J. (1982). The economics of hospital reimbursement, in *Advances in Health Economics and Health Services Research*, Vol. 3, R.M. Scheffler & L.F. Rossiter, eds. JAI Press, Greenwich, pp. 79–115.

[17] Johannesson, M. (1996). *Theory and Methods of Economic Evaluation of Health Care*. Kluwer, Dordrecht.

[18] Jones-Lee, M.W. (1976). *The Value of Life: an Economic Analysis*. Martin Robertson, London.

[19] Kaldor, N. (1939). Welfare propositions of economists and interpersonal comparisons of utility, *Economic Journal* **September**, 549–552.

[20] Klarman, H.E., Francis, O'S. & Rosenthal, G.D. (1968). Cost–effectiveness analysis applied to the treatment of chronic renal disease, *Medical Care* **6**, 48.

[21] Krahn, M. & Gafni, A. (1993). Discounting in the economic evaluation of health care interventions, *Medical Care* **5**, 403–418.

[22] Laupacis, A., Feeny, D., Detsky, A.S. & Tugwell, P.X. (1992). How attractive does a new technology have to be to warrant adoption and utilization? Tentative guidelines for using clinical and economic evaluations, *Journal of the Canadian Medical Association* **146**, 473–481.

[23] Logan, A.G., Milne, B.J., Achber, C., Campbell, W.P. & Haynes, R.B. (1981). Cost-effectiveness of work-site hypertension treatment program, *Hypertension* **3**, 211–218.

[24] Mehrez, A. & Gafni, A. (1989). Quality-adjusted life years, utility theory, and healthy-year equivalents, *Medical Decision Making* **9**, 142–149.

[25] Mishan, E.J. (1971). Evaluation of life and limb: a theoretical approach, *Journal of Political Economy* **75**, 139–146.

[26] Mishan, E.J. (1988). *Cost–Benefit Analysis*, 4th Ed. Unwin Hyman, London.

[27] Newhouse, J.P. (1978). Plan and market alternatives to the status quo: techniques for managing resource allocation in medical care, in *The Economics of Medical Care*, J.P. Newhouse, ed. Addison-Wesley, Menlo Park. Chapter 6.

[28] Newhouse, J.P. & Phelps, C.E. (1976). New estimates of price and income elasticities, in *The Role of Health Insurance in the Health Services Sector*, R.N. Rossett, ed. Universities–NBER Series 27. National Bureau of Economic Research, New York.

[29] Newhouse, J.P., Manning, W.G., Duan, N., Morris, C.N., Keeler, E.B., Leibowitz, A., Marquis, S.M., Rogers, W.H., Davies, A.R., Lohr, K.N., Ware, J.E. & Brook, R.E. (1987). The findings of the Rand Health Insurance Experiment: a reply to Welch et al., *Medical Care* **25**, 157–179.

[30] Phelps, C.E. & Mushlin, A.I. (1991). On the (near) equivalence of cost-effectiveness and cost–benefit analysis, *International Journal of Technology Assessment in Health Care* **7**, 12–21.

[31] Rice, D.P. (1966). *Estimating the Cost of Illness*. US Department of Heath, Education, and Welfare, Washington, pp. 16–19.

[32] Salkever, D.S., Skinner, E.A., Steinwachs, D.M. & Katz, H. (1982). Episode-based efficiency comparisons for physicians and nurse practitioners, *Medical Care* **20**, 143–153.

[33] Schelling, T.C. (1968). The life you save may be your own, in *Problems in Public Expenditure Analysis*, S.B. Chase, Jr, ed. Brookings Institution, Washington.

[34] Simon, G.E., VonKorff, M., Heiligenstein, J.H., Revicki, D.A., Grothaus, L., Katon, W. & Wagner, E.H. (1996). Initial antidepressant choice in primary care: effectiveness and cost of fluoxetine vs tricyclic antidepressants, *Journal of the American Medical Association* **275**, 1897–1902.

[35] Torrance, G.W. (1986). Measurement of health state utilities for economic appraisal: a review, *Journal of Health Economics* **5**, 1–30.

[36] Van Hout, B., Bansel, G., Habbema, D., van der Maas, P. & deCharro, F. (1993). Heart transplantation in the Netherlands; costs, effects and scenarios, *Journal of Health Economics* **12**, 73–93.

[37] Viscusi, W.K. (1978). Labor market valuations of life and limb: empirical estimates and policy implications, *Public Policy* **26**, 359–386.

[38] Viscusi, W.K., Magat, W.A. & Huber, J. (1991). Pricing environmental health risks: survey assessments of risk-risk and risk–dollar tradeoffs for chronic bronchitis, *Journal of Environmental Economics and Management* **21**, 32–51.

[39] Weinstein, M.C. & Stason, W.B. (1977). Foundations of cost–effectiveness analysis for health and medical practices, *New England Journal of Medicine* **296**, 716–720.

[40] Weisbrod, B. (1961). *The Economics of Public Health: Measuring the Economic Impact of Disease*. University of Pennsylvania Press, Philadelphia.

Douglas A. Conrad & Sean D. Sullivan

Health Examination Survey *see* Surveys, Health and Morbidity

Health Indices *see* Outcome Measures in Clinical Trials

Health Interview Survey *see* Surveys, Health and Morbidity

Health Ratio *see* Synergy of Exposure Effects

Health Services Data Sources in Canada

Canada has a predominantly publicly financed health insurance system that covers medically necessary hospital (inpatient and outpatient) and physician services for all residents. This system, popularly known as "Medicare", consists of 12 interlocking health plans administered by the 10 provinces and two territories. The system is referred to as "national" because plans are linked by the federal government's Canada Health Act principles.

Similarly, the provinces and territories have separate health information systems to serve their particular purposes. These are a complex assortment of components operating in different places and at different levels, often quite independently. However, through agreements, the provinces and territories, federal government departments, and other organizations have instituted national health information databases and registries, maintained according to national standards. These databases do not yet form a coherent whole, but they are accessible to decision makers, planners, epidemiologists, researchers, and others to improve health services, and ultimately the health of Canadians (*see* **Administrative Databases**).

In 1989, the Conference of Deputy Ministers of Health, concerned about the limited and fragmented nature of health information, approved the establishment of the National Health Information Council (NHIC). In 1990, a National Task Force on Health Information was created to assist the NHIC with identifying health information needs. In addition, the Task Force was asked to develop priorities and organizational structures to bring about improvements and changes. Following consultations, the Task Force recommended establishing a Canadian coordinating council for health information. In December 1993, the Canadian Institute for Health Information (CIHI) was established as an independent, nongovernmental, not-for-profit corporation and the Deputy Ministers of Health confirmed the CIHI board as its principal advisor on all health-information-related matters. The CIHI was established to serve as the national mechanism to coordinate the development and maintenance of a comprehensive and integrated health information system for Canada. In addition, the CIHI will provide and coordinate the provision of accurate and timely information required for the establishment of sound health policy; the effective management of the Canadian health system; and generate public awareness about factors affecting good health.

This article describes some of the major Canadian health-related data holdings which may be accessible to researchers or others. These are available from the CIHI, two federal government departments – Statistics Canada (STC) and Health Canada (HC) – and a smaller but important special purpose agency, the Canadian Centre for Occupational Health and Safety (CCOHS). Each of these agencies is described briefly in the section "National Health Information Organizations in Canada". There are other data sources in the provinces/territories but national series and comparisons are mostly available through the national agencies.

Framework for Health Information

The evolution of health information has mirrored paradigm shifts in the view of health care – largely administrative data at first, and over time moving towards information on a broader definition of health. Canadian health information consists mainly of information from government and hospital sources. **Sample surveys** are being used to augment the breadth of coverage and for special purposes. Canada has standardized and comprehensive national databases, and these have the potential for much further development. Currently, the availability of data is most complete in the areas of hospitals, identifiable diseases or conditions, and utilization and costing. For convenience in identifying current data sources and development activities for the future, Canadian health information is categorized into three main areas.

1. *Health determinants*. The factors that influence or determine health. They include the environment, human biology, lifestyles, behaviors and risk factors, demographics, occupation, and socioeconomic factors. Examples are satisfaction with job, cigarettes smoked, proportion of aged, elderly below low income cutoffs, and labor force participation, or lack of it.

2. *Health services*. Services, interventions, and systems (whether governmental or private sector) allocated for restoring, maintaining, or improving health. These are subdivided into morbidity, health human resources, environmental and **occupational health**, and financial and operational data areas. Examples include physician to population ratios and numbers of health care facility beds (*see* **Health Services Research, Overview**).

3. *Health status/population health*. Objective and subjective measures – including morbidity, disability, **life expectancy**, and **vital statistics** – of the health and well-being of populations as diagnosed by health care professionals or reported through self-assessment. Examples are life expectancy and **infant mortality**.

The remainder of the article discusses these broad areas of health information, listing major data holdings and indicating specific examples of information that may be derived from the sources. In addition, a sample of Canadian initiatives underway to widen the scope and fill the gaps in current information are described.

Health Determinants

Data for health determinants are mainly derived from general or special purpose population surveys, both periodic and occasional (*see* **Surveys, Health and Morbidity**). After the one-time Canada Health Survey in 1978, there was a gap until the mid-1980s when a number of federal and provincial surveys were initiated. These include surveys to provide information on current issues such as **AIDS**, tobacco control, and fitness. Other surveys have health-related components for population subgroups, including aboriginal Canadians, children and youth, disabled persons, seniors, and women. There have also been large provincial population sample surveys in Ontario and Quebec. Many of these activities are continuing.

A major ongoing survey is the biennial National Population Health Survey (NPHS) (1994–95, 1996–97, etc.). It includes a set of core population health status measures, longitudinal data on health determinants, and special, periodic **cross-sectional** information. This survey of 22 000 households as well as 3000 residents of chronic care facilities is conducted by Statistics Canada. The self-reported information helps to monitor the health objectives of the provinces and territories, focusing on conditions responsive to prevention, treatment or intervention and examining the states of good health – not just illness. Specific survey categories are **health status**, use of health services (*see* **Health Care Utilization, Data**), determinants of health, and demographic and economic information. The survey also allows the possibility of linking to the national health databases (*see* **Record Linkage**).

Other surveys which provide information either directly or indirectly on health determinants include: consumer income and expenditure; general social surveys; labor force surveys; the international literacy survey; environmental surveys, etc. These may either originate from or be conducted by Statistics Canada for another client (i.e. other government departments such as Industry Canada).

Examples of health determinants available from population surveys include:

1. Alcohol consumption (Statistics Canada – STC; Health Canada – HC).
2. Exercise frequency (STC, HC).
3. Measures taken to improve health (STC, HC).
4. Nutrition (HC).
5. Risk factors (lifestyle) (STC, HC).
6. Smoking/tobacco control and use (STC, HC).

Health Services

Health services data sources contain data elements on health-related curative, preventive, or promotional services provided to patients or to the general public. Many of these data have personal and/or institutional identifiers, so privacy, **confidentiality**, and security standards must be maintained. The major subcategories of data are morbidity, health human resources, environmental and occupational health, and financial and operational areas.

Morbidity

Morbidity databases include data from services provided in hospitals and those provided by physicians and other health practitioners. The Hospital Discharge Abstract Database (DAD) and its companion Hospital Morbidity Database at CIHI are major service event databases. DAD contains over 85% of all Canadian hospital patient discharges (about 3.6 million records annually). It provides data collection and processing services, reports to facilities, and carries out comparative reporting.

Major health care services data sources include:

1. Canadian Organ Replacement Register (Canadian Institute for Health Information – CIHI).
2. Hospital Discharge Abstract Database and Hospital Morbidity Database (CIHI, STC) – (i) most responsible diagnosis leading to hospital length of stay; (ii) interventions; and (iii) relative resource use by grouping of cases.
3. Health Promotion Surveys (HC).

Health Human Resources

Health human resources databases (*see* **Health Workforce Modeling**) track data elements related to medical and health practitioners, including numbers graduating and practicing, geographical distribution, services provided, and remuneration. The National Physician Database is a major source of information on the quantity of physician services, their costs, and limited patient information. It receives about 16 million records annually from the provincial/territorial health insurance (Medicare) system.

Major health human resources data sources include:

1. National Physician Database (CIHI).
2. Southam Medical Database (physician demographics) (CIHI).
3. Registered Nurses Database (CIHI).

Environment and Occupational Health

Environmental health databases (*see* **Environmental Epidemiology**) from Health Canada and Statistics Canada track chemical hazards (*see* **Risk Assessment for Environmental Chemicals**), product safety, medical devices, **radiation** protection, and tobacco control (*see* **Smoking and Health**). Occupational health and safety databases, mainly from CCOHS, include practical health and safety information on chemical and other contaminants and hazards, regulations, standards, and guidelines.

Major environmental health data sources include:

1. Environmental analysis databases (STC).
2. Environmental health databases (HC).
3. Occupational health and safety databases and information (CCOHS).

Financial and Operational Areas

Financial and Operational databases (*see* **Health Care Financing**) contain details on both governmental and nongovernmental areas, in particular sectors (including hospitals and residential care facilities) or geographic areas (provinces and territories) or at the national level. The main database is National Health Expenditures which contains data from 1960 to the present by spending category and source of funding. The data originate from diverse public documents, including public accounts and annual reports, and private sector sources.

Major health expenditures data sources include:

1. National Health Expenditures Database (CIHI) – actual, real, and per capita expenditures by sector and category.
2. Annual Hospital Survey (CIHI) – beds per 1000 population by type of care.
3. Residential Care Facilities Survey (STC) – finances, level of care, patient demographics.

Health Status/Population Health

Health status includes demographic information, general health status, health status of population subgroups, and illnesses or conditions by geographic or population groups.

The major sources of demographic information are the **census** (held every five years) and the regular reporting of vital statistics (historically – births, deaths, marriages, and divorces). These programs are managed by Statistics Canada. Vital statistics measures are traditional, if indirect, health status measures and may include such items as the age-specific fertility rate, births by **birthweight**, and age of mother (such as teenage births).

Health status data are derived from mandatory disease reporting systems (*see* **Disease Registers**), from general or special purpose population surveys (i.e. the National Population Health Survey), or from hospital or self-reported morbidity and general mortality databases (see details under the section "Health Determinants" above). Under the leadership of Health Canada, national **surveillance** networks are in place to create a picture of health risks, patterns, and trends across Canada. New early warning systems have been set up to detect **communicable diseases** of public health importance. These new surveillance networks represent combined laboratory and epidemiologic efforts. New surveillance systems are also in place to detect trends and risk factors in noncommunicable diseases. These include: acute coronary syndrome; myocardial infarction; childhood asthma; diabetes; congenital anomalies; breast, cervical, prostate, and brain cancer; perinatal health; and childhood injuries.

Selected data available include:

1. Demographic – birth rates (STC); fertility rates (STC); population size and distribution (STC).
2. General health status – health expectancy (STC); life expectancy (STC); health indicators (STC).
3. Health status of population subgroups – aboriginal health (HC, STC); children's health (HC, STC); seniors' health (HC, STC); women's health (HC, STC).
4. Illnesses and conditions – accidents and injuries/trauma (CIHI, HC); AIDS (HC, also in STC health indicators); cancer (STC, HC); cardiovascular disease (STC, HC); chronic diseases (HC); communicable diseases (HC, also in STC health indicators); congenital abnormalities (HC); disability (STC); hospital mental health (CIHI, STC); hospital morbidity (CIHI, STC); mortality/causes of death (STC); notifiable diseases (HC, also in STC health indicators); therapeutic abortions (CIHI/STC); tropical diseases (HC).

Further Initiatives

There are a number of initiatives underway to widen the scope and fill the gaps in current Canadian health information. Of considerable note is the federal government's decision to increase its spending on health information to improve **evidence-based** decision making. Private and public sectors are working on the development of an electronic health record, an initiative with the potential to yield rich data. Development continues at CIHI on programs to expand management information systems beyond the acute care hospital setting, in the areas of Ambulatory Care, Continuing Care, Mental Health, and Rehabilitation. Other Canadian priorities include the further development and tracking of population health. These projects are in various stages from planning to performing national pilot tests of data.

National Health Information Organizations in Canada

Canadian Institute for Health Information (CIHI)

CIHI's mandate is twofold. It is mandated to be a national coordinator for the development and maintenance of an integrated health information system in Canada. Also, it provides accurate and timely information needed to: establish sound health policies, effectively manage the Canadian health care system, and generate awareness of factors affecting good health. The Institute was established in 1993 as a nongovernmental, nonprofit agency. CIHI is responsible for data collection, processing, and analysis in wide areas of health, human resources, health care, and health expenditures. It also develops, promotes, and applies national standards to improve the accuracy and comparability of health statistics. Products and services are described in the Canadian Institute for Health Information *Catalogue of Products and Services* (1997) and on the World Wide Web.

Canadian Institute for Health Information. 377 Dalhousie Street, Suite 200, Ottawa, Ontario, Canada K1N 9N8. Tel. (613) 241-7860; fax. (613) 241-8120; internet: www.cihi.ca.

Statistics Canada (STC)

STC is recognized internationally for its expertise in statistics for all aspects of Canadian life. In health, it is responsible, mainly through its Health Statistics Division, for data in the areas of determinants of health, vital statistics, and health surveys to provide accurate and timely statistical information and analyses about the health of Canadians. Statistics Canada provides information on the health status of the population and other specialized information to diverse clients, including life insurance companies, health care associations, pharmaceutical companies, local health units, federal and provincial policy and program areas, and the general public. Products and services are described in the Statistics Canada *Catalogue and Supplement of Products and Services* (1994, 1995), and may also be found on the World Wide Web.

Statistics Canada. Director, Health Statistics Division, Statistics Canada, R.H. Coats Bldg., Tunney's Pasture, Ottawa, Ontario, Canada K1A 0T6. Tel. (613) 951-1746; fax. (613) 951-0792; internet: www.statcan.ca.

Health Canada

Within the Health Protection Branch of Health Canada, the Laboratory Centre for Disease Control (LCDC) is mandated to evaluate and monitor epidemiologic trends and feed information to both provinces and federal policy developers. Other parts of the Health Protection Branch have systems on food, drugs, and the environment in relation to human health. In addition, the Medical Services Branch has data and information on aboriginal people, and the Health Promotion and Programs Branch has data and information on health determinants and health services related to national programs on health promotion.

LCDC is the hub of a multijurisdictional network the role of which is the identification, investigation, prevention, and control of disease on a national basis. In conjunction with the Policy and Consultation Branch, LCDC is expanding its Population Health Intelligence Database with additional surveillance systems and approximately 250 survey data sets containing existing disease outcomes, risk factors, and health determinant data. Health intelligence as reported from this network supports the public health risk management role of Health Canada, and is used by the Department and other agencies and government jurisdictions for prevention, control, and policy formulation.

Health Canada. Assistant Deputy Minister, Health Protection Branch, Health Canada, Health Protection Bldg., Tunney's Pasture, Ottawa, Ontario, Canada K1A 0L2. Tel. (613) 952-7454; fax. (613) 957-4180; internet: www.hwc.ca.

Canadian Centre for Occupational Health and Safety (CCOHS)

CCOHS is a federal government agency under the Department of Human Resources Development. It is an internationally recognized resource in occupational health and safety and in electronic information delivery systems. It provides information and advice about occupational health and safety in order to promote safe and healthy working environments.

Canadian Centre for Occupational Health and Safety. Customer Service, 250 Main Street East, Hamilton, Ontario, Canada L8N 1H6. Tel. (905) 572-4400; fax. (905) 572-4500; internet: www.ccohs.ca.

Bibliography

Adams, O., Ramsey, T. & Millar, W. (1992). Overview of selected health surveys in Canada, 1985–1991. *Health Reports* **4**, 25–52 [Cat. 82-003].

Canadian Institute for Health Information (1997). *Catalogue of Products and Services*. CIHI, Ottawa.

Last, J.M. (1995). *A Dictionary of Epidemiology*, 3rd Ed. Oxford University Press, Oxford.

McCullough, R. & Stephens, T. (1995). Status report on completed and planned national and provincial health-related surveys in Canada, 1990–94, in *Health Data Sharing in Canada*. Canadian Institute for Health Information, Ottawa, Appendix 1.

Shah, C. P. (1994). *Public Health and Preventive Medicine in Canada*, 3rd Ed. University of Toronto Press, Toronto.

Statistics Canada (1994). *Statistics Canada Catalogue, 1994; Supplement, 1995*. Statistics Canada, Ottawa.

Statistics Canada (1995). *National Population Health Survey Overview*. Statistics Canada, Ottawa.

Sutherland, R.W. & Fulton, M.J. (1992). *Health Care in Canada: A Description and Analysis of Canadian Health Services*. The Health Group, Ottawa

Wilk, M.B. (1991). *Health Information for Canada: Report of the National Task Force on Health Information*. National Health Information Council, Health Canada, Ottawa.

Wolfson, M.C. (1995). Social Proprioception: Measurement, Data and Information from a Population Health Perspective, in *Why Are Some People Healthy And Others Not?* Evans, Barer & Marmor, eds. Aldine De Gruyter, New York.

S. TAILLON

Health Services Data Sources in Europe

Describing half a century of development for the more than 20 health systems of Europe, each of which has followed a somewhat different path, is difficult. However, one could summarize by noting that Europe's health systems, in general: (i) experienced a virtually unbridled expansion during the third quarter of the twentieth century; (ii) underwent a process of learning to operate under relative fiscal constraints between the mid-1970s and the late 1980s; and (iii) in the 1990s are experiencing a host of reforms that aim simultaneously at consolidating high but insufficient Equity achievements, and at doing more (Effectiveness) with fewer resources (Efficiency) while involving a broader array of participants in the decision processes (Empowerment) [3].

Europe's health systems are typically described as *Bismarckian* (i.e. predominantly nationwide public schemes to protect individuals against the financial risks associated with illness, through subsidized medical care benefits largely delivered through autonomous agents) or as *Beveridgian* (i.e. medical suppliers accessible to all residents at public expense, often publicly supplied, with out-of-pocket expenses limited – generously so in the early decades). In the Central and Eastern countries – not reviewed here – the appropriate label to describe collective production of, and universal entitlement to, a basic medical package was that of a *Semashko* model. That model nominally supported more preventive interventions than in the West but a considerably small array of high-technology procedures aimed at increasing survival rates in the older age strata. A fourth mixed model with heavier reliance on private insurance for sizable population segments and safety nets for frailer segments applies in a third of the Dutch population and, in a different way, in Swiss cantons. Although there is vocal advocacy for higher private insurance participation, this approach has not been a dominant model in the pattern of Europe's **health care financing** during the second half of the twentieth century.

There are, of course, many variations in European health systems within this broad classification scheme. For example, in Bismarckian France, insurees are required to pay their bills directly and are subsequently reimbursed, whereas in Bismarckian Germany vouchers relieve patients from the necessity of most cash transactions. These differences are more than cosmetic. Faced with broadly similar structural problems, some European public authorities opt for modest doses of reform in the apparent belief that structural adjustments can be painless, whereas others such as Britain choose to restructure on a large scale. Ambitious blueprints for a different system with competition among providers and among payers with a larger role for the insurees (the Dutch Dekker Plan in the late 1980s) appear to have yielded to more modest and politically easier ways using a small measure of competition. Stepwise priority setting, which started in the Netherlands and in the Nordic countries, is gaining ground in larger countries. After several decades of a pull towards public responsibility for medical care financing, a redefinition of the private–public mix is everywhere on the agenda, with population *well-being* still a dominant driver but with a strong concern for cost-effectiveness (*see* **Health Economics**) and greater codetermination.

European *averages* – used by necessity to describe expenditure trends and health states of the population to highlight the spread of real-world dispersions among the 22 countries – are published under the auspices of OECD (Organization for Economic Cooperation and Development)-Europe. Broadly similar measurement is available only for the 22 European country members of the OECD. OECD-Europe in 1997 comprised the 15 Member States of the European Union (formerly referred to as the European Community), which are Austria, Belgium, Denmark, Finland, France, Germany, Greece, Ireland, Italy, Luxembourg, Netherlands, Portugal, Spain, Sweden, and the UK, together with the Czech Republic, Hungary, Iceland, Norway, Poland, Switzerland, and Turkey. OECD's membership also includes Australia, Canada, Japan, Korea, Mexico, New Zealand, and the US (these non-European countries are not reviewed in this article).

In the 1990s the institutions governing the European health systems and the mix of incentives and regulations governing them have become more diverse. However, there appears to be an underlying trend towards a separation of finance and delivery. Health services in Europe involve monetary transactions, but by and large they are not an activity like all others and obey a distinct set of principles. Money increasingly follows the patient. Monolithic structures are yielding, as in Britain, in favor of fund-holding general practitioners or, as in Italy, in favor of hospitals run as still publicly owned but autonomous enterprises. The concern for quality has become pervasive, thereby generating closer monitoring and a growing demand for evaluation. External constraints (mainly of a financing nature, but also strained labor relations or ideologic debates as well as the time required to generate micromanagement models) slow down the transformation process of the multifaceted European health systems. An underlying converging current is, however, greatly facilitated by common external constraints (the need to abide by the discipline of a common currency unit, for instance, prompted Belgium, France, Italy, Spain, and others to accelerate reform proceedings) and by shared ethical principles, notably with respect to children, to ethnic minorities, and to underprivileged segments of the population. The OECD *Health Policy Studies* series (notably volumes 2, 5, 6, and 7) and the CD-ROM statistical compendium *OECD HEALTH DATA 97* embrace in a reasonably comprehensive way the health systems trends in the 22 countries referred to here.

In 1996 the European nations' *measured* effort to finance the range of medical goods and services varied by a 2 to 1 ratio (Germany, at 10.5% of GDP, leading Switzerland and France at the top; Poland and Turkey, at under 5% of GDP, at the bottom, with a sizable concentration at around 8% of GDP). Higher spending in some countries (about $2400 at purchasing power parity – a level of living exchange rate – in Switzerland, $2000 in Germany, and $2000 in France) primarily reflects higher per capita incomes but also higher costs of in-patient care episodes, physician contacts, and medicines. Poland and Turkey, whose *measured* expenditure on medical goods and services is closer to $300 per capita, are OECD-Europe's lowest real income countries. The elasticity of health expenditure to total domestic demand – which translates to a relative citizen and consumer preference for medical goods and services over all goods and services – has been well above unity during the second half of the twentieth century, although financing pressures have slowed this proclivity in most countries. Sizable public deficits and public debts have constrained the management of Europe's health systems in the 1990s while at the same time providing them with an opportunity to restructure.

The main driver of Europe's health systems is not simply a finance engine, but one which also has concerns for quantity and **quality of life**. Gains in **life expectancy** at birth have been greater than three months per year since the 1950s in Europe, with somewhat faster gains for disability-free life expectancy. Potential life years lost – a measure of avoidable mortality below 70 years of age – has shrunk by two-thirds, and morbidity from a number of causes has declined, even though the accelerating demand for services and the fluctuating indicators of patient satisfaction may convey the opposite perception. **Quality of care** and **outcomes** remain important concerns in the European health systems.

Europe's Health Systems Information

The intrinsic complexity of political and social organizations implies that – short of mammoth and virtually unmanageable integrated information systems – the data describing their features are compartmentalized and typically developed in isolated corners of the system. A catalog of data sources is required in each European country. No country releases information on inputs, on throughputs, on financing and on performance indicators, on health status and on outcome measurement, and on **population-based studies** in less than a dozen statistical collections. Multiplied by 22 (not to mention the **World Health Organization's** 50 European members), a combined catalog would reach booklet size. As **evidence-based medicine** and evidence-based health systems are only slowly maturing in most countries, the booklet would soon become a directory. A printout of the *OECD HEALTH DATA* sources and methods facility in hypertext – which ties to the 700–800 **time series** on 29 health systems contained in the software – exceeds 200 normal pages, but even that represents a considerable shortcut for a policy analyst in need of simultaneous access to information on several industrialized countries. Forerunners of the hypertext file have been published in conventional paper format [1, 2].

In particular, *OECD HEALTH DATA* covers macrohealth data pertaining to:

1. **Health status** (life expectancy, potential years of life lost, premature mortality, morbidity, and perceived health status)

2. Inputs and throughputs (health employment, medical education and training, high-technology medical facilities, health R&D, the pharmaceutical industry activity, and trade in medical goods)

3. Medical consumption and practice (average length of stay and admission/discharges by **case-mix** groupers or by **International Classification of Diseases (ICD)** categories, pharmaceutical deliveries by therapeutic classes, ambulatory surgical procedures, and other indicators of medical activity and their prices)

4. Lifestyle and environment (nutrition, nuisances and pollutions, behavioral parameters affecting health, and social protection arrangements)

5. Expenditure on health services and finance (*see* **Health Care Financing**) (total and public, outlays on medical functions and benefits: in-patient care, outpatient services, pharmaceuticals, therapeutic appliances; expenditure by age groups; and sources of funding)

6. Demographic and macroeconomic references related to the composition of the population and the labor force, general education, the national product, public finance, and monetary conversion rates.

A particular feature of the datafile is the inclusion of a hypertext facility that lists for every group of variables the intended content of each series, known deviations from the *standard* definition, and the sources of the data.

Other multicountry datafiles are available to the analyst. The European Office of the World Health Organization (WHO) periodically releases a *HEALTH FOR ALL* software which focuses on public health objectives set in the aftermath of the 1978 Alma Ata Conference. These include 38 targets designed to reduce substantially the toll of premature mortality and largely avoidable morbidity, resulting notably from lifestyle and environmental factors. These targets reinforce the continuous monitoring exercise of WHO in the areas of **communicable diseases** and of cancer and other chronic diseases. WHO supports a network of collaborating centers which collate information in their area of specialty, e.g. the **incidence** of **AIDS**. The total sum of these datafiles makes up a sizable amount of reasonably homogeneous data.

The Nordic Council, an informal institutional machinery set up by Denmark, Finland, Iceland,

Norway, and Sweden, pioneered a harmonized development of epidemiologic as well as activity nomenclatures, notably in surgery. *Health Statistics in the Nordic Countries*, specialized publications on medicines and on social protection, and the relevant tables in the *Yearbook of Nordic Statistics* provide a limited but harmonized supply of data with detailed indications on the sources in the five countries.

The Commission of the European Union, chiefly through its Statistical Office (Eurostat), has over time developed data files dealing with policy areas pursued by the European Union or related to these pursuits. One example is a large database on congenital anomalies, Eurocat. Another is a database related to the use of casemix (**diagnosis related groups** or related approaches) management. Many of these specific datasets are, like those developed under the auspices of the WHO collaborative work, the product of learned societies united by prospective economies of scale in pooling basic data. The European Union has an ambitious data development program on its agenda for the 5-year period 1997–2002 that expands its long-term concern for data on work accidents and occupational diseases, on the mobility of medical professionals, on trade in pharmaceuticals and medical equipment, and on selected areas of prevention, all domains in which the Treaties governing the Union provide the authority.

A few learned societies, like the European Dialysis and Transplant Association or the International Birth Defect Monitoring Association, have, over time, built sizable registries (*see* **Disease Registers**). These reasonably homogeneous datasets are similar to those generated by North American and Australasian bodies. Elsewhere, world associations, such as the International Dental Federation, which created a Working Party with participants from several continents, have instilled a world standard gradually disseminated through the national associations willing to take part in a survey of professional practice. Networks of social insurance administrators and payers and of public hospital managers etc. have instilled a culture in which their domestic reporting procedures are slowly converging.

The bulk of the data developmental effort lies, however, where the power to intervene lies: in public and in private national machineries. Health is virtually not defined anywhere; only its absence is recognized. In much the same way, the characteristics of health professionals and of delivery functions such as hospital care and the measurement of quality of life attributes are not shared. Referring to one of the most established nomenclatures, the ICD, half a century of practice has not sufficed to erase variations in coding practices, let alone in aggregation. Medical culture is not uniform across countries, nor sometimes within countries. Since cross-national compendia are built from national time series or surveys, important attributes or characteristics may vary among individual entries. Lengthy commentaries are thus required for virtually every single component.

International agencies which cooperate in limiting the costly multiplication of nomenclatures are not immune to the risk of using similar headings for different datasets since the criteria underlying the construction of these datasets may vary. The reporting of drinking habits supplies an illustration: the *Health for All* compendium seeks comprehensiveness and identity of concepts; it borrows the basic data from a distillers' compilation which rests on identical conversion of beer, wine, and spirits into pure alcohol. *OECD Health Data*, on the other hand, seeks consistency between the hundreds of data elements it collates from each country more than cross-national comparability.

The preponderance of national datasets over international ones relates to the obvious policy relevance of the former. Companies develop datasets or purchase them from specialized service outfits because of their contribution to corporate strategy; governments develop sizable datasets to plan, implement, and evaluate incentives and regulatory interventions in their health systems. The statistical instruments developed in European countries much resemble those found in the US, comprising one-off surveys, recurrent surveys, **administrative databases**, and elaborate statistical constructs. Because the governance culture of most countries comprising OECD-Europe has been on the whole less quantitative than that prevailing in North America, and notwithstanding sociopolitical choices conducive to considerably greater involvement of public authorities in the management of health care delivery and in health systems financing, European countries have historically been providing less quantitative information on their respective health systems than what may be readily accessible in the US. The quantity and the quality of information released in Europe has been progressing at a rapid pace, however, since the oil crisis of the mid-1970s forced countries to reappraise the cost-effectiveness

of public spending and since corporations operate less and less on captive markets but must live in a competitive environment. The list of these new statistical products is a long one – concerned analysts may turn to the *OECD Health Data* hypertext facility, to other international sources of quantitative information and, increasingly, to *Annual Statistical Yearbooks* or *Statistical Abstracts* of the countries in which they have a greater interest for preliminary indications of what is currently accessible. Furthermore, the stream of information is not drying up and, in several areas, new data collection activities have recently been started in Europe in support of evidence-based management systems.

References

[1]   OECD (1985). *Measuring Health Care*. OECD, Paris.
[2]   OECD (1993). *OECD Health Systems, Facts and Trends*. OECD, Paris.
[3]   Poullier, J.-P. (1997). Public health policies in Europe – doing better and feeling worse, in *Oxford Textbook of Public Health*, Vol. 1, Part III, 3rd Ed. Oxford University Press, Oxford, pp. 275–295.

JEAN-PIERRE POULLIER

Health Services Data Sources in the US

The ability of the health care system to respond to the dynamic needs of a nation, and the adequacy of that response, is governed by the availability of relevant data. The necessary information is used for purposes of planning, and to establish baselines and assess change. Sociodemographic, economic, medical utilization, health care expenditure, insurance coverage, health status, and diagnostic measures are critical health care indices that assist in the determination of the demand for health care by the health service user population. For effective administration of health services, information is also needed on manpower and facility requirements and supply, access to care, satisfaction with care, manpower shortage areas, and financial constraints [9].

In the US, federally sponsored health care **surveys** and other related data systems such as inventories of health care providers have served as the primary data sources to assess the nation's overall level of health and health care needs, and to help identify deficiencies in the health care delivery system. Resultant analytic databases (*see* **Administrative Databases**) have been used to formulate analyses with policy implications, to model the impact of proposed changes in programs, and to evaluate the impact of policies over time. Numerous health surveys have also been conducted by state and local governments to address comparable health system evaluations at the subnational level. Health services information systems have also been developed with funding from private foundations and industries, but their focus is usually quite specific in nature. A brief description of these health services data systems in the US is presented below.

Population-based Surveys: Measures of Health Care Use, Expenditures, Access, and Need

National data on the incidence of acute illness, the **prevalence** of chronic conditions and impairments, the extent of disability, and the utilization of health care services are obtained in the US through the National Health Interview Survey (NHIS). The survey is an annual **cross-sectional** survey of approximately 40 000 households selected to represent the civilian, noninstitutionalized population of the US. Sponsored by the **National Center for Health Statistics (NCHS)**, the sample data measure demographic and socioeconomic characteristics, health status, and the use of health care services. Periodic supplements in the area of utilization, behavior, and health status are used on a rotating basis to collect more detailed information.

The NHIS national core sample also serves as the sampling frame for the Medical Expenditure Panel Survey (MEPS), which replaces the periodic National Medical Expenditure Survey (NMES). The survey is cosponsored by the Agency for Health Care Policy and Research (AHCPR) and the National Center for Health Statistics. This **panel** survey collects data to provide national annual estimates of health care utilization, expenditures, insurance coverage, and sources of payment for the civilian noninstitutionalized population, and for an oversample of policy-relevant subgroups that include the poor and

near poor, the elderly, individuals with functional limitations, and individuals predicted to incur high levels of medical expenditures. Data collection for the redesigned MEPS was initiated in 1996, based on a sample of households from the 1995 NHIS. The MEPS survey is conducted annually, and obtains both cross-sectional and **longitudinal data** needed to monitor health care utilization, expenditures, and health insurance coverage continuously and to examine changes over time. The survey has sample size peaks, consisting of 13 000 households at five-year intervals starting in 1997, that satisfy national precision requirements for policy-relevant population subgroups. In the off-years of the survey (e.g. 1998–2001 and 2003–2006), the sample will be reduced in scale to approximately 9000 households, but with sufficient sample for national estimation and for large policy-relevant population subgroups. The survey obtains data necessary to make annual estimates and to model individual (and family-level) health status, access to care and use, expenditures, and insurance behavior over the two-year period [5]. Furthermore, the household data on utilization and expenditures is supplemented by linkage to data from medical providers [8] (*see* **Record Linkage**).

Person-specific data comparable to those collected in the MEPS are also obtained for a sample of the Medicare eligible population in the Medicare Current Beneficiary Survey (MCBS), sponsored by the Health Care Financing Administration (HCFA). The MCBS is an ongoing longitudinal panel survey of 12 000 individuals selected from Medicare administrative files, that collects health care data covering a three-year period. Household respondents provide data on health care utilization, expenditures, insurance coverage, and health status, which is supplemented by linkage to Medicare Claims Information.

Prevalence data for specific diseases and health conditions and measurements of the nutritional status of the US population are collected in the National Health and Nutrition Examination Survey (NHANES), which is also sponsored by NCHS [20]. Data for NHANES are collected through direct physical examinations, laboratory analyses, and interviews. In the most recent NHANES, completed in 1994, approximately 30 000 persons aged two months and older, were examined in standardized mobile examination centers to obtain a wide range of medical measurements. The measurements include dietary intake, hematologic and biochemical tests, a physical examination and a nutritional assessment. The resultant database allows for the monitoring of national trends with respect to heart disease, diabetes, lead exposure, iron deficiency, and children's growth and development in addition to the nutritional health of the nation.

National estimates of the incidence, prevalence, consequences, and patterns of substance use and abuse are obtained from the National Household Survey on Drug Abuse (NHSDA). This annual survey, sponsored by the Substance Abuse and Mental Health Services Administration (SAMHSA), consists of about 18 000 household interviews of the population aged 12 and older, using special procedures to assure privacy and anonymity.

Analytic data on the use of medical services for family planning, infertility, and prenatal care are obtained in the National Survey of Family Growth (NSFG), conducted by the National Center for Health Statistics. The survey collects information from a nationally representative sample of over 8000 women in the child-bearing ages (15–44) on fertility, factors affecting childbearing (such as contraception, sterilization, and infertility), and related aspects of maternal and infant health [15]. The survey is usually conducted approximately every five years, and the NSFG survey design is consolidated with the NHIS, which serves as the sampling frame for the study.

Another survey with a focus on children, the NCHS-sponsored annual National Immunization Survey (NIS, formerly referred to as the State and Local Immunization Coverage and Health Survey), has been designed to produce estimates of early childhood immunization rates [1]. The annual survey consists of a telephone screening interview with 800 000 households each year to identify approximately 32 000 households with children between the ages of 19–35 months of age, in order to obtain more detailed immunization data on this target population.

The **Centers for Disease Control** and Prevention (CDC) sponsors the Behavioral Risk Factor Surveillance System (BRFSS), which is designed to collect state-specific general population data on forms of behavior that are related to the leading causes of premature death. The survey is a general population telephone **surveillance** system, which obtains data of particular interest to state health departments in targeted risk reduction and disease prevention activities [29].

Another source of both national and community-specific population based data on health services utilization, access to care, insurance coverage, and consumer satisfaction will be forthcoming from the household survey component of the Community Tracking Survey (CTS). The survey is being conducted by the Center for Studying Health System Change and is funded by the Robert Wood Johnson Foundation [16]. The study is designed to track changes in the health care system and their effects on care delivery and individuals. The household survey sample consists of 36 000 households to be interviewed in 1996–1997, primarily selected in 60 communities, and includes a longitudinal component with data collection in 1998–1999.

Another set of more targeted person-specific surveys have been designed with a special emphasis on obtaining statistical information on the older population. The Longitudinal Study of Aging, sponsored by NCHS and the National Institute on Aging (NIA), was designed to measure changes in functioning and in living arrangements in a cohort of older Americans. The survey was based on a supplement on aging to the 1984 National Health Interview Survey and consisted of 7500 participants aged 70 or older, who were interviewed in 1984, 1986, 1988, and 1990 [17]. The Health and Retirement Survey, also sponsored by the National Institute on Aging, is a national panel survey consisting of a sample of individuals who were 51–61 in 1992 and their spouses (7600 households, over 12 600 persons) that are subsequently interviewed every two years over a 12-year period. The survey obtains information on health and cognitive conditions and status, retirement plans and perspectives, health insurance and pension plans, and income and net worth, to facilitate analyses of decisions affecting retirement [14]. In addition, the Asset and Health Dynamics Among the Oldest-Old (AHEAD) Survey, sponsored by the NIA, is a panel study of 10 000 persons born in 1923 or earlier that were primarily identified in the screening of 69 000 households for the Health and Retirement Survey. The survey obtains data on physical and functional health, cognitive functioning, economic status (assets and income), out-of-pocket costs for service use (community and nursing home), and other economic resources, in order to support analyses on the interplay of resources and late life health transitions [29]. Data collected in the AHEAD survey will be linked with information from the National Death Index.

The National Center for Health Statistics collects and publishes data on births, deaths, marriages, and divorces in the US through the National Vital Statistics System. In addition to demographic information, the death certificate data include items on educational attainment, Hispanic origin, and recent improvements in the medical certification information on **cause of death** [21] (*see* **Vital Statistics, Overview**).

A number of national household surveys that have been designed with a primary emphasis on socioeconomic issues also serve as important sources of health care estimates in the US. The Current Population Survey is an annual household survey consisting of approximately 60 000 housing units, sponsored by the Bureau of Labor Statistics and the Bureau of the Census, to obtain national estimates of employment, unemployment, and other socioeconomic characteristics of the general laborforce and the overall population [28]. The survey permits national and regional estimates of health insurance coverage for the US civilian noninstitutionalized population. The Survey of Income and Program Participation is a panel survey consisting of 36 700 households, sponsored by the Census Bureau, to produce national estimates on the economic situation of households, families and persons by detailed demographic characteristics covering a four-year period. The survey has included questions on work disability, functional limitations, and health insurance coverage which allow for the derivation of national population estimates for these health-related measures [28]. National household level estimates of out-of-pocket expenditures for health care can be obtained from the Consumer Expenditure Survey, sponsored by the Bureau of Labor Statistics [30]. The survey has been designed to provide data on the buying habits of American consumers, and consists of interviews with approximately 5000 consumer units each quarter.

Surveys of Health Care Institutions and Providers, and Hospital and Medical Information Systems

Surveys of medical providers and health care institutions both complement and enhance the information on health services utilization that are obtained from household surveys and serve as the primary source of clinical information on diagnostic and therapeutic services provided to patients (*see* **Health Care Utilization, Data**). Physician-specific surveys provide information on practice characteristics, perceptions regarding clinical autonomy, scope of care provided, financial incentives derived through association with managed care organizations, and the impact of managed care arrangements on the practice of medicine. Health services utilization data obtained from institutions, such as from hospital discharge records, provides essential information on surgical procedure rates to help inform whether unexplained geographic variation exists for specific conditions. Furthermore, surveys of institutions such as nursing homes provide data for national estimates of institutional health services utilization, related expenses, and sources of payment, further distinguished by characteristics of the facility, including structure, size, certification, staffing, revenues, and expenses.

The MEPS Medical Provider Survey (MPS), sponsored by the Agency for Health Care Policy and Research, reflects a design strategy to enhance data reported by households on health services utilization and related expenditures through a contact with the associated medical providers. Data from the survey will be used to reduce the **bias** in national health care expenditure estimates that would occur if solely derived from household reported data. Individuals enrolled in the Medicaid program, in which financial transactions occur only between the provider and the state Medicaid agency, and enrollees of managed care plans are often unaware of the total amount billed or how much the provider is paid for the services they received [6]. Furthermore, detailed information on the specific types and intensity of the services provided, such as physician procedure codes (CPT-4s), diagnosis codes (ICD-9s and DSM-IVs), and classification codes for inpatient stays (DRGs), need to be obtained directly from the medical providers (*see* **International Classification of Diseases (ICD)**). To satisfy these design objectives, the annual MEPS Medical Provider Survey targets a nationally representative sample of the physicians, facilities and home health providers that were reported to provide medical care to MEPS household respondents [7].

The National Ambulatory Medical Care Survey (NAMCS), sponsored by NCHS, is a perennial source of statistical data on the ambulatory medical care provided by office-based physicians to the US population. The target population consists of office based visits to physicians engaged in the provision of direct care to ambulatory patients. The survey data collected can be used for research on the use, organization, and delivery of medical care. For the physician practices selected into the sample, information is collected on patient visits, date and duration of visit, patient characteristics, diagnostic and therapeutic services provided, and the disposition and duration of the visit [25]. For the 1992 survey a sample of 3000 physicians was selected, with data obtained from approximately 34 000 patient records.

The National Hospital Ambulatory Medical Care Survey (NHAMCS), sponsored by NCHS, is an annual survey of visits by patients to emergency departments and outpatient departments of non-Federal short-stay or general hospitals. In 1993, utilization data were collected for approximately 36 000 patient visits to emergency departments and 35 000 patient visits to outpatient departments [21]. Non-Federal short-stay general hospitals that have a 24-hour emergency room are also eligible for the Drug Abuse Warning Network (DAWN) sample. The DAWN is an ongoing drug abuse data collection system sponsored by the Substance Abuse and Mental Health Services Administration, which obtains data on drug abuse occurrences that have resulted in a medical crisis or death. The primary objective of the data system is to facilitate the monitoring of drug abuse patterns and trends [21].

National estimates of the utilization of non-Federal short-stay hospitals can be obtained from data collected through the NCHS sponsored National Hospital Discharge Survey (NHDS), from a national sample of the hospital records of discharged patients. Estimates are provided by the demographic categories of the patients discharged, geographic regions of hospitals, conditions diagnosed, and surgical and nonsurgical procedures performed. Measurements of hospital use include frequency, rate and percent of discharges, and days of care and average length of stay [11]. For the 1991 survey, 466 hospitals participated and data were abstracted from about 235 000 medical records.

The Agency for Health Care Policy and Research's Healthcare Cost and Utilization Project (HCUP-3) uses encounter-level administrative data collected by state governments and state hospital associations to create research databases. There are two HCUP-3 inpatient databases. The State Inpatient Database (SID) contains discharge abstract records for all discharges from community hospitals in 17 states, comprising half the discharges in the

US. The Nationwide Inpatient Sample (NIS) is a sample of the SID and approximates a 20% sample of US community hospitals. The NIS contains all discharges from 900 hospitals. The HCUP-3 hospital inpatient databases include patient demographics, diagnoses, and procedures, length of stay, hospital charges, expected pay source, and hospital and physician identifiers. The databases are designed to support research in the following areas: variations in medical practice, diffusion in medical technology, effectiveness of medical treatments, quality of health services, hospital economic behavior, impacts of market structure, changes in delivery systems, and impact of state and federal health care reform initiatives. HCUP-3 also includes an Alternative Services Database that contains records for all hospital-based ambulatory surgeries in five states. The Alternative Services Database enables studies examining the shift of health services from inpatient to outpatient settings [10].

The US Department of Health and Human Services sponsors three distinct surveys of nursing homes: the institutional portion of the Medicare Current Beneficiary Survey (MCBS); the National Nursing Home Survey (NNHS), conducted by NCHS; and the National Nursing Home Expenditure Survey (NNHES), conducted by AHCPR. The MCBS includes an annual institutional component; the NNHS was last conducted in 1995; and the NNHES was fielded in 1996 as part of the MEPS. To complement the 1996 MEPS Household Survey, the National Nursing Home Expenditure Survey collected data from a sample of 800 nursing homes and more than 5000 residents nationwide on the characteristics of the facilities and services offered, expenditures, and sources of payment on an individual resident level, and resident characteristics, including functional limitation, cognitive impairment, age, income, and insurance coverage for calendar year 1996. The survey also collected information on the availability and use of community-based care prior to admission to nursing homes and data on the capacity, staffing, and services provided by the institutions [5, 24]. NCHS also sponsors the annual National Home and Hospice Care Survey, which obtains facility characteristics and patient specific health service utilization information from home health agencies and hospices.

Other related nongovernment data sources of health care providers and institutions in the

US include the American Medical Association's (AMA) Annual Physician Survey [4], which obtains information on practice characteristics, patient profiles, hours and weeks worked, professional income, professional expenses, and fees. The Community Tracking Survey (CTS), conducted by the Center for Studying Health System Change and funded by the Robert Wood Johnson Foundation [16], includes a physician survey to obtain data necessary to track changes in service delivery, access, and perceived ability to provide quality care. The sample design complements the CTS household survey, consisting of a sample of 12 600 physicians in 60 communities.

Health Insurance Data Systems

Coverage and Costs

In the US, the population's access to health services is influenced by the presence and generosity of their health insurance coverage (*see* **Health Care Financing**). Population-based surveys such as the MEPS and the NHIS provide critical data on the sources of insurance coverage that characterize the population. The 1997 Integrated MEPS-Insurance Component (IC), sponsored by AHCPR, will consist of interviews with approximately 9200 employers, 300 union officials, and 400 insurers, to obtain supplemental information on the health insurance held by respondents to the 1996 MEPS Household Survey. This linked survey will provide data to support analyses of individual behavior and choices made with respect to health care use and expenditures and insurance coverage (*see* **Health Care Utilization and Behavior, Models of**).

In a complementary fashion, the 1994 National Employer Health Insurance Survey (NEHIS), co-sponsored by the Agency for Health Care Policy and Research, the National Center for Health Statistics, and the Health Care Financing Administration, was designed to obtain national and state-level estimates of the number of employers offering health insurance, their costs, and the coverage and characteristics of their respective health plans. The 1997 MEPS-IC will include an establishment component that conducts interviews at more than 30 000 establishments to obtain national and regional estimates of the availability of health insurance at the workplace. The analytic objective is to derive estimates

of the amount, types, and costs of health insurance provided to Americans by their employers [5, 27].

The Community Tracking Survey (CTS) also includes an employer survey to measure changes in employers' offering of insurance, the types of insurance offered, premiums, and employees' share of premiums [16]. The sample design complements the CTS household survey, consisting of a sample of approximately 10 000 employers in 60 communities.

Utilization

In addition to survey data, **administrative databases** such as data on insurance claims provide another mechanism to measure health services utilization (*see* **Health Care Utilization, Data**). Claims data are generally gathered and maintained at the patient level in order to report charges and monitor the use of medical services and resources [2]. In the US there are three major sources of claims data: Medicare, Medicaid, and private insurers [19]. As of 1991, Medicare claims are available for all Medicare enrollees in the US. The Medicare claims database includes information on cost, diagnoses, and procedures. Alternately, state-specific Medicaid claims data are available as part of the Medicaid Statistical Information System (MSIS) for 21 states, although the level of detail provided on diagnosis and procedures varies widely, given the nonmandatory reporting requirements for these data elements. Complete Medicaid diagnosis and procedure coding is available in the Tape-to-Tape Medicaid database, but is limited to four states (California, Georgia, Michigan, and Tennessee). Claims data from private insurers are generally employer-based, and vary in the level of detail provided regarding information on cost, diagnoses and procedures, and enrollment data. Insurers such as Blue Cross/Blue Shield, United Health Care, and Kaiser Permanente maintain comprehensive claims databases, as do commercial vendors such as MEDSTAT/SysteMetrics, Inc. and Shared Medical Systems, Inc. [23]. These claims data also have been used in the conduct of cost analyses of clinical practice guidelines.

Health System Inventories and Related Federal Program Data

The US Department of Health and Human Services now obtains data on the level, characteristics, and distribution of the **health workforce** and the physical capital in the health system through a number of separate inventories and surveys, with several more in the early planning stages.

The Health Resources and Services Administration (HRSA) has developed and maintained the Area Resource File System (ARFS), which is designed to be used by health professionals seeking consistent, current, and compatible information for conducting research on the nation's health care delivery system [13] (*see* **Health Services Organization in the US**). The Area Resource File System consists of four major components: (i) the Area Resource File (ARF) which is a county-specific database that consolidates many disparate data elements useful in the analysis of health professions issues and developments on a geographic basis (*see* **Small Area Estimation**); (ii) a State/National Timeseries database; (iii) a microcomputer data series containing demographic, health facilities, and health professions data extracts for use on microcomputers; and (iv) detailed hospital data files. This data system provides the necessary information to allow for research and analysis of the geographic distribution and maldistribution of health manpower, the analysis of health manpower supply, utilization, requirements and cost, and the development of long-range **forecasts** of the health profession's supply and requirements [13].

The National Health Provider Inventory was developed and is maintained by the National Center for Health Statistics to provide counts of the number of health care facilities such as nursing homes and board and care homes in the United States. It also includes an inventory of all home health agencies and hospices in the US, and has served as a **sampling frame** for more detailed surveys of these facilities and agencies [26]. The inventory was last conducted in 1991. The American Medical Association maintains a master file containing data on physician specialty and current employment status for nearly every physician in the US [4]. Hospital-level inventory information is obtained in the American Hospital Association's annual survey of all non-Federal hospitals in the US [3]. A biennial inventory of mental health organizations and general hospital mental health services (IMHO/GHMHS) is maintained by the Substance Abuse and Mental Health Services Administration.

The Health Care Financing Administration maintains the Medicare Statistical System (MSS), which

provides data for examining the program's effectiveness and for tracking the eligibility of enrollees and the benefits that they use, the certification status of institutional providers, and the payments made for covered services. The MSS consists of four distinct databases: the health insurance master file, containing demographic and benefit utilization data for Medicare enrollees; the service provider file, which contains information on hospitals, home health care agencies, skilled nursing facilities, clinical laboratories, and suppliers of outpatient physical therapy services that participate in the Medicare program; the Hospital Insurance (HI) claims file, which includes information on the beneficiaries' entitlement and use of benefits for hospital, skilled nursing facility, and home health agency services; and the Supplementary Medical Insurance (SMI) payment records file, which provides information on whether the enrollee has met the deductible and on amounts paid for physician services and other SMI covered services and supplies [12, 21]. The Health Care Financing Administration also compiles estimates of health expenditures on an annual basis by type of expenditure and source of funds in their National Health Accounts [18].

Other administrative data systems with a health services focus are maintained by Federal government departments outside Health and Human Services, in order to satisfy program-specific objectives. The Department of Defense maintains several health-related data systems within the Office of the Deputy Assistant Secretary of Defense. One such system, the Defense Enrollment Eligibility Reporting System (DEERS), has information on eligibility for medical, dental, and other related benefits on approximately 13.8 million uniformed services beneficiaries [22]. The Defense Department also maintains the Defense Medical Information System (DMIS), which contains patient data with data elements comparable to those found on the Uniform Hospital Discharge Data Set or the UB-82 [2]. The clinical and administrative data in DMIS on all inpatient episodes at Defense Department facilities are obtained for the Automated Quality of Care Evaluation Support System (AQCESS).

The Department of Veterans Affairs (DVA) maintains four main health related data files: the Patient Treatment File (PTF), which includes patient-specific claims type data (admission date, diagnosis, and procedures) for care received at VA facilities; the Out Patient Care file (OPC), which includes patient specific outpatient utilization data; the Long-Term

Care Patient Assessment Instrument (PAI) file, which contains patient-specific demographic, treatment, and diagnostic data for residents of DVA hospital intermediate medicine wards or nursing home units; and the Annual Patient Census (APC) file, which contains utilization data on patients in DVA hospitals at the end of the fiscal year [2].

Summary

In totality, the set of health service information systems that are available in the US are quite comprehensive in their capacity to measure the demand for health services by the US population, and to assess the ability of the health system to satisfy that demand. Future efforts at health service information system expansions at the federal level will be directed to a broader systems view that allows for characterization of the health system as a whole, the analysis of interactions between supply and demand, and the analysis of the relationship between capacity, functioning of the system, and cost. Such information will allow modeling of the impact of change in one aspect of the system on others (e.g. the interaction of the private and public health systems under various health reform scenarios). Similarly, a stronger focus on systems-wide or community perspectives will allow for analysis of the overall structure of the system in terms of regionalization, organization, and redundancy [5].

References

[1]   Abt Associates, Inc. (1994). *State and Local Area Immunization Coverage Health Survey Final Sampling Plan.* Abt Associates, Inc., Chicago.

[2]   Agency for Health Care Policy and Research (1991). *Report to Congress: the Feasibility of Linking Research-related Data Bases to Federal and Non-Federal Medical Administrative Data Bases.* AHCPR Publ. No. 91-0003.

[3]   American Hospital Association (1993). *Hospital Statistics, 1993–94 Edition. Data from the American Hospital Association 1992 Annual Survey.* American Hospital Association, Chicago.

[4]   American Medical Association (1994). *Physician Characteristics and Distribution in the U.S.*, 1994 Ed. American Medical Association, Chicago.

[5]   Arnett, R.A., Hunter, E., Cohen, S., Madans, J. & Feldman, J. (1996). The Department of Health and Human Services' Survey Integration Plan, *American Statistical Association 1996 Proceedings of the Section on Government Statistics.* American Statistical Association, Alexandria, pp. 142–147.

[6]   Cohen, J.W., Monheit, A.C., Beauregard, K.M., Cohen, S.B., Lefkowitz, D.C. Potter, D.E.B., Sommers, J., Taylor, A. & Arnett, R.A. (1997). The National Medical Panel Survey: a national health information resource, *Inquiry* **33**, 373–389.

[7]   Cohen, S.B. (1996). Sample design of the MEPS medical provider survey, in *American Statistical Association 1996 Proceedings of the Section on Government Statistics.* American Statistical Association, Alexandria, pp. 152–157.

[8]   Cohen, S.B. (1997). The redesign of the Medical Expenditure Panel Survey – a component of the DHHS Survey Integration Plan, Seminar on Statistical Methodology in the Public Service, Statistical Policy Office, Office of Information and Regulatory Affairs, Office of Management and Budget, 211–249.

[9]   Cox, B.G. & Cohen, S.B. (1985). *Methodological Issues for Health Care Surveys.* Marcel Dekker, New York.

[10] Elixhauser, A. (1996). *Clinical Classifications for Health Policy Research, Version 2: Software and User's Guide.* AHCPR Publ. No. 96-0046.

[11] Graves, E.J. (1994). National Hospital Discharge Survey: annual summary, 1992, in *Vital and Health Statistics Series 13: Data from the National Health Survey No. 117.* DHHS Publ. No. (PHS) 94-1779.

[12] Health Care Financing Administration (1988). *Medicare Statistical File Manual.* HCFA Publ. No. 03272.

[13] Health Resources and Services Administration (1994). *The Area Resource File (ARF) System: Information for Health Resources Planning and Research.* Office of Health Professions Analysis and Research, OHPAR Report No. 4-94.

[14] Heeringa, S. & Conner, J. (1995). *Technical Description of the Health and Retirement Survey Sample Design.* Institute for Social Research, Ann Arbor.

[15] Judkins, D.R., Moser, W.D. & Botman, S. (1991). National Survey of Family Growth: design, estimation and inference, in *Vital and Health Statistics Series 2, Data Evaluation and Methods Research, No. 109.* DHHS Publ. (91-1386).

[16] Kemper, P., Blumenfeld, D., Corrigan, J., Felt, S., Grossman, J., Kohn, L., Metcalf, C., St. Peter, R., Strouse, R. & Ginsburg, P. (1996). The design of the Community Tracking Study: a longitudinal study of health system change and its effects on people, *Inquiry* **33**, 195–206.

[17] Kovar, M., Fitti, J. & Chyba, M. (1992). The Longitudinal study of aging, *Vital and Health Statistics, Series 1, No. 28* DHHS Publ.

[18] Lazenby, H., Levit, K.R. & Waldo, D.R. (1992). National health accounts: lessons from the U.S. experience, *Health Care Financing Review* **14** (4). Health Care Financing Administration, Washington.

[19] Mitchell, J.B. (1995). Cost analysis of clinical guidelines: which data to use and how to find them, in *Conference Proceedings: Cost Analysis for Clinical Practice Guidelines.* AHCPR Publ. No. 95-0001.

[20] National Center for Health Statistics (1994). Plan and operation of the Third National Health and Nutrition Examination Survey 1988–94, in *Vital and Health Statistics Series 1: Programs and Data Collection Procedures No. 32*. DHHS Publ. No. (PHS) 94-1308.

[21] National Center for Health Statistics (1995). *Health, United States, 1994*. DHHS Publ. No. (PHS) 95-1232.

[22] Office of the Deputy Assistant Secretary of Defence and Defence Medical Support Systems Center (1990). *Program Fact Book*.

[23] Paul, J.E., Weis, K.A. & Epstein, R.A. (1993). Data bases for variations research, *Medical Care* **31**, 96–102.

[24] Potter, D.E.B. (1996). The MEPS National Nursing Home Survey: design and preliminary round 1 field progress, in *American Statistical Association 1996 Proceedings of the Section on Government Statistics*. American Statistical Association, Alexandria, pp. 158–163.

[25] Schappert, S.M. (1994). National Ambulatory Medical Care Survey: 1991 summary, in *Vital and Health Statistics Series 13: Data from the National Health Survey No. 116*. DHHS Publ. No. (PHS) 94-1777.

[26] Sirocco, A. (1994). Nursing homes and board and care homes: data from the 1991 National Health Provider Inventory, in *Advance Data from Vital and Health Statistics, No. 244*. National Center for Health Statistics.

[27] Sommers, J. & Chapman, D. (1996). Sampling issues for the 1997 MEPS-IC, in *American Statistical Association 1996 Proceedings of the Section on Government Statistics*. American Statistical Association, Alexandria.

[28] US Bureau of the Census (1996). *Current Population Survey, March 1996 Technical Documentation*. Administrative and Customer Services Division, Microdata Access Branch. Washington.

[29] US Bureau of the Census (1996). *Data Base News in Aging*. Federal Interagency Forum on Aging-Related Statistics.

[30] Walden, D., Miller, R. & Cohen, S. (1994). Comparison of out of pocket health expenditure estimates from the 1987 National Medical Expenditure Survey with the Consumer Expenditure Survey, *Journal of Economic and Social Measurement* **20**, 139–158.

ROSS ARNETT

Health Services Organization in the US

This article describes several of the key features and components of the health care system in the US.

Integrated Health Systems

The medical care system in the US has many separate components including physicians' offices, nursing homes, hospitals, drug stores, laboratories, and insurance companies. Historically, the US has operated primarily under the fee-for-service system, whereby a physician or other practitioner bills the patient for each encounter or service rendered (*see* **Health Care Financing**). Under this system, the components of the medical care system have usually operated independently.

When various elements of the delivery system necessary for the provision of care are formally interrelated, they are referred to as an *integrated health system*. An integrated health system may own all the components of the system, or it may own some components and contract for the others to achieve a complete system. The degree of integration can vary greatly. Some integrated systems include a direct insurance function, offering packaged insurance benefits to an enrolled population, with all services delivered through the integrated system. Alternatively, an employer or insurer may contract with the integrated system to use the delivery mechanism only.

One early US example of a longstanding, highly integrated health care system is the Kaiser Health Plan of California, which has its own salaried doctors who are usually required to treat patients in Kaiser's outpatient facilities. In Europe, an example is the British National Health Service, which pioneered integration and coordination with the control of resources.

The rapid increase in the cost of medical care has accelerated interest in, and prompted increased development of, integrated health care systems. It is believed that integrated systems promote more efficient and effective health care, in part because comprehensive management information systems permit administrators to monitor the use of services, the referrals to specialists, and access to specific, and especially expensive, services. A large system can obtain discounts on supplies and drugs.

Numerous organizational arrangements exist for structuring the components of an organized system. The essential features of an integrated delivery system are the degree of coordination in its network and its potential for controlling physician and patient behavior.

The best-known structure for an integrated system in the US is the *Health Maintenance Organization (HMO)*. It is so called because each patient pays a premium amount prospectively for all covered services, independent of which services were actually provided, which gives a physician or system an incentive to maintain the patient's health. There are several variants of the HMO model. In a *Closed-Panel HMO*, the HMO owns the outpatient and inpatient facilities and owns or contracts for most other services, is paid a fixed amount for each patient covered (*capitation*), and pays the doctors (the panel) a salary or other predetermined compensation. This model allows a great degree of control over both physicians and patients.

Another common HMO structure is the *Independent Practice Association (IPA)*, which contracts with some or all community-based physicians, hospitals, and other providers for services provided to enrolled clients. More structure is offered by the organizational form termed "group practice without walls" in which community-based physicians form a single legal entity while practicing independently with common office management services and shared contracting.

Another category of integrated system is based on legal and organizational relations between hospitals and physicians. These include *Physician Hospital Organizations (PHOs)* and *Management Service Organizations (MSOs)*. PHOs are usually initiated by hospitals for the development of partially integrated systems of care that can contract with insurance companies and employers. PHOs may work with a restricted universe of physicians or may be more broadly based. The MSO tends to be more physician-oriented than the PHO, is sometimes initiated by physicians, and provides greater practice support services for the physicians who are participating.

Health services research is easier to perform within an integrated health care system than in independent facilities, because there are enrolled populations and often a unified information system. Considerable research has been done to determine whether one organizational system yields higher **quality of care**, higher satisfaction, or lower cost than other systems. The impact of such systems and differences between for-profit and not-for-profit systems will need a further evaluation as they evolve, although the evidence thus far is generally positive. For a further description of integrated health systems, see Brown [1].

Hospital and Health Systems

Hospitals were first termed "almshouses" or "poor houses" and provided care primarily to the homeless poor and chronically disabled. Wealthier people received care in their own residences. As medicine advanced, particularly after the turn of the century, and most notably after World War II, the hospital's role as a source of biomedical expertise and knowledge grew dramatically. In the US, the development of professional **nursing** and specialized technology and the increasing ability of physicians to intervene in disease and illness spurred on the growth of the nation's hospitals in the first half of the 1900s. The growth of private health insurance and government entitlement programs, and further advances in medical technology and the professional development of physicians in the years prior to and after World War II, gave a further thrust to hospital growth and development. In the US, health services are increasingly provided in an ambulatory setting, causing hospitals to become more a source of highly specialized services.

Hospitals and health systems may be organized and owned as government entities or as private for-profit or nonprofit entities. Hospital ownership and hospital management may be differentiated in that in some instances a hospital may be publicly owned, or owned by a nonprofit entity, but managed under contract by a for-profit corporation. Government hospitals may be owned by federal, state, or local entities. A for-profit hospital is typically part of a larger corporation, as may be the case also for a nonprofit entity. Publicly held, for-profit companies that own and operate or manage hospitals under contract are typically large corporations whose stock is traded on national stock exchanges.

In recent years, the for-profit hospital sector has experienced a high degree of turmoil with, most recently, increasing consolidation. Some controversy exists as to the extent to which for-profit hospitals are run more efficiently and have lower personnel-to-patient ratios. Economic pressures, however, are forcing all hospitals to improve their economic efficiency and management expertise and to focus on parameters of performance.

The traditional organizational structure of hospitals in the US includes three sources of power and authority. The governing board is ultimately responsible for all of the operations of the hospital.

Hospital administration is delegated responsibility for the day-to-day management of the facility. The hospital medical staff is typically separately organized with delegated responsibility from the board for clinical matters, including the credentialing of physicians and assessing and assuring the quality of health services provided. Hospitals that are part of larger health systems, however, typically lose managerial and governance autonomy.

Hospitals and health systems in the US are facing increasing competition and cost pressures. Managed care requires an assumption of risk and participation in various new forms of reimbursement that have a variety of controls associated with them. Increasing vertical integration is occurring throughout the US in the hospital industry. Concerns over quality of care, malpractice litigation, excess bed capacity, and provision of care to the medically underserved are also common in most communities throughout the US.

Research needs to focus on issues of efficiency, outcomes, and costs of care in the hospital and health systems. Also relevant are issues associated with the integration of the hospital with other services and with systems of care.

Further information on the organization of hospitals in the US can be found in [13].

Ambulatory Care Services

Ambulatory (outpatient) care encompasses those services provided to a noninstitutional patient, as opposed to inpatient services, which are provided to a patient who has been admitted, at least overnight, to a hospital or other health care facility. Ambulatory services include a wide range of settings, professionals, and specific health care clinical services. Technological advances and financial pressures are increasingly leading to a shift of services from inpatient to outpatient care.

The typical US citizen has approximately six physician contacts per year. The most common setting for ambulatory care services is the physician's office, incorporating solo practitioners, group practices, and hospital outpatient departments. Ambulatory services are also provided in a variety of other settings, including, most notably, ambulatory surgery centers, which have grown tremendously in importance and are now the setting for 70% of all surgery performed in the US, emergency rooms, and hospital clinics. Governmentally sponsored ambulatory care services include those in institutional settings such as Department of Veterans Affairs facilities and prisons, as well as military services and the Indian Health Service.

Ambulatory care plays an important role, particularly in managed care plans, in the coordination, organization, and control of all health care. Ambulatory care is usually less expensive than inpatient care.

Research has begun to address key issues such as the role of the gatekeeper in ambulatory care, appropriate use of services, coordination and access, and clinical practices and outcomes (*see* **Outcomes Research**).

Further details on ambulatory care services may be found in [12].

Group Practice

A group practice is a formal organizational arrangement for the affiliation of three or more health care professionals characterized by the sharing of income, expenses, medical records, staff, facilities, and other resources. The first physician group practice in the US was the Mayo Clinic in Rochester, Minnesota. Historically, most physicians were solo practitioners. With the advent of increasing specialization and administrative complexity, and, more recently, of insurance and prepayment, group practice has grown explosively, with approximately 40% of all physicians in the US practicing in a group.

Group practice provides professional management and shared financial and patient care responsibility. Group practice also limits a practitioner's clinical and financial freedom, requiring that practitioners conform to group norms and standards. Personal autonomy is exchanged for greater financial flexibility and contracting advantages.

Group practices may be organized as professional corporations, foundations, partnerships, and other legal forms. Other complex legal entities and contracting arrangements are used in groups that are involved in managed care. Some larger groups own their own hospitals, and most groups own ambulatory surgery, laboratory, and other specialized facilities. Under managed care, group practice assumes a particularly important role in managing physician resources and in controlling patient access to services.

Havlicek [5] provides further description of group practice.

Primary Care

Primary care is the provision of ongoing, day-to-day health care services, encompassing preventive services (*see* **Preventive Medicine**) as well as relatively routine and patient- and provider-initiated services. Primary care typically requires less intensive resources than more specialized care and can often be provided during a brief office visit. Primary care also includes follow-up and continuing care for chronic diseases.

Primary care is typically provided by a physician in the physician's office, but is also provided by other health professionals, such as nurse practitioners, especially in specialties such as pediatrics. Primary care is also available in hospital facilities and the patient's home.

Primary care provides an important entry into the health care system. It is the best setting for ongoing monitoring and coordination of care, and a reliable source of advice and guidance. It is the coordinating and controlling aspect of primary care, combined with increased reliance on primary care providers (i.e. general internists, family practitioners (*see* **General Practice**), pediatricians, and sometimes obstetrician/gynecologists), that is a key defining principle of many forms of managed care.

Wenzel [16] elaborates on the characteristics of primary care in the US.

Long-Term Care

Long-term care includes a broad array of physical health, mental health, and social services provided to individuals with significant, often permanent, illness and disability. In some instances, the need for long-term care may be only temporary, with eventual recovery. Long-term care services, in contrast to acute or short-term care, typically involve a broader array of social, and residential, services, as well as health services. The involvement of social and other services may present financial difficulties for many individuals due to lack of external subsidies such as health insurance.

Long-term care services include skilled nursing facilities, such as nursing homes; inpatient hospital services, including medical, surgical, psychiatric, and rehabilitation facilities; ambulatory care services, and mental health facilities; alcohol and drug abuse programs; adult day care; home health services; hospice care; and social services, including meals on wheels, homemaker and personal care services; transportation, communication, health promotion activity programs, and recreational activities; and, finally, housing programs, including congregate care, retirement communities, assisted living facilities, and other living arrangements.

Long-term care services are primarily devoted to individuals with chronic physical or mental disability. An important component of long-term care is the rehabilitation service, particularly for individuals suffering from chronic disease, trauma, and accidents. The older population of long-term care users typically have multiple physical and/or mental health problems, as well as various social and financial constraints. A growing population of individuals in both the long-term and mental health systems is characterized by mental and/or physical disability attributable to various forms of dementia, such as Alzheimer's disease.

Nursing homes are an important component of long-term care. Nursing homes that are Medicare-certified are eligible to accept patients covered under the Medicare program. Medicare coverage of long-term care services is extremely limited, and most patients are required to spend-down most of their personal financial resources before becoming eligible for Medicaid program coverage. The nursing home resident is typically aged 85 and above with multiple health, and often mental health, problems and with a variety of dependency requirements.

Hospice is a form of organizing services for individuals with terminal illness. Hospice may be provided in specifically designated facilities or in the patient's home and involves a coordinated, multidisciplinary approach to addressing the patient's needs as well as those of the family.

Home health services is another growth area in long-term care. Technological advances allow a wider range of services, such as infusion therapy, to be provided in patients' homes, thereby decreasing the need for inpatient care. Increasing coverage under Medicare and insurance plans has spurred the growth of home health care in the US.

Long-term care services are often fragmented and need integration to match services to patient needs.

Coordination requires integrated information systems (*see* **Administrative Databases**), care coordination, particularly by case managers, and integrated financing mechanisms. Current long-term care financing arrangements in the US limit this type of integration. Social services, in particular, are often inadequately coordinated with physical health and mental health needs. For further reading, see Evashwick [4].

Public Health and Preventive Services

Public health and preventive services are the front line of protection against injury, disease, and illness. Primary prevention and many public health services are population-based, such as the protection of food, water, and milk supplies, and the monitoring of disease (*see* **Surveillance of Diseases**) and disposal of wastes. Preventive services delivered to individuals with the purpose of avoiding illness include vaccinations and immunizations, physician examinations, and screening (*see* **Screening, Overview**). Of increasing importance in recent years is work site accident avoidance (*see* **Occupational Health and Medicine**).

Public health services are provided through state and local public health agencies. The core functions of public health agencies at all levels of government (see [7]), are: assessment, development, and assurance of public health services. State agencies have responsibility for the entire population in a state. Local agencies provide direct services, such as restaurant inspections and monitoring of food and water supplies. Provision of personal services such as immunization, venereal disease screening, and family planning clinics is a local function. State agencies intervene when local agencies do not perform adequately legally required public health services. In the US, federal agencies with responsibility for public health include the federal **Centers for Disease Control** and Prevention, which provides laboratory, epidemiologic, and advisory expertise. Federal grant support for selected priorities is provided to state and local agencies. Responsibility for protecting the nation's health is ultimately shared by governmental agencies with front-line providers and by every citizen as well. Research needs in this area include cost/benefit analysis of screening (*see* **Screening Benefit, Evaluation of**) and routine personal preventive services. There is controversy about the appropriateness and frequency of most preventive measures. Further discussion on this topic appears in [7] and [14].

Mental Health Services

Mental health services involve services provided for psychiatric and neurological disease and illness pertaining to the brain and its function, as well as to emotional and behavioral deviance (*see* **Psychiatry; Neurology**).

Until the second half of the twentieth century, mental illness and dysfunctional behavior were treated by institutionalization and isolation as well as persecution. Developmental and experiential origins for behavior, codified by Freud and others, led to the establishment of psychiatry and psychoanalysis to diagnose and treat mental illness. Biomedical research is now vastly improving the identification and treatment of such illnesses as depression, schizophrenia, obsessive–compulsive behavior, and addictions.

Increasingly, physiologic etiologies are being identified for many forms of mental illness and aberrant behavior, leading to enhanced pharmacologic intervention. The introduction of psychotropic drugs in the 1950s, along with community-based outpatient services, led to the deinstitutionalization of mental health patients in the US. However, inadequate resources and lack of an integrated and comprehensive delivery system have also caused increases in the homeless population in many cities, multiple hospitalization episodes, and increased criminal activity by and against those with mental illness.

The US has both public and private mental health systems. The public system is the provider of last resort and is characterized by governmental facilities, while the private system cares for individuals with insurance, the ability to self-pay, or coverage under entitlement programs. The private system is characterized by private psychiatric hospitals and a greater role for psychiatrists as opposed to psychologists, who are more prevalent in the public system. Mental health services tend to be limited under private health insurance. Where physiologic origins for mental disorders are identified, prospects for enhanced coverage are brighter, as are the social advantages. However, problems such as developmental disabilities and severe organic brain disorders, dementia, including Alzheimer's disease, substance abuse, and criminal activity remain complex challenges. Mental health problems also raise numerous complex legal, ethical, and moral issues regarding individuals' rights to privacy, to treatment, and to involvement in society, as well as issues of access to care, appropriateness of various professional providers, and avenues for financing.

Research needs include continued epidemiologic investigations of the nature of illness and determination of cost-effective interventions (*see* **Health Economics**), as well as determination of the most appropriate sites for care, best practitioners to utilize, and financing arrangements.

The reader is referred to [6] and [11] for more detailed description of mental health services in the US.

Health Care Personnel

Approximately 8% of US, civilian employment is involved in the health care system as providers of care or in organizing or managing the system. Physicians are the key clinical decision-makers in the health care system. In the US, federal and state government initiatives in the mid-1960s led to substantial increases in the number of medical schools, as well as medical school graduates from existing schools. In addition, during the late 1960s and 1970s, federal policy allowed for an influx of substantial numbers of foreign medical school graduates. The result of these policy actions is a substantial increase in the number of physicians in training and in practice. Geographic dispersion of physician supply has also improved greatly over the past 30 years. Significant attention has been directed toward specialty distribution, to focus recently on increasing the supply of primary care practitioners at the expense of many surgical subspecialities. Managed care has endorsed this shift with an emphasis on providing care through primary care practitioners wherever possible.

There are over 2 000 000 registered nurses in the US. In recent years, there has been a dramatic shift in the education of individuals eligible to become registered nurses from hospital-based diploma programs to baccalaureate and associate degree programs based in colleges and universities. The nursing field also includes many other roles, including various forms of nursing assistants and licensed practical nurses,

as well as more heavily credentialed nurses, such as nurse practitioners.

Numerous other specialty professionals contribute to health services. For example, improvements in oral health combined with greater efficiency in dental practice have impacted demand for dental services and education; the number of dental schools and graduating dentists has begun to decline. However, dental services are still inequitably distributed due to financial constraints.

Research issues for the future are complex and include the increasing role of specialists in many areas, competition between different practitioners for employment and clinical roles, credentialing and licensure of professionals, and matching availability of personnel to the need for such individuals in an increasingly fiscally constrained environment. Issues of quality, cost, and appropriateness of utilization, will also need to be addressed in the future (*see* **Health Workforce Modeling**).

For further information on health care personnel in the US, see [2], [3], and [8].

Managed Care

Managed care is a general term representing the realignment of health care services and reimbursement in such a manner as to shift the risk, both financially and in other forms, from insurers to providers and consumers. Managed care is the more current form of what was previously termed prepaid health care. Although managed care is in a state of flux, some specific organizational structures are beginning to evolve.

Managed care plans are designed to reduce utilization, particularly of inpatient services, and at the same time often to provide a broader benefit structure with some degree of emphasis on preventive services in view of their potential long-term cost benefits. One important feature of managed care plans is the establishment of contractual arrangements with providers to allow the plan and its management to impose various forms of oversight and control over providers. Provider risk-sharing through contractual arrangements that provide incentive compensation is also common. Reduced consumer administrative burdens are typical of many forms of managed care, although various barriers are also introduced to reduce consumer incentives for utilization as well.

Managed care provides services in a more financially constrained framework, whereby both providers and consumers have greater incentive to control use of services and hence costs. Substitution of lower-cost clinical alternatives, rationing of services, coordination of care, reduction of duplication of services, and managerial efficiencies are among the approaches utilized in implementing managed care systems. Use of quantitative databases to monitor and evaluate clinical patterns of care, financial experience, and quality and utilization is an important component of managed care, which drives the need for a structured information system (*see* **Administrative Databases**) and for statistical evaluation methods for assessing use and patterns of care.

Managed care often incorporates various forms of HMOs. The percentage of the population enrolled in managed care plans has increased dramatically in the past decade. In the US, entitlement programs such as Medicare and Medicaid increasingly incorporate managed care principles and contractors to instill efficiencies and cost savings.

Managed care plans, through contractual arrangements with providers, establish networks of individual and institutional care sources. Less restrictive plans, such as Preferred Provider Organizations and Point-of-Service HMO plans use networks but allow out-of-plan use at higher cost. More restrictive forms of managed care, such as Closed-Panel HMOs often do not allow out-of-plan use of services. Other incentives and controls affecting consumers include copayments and deductibles, case management, benefit limitations and exclusions, and access barriers in various forms.

An increasingly popular mechanism for controlling utilization by consumers in managed care plans, particularly HMOs is the gatekeeper. The gatekeeper is a primary care physician who must either provide or approve referrals for any services within the plan. The gatekeeper concept has assigned much greater responsibility to the primary care physician and has reduced direct access to specialists by consumers.

In managed care plans, financial incentives for providers are often designed to provide rewards for the careful management of dollars. Various forms of incentives, such as bonuses and profit-sharing pools, are used to encourage physicians to control carefully the use of services, particularly expensive inpatient and specialty care. Reimbursement of physicians has also shifted in many plans from traditional fee-for-service payment to salary and capitation, whereby incentives are much more clearly focused on rationing and control of utilization.

Further research is needed to test many of the principles of managed care and their long-term effects on cost, quality, and patient and provider satisfaction. Possible underutilization, lack of access, and adverse effects of financial incentives for physicians are other research issues.

Kongstvedt [9, 10] provides a good source for further reading regarding managed care.

Regulation and Controls

Regulatory mechanisms to control health care services may be imposed by governmental entities or by payers under contractual arrangements. Government intervention is usually designed to protect health and safety or to influence the health care market when the market fails to achieve those social goals desired by political forces.

Examples of US governmental regulations pertaining to health and safety include fire, health, and safety codes imposed by state and local governments. State regulation of health care personnel includes licensure of physicians, nurses, and other categories of professionals. Payers may also implement limited regulation of this nature, such as evaluation of participating physicians' qualifications and credentials.

Marketplace regulations in the US, particularly by government, date back to the Hill–Burton legislation, which allocated federal funds for hospital construction and renovation after World War II on the basis of simple health planning computations. The more recent era of government intervention dates to the Great Society in the mid-1960s. Numerous interventions attempted to influence costs and allocation of resources. Examples include subsidies aimed at individuals and institutions, such as grant and loan program tax exemptions. Entitlement programs such as Medicare and Medicaid represent large-scale, subsidy-type interventions. Restrictions on entry into professional fields through licensure requirements and facility licensure and capital expenditure controls are additional examples of interventions. Regulation through payment mechanisms includes requirements under the Medicare and Medicaid programs, rate-setting commissions, wage and price controls, payment restrictions under insurance programs, including contractual arrangements under managed care, and the determination of fee schedules.

Controls to assure the **quality of care** are also common in health services. These are usually associated with entitlement programs or with contractual obligations under insurance plans, particularly under managed care. These mechanisms have included professional review organizations, utilization review, preadmission authorization, second opinions for surgery, and other programs to assess quantitatively various aspects of the quality and utilization of services, and the control of use of services by providers and patients.

Numerous other regulatory mechanisms have been utilized in the past or are currently in place. These include: financial controls on consumers, including benefit limitations, deductibles, coinsurance exclusions, and other provisions of insurance plans; limitations on the supply of services through rationing, queues, and other restrictions on access; reviews of provider services, including claims reviews, medical audits, institutional reviews; and legal, regulatory, and practice-influencing effects from medical malpractice litigation.

Regulation and control of health services has historically had a focus on either affecting utilization and costs or influencing perceived inadequacies and misallocations of resources within the health care system. Although many regulatory efforts in the past have failed to provide adequate results or have simply not been cost-effective, marketplace mechanisms continue to be the primary focus at the present time with an emphasis on reduction in cost increases, on influencing patient expectations of behavior, and on affecting physician practice patterns and use of resources. Regulatory control mechanisms are increasingly focusing on economic considerations with some added focus on monitoring various aspects of the quality of care provided. Evaluation of consumers and providers by managed care organizations and self-evaluation of such managed care organizations themselves and by external organizations have grown substantially in recent years. Under the pro-competitive market approach in the US of recent years, the federal government's direct role in the regulation and control of health services has focused primarily on costs, access, and quality issues in government entitlement programs with a less

substantive contribution to the assessment of various aspects of the larger system.

The reader is referred to [17] for more details regarding regulating and controlling health services in the US.

Technology Assessment

Advances in technology can improve the diagnosis, treatment, and cure of disease and illness. However, important issues related to the diffusion and evaluation of technology impinge on policy-making regarding the role of technology in health services.

The evaluation of technology involves complex considerations including costs and benefits, regulation, efficacy, and clinical effectiveness. Diffusion of new technology is driven by financial considerations. Under fee-for-service reimbursement, technological advances have a tendency to be utilized as quickly as regulatory approval is achieved, while in a managed care environment the potential for some hesitation exists.

The principal federal agency responsible for technology assessment in the US is the **Food and Drug Administration (FDA)**. Drugs and medical devices must be demonstrated to be safe and efficacious to achieve FDA approval for clinical application. This complex and controversial process requires considerable time and financial resources.

Clinical research studies are usually necessary to determine the appropriate clinical situations when each technology should be utilized. Technologies that lead to overall cost reductions in health services due to their substitution for more expensive therapies are of particular research interest. Managed care organizations are interested in the appropriateness of various technologies and their associated costs. Controversy is building over the potential restriction of some technologies under insurance and entitlement programs due to costs and limited benefits. Ultimately, rationing of resources necessitates making judgments as to whether particular technologies are warranted in individual cases.

Further details may be found in Skorup [15].

References

[1]   Brown, M. (1996). *Integrated Health Care Delivery.* Aspen, Gaithersburg.

[2]   Bureau of Health Professions, Health Resources and Services Administration (1993). *Factbook: Health*

Personnel U.S. (DHHS Pub. No. HRSA-P-AM-93-1). US Government Printing Office, Washington.

[3]   Council on Graduate Medical Education (1995). *Seventh Report to Congress and the Department of Health & Human Services Secretary: Recommendations for Department of Health and Human Services' Programs.* US Government Printing Office, Washington.

[4]   Evashwick, C.J. (1996). *The Continuum of Long-Term Care: An Integrated Systems Approach.* Delmar, Albany.

[5]   Havlicek, P.L. (1996). *Medical Groups in the U.S.: A Survey of Practice Characteristics.* American Medical Association, Chicago.

[6]   Howard, K.I., Cornille, T.A., Lyons, J.S., Vessey, J.T., Lueger, R.J. & Saunders, S.M. (1996). Patterns of mental health services utilization, *Archives of General Psychiatry* **53**, 696–703.

[7]   Institute of Medicine (1988). *The Future of Public Health.* National Academy Press, Washington.

[8]   Institute of Medicine (1996). *The Nation's Physician Workforce: Options for Balancing Supply and Requirements.* National Academy Press, Washington.

[9]   Kongstvedt, P.R. (1997). *Essentials of Managed Care,* 2nd Ed. Aspen, Gaithersburg.

[10] Kongstvedt, P.R. (1996). *The Managed Health Care Handbook,* 3rd Ed. Aspen, Gaithersburg.

[11] Robins, L.N., Locke, B.Z. & Regier, D.A. (1991). An overview of psychiatric disorders in America, in *Psychiatric Disorders in America.* Free Press, New York.

[12] Ross, A., Williams, S.J. & Pavlock, E.J. (1997). *Ambulatory Care Management,* 3rd Ed. Aspen, Gaithersburg.

[13] Rowland, H.S. & Rowland, B.L. (1992). *Manual of Hospital Administration.* Aspen, Gaithersburg.

[14] Scutchfield, F. & Keck, C.W. (1996). *Principles of Public Health Practice.* Delmar, Albany.

[15] Skorup, T.E. (1994). Technology assessment and management, in *The AUPHA Manual of Health Services Management,* R.J. Taylor & S.B. Taylor, eds. Aspen, Gaithersburg.

[16] Wenzel, F.J. (1994). Primary care services, in *The AUPHA Manual of Health Services Management,* R.J. Taylor & S.B. Taylor, eds. Aspen, Gaithersburg.

[17] Williams, S.J. & Torrens, P.R. (1993). Influencing, regulating, and monitoring the health care system, in *Introduction to Health Services,* 4th Ed. Delmar, Albany.

STEPHEN J. WILLIAMS

Health Services Research, Overview

Health services research (HSR) is a "multidisciplinary field of inquiry, both basic and applied, that examines the use, costs, quality, accessibility, delivery, organization, financing, and outcomes of health care services to increase knowledge and understanding of the structure, processes, and effects of health services for individuals and populations" [9]. The origins of health services research can be traced to the 1920s in the US, and several experts since the 1970s have developed descriptions or definitions of the field [3, 4, 11, 12, 15]. HSR has grown most prominent in the 1990s in both the US and abroad, where it is sometimes referred to as health systems research, or simply health research.

Definitional Concepts

Several important concepts set the field of health services research apart from more academic or clinical disciplines. First, health services research is multidisciplinary in that it involves a wide range of disciplines, clinical specialties, and distinct academic fields; those who work in health services research tend to be identified not by their academic training but rather by the nature of the research they conduct. Core areas generally include the clinical specialties (e.g. medicine, nursing, dentistry, and public health), economics (or **health economics**), epidemiology, statistics, and biostatistics, but depending on the research or policy question at hand a considerable range of fields can play major roles in HSR, including anthropology, bioengineering, business administration, computer sciences, decision analysis, ethics and bioethics, history, law, management sciences and administration, psychology, **operations research**, and sociology.

Secondly, HSR involves investigations into basic questions of the behavior of individuals, organizations, and systems within health care; more commonly, HSR comprises applied studies concerned with practical questions of health policy, health care delivery and management, evaluation of health care interventions, and the use of information for public and private health care decisionmaking. Thirdly, HSR directly generates new or better knowledge about this range of topics, and it also contributes to conceptual, theoretic, and methodological structures by which empirical work can be framed, conducted, and interpreted. Fourthly, HSR is concerned with issues of health services that are broadly defined and involve populations (i.e. members of groups defined by sociodemographic characteristics, health conditions or diagnoses, cultural or ethnic factors, geography or geopolitical jurisdictions, or public or private health insurance plans); it is not focused solely on personal health care for individuals.

Finally, HSR is an expansive field that can include clinical evaluative studies (*see* **Clinical Trials, Overview**), **outcomes research**, and health technology assessment; it is sometimes characterized as boundary-crossing [2] when multiple fields, disciplines, and methods are brought to bear on a single question. HSR is distinguished, however, from basic biomedical research and clinical investigation in that it is concerned more with the effectiveness of health care interventions (what works in health care in average or day-to-day practice and health care delivery) than with their efficacy (what works and how safely in ideal settings or controled trial circumstances). Thus, for many decisions about allocation of resources in the health care sector and day-to-day clinical practice, HSR often provides the critical information that biomedical research cannot [10].

Topics Addressed by Health Services Research

The breadth of health services research is explained by the fact that the field endeavors to understand and improve all aspects of the processes and outcomes of health care delivery and to overcome significant problems of making high-quality health care available to all members of a given society at an affordable cost to that society. The costs and the quality of health care have been the subject of study for the longest period (several decades); more recently, HSR has also been concerned with access to care, health care reform and restructuring of public- and private-sector health care systems, computer-based and electronic communications and information systems, and the size and changing roles of the health care workforce.

Costs of Health Services

The costs of health care and public (e.g. national) and private (e.g. individual) levels of expenditures on care have long been an important area of investigation in health services research (*see* **Health Care Financing; Health Economics**). Most basic are studies of the total expenditures on health care, often described in terms of the percentage of gross domestic product

(GDP) of a country that is devoted to health care. The effects of various elements of private or public health insurance, including the impact of so-called cost-sharing (coinsurance and deductibles), have been a major area of research; the most prominent HSR investigation of these issues was the Health Insurance Experiment, conducted by the RAND Corporation in the 1970s and 1980s [13]. Related issues concern what services or benefits are included in health insurance packages, how insurance is priced, how health insurance plans reinsure themselves against catastrophic loss, and how insurance plans should be regulated. Because consumer choice of health insurance plans can significantly affect how well and how extensively health care costs are shared across healthy and sick individuals, and even undermine the basic idea of insurance, HSR has directed considerable attention to biased (i.e. adverse or favorable) selection of risk and **risk** (or **case-mix**) adjustment techniques. HSR also involves studies of who pays for what portions of the cost of different types of services (such as health care for physical ailments, as contrasted with mental or emotional disorders, or sociomedical problems such as substance abuse).

Organization of Health Care

Closely tied to questions of the costs of health care are issues of how health care delivery is organized and financed (*see* **Health Services Organization in the US**). Health services researchers investigate a wide range of ways in which to structure health care systems: for example, national health systems (or universal national or provincial health insurance), systems in which some portions of a population are enrolled in publicly supported health plans or insurance schemes, private-sector approaches based largely on fee-for-service reimbursement, and private-sector entities of various sorts that are characterized as health maintenance or managed care organizations. HSR illuminates how the structure of health care delivery systems affects the practices and performance of clinicians and of persons seeking or obtaining care, and it documents how different organizational structures and ways of reimbursing health care facilities or clinicians pose incentives for inducing or constraining the provision of services. It is also concerned with the effects of different attempts to control national health care spending through various regulatory controls and, more recently, through the use of competition and free-market principles. In the late 1990s, much of HSR has been directed at studies of "health care reform", such as the shift in the US from a fee-for-service to a prepaid, capitated, or managed care orientation, and the movement in countries with national health systems to introduce various aspects of private-sector health care delivery or insurance.

Quality of Care and Satisfaction with Care

An important component of HSR is the study of how populations and individuals can obtain efficacious, effective, appropriate, competent, and compassionate health care services – in short, high-quality health care. **Quality of care** has been defined as "the degree to which health services for individuals and populations increase the likelihood of desired health outcomes and are consistent with current professional knowledge" [6]. HSR aims to identify problems with quality of care, such as overuse of unnecessary or inappropriate services, underuse of needed and appropriate care, and good or poor technical and interpersonal care. It measures the structural aspects of care (e.g. professional credentials or characteristics of facilities), processes of care (e.g. what is done to and for patients and consumers), and outcomes of care (e.g. death, disease, disability, or discomfort). Investigators in this field also study patient or consumer satisfaction with health care amenities, delivery system procedures, and/or outcomes. HSR studies that combine issues of costs and quality are said to be concerned with the "value" of health care.

HSR also contributes to the measurement and improvement of the quality of health care by providing data collection and analysis tools for programs of quality assurance and continuous quality improvement or total quality management. Because some of these programs rely heavily on gathering and disseminating information to patients and consumers, HSR has in the mid-1990s been much concerned with devising reliable, valid, and practical means by which information can be obtained, synthesized, and made available in forms such as so-called report cards to purchasers and consumers. Such efforts typically imply comparisons among health care providers and plans, so HSR has been expected to develop techniques by which differences in patient severity of illness, presence of other health problems ("**co-morbidity**"), or other factors can be taken into

account. These **"risk adjustment"** questions are considered to pose among the most difficult research questions facing the field in the late 1990s.

To provide adequate guidance on these quality-of-care issues, HSR is also deeply involved in evaluating the clinical effectiveness (e.g. expected benefit of a health care intervention under average conditions of use) of health services. Such studies typically focus on the expected benefits and harms of alternate approaches to prevent, diagnose, treat, or palliate illnesses in different patient populations; they may specifically address the cost–effectiveness of alternate health care interventions [5]. These activities may involve assessing and comparing specific health care technologies (i.e. technology assessment) or developing clinical practice guidelines ("systematically developed statements to assist practitioner and patient decisions about appropriate health care for specific clinical circumstances" [7]). HSR directed at these areas also targets questions of how patients (and their families) and clinicians make treatment decisions (*see* **Health Care Utilization and Behavior, Models of**) and what appropriate roles are for **medical informatics** and decision support systems.

Access to Health Care

Health services research has for decades also been concerned with the extent to which individuals can seek and successfully obtain health care when it is needed – in short, access to care, defined as the timely receipt of appropriate care [8]. Among the topics studied are the numerous financial and nonfinancial barriers that confront individuals or groups in gaining access to care. These can include costs (especially for those who have no public or private health insurance), geographic difficulties (travel distances or times to obtain care, especially for persons in rural or frontier areas), **ethnic** and racial factors, cultural and attitudinal barriers, and language or literacy impediments. Investigators study the demographic, cultural, financial, and other factors that influence people to choose among health insurance plans, to seek preventive services and health care, to follow healthy lifestyle or treatment recommendations and regimens, and to acquire information about illnesses and problems. Also of concern to HSR investigators are mechanisms for expanding access to care and the effects on access (and hence health) of the lack or loss of public or private health insurance coverage.

Information Systems, Informatics, and Clinical Decision Making

HSR depends heavily on computer-based health services information systems (*see* **Administrative Databases**). These supply health care providers and researchers with faster and easier access to better and more complete health care information on both individuals and groups than was ever possible in the past. Many different information systems are now available to clinicians and to patients and consumers, and these provide information on clinical problems, practice guidelines, and other data needed to make informed decisions about clinical care. In addition, computer-based systems often include tools to assist clinicians in real-time decision making, such as automatic alerts or reminders at the time of patient visits or when the results of laboratory tests or diagnostic procedures are obtained. How such clinical decision making tools should be developed, deployed, and evaluated in terms of costs and quality of care are questions of considerable interest to HSR (*see* **Decision Analysis in Diagnosis and Treatment Choice**).

Computer-based information and telecommunications systems also permit individuals to communicate with others about health problems of concern to them and to learn about different treatment options. The impact of all these resources and communications technologies on the attitudes and behavior of clinicians and patients or consumers, and ultimately on health care systems, is another important area of HSR.

Health Care Professions and Workforce

Investigators in the HSR field also track the supply of and demand for different types of health care professionals and workers, including the development of various types of models that permit educators and policy makers to predict the need for and plan for education and training of health personnel (*see* **Health Workforce Modeling**). In addition, researchers examine how individual and team education and training, professional socialization, and cultural and ethnic background affect practitioner attitudes, behavior, and performance. HSR also concerns itself with ethical and bioethical questions involving the health professions, such as how health care professionals, particularly physicians, reconcile their professional duties to act in their patients' best interests with their responsibility to society as a whole, especially when resources are scarce and economic incentives pose difficult or conflicting obligations.

Methods Used in Health Services Research

Health services research employs virtually all quantitative and qualitative methods found in statistics and biostatistics, economics (*see* **Health Economics**), sociology (*see* **Social Sciences**) and anthropology (*see* **Anthropometry**), psychology, epidemiology (*see* **Analytic Epidemiology; Descriptive Epidemiology**), **operations research**, **actuarial** sciences; finance, management, political science, policy analysis, and law. The types of studies done in HSR can include randomized controlled trials (*see* **Clinical Trials, Overview**), a wide array of **quasi-experimental** investigations involving simple or complex **case–control studies, observational studies** and descriptive studies, and community-based demonstrations and evaluations (*see* **Community Intervention Trials**); the **units of analysis** can be nations; regions, states, or provinces; municipalities of all sizes, and communities or neighborhoods (*see* **Small Area Variation Analysis**); groups of individuals defined according to many different sociodemographic (*see* **Social Classifications**), cultural, or health characteristics; health care providers, specified according to type of clinician or facility, health care plan, or setting of care; and families or individuals. HSR places significant emphasis on understanding the end results of health care programs and health care delivery and on obtaining self-reported information on processes and outcomes of care from patients and consumers (*see* **Quality of Life and Health Status; Outcomes Research; Quality of Care**), and the field has generated many reliable and valid instruments for obtaining such information (*see* **Health Status Instruments, Measurement Properties of**). HSR studies employ many sources of information (*see* **Health Services Data Sources in Canada; Health Services Data Sources in Europe; Health Services Data Sources in the US**), including various types of interviews and questionnaires, focus groups, **surveys** and polls, so-called **administrative data** from various types of computer-based information systems (e.g. insurance billing claims, or hospital discharge abstracts), administrative records of health care programs and plans in the private or public sector, community health information networks, and patient medical records – both paper- and computer-based. Generally, the biostatistical methods required in HSR are similar to those used in biomedical research, except that the sets of variables of interest in HSR tend to be more broadly defined, more concerned with functional and quality-of-life outcomes of interest to patients, families, consumers, and policy makers, and sometimes more difficult or costly to measure than variables of interest in biomedical or clinical investigations.

Major Funders of Health Services Research

Globally, the US funds and produces the great majority of health services research work: of this, the largest portions are supported by agencies of the US federal government. Since the late 1960s, the leading agency has been the National Center for Health Services Research (variously titled over the years), a unit of the Department of Health and Human Services (DHHS, formerly the Department of Health, Education and Welfare). In 1989, the Agency for Health Care Policy and Research (AHCPR) was created from this Center, and continues to this day to be the central public-sector funding source for HSR. As of 1996, AHCPR had centers focused on clinical practice guidelines, health care technology, outcomes and effectiveness research, primary care, organization and delivery of health care, cost and financing of health care, quality of health care, and health information systems.

Other DHHS agencies, notably several in the **National Institutes of Health** (especially the National Institute for Mental Health, National Institute for Drug Abuse, and the National Institute for Alcoholism and Alcohol Abuse) and the Health Care Financing Administration, also support projects that fall within the HSR rubric. The US Department of Veterans Affairs has a formal program to support HSR, and increasingly elements of the US Department of Defense (such as the Office of Prevention and Health Services Assessment of the US Air Force) conduct activities focused on HSR issues (such as quality or efficient delivery of services) using HSR concepts and methods. Numerous private philanthropic organizations (foundations) also support research (or demonstrations and evaluations) on HSR topics, especially in areas related to access to care, quality of care, and organization and financing of care; often their focus is on state or local, rather than national or international, issues. Internationally, some governments have programs of health systems research within their national health services (e.g. the UK) or support related efforts in health technology assessment (e.g. Sweden and Canada).

Compared with levels of spending on health care or on biomedical research, the support for HSR is small. In the mid-1990s in the US, approximately $470 million (US dollars) was spent on HSR, a figure that approached only 0.05% of the $1 trillion spent that year on health care in that country. Few if any other nations support HSR at these or higher levels.

Personnel Engaged In or Trained In Health Services Research

The number of professionals in the HSR workforce has always been difficult to estimate, for it consists of researchers trained to design, supervise or carry out, and report on HSR work, individuals who assist in such investigations, and users who analyze HSR information or apply HSR for management and policy purposes. A mid-1990s estimate put the number of current health services researchers at 5000, largely in the US; of these, about one-half are trained at the doctoral level and just over one-quarter (mostly physicians) have clinical degrees [9]. This workforce has been trained through many different organizations and programs supported by both public and private funds; only a small minority of these programs are formally established to train individuals at the doctoral level in health services research *per se*.

Professional Organizations and Publications

The most prominent professional organization for health services researchers is the private, nonprofit Association of Health Services Research (AHSR), established in 1981 and based in Washington, DC. Related organizations include international societies focused on specific areas that HSR studies, including quality of care (International Society for Quality in Health Care) and technology assessment (International Society for Technology Assessment in Health Care). An emerging international effort is the **Cochrane Collaboration**, started originally in the UK and now with centers in several other countries including Australia, Canada, Denmark,

France, Italy, the Netherlands, Norway, and the US; these centers prepare, maintain, and disseminate systematic reviews of the effectiveness of health care, generally using information from randomized controled trials or other reliable evidence (*see* **Meta-Analysis of Clinical Trials**).

Journals available internationally that exclusively or frequently publish on HSR-related topics include *Health Care Financing Review, Health Economics, Health Services Research, Inquiry, Journal of Health Economics, Medical Care*, and *Medical Care Review*; some have been publishing since the 1960s. Newer journals include *Health Services Management Research, Journal of Evaluation in Clinical Practice, Journal of Health Services Research & Policy*, and *Quality of Life Research*. Health policy publications, which also typically feature HSR-related work, include *Health Affairs, International Journal of Health Services, Journal of Health Politics, Policy and Law*, and the *Milbank Memorial Fund Quarterly*. Journals with a public health, epidemiologic, or clinical orientation that also publish HSR-related work include the *American Journal of Public Health, Annals of Internal Medicine, British Medical Journal, Journal of the American Medical Association, Journal of Clinical Epidemiology, Journal of General Internal Medicine, Lancet, Medical Decisionmaking, New England Journal of Medicine*, and publications of other professional and clinical societies in the United States and other nations. HSR is often at the core of material published in the journals of international societies, such as the *International Journal for Quality in Health Care* and the *International Journal of Technology Assessment in Health Care*. Several monographs published since 1990 provide substantial overviews of the primary issues that HSR has covered since that time [1, 4, 9, 14].

References

[1]   Altman, S.H. & Reinhardt, U.E., eds (1996). *Strategic Choices for a Changing Health Care System*. AHSR and Health Administration Press, Chicago,

[2]   Brook, R.H. & Lohr, K.N. (1985). Efficacy, effectiveness, variations, and quality: boundary-crossing research, *Medical Care* **23**, 710–722.

[3]   Flook, E.E. & Sanazaro, P.J. (1973). Health services research: origins and milestones, in *Health Services Research and R&D in Perspective*, E.E. Flook & P.J. Sanazaro, eds. Health Administration Press, Ann Arbor, pp. 1–81.

[4]   Ginzberg, E. (1991). The challenges ahead, in *Health Services Research. Key to Health Policy*, E. Ginzberg, ed. Harvard University Press, Cambridge, Mass., pp. 315–331.

[5]   Gold, M.R., Siegel, J.E., Russell, L.B. & Weinstein, M.C., eds (1996). *Cost-Effectiveness in Health and Medicine*. Oxford University Press, New York.

[6]   Institute of Medicine (1990). *Medicare: a Strategy for Quality Assurance*, Vol. I, K.N. Lohr, ed. National Academy Press, Washington.

[7]   Institute of Medicine (1992). *Guidelines for Clinical Practice: From Development to Use*, M.J. Field & K.N. Lohr, eds. National Academy Press, Washington.

[8]   Institute of Medicine (1993). *Access to Health Care in America*, M. Millman, ed. National Academy Press, Washington.

[9]   Institute of Medicine (1995). *Health Services Research. Work Force and Educational Issues*, M.J. Field, R.E. Tranquada & J.C. Feasley, eds. National Academy Press, Washington.

[10]   Lohr, K.N. (1996). The role of research in setting priorities for health care, *Journal of Evaluation in Clinical Practice* **2**, 79–82.

[11]   Marshall, J.E. (1985). Introduction, *Medical Care* **23**, 381–382.

[12]   Neuhauser, D. (1985). Health services research, 1984, *Medical Care* **23**, 739–742.

[13]   Newhouse, J.P. and the Health Insurance Group (1993). *Free for All? Lessons from the RAND Health Insurance Experiment*. Harvard University Press, Cambridge, Mass.

[14]   Shortell, S.M. & Reinhardt, U.E., eds (1992). *Improving Health Policy and Management: Nine Critical Research Issues for the 1990s*. Health Administration Press, Ann Arbor.

[15]   Steinwachs, D.M. (1991). Health services research: its scope and significance, in *Promoting Health Services Research in Academic Health Centers*, P. Forman, ed. Association of Academic Health Centers, Washington, pp. 9–19.

KATHLEEN N. LOHR

Health Status Instruments, Measurement Properties of

In this article we present the key measurement properties necessary for a useful health status instrument. This article also includes a comment on the issue of respondent and administrative burden. The discussion is drawn largely from a previous publication [5]. The concepts are most relevant for measurement of health status, but apply to measurements of any human attribute or characteristic.

The Structure of Health Status Measures

Since semantic issues in health status measurement are both controversial and important, we will clarify how we shall use words in our discussion. Some measures consist of a single question which essentially asks "How would you rate the quality of your life?" [18]. This question may be asked in a simple or a very sophisticated fashion, but either way yields limited information. More commonly, health status instruments are questionnaires made up of a number of *items*, or questions. These items are added up in a number of *domains* (also sometimes called *dimensions*). A domain or dimension refers to the area of behavior or experience that we are trying to measure. Domains might include mobility and self-care, which could further be aggregated into physical function, or depression, anxiety, and well-being, which could be aggregated to form an emotional function domain. For some instruments, investigators have undertaken rigorous valuation exercises in which the importance of each item is rated in relation to the others. More often, items are equally weighted, implying an assumption that their value is equal.

What Makes a Good Health Status Instrument?

Current strategies for evaluating health status measures build on close to 100 years' work in

the measurement of attributes such as intelligence and attitudes [15]. These strategies have evolved, incorporating insights from studies directly relating to health status and **quality of life** [14].

Measuring at a Moment in Time vs. Measuring Change

The goals of health status measures include differentiating between people who have a better health status and those who have a worse health status (a *discriminative instrument*), and measuring how much health status has changed (an *evaluative instrument*) [10]. The construction of instruments for these two purposes can be quite different. For instance, let us take the example of thyroid disease. If we are trying to discriminate between those with and without thyroid disease, we would be unlikely to include fatigue as an item, because fatigue is too common among people who do not have thyroid disease. On the other hand, in measuring improvement in health status with treatment, fatigue, because of its importance in the day-to-day lives of people with thyroid disease, would be a key item. In the next sections, concerned with what makes a good health status instrument, we list key measurement properties separately for discriminative and evaluative instruments. The properties that make useful discriminative and evaluative instruments are presented in Table 1.

Signal and Noise

Investigators examining physiologic endpoints have long been aware that reproducibility and validity are the necessary attributes of a good test. For health status instruments, reproducibility translates into having a high ratio of signal to noise, and validity translates

Table 1 What makes a good health status measure

Instrument property	Evaluative instruments (measuring differences within subjects over time)	Discriminative instruments (measuring differences between subjects at a moment in time)
High signal-to-noise ratio	Responsiveness	Reliability
Validity	Correlations of changes in measures over time consistent with theoretically-derived predictions	Correlations between measures at a moment in time consistent with theoretically-derived predictions
Interpretability	Differences within subjects over time can be interpreted as trivial, small, moderate, or large	Differences between subjects at a moment in time can be interpreted as trivial, small, moderate, or large

into whether they are really measuring what they are intended to measure. For discriminative instruments, the way of quantifying the signal-to-noise ratio is called *reliability*. If the variability in scores between subjects (the signal) is much greater than the variability within subjects (the noise), an instrument will be deemed reliable. Reliable instruments will generally demonstrate that stable subjects show more or less the same results on repeated administration. For evaluative instruments, those designed to measure changes within individuals over time, the way of determining the signal-to-noise ratio is called *responsiveness*. Responsiveness refers to an instrument's ability to detect change. If a treatment results in an important difference in health status, investigators wish to be confident that they will detect that difference, even if it is small. Responsiveness will be directly related to the magnitude of the difference in score in patients who have improved or deteriorated (the signal) and the extent to which patients who have not changed obtain more or less the same scores (the noise).

Validity When There is a Gold Standard

If we have a **gold standard** or criterion standard for some aspect of health, it implies that we have endorsed a particular measurement tool as providing the underlying truth about that aspect. The concept of a reference, gold, or criterion standard is most easily applied for physiologic measures. For instance, experts may agree that the cardiac angiogram is a gold standard for measurement of various aspects of cardiac anatomy and function, and noninvasive tests should be judged in relation to this criterion. Although there is no gold standard for health status, there are instances in which there is a specific target for a health status measure that can be treated as a criterion or gold standard. Under these circumstances, one determines whether an instrument is measuring what is intended using *criterion validity*, according to which an instrument is valid insofar as its results correspond to those of the criterion standard. For instance, criterion validity is applicable when a shorter version of an instrument (the test) is used to predict the results of the full-length index (the gold standard). Another example is using a health status instrument to predict mortality. In this instance, to the extent that variability in survival between patients (the gold standard) is explained by the questionnaire results (the test), the instrument will be valid.

Self-ratings of health such as more comprehensive and lengthy measures of general health perceptions, include an individual's evaluation of her or his physiologic, physical, psychologic, and social well-being. Perceived health, measured through self-ratings, is an important predictor of mortality [12].

Validity When There is No Gold Standard

Validity has to do with whether the instrument is measuring what it is intended to measure. When there is no gold or criterion standard, health status investigators have borrowed validation strategies from clinical and experimental psychologists, who have for many years been dealing with the problem of deciding whether questionnaires examining intelligence, attitudes, and emotional function are really measuring what they are supposed to measure. The types of validity that psychologists have introduced include face, content, and construct validity. *Face validity* refers to whether an instrument appears to be measuring what it is intended to measure, while *content validity* refers to the extent to which the domain of interest is comprehensively sampled by the items, or questions, in the instrument. Quantitative testing of face and content validity are rarely attempted. Feinstein [3] has reformulated these aspects of validity by suggesting criteria for what he calls the *sensibility*, including the applicability of the questionnaire, its clarity and simplicity, likelihood of **bias**, comprehensiveness, and whether redundant items have been included. Some of these criteria compete with one another: redundant items may help to ensure comprehensiveness, and reduce the likelihood of bias, while increasing the burden on respondents. Because of their specificity, Feinstein's criteria facilitate quantitative rating of an instrument's face and content validity [13].

The most rigorous approach to establishing validity is called *construct validity*. A construct is a theoretically derived notion of the domain(s) that we wish to measure. An understanding of the construct will lead to expectations about how an instrument should behave if it is valid. Construct validity therefore involves comparisons between measures, and examination of the logical relationships that should exist between a measure and characteristics of patients and patient groups.

The first step in construct validation is to a establish a "model" or theoretic framework, which represents an understanding of what investigators are trying to measure. That theoretic framework provides a basis for understanding how the system being studied behaves, and allows hypotheses or predictions about how the instrument being tested should relate to other measures. Investigators then administer a number of instruments to a population of interest, and examine the data. Validity is strengthened or weakened according to the extent to which the hypotheses are confirmed or refuted.

For example, a discriminative health status instrument may be validated by comparing two groups of patients; those who have undergone a very toxic chemotherapeutic regimen and those who have undergone a much less toxic chemotherapeutic regimen. A health status instrument should distinguish between these two groups, and if it does not it is very likely that something has gone wrong. Alternately, correlations between symptoms and functional status can be examined, the expectation being that those with a greater number and severity of symptoms will have lower functional status scores on a health status instrument. Another example is the validation of an instrument discriminating between people according to some aspect of emotional function. Results from such an instrument should show substantial **correlations** with existing measures of emotional function.

The principles of validation are identical for evaluative instruments, but their validity is demonstrated by showing that *changes* in the instrument being investigated correlate with *changes* in other related measures in the theoretically derived predicted direction and magnitude. For instance, the validity of an evaluative measure of health status for patients with chronic lung disease was supported by the finding of moderate correlations with changes in walk test scores [7].

Validation is not an all-or-nothing process. We may have varying degrees of confidence that an instrument is really measuring what it is supposed to measure. A priori predictions of the strength of relationship with other measures that one would expect if a new instrument is really measuring what is intended strengthen the validation process. Without such predictions, it is generally easy to rationalize whatever correlations between measures are observed.

Validation does not end when the first study with data concerning validity is published, but continues with repeated use of an instrument. The more frequently an instrument is used, and the wider the situations in which it performs as we would expect if it were really doing its job, the greater is our confidence in its validity. Perhaps we should never conclude that a questionnaire has "been validated"; the best we can do is to suggest that strong evidence for validity has been obtained in a number of different settings and studies.

Interpretability

A final key property of a health status measure is *interpretability*. For a discriminative instrument, we could ask whether a particular score signifies that a patient is functioning normally, or has mild, moderate, or severe impairment of health status. For an evaluative instrument we might ask whether a particular change in score represents a trivial, small but important, moderate, or large improvement or deterioration.

A number of strategies are available for trying to make health status scores interpretable [6]. For an evaluative instrument, one might classify patients into those who had important improvement and those who did not, and examine the changes in score in the two groups; interpret observed changes in health status measures in terms of elements of those measures that will be familiar to readers (for instance, descriptions of changes in mobility); or determine how scores in health status measures relate to marker states which are familiar and meaningful to clinicians. Health status measurement instruments often use seven-point scales as response options. Evidence suggests that a change in mean score of 0.5 per question represents a small but important effect, while changes of 0.75–1.0 and over 1.0–1.5 per question represent medium and large changes [9]. Investigators have used this information to interpret a recent trial that showed that bronchodilators result in small but clinically important improvement in dyspnea, fatigue, and emotional function in patients with chronic airflow limitation [8]. In another study, investigators demonstrated that patients who could walk but had physical limitations had scores 0.02 points higher than patients who could move about in a wheelchair without help, but could not walk. This finding helped to interpret the results of a study of patients with arthritis [17].

In its use as a discriminative instrument, we know how patients in various health states score on the

Sickness Impact Profile (SIP): patients shortly after hip replacement have scores of 30, which decrease to less than 5 after full convalescence [1]; scores in patients with chronic airflow limitation severe enough to require home oxygen are approximately 24 [11]; scores in patients with chronic, stable angina are approximately 11.5 [4]; scores in those with arthritis vary from 8.2 in patients with American Rheumatism Association arthritis class I to 25.8 in class IV [2]. The availability of data that improve the interpretability of health status measures is likely to increase exponentially in the next decade.

Respondent and Administrative Burden

Alternate approaches to obtaining information from patients have different resource implications. The strengths and weaknesses of the different modes of administration are summarized in Table 2. Health status questionnaires are either administered by trained interviewers or self-administered. The former method is resource intensive, but ensures compliance and minimizes errors and missing items. The latter approach is much less expensive, but increases the number of missing patients and missing responses. A compromise between the two approaches is to have the instrument completed under supervision. Another compromise is the telephone interview, which minimizes errors and missing data but may necessitate a relatively simple questionnaire structure. Investigators have conducted initial experiments with computer administration of health status measures, but this is not yet a common method of questionnaire administration (*see* **Computer-Assisted Interviewing**).

Another issue in administrative and respondent burden is the length of the questionnaires. This may be less of an issue in research settings in which, once one has invested the resources in setting up the interview, the incremental resource expenditure of a longer interview is relatively minor. On the other hand, it may be necessary to find a short questionnaire for clinical settings in which one needs to obtain information at regular intervals (*see* **Questionnaire Design**).

Under these circumstances, distilling the measurement of health status into a few key questions would be a dream come true. One approach to achieving this goal is to develop a long instrument, test it, and use its performance to choose key questions to include in a shorter index. This approach has been used, for example, to create shorter questionnaires based on the lengthy instruments from the Medical Outcomes Studies [16].

How would one determine if the shortened questionnaire is an adequate substitute for the full version? The issue for discriminative purposes is the extent to which people are classified similarly by the short and long forms of the questionnaire. Statistically, one would examine the extent to which **variance**, or variability in scores, in the full instrument is predicted or explained by scores of the abbreviated version: the greater the extent to which the rating of people's quality of life by the shorter instrument corresponds

Table 2 Modes of administration of health status measures

Mode of administration	Strengths	Weaknesses
Interviewer-administered	Maximizes response rate Few, if any, missing items Minimizes errors of misunderstanding	Requires considerable resources, training of interviewers May reduce willingness to acknowledge problems
Telephone-administered	Few, if any, missing items Minimizes errors of misunderstanding Less resource-intensive than interviewer-administered	Limits format of instrument
Self-administered	Minimal resources required	Greater likelihood of low response rate, missing items, or misunderstandings
Surrogate responders	Reduces stress for target group (very elderly or sick)	Perceptions of surrogate may differ from those of target group

to ratings by the longer version, the more comfortable we should be with the substitution.

For evaluative purposes, the responsiveness and validity of the shorter version should be tested against the full instrument. If both correlations of change with independent measures and instrument responsiveness were comparable, substitution of the shorter instrument would be desirable. If measurement properties deteriorated, the investigator would face a decision about trading off respondent burden with increases in sample size necessitated by a less responsive instrument.

References

[1] Bergner, M., Bobbitt, R.A., Carter, W.B. & Gilson, B.S. (1981). The sickness impact profile: development and final revision of a health status measure, *Medical Care* **19**, 787–805.

[2] Deyo, R.A., Inui, T.S., Leininger, J.D. & Overman, S.S. (1983). Measuring functional outcomes in chronic disease: a comparison of traditional scales and a self-administered health status questionnaire in patients with rheumatoid arthritis, *Medical Care* **21**, 180–192.

[3] Feinstein, A.R. (1987). *Clinimetrics*. Yale University Press, New Haven, pp. 141–166.

[4] Fletcher, A., McLoone, P. & Bulpitt, C. (1988). Quality of life on angina therapy: a randomised controlled trial of transdermal glyceryl trinitrate against placebo, *Lancet* **2**, 4–7.

[5] Guyatt, G.H., Feeny, D.H. & Patrick, D.L. (1993). Measuring health-related quality of life: basic sciences review, *Annals of Internal Medicine* **70**, 225–230.

[6] Guyatt, G.H., Feeny, D. & Patrick, D. (1991). Proceedings of the International Conference on the Measurement of Quality of Life as an Outcome in Clinical Trials: postscript, *Controlled Clinical Trials* **12**, 266S–269S.

[7] Guyatt, G.H., Berman, L.B., Townsend, M., Pugsley, S.O. & Chambers, L.W. (1987). A measure of quality of life for clinical trials in chronic lung disease, *Thorax* **42**, 773–778.

[8] Guyatt, G.H., Townsend, M., Pugsley, S.O., Keller, J.L., Short, H.D., Taylor, D.W. & Newhouse, M.T. (1987). Bronchodilators in chronic airflow limitation, effects on airway function, exercise capacity and quality of life, *American Review of Respiratory Disease* **135**, 1069–1074.

[9] Jaeschke, R., Guyatt, G., Keller, J. & Singer, J. (1989). Measurement of health status: ascertaining the meaning of a change in quality-of-life questionnaire score, *Controlled Clinical Trials* **10**, 407–415.

[10] Kirshner, B. & Guyatt, G.H. (1985). A methodologic framework for assessing health indices, *Journal of Chronic Diseases* **38**, 27–36.

[11] McSweeney, A.J., Grant, I., Heaton, R.K. et al. (1982). Life quality of patients with chronic obstructive pulmonary disease, *Archives of Internal Medicine* **142**, 473–478.

[12] Mossey, J. & Shapiro, E. (1982). Self-rated health: a predictor of mortality among the elderly, *American Journal of Public Health* **72**, 800–809.

[13] Oxman, A. & Guyatt, G.H. (1991). Validation of an index of the quality of review articles, *Journal of Clinical Epidemiology* **44**, 1271–1278.

[14] Scientific Advisory Committee, Medical Outcomes Trust (1995). Instrument review criteria, *Medical Outcomes Trust Bulletin* **3**.

[15] *Standards for Educational and Psychological Testing* (1985). American Psychological Association, Washington.

[16] Stewart, A.L., Hays, R.D. & Ware, J.E. (1988). The MOS short-form general health survey, *Medical Care* **26**, 724–731.

[17] Thompson, M.S., Read, J.L., Hutchings, H.C., Paterson, M. & Harris, E.D., Jr (1988). The cost effectiveness of auranofin: results of a randomized clinical trial, *Journal of Rheumatology* **15**, 35–42.

[18] Torrance, G.W. (1986). Measurement of health state utilities for economic appraisal, *Journal of Health Economics* **5**, 1–30.

GORDON GUYATT & ELIZABETH JUNIPER

Health Workforce Modeling

Health workforce modeling is generally concerned with projecting the future supply of and requirements for a particular type of health professional. The objective of such an effort is to assess the relative balance between supply and requirements under various assumptions and alternative future workforce policies. *Health workforce modeling* is a term that has come into usage over the last two decades as a more gender-neutral formulation of what had traditionally been called *health manpower* planning [6]. In addition, modelers have in more recent years used the more neutral term *requirements* as a generic term which may reflect, depending on the disciplinary background and/or political orientation of the modeler, the "needs", "wants", "demand", or "expected utilization" for health services of a relevant population (*see* **Health Care Utilization, Data**). Health workforce modeling, when employed at a regional or national level, is directed toward alerting policy makers to current or potential future imbalances between supply and requirements or to identifying maldistributions of professionals by geographic region, specialty, or practice setting which may adversely affect access to care, **quality of care**, or health care costs. The deceptively simple goal of these analyses is to develop policies, typically affecting the supply side, to ensure that the proper number and type of health professionals will be available to deliver required services to a specified future population. In practice, the achievement of this goal is complicated by the incompleteness of data necessary to implement the models, lack of agreement on essential definitions, competing perspectives of diverse stakeholders, and lack of agreement on what constitutes the "correct" balance between supply and requirements.

Workforce modeling has become of greater interest as governments wrestle with fundamental reforms of the structure and financing of their health care systems (*see* **Health Care Financing**). The undersupply of health professionals can adversely affect the health status and economic viability of populations. Alternatively, because the education of health professionals is supported in large part by public funds, the oversupply of highly trained professionals wastes scarce societal resources that could be better employed elsewhere. The unemployment or underutilization of health professionals carries enormous personal costs as well. However, it has been persuasively argued by Reinhardt [11] that the role of governments in attempting to bring supply in line with requirements ought to be limited to making information on health professions markets freely available to all affected parties so that the market can adjust supply and demand as it does in most other professions.

Invariably, a health professions model will develop a forecast of the future supply of one or more types of personnel and a forecast of the requirements for the personnel in a future time period. Occasionally, modelers will verify their models by "backcasting" to determine if the model, under known conditions and parameter settings, would have predicted correctly a previously recorded level of supply. Some intrepid researchers have assessed the historical performance of alternate forecasts made in prior periods to actual data after they became available [1].

At the national or regional level, three categories of models have been employed:

1. Supply models which forecast the number of a particular kind of health professional expected to be practicing at some future time period (usually expressed either in full-time equivalent persons or in head count).
2. Requirements models which translate the expected utilization or need for specified health services into requirements for a particular kind of professional.
3. Integrated models which explicitly represent the interaction of supply and requirements and other exogenous factors such as disposable personal income, health insurance coverage, and managed care penetration simultaneously to develop estimates of supply and requirements.

Health Workforce Supply Models

Health professions supply models have taken several forms. Conceptually, the most simple is a model that forecasts the future stock of particular kinds of health professionals by obtaining from professional associations or licensure data a count of those practicing in one year, adding to it the expected entrants and subtracting those who leave the profession owing to retirement or death, to produce an estimate of the active workforce in a future period. Rates of addition, separation, and labor force participation in a cohort will depend on age, gender, and geographical location, among other factors. These labor stock models are appealing for policy analysis because training program enrollments, graduation rates, class composition, and licensure or certification rates are at least partially controllable through policy interventions. As described below, the US Bureau of Health Professions has developed a set of labor stock models to estimate supply [13].

The Bureau of Labor Statistics (BLS) of the US government uses a complex econometric model to estimate the occupational employment of 507 occupations in 258 industrial groupings. The model depends in part on projections of the gross domestic product (GDP) contributions of various industry sectors, the interrelationships between sectors, demand for goods and services, personal income, and other factors. The GDP, demand, and income projections alone require the solution of 400 equations with 213 exogenous variables. Despite the complexity of the BLS models at the macro level, these techniques cannot capture the micro-level details of training program structure and career choice that are found in workforce stock models which frequently drive the production of health professionals.

Bureau of Health Professions Physician Supply Models

Because the investment by society into the training of physicians is greater than for any other health profession and because the length of the supply "pipeline" is the longest of any health profession, considerable effort has been devoted to modeling the physician supply process. At the US federal level, the Bureau of Health Professions [3] utilizes a physician supply forecasting model that consists of five submodels: three at the national level and two at the level of states and census regions. An aggregate supply model forecasts the total national supply of physicians by age, gender, and country of medical education. A specialty model allocates the total supply among 36 specialties in eight practice settings (inpatient, outpatient, long-term care, etc.) and to nonpatient care activities (administration, teaching, and research). A model of the graduate medical education process projects the distribution of residents by specialty and by year of training for future years. The results of the graduate medical education model may be influenced by changing the size, fill rates, and proportions of US and international medical graduates in residency programs. These, and the dynamics of specialty choice and specialty switching, are policy variables that can be influenced, in part, by government initiatives.

Health Workforce Requirements Models

Unlike supply models, which are relatively transparent in their assumptions, requirements modeling is influenced at least as much by the philosophical perspective taken by the model as by the analytic approach. Supply models are largely descriptive. Requirements models are either explicitly or implicitly normative in that they describe what the number and type of health care professionals should be to provide health care to a given population. The simplest (and least useful) kind of requirements model is to form a ratio of providers-to-population, e.g. dentists per 100 000 persons. These provider-to-population ratios give a gross measure of supply which can

be used to compare one nation with another or one region with another but tell us nothing about what care is delivered, how it is delivered, to whom it is delivered, and in what facilities it is delivered.

A utilization-based model will forecast health services utilization for a particular population, usually in the form of office visits, inpatient episodes of care, nursing home days, etc. Each encounter type can then be described in terms of who is involved and how long a particular person or team is typically involved. Person-hours are then aggregated over all delivery venues applicable to a given health profession to determine the number of full-time equivalent providers required to deliver an assumed volume of services. In their pure form, utilization-based models forecast only what *will* be rather than what *should* be the number and types of providers required under certain utilization and task allocation assumptions. Utilization models will account for variation in utilization of services by age, gender, and geographic region and they may account for differential access owing to insurance status, provider availability, travel distance, and social and economic factors. Utilization models do not attempt to provide estimates of the number and kind of services needed by a population to maintain that population in optimum health.

Need-based models, on the other hand, start from the perspective of a population's need for a certain mix of health services as recommended by knowledgeable health professionals usually convened in consensus panels. Gaining consensus on what should be done, to whom it should be done, and by whom it should be done is not an easy process, especially when competing specialties and professions are involved. The term *adjusted need-based model* refers to an approach that tempers the requirements estimate with information about how populations actually use services based on assumptions relating price and accessibility.

In the US in the early 1980s, the Graduate Medical Education National Advisory Committee (GMENAC) [14] developed an adjusted need-based model from the work of a number of disease area expert panels representing medical or surgical specialists, primary care providers, and nonphysician providers (such as physician assistants and nurse practitioners). A modeling panel integrated the findings of the disease area panels to resolve problems with overlap and variations in assumptions.

The opportunity for enormous variation in requirements estimates exists at two points in the process. First, professionals (and clinical evidence) may not agree on what services should be provided. Secondly, the rate of service provision and the mix of professionals providing the service can be affected greatly by health system organization (*see* **Health Services Organization in the US**) and financing structures. Analysts have, for example, found variations of 25% or more in the number of physicians required, depending on whether traditional fee-for-service or aggressive managed care utilization rates and staffing ratios are assumed [12, 16]. Unless one is willing to accept wildly unrealistic estimates of the number of health professionals required, estimates must be based on supportable assumptions regarding the utilization and delivery patterns that will actually occur at the specified future time [10]. Presentation of supply and requirements estimates under alternative future scenarios is one way to illustrate the sensitivity of estimates to changes in the settings of model parameters or policy options.

Another recent development is the Bureau of Health Professions' Integrated Requirements Model for Primary Care for Physicians' Assistants (PAs), Nurse Practitioners (NPs), and Certified Nurse-Midwives (CNMs) [9]. Known as the IRM, this system has been used to forecast US requirements for physicians and other nonphysician primary care providers for the delivery of primary health care services, using a variety of assumptions (or scenarios). These assumptions can be adjusted by the users and are designed so that users can also forecast requirements under an unlimited number of scenarios by varying model inputs and parameters. At the heart of the model is the assumption that requirements will differ depending on how certain primary care tasks are allocated to the various health professions and where the boundaries of "primary care" tasks lie within the health services domain.

A Recent Application of Requirements Forecasting in an Integrated Delivery System

To determine the number and kinds of physicians required to staff the US Department of Veterans' Affairs (VA) health care delivery system, the Institute of Medicine [7] utilized three distinct but complementary approaches: (i) empirical models based on current practice in the VA; (ii) expert judgment models; and (iii) comparisons to other large integrated systems operating in the US. In practice, these three approaches interacted to a great extent, and the final recommendation was for an informed blending of alternative requirements forecasts.

The empirical models developed were of two forms: (i) production functions (PF), in which physicians were one of several factors leading to the production of patient care workload, and (ii) inverse production functions (IPF), in which the required number of physicians in a given specialty was estimated directly from workload and other staffing inputs. In the PF variant, the patient workload (measured, for example, in weighted workload units) for one of 14 patient care areas (e.g. inpatient psychiatric service) was hypothesized to be related to the number of physician FTEs by specialty allocated to the area, the number of residents by year of training, nurse FTE per physician, other support FTE per physician, and other institutional factors possibly affecting productivity.

In the IPF variant the required number of physicians in 11 specialties for a given facility was assumed to be a function of the estimated required workload in all settings (inpatient, outpatient, and long-term care), the number of residents assigned in the specialty by year of training, support staff allocated to the specialty, and other productivity-related factors such as hospital type.

The second major approach to forecasting physician requirements was to use 11 expert panels organized around specialty (e.g. neurology, rehabilitation medicine, and radiation oncology) or multidisciplinary care area (e.g. long-term care). Rather than simply critiquing the empirically derived estimates, the panels developed independent quantitative estimates of physician requirements under a variety of alternative scenarios of care provision. The work of the panels was informed by the results of the empirical models and external norm data from other organizations.

Ultimately, estimates of requirements from the empirical models were formally reconciled with estimates from the expert judgment methods through a weighting and smoothing process. In the end, no "cook book" approach was developed. Rather, it was recommended that the empirical, expert judgment, and external norm approaches be continually enhanced and coordinated to produce demand-driven staffing requirement estimates that would guide management decisions and resource allocation. On the basis of the Institute of Medicine (IOM) experience, Lipscomb et al. [8] have developed a **Bayesian** statistical approach to combine expert panel judgments through **hierarchical models**.

Integrated Supply and Requirements Models

One currently used example of an integrative model is the Econometric Model of the Dental Sector (EMODS) developed at the US Bureau of Health Professions [1]. EMODS employs an interactive system of equations explicitly to represent the impact of population changes, disease etiology, dental insurance, cost of services, and personal income on demand for dental care. Also included on the production side is the technology of care delivery, use of auxiliaries, hours of work, and the labor content of procedures. Supply equations (exogenous to the model) include not only the stock of dentists, but also the stock of various auxiliaries as well. Prices for care affect consumption of services, which in turn affects employment of dentists. The full model contains a set of 195 equations that represent the interactions in the dental care sector. The model has been tested and **calibrated** by comparing model estimates to actual data over a period of several years (*see* **Model Checking**). Among the complex econometric models that have been formulated for various health professions, the most highly developed is the model of the dental sector, which is self-contained and relatively easy to describe. Even in dentistry, however, it is difficult to obtain adequate data to permit full utilization of econometric models. In fact, to reduce the data burdens, researchers have found that a single-equation **regression** model, while not providing the richness of insight available in the full model, does permit adequate forecasts of dental prices and expenditures [1].

Data Requirements for Workforce Modeling

Figure 1, adapted from *Data Systems to Support State Health Personnel Planning and Policy making: A Resource Guide for State Agencies* [15], outlines three different levels of sophistication in both the supply and requirements domains and identifies the kinds of data required at each level. An important feature of this approach is that it allows one to move from the simplest approaches to the more complex approaches. This is essential because one can get lost quite easily in sophisticated details of modeling and equations before one has had a chance to answer the more basic questions about supply and requirements. From a practical perspective, modeling efforts should proceed sequentially, collecting data specified in the innermost portions of Figure 1 and then proceeding outward in both the supply and requirements directions consistent with not only the required precision and planning time horizon, but also the resources available to the task.

On the supply side, these basic analyses and data include the counts of licensees in state and employment counts. Such basic data can be augmented by national and state trends in the number of practitioners, as indicated by the growth in newly licensed persons in the state or nation and trends in employment. Professional association data can be useful in understanding and projecting supply, but, because of duplication in licenses, national estimates of supply remain problematic. Such an approach, however, can be used at the state or regional level, where universal unduplicated licensure ensures that supply can be adequately measured and trends can give us a hint as to what the underlying demand might be.

A comprehensive licensure data system – such as maintained in the state of North Carolina – takes time to implement, but, with periodic resurveys, the quality of data improves. Additional items can be added to increase the usefulness of the database. Data generated in North Carolina using this model are now available on location, employment setting, and type of employment. These data provide helpful information by projecting demand as well as supply, as mobility in and out of employment sectors can be quite sensitive to economic trends.

One of the ways in which demand can be estimated from supply data is by looking at the different sectors in which health professionals are employed, and by comparing the kinds of employment for the entire workforce with those of the newly licensed individuals in a given year. For example, in North Carolina, 36.8% of the currently licensed individuals in physical therapy are working primarily in hospitals. This figure has fluctuated between 35% and 40% over

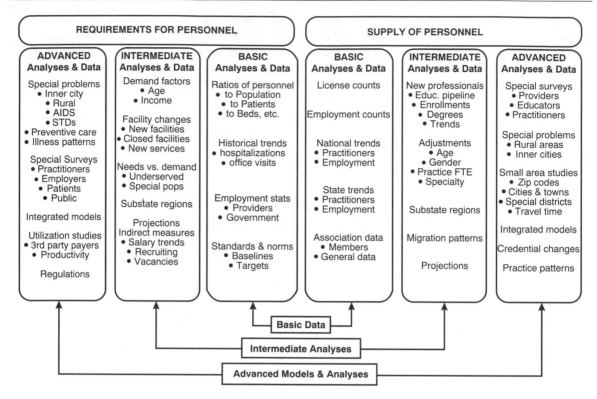

Figure 1 The health workforce data analysis hierarchy. Adapted from [4], based on [15, Figure 1]. Reproduced from *Physical Therapy* by permission of the American Physical Therapy Association

the past decade, even as the total number of therapists has increased. Among newly licensed personnel in 1994, including both new graduates and immigrants to the state, the proportion employed in hospitals is 64%. This proportion suggests that hospital employment is especially attractive to new graduates and immigrants. By examining employment trends, it may be possible to determine whether this percentage increase will continue (representing an increase in employment in that particular sector) or whether it represents the employment patterns of new entrants who subsequently move to other sectors.

The methods used here to assess requirements emphasize trends rather than needs or demands. Obviously, such an approach is subject to misinterpretation, but it uses available data from supply to assess changes in different sectors to provide "reality checks" on the more idealistic need-based models and the more abstract and data-intensive demand-based models. Such an approach also provides information at the state and local levels, where decisions about

expansion in the number and size of training institutions are likely to occur.

Emerging Issues

As the data requirements for both supply and demand models become more complex and sophisticated, and as various elements in national health systems are becoming decentralized and privatized, new issues are coming to the fore. Chief among these are how to resolve inherent tensions between the need for regulation and accountability expressed by central health authorities, credentialling bodies, national payment systems, and health professional educational systems, and the need for privacy and **confidentiality** expressed by individual health professionals, their associations, and health service delivery systems, which increasingly employ health professionals. As data requirements for workforce planning become more complex, they also become more onerous to individuals. Health workforce planners of the next generation will be faced with the challenge to use creative and innovative strategies to acquire data at increasingly detailed levels while preserving the confidentiality of the sources.

New information technologies also provide unprecedented opportunities for health workforce modeling. For example, the availability of various kinds of **simulation** software for microcomputers allows the development and display of simulations and **sensitivity analyses** in real time. In addition, the use of geographic information systems (GIS) allows cartographic presentation of databases containing disease patterns (*see* **Mapping Disease Patterns**) and demographic data. Overlaying the location of health professions or activity space data on such maps can provide dramatic opportunities to identify issues of distribution which might well remain opaque in the absence of such visual displays. Creatively applied, such processes can be conducted in group settings with panels of health professions, education administrators, and health policy analysts in attendance in such a way that not only engages their attention, but also serves to close the loop between planning and policy.

Conclusion

Health workforce modeling has been employed at a variety of organizational levels and has either concentrated on a single health profession or considered multiple health professions interacting to provide a spectrum of health care services. At the micro level, models have been developed to analyze one or more specific types of personnel in a specific delivery setting (e.g. physician assistants employed in the office of a generalist physician). Models have been developed to analyze various kinds of personnel in an organized delivery system (e.g. all physician specialties in an integrated health care delivery system which includes inpatient, outpatient, long-term, and home health care). Some models have covered specific kinds of personnel in a regional, state, or national framework with the purpose of forecasting future workforce structure and affecting health workforce policy (e.g. physical therapists in the US or all licensed health professions practicing within the boundaries of a given state, perhaps at a county level of disaggregation).

Although not formally workforce modeling, population-based "benchmarking" also has been applied recently in health workforce studies as a way to get at the notion of "requirements", while avoiding the question of whether "needs" or "demands" are being met. This approach compares a priori standard ratios of health professionals to populations (either normative or those extant in particular health systems) to the range of these ratios across **hospital market areas**, broad regions, or national health systems. A recent application of this approach used managed care ratios in the US to examine how variations in supply and composition of the physician workforce relate to the organization of the health care delivery system in different areas [2]

This article concentrates on applications at the health system or national levels because most of the recently published material is directed at macro-level analyses. This concentration of published material at higher levels of aggregation is a result of the recent emphasis on workforce reform as a part of health system reform proposals, and is also a consequence of single-site studies being described most frequently in less accessible internal documents of the firms in which the analyses were performed. An excellent earlier summary of **operations research** applications that spanned this entire spectrum appears in [6]. In addition, Hall & Mejia [5] provided a comprehensive monographic summary of the various approaches up to the mid-1970s, with a special focus on techniques applicable to developing countries and feasible for health workforce planning as a component of more general health and development strategies.

References

[1]   Capilouto, E. (1995). A review of methods used to project the future supply of dental personnel and the future demand and need for dental services, *Journal of Dental Education* **59**, 237–257.

[2]   Goodman, D.C. (1996). Benchmarking the US physician workforce: An alternative to needs-based or demand-based planning, *Journal of the American Medical Association* **276**, 1811–1817.

[3]   Greenberg, L. (1992). *Forecasting the Future Supply of Physicians: Logic and Operation of the BHPr Physician Supply Model*. OHPAR Report No. 3-93, BHPr. Rockville.

[4]   Hack, L.M. & Konrad, T.R. (1995). Determination of supply and requirements in physical therapy: Some considerations and examples, *Physical Therapy* **75**, 52.

[5]   Hall, T.L. & Mejia, A. (1978). *Health Manpower Planning: Principles, Methods, Issues*. World Health Organization, Geneva.

[6]   Levin, E. & Kahn, H.D. (1975). Health manpower models, in *Operations Research in Health Care: A Critical Analysis*, L.J. Shulman, R.D. Speas, Jr & J.P. Young, eds. The Johns Hopkins University Press, Baltimore, pp. 337–364.

[7]   Lipscomb, J. & Alexander, B.J. eds (1992). *Institute of Medicine, Physician Staffing for the VA*, Vol. II. National Academy Press, Washington.

[8]   Lipscomb, J., Parmigiani, G. & Hasselbad, V. (1997). Combining expert judgment by hierarchical modeling: an application to physician staffing, *Management Science* (to appear).

[9]   Moses, E. & Sekscenski, T. (1997). Bureau of Health Professions' integrated requirements model, in *Combined Proceedings of the Seventh and Eighth Federal Forecasters' Conferences*, D.E. Gerald, ed. US Department of Education, National Center for Educational Statistics, Washington, pp. 69–77.

[10]   Reinhardt, U.E. (1981). The GMENAC forecast: An alternative view, *American Journal of Public Health* **71**, 1149–1157.

[11]   Reinhardt, U.E. (1996). The economic and moral case for letting the market determine the health workforce, in *The U.S. Health Workforce: Power, Politics, and Policy*. M. Osterweis et al. eds. Association of Academic Health Centers, Washington, pp. 3–13.

[12]   Schwartz, W.B. (1988). Why there will be little or no physician surplus between now and the year 2000, *New England Journal of Medicine* **318**, 892–897.

[13]   Traxler, H. (1994). Physician supply modeling in the United States of America and its uses in assisting policy making, *World Health Statistics Quarterly* **47**, 118–125.

[14]   US Department of Health and Human Services (1981). *Summary Report of the Graduate Medical Education National Advisory Committee to the Secretary, Department of Health and Human Services*, Vol. I (GMENAC Summary Report), DHHS Publ. No. (HRA) 81-651, Government Printing Office, Washington.

[15]   US Department of Health and Human Services, Public Health Service, Health Resources and Services Administration, Bureau of Health Professions, Office of Health Professions (1992). *Data Systems to Support State Health Personnel Planning and Policymaking: A Resource Guide for State Agencies, Washington*. Analysis and Research Report No. 2-93. Washington.

[16]   Weiner, J.P. (1994). Forecasting the effects of health reform on US physician workforce requirements. Evidence from HMO staffing patterns, *Journal of the American Medical Association* **272**, 222–230.

KERRY E. KILPATRICK & THOMAS R. KONRAD

Health-Related Quality of Life *see* Quality of Life and Health Status

Healthy Migrant Effect *see* Migrant Studies

Healthy Worker Effect *see* Occupational Epidemiology

Healthy-Year Equivalent *see* Health Economics

Heaping *see* Grouped Data

Heart Rate *see* Clinical Signals

HEDIS *see* Health Care Utilization, Data Analysis

Helminths *see* Epidemic Models, Deterministic

Hepatology

Hepatology is the study of diseases of the liver. These can be mainly classified as hepatitis, hepatocellular carcinoma (or liver cancer), and liver cirrhosis.

Hepatitis

Several distinct infections are included under the generic title of hepatitis. There are many similarities between these different forms of hepatitis, but their epidemiologies and methods of prevention and control vary. These infections are labeled as hepatitis A, B, C, D, and E. Hepatitis D is sometimes called delta hepatitis [3]. Most statistical work has been done on hepatitis A and B, with little on other forms of hepatitis.

Hepatitis A and B occur worldwide. Outbreaks of hepatitis A are patchy and tend to occur in regular cycles. For developed countries disease spreads in day-care centres for children in diapers, to household and sexual contacts of acute cases, intravenous drug users, and travelers to endemic countries. Hepatitis A is spread by the fecal–oral route. Contaminated water supplies, handling and preparation of food by infected foodhandlers, and shellfish have all been responsible for outbreaks. Hepatitis B is endemic with little seasonal variation in incidence. In developed countries such as the US, infection is most common in young adults, whereas in developing countries widespread infection occurs in infancy. Hepatitis B infection is common in certain high risk groups: intravenous drug injectors, promiscuous heterosexuals, male homosexuals, and workers in some health care and public safety occupations. It is spread by infectious blood, saliva, semen, and vaginal fluids.

Hepatitis C is transmitted by infected blood and blood products, and occurs virtually everywhere in the world. It accounts for 15%–40% of community-acquired hepatitis cases. High-risk groups include transfusion recipients, intravenous drugabusers, and dialysis patients. Hepatitis D closely resembles and is often associated with hepatitis B infection. Its mode of transmission is also very similar. Hepatitis E closely resembles hepatitis A in both its clinical symptoms and its epidemiology. The attack rate is highest amongst young adults, especially males.

Hepatitis A

Frösner et al. [8] discussed the decrease in incidence of hepatitis A infections in Germany using serological data. They used a catalytic model (*see* **Communicable Diseases**) with a sigmoidal decrease in the force of infection (*see* **Hazard Rate**). The force of infection fell from 0.04 per year in 1945 to 0.005 per year in 1965. Frösner et al. [9] and Schenzle et al. [23] discussed antibodies against hepatitis A in seven European countries. Prevalence was highest in Greece and France and lowest in Scandinavia. The force of infection had declined almost everywhere in the period leading up to 1979. Keiding [14] considered nonparametric estimation (*see* **Nonparametric Methods**) of the age-specific force of infection applied to serological hepatitis A data for Bulgaria. These data are ideal for statistical **estimation** as they were collected before the advent of mass vaccination. Keiding estimated the proportion

of people of different ages who must be vaccinated to eliminate hepatitis A in Bulgaria. Greenhalgh & Dietz [10] extended this work to an age-structured model and vaccination at several different ages. They examined the effect of different mixing patterns on vaccination campaigns.

Hadeler et al. [11, 12] performed a statistical analysis of the outbreaks of hepatitis A in Maricopa County, Arizona. These studies strongly link the spread of hepatitis A in the US to very young children in day-care centres and provide a framework for designing disease control strategies. Sattenspiel [20] developed a matrix-migration model for the spread of hepatitis A in US day-care centers using these results. The theoretical results of Sattenspiel's model were applied to data on the incidence of hepatitis A in Alberquerque, New Mexico, in 1979. Analysis of the data suggested that local clusters were at higher risk for epidemics. Close social ties linked up these centers in small local clusters which helped explain the disproportionate number of cases associated with these centers. Sattenspiel [21] described two stochastic **simulation** models which supported these results. Sattenspiel & Simon [22] pushed the theoretical development of the model further.

Liu [15] considered a differential equation **epidemic model** for hepatitis A where the duration of the **latent period** depends on the number of infectious individuals. He showed that nonlinearity due to a dose-dependent latent period can cause periodicity. This model was compared with US hepatitis data.

Hepatitis B

Hepatitis B infects people worldwide. The highest rates of infection are in sub-Saharan Africa and East Asia. Early mathematical models for hepatitis B were due to Cvetanovic et al. [5] and Pasquini & Cvetanovic [19], who used a compartment model (*see* **Pharmacokinetics and Pharmacodynamics**) in which the host population was stratified clinically and epidemiologically to investigate a variety of control strategies in Mediterranean countries. Anderson & May [1] developed a differential equation model for the spread of hepatitis B. A key feature was that around 1% of infected individuals became carriers and continued to transmit the disease for the rest of their lives. These carriers are an important reservoir of infection and their presence represents a complication for immunization programs. Anderson et al. [2] described a model for the sexual transmission of hepatitis B in developed countries which included heterogeneous mixing with respect to age and sexual activity class. They used this model to assess the effects of vaccination campaigns. The first dynamic model of hepatitis B transmission in developing countries has been developed by McLean & Blumberg [18].

Edmunds et al. [7] discussed the influence of age on the development of the carrier state. A model was fitted to the data using **maximum likelihood**. Infants infected perinatally were found to have a high probability, 0.885, of becoming carriers. Over early childhood there is a sharp decrease in the proportion of infections which lead to the carrier state. By adulthood the probability of becoming a carrier was about 0.1. Implications for vaccination programs were also discussed. Edmunds et al. [6] outlined a deterministic compartmental model to describe the transmission dynamics and control of hepatitis B in the Gambia. The model included a class of carriers. They examined the impact of mass vaccination on the incidence of liver cancer (as carriers have a higher than average chance of developing liver cancer). They used age-structured serological data to estimate parameters. Two models were outlined which assumed that infection in adults was due to horizontal and sexual transmission, respectively.

Cirrhosis

Liver cirrhosis is a chronic disease of the liver, normally suffered by alcoholics, but it can also be caused by chronic hepatitis C infection. Carriers of hepatitis B also have a higher risk of developing cirrhosis [3]. Hepatocellular carcinoma occurs in 10%–25% of cirrhotic patients [17]. The prevalence of cirrhosis in the population is not known exactly. This is partly due to the fact that many cases are clinically silent. Up to 30% or even 40% of cases may be discovered at autopsy, and an unknown proportion remains clinically silent. There may be marked geographical differences in incidence from one country to another, or even between different regions in the same country [16]. Moreover, the proportion of alcoholic and nonalcoholic cirrhosis differs from one country to another, the prevalence of alcoholic cirrhosis being highest generally in wine-producing countries [17].

Hepatocellular Carcinoma

Primary hepatocellular cancer (PHC) or hepatocellular carcinoma (HCC) is recognized worldwide. It is among the most common malignant neoplasms in China, many parts of Asia, and Africa. It is relatively uncommon in the US and Europe. Chronic infection with hepatitis B virus is an important risk factor in most cases; hepatitis C may also be involved. Most patients go through a stage of liver cirrhosis before development of the tumor [3].

Berman [4] and later Higginson [13] called world attention to the extremely high incidence rate of HCC amongst the black male population in Mozambique. From the statistical data from various geographical locations it seems that the greater the incidence rate, the younger the peak age. Among Mozambican males the peak age is between 25 and 34 years, the average age in Japan is 56.8 years in males and 59.9 years in females, and it is higher in Northern Europe [17]. HCC occurs in more advanced ages in alcoholic cirrhosis.

References

[1]   Anderson, R.M. & May, R.M. (1991). *Infectious Diseases of Humans: Dynamics and Control*. Oxford University Press, Oxford.

[2]   Anderson, R.M., Medley, G.F. & Nokes, D.J. (1992). Preliminary analyses of the predicted impacts of various vaccination strategies on the transmission of hepatitis B virus, in *The Control of Hepatitis B: the Role of Prevention in Adolescence*, D.L. Bennett, ed. Gower Medical Publishing, London, pp. 95–130.

[3]   Beneson, A.S. (1990). *Control of Communicable Diseases in Man*, 16th Ed. American Public Health Association, Washington.

[4]   Berman, C. (1951). *Primary Carcinoma of the Liver*. Lewis, London.

[5]   Cvetanovic, B., Delimar, B., Kosicek, M., Likar, M. & Spoljaric, B. (1984). Epidemiological model of hepatitis B, *Annals of the Academy of Medicine* **13**, 175–184.

[6]   Edmunds, W.J., Medley, G.F. & Nokes, D.J. (1997). The transmission dynamics and control of hepatitis B in The Gambia, *Statistics in Medicine* **15**, 2215–2234.

[7]   Edmunds, W.J., Medley, G.F., Nokes, D.J., Hall, A.J. & Whittle, H.C. (1993). The influence of age on the development of the hepatitis B carrier state, *Proceedings of the Royal Society of London, Series B* **253**, 197–201.

[8]   Frösner, G., Willers, H., Müller, R., Schenzle, D., Deinhardt, F. & Höpken, W. (1978). Decrease in incidence of hepatitis A infections in Germany, *Infection* **6**, 259–260.

[9]   Frösner, G., Papavangelou, G., Butler, R., Iwarson, S., Lindholm, A., Courouce-Pauty, A., Hass, H. & Deinhardt, F. (1979). Antibodies against hepatitis A in seven European countries, *American Journal of Epidemiology* **110**, 63–69.

[10] Greenhalgh, D. & Dietz, K. (1994). Some bounds on estimates for reproductive ratios derived from the age-specific force of infection, *Mathematical Biosciences* **124**, 9–57.

[11] Hadeler, S.C., Erben, J.J., Francis, D.P., Webster, H.M. & Maynard, J.E. (1982). Risk factors for hepatitis A in day-care centers, *Journal of Infectious Diseases* **145**, 255–261.

[12] Hadeler, S.C., Webster, H.M., Erben, J.J., Swanson, J.E. & Maynard, J.E. (1980). Hepatitis A in day-care centres, *New England Journal of Medicine* **302**, 1222–1227.

[13] Higginson, J. (1963). The geographical pathology of primary liver cancers, *Cancer Research* **23**, 1624–1633.

[14] Keiding, N. (1991). Age-specific incidence and prevalence: a statistical perspective, *Journal of the Royal Statistical Society, Series A* **154**, 371–412.

[15] Liu, W. (1993). Dose-dependent latent period and periodicity of infectious diseases, *Journal of Mathematical Biology* **31**, 487–494.

[16] Marubini, E. (1987). Epidemiology of cirrhosis, in *Cirrhosis of the Liver*, N. Tygstrup & F. Orlandi, eds. Elsevier, Amsterdam, pp. 275–294.

[17] McIntyre, N., Benhamou, J.-P., Bircher, J., Rizetto, M. & Rhodes, J. (1991). *Oxford Textbook of Clinical Hepatology*, Vols 1 and 2. Oxford University Press, Oxford.

[18] McLean, A.R. & Blumberg, B.S. (1994). Modelling the impact of mass vaccination against hepatitis B. I. Model formulation and parameter estimation, *Proceedings of the Royal Society of London, Series B* **256**, 7–15.

[19] Pasquini, P. & Cvetanovic, B. (1988). Mathematical models of hepatitis infection, *Annali Istituto Superiore di Sanita* **24**, 245–250.

[20] Sattenspiel, L. (1987). Population structure and the spread of disease, *Human Biology* **59**, 411–438.

[21] Sattenspiel, L. (1987). Epidemics in nonrandomly mixing populations: a simulation, *American Journal of Physical Anthropology* **73**, 251–261.

[22] Sattenspiel, L. & Simon, C.P. (1988). The spread and persistence of infectious diseases in structured populations, *Mathematical Biosciences* **90**, 341–366.

[23] Schenzle, D., Dietz, K. & Frösner, G. (1979). Hepatitis A antibodies in European countries. II. Mathematical analysis of cross-sectional surveys, *American Journal of Epidemiology* **110**, 70–76.

DAVID GREENHALGH

Herd Immunity *see* Communicable Diseases

Heritability

Before discussing what genetic heritability is, it is important to be clear about what it is not. For a binary trait, such as whether or not an individual has a disease, heritability is not the proportion of disease in the population attributable to, or caused by, genetic factors. For a continuous trait, genetic heritability is not a measure of the proportion of an individual's score attributable to genetic factors. Heritability is not about cause *per se*, but about the causes of variation in a trait across a particular population.

Definitions

Genetic heritability is defined for a quantitative trait. In general terms it is the proportion of variation attributable to genetic factors. Following a genetic and environmental variance components approach, let Y have a mean μ and variance σ^2, which can be partitioned into genetic and environmental components of variance, such as additive genetic variance σ_a^2, dominance genetic variance σ_d^2, common environmental variance σ_c^2, individual specific environmental variance σ_e^2, and so on.

Genetic heritability in the narrow sense is defined as

$$\sigma_a^2/\sigma^2, \tag{1}$$

while genetic heritability in the broad sense is defined as

$$\sigma_g^2/\sigma^2, \tag{2}$$

where σ_g^2 includes all genetic components of variance, including perhaps components due to epistasis (gene–gene interactions; *see* **Genotype**) [3]. In addition to these random genetic effects, the total genetic variation could also include that variation explained when the effects of measured **genetic markers** are modeled as a **fixed effect** on the trait mean.

The concept of genetic heritability, which is really only defined in terms of variation in a quantitative trait, has been extended to cover categorical traits by reference to a **genetic liability model**. It is assumed that there is an underlying, unmeasured continuous "liability" scale divided into categories by "thresholds". Under the additional assumption that the liability follows a **normal distribution**, genetic and environmental components of variance are estimated from the pattern of associations in categorical traits measured in relatives. The genetic heritability of the categorical trait is then often defined as the genetic heritability of the presumed liability (latent variable), according to (1) and (2).

Comments

There is no unique value of the genetic heritability of a characteristic. Heritability varies according to which factors are taken into account in specifying both the mean and the total variance of the population under consideration. That is to say, it is dependent upon modeling of the mean, and of the genetic and environmental variances and covariances (*see* **Genetic Correlations and Covariances**). Moreover, the total variance and the variance components themselves may not be constants, even in a given population. For example, even if the genetic variance actually increased with age, the genetic heritability would decrease with age if the variation in nongenetic factors increased with age more rapidly. That is to say, genetic heritability and genetic variance can give conflicting impressions of the "strength of genetic factors".

Genetic heritability will also vary from population to population. For example, even if the heritability of a characteristic in one population is high, it may be quite different in another population in which there is a different distribution of environmental influences.

Measurement error in a trait poses an upper limit on its genetic heritability. Therefore traits measured with large measurement error cannot have substantial genetic heritabilities, even if variation about the mean is completely independent of environmental factors. By the definitions above, one can increase the genetic heritability of a trait by measuring it more precisely, for example by taking repeat measurements and averaging, although strictly speaking the definition of the trait has been changed also. A trait that is measured poorly (in the sense of having low **reliability**) will inevitably have a low heritability because much of the total variance will be due to measurement error (σ_e^2). However, a trait with relatively little measurement error will have a high heritability if all the nongenetic factors are known and taken into account in the modeling of the mean.

Fisher [1] recognized these problems and noted that

> whereas ... the numerator has a simple genetic meaning, the denominator is the total variance due to errors of measurement [including] those due to uncontrolled, but potentially controllable environmental variation. It also, of course contains the genetic variance ... Obviously, the information contained in [the genetic variance] is largely jettisoned when its actual value is forgotten, and it is only reported as a ratio to this hotch-potch of a denominator.

Historically, other quantities have also been termed heritabilities, but it is not clear what parameter is being estimated, e.g. Holzinger's $H = (r_{MZ} - r_{DZ})$ (the correlation between monozygotic twins minus the correlation between dizygotic twins) (*see* **Twin Analysis**) [2], Nichol's $HR = 2(r_{MZ} - r_{DZ})/r_{MZ}$ [5], the E of Neel & Schull [4] based on twin data alone, and Vandenburg's $F = 1/[1 - \sigma_a^2/\sigma^2)]$ [6]. Furthermore, the statistical properties of these estimators do not appear to have been studied.

References

[1]   Fisher, R.A. (1951). Limits to intensive production in animals, *British Agricultural Bulletin* **4**, 217–218.
[2]   Holzinger, K.J. (1929). The relative effect of nature and nurture influences on twin differences, *Journal of Educational Psychology* **20**, 245–248.
[3]   Lush, J.L. (1948). Heritability of quantitative characters in farm animals, *Suppl. Hereditas* **1948**, 256–375.
[4]   Neel, J.V. & Schull, W.J. (1954). *Human Heredity*. University of Chicago Press, Chicago.
[5]   Nichols, R.C. (1965). The National Merit twin study, in *Methods and Goals in Human Behaviour Genetics*, S.G. Vandenburg, ed. Academic Press, New York.
[6]   Vandenberg, S.G. (1966). Contributions of twin research to psychology, *Psychological Bulletin* **66**, 327–352.

JOHN L. HOPPER

Hermite Distribution *see* Contagious Distributions

Hermite Polynomials *see* Polynomial Approximation

Heterogeneity Test *see* Poisson Distribution

Heteroscedasticity *see* Scedasticity

Heterozygosity

Genes can exist in different allelic forms and there are several ways to quantify the degree of allelic variation in a population. One way is simply to report the frequencies of the different alleles. Other parameters are used to address specific genetic questions. Individuals with two different alleles for some gene are said to be heterozygous for that gene, whereas those with two alleles that are the same are homozygous. The continued existence of heterozygotes implies continued genetic variation, and there have been several reports of correlation between growth rate and heterozygosity (see [2]).

If a gene has alleles a_i, then the frequencies of **genotypes** $a_i a_i$ and $a_i a_j$, $j \neq i$, are written as P_{ii} and P_{ij}, and the frequency of allele a_i is written as p_i. For large random mating populations, the **Hardy–Weinberg** law states that

$$P_{ii} = p_i^2,$$
$$P_{ij} = 2 p_i p_j, \quad i \neq j.$$

When it is of interest to be able to quantify H, the total frequency of heterozygotes, under the Hardy–Weinberg situation this requires only the following allele frequencies:

$$H = \sum_i \sum_{j \neq i} P_{ij}$$
$$= \sum_i \sum_{j \neq i} p_i p_j$$
$$= 1 - \sum_i p_i^2.$$

This last expression is often referred to as *heterozygosity*, but this is a misnomer since it provides the frequency of heterozygotes only under Hardy–Weinberg equilibrium. It is more appropriate to define "gene diversity" D by

$$D = 1 - \sum_i p_i^2.$$

For populations with an **inbreeding** coefficient of f, heterozygote frequencies are modified to

$$P_{ij} = 2 p_i p_j (1 - f),$$

so that

$$H = (1 - f)D.$$

The most likely cause of a difference between H and D in human populations is population **admixture**. If a proportion α_k of the population belongs to subpopulation k, in which frequencies for alleles a_i are p_{ki}, then the frequency of $a_i a_{i'}$ heterozygotes in the whole population is

$$P_{ii'} = 2 p_i p_{i'} + \sum_k \alpha_k (p_{ki} - p_i)(p_{ki'} - p_{i'}),$$

where the total allele frequencies are given by

$$p_i = \sum_k \alpha_k p_{ki}.$$

This result assumes Hardy–Weinberg frequencies within each subpopulation. There may be more or less of a particular heterozygote than expected from the Hardy–Weinberg law in the whole population, although the overall heterozygosity is diminished:

$$H = D - \sum_i \sum_k \alpha_k (p_{ki} - p_i)^2.$$

In linkage studies it is necessary to determine whether or not recombination has occurred between two loci, and this in turn puts constraints on the genotypes of individuals in successive generations. The **polymorphism information content** (PIC) characterizes the extent to which a marker gene (*see* **Genetic Markers**) is useful for linkage studies, with higher values being better. It cannot be greater than H.

Variance of Heterozygosity

If sample allele and genotype frequencies are written as $\tilde{p}_i$ and $\tilde{P}_{ij}$, the sample heterozygosity is

$$\tilde{H} = \sum_i \sum_{j \neq i} \tilde{P}_{ij}.$$

Taking expectation $\mathcal{E}$ over repeated samples of n individuals from the same population, assuming genotype counts are **multinomially distributed**, provides

$$\mathcal{E}(\tilde{H}) = H,$$

whereas the expected value of sample diversity,

$$\tilde{D} = 1 - \sum_i \tilde{p}_i^2,$$

is

$$\mathcal{E}(\tilde{D}) = \left(1 - \frac{1+f}{2n}\right) D$$

The variance over repeated samples from the same population is just the **binomial** variance for $\tilde{H}$,

$$\mathrm{var}(\tilde{H}) = \frac{1}{n}H(1-H),$$

whereas for diversity [3],

$$\mathrm{var}(\tilde{D}) = \frac{2(1+f)}{n}\left[\sum_i p_i^3 - \left(\sum_i p_i^2\right)^2\right].$$

If heterozygosity is averaged over loci, then the variance of the average depends on two-locus heterozygosities. If $H_{ll'}$ is the probability of an individual being heterozygous at loci l and l', then the sample single-locus heterozygosities are correlated:

$$\mathrm{cov}(\tilde{H}_l, \tilde{H}_{l'}) = \frac{1}{n}(H_{ll'} - H_l H_{l'}),$$

so that the variance within populations of heterozygosity averaged over m loci is

$$\mathrm{var}(\tilde{H}) = \frac{1}{nm^2}\sum_l H_l(1-H_l)$$

$$+ \frac{1}{nm^2}\sum_l \sum_{l'\neq l}(H_{ll'} - H_l H_{l'}).$$

Brown et al. [1] pointed out that the two-locus heterozygosity depends on **linkage disequilibrium** between the loci, and the variance of average single-locus heterozygosity therefore serves as a summary statistic for linkage disequilibrium. The same holds for average gene diversity.

References

[1] Brown, A.H.D., Feldman, M.W. & Nevo, E. (1980). Multilocus structure of natural populations of *Hordeum spontaneum, Genetics* **96**, 523–530.

[2] Hartl, D.L. & Clark, A.G. (1989). *Principles of Population Genetics*, 2nd Ed. Sinauer, Sunderland.

[3] Weir, B.S., Reynolds, J. & Dodds, K.G. (1990). The variance of sample heterozygosity, *Theoretical Population Biology* **37**, 235–253.

B.S. WEIR

Hidden Bias *see* Propensity Score

Hidden Markov Models

Hidden Markov models (HMMs) are a class of stochastic models that have proven to be useful in a wide range of applications for modeling highly structured sequences of data. Some applications of HMMs include machine speech recognition [15], ion channel kinetics [9, 10], and biomolecular sequence analysis [1, 4–6, 8] (*see* **DNA Sequences**).

A hidden Markov model can be viewed as a black box that generates sequences of observations. The unobservable internal state of the box is stochastic and is determined by a finite state **Markov chain**. The observable outputs of the black box are stochastic, with distribution determined by the current state of the hidden Markov chain. In more detail, let $(s_t, t = 0, 1, 2, \ldots)$ be an unobserved Markov chain on the state space $(1, 2, \ldots, L)$ and let $(y_t, t = 0, 1, 2, \ldots)$ be an observed process that takes values in the set $(1, 2, \ldots, K)$. The restriction to discrete observations is not essential but it is adequate for the applications considered here.

There are three inference problems that arise in the development or application of hidden Markov models: **estimation** of model parameters, restoration of the hidden states, and model selection (*see* **Model, Choice of**). In this article we define an HMM as a stochastic model that generates sequences of observations, provide examples of HMMs that are used in applications, and discuss approaches to the first two inference problems.

Model Specification

An HMM with L hidden states and K observable outputs is specified by three sets of distributions. First is the *initial distribution* of the hidden Markov chain

$$\Pr(s_0 = i), \quad i \in \{1, \ldots, L\}. \tag{1}$$

Second is the *transition distribution* of the hidden Markov chain as represented by the $L \times L$ matrix $\Lambda = [\lambda_{ij}]$ with elements

$$\lambda_{ij} = \Pr(s_{t+1} = j | s_t = i),$$
$$i \in \{1, \ldots, L\}, \quad j \in \{1, \ldots, L\}. \tag{2}$$

Third is the set of *output distributions* of the hidden states as represented by the $L \times K$ matrix $\Pi = [\pi_{ij}]$ with elements

$$\pi_{ij} = \Pr(y_t = j | s_t = i),$$
$$i \in \{1, \ldots, L\}, j \in \{1, \ldots, K\}. \tag{3}$$

Both of the matrices Λ and Π are stochastic, i.e. they are formed by nonnegative numbers and their row sums are equal to one. Thus the parameter $\theta \equiv (\Lambda, \Pi)$ takes values in a compact set Θ which is a direct product of L L-dimensional and L K-dimensional simplexes.

Models with continuous output distributions can be developed by replacing the probability mass function in (3) with an appropriate density function, e.g. **normal**. With some minor modifications, the results below can be applied to continuous data.

The number of hidden states and their connectivity, i.e. the set of nonzero λ_{ij}, define the *architecture* of an HMM. The choice of an architecture is typically driven by an application for which the HMM is intended. In some cases the architecture is an attempt to model a physical system (e.g. ion channels) and in other cases the HMM is merely a convenient fiction that is useful for **classification** or **prediction** (e.g. speech recognition). The states of the hidden Markov chain may be recurrent or transient. It is worthwhile to consider two classes of architectures. First is the *recurrent* architecture in which any hidden state may be reached from any other hidden state. Second is the *left-to-right* architecture, in which the hidden states are transient. Of course, arbitrarily complex HMMs can be constructed with both recurrent and nonrecurrent components.

It is often convenient to consider transient chains and to introduce two states *begin* (B) and *end* (E) that do not produce any output. Without loss of generality we assume that the initial distribution is concentrated in the state B. Thus $\Pr(s_0 = B) = 1$. The state transition matrix Λ, whose dimension becomes $(L + 2) \times (L + 2)$, is modified as follows:

1. The state B is unattainable from any state including itself; $\lambda_{iB} = 0$, for all i.
2. State E is absorbing, so that $\lambda_{EE} = 1$ and is recurrent, so there is a stopping time $n^* = \min(k : s_k = E, k \geq 0)$ such that $\Pr(n^* \leq \infty) = 1$.
3. The direct transition from state B to state E is not allowed; $\lambda_{BE} = 0$.

Introduction of the absorbing state E allows us to deal with finite realizations of the HMM up to the stopping time n^*. We put $n = n^* - 1$ and use the following notation for the sequence of hidden states and the corresponding sequence of outputs

$$\mathbf{s} \equiv s_1 s_2 \ldots s_n,$$
$$\mathbf{y} \equiv y_1 y_2 \ldots y_n.$$

The states $s_0 = B$ and $s_{n+1} = E$ will be suppressed in the notation, except where they are explicitly needed below.

Suppose we observe N independent realizations of an HMM and denote the set of observed outputs by

$$\mathbf{Y} \equiv \left\{ \begin{array}{ll} \mathbf{y}_1 = y_{1,1} y_{1,2} \cdots, y_{1,n_1} \\ \vdots \quad \vdots \\ \mathbf{y}_N = y_{N,1} y_{N,2} \cdots, y_{N,n_N} \end{array} \right\}.$$

The sequences of paths through the hidden Markov chain that produced $\mathbf{Y}$ will be denoted by

$$\mathbf{S} \equiv \left\{ \begin{array}{ll} \mathbf{s}_1 = s_{1,1} s_{1,2} \cdots, s_{1,n_1} \\ \vdots \quad \vdots \\ \mathbf{s}_N = s_{N,1} s_{N,2} \cdots, s_{N,n_N} \end{array} \right\}.$$

In this formulation there is a one-to-one correspondence between the states of the hidden Markov chain and the elements of the observed sequence. The model can be generalized to include null states (other than B and E). Null states may be visited by the hidden Markov chain but do not produce any observable output.

Hidden Markov models can have large parameter spaces because there may be many possible state transitions and because each state can have its own unique output distribution. Depending on the application, it may be desirable to allow all nonzero parameter values to vary freely. At the other extreme, we may require that some subsets of parameters take identical values. Constraints of this type are referred to as "tied" parameterizations. A less extreme form of combining information can be achieved by imposing a hierarchical model on the parameters in which sets of parameter values are assumed to be drawn from a common distribution [7, 19].

There are known **identifiability** problems with the recurrent HMM model due to the labeling of the states, and some convention for state labeling is needed. There can also be identifiability problems if the output distributions in different states are not distinct. These issues are discussed by Leroux [15]. We note that, for the two-state model, identifiability problems also arise when $\lambda + \mu = 1$. This result suggests that further investigation into the identifiability of HMMs may be worthwhile.

Examples of HMMs

Finite-State Recurrent Architecture

Consider a hidden Markov chain with two main states denoted by 0 and 1. The two-state recurrent architecture is illustrated in Figure 1. Its transition probability matrix, defined on the extended state space (B, 0, 1, E), is

$$\Lambda = \begin{bmatrix} 0 & \lambda_{B0} & \lambda_{B1} & 0 \\ 0 & \lambda_{00} & \lambda_{01} & \lambda_{0E} \\ 0 & \lambda_{10} & \lambda_{11} & \lambda_{1E} \\ 0 & 0 & 0 & 1 \end{bmatrix}.$$

For the case of binary (0, 1) data sequences, the output distribution is given by

$$\Pi = \begin{bmatrix} \pi_{00} & \pi_{01} \\ \pi_{10} & \pi_{11} \end{bmatrix}.$$

This HMM generates nonhomogeneous binary sequences that consist of homogeneous regions of two types, with distinct frequencies of zeros and ones. This model and the more general L-state, K-output recurrent model were applied by Churchill [4, 5] to identify regions with distinct functions in DNA sequences based on differences in local base frequencies.

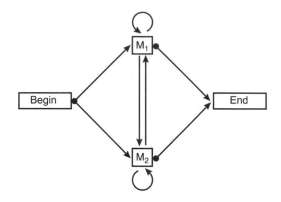

Figure 1   Two-state recurrent HMM architecture

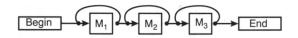

Figure 2   A simple left-to-right HMM architecture

Left-to-Right Architectures

An example of a left-to-right architecture is shown in Figure 2. Left-to-right models are used in applications to speech recognition as "word" models. Each state has an output distribution that characterizes part of the acoustic signal that defines a word. The state transitions follow the evolution of the word from left to right and allow for compression or expansion of the duration of the signal over time. Collections of word models can be nested inside a larger HMM for purposes of word classification and recognition. Further details and references on HMM applications to speech recognition can be found in [13].

Biomolecular Models

Another example of a left-to-right architecture is the mutation–deletion–insertion (MDI) model shown in Figure 3. The MDI model has become a very popular tool for the problem of aligning multiple DNA or protein sequences [1, 14]. In this model, there are three different types of states. The backbone of the model consists of *mutation* states ($M_1, M_2, \ldots, M_L$). Each mutation state M_i has a corresponding *deletion* state D_i. Following the state B there is an *insertion* state I_0, and following each of the mutation states M_i there is an insertion state I_i. There are two sets of output distributions in the MDI model. Outputs from M-states are generated according to $\Pr(j|M_i)$. These distributions will typically vary from state to

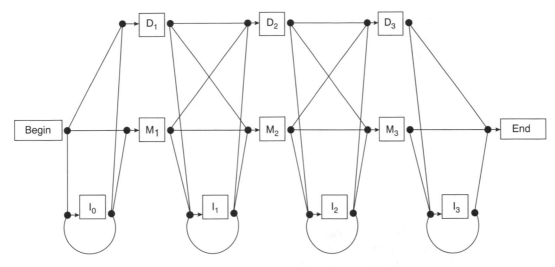

Figure 3 Mutation–deletion–insertion (MDI) architecture with three M-states

state and reflect the position-specific frequencies of nucleotide or amino acid subunits as they occur along the length of a molecule. Outputs from I-states are generated according to $\Pr(j|I_i)$. These states allow for site-specific insertion of letters into the sequence. The D-states are silent and do not produce any output. These states allow specific positions (modeled by M-states) to be skipped in the generation of an output sequence. The length of an output sequence will typically be close to the number of M-states in the model, but any realization may be shorter or longer due to insertion and deletion events.

The presence of silent states in the MDI model introduces a minor complication into our description of these HMMs. It was implicit in our earlier definition of an HMM that there is a one-to-one correspondence between outputs and hidden states. However, in the MDI model, as it is typically implemented, there may be hidden states (D-states) that are visited but have no corresponding output. Thus the length of **y** may be less than the length of the corresponding hidden state sequence **s**. We note that the output of an MDI model can be viewed as the output of a standard HMM consisting of only M-states and I-states. This MI chain is embedded within the MDI chain and can be constructed by simply removing the D-states. The architecture of the MI chain includes additional transitions to replace the removed D-states. Unfortunately the additional transition parameters must be constrained in a rather complicated fashion to recover exactly the original MDI model. The output distributions of the MI model are identical to those of

the MDI model. It follows that results derived for standard HMMs apply equally to MDI models.

A hidden Markov model has been developed for the problem of DNA sequence assembly [6, 7]. We consider a collection of DNA sequences (see Table 1) that are independently copied from a common *prototype* sequence, $\mathbf{r} = r_1, \ldots, r_L; r_i \in (A,C,G,T)$, by a process that introduces errors in the form of *substitutions, deletions*, and *insertions*. Each realization, $i = 1, \ldots, N$, of the MDI chain will generate a sequence $\mathbf{y}_i$ with elements $y_{ij} \in (A,C,G,T,N)$. The output character N is sometimes generated by DNA sequencing devices to represent ambiguous determination of a base. Each M-state in the MDI chain is associated with an element of the prototype sequence, i.e. M_i is associated with r_i. This association will determine the output distribution of the M-state. For example, if the state M_i is associated with $r_i = A$, the most likely output of state M_i is the letter A. A substitution error occurs when the output is a letter other than A. A deletion error occurs when the state D_i is visited, thus bypassing M_i, and no letter is generated as output. An insertion error occurs when the state I_i is visited, thus generating extraneous letters in the output sequence. To summarize, a visit of the D_i-state results in a deletion of r_i in the copying process; k successive visits of the I_i-state result in an insertion of k letters after the ith position in the prototype; a visit of the M_i-state results in copying r_i, with possible substitution error.

The output from N realizations of an MDI chain will be a set of sequences of letters. The

Table 1   An unaligned set of DNA sequences

```
TAGACAGGNGCCCCACTGGAGGAATGAGGTCACCAACCAACCTTCAAAAACTT
TAGACAGGGNCCCACTGGAGGAATGAGGTCACCAACCAACCTTCAAAAACTT
TAGANAGGGCCTCCACTGGGGAAATGAAGGTACCNACCAACCTTCAAAACTT
TAGACCAGGNGCTCCACTGGAGGAATGAGGTCACCAACCAACCTTCAAAAACTT
TAGACAGGGCCTCCACTGGAGATNTGAGGTCACCAACCAACCTTCAAAAACTT
TAGACAGGGGCTCCACTGGAGGAATGAGGTCACCAACCAACCTTCAAAAACTT
```

sequences will generally be similar to one another but may vary in length as well in the identity of specific letters. Often the goal of applying an MDI model to a sequence is to restore the hidden state sequence. Restoration of s_i establishes a correspondence between the elements of y_i and the states of the MDI model. Furthermore, the multiple path restoration of S establishes a correspondence among all elements of all the DNA sequences via their correspondence with the M-states. This correspondence is a *multiple sequence alignment* [21]. An example of an HMM-generated sequence alignment of the DNA sequences from Table 1 is shown in Figure 4.

Inference for HMMs

Likelihood

In this section, we describe an **algorithm** to compute the **likelihood** of an observed sequence y, i.e. $\Pr(y|\theta)$. In the case of multiple independent observations, the likelihood is simply the product $\Pr(Y|\theta) = \prod_{i=1}^{N} \Pr(y_i|\theta)$.

We can express the likelihood as a summation over all possible hidden state sequences

$$\Pr(\mathbf{y}|\boldsymbol{\theta}) = \sum_{s} \Pr(\mathbf{y}|\mathbf{s}, \boldsymbol{\Pi})\Pr(\mathbf{s}|\boldsymbol{\Lambda}), \qquad (4)$$

where

$$\Pr(\mathbf{y}|\mathbf{s}, \boldsymbol{\Pi}) = \pi_{s_1, y_1} \cdot \pi_{s_2, y_2} \ldots \pi_{s_n, y_n} \qquad (5)$$

and

$$\Pr(\mathbf{s}|\boldsymbol{\Lambda}) = \lambda_{Bs_1} \cdot \lambda_{s_1 s_2} \ldots \lambda_{s_n E}. \qquad (6)$$

However, this summation is generally intractable, and an alternative approach is needed to compute the likelihood.

The likelihood can also be written in the form

$$\Pr(\mathbf{y}|\boldsymbol{\theta}) = \prod_{t=1}^{n} \Pr(y_t|\mathbf{y}^{t-1})$$

$$= \prod_{t=1}^{n} \sum_{s_t=1}^{L} \Pr(y_t|s_t)\Pr(s_t|\mathbf{y}^{t-1}), \qquad (7)$$

where $\mathbf{y}^{t-1} = y_1, \ldots, y_{t-1}$. We assume that the distribution of y_t depends only on s_t. The first term

```
            TAGACAGGGCC-CCACTGGAGGAATGAGGTCACCAACCAACCTTCAAAAACTT
                  N
            TAGACAGGGNC-CCACTGGAGGAATGAGGTCACCAACCAACCTTCAAAAACTT
            TAGANAGGGCCTCCACTGG-GGAATGAGGT-ACCNACCAACCTTC-AAAACTT
                            A A
            TAGACAGGNGCTCCACTGGAGGAATGAGGTCACCAACCAACCTTCAAAAACTT
                  C
            TAGACAGGGCCTCCACTGGAG-ATTGAGGTCACCAACCAACCTTCAAAAACTT
                          N
            TAGACAGGGGCTCCACTGGAGGAATGAGGTCACCAACCAACCTTCAAAAACTT
```
Consensus   TAGACAGGGNCTCCACTGGAGGAATGAGGTCACCAACCAACCTTCAAAAACTT

Figure 4   A multiple sequence alignment of the DNA sequences in Table 1. The alignment was generated using an MDI architecture with 52 M-states. Letters aligned in each column correspond to the same M-states. Insertions are shown above the main sequence and deletions are shown as dashes. An estimated consensus or prototype sequence is shown below the multiple alignment

in (7) is the output distribution and the second term is the predictive density. The predictive density can be computed using the *forward pass algorithm*. This algorithm is the basis for a number of other computations and is presented here.

The Forward Pass Algorithm.   To begin, suppose that $\Pr(s_{t-1}|\mathbf{y}^{t-1})$ is known. A prediction of the state at time t can be computed, using the law of total probability, as

$$\Pr(s_t|\mathbf{y}^{t-1}) = \sum_{s_{t-1}=1}^{L} \Pr(s_t|s_{t-1}, \mathbf{y}^{t-1})$$

$$\times \Pr(s_{t-1}|\mathbf{y}^{t-1}). \qquad (8)$$

This conditional distribution is called the *predictive density*. Next, the information in the current observation is incorporated by updating the predictive density. The so-called *filtered density* is

$$\Pr(s_t|\mathbf{y}^t) = \frac{\Pr(y_t|s_t, \mathbf{y}^{t-1})\Pr(s_t|\mathbf{y}^{t-1})}{\Pr(y_t|\mathbf{y}^{t-1})}, \qquad (9)$$

by **Bayes' theorem**, where

$$\Pr(y_t|\mathbf{y}^{t-1}) = \sum_{s_t=1}^{L} \Pr(y_t|s_t, \mathbf{y}^{t-1})\Pr(s_t|\mathbf{y}^{t-1}).$$

Restoration of the Hidden Markov Chain

The problem of restoring the hidden state sequence **s** from a given observation sequence **y** is addressed here. We assume that the model parameters θ are given and suppress θ in the notation of this section.

There are two general approaches to the state restoration problem. A local restoration uses the marginal conditional densities to find the most probable state at each point t. This marginal restoration is given by

$$s_{i,t}^* = \text{argmax}_{s_t} \Pr(s_t|\mathbf{y}_i).$$

A global restoration maximizes the full conditional density to find a most probable restoration. Thus,

$$\mathbf{s}_t^* = \text{argmax}_s \Pr(\mathbf{s}|\mathbf{y}_i).$$

These two approaches can result in quite different solutions. The first problem is solved using the *backward algorithm* and the second is solved using the *Viterbi algorithm* [20].

The Backward Algorithm.   The backward algorithm uses the results of the forward algorithm to compute the conditional distribution of the hidden state sequence given the complete sequence of observed data. It is sufficient to specify the distribution of pairs of adjacent states because we assume the Markov property.

The joint distribution of two adjacent states is computed recursively, starting with the last step of the forward algorithm

$$\Pr(s_t, s_{t+1}|\mathbf{y}) = \frac{\Pr(s_{t+1}|\mathbf{y})\Pr(s_{t+1}|s_t)\Pr(s_t|\mathbf{y}^t)}{\Pr(s_{t+1}|\mathbf{y}^t)}$$

The marginal distribution can be obtained by summing the expression over s_{t+1}. Thus

$$\Pr(s_t|\mathbf{y}) = \Pr(s_t|\mathbf{y}^t) \sum_{s_{t+1}=1}^{L} \frac{\Pr(s_{t+1}|\mathbf{y})\Pr(s_{t+1}|s_t)}{\Pr(s_{t+1}|\mathbf{y}^t)}.$$

See Rabiner [17] or Churchill [4] for more detail.

The Viterbi Algorithm.   Our goal is to find the sequence of states **s** that maximizes over the space of all state sequences the conditional probability of **s** given the observation sequence **y** and known model parameters. Notice that

$$\Pr(\mathbf{s}|\mathbf{y}) = \frac{\Pr(\mathbf{s}, \mathbf{y})}{\Pr(\mathbf{y})}, \qquad (10)$$

and thus it is sufficient to find the sequence of states which maximizes $\Pr(\mathbf{s}, \mathbf{y})$.

The joint probability can be factored as

$$\Pr(\mathbf{s}, \mathbf{y}) = \prod_{t=1}^{n} \Pr(s_t, y_t|\mathbf{s}^{t-1}, \mathbf{y}^{t-1})$$

$$= \prod_{t=1}^{n} \Pr(y_t|\mathbf{s}^t, \mathbf{y}^{t-1})\Pr(s_t|\mathbf{s}^{t-1}, \mathbf{y}^{t-1})$$

$$= \prod_{t=1}^{n} \Pr(y_t|s_t)\Pr(s_t|s_{t-1}). \qquad (11)$$

Let $\delta_t(i)$ denote the maximum probability up to time t over all state sequences which end at the state $s_t = i$,

$$\delta_t(i) = \max_{s^{t-1}} \Pr(\mathbf{s}^{t-1}, s_t = i, \mathbf{y}^t). \qquad (12)$$

The joint probability, (11), can be maximized by the following procedure:

1. initialization,

$$\delta_1(i) = \Pr(s_1 = i)\Pr(y_1|s_1 = i), \ 1 \le i \le r; \tag{13}$$

2. recursion,

$$\delta_t(j) = \max_{1 \le i \le r} [\delta_{t-1}(i)\lambda_{ij}]\Pr(y_t|s_t = j); \tag{14}$$

3. termination,

$$\max_{\mathbf{s}} \Pr(\mathbf{s}, \mathbf{y}) = \max_{1 \le i \le r} \delta_n(i). \tag{15}$$

We are asking at each time point t, if the present state is $s_t = j$, which state at time $t - 1$ maximizes the joint probability over all past state sequences. Roughly, if we are in state j at time t, where did we come from at time $t - 1$?

For each state $1 \le j \le r$ at time t we wish to keep track of the state at time $t - 1$ which gives us the maximum. To do this, we define the quantity

$$\psi_t(j) = \arg \max_{1 \le i \le r} [\delta_{t-1}(i)\lambda_{ij}]. \tag{16}$$

When the process is terminated, we have computed $\delta_n(i)$ and $\psi_n(i)$ for $1 \le i \le r$. A state sequence which attains the maximal probability can be constructed by a traceback. Let

$$s_n^* = \arg \max_{1 \le i \le r} [\delta_n(i)] \tag{17}$$

be the best final state. The traceback is completed by the recursion

$$s_t^* = \psi_{t+1}(s_{t+1}^*), \ t = n - 1, \ n - 2, \dots, 1. \tag{18}$$

Note that $\delta_t(j) \to 0$ fast. Thus computations are more easily executed on a log scale. The recursion, (13), will look like

$$\log \delta_t(j) = \max_{1 \le i \le r} [\log \delta_{t-1}(i) + \log \lambda_{ij}]$$
$$+ \log \Pr(y_t|s_t = j). \tag{19}$$

Parameter Estimation

In the **maximum likelihood** approach to HMM restoration, no prior information on the parameter θ is assumed and the inference problems of parameter estimation and state restoration are addressed by first finding an estimator for θ and then restoring $\mathbf{S}$ conditionally given the estimated value.

In general, the likelihood is intractable for direct maximization. However, given a state sequence $\mathbf{S}$, the augmented data likelihood,

$$\Pr(\mathbf{Y}, \mathbf{S}|\theta) = \prod_{i=1}^{N} \Pr(\mathbf{y}_i, \mathbf{s}_i|\theta)$$

$$= \prod_{i=1}^{N} \Pr(\mathbf{y}_i|\mathbf{s}_i, \boldsymbol{\Pi})\Pr(\mathbf{s}_i|\boldsymbol{\Lambda}), \tag{20}$$

is quite well behaved. The problem of maximizing the augmented data likelihood is trivial. The augmented data **sufficient statistics** for this problem are matrices $\mathbf{C}^{\boldsymbol{\Lambda}} \equiv [c_{ij}^{\boldsymbol{\Lambda}}]$ and $\mathbf{C}^{\boldsymbol{\Pi}} \equiv [c_{ij}^{\boldsymbol{\Pi}}]$, where $c_{ij}^{\boldsymbol{\Lambda}}$ is the number of transitions to the j-state from the i-state and $c_{ij}^{\boldsymbol{\Pi}}$ is the number of outputs j from state i. When some parameter values are tied, the dimensions of the sufficient statistics can be reduced.

The problem of maximizing the observed data likelihood is solved by the *Baum–Welch* algorithm [2, 3, 17]. An initial estimate θ^0 is chosen. The algorithm iterates the following steps:

1. Use the forward and backward algorithms to compute the conditional expectation of $\mathbf{C}^{\boldsymbol{\Lambda}}$ and $\mathbf{C}^{\boldsymbol{\Pi}}$ with respect to $\Pr(\mathbf{S}|\mathbf{Y}, \theta^m)$.
2. Use the expected sufficient statistics from step 1 to obtain a new estimate θ^{m+1}. The MLEs for $\boldsymbol{\Pi}$ and $\boldsymbol{\Lambda}$ are simply the row-normalized expectations of $\mathbf{C}^{\boldsymbol{\Lambda}}$ and $\mathbf{C}^{\boldsymbol{\Pi}}$, respectively.

As $m \to \infty$ the sequence of parameter estimates θ^m will converge to a point of maximum, not necessarily global, of the likelihood function [3, Eq. (4)]. HMM likelihoods can be multimodal, and thus it is recommended to try several starting values for the estimation algorithm.

From a computational point of view the first step can be carried out in time proportional to $N \times L^2 \times$ (average sequence length) and the estimator in step 2 can be obtained in closed form. However, the implementation can be rather tedious and in many applications a *modified* version, called the segmental *k*-means algorithm [12], is used. Step 1 is replaced by:

1. Obtain a most probable path $s_i^{m+1} = \text{argmax}_\mathbf{s}$ $\Pr(\mathbf{s}|\mathbf{y}_i, \theta^m)$ for each $i = 1, \dots, N$.
2. Obtain a new estimate θ^{m+1} that maximizes the augmented data likelihood $\Pr(\mathbf{Y}, \mathbf{S}^{m+1}|\theta)$.

The first step can be accomplished by dynamic programming [20], and a closed-form estimator is available for step 2. This algorithm produces an estimator $\tilde{\theta}$ that maximizes the objective function $\max_{\mathbf{s}} \Pr(\mathbf{y}, \mathbf{s}|\theta)$. Although this is not a maximum likelihood estimator, the two estimators will generally be very similar [16].

Having obtained some parameter estimate θ^*, we can restore $\mathbf{S}$ using either of the methods in the section, "Restoration of the Hidden Markov Chain".

A Bayesian Approach

A weakness of the likelihood approach to the state restoration problem is that the final solution is based on the point estimator of θ and fails to take into account other "reasonable" values of θ. Furthermore, it may be of interest to find not only an *optimal* multiple path but also to have access to reasonable alternative restorations. These concerns motivate a **Bayesian** approach to the state restoration problem.

We assume a **prior distribution** $P_0(\theta)$ for the parameter $\theta \equiv (\mathbf{\Lambda}, \mathbf{\Pi})$ so that the posterior distribution of the pair $(\mathbf{S}, \theta)$ is

$$\Pr(\mathbf{S}, \theta|\mathbf{Y}) \propto P_0(\theta) \prod_{i=1}^{N} \Pr(\mathbf{y}_i|\mathbf{s}_i, \mathbf{\Pi})\Pr(\mathbf{s}_i|\mathbf{\Lambda}), \quad (21)$$

where the last two terms are defined in (5) and (6), respectively. Integrating out the parameter θ in (21) we obtain the marginal posterior $\Pr(\mathbf{S}|\mathbf{Y})$, which will be our primary interest. Similarly, summing over all multiple paths, we obtain the marginal posterior of $\Pr(\theta|\mathbf{Y})$. These marginal posterior distributions are not practically computable, in part because of unassessable normalizing constants.

Two slightly different solutions have been proposed for this problem. Both approaches use a Gibbs sampler (e.g. [11]) to approximate the desired posterior distributions (*see* **Markov Chain Monte Carlo**). The Gibbs sampler alternately generates random samples from the full conditional distributions $\Pr(\mathbf{s}|\mathbf{y}, \theta)$ and $\Pr(\theta|\mathbf{y}, \mathbf{s})$. In Robert et al. [18] the hidden state sequence is sampled elementwise. In Churchill & Lazareva [7], the full sequence is sampled in one step at each iteration of the Gibbs sampler. Sampling of θ is trivial when conjugate Dirichlet or Dirichlet mixture priors are used (*see* **Loglinear Models**).

Summary

Hidden Markov models provide a powerful class of models that can be applied to analyze data that consist of sequences of dependent observations with an underlying heterogeneous structure. The inference problems of parameter estimation and state restoration can be addressed using algorithms described in this article, but many subtle and difficult issues may arise in any particular application. The widespread use and success of hidden Markov models in speech recognition and molecular sequence analysis suggest that there may be many fruitful areas of application to which these methods can be applied.

References

[1] Baldi, P., Chauvin, Y., Hunkapillar, T. & McClure, M.A. (1994). Hidden Markov models of biological primary sequence information, *Proceedings of the National Academy of Sciences* **91**, 1059–1063.

[2] Baum, L.E. & Petrie, T. (1966). Statistical inference for probabilistic or finite state Markov chains, *Annals of Mathematical Statistics* **37**, 1554–1563.

[3] Baum, L.E., Petrie, T., Soules, G. & Weiss, N. (1970). A maximization technique occurring in the statistical analysis of probabilistic functions of Markov chains, *Annals of Mathematical Statistics* **41**, 164–171.

[4] Churchill, G.A. (1989). A stochastic model for heterogeneous DNA sequences, *Bulletin of Mathematical Biology* **51**, 79–94.

[5] Churchill, G.A. (1992). Hidden Markov chains and the analysis of genome structure, *Computers and Chemistry* **16**, 107–115.

[6] Churchill G.A. (1995). Accurate restoration of DNA sequences, in *Case Studies in Bayesian Statistics*, Vol. II, C. Gatsaris, J.S. Hodges, R.E. Kass & N.D. Singpurwalla, eds. Springer-Verlag, New York, pp. 90–148.

[7] Churchill, G.A. & Lazareva, B. (1998). Bayesian restoration of a hidden Markov chain with applications to DNA sequencing, unpublished manuscript.

[8] Eddy, S.R. (1996). Hidden Markov models, *Current Opinion in Structural Biology* **6**, 361–365.

[9] Fredkin, D.R. & Rice, J.A. (1992). Maximum likelihood estimation and identification directly from single-channel recordings, *Proceedings of the Royal Society of London, Series B* **249**, 125–132.

[10] Fredkin, D.R. & Rice, J. (1992). Bayesian restoration of single channel patch clamp recordings, *Biometrics* **48**, 427–448.

[11] Gelfand, A.E. & Smith, A.F.M. (1990). Sampling based approaches to calculating marginal densities, *Journal of the American Statistical Association* **85**, 398–409.

[12] Juang, B.H. & Rabiner, L.R. (1990). The segmental *k*-means algorithm for estimating parameters of hidden Markov models, *IEEE Transactions on Acoustics, Speech and Signal Processing* **38**, 1639–1641.

[13] Juang, B.H. & Rabiner, L.R. (1991). Hidden Markov models for speech recognition, *Technometrics* **33**, 251–272.

[14] Krogh, A., Brown, M., Mian, I.S., Sjölander, K. & Haussler, D. (1994). Hidden Markov models in computational biology: applications to protein modeling, *Journal of Molecular Biology* **235**, 1501–1531.

[15] Leroux, B.G. (1992). Maximum-likelihood estimation for hidden Markov models, *Stochastic Processes and their Applications* **40**, 127–143.

[16] Merkav, N. & Ephraim, Y. (1991). Maximum likelihood hidden Markov modeling using a dominant sequence of states, *IEEE Transactions on Signal Processing* **39**, 2111–2115.

[17] Rabiner, L.R. (1989). A tutorial on hidden Markov models and selected applications in speech recognition, *Proceedings of the IEEE* **77**, 257–286.

[18] Robert, C.P., Celeux, G. & Diebolt J. (1994). Bayesian estimation of hidden Markov chains: a stochastic implementation, *Statistics and Probability Letters* **16**, 77–83.

[19] Sjölander, K., Karplus, K., Brown, M., Hughey, R., Krogh, A., Main, I.S. & Haussler, D. (1996). Dirichlet mixtures: a method for improved detection of weak but significant protein sequence homology, *CABIOS* **12**, 327–345.

[20] Viterbi, J. (1967). Error bounds for convolutional codes and an asymptotically optimal decoding algorithm, *IEEE Transactions on Information Theory* **13**, 260–269.

[21] Waterman, M.S. (1995). *Introduction to Computational Biology*. Chapman & Hall, London.

GARY A. CHURCHILL

or nested, then special procedures are required (*see* **Separate Families of Hypotheses**).

The term "hierarchical" can also be used to refer to a single model, usually in the context of **regression** or **analysis of variance**. In this usage, a model is said to be hierarchical if the presence of an **interaction** term implies the inclusion of all lower-order interactions and main effects for the explanatory variables involved in the interaction. The model is hierarchical in the sense that it includes all submodels in a hierarchy as special cases. It has been argued that only such models should be considered [1], but this is not universally accepted. Significance tests for the presence of interactions are, however, best considered in the context of hierarchical models.

Another usage of the term "hierarchical models" is as a synonym for **multilevel models**. This usage derives from the hierarchical nature of data in which observations are nested within higher level classifications. For example, individuals may be nested within families, or patients may be nested within clinics. **Bayesian** hierarchical models provide another use of the term. **Markov chain Monte Carlo** methods are very important in this context.

Reference

[1] Nelder, J.A. (1977). A reformulation of linear models (with discussion), *Journal of the Royal Statistical Society, Series A* **140**, 48–77.

V.T. FAREWELL

Hierarchical Models

This term is currently used in a variety of contexts. The most traditional one is in the sense that two statistical models are said to be hierarchical if one is a submodel of the other. A set of models, $H_1, H_2, \ldots, H_k$, is similarly called a hierarchy if

$$H_1 \subset H_2 \subset \ldots \subset H_k.$$

Hierarchical models specified by a finite set of parameters are of particular importance, because the comparison of models can be based on standard likelihood ratio tests. When models are not hierarchical,

Hierarchical Models in Health Services Research

Hierarchical models provide a natural framework for conceptualizing and quantifying systematic and random components of variation in **multilevel** data. For example, hierarchical nested structures are present in data describing **health care utilization**, cost (*see* **Health Economics**), and **outcomes** for patients treated in specific hospitals, which may in turn belong to particular health care systems or may be clustered by geographic or **hospital market areas** (*see* **Small Area Variation Analysis**).

The analysis of variations in health care processes and outcomes seeks to quantify and characterize variability across clusters, such as physicians, hospitals, and geographic or market areas, at each level of the hierarchical data structure. In particular, the analysis seeks to determine whether comparable patients receive similar treatment and experience similar outcomes across clusters. If differences exist, the analysis turns to the examination of how patient, hospital, or regional characteristics may be related to these differences. In addition, the analysis examines the link between measures of outcome, such as patient mortality, morbidity, and functioning and indicators of process, such as descriptors of regional or provider practice patterns. When the focus of the analysis is on comparative measures of performance of health care providers, the term *profiling* analysis is often used (*see* **Profiling Providers of Medical Care**).

A number of methodologic issues confront the investigator in the analysis of variations in health care. First, sample size can vary across clusters, resulting in substantially different precision of cluster-specific estimates. For example, the number of patients with a particular condition in each hospital may vary from a handful to several hundred in a typical analysis of hospital variations. Secondly, the analytic strategy needs to take into account the **correlation** of the responses within each cluster (*see* **Clustering**). Failure to do so may result in understating the error associated with the estimates of effects of case-specific **covariates**, such as the effect of patient characteristics on medical procedure utilization across different geographic areas. Thirdly, the analyst needs to derive reliable cluster-specific estimates, such as mortality rates for each hospital, and also to estimate the effects of cluster-level covariates, such as hospital characteristics. The usual approach of fitting a single **regression** model to the entire data set does not account for correlations and cannot accommodate both cluster-specific indicator variables and cluster-level covariates.

Hierarchical regression modeling goes a long way toward meeting these methodologic challenges. The approach enables the analyst to separate sampling variability from variability across clusters. It also allows the latter to be further partitioned into a *systematic* component (*see* **Fixed Effects**), which is linked to cluster characteristics, and a *random* component (*see* **Random Effects**). The hierarchical model accommodates within-cluster correlations and

makes it possible to estimate case- and cluster-level covariate effects and **variance components** simultaneously. The model also makes it possible to pool information across clusters in order to derive more precise estimates of cluster-specific parameters and cluster-level effects.

Examples

Although hierarchical models have been extensively discussed in the statistical literature (see [4], [7], [8], and [14], and references in **Multilevel Models**), their use in **health services research** is relatively recent [1–3, 5, 6, 9, 10, 12, 13]. In a particular study, the complexity of the hierarchical model will be commensurate with the research question and the level of detail in the data. The following examples illustrate two typical scenaria.

Aggregate Responses: Hierarchical Poisson Model

Consider studies in which a **Poisson** count, Y_i, of events is observed in the ith of K clusters. For example, Y_i can be the number of patients who experience complications after undergoing a specific operation in the ith hospital during a particular year. The number of patients receiving the operation in the ith hospital is denoted by n_i. If there is no reason to suspect systematic differences across hospitals, the following hierarchical model with an **exchangeable** second-level structure can be considered:

Level I (within-hospital). $Y_i|\theta_i \sim$ Poisson $(\theta_i n_i)$.

Level II (between-hospitals). $\log(\theta_i) \sim N(\mu, \sigma)$.

Fully **Bayesian** formulations of the hierarchical model include a third level, in which **priors** on the population parameters μ and σ are specified. Vague (but proper) priors are often used at this stage.

A model of this type was employed in a recently published analysis of teenage conception rates for different health boards in Scotland [5]. The model was used to derive estimates and posterior intervals of the individual health board rates (θ_i) and of the relative ranking for each health board. Similar models have been used with **binomial** outcomes in Level I and with cluster-level covariates in Level II of the hierarchy.

Case-level Responses: Hierarchical Logistic Model

The models for binomial and Poisson responses are applicable to studies in which only aggregate data are available on each cluster. If case-specific data are available, more intricate hierarchical regression models can be employed. In many studies a **binary** response, Y_{ij}, is observed on the jth case in cluster i, where $j = 1, \ldots, n_i$ and $i = 1, \ldots, N$. The available data include a K-dimensional vector of covariate values X_{ij} on the ijth case and an L-dimensional vector of covariate values Z_i on cluster i. For example, in a study of geographic patterns of utilization of coronary angiography in elderly patients who had a heart attack, the binary response of interest was the indicator of whether angiography was performed on a patient within a specific time interval after the infarction. Data on patient sociodemographics (such as age, gender, and race) and **co-morbid** conditions were represented by the vector X_{ij}, and characteristics of the geographic area (such as location, and availability of angiography in local hospitals) were represented by Z_i [2]. As a second example, in a profiling analysis of the performance of hospitals which treat heart-attack patients, the binary response of interest was the indicator of whether a patient survived past the initial 30-day period after the heart attack. Data on patient sociodemographic characteristics and severity at hospital entry were represented by the vector X_{ij} and selected hospital characteristics by the vector Z_i [12]. As a third example, in an analysis of data from the National Health Interview Survey, the binary response was an indicator of whether an individual had a physician visit in the past year. The analysis included data on characteristics of the individual and the county of the individual's residence [9].

The following hierarchical **logistic regression** model was used in the analysis of the angiography data:

Level I (within-area variability). A logistic model was assumed within each area. Specifically, if $p_{ij} = \Pr(Y_{ij} = 1)$, then

$$\mathrm{logit}(p_{ij}) = \beta_{0i} + \beta_{1i}X_{1ij} + \beta_{2i}X_{2ij}$$
$$+ \cdots + \beta_{Ki}X_{Kij}.$$

Level II (between-areas variability). The variation across areas was partitioned into a systematic and a random component. The systematic component was expressed by a **multiple linear regression** model linking the within-area logistic coefficients to area-level covariates. Specifically,

$$\beta_{ki} = \gamma_{k1}Z_{1i} + \cdots + \gamma_{kL}Z_{Li} + \varepsilon_{ki}.$$

The error terms ε_{ki} were assumed to have a **multivariate normal distribution** with mean zero and covariance structure such that (i) the error terms for different units are independent, and (ii) the within-unit $(K + 1) \times (K + 1)$ **covariance matrix** D is the same for all units. Heavier-tailed distributions, such as **multivariate t** may also be used for modeling the variability of the β_i [1]. In a third and final level, vague proper priors can be assumed on the components of γ and on the covariance matrix D.

The above hierarchical logistic model makes it possible to combine data across geographical areas in order to derive smoothed estimates of the effects of patient characteristics, such as sociodemographics and co-morbidity, both over the entire country and within each area. Therefore, we can determine whether a specific patient characteristic (such as race) has a differential impact on practice patterns in different areas of the country. The process of combining information across areas takes into account differences in sample size and results in improved precision of estimates for areas with small sample sizes. The hierarchical model estimates of the logistic coefficients can be conceptually described (and numerically approximated) as a weighted combination of (i) the coefficients resulting from fitting the logistic model solely to the data of the particular area and (ii) average values of these coefficients across areas, as determined by the area-level characteristics. In the angiography example, the hierarchical model estimates are effectively obtained by shrinking the coefficients from the fully stratified analysis towards a regression line determined by the area characteristics included in the vector **Z**. The degree of **shrinkage** is different for each covariate, being influenced by (i) the accuracy with which the particular covariate can be estimated via the stratified analysis (*see* **Stratification**) and (ii) by the degree to which the estimate for a particular area differs from the estimates for the other areas. Shrinkage is generally going to be higher for coefficients of areas with smaller overall sample sizes and/or small cell counts for a particular covariate.

The hierarchical model also makes it possible to derive area-specific estimates of the probability of the outcome (in this case, performance of angiography) for each stratum of patients that can be defined using the covariate vector **X**. These probabilities can be presented graphically using maps (*see* **Mapping Disease Patterns**). In addition, the model makes it possible to examine the relation between area-level covariates (**Z**) and area-specific event rates or area-specific effects of patient characteristics. In the angiography analysis, for example, it was determined that an area's rate of angiography for an average patient was positively related to an index measuring the availability of the procedure to patients in that area. It was also found that the effect of race differed across census regions in the country.

There are two simpler *fixed-effects* alternatives to the hierarchical logistic model of the analysis of variations across areas: (i) regression analysis stratified by area, and (ii) regression analysis using a single logistic model for the entire country, with indicator variables for each area and their interactions. The fully stratified analysis is close to the spirit of Level I of the hierarchical model. However, such an analysis may not be an efficient approach and may lead to highly imprecise estimates of effects, especially in areas with small sample sizes overall or in some categories of patients. The analysis via a single logistic regression model is more common in practice. However, the **standard errors** of the coefficients from this analysis do not account for the effects of clustering of patients within areas and will, therefore, need to be adjusted. This correlation is accounted for by the hierarchical analysis. In addition, the analysis via a single regression model for the entire country cannot incorporate both patient-level and area-level covariates without leading to model indeterminacy. For example, if **dummy variables** for areas are included then it is no longer possible to include variables indicating the location of the area and other area characteristics. Such area characteristics can be accommodated via the hierarchical model or via a two-stage approach in which a fully stratified analysis is first carried out and the resulting coefficients are used as the dependent variable in regression models similar to those in Level II of the hierarchical model. The two-stage analysis will generally lead to consistent estimates of the second-stage coefficients but is likely to understate the standard error of the estimates without careful adjustment.

Further Applications

Hierarchical regression modeling techniques are by now available for most response data of interest in health services and outcomes research. In particular, the response may be binary or a count as above; **polytomous**, e.g. utilization of one of several alternative treatments [1]; **ordered categorical**, e.g. appropriateness of care; or continuous. The latter may be observed completely, e.g. cost of care; or above a threshold, e.g. vulnerability to malpractice claim [3]. For each type of response the models can include cluster-level covariates, such as hospital size and teaching status. Aggregate data on patient mix can also be included in Level II of the model, but that would provide only a rudimentary method for **case-mix** adjustment. More substantial case-mix adjustment can be implemented with models such as the hierarchical logistic model above. The approach requires the use of patient-level information and can be accomplished with hierarchical models in which Level I describes the relation of the response on an individual patient to patient characteristics. However, it should be noted that the use of hierarchical modeling does not necessarily address the effects of **selection bias**, especially if such bias is related to covariates that are not represented in the database.

Further levels can be added to the above hierarchical models in order to accommodate additional structure in the data. In the Poisson example, longitudinally observed counts may be available on each cluster over several years (*see* **Longitudinal Data Analysis, Overview**). In the logistic example, primary clusters such as hospitals may be further grouped by geographic region or market area. In each case, the incorporation of further levels and corresponding covariates is straightforward. In addition to cluster-level covariates, the hierarchical structure may also be used to model spatial dependence. Such models have already been developed and used in epidemiologic studies and can be readily adapted for health services research data.

Model Fitting and Checking

Simulating observations from the posterior distribution of the parameters is generally recognized to be the most flexible and broadly applicable approach to fitting hierarchical regression models.

This fully Bayesian framework provides a more realistic account of uncertainty in the estimates without the need for rather complex adjustments. A key practical advantage of the approach is that it makes it possible to **simulate** values and derive estimates of any function of the parameters, with little additional computational burden. For example, in profiling analyses, it is generally straightforward to simulate values from the posterior distribution of any measure of hospital performance, to derive estimates and to account for the uncertainty in these estimates. The most common algorithms for generating simulated values involve **Markov chain Monte Carlo** (MCMC) methodology [4]. Although special programs may have to be developed for some of the more complex, multilevel models, a large class of problems can be analyzed using the publicly available software BUGS [11]. A number of recent authors have proposed **diagnostics** for checking the convergence of MCMC runs [4]. Some of these diagnostics are now available in BUGS and other MCMC software. A recent account of approaches to checking model fit (*see* **Model Checking**) and comparing alternative models can be found in [4].

An alternative computational approach to posterior simulation has been developed using weighted **least squares** methods and can be implemented via the software package MLn (*see* **Multilevel Models**). Some classes of hierarchical regression models can also be fitted using special SAS subroutines (*see* **Software, Biostatistical**) for mixed models as well as a plethora of more specialized software.

References

[1] Daniels, M. & Gatsonis, C. (1997). Hierarchical polytomous regression models with applications to health services research, *Statistics in Medicine* **16**, 2311–2325.

[2] Gatsonis, C.A., Epstein A.M., Newhouse, J.P., Normand, S.L. & McNeil, B.J. (1995). Variations in the utilization of coronary angiography for elderly patients with an acute myocardial infarction: An analysis using hierarchical logistic regression, *Medical Care* **33**, 625–642.

[3] Gibbons, R.D., Hedeker, D., Charles, S.C. & Frisch P. (1994). A random-effects probit model for predicting medical malpractice claims, *Journal of the American Statistical Association* **89**, 760–767.

[4] Gilks, W.R., Richardson, S. & Spiegelhalter, D.J. (1996). *Markov Chain Monte Carlo in Practice.* Chapman & Hall, London.

[5] Goldstein, H. & Spiegelhalter, D. (1996). League tables and their limitations: statistical issues in comparisons of institutional performance, *Journal of the Royal Statistical Society, Series A* **159**, 385–444.

[6] Jenks, S.F., Daley, J., Draper, D., Thomas, N., Lehnart, G. & Walker, J. (1988). Interpreting hospital mortality data: the role of clinical risk adjustment, *Journal of the American Medical Association* **260**, 3611–3616.

[7] Kass, R.E. & Steffey, D. (1989). Approximate Bayesian inference for conditionally independent hierarchical models, *Journal of the American Statistical Association* **84**, 717–726.

[8] Lindley, D. & Smith, A. (1972). Bayes estimates for the linear model, *Journal of the Royal Statistical Society, Series B* **34**, 1–41.

[9] Malec, D., Sedransk, J. & Tompkins, L. (1993). Bayesian predictive inference for small areas for binary variables in the National Health Interview Survey, in *Case Studies in Bayesian Statistics*, C. Gatsonis, J. Hodges, R. Kass & N. Singpurwall, eds. Springer-Verlag, New York, pp. 377–389.

[10] McNeil, B.J., Pederson, S. & Gatsonis, C. (1992). Current issues in profiling quality of care, *Inquiry* **29**, 298–307.

[11] MRC Biostatistics Unit (1996). *BUGS Manual.* Institute of Public Health, Cambridge.

[12] Normand, S.L., Glickman, M. & Gatsonis, C. (1997). Statistical methods for profiling providers: issues and applications. *Journal of the American Statistical Association* **92**, 803–814.

[13] Shwartz, M., Ash, A., Anderson, J., Iezzon, L., Payne, S. & Restuccia, J. (1994). Small area variation in hospitalization rates: how much you see depends on how you look, *Medical Care* **32**, 189–201.

[14] Wong, G. & Mason, W.M. (1991). Contextually specific effects and other generalizations of the hierarchical linear model for comparative analysis, *Journal of the American Statistical Association* **86**, 487–503.

CONSTANTINE GATSONIS

Hill's Criteria for Causality

Despite philosophic criticisms of inductive **inference**, inductively oriented causal criteria have commonly been used to make such inferences. If a set of necessary and sufficient causal criteria could be used to distinguish causal from noncausal **associations** in **observational studies**, the job of the scientist would be eased considerably. With such criteria, all the concerns about the logic or lack thereof in causal inference could be forgotten: it would only be necessary to consult the checklist of criteria to see if a relation were causal. We know from philosophy that a set of sufficient criteria does not exist [3, 6]. Nevertheless, lists of causal criteria have become popular, possibly because they seem to provide a road map through complicated territory.

A commonly used set of criteria was proposed by **Sir Austin Bradford Hill** [1]; it was an expansion of a set of criteria offered previously in the landmark Surgeon General's report on Smoking and Health [11], which in turn were anticipated by the inductive canons of John Stuart Mill [5] and the rules of causal inference given by Hume [3]. Hill suggested that the following aspects of an association be considered in attempting to distinguish causal from noncausal associations: strength, consistency, specificity, temporality, biologic gradient, plausibility, coherence, experimental evidence, and analogy. The popular view that these criteria should be used for causal inference makes it necessary to examine them in detail:

Strength

Hill's argument is essentially that strong associations are more likely to be causal than weak associations because, if they could be explained by some other factor, the effect of that factor would have to be even stronger than the observed association and therefore would have become evident (*see* **Cornfield's Inequality**). Weak associations, on the other hand, are more easily explained by undetected **biases**. To some extent this is a reasonable argument, but, as Hill himself acknowledged, the fact that an association is weak does not rule out a causal connection. A commonly cited counterexample is the relation between cigarette smoking and cardiovascular disease.

Counterexamples of strong but noncausal associations are also not hard to find; any study with strong **confounding** illustrates the phenomenon. For example, consider the strong but noncausal relation between Down syndrome and birth rank, which is confounded by the relation between Down syndrome and maternal age. Of course, once the confounding factor is identified, the association is diminished by adjustment for the factor. These examples remind

us that a strong association is neither necessary nor sufficient for causality, nor is weakness necessary nor sufficient for absence of causality. In addition to these counterexamples, we have to remember that neither **relative risk** nor any other measure of association is a biologically consistent feature of an association; as described by many authors [4, 7], it is a characteristic of a study population that depends on the relative **prevalence** of other causes. A strong association serves only to rule out hypotheses that the association is entirely due to one weak unmeasured **confounder** or other source of modest bias.

Consistency

Consistency refers to the repeated observation of an association in different populations under different circumstances. Lack of consistency, however, does not rule out a causal association, because some effects are produced by their causes only under unusual circumstances. More precisely, the effect of a causal agent cannot occur unless the complementary component causes act, or have already acted, to complete a sufficient cause. These conditions will not always be met. Thus, transfusions can cause HIV infection but they do not always do so: the virus must also be present. Tampon use can cause toxic shock syndrome, but only when other conditions are met, such as presence of certain bacteria. Consistency is apparent only after all the relevant details of a causal mechanism are understood, which is to say very seldom. Even studies of exactly the same phenomena can be expected to yield different results simply because they differ in their methods and **random errors**. Consistency serves only to rule out hypotheses that the association is attributable to some factor that varies across studies.

Specificity

The criterion of specificity requires that a cause leads to a single effect, not multiple effects. This argument has often been advanced to refute causal interpretations of exposures that appear to relate to myriad effects, especially by those seeking to exonerate smoking as a cause of lung cancer. The criterion is wholly invalid, however. Causes of a given effect cannot be expected to lack other effects on any logical grounds. In fact, everyday experience teaches us repeatedly that single events or conditions may have many effects. Smoking is an excellent example: it leads to many effects in the smoker. The existence of one effect does not detract from the possibility that another effect exists. Thus, specificity does not confer greater validity to any causal inference regarding the exposure effect. Hill's discussion of this criterion for inference is replete with reservations, and many authors regard this criterion as useless and misleading [8, 9].

Temporality

Temporality refers to the necessity that the cause precede the effect in time. This criterion is unarguable, insofar as any claimed observation of causation must involve the putative cause C preceding the putative effect D. It does *not*, however, follow that a reverse time order is evidence against the hypothesis that C can cause D. Rather, observations in which C followed D merely shows that C could not have caused D in these instances; they provide no evidence for or against the hypothesis that C can cause D in those instances in which it precedes D.

Biologic Gradient

Biologic gradient refers to the presence of a monotone (unidirectional) **dose–response** curve. We often expect such a monotonic relation to exist. For example, more smoking means more carcinogen exposure and more tissue damage, hence more carcinogenesis. Such an expectation is not always present, however. The somewhat controversial topic of alcohol consumption and mortality is an example. Death rates are higher among nondrinkers than among moderate drinkers, but ascend to the highest levels for heavy drinkers. Because modest alcohol consumption can have beneficial effects on serum lipid profiles, such a J-shaped dose–response curve is at least biologically plausible.

Conversely, associations that do show a monotonic trend in disease frequency with increasing levels of exposure are not necessarily causal; confounding can result in a monotonic relation between a noncausal risk factor and disease if the confounding factor itself demonstrates a biologic gradient in its relation with disease. The noncausal relation between birth rank and Down syndrome mentioned above shows a biologic gradient that merely reflects the progressive

relation between maternal age and the occurrence of Down syndrome.

Thus the existence of a monotonic association is neither necessary nor sufficient for a causal relation. A nonmonotonic relation only conflicts with those causal hypotheses specific enough to predict a monotonic dose–response curve.

Plausibility

Plausibility refers to the biologic plausibility of the hypothesis, an important concern but one that is far from objective or absolute. Sartwell [9], emphasizing this point, cited the remarks of Cheever, in 1861, who was commenting on the etiology of typhus before its mode of transmission (via body lice) was known:

> It could be no more ridiculous for the stranger who passed the night in the steerage of an emigrant ship to ascribe the typhus, which he there contracted, to the vermin with which bodies of the sick might be infested. An adequate cause, one reasonable in itself, must correct the coincidences of simple experience.

What was to Cheever an implausible explanation turned out to be the correct explanation, since it was indeed the vermin that caused the typhus infection. Such is the problem with plausibility: it is too often not based on logic or data, but only on prior beliefs. This is not to say that biological knowledge should be discounted when evaluating a new hypothesis, but only to point out the difficulty in applying that knowledge.

The **Bayesian** approach to inference attempts to deal with this problem by requiring that one quantify, on a probability (0 to 1) scale, the certainty that one has in prior beliefs, as well as in new hypotheses. This quantification displays the dogmatism or open-mindedness of the analyst in a public fashion, with certainty values near 1 or 0 betraying a strong commitment of the analyst for or against a hypothesis. It can also provide a means of testing those quantified beliefs against new evidence [2]. Nevertheless, the Bayesian approach cannot transform plausibility into an objective causal criterion.

Coherence

Taken from the Surgeon General's report on Smoking and Health [11], the term *coherence* implies that a cause and effect interpretation for an association does not conflict with what is known of the natural history and biology of the disease. The examples Hill gave for coherence, such as the histopathologic effect of smoking on bronchial epithelium (in reference to the association between smoking and lung cancer) or the difference in lung cancer incidence by sex, could reasonably be considered examples of plausibility as well as coherence; the distinction appears to be a fine one. Hill emphasized that the absence of coherent information, as distinguished, apparently, from the presence of conflicting information, should not be taken as evidence against an association being considered causal. On the other hand, presence of conflicting information may indeed undermine a hypothesis, but one must always remember that the conflicting information may be mistaken or misinterpreted [12].

Experimental Evidence

It is not clear what Hill meant by experimental evidence. It might have referred to evidence from laboratory experiments on animals, or to evidence from human experiments. Evidence from human experiments, however, is seldom available for most epidemiologic research questions, and animal evidence relates to different species and usually to levels of exposure very different from those that humans experience. From Hill's examples, it seems that what he had in mind for experimental evidence was the result of removal of some harmful exposure in an intervention or prevention program, rather than the results of laboratory experiments [10]. The lack of availability of such evidence would at least be a pragmatic difficulty in making this a criterion for inference. Logically, however, experimental evidence is not a criterion but a test of the causal hypothesis, a test that is simply unavailable in most epidemiologic circumstances.

Although experimental tests can be much stronger than other tests, they are not as decisive as often thought, because of difficulties in interpretation. For example, one can attempt to test the hypothesis that malaria is caused by swamp gas by draining swamps in some areas and not in others to see if the malaria rates among residents are affected by the draining. As predicted by the hypothesis, the rates will drop in the areas where the swamps are drained. As Popper

emphasized, however, there are always many alternative explanations for the outcome of every experiment. In this example, one alternative, which happens to be correct, is that mosquitoes are responsible for malaria transmission.

Analogy

Whatever insight might be derived from analogy is handicapped by the inventive imagination of scientists who can find analogies everywhere. At best, analogy provides a source of more elaborate hypotheses about the associations under study; absence of such analogies only reflects lack of imagination or experience, not falsity of the hypothesis.

Conclusion

As is evident, the standards of epidemiologic evidence offered by Hill are saddled with reservations and exceptions. Hill himself was ambivalent about the utility of these "standards" (he did not use the word *criteria* in the paper). On the one hand he asked "in what circumstances can we pass from this observed *association* to a verdict of *causation?*" (original emphasis). Yet, despite speaking of verdicts on causation, he disagreed that any "hard-and-fast rules of evidence" existed by which to judge causation:

> None of my nine viewpoints [criteria] can bring indisputable evidence for or against the cause-and-effect hypothesis and none can be required as a *sine qua non.*

Actually, the fourth criterion, temporality, is a *sine qua non* for causality: If the putative cause did not precede the effect, that indeed is indisputable evidence that the observed association is not causal (although this evidence does not rule out causality in other situations, for in other situations the putative cause may precede the effect). Other than this one condition, however, which may be viewed as part of the definition of causation, there is no necessary or sufficient criterion for determining whether an observed association is causal.

Acknowledgment

This article is adapted from Chapter 2 of *Modern Epidemiology* 2nd Ed. [8], with permission from the publisher.

References

[1] Hill, A.B. (1965). The environment and disease: association or causation?, *Proceedings of the Royal Society of Medicine* **58**, 295–300.

[2] Howson, C. & Urbach, P. (1993). *Scientific Reasoning. The Bayesian Approach*, 2nd Ed. Open Court, LaSalle.

[3] Hume, D. (1978). *A Treatise of Human Nature* (originally published in 1739). Oxford University Press edition, with an Analytical Index by L. A. Selby-Bigge, published 1888. 2nd Ed. with text revised and notes by P.H. Nidditch, published 1978.

[4] MacMahon, B. & Pugh, T.F. (1967). Causes and entities of disease, in *Preventive Medicine*, D.W. Clark & B. MacMahon, eds. Little, Brown & Company, Boston.

[5] Mill, J.S. (1862). *A System of Logic, Ratiocinative and Inductive*, 5th Ed. Parker, Son and Bowin, London.

[6] Popper, K.R. (1968). *The Logic of Scientific Discovery*. Harper & Row, New York.

[7] Rothman, K.J. (1976). Causes, *American Journal of Epidemiology* **104**, 587–592.

[8] Rothman, K.J. & Greenland, S. (1997). *Modern Epidemiology*, 2nd Ed. Lippincott, Philadelphia, Chapter 8.

[9] Sartwell, P. (1960). On the methodology of investigations of etiologic factors in chronic diseases – further comments, *Journal of Chronic Diseases* **11**, 61–63.

[10] Susser, M. (1988). Falsification, verification and causal inference in epidemiology: reconsiderations in the light of Sir Karl Popper's philosophy, in *Causal Inference*, K.J. Rothman, ed. Epidemiology Resources, Inc., Boston.

[11] US Department of Health, Education and Welfare (1964). Smoking and Health: Report of the Advisory Committee to the Surgeon General of the Public Health Service, *Public Health Service Publication No. 1103*. Government Printing Office, Washington.

[12] Wald, N.A. (1985). Smoking, in *Cancer Risks and Prevention*, M.P. Vessey & M. Gray, eds. Oxford University Press, New York, Chapter 3.

(*See also* **Causation**)

KENNETH J. ROTHMAN &
SANDER GREENLAND

Hill, Austin Bradford

Born: July 8, 1897, in Hampstead, London, UK.
Died: April 18, 1991, in Cumbria, UK.

Austin Bradford Hill was Professor of Medical Statistics and Director of the Medical Research

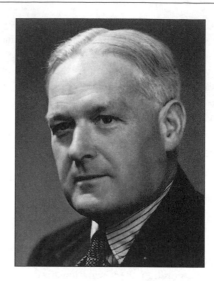

Reproduced by permission of the Royal Statistical Society

Council's Statistical Research Unit at the London School of Hygiene and Tropical Medicine, 1946–61; he introduced the principle of **randomization** into the conduct of controlled trials (*see* **Clinical Trials, Overview**) in clinical medicine and established particularly clearly the role of smoking in the production of lung cancer and, subsequently, many other diseases (*see* **Smoking and Health**). As a result of the experience gained in interpreting the observed association between smoking and lung cancer, Hill drew up "guidelines" to help reach a positive conclusion about causality that have come to be used widely in epidemiology and, on occasions, in the law (*see* **Hill's Criteria for Causality**).

Career

Hill, who was always known as Bradford Hill in scientific circles and as Tony to his friends, had wanted to study medicine, but he was diverted from doing so by the outbreak of World War I. He enlisted, at the first opportunity, in 1916 and opted for a commission in the Royal Naval Air Service. After being posted to the Greek islands in support of the attack on the Dardanelles, he developed pulmonary tuberculosis and, in November 1917, was invalided out of the service and sent home. Instead of causing his death, which was the anticipated outcome, the development of pulmonary tuberculosis probably saved his life, for the expectation of life of fighter pilots in World

War I was measured in weeks. The downhill progress of the disease was, however, arrested after he was given an artificial pneumothorax to rest his lung, and by 1919 he was sufficiently recovered to think again about his future. Medicine was out of the question and he decided to study economics as an external student of London University. With the aid of a correspondence course and by reading in bed, he succeeded in obtaining a second class honours degree in 1922, having attended the university itself only to take examinations.

Hill had no desire to make a career of economics and he managed to enter medicine with the help of **Major Greenwood**, a friend of his father and one of the few medical statisticians of the day. He obtained a grant from the **Medical Research Council** to investigate the reasons for the high mortality of young adults in rural areas and, whilst holding it, attended part of **Karl Pearson's** course on statistics for the London B.Sc. at University College. From then on he worked consistently with Greenwood in a variety of capacities in the conduct of epidemiologic research and, later, in the teaching of medical statistics at the London School of Hygiene and Tropical Medicine, where Greenwood had been appointed to the professorship of Medical Statistics. On the outbreak of World War II he was seconded to the Research and Experimental Department of the Ministry of Home Security and subsequently to the Medical Directorate of the Royal Air Force. In 1946 Greenwood retired and Hill was appointed to succeed him, both as professor at the School and as director of the MRC's unit.

Teaching Medical Statistics

Hill described himself as an arithmetician rather than a statistician, and it was the clarity of his exposition of simple arithmetic and statistical procedures and of the logic that justified conclusions from epidemiologic studies, combined with his sensitivity to the ethical concerns of practicing clinicians, that enabled him to influence British academic medicine as greatly as he did. From his first appointment at the London School of Hygiene in 1933 he found himself responsible for **teaching** the elements of statistics to medical postgraduates who, as a group, had little liking or aptitude for mathematics in any form. At that time, the need for some sort of statistical analysis had been recognized in the field of public health and had begun to be appreciated in laboratory medicine, but it was

hardly understood in clinical medicine at all. Hill responded, not by pressing the need for deferring to a statistical consultant, but by urging research workers in all branches of medicine to learn enough about statistical techniques to appreciate their value in both the planning of experiments (*see* **Experimental Design in Biostatistics**) and in the interpretation of figures and so to accept the statistician as a partner in their research, while the statistician, for his part, had to steep himself in the realities of medical practice. His lectures on medical statistics proved to be so effective that he was asked to publish them in a series of articles in the *Lancet* and to republish them in book form. The book, entitled *Principles of Medical Statistics*, was published in 1937 [4] and republished and expanded in a further 10 editions, some of which were translated into Spanish, Korean, Indonesian, Polish, and Russian, before a twelfth enlarged edition appeared shortly after his death, with his son, I.D. Hill, as joint author [8]. The fact that statistical analysis is now an integral part of almost every medical publication is a result of the work of many gifted statisticians throughout the world (*see* **Statistical Review for Medical Journals, Journal's Perspective**). The fact that the medical profession awoke to its need in the middle of the century was largely due to its exposition by Hill.

The Introduction of Randomization

In the first edition of his book, Hill made no reference to randomization in the planning of controlled trials. He urged only the need for concurrent controls, obtained, for example, by giving different treatment to alternate patients, a technique that had been recommended since the end of the nineteenth century, but was still the exception rather than the rule. This method was, however, far from ideal, as practice proved that a doctor's decision to enter a patient into a trial could be **biased** if he knew what treatment he or she would receive. Hill appreciated this, but he explained, shortly before his death, that he had deliberately omitted any reference to randomization in his 1937 articles

> because I was trying to persuade doctors to come into controlled trials in the very simplest form and I might have scared them off. I think the concepts of "randomization" and "random sampling numbers" are slightly odd to the layman or, for that matter, to the lay doctor, when it comes to statistics. I thought

it would be better to get doctors to walk first, before I tried to get them to run [6].

By the end of World War II, the situation had changed and Hill felt able to introduce physicians to the idea, and in 1946 he persuaded two committees of the Medical Research Council to adopt the method: first, to test the value of a pertussis vaccine to prevent whooping cough [11] and second, a few months later, to test the efficacy of streptomycin in the treatment of pulmonary tuberculosis (*see* **Medical Research Council Streptomycin Trial**) [10]. The results of the latter study were, however, published first and it is usually, but undeservedly, described as the first randomized clinical trial.

The idea of randomization in biological experiments was not new. It had been introduced by **R.A. Fisher** 20 years before as a basic principle of experimental design in agriculture; but it was unheard of in clinical medicine and was anathema on first presentation to many clinicians who thought it conflicted with their responsibility for doing the best they could for individual patients and resulted in beneficial effects being diluted by giving the new treatment to patients who were unsuitable for it. Neither objection was, of course, valid, as entry to the trial was in the clinician's own hands and required him or her not to know which was the better treatment and to exclude patients if they were thought to be unsuitable for either of the therapies under trial (*see* **Ethics of Randomized Trials; Medical Ethics and Statistics**). Gradually clinical opposition was overcome, largely, in the UK, as a result of Hill's emphasis on ethical considerations, which won the respect of practising clinicians, and within 10 years randomization had become the standard technique for the conduct of controlled clinical trials. Recent claims that randomization had been introduced earlier by others as, for example, in the trial of patients for the treatment of the common cold, do not bear close investigation [9].

Smoking and Lung Cancer

Of Hill's many epidemiologic studies the most outstanding are those that demonstrated the importance of cigarette smoking as a cause of lung cancer. In one, comparisons were made between the smoking habits of patients with lung cancer admitted to 20 London hospitals and the habits of other patients of the same sex and age admitted to the same hospitals with other diseases (*see* **Case–Control Study, Hospital-Based**). The results showed sharp differences between the two groups and led to the conclusion that cigarette smoking was an important cause of the disease [1]. This was not the first study to have shown that patients with lung cancer tended to have smoked more than other patients, but it was the first in which a firm conclusion about causality had been reached on logical grounds and it set out clearly the basis for it. The conclusion was not, however, widely accepted, and Hill set out to test it by means of a prospective study, in which information was obtained about the smoking habits of 40 000 British doctors, who were then followed to determine the mortality rates in different groups of men and women who smoked different amounts. Within a few years, results were obtained that were almost identical to those predicted from the case–control study [2, 3] and the validity of the earlier conclusion quickly came to be accepted. Neither the case–control study nor the prospective, or **cohort study** as it has come to be called, was the first of their type to have been carried out; but they set standards of design and analysis by which subsequent similar studies have come to be assessed.

Guidelines for Determining Causality

In reaching the conclusion that the association observed between smoking habits and the development of lung cancer reflected cause and effect, Hill had first to exclude chance, bias, and **confounding** as alternative explanations. The first two were not difficult to exclude, but the third was, and positive evidence had to be sought that would justify the choice of causality. Koch's postulates that had been valuable in determining the microbiological causes of infectious disease were not appropriate for other types of disease that could have multiple causes, and Hill suggested a set of guidelines to replace them, based on his experience in interpreting the results of his studies of lung cancer [5]. Only one feature had to be present (the temporal relationship of the suspected cause and its effect), none alone was conclusive, and Hill emphasized that the guidelines were no more than a help to constructive thought and that each case had to be considered on its merits. For this purpose, they have proved to have lasting value to both scientists and lawyers.

Hill, the Man

Hill was not a prolific writer of scientific papers. Apart from his lecture series on medical statistics and the many editions of his textbook, his bibliography lists only 140 publications, including 28 letters to journals and 13 reviews or historical notes [7]. His influence on British medicine was, however, disproportionately great; not only because of the importance of some of the papers, but because of his teaching, the advice he gave personally to the many individuals who sought it, and his contribution to the work of the Medical Research Council through membership of many committees and, in 1954, membership of the Council itself. In committee, he expressed his opinion cogently and firmly, but he never imposed it and he was, in consequence, always listened to with respect and his advice was almost always taken. In public he avoided controversy and, though distressed by Sir Ronald Fisher's attacks on his interpretation of the association between smoking and the development of lung cancer, he preferred to let the facts speak for themselves rather than embark on a public dispute. He took immense trouble over his lectures, which he gave without the use of visual aids and rehearsed so often and read so well that his audience often thought that he spoke without a text. Even those whose interest flagged were kept attentive by the occasional witty aside. As a department head, he kept his door open to any junior who sought his advice and he saw his job as providing the conditions under which his university and research staff could be most productive. No one who worked in his department ever wanted to leave, and it was only with the greatest difficulty that they could be persuaded to take up more senior positions elsewhere.

References

[1]   Doll, R. & Hill, A.B. (1950). Smoking and carcinoma of the lung. Preliminary report, *British Medical Journal* **2**, 739–748.

[2]   Doll, R. & Hill, A.B. (1954). The mortality of doctors in relation to their smoking habits. A preliminary report, *British Medical Journal* **1**, 1451–1455.

[3]   Doll, R. & Hill, A.B. (1956). Lung cancer and other causes of death in relation to smoking. A second report on the mortality of British doctors, *British Medical Journal* **2**, 1071–1076.

[4]   Hill, A.B. (1937). *Principles of Medical Statistics.* The Lancet, London.

[5]   Hill, A.B. (1965). The environment and disease: association or causation?, *Proceedings of the Royal Society of Medicine* **58**, 295–300.

[6]   Hill, A.B. (1990). Memories of the British Streptomycin Trial in Tuberculosis, *Controlled Clinical Trials* **11**, 77–79.

[7]   Hill, A.B. (1993). Bibliography: publications (in English) of Sir Austin Bradford Hill, *Statistics in Medicine* **12**, 797–806.

[8]   Hill, A.B. & Hill, I.D. (1991). *Bradford Hill's Principles of Medical Statistics.* Edward Arnold, London.

[9]   Medical Research Council Patulin Trials Committee (1944). Clinical trial of patulin in the common cold, *Lancet* **ii**, 373–374.

[10]   Medical Research Council Streptomycin in Tuberculosis Trials Committee (1948). Streptomycin treatment for pulmonary tuberculosis, *British Medical Journal* **2**, 769–782.

[11]   Medical Research Council Whooping-Cough Immunization Committee (1951). The prevention of whooping-cough by vaccination, *British Medical Journal* **1**, 1463–1471.

R. DOLL

Hinge *see* Exploratory Data Analysis

Histogram *see* Frequency Distribution

Historical Controls in Survival Analysis

The use of historical controls in treatment evaluation is a large and controversial topic, and a general discussion is given elsewhere (*see* **Bias from Historical Controls**). The purpose of this article is the more technical one of surveying current contributions to the centuries-old statistical tradition [10] of comparing the observed mortality of a study group with that expected under "standard" (historical) rates.

If the historical rates are derived from a specific statistical analysis, then the straightforward modern approach would usually be to formulate a general statistical model containing the current data as well as the historical information, and then simply test the hypothesis of equality of the relevant mortality rates, perhaps taking into account **covariates**. Partly because the historical information is not always available as concrete statistical estimators, but also to some extent motivated by tradition, there is considerable interest in rephrasing the question as "how would these individuals have survived had they been subject to standard (historical) conditions?" Note that the so-called Peters–Belson approach in regression analysis similarly predicts study group responses from a statistical model fitted only to a control group, and then compares observed with expected [3, 4, 7].

The next section recalls the classical calculation of **expected number of deaths** and contrasts it with a sometimes more easily interpretable calculation called the "prospective method", which however requires knowledge of the potential **censoring** time for each individual, including those who died during the study. The following section surveys several recent approaches to defining an expected survival curve, all of which have been illustrated through asymptotic statistical results of Nielsen [18], quoted later. The final sections briefly record some further topics and pitfalls in using **Cox regression models** in this area.

The "Prospective" and the "Person-years" Methods

Consider n independent individuals with survival functions $S_i = 1 - F_i$ and hazards $\lambda_i = F_i'/S_i$ (see **Survival Distributions and Their Characteristics**). Individual i is followed from u_i to t_i, where u_i and t_i here are taken as deterministic, and dies at X_i. If $D_i = I(u_i < X_i \le t_i)$, an indicator variable (see **Dummy Variables**) – and

$$A_i = \int_{u_i}^{X_i \wedge t_i} \lambda_i(s)\,\mathrm{d}s,$$

then defining

$$p_i = \frac{S_i(u_i) - S_i(t_i)}{S_i(u_i)},$$

it holds that

$$\mathrm{E}(D_i | X_i > u_i) = p_i = \mathrm{E}(A_i | X_i > u_i),$$

where the first equality is elementary, while the second requires a little calculation, or reference to the **counting process** approach to survival analysis.

The observed number of deaths is $D = \sum D_i$. There are two obvious ways of predicting the number of deaths that would have applied if individual i had death intensity λ_i, $i = 1, \dots, n$ [14].

The "*prospective*" method uses the expected number $\mathrm{E}(D) = \sum p_i$, which requires knowledge of the *potential follow-up time* t_i for all individuals, i.e. even for those who died before t_i. For many censoring patterns this is unrealistic.

The "**person-years**" method uses the total exposure $A = \sum A_i$. This has the correct expectation under the standard "historical" death rates, but it is biased if study rates differ from standard rates. The *total exposure A* is the classical *expected number of deaths* [10], and D/A is the classical *standardized mortality ratio* (see **Standardization Methods**). An important advantage of A is that it requires knowledge of the censoring times t_i only for the survivors ($X_i > t_i$).

Expected Survival Curves

Now generalize the purpose from calculating an expected number of deaths to calculating an expected survival curve [how would these patients have survived under standard (or historical) conditions?], where the standard or historical conditions are available as a survival curve $S_i(t)$ for each patient i individually, perhaps based on estimates in a regression model for survival data. The *direct adjusted survival curve* $\bar{S}(t)$ was discussed by Makuch [16], Gail & Byar [6], Markus et al. [17] and Thomsen et al. [19] as

$$\bar{S}(t) = \frac{1}{n} \sum S_i(t).$$

An important objection to the use of the direct adjusted survival function is that it does not take the realized censoring pattern into account – on the contrary, it depends strongly on an assumption of independent censoring and involves an averaging operation across the censoring pattern. Invoking each patient's *potential follow-up time*, Bonsel et al. [2] proposed what in continuous time would amount to the following estimator. Let $0 < f_1 < \dots < f_n$ be the potential follow-up times for the n patients, and define iteratively, for $f_j < t \le f_{j+1}$, *Bonsel's estimator,*

$$S_B(t) = S_B(f_j)\frac{\sum\limits_{j+1}^{n} S_i(t)}{\sum\limits_{j+1}^{n} S_i(f_j)}.$$

(A slightly different definition was proposed by Væth [21], cf. Thomsen et al. [20], Keiding [11], and Keiding & Thomsen [13].)

As was discussed earlier, in the simple context of expected number of deaths, it is often unrealistic to assume the potential follow-up times known (possible occurrence of ordinary loss to follow-up gives unknown potential follow-up times), and it may be preferable to base the calculation of the *expected survival curve*, S^*, on exposing each study individual to his/her standard mortality rate over the actually experienced period at risk. One such proposal [19] generalized the classical calculation of expected number of deaths as follows. Assume that the historical mortality is given as a Cox regression model so that patient i has hazard $\lambda_i(t) = \lambda_0(t)\exp(\boldsymbol{\beta}'\mathbf{z}_i)$. Let $Y_i(t) = I$ (patient i still at risk at time t), $Y(t) = \sum Y_i(t)$. Then, under the historical hypothesis on the mortality, the average hazard of the patients still under observation at time t would be

$$\lambda^*(t) = \sum Y_i(t)\lambda_0(t)\exp(\boldsymbol{\beta}'\mathbf{z}_i)/Y(t).$$

Defining the cumulative hazard as $\Lambda^*(t) = \int_{u=0}^{t} \lambda^*(u)\,du$, the survival function $S^*(t) = \exp[-\Lambda^*(t)]$ is a continuous-time version of the "expected survival rate" [5] or "expected survival curve" [9]. Andersen & Væth [1] pointed out that it has the following desirable property: let the standard Nelson–Aalen estimator of $\Lambda(t)$ be defined by

$$\hat{\Lambda}(t) = \sum_{T_j \leq t} \frac{1}{Y(T_j)},$$

where $T_1 < T_2 < \dots$ are the times of (observed) deaths. Then $\Lambda^*(t) - \hat{\Lambda}(t)$ has expectation zero, under the null hypothesis that patient i has hazard $\lambda_i(t)$. Therefore $S^*(t)$ represents, under the null hypothesis, an *expected survival curve*. Outside of the **null hypothesis** it is not so easy to interpret $S^*(t)$, containing as it does information on study group

mortality, through $Y_i(t)$, as well as standard mortality, through $\lambda_i(t)$. For similar reasons as explained earlier for the person-years method, $S^*(t)$ therefore cannot be recommended as an expected survival function, despite its wide use for this purpose.

$S^*(t)$ is, however, useful for inference on **excess mortality**, as follows. In the particular case where the study group has an *additive* excess mortality $\alpha(t)$ over the standard, that is, patient i has hazard $\alpha(t) + \lambda_i(t)$, one may obtain an estimate of the corresponding "survival" function

$$\exp\left[-\int_0^t \alpha(u)\,du\right]$$

as the so-called *relative* survival function $\hat{S}(t)/S^*(t)$. Andersen & Væth [1] showed that results on **unbiasedness, consistency**, and asymptotic normality are available. Thomsen et al. [19, 20] compared this "expected survival curve" to the previously discussed estimators.

These matters were discussed earlier by Hakulinen [8], who considered three estimators of "the expected survival rate". He divided the study population into homogeneous subgroups and considered a weighted average of the group-specific survival functions [his Eq. (2.2)] and the survival functions corresponding to the two different weighted averages of the standard mortality rates [his Eqs (2.3) and (2.4)]. When each subgroup consists of a single patient, his Eq. (2.2) equals the direct adjusted survival curve and his Eq. (2.3) equals S^*. Finally, the mortality rate in his Eq. (2.4) equals the mortality rate corresponding to Bonsel's estimator.

Nielsen's Asymptotic Results

Nielsen [18] considered the observed survival curve, $\hat{S}$, estimated by the **Kaplan–Meier** method, and estimated survival curves based on the Cox regression model. He showed the following asymptotic results under the null hypothesis of standard mortality, where $\|\cdot\|$ is $\sup_{\tau \leq t}|\cdot|$:

1. Under standard boundedness regularity conditions, $\|S^* - \hat{S}\| \xrightarrow{p} 0$.
2. Assume, in addition, conditional independence between survival time and censoring time given covariates; then $\|S_B - \hat{S}\| \xrightarrow{p} 0$.

3. Assume, in addition to the assumptions in 1 and 2, that the censoring times are identically distributed and marginally independent of covariates (and hence survival times); then $||\bar{S} - \hat{S}|| \xrightarrow{p} 0$.

Nielsen also proved asymptotic normality and gave martingale-based test statistics for the historical hypothesis (see **Convergence in Distribution and in Probability**).

Thus, the use of the direct adjusted survival curve requires marginally independent censoring, but no information about actual survival or potential follow-up is needed. In addition, it has the simple interpretation as the expected survival curve of the study population under standard mortality in absence of censoring. The use of Bonsel's method requires conditional independence and information on all potential follow-up times. S^* requires neither restrictive assumptions on the censoring pattern nor any knowledge of the potential follow-up times; only information about the actual time at risk is needed. However, the latter depends on both the actual survival of the study group and the standard mortality rates and, therefore, has no interpretation outside the null hypothesis.

Individual Comparison of Prognosis for New vs. Old Treatment

Keiding et al. [15] extended the above framework to also include a fitted regression model for the study patients. Under the Cox model for the historical hypothesis, the survival probability of patient i would be (in obvious notation)

$$S_H^i(t) = \exp[-\Lambda_H(t)\exp(\boldsymbol{\beta}_H'\mathbf{z}_i)],$$

while under the Cox model for current treatment, the survival probability would be

$$S_T^i(t) = \exp[-\Lambda_T(t)\exp(\boldsymbol{\beta}_T'\mathbf{z}_i)].$$

Since the prognostic indices $\boldsymbol{\beta}_H'z_i$ and $\boldsymbol{\beta}_T'z_i$ as well as the underlying intensities $\Lambda_H(t)$ and $\Lambda_T(t)$ will usually be rather different, the relative survival at time t,

$$\gamma_i(t) = S_H^i(t)/S_C^i(t),$$

will usually depend strongly on patient i and time t. Keiding et al. [15, Figure 5] proposed using $\gamma_i(t)$ as one aid in deciding on the best treatment for each individual patient, and developed a diagram to illustrate the rather dramatic variation of $\hat{\gamma}_i(t)$ when comparing transplantation to conservative treatment in a set of Nordic primary biliary cirrhosis patients (see **Prognostic Factors for Survival**).

Difficulties in Applying Non- or Semiparametric Models for the Historical Controls

Two largely unnoticed difficulties in applying the Cox regression model and similar non- or semiparametric models as historical controls concern the *interpretation of the time variable* in the underlying intensity and the use of **time-dependent covariates**.

The first point is most easily explained through specific reference to the transplantation example hinted to above. The model based on the historical data specifies that the death intensity at duration t after entrance into the clinical trials is $\lambda_0(t)\exp(\boldsymbol{\beta}'\mathbf{z})$. This is to be compared to survival *since transplantation* for the study patients. Patients would usually be assumed to be at a more advanced stage of disease at transplantation than at entry into a trial, so the conventional choice of $t = 0$ at transplantation (that is, underlying intensity $\lambda_0(t)$ at time t since transplantation) is ill-motivated. Only if $\lambda_0(t)$ is constant over t does the conventional application seem justified, and one ought indeed always to postulate this and (if possible) refit this parametric model to the historical data before the comparison.

The other difficulty is related to the use of time-dependent covariates, in particular when a natural time origin is available prior to the entry of the study patients. Delayed entry (left truncation) methods are then appropriate (see **Delayed Entry**) but, as pointed out by Keiding & Knuiman [12], it is then usually impossible to incorporate time-dependent covariates into the Cox regression model.

References

[1]   Andersen, P.K. & Væth, M. (1989). Simple parametric and nonparametric models for excess and relative mortality, *Biometrics* **45**, 523–535.

[2]   Bonsel, G.J., Klompmaker, I.J., van't Veer, F., Habbema, J.D.F. & Sloof, M.J.H. (1990). Use of prognostic models for assessment of value of liver transplantation in primary biliary cirrhosis, *Lancet* **335**, 493–497.

[3]   Cochran, W.G. (1969). The use of covariance in observational studies, *Applied Statistics* **18**, 270–275.

[4]   Cochran, W.G. & Rubin, D.B. (1973). Controlling bias in observational studies: a review, *Sankhyā, Series A* **35**, 417–446.

[5]   Ederer, F., Axtell, L.M. & Cutler, S.J. (1961). The relative survival rate: a statistical methodology, *National Cancer Institute Monographs* **6**, 101–121.

[6]   Gail, M.H. & Byar, D.B. (1986). Variance calculations for direct adjusted survival curves with applications to testing for no treatment effect, *Biometrical Journal* **28**, 587–599.

[7]   Gastwirth, J.L. & Greenhouse, S.W. (1994). Biostatistical concepts and methods in the legal setting, *Statistics in Medicine* **14**, 1641–1653.

[8]   Hakulinen, T. (1982). Cancer survival corrected for heterogeneity in patient withdrawal, *Biometrics* **38**, 933–942.

[9]   Hill, C., Laplanche, A. & Rezvani, A. (1985). Comparison of the mortality of a cohort with the mortality of a reference population in a prognostic study, *Statistics in Medicine* **4**, 295–302.

[10]   Keiding, N. (1987). The method of expected number of deaths, 1786–1886–1986, *International Statistical Review* **55**, 1–20.

[11]   Keiding, N. (1995). Historical controls and modern survival analysis, *Lifetime Data Analysis* **1**, 19–25.

[12]   Keiding, N. & Knuiman, M.W. (1990). Letter to the editor on "Survival analysis in natural history studies of disease" by A. Cnaan and L. Ryan, *Statistics in Medicine* **9**, 1221–1222.

[13]   Keiding, N. & Thomsen, B.L. (1998). Survival curves, Bonsel and Væth estimators of, in *Encyclopedia of Statistical Sciences Update*, Vol. 2, S. Kotz, C. Read & D. Banks, eds. Wiley, New York, to appear.

[14]   Keiding, N. & Væth, M. (1986). Calculating expected mortality, *Statistics in Medicine* **5**, 327–334.

[15]   Keiding, S., Ericzon, B.-G., Eriksson, S., Flatmark, A., Höckerstedt, K., Isoniemi, H., Karlberg, I., Keiding, N., Olsson, R., Samela, K., Schrumpf, E. & Söderman, C. (1990). Survival after liver transplantation of patients with PBC in the Nordic countries: comparison to expected survival from another series of transplantations and from an international trial of medical treatment, *Scandinavian Journal of Gastroenterology* **25**, 11–18.

[16]   Makuch, R.W. (1982). Adjusted survival curve estimation using covariates, *Journal of Chronic Diseases* **3**, 437–443.

[17]   Markus, B.H., Dickson, E.R., Grambsch, P.M., Fleming, T.R., Mazzaferro, V., Klintmalm, B.G.B., Wiesner, R.H., van Thiel, D.H. & Starzl, T.E. (1989). Efficacy of liver transplantation in patients with primary biliary cirrhosis, *New England Journal of Medicine* **320**, 1709–1713.

[18]   Nielsen, B. (1997). Expected survival in the Cox model, *Scandinavian Journal of Statistics* **24**, 275–287.

[19]   Thomsen, B.L., Keiding, N. & Altman, D.G. (1991). A note on the calculation of expected survival, *Statistics in Medicine* **10**, 733–738.

[20]   Thomsen, B.L., Keiding, N. & Altman, D.G. (1992). Reply to a letter to the editor, cf. Thomsen et al. (1991), *Statistics in Medicine* **11**, 1528–1529.

[21]   Væth, M. (1992). Letter to the editor re. Thomsen et al. (1991), *Statistics in Medicine* **11**, 1527–1528.

(*See also* **Survival Analysis, Overview**)

NIELS KEIDING

History of Biostatistics

From the seventeenth century to the present day, basic biologic phenomena (most notably mortality and morbidity) have been a central concern of those who collected and analyzed statistical data. For this reason, **John Graunt's** pioneering 1662 work *Observations upon the Bills of Mortality* sounds notes that are very similar in kind to biostatistical reports issued today – even though present-day statistical works make use of more sophisticated mathematical methods than their predecessors in earlier centuries. Consequently, the history of biostatistics can best be understood in terms of methodologic developments within statistical thinking. For analytical purposes, these methodologic developments can be divided into four phases: (i) the work of nineteenth-century statisticians who pioneered the concept that social patterns (including incidence of disease) could be shown to have "lawlike" characteristics [13, 15]; (ii) the mathematical work of **Karl Pearson** and his biometric associates at University College London in the early twentieth century; (iii) the interwar years when the methods of **hypothesis testing** (associated initially with the agricultural research of **R.A. Fisher**) were extended into the field of biomedicine; and (iv) the postwar rise of epidemiologic studies focusing on such celebrated discoveries as the association between cigarette smoking and lung cancer (*see* **Smoking and Health**) and the **Framingham study** of heart disease. Each of these four phases will be discussed in turn.

Nineteenth-Century Developments

As its name implies, statistics developed as a science concerned with information important to the state. With the rise of industrialization and democratic reforms in the early nineteenth century, Western governments became overwhelmed with what Hacking [7] has called an "avalanche of printed numbers" about their citizens, thereby leading writers to associate the term "statistics" specifically with information expressed in numeric form. One of the earliest examples from a biomedic context was **Bisset Hawkins'** [8] 1829 work *Elements of Medical Statistics*, which was concerned with "the application of numbers to illustrate the natural history of man in health and disease".

Throughout the course of the nineteenth century this numeric conception of statistics became institutionalized through the founding of statistical societies and the holding of international statistical conferences. In the English-speaking world, two of the most prominent societies were Section F of the British Association for the Advancement of Science (founded in 1833) and the Statistical Society of London (founded in 1834 (*see* **Royal Statistical Society**)). In both of these societies (and in many of the international conferences) one of the leading figures was the Belgian astronomer turned social statistician **Adolphe Quetelet** who helped to pioneer the concept that society had distinctly lawlike characteristics which could be revealed through the amassing of statistical evidence.

Most of the members of these statistical societies were not trained in the physical sciences like Quetelet; rather, they often came from the medical profession. As Lécuyer [10] has argued, several factors may account for the high proportion of physicians within these societies, namely the emergence of public health as a goal through the method of improved hygiene, the medical tradition of local investigation to improve the conditions of the poor, and the physicians' obvious professional association with the phenomena of death and sickness. All of these concerns lent themselves naturally to the amassing of numeric evidence.

In this period, two of the most prominent physicians to study public health problems statistically were the French physician, Louis René Villermé (1782–1863), and the English physician, **William Farr** (1807–1883). As William Coleman [4] has shown, Villermé corresponded with Quetelet as a result of their shared interest in describing society in numeric terms. In 1828, Villermé published a memoir positing a relationship between mortality and economic status, thereby firmly establishing his reputation as an advocate for a statistically based approach to public health problems. Similar concerns informed the work of William Farr who studied medicine in Paris under **P.-C.-A. Louis**, the advocate of the "numerical method". In 1839, Farr was appointed compiler of abstracts to the newly established General Register Office which had been founded to record all births and deaths within Great Britain. During Farr's long 41-year tenure at that institution, he made considerable contributions to the field of **vital statistics** and developed multiple disease and occupational taxonomies to be used in the collecting of statistical evidence (*see* **History of Health Statistics**).

The statistical record-keeping of individuals like Farr and his associates at the General Register Office proved to be indispensable for one of the major epidemiologic discoveries of the mid-nineteenth century, namely John Snow's [14] demonstration that cholera was a water-borne disease. After an outbreak of cholera near the Broad Street pump in London in 1854, Snow used data collected by the General Register Office to determine that there had been 83 deaths attributed to the disease during a three-day period. On closer examination Snow determined that in all but 10 of these cases the individuals had lived in households that were closer to the Broad Street pump than any other water source. Furthermore, in five of the households that could get water elsewhere, Snow interviewed the family members and discovered that they did indeed use the water from the Broad Street pump. Of the remaining five cases, three were children who probably also drank water emanating from this source since they attended a nearby school; the remaining two cases were dismissed by Snow as representing "only the amount of mortality from cholera that was occurring before the irruption took place". Although Snow's idea regarding the waterborne nature of cholera received little support during his lifetime (with the notable exception of William Farr), his paper has subsequently attained classic status as one of the most important epidemiologic discoveries prior to the discovery of the germ theory of disease.

The Biometrical School and the Mathematization of Statistics

Throughout the nineteenth century, statisticians conceived of their work as largely descriptive in nature with comparatively little emphasis placed on mathematical reasoning. This orientation was fundamentally changed by the creation of the biometrical school at University College London under the direction of the applied mathematician Karl Pearson (1857–1936). Pearson developed this school with the blessing (and financial backing) of the scientist **Francis Galton**, an English scientist who espoused the view that heredity played a decisive role in individual development. Thus, the primary *raison d'être* of Pearson's research was to provide scientific warrant to Galton's views through statistical analysis. Although Pearson clearly shared the views of his main financial backer, he also developed a full-blown philosophy of statistical reasoning arguing that, since all **inference** is based on the association of antecedents and consequents, all scientific reasoning is at its core fundamentally statistical. As a result, Pearson argued for the extension of statistical methods into potentially all domains of scientific endeavor, actively engaged in debates with other researchers over the proper interpretation of statistical data, and trained students in the biometric techniques that he pioneered.

In the field of biostatistics specifically, Pearson is remembered for engaging in a dispute with Alrmoth Wright (1861–1947) over the meaning of the statistics Wright had collected to demonstrate that antityphoid inoculation reduced the chance of infection for soldiers in the British Army. In critiquing Wright's conclusions, Pearson made use of one of the statistical constructs for which he is remembered today, namely the **correlation** coefficient, which was designed to measure the degree of association between two phenomena. Specifically, Pearson [12] found that the average correlation between immunity and inoculation was about 0.23, with individual results as high as 0.445 and as low as 0.021 (a one-to-one positive association would have generated a value of 1 and no relationship would have generated a value of 0). Since this was a very low correlation coefficient relative to other common therapeutic interventions (the protective character of vaccination at preventing mortality from smallpox was found to have a correlation coefficient of approximately 0.6), Pearson argued against the introduction of antityphoid inoculation as a standard practice. Although Pearson's criticisms did not convince the leaders of the British Army, who continued to test and use Wright's inoculation procedure, the episode is illustrative of Pearson's desire to show the applicability of his biometric techniques in the biomedical arena.

In addition to his theoretical innovations, Pearson was also important for training the physician **Major Greenwood** (1880–1949) in biometric methods; Greenwood launched his career by criticizing Wright's use of the so-called "opsonic index" for diagnostic purposes. Wright believed that there was a substance in blood serum (opsonin) which prepared bacteria to be ingested by the white blood corpuscles. Wright was able to measure the amount of opsonin that was present in the blood by comparing the average number of microbes per leucocyte in a blood sample from a normal individual with the average number of microbes per leucocyte from an individual suspected of having a bacterial infection; subsequently, Wright computed the ratio of these two mean values which he called the "opsonic index". In general, Wright believed that if the opsonic index were higher than 1.2 or lower than 0.8, then this would indicate bacterial infection. In his critique of Wright, Greenwood [6] plotted the **frequency distribution** of the number of microbes per leucocyte and found the distribution to be markedly asymmetric or skew. Thus, Greenwood advocated that the **mode**, or most frequently occurring value, would be a better constant with which to measure the opsonic index than the mean. Although Greenwood did not convince Wright, his work did succeed in impressing Charles James Martin who was then director of the Lister Institute of Preventive Medicine; late in 1909 Martin offered Greenwood a position as medical statistician at the Lister Institute thereby helping to legitimate the use of biometric techniques in the analysis of medical statistical results.

Greenwood was not the only individual to draw on Pearsonian methods to study biomedical phenomena; another prominent follower was **John Brownlee**. Brownlee [3] utilized Pearson's insight that the Gauss–Laplace or **normal distribution** curve was, in fact, just a particular case of an entire family of frequency distribution systems. By attempting to fit Pearson's various frequency distributions to medical statistics of disease incidence during an epidemic, Brownlee hoped to classify epidemics according to the type of frequency distributions they approximated; he often found that the type of distribution produced was nearly symmetric (*see* **Epidemic Curve**).

The Interwar Years and the Birth of Experimental Epidemiology

On both sides of the Atlantic the interwar years saw an attempt to forge a new and experimental approach to epidemiology. Rather than continuing to rely solely on vital statistics of human populations, systematic attempts were made to study the rise and fall of epidemic diseases within populations of laboratory animals – most notably mice. In the UK, this work was based at the **Medical Research Council** and consisted of a collaborative endeavor between the bacteriologist W.W.C. Topley and Major Greenwood; Greenwood had become head of the statistical research unit of the Medical Research Council in 1927. In the US, the principal investigator was L.T. Webster and his associates at the Rockefeller Institute. In both countries, researchers focused on mouse typhoid in an attempt to understand the relative importance of environment, host, and agent factors in disease occurrence.

In addition to these experiments on populations of laboratory animals, the interwar years also saw important theoretic developments in the methods of statistical **inference** as pioneered initially by Ronald A. Fisher. Whereas Pearson and the early biometricians had been associated primarily with classifying **observational** data, Fisher was more directly concerned with **experimental** data and **hypothesis testing**. Fisher developed his statistical ideas after being appointed to the Rothamsted Experimental Station where he studied the differing productivity of various types of grain in agricultural field experiments. Drawing on these scientific findings, Fisher published a series of books on statistical methodology. In his 1935 work *The Design of Experiments* [5], he outlined the key importance of **randomization** in assigning different grain types to various tracts of land in order to remove subjective experimenter **bias**.

Fisher's focus on randomization proved to have profound implications for research medicine – especially for the development of the modern **clinical trial** (*see* **History of Clinical Trials**). When faced with a shortage of the drug streptomycin during

World War II, **Austin Bradford Hill** (who had succeeded Greenwood as head of the statistical division of the Medical Research Council) chose to design a rigorous clinical trial of the effect of this drug on bilateral pulmonary tuberculosis. Bradford Hill used random numbers to determine which patients received the experimental drug and which patients were to be controls. Although the trial contained a relatively small number of patients (107 overall with 55 allocated to the streptomycin group and the remaining 52 allocated to the control group), Hill's attention to methodologic detail meant that the results were decisive: 7% of the streptomycin patients died and 27% in the control group died. As Hill and his associates [11] observed in the 1948 report on the trial, "The difference between the two series is statistically significant; the probability of it occurring by chance is less than one in a hundred" (*see* **Medical Research Council Streptomycin Trial**). Hill's streptomycin trial has often been seen as the standard against which all subsequent clinical trials have been judged.

The Rise of Postwar Epidemiology

Even though the study of epidemiology (or disease within populations) has a long history, the postwar era is significant in at least two respects: the use of more sophisticated statistical techniques in analyzing the etiology of disease; and the increasing shift in focus from infectious to chronic conditions. Although these twin facets of postwar epidemiology are distinguishable for analytical purposes, they actually were historically interwoven. With the transition from infectious to chronic disease as the principal reason for mortality and morbidity, research became centered less on the search for a specific agent (or germ) and more on the analysis of (multiple) environmental factors. Since multiple factors presented the problem of **confounding** causal relationships (*see* **Causation**), epidemiologists increasingly turned to the statistically trained who had dealt with similar issues in the context of social surveys. Of the many epidemiologic claims established through these methods, the two most famous examples were the researches establishing a link between cigarette smoking and lung cancer and the study of cardiovascular disease.

As discussed in Brandt [2], epidemiologic studies began to appear in the late 1940s and early 1950s indicating that cigarette smokers were at a higher risk of lung cancer than nonsmokers. Most of these studies were **retrospective** in nature – meaning that individuals who had already developed lung cancer were interviewed about their smoking habits after the fact; their responses were then compared with a control group of individuals who did not smoke (*see* **Case–Control Study**). However, two pioneering prospective studies were also launched at this time (*see* **Cohort Study**). In 1951, Richard Doll and Bradford Hill sent questionnaires to all British physicians inquiring about their smoking habits. When individuals who responded to their survey died, Doll and Hill obtained data about their cause of death. At about the same time, a similar study was being conducted in the US by E. Cuyler Hammond with the support of the American Cancer Society. Both studies implied conclusions consistent with retrospective studies: cigarette smoking increased one's risk of contracting cancer.

In the US, the most famous postwar epidemiologic investigation has been the Framingham Study, which was initiated in October 1947. As Susser [16] has argued, the Framingham Study has often been cited as the paradigmatic example of a prospective or "cohort study" which follows a specific group (or cohort) of individuals over their life courses to see what factors influence disease development. As its name implies, the researchers selected their study population from the residents of the town of Framingham, Massachusetts. By examining a sample of 30- to 59-year-old persons biennially, the researchers were able to test the role of such factors as cholesterol level, physical activity, diet, and life stress on the development of heart disease. In addition to specific empirical findings, the Framingham Study also generated important methodologic insights of how to deal with the variability of repeated measurements over time (*see* **Longitudinal Data Analysis, Overview**); however, the researchers could not solve the problem of when to terminate the study. As a result, more recent findings have centered on diseases related to aging (e.g. stroke) and follow-up studies of the offspring of the original participants.

Since the 1960s, several factors gave increasing prominence to statistically based ways of studying biomedic phenomena. After the Thalidomide scandal raised the specter of infant deformity, the clinical trial became a standard requirement before experimental drugs could be administered to the general public.

In 1965, the *American Journal of Hygiene* changed its name to the *American Journal of Epidemiology* [1] reflecting the "greatly increased importance" of the "epidemiologic approach to disease". Finally, the discipline of epidemiology was put on a secure conceptual foundation by researchers on both sides of the Atlantic who articulated causality criteria for epidemiologic studies; these criteria were designed to serve as the chronic disease analog to Robert Koch's famous postulates for establishing causality for infectious disease. In the US, the most famous list of epidemiologic causality criteria was published as part of the Surgeon-General's 1964 [17] report positing a link between cigarette smoking and lung cancer; in the UK, the most famous list of causality criteria was published by Austin Bradford Hill [9] early in 1965 (*see* **Hill's Criteria for Causality**).

References

[1]   "Change in Name" (1965). *American Journal of Epidemiology* **81**, 1.

[2]   Brandt, A.M. (1990). The cigarette, risk, and American culture, *Daedalus: Journal of the American Academy of Arts and Sciences* **119**, 155–176.

[3]   Brownlee, J. (1918). Certain aspects of the theory of epidemiology in special relation to plague, *Proceedings of the Royal Society of Medicine (Section Epidemiology and State Medicine)* **11**, 85–132.

[4]   Coleman, W. (1982). *Death is a Social Disease: Public Health and Political Economy in Early Industrial France*. University of Wisconsin Press, Madison.

[5]   Fisher, R.A. (1935). *The Design of Experiments*. Oliver & Boyd, Edinburgh

[6]   Greenwood, M. (1909). A statistical view of the opsonic index, *Proceedings of the Royal Society of Medicine* **2**, 145–155.

[7]   Hacking, I. (1987). Was there a probabilistic revolution, 1800–1930?, in *The Probabilistic Revolution: Ideas in History*, Vol. 1, L. Krüger, L.J. Daston & M. Heidelberger, eds. MIT Press, Cambridge, Mass., pp. 45–55.

[8]   Hawkins, B. (1829). *Elements of Medical Statistics*. Longman, Rees, Orme, Brown & Green, London.

[9]   Hill, A.B. (1965). The environment and disease: association or causation?, *Proceedings of the Royal Society of Medicine* **58**, 295–300.

[10]   Lécuyer, B.-P. (1987). Probability in vital and social statistics: Quetelet, Farr, and the Bertillons, in *The Probabilistic Revolution: Ideas in History*, Vol. 1, L. Krüger, L.J. Daston & M. Heidelberger, eds. MIT Press, Cambridge, Mass., pp. 317–335.

[11]   Medical Research Council Streptomycin in Tuberculosis Trials Committee (1948). Streptomycin treatment

of pulmonary tuberculosis, *British Medical Journal* **2**, 769–782.

[12]   Pearson, K. (1904). Report on certain enteric fever inoculation statistics, *British Medical Journal* **2**, 1243–1246.

[13]   Porter, T.M. (1986) *The Rise of Statistical Thinking, 1820–1900*. Princeton University Press, Princeton.

[14]   Snow, J. (1855). *On the Mode of Communication of Cholera*, 2nd Ed. London.

[15]   Stigler, S.M. (1986) *The History of Statistics: The Measurement of Uncertainty Before 1900*. The Belknap Press of Harvard University Press, Cambridge, Mass.

[16]   Susser, M. (1985). Epidemiology in the United States after World War II: the evolution of technique, *Epidemiologic Reviews* **7**, 147–177.

[17]   US Department of Health, Education, and Welfare (1964). *Surgeon General's Report, Smoking and Health: Report of the Advisory Committee to the Surgeon General of the Public Health Service*, PHS Publication No. 1103. Government Printing Office, Washington.

J.R. MATTHEWS

History of Clinical Trials

Aspects of the history of **clinical trials** have been reviewed by, among others, Bull [10], Lilienfeld [49], Armitage [4], Meinert [59], and Gail [31]. In this article we survey the historical progression toward the modern clinical trial, as this method of research is practiced at the end of the twentieth century, by tracing the development of five of its requisite elements: **controls** (a comparison group), **randomization, blinding or masking, ethics**, and interim statistical analysis (*see* **Data and Safety Monitoring**).

Controls

The essence of the clinical trial is the control group, which provides the basis for comparing the outcomes of two or more treatments. The comparative concept of assessing therapeutic efficacy has been known from ancient times. Lilienfeld [49] cites a description of a nutritional experiment involving a control group in the Book of Daniel from the Old Testament:

1.   In the third year of the reign of Jehoiakim king of Judah came Nebuchadnezzar king of Babylon unto Jerusalem, and besieged it...

2.   And the king spoke unto Ashpenaz his chief officer, that he should bring in certain of the children of Israel, and of the seed royal, and of the nobles...

5.   And the king appointed for them a daily portion of the king's food and of the wine which he drank that they should be nourished for three years...

8.   But Daniel purposed in his heart that he would not defile himself with the king's food, nor with the wine which he drank; therefore he requested of the chief of the officers that he might not defile himself...

10. And, the chief of officers said unto Daniel: "I fear my lord the king who hath appointed your food and your drink; for why should he see your faces sad in comparison with the youths of your own age?"...

11. Then said Daniel to the steward...

12. Try thy servants, I beseech thee, ten days; and let them give us pulse (leguminous plants) to eat and water to drink...

13. Then let our countenances be looked upon before thee, and the countenances of the youths that eat of the king's food...

14. So, he hearkened unto them and tried them in this matter, and tried them ten days...

15. And at the end of ten days their countenances appeared fairer, and they were fatter in the flesh, than all the youths that did eat of the king's food [72].

In this early example of a clinical trial, we note the presence not merely of a control group, but of a concurrent control group. These fundamental elements of clinical research did not begin to be widely practiced until the latter half of the twentieth century.

There appear to be no other recorded examples of thinking in comparative terms about the outcome of medical treatment in ancient or medieval times. Lilienfeld [49] provides an example from the fourteenth century, a letter from Petrarch to Boccaccio:

I solemnly affirm and believe, if a hundred or a thousand of men of the same age, same temperament and habits, together with the same surroundings, were attacked at the same time by the same disease, that if one followed the prescriptions of the doctors of the variety of those practicing at the present day, and that the other half took no medicine but relied on Nature's instincts, I have no doubt as to which half would escape [78].

The Renaissance provides an example of an unplanned experiment in the treatment of battlefield wounds. The surgeon Ambroise Paré was using the standard treatment of pouring boiled oil over the wound during the battle to capture the castle of Villaine in 1537. When he ran out of oil, he resorted to the alternative of a digestive made of egg yolks, oil of roses, and turpentine. The superiority of the new treatment became evident the next day.

> I raised myself very early to visit them, when beyond my hope I found those to whom I applied the digestive medicament feeling but little pain, their wounds neither swollen nor inflamed, and having slept through the night. The others to whom I had applied the boiling oil were feverish with much pain and swelling about their wounds. Then I determined never again to burn thus so cruelly by arquebusses [63] (as cited in [10]).

An oft-cited eighteenth-century example of a planned controlled clinical trial is the ship-board experiment in which Lind found oranges and lemons to be the most effective of six dietary treatments for scurvy.

> On the 20th of *May*, 1747, I took twelve patients in the scurvy, on board the *Salisbury* at sea. Their cases were as similar as I could have them. They all in general had putrid gums, the spots and lassitude, with weakness of their knees. They lay together in one place, being a proper apartment for the sick in the fore-hold; and had one diet common to all, viz. water-gruel sweetened with sugar in the morning; fresh mutton-broth often times for dinner; at other times puddings, boiled biscuit with sugar etc. And for supper, barley and raisins, rice and currants, sago and wine, or the like. Two of these were ordered each a quart of cyder a day. Two others took twenty-five gutts of *elixir vitriol* three times a day, upon an empty stomach; using a gargle strongly acidulated with it for their mouths. Two others took two spoonfuls of vinegar three times a day, upon an empty stomach; having their gruels and their other food well acidulated with it, as also the gargle for their mouths. Two of the worst patients, with the tendons in the ham rigid (a symptom none of the rest had) were put under a course of sea-water. Of this they drank half a pint every day, and sometimes more or less as it operated, by way of gentle physic. Two others had each two oranges and one lemon given them every day. These they eat with greediness, at different times, upon an empty stomach. They continued but six days under this course, having consumed the quantity that could be spared. The two remaining patients, took the bigness of a nutmeg three times a day of an electuary recommended by a hospital-surgeon, made of garlic, mustard-feed,

> *rad. raphan*, balsam of *Peru*, and gum myrrh; using for common drink barley-water well acidulated with tamarinds; by a decoction of which, with the addition of *cremor tartar*, they were greatly purged three or four times during the course.
> The consequence was, that the most sudden and visible good effects were perceived from the use of the oranges and lemons; one of those who had taken them, being at the end of six days fit for duty. The spots were not indeed at that time quite off his body, nor his gums sound; but without any other medicine, than a gargle of *elixir vitriol*, he became quite healthy before we came into Plymouth, which was on the 16th June. The other was the best recovered of any in his condition; and being now deemed pretty well, was appointed nurse, to the rest of the sick [50] (as cited in [10], [37], [49], and [59]).

Pierre-Charles-Alexandre Louis, a nineteenth-century clinician and pathologist, introduced the "numerical method" for comparing treatments. His idea was to compare the results of treatments on groups of patients with similar degrees of disease, i.e. to compare "like with like":

> I come now to therapeutics, and suppose that you have some doubt as to the efficacy of a particular remedy: How are you to proceed?... You would take as many cases as possible, of as similar a description as you could find, and would count how many recovered under one mode of treatment, and how many under another; in how short a time they did so; and if the cases were in all respects alike, except in the treatment, you would have some confidence in your conclusions; and if you were fortunate enough to have a sufficient number of facts from which to deduce any general law, it would lead to your employment in practice of the method which you had seen oftenest successful [51] (as cited in [10], [49], [3], and [59]).

It remained for **Bradford Hill** more than a century later to use a formal method for creating groups of cases that were "in all respects alike, except in the treatment".

Randomization

The use of randomization as a scientific tool was a brilliant contribution by the famous statistician **Ronald A. Fisher** [22, 23]. Fisher's early applications of randomization were in agriculture. To determine which fertilizers effected the greatest crop yields, Fisher divided agricultural areas into plots, and randomly assigned the plots to experimental fertilizers. A goal of Fisher's was to obtain, through independent replications, a valid test of statistical significance (*see* **Randomization Tests**). In previous systematic designs, the fertilities of adjoining plots, to which different treatments had been applied, were not independent.

In clinical trials there were early schemes to use "**group randomization**": after dividing the patients into two groups, the treatment for each group was randomly selected. This method does not involve replication, and therefore precludes estimation of error. Armitage [3] cites a challenge based on the notion of random assignment, though not of individuals, issued as early as 1662 by the Belgian medicinal chemist van Helmont:

> Let us take out of the hospitals, out of the Camps, or from elsewhere, 200, or 500 poor People that have Fevers, Pleurisies, &c, Let us divide them into halfes, let us cast lots, that one half of them may fall to my share, and the others to yours,... we shall see how many funerals both of us shall have: *But* let the reward of the contention or wager, be 300 florens, deposited on both sides [75].

Group randomization was used by Amberson et al. in a trial of sanocrysin in the treatment of pulmonary tuberculosis published in 1931 [1].

A great step forward was the use of systematic assignment by Fibiger [21], who alternately assigned diphtheria patients to serum treatment or an untreated control group. As noted by Armitage [3], alternate assignment "would be deprecated today on the grounds that foreknowledge of the future treatment allocations may selectively bias the admission of patients into the treatment groups". Diehl et al. [18] reported in 1938 a common cold vaccine study with University of Minnesota students as subjects:

> At the beginning of each year... students were assigned at random... to a control group or an experimental group. The students in the control groups... received placebos... All students thought they were receiving vaccines... Even the physicians who saw the students... had no information as to which group they represented.

Gail [31] points out that, although on its face this appears to be the first published report of a modern randomized clinical trial, a typewritten manuscript by Diehl clarifies that this is another instance of systematic assignment:

> At the beginning of the study, students who volunteered to take these treatments were assigned alternately and without selection to control groups and experimental groups.

Hill, in the study of streptomycin in pulmonary tuberculosis [53], used random sampling numbers in assigning treatments to subjects in clinical trials, so that the subject was the unit of randomization (*see* **Medical Research Council Streptomycin Trial**). This study is now generally acknowledged to be the "first properly randomized clinical trial" [3]. It is of interest to note, as did Meier [58], that what Fisher saw important in randomization was that it made possible a valid test of significance (*see* **Hypothesis Testing**), whereas what Hill found important was the creation of comparable groups.

After the streptomycin-pulmonary tuberculosis trial, Bradford Hill and the British **Medical Research Council** continued with further randomized trials: chemotherapy of pulmonary tuberculosis in young adults [55], antihistaminic drugs in the prevention and treatment of the common cold [54], cortisone and aspirin in the treatment of early cases of rheumatoid arthritis [56, 57], and long-term anticoagulant therapy in cerebrovascular disease [39].

In the US, the **National Institutes of Health** followed the lead of the British Medical Research Council, starting in 1951 its first randomized trial [34], a National Heart Institute study of ACTH, cortisone, and aspirin in the treatment of rheumatic heart disease [68] (*see* **Clinical Trials, Early Cancer and Heart Disease**). This was followed in 1954 by a randomized trial of retrolental fibroplasia (now known as retinopathy of prematurity), sponsored by the National Institute of Neurological Diseases and Blindness [44]. In that same year, members of the US Congress asked officials of the National Cancer Institute to organize a comprehensive program for research in cancer chemotherapy, which led the next year to the development of a rapidly growing program of clinical trials under the Cancer Chemotherapy National Service Center [32]. By fiscal year 1986, the annual cost of randomized clinical trials sponsored by 10 categorical institutes of the National Institutes of Health amounted to 300 million dollars; the National Cancer Institute bore 58% of that cost [35]. During the four decades following the pioneering trials of the 1940s and 1950s, there was a large growth in the number of randomized trials not only in Britain and the US, but also in Canada and on the European continent. This growth gave impetus to the formation in the 1970s of two societies, the **International Society of Clinical Biostatistics** and the Society for Clinical Trials, and the publication of two new journals, **Controlled Clinical Trials** and **Statistics in Medicine**.

Masking

The purpose of masking, or blinding, in experiments is to prevent personal **bias** from influencing study observations. An awareness that personal bias can affect observation and judgment has existed for at least 400 years. Francis Bacon (1561–1626) noted "for what a man would like to be true, he more readily believes" [5]. Investigator bias caused a remarkable scientific delusion in the early years of the twentieth century: n-rays [76]. N-rays were "discovered" in 1902 by the eminent French physicist Blondlot, who in *Comptes rendus*, the leading French scientific journal, reported properties of these rays that far transcended those of X-rays. According to Blondlot, n-rays were given off spontaneously by many metals, such as copper, zinc, lead, and aluminum, and when the rays fell upon the eye, they increased the eye's ability to see objects in a nearly dark room. The existence of n-rays was soon confirmed in laboratories in various parts of France, and a number of noted French scientists soon applied n-rays to research in chemistry, botany, physiology, and neurology. In 1904, *Science Abstracts* listed 77 n-ray papers. The French Academy awarded Blondlot the Lalande prize of 20 000 francs and its gold medal "for the discovery of n-rays". That same year, however, the American Physicist R.W. Wood visited Blondlot in his laboratory to test the experiments:

> He [Blondlot] first showed me a card on which some circles had been painted in luminous paint. He turned down the gas light and called my attention to their increased luminosity when the n-ray was turned on. I said that I saw no change. He said that was because my eyes were not sensitive enough, so that proved nothing. I asked him if I could move an opaque lead screen in and out of the path of the rays while he called out the fluctuations of the screen. He was almost 100 percent wrong and called out fluctuations when I made no movement at all, and that proved a lot, but I held my tongue. He then showed me the dimly lighted clock, and tried to convince me that I could see the hands when he held a large flat file just above his eyes. I asked if I could hold the file, for

I had noticed a flat wooden ruler on his desk, and remembered that wood was one of the substances that *never* emitted n-rays. He agreed to this, and I felt around for the ruler and held it in front of his face. Oh, yes, he could see the hands perfectly. This also proved something [70, 76].

After Wood published his account, n-ray publications diminished in number. *Science Abstracts* listed only eight n-ray papers in 1905, and none in 1909. The French Academy changed its announced reason for the award to Blondlot "for his life work taken as a whole". According to Seabrook [70], the exposure of the blunder led to Blondlot's madness and death.

A masked experiment by the Austrian physicist Pozdena contributed to the disproof of the existence of n-rays. At haphazard intervals Pozdena's assistant soundlessly operated a shutter which in its closed position blocked the transmission of the hypothetical n-rays. During a pretest, the assistant wrote "o" for *offen* (open) and "g" for *geschlossen* (closed) while Pozdena indicated when he could detect increased luminosity. Whereas the shutter's movements were silent, the assistant's pencil scratches were not. Pozdena was able to hear the difference between an "o" and a "g". In the definitive experiment the assistant switched to a coded notation, and in 150 trials Pozdena reported increased luminosity about as often when the shutter was open as when it was closed [67].

The common cold vaccine study published by Diehl et al. [18] in 1938 cited earlier, in which University of Minnesota students were alternately assigned to vaccine or placebo, was a masked clinical trial.

> The students in the control groups . . . received placebos . . . All students thought they were receiving vaccines . . . Even the physicians who saw the students . . . had no information as to which group they represented.

Masking was used in the early Medical Research Council trials in which Bradford Hill was involved. Thus, in the first of those trials, the study of streptomycin in tuberculosis, the X-ray films were

> viewed by two radiologists and a clinician, each reading the films independently and not knowing if the films were of C [bed-rest alone] or S [streptomycin and bed-rest] cases [53].

Hill's lesson from the experience:

If it [the clinical assessment of the patient's progress and of the severity of the illness] is to be used effectively, without fear and without reproach, the judgments must be made without any possibility of bias, without any overcompensation for any possible bias, and without any possible accusation of bias [37].

In the second trial, the antihistamine–common cold study [54], placebos ("dummies indistinguishable" from the drug under test) were used. Hill's lesson:

...in [this] trial..., feelings may well run high in the bosom (or should I say the mucosa?) either of the recipient of the drug or the clinical observer, or indeed of both. If either were allowed to know the treatment that had been given, I believe that few of us would without qualms accept that the drug was of value – if such a result came out of the trial [37].

The terms "blind" and "double-blind" have been used commonly in clinical trials, the latter indicating that neither the doctor nor the patient knows what treatment the patient is getting. When these terms were recognized as being awkward in trials of eye disease, the terms "masking" and "double-masking" were introduced [19].

Ethics

Medical Research Abuses

Experimentation in medicine is as old as medicine itself, and since antiquity some experiments on humans have been conducted without concern for the welfare of the subjects, who were often prisoners or disadvantaged people [52]. Thus, in the flourishing days of intellectual and scientific achievement in ancient Alexandria, anatomists used criminals for dissection alive [6]. Katz [42] provides examples of 19th century studies in Russia and Ireland of the consequences of infecting persons with syphilis and gonorrhea. During the same time, in the US,

physicians put slaves into pit ovens to study heat stroke, and poured scalding water over them as an experimental cure for typhoid fever. One slave had two fingers amputated in a "controlled trial", one finger with anesthesia and one finger without, to test the effectiveness of anesthesia [52].

Unethical experiments on human beings have continued into the twentieth century [7, 24, 52]. In

1932 the US Public Health Service began a study in Tuskegee, Alabama, of the natural progression of untreated syphilis in 400 black men. The study continued until 1972, when a newspaper reported that the subjects were uninformed or misinformed about the purpose of the study. Participants were told that painful lumbar punctures were given as treatment, when in fact treatment for syphilis was withheld even after penicillin became available [24].

During the Nazi regime, 1933–1945, German doctors conducted sadistic medical experiments, mainly on Jews, but also on Gypsies, mentally disabled persons, Russian prisoners of war, and Polish concentration camp inmates:

The "experiments" were quite varied. Prisoners were placed in pressure chambers and subjected to high-altitude tests until they stopped breathing. They were injected with lethal doses of typhus and jaundice. They were subjected to "freezing" experiments in icy water or exposed naked in the snow outdoors until they froze to death. Poison bullets were tried out on them as was mustard gas... [71].

Codes of Ethics, Informed Consent

The fact that in 1931, two years before the Nazis acceded to power, Germany had enacted "Richtlinien" (regulations) to control human experiments adds irony to the German doctors' cruel abuse and exploitation of human subjects.

Issued by the Reich's Health Department, these regulations remained binding law throughout the period of the Third Reich. Consent requirements formed two of fourteen major provisions in the guidelines, one dealing with "New Therapy" and the other with "Human Experimentation". It was demanded that in both cases consent (first party or proxy consent, as appropriate) must always be given "in a clear and undebatable manner" [20].

The Nazi doctors were tried for their atrocities by the Allied Forces in 1946–1947 at Nuremberg. Three US judges at the trial promulgated the Nuremberg Code [47], the first international effort to codify ethical principles of clinical research. Principle 1 of the Nuremberg Code states:

The voluntary consent of the human subject is absolutely essential. This means that the person involved should have legal capacity to give consent; should be so situated as to be able to exercise free power of choice, without the intervention of any element of force, fraud, deceit, duress, over-reaching, or other ulterior form of constraint or coercion; and should have sufficient knowledge and comprehension of the elements of the subject matter involved as to enable him to make an understanding and enlightened decision [74] (cited in [47, Appendix 3]).

Other principles of the Code are that the experiment should yield results for the good of society, that unnecessary suffering and injury should be avoided, and that the subject should be free to end the experiment.

Informed consent (*see* **Ethics of Randomized Trials**) was used by Walter Reed in his studies of yellow fever at the turn of the twentieth century [6, 69]. Mosquitoes were known to be involved in the transmission of the disease, but their precise role was not clear. To clarify the mode of transmission, members of Reed's research team had themselves been bitten by mosquitoes. After a fellow worker died of yellow fever from a purposeful bite, Reed recruited American servicemen and Spanish workers for the experiments, and drew up a contract with the Spanish workers:

> The undersigned understands perfectly well that in the case of the development of yellow fever in him, that he endangers his life to a certain extent but it being entirely impossible to avoid the infection during his stay on this island he prefers to take the chance of contracting it intentionally in the belief that he will receive... the greatest care and most skillful medical service [6, 69].

The contract specified that volunteers would each receive $100 in gold, and a $100 bonus if they contracted yellow fever. In the event 25 volunteers became ill, but none died.

In addition to Reed, other early advocates of informed consent were Charles Francis Withington and William Osler. Withington, noting in 1886 the "possible conflict between the interests of medical science and those of the individual patient", sided with "the latter's indefensible rights" [77]. Osler in 1907 insisted on informed consent in medical experiments: "For man absolute safety and full consent are the conditions which make such tests allowable" [62]. Despite this early advocacy, and despite the promulgation of the 1931 German doctors' code and the 1946–1947 Nuremberg Code, the application of informed consent to medical experiments did not take

foothold during the first six decades of the twentieth century. Bradford Hill [38], based on his experience in a number of early randomized clinical trials sponsored by the Medical Research Council, believed that it was not feasible to draw up a detailed code of ethics for clinical trials that would cover the variety of ethical issues that came up in these studies, and that the patient's consent was not warranted in all clinical trials. Although the judges at Nuremberg evidently intended the Code to apply not only to the case before them, but "for the practice of human experimentation wherever it is conducted" [43], European and American clinical investigators were slow to adopt it [7]. Gradually the medical community came to recognize the need to protect the reputation and integrity of medical research. In 1955 a human experimentation code was adopted by the Public Health Council in the Netherlands [60], cited in [15], and in 1964 the World Medical Association issued the Declaration of Helsinki [47], essentially adopting the ethical principles of the Nuremberg Code, with consent "a central requirement of ethical research" [20].

Justification to Begin

The view of Bradford Hill [38] was that in starting a randomized clinical trial the doctor accepts that "he really has no knowledge that one treatment [in the trial] will be better or worse [than the other treatments]". This state of uncertainty, which has come to be known as "equipoise" [28], has remained the ethical standard for starting a randomized clinical trial. For completeness, Levine [47] has added the proviso that there must not be a treatment, other than those to be studied in the trial, that is known to be superior to the study treatments.

Peer Review

One can trace back to 1803 the notion that therapeutic innovation must be preceded by peer review:

> And no such trials [of new remedies and new methods of chirurgical treatment] should be instituted, without a previous consultation of the physicians or surgeons ... [64] (cited in [47]).

According to Levine [47], "not much more was said about peer review for about 150 years".

Research ethics committees, the US history of which is traced by McNeill [52] and Levine [48], came into being in the US in the 1950s. The 1946–1947 Nuremberg Code and the 1964 Declaration of Helsinki do not mention committee review. A requirement for such review was imposed in 1953 at the newly established Clinical Center at the National Institutes of Health, and peer review of clinical research was also practiced at some US medical schools in the 1950s. By the early 1960s, one-third of US university medical schools responding to a survey had established research ethics committees. Public outrage at highly publicized research abuses, such as those published by Beecher [7], or those committed in the Tuskegee syphilis study, gave impetus to the adoption of requirements for informed consent and peer review in research on human beings in the US [52]. In 1966 the US Public Health Service issued a policy requiring recipients of Public Health Service research grants to provide for prior committee review of studies involving human subjects to ensure that the study plans conform to ethical standards. Because the Public Health Service was then (and still is) sponsoring a large majority of medical research in the US, research ethics committees were established at medical schools throughout the US soon after 1966. National recommendations, guidelines, or regulations for the establishment of research ethics committees in other countries soon followed: Canada in 1966, the UK in 1967, Australia in 1973, New Zealand in 1975, and Ireland in 1987 [52].

Data Monitoring by Peers

In the modern randomized clinical trial, the accumulating data are usually monitored for safety and efficacy by an independent *data monitoring committee* – also called *data and safety monitoring committee*, or **data and safety monitoring board**. In 1968 the first such committee was established, serving the Coronary Drug Project, a large multicenter trial sponsored in the United States by the National Heart Institute of the National Institutes of Health [11, 29]. The organization of the Coronary Drug Project included a policy board – a senior advisory group made up of five scientists who were not otherwise participating in the study. In 1967, after a presentation of interim outcome data by the study leadership to all participating investigators of the Coronary Drug Project, **Thomas Chalmers** addressed a letter to the policy board chairman expressing concern:

that knowledge by the investigators of early nonstatistically significant trends in mortality, morbidity, or incidence of side effects might result in some investigators – desirous of treating their patients in the best possible manner, ie, with the drug that is ahead – pulling out of the study or unblinding the treatment groups prematurely [11].

In 1968 a data and safety monitoring committee was established for the Coronary Drug Project (apparently by the policy board) consisting of scientists who were not contributing data to the study, and thereafter the practice of sharing accumulating outcome data with the study's investigators was discontinued. The data safety and monitoring committee assumed responsibility for deciding when the accumulating data warranted changing the study treatment protocol or terminating the study (*see* **Data and Safety Monitoring**).

In 1971, for the first randomized clinical trial it sponsored, the recently established National Eye Institute of the US National Institutes of Health adopted the model of the Coronary Drug Project by including in its organization a policy board and data monitoring committee; the trial was the multicenter Diabetic Retinopathy Study [17]. In this study, as in the Coronary Drug Project, the accumulating outcome data were not shared with data-contributing investigators.

In subsequent trials sponsored by the National Heart Institute (later named National Heart, Lung, and Blood Institute) and the National Eye Institute the functions of the policy board and data and safety monitoring committee were combined in a single data monitoring committee. The example set by the Coronary Drug Project and the Diabetic Retinopathy Study established a pattern for monitoring interim clinical trials data by an independent committee that was gradually adopted by many trials in North America and Europe.

Interim Analysis

In the conduct of the modern randomized clinical trial, the ethical requirement for interim analysis of study outcomes is widely recognized, and the responsibility for such analysis is commonly delegated to an independent data monitoring committee. Bradford Hill does not mention interim analysis in his extensive writings about the clinical trials he worked on during the late 1940s and 1950s [37].

The first formal recognition of the need for interim analyses, and that such analyses affect the probability of the type I error (*see* **Hypothesis Testing**), came with the publication in the 1950s of papers on sequential clinical trials by Bross [9] and Armitage [2] (*see* **Sequential Analysis**). In sequential trials of two treatments, patients are enrolled in pairs, with members of each pair randomly assigned to one or the other treatment. The data are analyzed each time that both members of a pair reach an endpoint (e.g. treatment failure). The overall probability of the type I error is controlled at a predetermined level. The principal advantage of a sequential trial over a fixed-sample-size trial, apart from that of correcting the significance level for repeated data analyses, is that when the length of time needed to reach an endpoint is short, e.g. weeks or months, the sample size required to detect a substantial benefit from one of the treatments is less. Applications of sequential trials have been limited because when follow-up is long-term, as is required by most trials, the sequential design is less effective.

In the 1960s **Cornfield** argued that data analysis in clinical trials, because it is often marked by unforeseen developments, does not lend itself well to predetermined stopping rules [13, 16]. For the dilemma of repeated interim analyses of the accumulating data, and to address the issue of **multiplicity in clinical trials** in general, he proposed use of the **likelihood ratio**. In particular, he proposed a **Bayesian** solution in the form of "relative betting odds" [12] – a method that was applied alongside conventional frequentist methods in two trials [14, 73].

In the 1970s and 1980s frequentist solutions to interim analysis came about in the form of "group sequential trials" and "stochastic curtailment" [4, 30, 66]. In the group sequential trial, an analogue of the classical sequential trial [2, 9], the frequency of interim analysis is usually limited to a small number, say, between 3 and 6, while the overall type I error probability is controlled at a predetermined level. Pocock's boundaries use constant nominal significance levels for the individual tests; the Haybittle–Peto boundary [36, 65] uses stringent significance levels, except for the final test; in the O'Brien–Fleming boundary, stringency gradually decreases [61]; in the model by Lan & DeMets [45], the total type I error probability is gradually spent in a manner that does not require the timing of analyses be prespecified; there have also been proposals

for methods of repeated **confidence intervals** [40]. Whereas group sequential designs are used to determine whether a trial should be stopped early because a treatment is efficacious, stochastic curtailment, which involves prediction of future events, is invoked when it appears that a treatment is unlikely to be shown to be efficacious even if the trial is continued to its planned conclusion [46]. Both group sequential methods and stochastic curtailment have been frequently applied to trials in the 1980s and 1990s.

Despite a renewed interest in Bayesian clinical trials since the 1980s [8, 25, 26, 33, 41], there have been few applications. Freedman et al. [27] provide an overview of Bayesian approaches to interim analysis, including a Bayesian analogue to stochastic curtailment.

References

[1] Amberson, B. & McMahon, P.M. (1931). A clinical trial of sanocrysin in pulmonary tuberculosis, *American Review of Tuberculosis* **24**, 401.

[2] Armitage, P. (1954). Sequential tests in prophylactic and therapeutic trials, *Quarterly Journal of Medicine* **23**, 255–274.

[3] Armitage, P. (1983). Trials and errors: the emergence of clinical statistics, *Journal of the Royal Statistical Society, Series A* **146**, 321–334.

[4] Armitage, P. (1991). Interim analysis in clinical trials, *Statistics in Medicine* **10**, 925–937.

[5] Bacon, F.V.S. (1961–1963). Novum organum, in *The Works of Francis Bacon* (transl. James Spedding, orig. publ. Longman, London, 1858–1874). Facsimile reprint, Frommann, Stuttgart, 1961–1963. Also cited in *The Oxford Dictionary of Quotations*, 3rd Ed. Oxford University Press, 1979.

[6] Bean, W.B. (1995). Walter Reed and the ordeal of human experiments, in *Ethics in Epidemiology and Clinical Research*, S.S. Coughlin, ed. Epidemiology Resources Inc., Newton, pp. 3–22.

[7] Beecher, H.K. (1966). Ethics and clinical research, *New England Journal of Medicine* **274**, 1354–1360.

[8] Berry, D.A. (1987). Interim analyses in clinical research, *Cancer Investigation* **5**, 469–477.

[9] Bross, I. (1952). Sequential medical plans, *Biometrics* **8**, 188–295.

[10] Bull, J.P. (1959). The historical development of clinical therapeutic trials, *Journal of Chronic Disease* **10**, 218–248.

[11] Canner, P. (1983). Monitoring of the data for adverse or beneficial treatment effects, *Controlled Clinical Trials* **4**, 467–483.

[12] Cornfield, J. (1969). The Bayesian outlook and its applications, *Biometrics* **24**, 617–657.

[13] Cornfield, J. (1976). Recent methodological contributions to clinical trials, *American Journal of Epidemiology* **104**, 408–421.

[14] Coronary Drug Project Research Group (1970). The Coronary Drug Project. Initial findings leading to a modification of its research protocol, *Journal of the American Medical Association* **214**, 1303–1313.

[15] Curran, W.J. & Shapiro, E.D. (1970). *Law, Medicine, and Forensic Science*, 2nd Ed. Little, Brown & Company, Boston.

[16] Cutler, S.J., Greenhouse, S.W., Cornfield, J. & Schneiderman, M.A. (1966). The role of hypothesis testing in clinical trials. Biometrics seminar, *Journal of Chronic Diseases* **19**, 857–882.

[17] The Diabetic Retinopathy Study Research Group (1981). Photocoagulation treatment of diabetic retinopathy. Design, methods, and baseline results. Report 6, *Investigative Ophthalmology and Visual Science* **21**, Part 2, 149–209.

[18] Diehl, H.S., Baker, A.B. & Cowan, D.W. (1938). Cold vaccines: an evaluation based on a controlled study, *Journal of the American Medical Association* **111**, 1168–1173.

[19] Ederer, F. (1975). Patient bias, investigator bias and the double-masked procedure, *American Journal of Medicine* **58**, 295–299.

[20] Faden, R.R., Beauchamp, T. & King, N.M.P. (1986). *A History of Informed Consent*. Oxford University Press, New York.

[21] Fibiger, J. (1898). Om Serum Behandlung of Difteri, *Hospitalstidende* **6**, 309–325, 337–350.

[22] Fisher, R.A. (1926). The arrangement of field experiments, *Journal of the Ministry of Agriculture* **33**, 503–513.

[23] Fisher, R.A., & McKenzie, W.A. (1923). Studies in crop variation: II. The manurial response of different potato varieties, *Journal of Agricultural Science* **13**, 315.

[24] Freedman, B. (1995). Research, unethical, in *Encyclopedia of Bioethics*, W.T. Reich, ed. Free Press, New York, pp. 2258–2261.

[25] Freedman, L.S. & Spiegelhalter, D.J. (1983). The assessment of subjective opinion and its use in relation to stopping rules for clinical trials, *Statistician* **32**, 153–160.

[26] Freedman, L.S., Lowe, D. & Macaskill, P. (1984). Stopping rules for clinical trials incorporating clinical opinion, *Biometrics* **40**, 575–586.

[27] Freedman, L.S., Spiegelhalter, D.J. & Parmar, M.K.B. (1994). The what, why, and how of Bayesian clinical trials monitoring, *Statistics in Medicine* **13**, 1371–1383.

[28] Fried, C. (1974). *Medical Experimentation: Personal Integrity and Social Policy*. North-Holland, Amsterdam.

[29] Friedman, L. (1993). The NHLBI model: a 25-year history, *Statistics in Medicine* **12**, 425–431.

[30] Friedman, L.M., Furberg, C.D., & DeMets, D.L. (1985). *Fundamentals of Clinical Trials*, 2nd Ed. Wright, Boston.

[31] Gail, M.H. (1996). Statistics in action, *Journal of the American Statistical Association* **91**, 1–13.

[32] Gehan, E.A. & Lemak, N.A. (1994). *Statistics in Medical Research: Developments in Clinical Trials*. Plenum Medical Book Company, New York.

[33] George, S.L., Chengchang, L., Berry, D.A. & Green, M.R. (1994). Stopping a trial early: frequentist and Bayesian approaches applied to a CALGB trial of non-small-cell lung cancer, *Statistics in Medicine* **13**, 1313–1328.

[34] Greenhouse, S.W. (1990). Some historical and methodological developments in early clinical trials at the National Institutes of Health, *Statistics in Medicine* **9**, 893–901.

[35] Hawkins, B.S. (1988). The National Institutes of Health and their sponsorship of clinical trials, *Controlled Clinical Trials* **9**, 103–106.

[36] Haybittle, J.L. (1971). Repeated assessment of results of cancer treatment, *British Journal of Radiology* **44**, 793–797.

[37] Hill, A.B. (1962). *Statistical Methods in Clinical and Preventive Medicine*. E & S Livingstone, Edinburgh.

[38] Hill, A.B. (1963). Medical ethics and controlled trials, *British Medical Journal* **1**, 1043–1049.

[39] Hill, A.B., Marshall, J. & Shaw, D.A. (1960). A controlled clinical trial of long-term anticoagulant therapy in cerebrovascular disease, *Quarterly Journal of Medicine* **29** (NS), 597–608.

[40] Jennison, C. & Turnbull, B.W. (1989). Interim analysis: the repeated confidence interval approach, *Journal of the Royal Statistical Society, Series B* **51**, 305–361.

[41] Kadane, J.B. (1995). Prime time for Bayes, *Controlled Clinical Trials* **16**, 313–318.

[42] Katz, J. (1972). *Experimentation with Human Beings: The Authority of the Investigator, Subject, Professions, and State in the Human Experimentation Process*. Russell Sage Foundation, New York.

[43] Katz, J. (1996). The Nuremberg Code and the Nuremberg Trial. A reappraisal, *Journal of the American Medical Association* **276**, 1662–1666.

[44] Kinsey, V.E. (1956). Retrolental fibroplasia, *AMA Archives of Ophthalmology* **56**, 481–543.

[45] Lan, K.K.G., & DeMets, D.L. (1983). Discrete sequential boundaries for clinical trials, *Biometrika* **70**, 659–663.

[46] Lan, K.K.G., Simon, R. & Halperin, M. (1982). Stochastically curtailed tests in long-term clinical trials, *Communications in Statistics – Sequential Analysis* **1**, 207–219.

[47] Levine, R.J. (1986). *Ethics and Regulation of Clinical Research*, 2nd Ed. Urban & Schwarzenberg, Baltimore, pp. 187–190.

[48] Levine, R. (1995). Research ethics committees, in *Encyclopedia of Bioethics*, W.T. Reich, ed. Free Press, New York, pp. 2258–2261.

[49] Lilienfeld, A.M. (1982). Ceteris paribus: The evolution of the clinical trial, *Bulletin of the History of Medicine* **56**, 1–18.

[50] Lind, J. (1753). *A Treatise of the Scurvy*. Sands Murray Cochran, Edinburgh, pp. 191–193.

[51] Louis, P.C.A. (1837). The applicability of statistics to the practice of medicine, *London Medical Gazette* **20**, 488–491.

[52] McNeill, P.M. (1993). *The Ethics and Politics of Human Experimentation*. Press Syndicate of the University of Cambridge, Cambridge.

[53] Medical Research Council (1948). Streptomycin treatment of pulmonary tuberculosis, *British Medical Journal* **2**, 769–782.

[54] Medical Research Council (1950). Clinical trials of antihistaminic drugs in the prevention and treatment of the common cold, *British Medical Journal* **ii**, 425–431.

[55] Medical Research Council (1952). Chemotherapy of pulmonary tuberculosis in young adults, *British Medical Journal* **i**, 1162–1168.

[56] Medical Research Council (1954). A comparison of cortisone and aspirin in the treatment of early cases of rheumatoid arthritis - I, *British Medical Journal* **i**, 1223–1227.

[57] Medical Research Council (1955). A comparison of cortisone and aspirin in the treatment of early cases of rheumatoid arthritis - II, *British Medical Journal* **ii**, 695–700.

[58] Meier, P. (1975). Statistics and medical experimentation, *Biometrics* **31**, 511–529.

[59] Meinert, C.L. (1986). *Clinical Trials. Design, Conduct, and Analysis*. Oxford University Press, New York.

[60] Netherlands Minister of Social Affairs and Health (1957). *4 World Medical Journal*, 299–300.

[61] O'Brien, P.C. & Fleming, T.R. (1979). A multiple testing procedure for clinical trials, *Biometrics* **35**, 549–556.

[62] Osler, W. (1907). The evolution of the idea of experiment, *Transactions of the Congress of American Physicians and Surgeons* **7**, 1–8.

[63] Packard, F.R. (1921). *The Life and Times of Ambroise Paré*, 2nd Ed. Paul B. Hoeber, New York, pp. 27, 163.

[64] Percival, T. (1803). *Medical Ethics*. Russell, London.

[65] Peto, R., Pike, M.C., Armitage, P., Breslow, N.E., Cox, D.R., Howard, S.V., Mantel, N., McPherson, K., Peto, J. & Smith, P. (1976). Design and analysis of randomized clinical trials requiring prolonged observation of each patient. 1. Introduction and design, *British Journal of Cancer* **34**, 585–612.

[66] Pocock, S.J. (1983). *Clinical Trials: A Practical Approach*. Wiley, Chichester.

[67] Pozdena, R.F. (1905). Versuche über Blondlot's "Emission Pesante", *Annalen der Physik* **17**, 104.

[68] Rheumatic Fever Working Party (1960). The evolution of rheumatic heart disease in children: five-year report of a cooperative clinical trial of ACTH, cortisone, and aspirin, *Circulation* **22**, 505–515.

[69] Rothman, D.J. (1995). Research, human: historical aspects, in *Encyclopedia of Bioethics*, W.T. Reich, ed. Free Press, New York, pp. 2258–2261.

[70] Seabrook, W. (1941). *Doctor Wood*. Harcourt, Brace & Company, New York, p. 234.

[71] Shirer, W.L. (1960). *The Rise and Fall of the Third Reich*. Simon & Schuster, New York.

[72] Slotki, J.J. (1951). *Daniel, Ezra, Nehemia, Hebrew Text and English Translation with Introductions and Commentary*. Soncino Press, London.

[73] Urokinase-Pulmonary Embolism Trial (1973). A National Cooperative Study, A.A. Sasahara, T.M. Cole, F. Ederer, J.A. Murray, N.K. Wenger, S. Sherry & J.M. Stengle, eds. *Circulation* **47**, Supplement 2, pp. 1–108.

[74] US Government Printing Office (1949). *Trials of War Criminals before the Nuremberg Military Tribunals under Control Council Law No. 10*, Vol. 2. US Government Printing Office, Washington, pp. 181–182.

[75] Van Helmont, J.B. (1662). *Oriatrike or Physik Refined* (translated by J. Chandler). Lodowick Loyd, London.

[76] Vogt, E.Z. & Hyman, R. (1959). *Water Witching, USA*. University of Chicago Press, Chicago, p. 50.

[77] Withington, C.F. (1886). *The Relation of Hospitals to Medical Education*. Cupples Uphman, Boston.

[78] Witkosky, S.J. (1889). *The Evil That Has Been Said of Doctors: Extracts From Early Writers*, Trans. with annotations by T.C. Minor. The Cincinnati Lancet-Clinic, Vol. 41, New Series Vol. 22, pp. 447–448.

FRED EDERER

History of Health Statistics

The field of statistics in the twentieth century (*see* **Statistics, Overview**) encompasses four major areas; (i) the **theory of probability** and mathematical statistics; (ii) the analysis of uncertainty and errors of measurement (*see* **Measurement Error in Epidemiologic Studies**); (iii) design of experiments (*see* **Experimental Design in Biostatistics**) and **sample surveys**; and (iv) the collection, summarization, display, and interpretation of observational data (*see* **Observational Study**). These four areas are clearly interrelated and have evolved interactively over the centuries. The first two areas are well covered in many histories of mathematical statistics while the third area, being essentially a twentieth-century development, has not yet been adequately summarized. Although the fourth area has been going on since man first learned to think inductively, it relies on the state of the art in the first three areas. In this brief survey of health statistics during the past five centuries, emphasis will be given to the development of official health statistics systems in Europe and the US.

Early Interest in Statistics

At the end of the fifteenth century, mathematics was at a rather primitive stage and the threshold of the "scientific revolution" was still two generations away. The mathematics of the Greeks had only re-entered European thinking in the twelfth century, and although some progress had been made in practical applications in navigation and commercial arithmetic, the burgeoning of numeracy was only beginning. Mathematicians still did not recognize the number zero or know how to deal with negative numbers. Except for a few examples of probabilistic thinking such as that in the talmudic literature [10], there was scant evidence of the use of a mathematical approach to probabilities to estimate **risks** or assess the reliability of measurements until the mid-seventeenth century.

Most historians of statistics trace the origins of modern probability theory to the efforts to solve certain gambling problems [e.g. Pacioli (1494), Cardano (1539), and Forestani (1603)] which were first solved definitively by Pierre de Fermat (1601–1665) and Blaise Pascal (1623–1662). These efforts gave rise to the mathematical basis of probability theory, statistical distribution functions (*see* **Sampling Distribution**), and statistical **inference**.

The analysis of uncertainty and errors of measurement had its foundations in the field of astronomy which, from antiquity until the eighteenth century, was the dominant area for use of numerical information based on the most precise measurements that the technologies of the times permitted. The fallibility of their observations was evident to early astronomers, who took the "best" observation when several were taken, the "best" being assessed by such criteria as the quality of observational conditions, the fame of the observer, etc. But, gradually an appreciation for averaging observations developed and various techniques for fitting the observational data to

parametric models evolved. Many of the founders of modern statistics contributed to the early development of the theory of measurement errors including **Jacob Bernoulli** (1654–1705), **Abraham De Moivre** (1667–1754), **Pierre Simon Laplace** (1749–1827), and **Carl Friedrich Gauss** (1777–1855).

A systematic approach to the collection of data and tabulating observations in a rational manner began with the teachings of Francis Bacon (1561–1626). In his influential treatise *Novum Organum* (1620), he attacked the scholastic philosophy which had developed in the Middle Ages on the basis of the methods of Aristotle. One of the first areas influenced by Bacon's approach was **demography** and **vital statistics** and the social utility of systematic observations is clearly reflected in these early efforts.

The utilitarian nature of statistics is evident in the origins of the word from the Italian *stato* (state), and the original meaning of statistics was a collection of facts of interest to a statesman. Initially such facts were not primarily numerical, but included information on geography, politics, and customs of a region. The compilers of such facts were called statists, a term which survived into the nineteenth century, when the word statistics came to be used for numerical data only, replacing the term "political arithmetic", and the word "statistician" came into vogue.

The Origins of Demography and Vital Statistics

Since ancient times, sporadic surveys of people and property were done to set tax assessments and levies for military service. But after the fall of the Roman empire, regular **censuses** covering an entire state did not occur until the eighteenth century. However, there were intermittent attempts to keep track of the births and deaths in some areas through church records of weddings, christenings, and burials. The City of London was one of the first to regularize the maintenance of such records in 1538, but only within the Church of England. Also at about this time a **surveillance** or early warning system of plague deaths was started in London. To detect the onset of a plague epidemic, parish clerks submitted weekly reports on the numbers and causes of deaths. These weekly *Bills of Mortality* were noted by the authorities who were to take actions if they detected the onset of an epidemic, and by the wealthier citizens for "an indication of when to leave the city for the fresh air of the country" [7]. The weekly bills were published regularly from 1604 until 1842 when they were superseded by reports from the Registrar General.

In 1662, **John Graunt** (1620–1674), a London tradesman who had been active in local politics and intellectual society, published his *Natural and Political Observations Made Upon the Bills of Mortality*, which historians of statistics have referred to as "a remarkable book [12]", "one of the great classics of science [6]", and "a paragon for descriptive statistical analysis of demographic data [7]". Hald summarizes Graunt's contributions to the origins of statistics thus:

> Graunt's critical appraisal of the rather unreliable data, his study of mortality by cause of death, his estimation of the same quantity by several different methods, his demonstration of the stability of statistical ratios, and his life table set up new standards for statistical reasoning. Graunt's work led to three different types of investigations: political arithmetic; testing the stability of statistical ratios; and calculation of expectations of life and survivorship probabilities [7].

At a time when denominator data on the size of the population by age were not available, Graunt used several ingenious lines of reasoning to generate the first **life table** ever published, perhaps his most famous contribution.

Owing to the widespread influence of Graunt's work, bills of mortality similar to the London bills were introduced in Paris in 1667, and soon after in other cities in Europe.

Graunt's life table was brought to the attention of Christiaan Huygens (1629–1695) and his brother Ludwig (1631–1699) who proceeded to develop a probabilistic interpretation of the life table, which was rediscovered independently by **Nicholas Bernoulli** (1687–1759). These investigations, together with the more applied techniques of **Edmond Halley** (1656–1742) based on the births and funerals in the City of Breslau (1693), and the work of Deparcieux (1703–1768) in France who used data from tontines to construct the first correct life tables, formed the foundation of the **actuarial** sciences for life insurance and annuities. These were developed further by Abraham DeMoivre (1667–1754), Thomas Simpson (1710–1761), Benjamin Gompertz (1779–1865), and William Makeham (1826–1891).

It was not until 1766 in Sweden that Per Wargentin (1717–1783) published the first mortality tables for a whole country based on enumerations of the living population as well as on deaths. These mortality tables demonstrated for the first time in a general population that the mortality rate of females was less than that of males.

Graunt's methods of statistical analysis were widely adopted by seventeenth-century statists. **William Petty** (1623–1687), who was a protégé of Graunt, and after Graunt's financial bankruptcy in 1666, his patron, coined the term "political arithmetick" and was one of the founders of the field of political economy. Gregory King (1648–1712) and Charles Davenant (1656–1714) contributed to improvements in the estimates of the population of England. Sebastien de Vauban (1633–1707) described the extent of poverty in France, for which he suffered public disgrace because of its embarrassment of the royal government. Nicholas Struyck (1678–1769) instituted town censuses in the Netherlands and improved the recording of births and deaths. The revelations of statistical data were also used to support religious positions such as the claim of John Arbuthnott (1667–1735), who was a vigorous proponent of political arithmetic, that the stability of the sex ratio "is not the effect of chance but divine providence". Somewhat later, Johann Peter Suessmilch (1707–1767) in Germany gathered vital statistics from virtually every source then available as evidence of certain tenets of orthodox Lutheran theology. He maintained that the life span (*see* **Life Expectancy**) was constant and that little could be done to improve mortality rates. His work directly influenced the thinking of **Thomas Robert Malthus** (1766–1834). These diverse endeavors eventually led to the establishment of governmental statistical offices in the nineteenth century.

Among the developments in mathematical statistics that occurred during the eighteenth century, two had special relevance for health statistics. **Daniel Bernoulli** (1700–1782), who first developed the **normal** approximation to the **binomial distribution** and used it in studies of the stability of the sex ratio at birth, applied the methods of calculus to mortality rates by treating them as continuous functions. This enabled him to obtain a solution in 1760 to an important public health question of his day: to estimate the impact on life expectancy of eliminating smallpox through a proposed program of mandatory vaccination. His invention of the method of **competing risks**, with some improvement by d'Alembert (1761) and by Makeham (1874), still forms the basic tool for such analyses.

A second development expanded the techniques used by Vauban. Laplace proposed a nonrandom sampling method to estimate the size of the population in 1786. It was based on a notion similar to that of current **ratio estimates**, i.e. that the size of the population of a region was proportional to the annual number of births in that region and that the constant of proportionality could be determined from a purposive sample of subregions. Graunt had used a similar assumption implicitly a century earlier.

Laplace's method was severely criticized, most notably by Baron de Keverberg (1827) [11, p. 164]. These criticisms clearly reflected an appreciation that there were a multitude of factors that could influence any chosen characteristic of a population, that subgroups of the population were not homogeneous with regard to the array of factors influencing the characteristic, and, therefore, purposive samples of the population could not reflect the total population. Only complete censuses of the population would do, and these would have to amass immense amounts of information. At this time there was not yet an appreciation for the power of random sampling methods (*see* **Probability Sampling**).

Applying Statistics to Medical and Social Issues

Just as **demographic** and economic statistics began with the name of "political arithmetic" in the seventeenth century, medical statistics began with the name of "the numerical method" early in the nineteenth century. Although some of his methods were evident in the works of **Phillipe Pinel** (1745–1826) and other French physicians, **Pierre-Charles-Alexandre Louis** (1787–1872) has been described "as the first modern clinician, the man who made bedside medicine a science as well as an art, and who established the principle of learning medicine from thoughtful observation of patients [1]." His studies on the inefficacy of blood letting were the beginning of quantitative medicine and earned him the title of "father of medical statistics" [12]. Louis's hopes for his numerical method were echoed by Giacomo Tommasini (1768–1846)

in Italy, and **F. Bisset Hawkins** (1796–1894) in England, who published in 1829 the first English textbook on medical statistics with the rather grand title of *Elements of Medical Statistics; Containing the Substance of the Gulstonian Lectures Delivered at the Royal College of Physicians with Numerous Additions Illustrative of the Comparative Salubrity, Longevity, Mortality, and Prevalence of Diseases in the Principal Countries and Cities of the Civilized World.* Although by later standards Louis's statistical attempts were often inadequate, suffering particularly from sparse numbers, he had a crucial influence on **William Farr** who attended his lectures during his two years in Paris, as did several American physicians who were influential in the early development of public health and epidemiology.

Louis's methods were not immediately accepted for many of the same reasons that Laplace's methods were not: the variability between cases was thought to be highly individualistic and not subject to statistical summarization. For example, **William A. Guy** (1810–1885), who contributed much to public health and occupational statistics, felt "the formulae of the mathematician have a very limited application to the results of observation" [12, p. 151].

The Belgian, **Adolphe Quetelet** (1796–1874), who dominated the field of social statistics for half a century, may have gone too far in the other direction. Impressed by the **central limit theorem** and believing that averages based on large numbers of observations from a population had remarkable stability, he introduced the concept of the "average man" (*l'homme moyen*) which had considerable popular appeal. He was also enamored of the normal distribution and fitted it to many characteristics, marvelling at the statistical homogeneity of large bodies of data which detracted from further exploration of valid heterogeneities. However, he influenced a large number of statisticians including **Louis Adolphe Bertillon** (1821–1883), Wilhelm Lexis (1837–1914), **Francis Galton** (1822–1911), **Karl Pearson** (1857–1936), and **Ronald A. Fisher** (1890–1962) [11].

Development of Health Statistics in England

During the eighteenth century many physicians and registrars in England recognized the inadequacies of the bills of mortality. There were frequent calls for reforms but because of concerns about personal liberties, religious arguments, and beliefs that population figures were crucial state secrets, it was not until 1800 that Parliament passed a population act that set up the census of 1801. By the 1830s, as in the mid-seventeenth century (with Graunt and Petty), London "witnessed a flash of enthusiasm for vital statistics and political arithmetic" [5, p. 13]. The Statistical Society of London was founded in 1834 by the same group that had founded the statistics section (Section F) of the British Association for the Advancement of Science in 1833, and started publication of its Journal in 1838. These and other early statistical societies in England were greatly concerned with social problems, conducting several surveys to document conditions in England and continuing to push for social reforms long after the surveys proved too expensive to continue. Although they claimed scientific objectivity, these statists were superficial in their use of mathematical methods, paid little attention to the validity or accuracy of their data, but were aware that using numeric data gave credibility to political arguments [5].

A more balanced contribution was made by William Farr (1807–1883) in the area of vital statistics. Starting his career as an unsuccessful London clinician, he quickly became an acknowledged authority on vital and health statistics with a strong interest in medical and social reform. He founded his own weekly journal, *British Annals of Medicine, Pharmacy, Vital Statistics, and General Science*, which lasted only eight months, January to August 1837, but allowed him to write major articles on medical reform and vital statistics. The Births and Deaths Registration Act of 1836 had inaugurated the modern system of civil registration and led to the establishment of the General Register Office in 1837. Farr joined the staff of the General Register Office in 1839, serving forty years, first as compiler of abstracts and then as superintendent of the Statistical Department.

Farr "insisted that the statistician adopt a critical approach, investigating the accuracy of his data, questioning the appropriateness of the units used, and attempting with the help of ratios, logarithms, and the calculus of probabilities to discover relationships and regularity in order to make predictions" [5, p. 29]. Farr's philosophy had an almost immediate impact on improving British statistics. The first four censuses were fraught with many problems. The 1841 census

was the first conducted under the supervision of the General Register Office and Farr was one of the key advisors. It was a great improvement over its predecessors and, together with the annual vital statistics data, enabled Farr to put together tables and analyses which placed England at the forefront of this discipline. Between 1836 and the Registration Act of 1874, Farr was largely responsible for establishing the procedures for collecting and analyzing the official mortality statistics. He introduced the standard **death certificate** in 1845 which saw almost no change until 1902. Through Farr's influence the census of 1851 introduced questions on physical disabilities and other medical items which were continued through 1911.

Farr was greatly interested in statistical nosology, introducing his first classification of diseases in 1839. The first International Statistical Congress in 1853 took up the issue, but Farr's nosology did not win the support of other European countries. It was not until 1893 that Jacques Bertillon (1851–1922) proposed a system that became the International List of Causes of Death (*see* **International Classification of Diseases (ICD)**).

Problems noted in the vital registration system in the mid-nineteenth century are still of concern at the end of the twentieth, namely accuracy of diagnoses was not reliable, selection of a single underlying cause of death (*see* **Cause of Death, Underlying and Multiple**) from among several listed conditions, "the temptation of practitioners to obscure or falsify the cause of death to save respectable families embarrassment in certain sorts of death" [5, p. 62]. Henry Wyldbore Rumsey (1809–1876), one of the chief proponents of sound vital statistics, was vigorous in pointing out statistical fallacies and shortcomings of the existing systems that bear rereading today.

Many of Farr's statistical methods have had a lasting impact: defining mortality rates precisely and basing them on **person-years at risk**, establishing the standard expression of mortality as "deaths per thousand", using the life table and life expectancy as key instruments to assess mortality, using the method of indirect standardization (*see* **Standardization Methods**) to compare mortality rates of localities (although he seems to have made little use of the direct method first demonstrated by F.G.P. Neison in his refutation of the proposal of Edwin Chadwick (1800–1890) to use **average age at death** as a criterion for the health of communities), recommending the establishment of longitudinal **cohort studies** [9], and proposing a paradigm for the estimation of the economic value of human life at each age and social class. Farr's association with **Florence Nightingale** (1820–1910) also resulted in contributions to the use of statistical information for health policy purposes, particularly in respect to the graphic presentation of data (*see* **Graphical Displays**).

Development of Vital Statistics in the United States

As interest in statistical information burgeoned in Europe in the first third of the nineteenth century, a similar phenomenon was occurring on the other side of the Atlantic [4]. Although medicine, statistics, and science generally, in the US lagged behind that in Europe, America had actually preceded other countries in two important respects. Whereas other areas relied on church-maintained records of christenings and burials as the basis for vital statistics, the Massachusetts Bay Colony enacted a law in 1639 requiring the reporting of every birth and death within its jurisdiction, thus establishing the collection of vital statistics as a governmental function covering the entire population. The other colonies gradually adopted similar regulations but for at least the next two hundred years the quality and completeness of the reports were decidedly deficient. The second precedent was when the US became the first nation to establish by constitutional mandate a periodic census requiring complete enumeration of the entire population, conducting its first census in 1790.

At about this time death reports were being used on occasion in port cities to institute quarantine measures in efforts to control epidemics of cholera, yellow fever, and typhus. As the Benthamite social reform interests reached America and evidence for the harmful effects of poverty, industrialization, and unsanitary conditions was sought from vital statistics, the inadequacies of the city and local registration systems became evident. In 1826, Walter Channing (1786–1876) in Boston outlined some of the requirements for valid data on causes of death, including the requisite for medical certification. In 1827 Nathaniel Niles and John D. Russ published the first report on public health statistics in a comparison of mortality data from New York, Philadelphia, Baltimore, and Boston. Other analyses soon followed which became

models for the quantitative health reports produced by subsequent generations of health officials which led to increasing pressures for improving the quality of the information. In 1842 Massachusetts again achieved a first by establishing a statewide vital registration system. The effort to establish similar systems in other states marked the beginning of an organized public health movement and contributed to the professionalization of statisticians in this country [2, 3].

Following on the foundation of the Statistical Society of London, statistical societies were started in New York and other American cities. Most did not last very long but the **American Statistical Association**, founded in Boston in 1839, proved to be enduring. It is significant that 14 of the original 54 local members were physicians. But it was a publisher and bookseller, Lemuel Shattuck (1793–1859), who was the Society's key "statist" for health-related issues. He consulted with, among others, Quetelet and was a prime mover for the Massachusetts Registration Act of 1842. He also played a role in the origins of national vital statistics by having mortality queries included in the 1850 census.

In 1846, the first national medical convention (which led to the founding of the American Medical Association) formed two committees relevant to health statistics: (i) a committee on registration whose report "provided for the convention to formally petition every state government to enact effective registration legislation and to request state and local medical societies to take the lead in lobbying for such laws" [3, p. 201], and (ii) a committee on disease nomenclature which adopted a modification of Farr's classification. Neither of these recommendations was widely adopted for at least 50 years. Although there were many attempts, these efforts were often failures since "the registration movement had moved too far ahead of its base of community support" [3, p. 204]. At the end of the century, no state had a system as good as those in several European countries.

During the last two decades of the nineteenth century, the initiative for improving vital statistics shifted to the Federal government [8]. Under Dr John Shaw Billings (1838–1913), who directed vital statistics in the 1880 and 1890 US censuses, improvements were made in gathering mortality data. The **American Public Health Association** joined with the Census Bureau, which was established in 1902, in drafting a model vital statistics law and standard birth and death certificates that each state could adopt. Because of the early efforts of Cressy L. Wilbur (1865–1928), Chief Statistician for Vital Statistics from 1906 to 1914, the birth- and death-registration areas grew, reaching completeness in 1933, nearly a century after several European countries. The Division of Vital Statistics of the Bureau of the Census was transferred to the Public Health Service in 1946, becoming the National Office of Vital Statistics, with Dr Halbert L. Dunn (1896–1975) as Director. In 1960, NOVS was combined with the National Health Survey to become the **National Center for Health Statistics** with **Forrest E. Linder** (1906–1988) as its first Director.

Development of Health Surveys in the United States

The establishment of the National Health Survey in 1957 marked a milestone in health statistics. With only a few exceptions, previous data relating to health came from vital statistics or from diagnosed diseases seen in hospitals or included in various notifiable **diseases registers**. As public health concerns in the US shifted from the surveillance and control of acute **communicable diseases** to the prevention of chronic diseases, it was necessary to develop data systems that would better describe the current health status of the population (*see* **Quality of Life and Health Status**) and shed some light on health-associated behaviors and use of health care services (*see* **Health Services Organization in the US**). The National Health Survey was the first continuous nationwide survey to gather information from randomly drawn representative samples (*see* **Probability Sampling**) of the noninstitutionalized population of the country to accomplish these aims (*see* **Surveys, Health and Morbidity**). It consists of two distinct surveys: the National Health Interview Survey (NHIS) and the National Health Examination Survey, the latter subsequently expanded to the National Health and Nutrition Examination Survey (NHANES). The NHIS conducts interviews in about 1000 households each week to obtain information on acute illnesses, chronic conditions, health-related knowledge and behaviors, and use of health services. The NHANES involves detailed standardized medical examinations, including laboratory studies and special tests such as ECGs

and X-rays, and extensive questionnaires on nutrition and previous health conditions. The NHANES is a periodic survey and NHANES III (actually the sixth cycle of these surveys), being carried out from 1988 to 1994, examined a sample of about 30 000 persons aged 6 months and over. Health interview surveys have now been conducted in many countries and examination surveys have been used effectively in several developing countries to assess the population's health.

These surveys would not have been feasible without the development of survey methodologies which occurred in the twentieth century. Anders N. Kiaer (1838–1919), the first director of the Norwegian Central Bureau of Statistics, reintroduced the idea of a survey sample in what he called the "representative method", in which the sample was to be selected purposively as Laplace had suggested a century earlier, rather than randomly. Arthur Lyon Bowley (1869–1957) is credited with being the first statistician to use random sampling (1906). The seminal breakthrough for sampling methodology came in 1934 when **Jerzy Neyman** (1894–1981) established the theoretical basis for **stratified sampling** with unequal inclusion probabilities. He made another major contribution when he introduced the use of cost functions into survey sampling theory (1938). In the early 1940s, Morris Hansen (1910–1990) and William Hurwitz (1908–1969) at the Bureau of the Census perfected the methodologies for complex **multistage sampling** designs that are the basis for most modern large-scale surveys.

Conclusion

At the end of the twentieth century, most industrialized countries have effective vital statistics systems in place and many have established periodic interview surveys to assess the health status and needs of their citizens. Much remains to be done in developing countries to institute health services information systems (*see* **Administrative Databases**) that can guide public policies and programs. As the public health burden continues to shift from infectious diseases to problems of an aging population, to concerns about health promotion and disease prevention, and to assuring adequate health care for all citizens, the needs for reliable, relevant, and timely health statistics become ever greater. Fortunately, the methodologies developed over several centuries and the data systems that have been established can, if appropriate resources are provided, meet these needs.

References

[1] Bollet, A.J. (1973). Pierre Louis: the numerical method and the foundation of quantitative medicine, *American Journal of Medical Science* **266**, 92–101.
[2] Cassedy, J.H. (1969). *Demography in Early America. Beginning of the Statistical Mind. 1600–1800*. Harvard University Press, Cambridge, Mass.
[3] Cassedy, J.H. (1984). *American Medicine and Statistical Thinking 1800–1860*. Harvard University Press, Cambridge, Mass.
[4] Cohen, P.C. (1982). *A Calculating People. The Spread of Numeracy in Early America*. University of Chicago Press, Chicago.
[5] Eyler, J.M. (1979). *Victorian Social Medicine: The Ideas and Methods of William Farr*. Johns Hopkins University Press, Baltimore.
[6] Greenwood, M. (1941–1943). Medical statistics from Graunt to Farr. *Biometrika* **32**, (1941), 101–127; **32** (1942), 203–225; **33** (1943), 1–24. Published by Cambridge University Press, Cambridge, 1948, as the Fitzpatrick Lectures for 1941 and 1943.
[7] Hald, A. (1990). *A History of Probability and Statistics and Their Applications Before 1750*. Wiley, New York.
[8] Lawrence, P.S. (1976). The health record of the American People, in *Health in America: 1776–1976*. US Department of Health, Education, and Welfare, DHEW Pub. No. (HRA)76-616.
[9] Nissel, M. (1987). *People Count. A History of the General Register Office*. Office of Population Censuses and Surveys, HMSO, London.
[10] Rabinovitch, N.L. (1973). *Probability and Statistical Inference in Ancient and Medieval Jewish Literature*. University of Toronto Press, Toronto.
[11] Stigler, S.M. (1968). *The History of Statistics. The Measurement of Uncertainty Before 1900*. Harvard University Press, Cambridge, Mass.
[12] Westergaard, H. (1932). *Contributions to the History of Statistics*. King, London.

MANNING FEINLEIB

HLA System

The HLA (human leukocyte antigen) **gene** complex on the short arm of chromosome 6 has been of widespread interest to scientists and physicians for more than 25 years. The most well-characterized genes are HLA-A, B, C, DR, DQ, and DP [4, 9, 14]. These code for transmembrane glycoproteins which function as receptors. They bind degraded pieces of proteins (peptides, 8–15 amino acids long) and present them to T lymphocytes to initiate immune responses.

The HLA-A, B, and C genes were identified first and are often referred to as class I genes. They are expressed on nearly all nucleated cells of the body where they allow cytotoxic T cells to recognize and eliminate tumor cells or cells infected with viruses or other intracellular pathogens [8, 10]. HLA-DR, DQ, and DP molecules (class II molecules) are expressed only on B cells, macrophages, and antigen-presenting cells. These present peptides to T helper cells to induce inflammatory immune responses [5, 8, 10].

The HLA molecules are extremely **polymorphic**. The number of alleles at each locus currently ranges from 38 to over 100 [1, 3]. Widespread amino acid substitutions occur around the molecule's peptide binding groove, and it is thought that the maintenance of polymorphism is due to selection and the evolutionary advantage of **heterozygotes** in combatting infection [7, 11, 12].

The polymorphism and immunologic function of the HLA molecules has made them of considerable interest in transplantation and disease pathogenesis. HLA molecules can induce rejection of HLA-mismatched cells and organs; matching is currently performed for kidneys and bone marrow transplants [6]. Some HLA-DR and HLA-DQ alleles show strong associations with susceptibility to autoimmune and inflammatory diseases such as rheumatoid arthritis, type I insulin-dependent diabetes mellitus, and multiple sclerosis [2, 13]. The reasons for the disease associations are not clear, but presumably relate to peptide-binding.

HLA allele frequencies can vary dramatically between **ethnic groups** [3]. Differences in allele frequencies have been used to monitor population movements and trace ancestral derivations. Some combinations of alleles at adjacent loci are inherited together on a haplotype (*see* **Haplotype Analysis**) more frequently than expected. Such **linkage disequilibrium** is often observed between HLA-B and HLA-C and between HLA-DR and HLA-DQ, and sometimes for longer distances or across the entire gene complex.

For population studies, HLA gene frequencies and two locus linkage disequilibrium coefficients can be determined by standard methods. HLA and disease associations are evident as statistically significant differences in allele frequency between patients and controls. The controls must be matched for ethnic group and adjustment made for **multiple comparisons** (*see* **Disease–Marker Association**).

Although most interest has centered on HLA-A, B, C, DR, DQ, and DP, the HLA region actually covers more than 4 million base pairs of DNA and includes numerous other genes, including those for cytokines, complement components, olfactory receptors, chaperones, and many with still undefined functions [14]. Analogous gene complexes are found in other mammals [9]. The generic term *major histocompatibility complex* or MHC is frequently used to designate these gene complexes irrespective of species.

References

[1]   Bodmer, J.G., Marsh, S.G.E., Albert, E.D., Bodmer, W.F., Dupont, B., Erlich, H.A., Mach, B., Mayr, W.R., Parham, P., Sasazuki, T., Schreuder, G.M. Th., Strominger, J.L., Svejgaard, A. & Terasaki, P.I. (1994). Nomenclature for factors of the HLA system, *Tissue Antigens* **44**, 1–18.
[2]   Campbell, R.D. & Milner, C.M. (1993). MHC genes in autoimmunity, *Current Opinion in Immunology* **5**, 887–893.
[3]   Charon, D. ed. (1997). Genetic diversity of HLA: functional and medical implications, in *Proceedings of the Twelfth International Histocompatibility Workshop and Conference*, to appear.
[4]   Corzo, D., Salazar, M., Granja, C.B., & Yunis, E.J. (1995). Advances in HLA genetics, *Experimental and Clinical Immunogenetics* **12**, 156–170.
[5]   Cresswell, P. (1995). Assembly, transport and function of MHC class II molecules, *Annual Review of Immunology* **12**, 259–293.
[6]   Field, H. & Garavoy, M.R. (1994). Positive impact of DNA typing on solid organ transplantation, *Transplantation Review* **8**, 151–173.
[7]   Hill, A.V. (1996). Genetic susceptibility to malaria and other infectious diseases: from the MHC to the whole genome, *Parasitology* **112**, Supplement, S75–S84.
[8]   Germain, R.N. (1994). MHC-dependent antigen processing and peptide presentation: providing ligands for T lymphocyte activation, *Cell* **76**, 287–299.
[9]   Klein, J. (1986). *Natural History of the Major Histocompatibility Complex*. Wiley, New York.
[10] Morris, A., Hewitt, C. & Young, S. (1994). The major histocompatibility complex: its genes and their roles in antigen presentation, *Molecular Aspects of Medicine* **15**, 377–503.
[11] Nei, M. & Hughes, A.L. (1991). Polymorphism and evolution of the major histocompatibility complex

in mammals, in *Evolution at the Molecular Level*, R.K. Selander, A.G. Clark & T.S. Whittam, eds. Sinauer, Sunderland, pp. 222–247.
[12] Parham, P., Adams, E.J. & Arnett, K.L. (1995). The origins of HLA-A,B,C polymorphism, *Immunology Reviews* **143**, 141–180.
[13] Thomson, G. (1995). HLA disease associations: models for the study of complex human genetic disorders, *Critical Reviews in Clinical Laboratory Science* **32**, 183–219.
[14] Trowsdale, J. (1993). Genomic structure and function in the MHC, *Trends in Genetics* **9**, 117–122.

DONNA D. KOSTYU

Hodges–Lehmann Estimator *see* Median Effective Dose

Hogben, Lancelot Thomas

Born: December 9, 1895.
Died: August 22, 1975.

Hogben had a brilliant academic career in biology, with chairs at the London School of Economics, Aberdeen, and Birmingham, and election to Fellowship of the Royal Society in 1936. He wrote popular books on mathematics, science, and linguistics. During the 1939–1945 war he became Acting Director of Medical Statistics at the War Office, and from 1947 to 1961 he was Professor of Medical Statistics at the University of Birmingham. His main interests were in procedures for recording and tabulating medical data, and in the philosophical basis of statistics. In the latter context, he was critical of the claims made for randomized **clinical trials,** and, in a 1957 book on *Statistical Theory,* he expressed dissatisfaction with probabilistic **inference** as a basis for the interpretation of statistics. A very full biography and a complete bibliography are given in [1].

Reference

[1.] Wells, G.P. (1978). Lancelot Thomas Hogben, *Biographical Memoirs of Fellows of the Royal Society* **24**, 183–221.

Holm's Procedure *see* Bonferroni Inequalities and Intervals

Holzinger's *H* *see* Heritability

Homoscedasticity *see* Scedasticity

Homozygosity *see* Genotype

Homozygosity Mapping *see* Linkage Analysis, Model-Based

Horizon Models *see* Adaptive and Dynamic Methods of Treatment Assignment

Horvitz–Thompson Estimator

The estimator known as the *Horvitz–Thompson estimator* (HTE) was developed by Horvitz & Thompson in their classic 1952 paper [4]. In that article they propose the following estimator of a population total, X, that is valid for any **sampling design with or without replacement**:

$$x'_{\text{hte}} = \sum_{i=1}^{v} \frac{x_i}{\pi_i},$$

where x_i is the value of the variable for the ith enumeration unit in the sample, π_i is the probability of the ith enumeration unit being selected into the sample and v is the number of distinct enumeration units sampled (as distinguished from n, which is the total sample size). Clearly, $n = v$ when sampling is without replacement.

In that same paper, the authors showed that the HTE is **unbiased** with **standard error** given by the following expression:

$$\text{se}(x'_{\text{hte}}) = \left[\sum_{i=1}^{N} \left(\frac{1 - \pi_i}{\pi_i} \right) x_i^2 \right.$$
$$\left. + \sum_{i=1}^{N} \sum_{j \neq i} \left(\frac{\pi_{ij} - \pi_i \pi_j}{\pi_i \pi_j} \right) x_i x_j \right]^{1/2},$$

where N is the number of enumeration units in the population and π_{ij} is the probability that both enumeration units i and j are included in the sample.

In addition, they showed that the estimator, $\bar{v}(x'_{\text{hte}})$, given by the expression

$$\bar{v}(x'_{\text{hte}}) = \sum_{i=1}^{v} \frac{1 - \pi_i}{\pi_i^2} x_i^2$$
$$+ \sum_{i=1}^{v} \sum_{j \neq i} \left(\frac{\pi_{ij} - \pi_i \pi_j}{\pi_i \pi_j} \right) \frac{x_i x_j}{\pi_{ij}},$$

is an unbiased estimator of the **variance** of x'_{hte}.

The Horvitz–Thompson estimator differs from an earlier unbiased estimator generally referred to as the *Hansen–Hurwitz estimator*:

$$x'_{\text{hh}} = \frac{1}{n} \sum_{i=1}^{n} \frac{x_i}{\pi'_i}$$

proposed by Hansen & Hurwitz [2] which is valid when sampling is with replacement, and where π'_i is the probability of selecting the ith enumeration unit at any drawing of the sample.

These estimators are illustrated in Table 1, in which $N = 3$, $n = 2$, $X_1 = 1$, $X_2 = 3$, $X_3 = 4$, $\pi'_1 = 1/6$, $\pi'_2 = 2/6$, $\pi'_3 = 3/6$, and the sampling is with replacement. As can be seen, the two estimators do not necessarily produce the same numerical estimate for the same sample, and both are unbiased estimators of the population total. Both estimators are used in unequal probability sampling, including widely used applications such as **sampling with probability proportionate to size** and **network sampling**. Because the Horvitz–Thompson estimator is appropriate for situations in which sampling is without replacement, however, it has been especially important in the development of design-based **estimation** theory and methodology for **sample surveys**.

Table 1 Comparison of estimators

Enumeration units in sample (ordered)	Probability of sample occurring	Horvitz–Thompson estimator	Hansen–Hurwitz estimator
X_1, X_1	0.0278	3.27	6.0
X_1, X_2	0.0556	8.67	7.5
X_1, X_3	0.0833	8.61	7.0
X_2, X_1	0.0556	8.67	7.5
X_2, X_2	0.1111	5.40	9.0
X_2, X_3	0.1667	10.73	8.5
X_3, X_1	0.0833	8.61	7.0
X_3, X_2	0.1667	10.73	8.5
X_3, X_3	0.2500	5.33	8.0

For more detailed discussions of the Horvitz–Thompson estimator, we refer the reader to the texts by Hedayat & Sinha [3] and Thompson [5]. Also, **Cochran** discusses this estimator in the *Encyclopedia of Statistical Sciences* [1] (this was one of Professor Cochran's last articles before his death in 1980).

References

[1] Cochran, W.G. (1983). Horvitz–Thompson estimator, in *Encyclopedia of Statistical Sciences*, Vol. 3. S. Kotz & N.L. Johnson, eds. Wiley, New York, pp. 665–668.

[2] Hansen, M.M. & Hurwitz, W.N. (1943). On the theory of sampling from finite populations, *Annals of Mathematical Statistics* **14**, 333–362.

[3] Hedayat, A.S. & Sinha, B.K. (1991). *Design and Inference in Finite Population Sampling*. Wiley, New York.

[4] Horvitz, D.G. & Thompson, D.J. (1952). A generalization of sampling without replacement from a finite universe, *Journal of the American Statistical Association* **47**, 663–685.

[5] Thompson, S.K. (1992). *Sampling*. Wiley, New York.

PAUL S. LEVY

Hospital and Health Systems *see* Health Services Organization in the US

Hospital Market Area

A hospital market area (HMA) is the geographic area served by a hospital or a group of hospitals.

Market areas are usually defined on the basis of patient origin studies, which examine the zip (postal) codes in which the patients of a hospital reside. HMAs are used in **health services research** to define the populations which provide the denominator for hospital admission rates. For example, one might use the number of back surgeries performed on people who live in a particular HMA, divided by the HMA population, as the admission rate for that area's hospital. In **small-area variation analysis**, one would examine the admission rates for different HMAs to find areas with particularly high or low admission rates, suggesting inappropriate use of services, perhaps attributable to the hospital in that HMA. Unfortunately, however, several hospitals may serve the same area, and a particular hospital may draw patients from many areas, especially in urban and suburban areas. These considerations make a hospital's admission rate both conceptually unclear and technically difficult to estimate.

Two methods have been proposed for defining HMAs and their corresponding hospital-based admission rates from population-based data. The plurality rule of Wennberg & Gittelsohn [3] assigns the population and the hospital admissions from each zip code to the hospital which is the recipient of the plurality of the admissions from the area. While simple to apply, this method is flawed by considerable **misclassification error** since many (potentially even a majority) of the persons and admissions from any given small area will be assigned to one hospital when, in truth, they "belong" to another. Furthermore, this method underemphasizes the utilization of small hospitals, since small hospitals infrequently constitute a plurality in any small area.

Griffith et al. [1] propose a "proportional allocation" method, which allocates a proportion of each small area's population to each hospital based on the proportion of that area's admissions to each hospital. Thus, if Hospital X received 24% of area A's admissions, it would be allocated 24% of Area A's population as well. By summing the populations allocated to Hospital X across all small areas, one can estimate a theoretical catchment population for Hospital X. Dividing this theoretic denominator into Hospital X's admissions yields an "admission rate" for Hospital X. The principal flaw in this method is that, because the population at risk is allocated in proportion to the numerator, it tends to diminish any true differences between hospitals in their propensity to admit.

There are other problems in defining hospital market areas. HMAs based on one patient origin study may not be appropriate for all conditions that might be studied. For example, HMAs defined by a patient origin study of all hospital admissions would not be appropriate for a study of trauma admission rates if one of the hospitals had a renowned trauma center that attracted patients from a large area. Origin studies are often based on Medicare data [2], which, since it is available primarily for people over age 65, may not be appropriate for services for younger people.

References

[1]   Griffith J.R., Restuccia, J.D. Tedeschi, P.J., Wilson, P.A. & Zuckerman, H.S. (1981). Measuring community hospital services in Michigan, *Health Services Research* **16**, 135–160.

[2]   Makuc, D.M., Haglund, B., Ingram, D.D., Kleinman, J.C. & Feldman, J.J. (1991). Health service areas for the United States, *Vital and Health Statistics, Series 2: Data Evaluation and Methods Research* **112**, 1–102.

[3]   Wennberg, J. & Gittelsohn, A. (1973). Small area variations in health care delivery, *Science* **182**, 1102.

PAULA DIEHR

Host Variability *see* Infectivity Titration

Hot Deck Methods *see* Missing Data Estimation, "Hot Deck" and "Cold Deck"

Hotelling's T^2

The Hotelling T^2 statistic is a generalization of the squared univariate t (*see* **Student's t Distribution**) for testing hypotheses on the normal distribution mean, when the population variance is unknown and must be estimated from the sample observations. For a single random sample of N p-dimensional observations from the **multivariate normal distribution**, the Hotelling statistic for testing the hypothesis $H_0 : \boldsymbol{\mu} = \boldsymbol{\mu}_0$ on the mean vector $\boldsymbol{\mu}$ is

$$T^2 = N(\overline{x} - \boldsymbol{\mu}_0)' S^{-1} (\overline{x} - \boldsymbol{\mu}_0).$$

In the squared univariate statistic the means have been replaced by mean vectors and the reciprocal of the sample variance has become the inverse of the sample **covariance matrix** S. T^2 is thus a measure of the distance of the sample mean vector from the hypothesized population vector, but in the metric of S. This case of Hotelling's T^2 test, its general derivation, and its application to two independent samples and repeated measures designs are covered in this article.

The Hotelling T^2 Test

Derivation

The T^2 statistic was originally proposed by Hotelling [3]. Hotelling's account of its derivation by the invariance properties of the roots of a certain determinantal equation is contained in [4]. T^2 is also the sample analog of **Mahalanobis distance** [5] of $\overline{x}$ and $\boldsymbol{\mu}_0$. Construction of the hypothesis test by the generalized **likelihood ratio** principle gives a statistic that is a monotonic function of T^2 [1]. Roy [10, 11] derived the T^2 statistic by his **union–intersection principle**; the explicit single-sample case has been given by Morrison [7].

Distribution of T^2

Hotelling [3] first found the distribution of T^2 by a geometrical argument. More recently, Rao [9] has given an ingenious and simple derivation of the distribution for both the null and alternative hypotheses.

We give a very general definition of T^2, state its distribution, and then apply it to cases of T^2 computed from sample observations. Let $\mathbf{Y}$ be a $p \times 1$ random vector with the multivariate normal distribution $N(\boldsymbol{\mu}, \boldsymbol{\Sigma})$. The sums of squares and products matrix $n\mathbf{S}$ has the **Wishart distribution** [1, Chapter 7] with parameters degrees of freedom n and covariance matrix $\boldsymbol{\Sigma}$, and is distributed independently of $\mathbf{Y}$. Then the general Hotelling statistic is

$$T^2 = \mathbf{Y}'\mathbf{S}^{-1}\mathbf{Y},$$

and its linear transformation,

$$F = [(n - p + 1)/n\,p]T^2,$$

has the noncentral F **distribution** with degrees of freedom p, $n - p + 1$, and noncentrality parameter $\boldsymbol{\mu}'\boldsymbol{\Sigma}^{-1}\boldsymbol{\mu}$. If $\mathbf{E}(Y) = \boldsymbol{\mu} = \mathbf{0}$, F has the usual central F distribution with p and $n - p + 1$ degrees of freedom. In the context of a single random sample and a test of the null hypothesis $H_0 : \boldsymbol{\mu} = \boldsymbol{\mu}_0$, $\mathbf{Y} = \bar{\mathbf{y}} - \boldsymbol{\mu}$ and $n = N - 1$. Under $H_0 : \boldsymbol{\mu} = \boldsymbol{\mu}_0$, $\bar{\mathbf{y}}$ is $N[\boldsymbol{\mu}_0, (1/N)\boldsymbol{\Sigma}]$, $T^2 = N(\bar{\mathbf{y}} - \boldsymbol{\mu}_0)'\mathbf{S}^{-1}(\bar{\mathbf{y}} - \boldsymbol{\mu}_0)$, and $F = [(N - p)/(N - 1)p]T^2$ has the central F distribution with p and $N - p$ degrees of freedom. For the general alternative hypothesis $H_0 : \boldsymbol{\mu} = \boldsymbol{\mu}_1$, $[(N - p)/(N - 1)/p]T^2$ has the noncentral F distribution with p and $N - p$ degrees of freedom and noncentrality parameter $\delta^2 = N(\boldsymbol{\mu}_1 - \boldsymbol{\mu}_0)'\boldsymbol{\Sigma}^{-1}(\boldsymbol{\mu}_1 - \boldsymbol{\mu}_0)$. **Power** probabilities of the T^2 test can be found from the Pearson–Hartley charts of the noncentral F distribution [7, 8], or by statistical *software* (e.g. [2] and [6]). **Sample size determination** for a given α-level test and power probability must, of course, be made iteratively, since the sample size appears both in the second degrees of freedom and in the noncentrality parameter.

Affine Invariance Property

The T^2 statistic has an important invariance property: it is unaffected by affine **transformations**

$$\mathbf{W} = \mathbf{A}\mathbf{Y} + \mathbf{h},$$

in which $\mathbf{A}$ is a $p \times p$ matrix of real constants with a nonzero determinant, and $\mathbf{h}$ is a $p \times 1$ vector of constants. The transformation must be applied to the sample mean vector $\bar{\mathbf{y}}$ as well as the population mean vector $\boldsymbol{\mu}_0$. Use of the transformation in the single-sample Hotelling statistic gives

$$
\begin{aligned}
T_{\mathrm{W}}^2 &= N(\mathbf{A}\bar{\mathbf{y}} + \mathbf{h} - \mathbf{A}\boldsymbol{\mu}_0 - \mathbf{h})'(\mathbf{A}\mathbf{S}\mathbf{A}')^{-1} \\
&\quad \times (\mathbf{A}\bar{\mathbf{y}} + \mathbf{h} - \mathbf{A}\boldsymbol{\mu}_0 - \mathbf{h}) \\
&= N(\bar{\mathbf{y}} - \boldsymbol{\mu}_0)'\mathbf{A}'(\mathbf{A}\mathbf{S}\mathbf{A}')^{-1}(\bar{\mathbf{y}} - \boldsymbol{\mu}_0) \\
&= T_{\mathrm{Y}}^2,
\end{aligned}
$$

and, of course, the affine invariance property can be verified for other more general forms of T^2. The statistic is not only unaffected by scale and location changes, but is also unchanged by oblique linear transformations of the coordinate system as well.

Tests of Hypotheses

Single Sample

We have already introduced the single-sample T^2 test of $H_0 : \boldsymbol{\mu} = \boldsymbol{\mu}_0$ against $H_1 : \boldsymbol{\mu} \neq \boldsymbol{\mu}_0$: reject H_0 at the α level if $F = [(N - p)/(N - 1)p]T^2 > F_{\alpha; p, N-p}$. The hypothesized mean vector $\boldsymbol{\mu}_0$ is given by the analyst from a substantive context: psychological test score means, dimension, or other specification means in quality assurance, or normative values of the random vector components.

Two Samples

The model for the two-sample T^2 test for equality of multivariate normal mean vectors assumes that independent random samples have been drawn from each population, and that the populations have a common covariance matrix $\boldsymbol{\Sigma}$. The observation vectors in the respective samples will be denoted by $\mathbf{x}_{11}, \ldots, \mathbf{x}_{N1}$, $\mathbf{x}_{12}, \ldots, \mathbf{x}_{M2}$. The sample mean vectors are

$$\bar{\mathbf{x}}_1 = \left(\frac{1}{N}\right)\sum_{i=1}^{N} \mathbf{x}_{i1}, \qquad \bar{\mathbf{x}}_2 = \left(\frac{1}{M}\right)\sum_{i=1}^{M} \bar{\mathbf{x}}_{i2}$$

and the pooled, or within-sample, covariance matrix estimating $\boldsymbol{\Sigma}$ is

$$
\mathbf{S} = \left(\frac{1}{N + M - 2}\right)\left[\sum_{i=1}^{N}(\mathbf{x}_{i1} - \bar{\mathbf{x}}_1)(\mathbf{x}_{i1} - \bar{\mathbf{x}}_1)' \right.
$$
$$
\left. + \sum_{i=1}^{M}(\mathbf{x}_{i2} - \bar{\mathbf{x}}_2)(\mathbf{x}_{i2} - \bar{\mathbf{x}}_2)'\right].
$$

The two-sample T^2 statistic is

$$T^2 = \left(\frac{NM}{N+M}\right)(\bar{\mathbf{x}}_1 - \bar{\mathbf{x}}_2)'\mathbf{S}^{-1}(\bar{\mathbf{x}}_1 - \bar{\mathbf{x}}_2).$$

When $H_0: \boldsymbol{\mu}_1 = \boldsymbol{\mu}_2$ is true, $F = [(N+M-p-1)/(N+M-2)p]T^2$ has the F distribution with p and $N+M-p-1$ degrees of freedom. The null hypothesis is rejected if $F > F_{\alpha;p,N+M-p-1}$. When the alternative $H_1 : \boldsymbol{\mu}_1 \neq \boldsymbol{\mu}_2$ holds, F has the noncentral F distribution with degrees of freedom $p, N+M-p-1$, and noncentrality parameter $\delta^2 = [NM/(N+M)](\boldsymbol{\mu}_1 - \boldsymbol{\mu}_2)'\boldsymbol{\Sigma}^{-1}(\boldsymbol{\mu}_1 - \boldsymbol{\mu}_2)$.

Repeated Measurements

Frequently, p observations are taken successively on each of N independent sampling units for a test of the hypothesis that the p means are equal (*see* **Longitudinal Data Analysis, Overview**). For example, plasma-free fatty acid levels might be measured in blood samples taken at $p = 6$ 15-min intervals from normal subjects after they had ingested a particular food or drug. The hypothesis of a common-mean-free fatty acid level at six times might be of interest, and could be tested by Hotelling's T^2 statistic.

The repeated-measures test is equivalent to testing the hypothesis that the $p - 1$ successive differences of the variables have zero means. We begin by transforming the p response variables $X_1, \ldots, X_p$ to the successive differences $Y_1, \ldots, Y_{p-1}$ by the linear transformation

$$\mathbf{Y} = \begin{bmatrix} Y_1 \\ Y_2 \\ \cdot \\ \cdot \\ \cdot \\ Y_{p-1} \end{bmatrix}$$

$$= \begin{bmatrix} -1 & 1 & 0 & . & . & . & 0 & 0 \\ 0 & -1 & 1 & . & . & . & 0 & 0 \\ . & . & . & . & & . & . & . \\ 0 & 0 & 0 & . & . & . & -1 & 1 \end{bmatrix} \begin{bmatrix} X_1 \\ X_2 \\ \cdot \\ \cdot \\ \cdot \\ X_p \end{bmatrix}$$

$$= \mathbf{C}\mathbf{X}.$$

We test $H_0 : E(Y_1) = \cdots = E(Y_{p-1}) = 0$ by

$$T^2 = N\bar{\mathbf{y}}'\mathbf{S}^{-1}\bar{\mathbf{y}},$$

or equivalently in terms of the observations on the original variables,

$$T^2 = N\bar{\mathbf{x}}'\mathbf{C}'(\mathbf{C}\mathbf{S}\mathbf{C}')^{-1}\mathbf{C}\bar{\mathbf{x}},$$

where $\mathbf{C}$ is the $(p-1) \times p$ matrix of the successive difference transformation. As in the single-sample case, $F = [(N-p+1)/(N-1)(p-1)]T^2$ has the F distribution with $p-1$ and $N-p+1$ degrees of freedom, and we reject the null hypothesis of equal response variable means if $F > F_{\alpha;p-1,N-p+1}$.

Paired Response Variables

Some repeated-measurements experiments consist of the same p response variables observed at two different times or conditions on the same subjects or other sampling units. If we represent the $p \times 1$ response vectors at the two times by $\mathbf{X}_1$ and $\mathbf{X}_2$ we can test the hypothesis $H_0 : E(\mathbf{X}_1) = E(\mathbf{X}_2)$ by the T^2 statistic. A random sample of N independent observation vectors partitioned according to the two times as $[\mathbf{x}'_{i1}, \mathbf{x}'_{i2}]$ yields the respective partitioned sample mean vector and covariance matrix

$$\begin{bmatrix} \bar{\mathbf{x}}'_1 \\ \bar{\mathbf{x}}'_2 \end{bmatrix}, \qquad \begin{bmatrix} \mathbf{S}_{11} & \mathbf{S}_{12} \\ \mathbf{S}'_{12} & \mathbf{S}_{22} \end{bmatrix},$$

where

$$\mathbf{S}_{ij} = \sum_{h=1}^{N}(\mathbf{x}_{hi} - \bar{\mathbf{x}}_i)(\mathbf{x}_{hj} - \bar{\mathbf{x}}_j)', \quad i, j = 1, 2.$$

The Hotelling statistic is

$$T^2 = N(\bar{\mathbf{x}}_1 - \bar{\mathbf{x}}_2)'(\mathbf{S}_{11} + \mathbf{S}_{22} - \mathbf{S}_{12} - \mathbf{S}'_{12})^{-1}$$
$$\times (\bar{\mathbf{x}}_1 - \bar{\mathbf{x}}_2),$$

and reflects the correlations between the two times through the elements of the submatrix $\mathbf{S}_{12}$. T^2 is merely the extension of the **paired t test** to p pairs of response variables. If the data were transformed to an $N \times p$ matrix of paired differences, then the T^2 statistic would reduce to the single-sample T^2 described previously. When H_0 is true, $F = [(N -$

$p)/(N-1)p]T^2$ has the F distribution with p and $N-p$ degrees of freedom. H_0 would be rejected when F exceeds the right-tail α-level critical value for that distribution.

Confidence Statements Obtained from T^2

Confidence Region for a Single Mean Vector

The distribution of T^2 for a single random sample from the multinormal distribution can be used to obtain this ellipsoidal $100(1-\alpha)\%$ confidence region for the population mean vector $\boldsymbol{\mu}$:

$$N(\boldsymbol{\mu} - \bar{\mathbf{x}})'\mathbf{S}^{-1}(\boldsymbol{\mu} - \bar{\mathbf{x}})$$
$$\leq [(N-1)p/(N-p)]F_{\alpha;p,N-p}$$

(*see* **Confidence Intervals and Sets**).

Simultaneous Confidence Intervals

Rejection of the null hypothesis by the T^2 test still does not indicate *which* of the p responses may have contributed to that decision. Roy's union–intersection derivation of T^2 [10] leads directly to simultaneous tests and confidence intervals for linear compounds of the population means (*see* **Simultaneous Inference**). "Simultaneous" means that one may construct an unlimited number of confidence intervals and still have an overall coverage probability of $1-\alpha$, or test infinitely many hypotheses and still enjoy an overall type I error rate no greater than α. For the single-sample case the $100(1-\alpha)\%$ Roy–Bose [12] simultaneous confidence interval for the linear compound $\mathbf{a}'\boldsymbol{\mu}$ is

$$\mathbf{a}'\bar{\mathbf{x}} - \left\{ (1/N)\mathbf{a}'\mathbf{S}\mathbf{a} \right.$$
$$\times [(N-1)p/(N-p)]F_{\alpha;p,N-p} \Big\}^{1/2}$$
$$\leq \mathbf{a}'\boldsymbol{\mu} \leq \mathbf{a}'\bar{\mathbf{x}} + \left\{ (1/N)\mathbf{a}'\mathbf{S}\mathbf{a} \right.$$
$$\times [(N-1)p/(N-p)]F_{\alpha;p,N-p} \Big\}^{1/2},$$

where $\mathbf{a}$ is any $p \times 1$ vector of constants chosen by the investigator. For the two-sample situation the $100(1-\alpha)\%$ simultaneous confidence interval for the linear compound $\mathbf{a}'(\boldsymbol{\mu}_1 - \boldsymbol{\mu}_2)$ of the differences of the mean vector elements is

$$\mathbf{a}'(\bar{\mathbf{x}}_1 - \bar{\mathbf{x}}_2) - \left\{ [(N+M)/NM]\mathbf{a}'\mathbf{S}\mathbf{a} \right.$$

$$\times [(N+M-2)p/(N+M-p-1)]$$
$$\times F_{\alpha;p,N+M-p-1} \Big\}^{1/2} \leq \mathbf{a}'(\boldsymbol{\mu}_1 - \boldsymbol{\mu}_2)$$
$$\leq \mathbf{a}'(\bar{\mathbf{x}}_1 - \bar{\mathbf{x}}_2) + \left\{ [(N+M)/NM]\mathbf{a}'\mathbf{S}\mathbf{a} \right.$$
$$\times [(N+M-2)p/(N+M-p-1)]$$
$$\times F_{\alpha;p,N+M-p-1} \Big\}^{1/2}.$$

If the interval contains zero, then the hypothesis $H_0: \mathbf{a}'\boldsymbol{\mu}_1 = \mathbf{a}'\boldsymbol{\mu}_2$ is tenable at the α level in the simultaneous testing sense. Alternatively, in both cases families of hypotheses can also be tested with an overall type I error rate no greater than α.

References

[1] Anderson, T.W. (1984). *An Introduction to Multivariate Statistical Analysis*, 2nd Ed. Wiley, New York.

[2] Galen Research, Inc. (1990). *Electronic Tables*. Galen Research, Inc., Salt Lake City.

[3] Hotelling, H. (1931). The generalization of Student's ratio, *Annals of Mathematical Statistics* **2**, 360–378.

[4] Hotelling, H. (1954). Multivariate analysis, in *Statistics and Mathematics in Biology*, O. Kempthorne, T. Bancroft, J. Gowen & J.L. Lush, eds. Hafner, New York, pp. 67–80.

[5] Mahalanobis, P.C. (1936). On the generalized distance in statistics, *Proceedings of the National Institute of Sciences of India* **2**, 49–55.

[6] Mehta, C.R. & Patel, N.R. (1994). *StaTable^{TM} Electronic Tables for Statisticians and Engineers*. Cytel Software Corporation, Cambridge, Mass.

[7] Morrison, D.F. (1990). *Multivariate Statistical Methods*, 3rd Ed. McGraw-Hill, New York.

[8] Pearson, E.S. & Hartley, H.O. (1951). Charts of the power function of the analysis of variance tests, derived from the non-central F distribution, *Biometrika* **38**, 112–130.

[9] Rao, C.R. (1973). *Linear Statistical Inference and Its Applications*, 2nd Ed. Wiley, New York.

[10] Roy, S.N. (1953). On a heuristic method of test construction and its use in multivariate analysis, *Annals of Mathematical Statistics* **24**, 220–238.

[11] Roy, S.N. (1957). *Some Aspects of Multivariate Analysis*. Wiley, New York.

[12] Roy, S.N. & Bose, R.C. (1953). Simultaneous confidence interval estimation, *Annals of Mathematical Statistics* **24**, 513–536.

(*See also* **Multivariate Analysis of Variance; Multivariate Analysis, Overview**)

DONALD F. MORRISON

Hotelling, Harold

Born: September 29, 1895, in Fulda, Minnesota.
Died: December 26, 1973, in Chapel Hill, North Carolina.

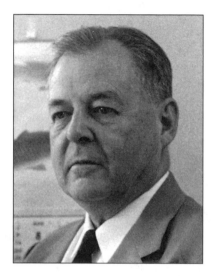

Reproduced by permission of the Royal Statistical Society

Harold Hotelling was responsible for much original theoretical work in both statistics and mathematical economics and did much to advance the teaching of statistics at US universities, including Columbia and the University of North Carolina. Hotelling's undergraduate degree was a B.A. in journalism from the University of Washington in 1919, but his mathematical talent was recognized and encouraged by Eric T. Bell. Hotelling received an M.S. degree in Mathematics at the University of Washington in 1921 and a Doctorate of Philosophy at Princeton University in 1924, with a dissertation in the field of topology.

Following his doctorate, he spent seven years at Stanford University, first as Research Associate in the Food Research Institute and later as a Associate Professor of Mathematics. During his time at Stanford, he applied mathematical ideas to problems in journalism and political science, population and food supply, and theoretic economics. In 1929, he spent six months with **R.A. Fisher** at the Rothamstead Experimental Station at Harpenden in England which helped to develop his strong interest in mathematical statistics. In 1931 he published perhaps his most important contribution to statistics when he generalized to the multivariate case **Student's t** test for the **mean** of a univariate **normal distribution** [4] (*see* **Multivariate t Distribution**). This test has become known as **Hotelling's generalized T^2** test and was later recognized as having wide applicability in statistics.

In 1931 Hotelling was appointed Professor of Economics at Columbia University where he stayed for 15 years. During World War II he organized the Statistical Research Group, which was engaged in statistical work relating to military problems. The group included **Abraham Wald**, W. Allen Wallis, and Jacob Wolfowitz. During this time Wald developed his theory of **sequential analysis**. In 1946 Hotelling was invited by **Gertrude Cox** to organize a Department of Mathematical Statistics at the University of North Carolina at Chapel Hill (UNC-Chapel Hill), which became an important center for statistical research and teaching. He recruited many outstanding statisticians, including R.C. Bose, S.N. Roy, W. Hoeffding, W.G. Madow, H.E. Robbins, W.L. Smith, and N.L. Johnson. Hotelling remained at UNC–Chapel Hill until his death.

Hotelling proposed a method of **principal components** [6] which is applicable to problems of **factor analysis** arising in educational testing. Using ideas of n-dimensional geometry, the principal components are linear functions of multivariate observations, the first of which has the greatest variability and each subsequent one less variability. A similar mathematical idea underlies Hotelling's theory of **canonical correlations** [7]. Among Hotelling's other contributions to statistics are his paper on differential equations subject to error [3], one of the first dealing with statistical problems related to **stochastic processes**; a paper (jointly with H. Working) on the interpretation of trends [18] which had one of the first examples of a **confidence region** and the idea of **multiple comparisons**; the derivation of the distribution of Spearman's **rank correlation** coefficient [11]; and the experimental determination of the maximum of a function [10].

In economic theory, he dealt with problems in depreciation and the importance of maximizing principles [2]; the interrelated demand and supply functions of profit maximizers [5]; and welfare economics [8], possibly his most important contribution to mathematical economics.

Hotelling had a talent for attracting excellent faculty members, both at Columbia and the University of

North Carolina, and played an important role in raising standards in statistical research and developing mathematical statistics as a respected academic discipline. He was a strong advocate of the importance of **teaching statistics** [9], which had an impact on the academic community and aided in the establishment of departments of statistics at American universities. Levene paid tribute to his excellence as a teacher and lecturer [12].

In 1955 Hotelling received an honorary LL.D. from the University of Chicago. In 1963 he received an honorary D.Sc. from the University of Rochester and was an Honorary Fellow of the **Royal Statistical Society** and a Distinguished Fellow of the American Economic Association. In 1936–37 he was the President of the Econometric Society and in 1941 of the Institute of Mathematical Statistics. In 1970 he was elected to the National Academy of Sciences and in 1972 received the North Carolina Award for Science. His final award, in 1973, was his election to membership of the Accademia Nazionale dei Lincei in Rome, which occurred shortly before his death.

Hotelling's contributions to statistics have been memorialized by Anderson [1], Madow [13, 14], **Neyman** [15], and Olkin [16], and to mathematical economics by Samuelson [17].

References

[1]   Anderson, T.W. (1960). Harold Hotelling's research in statistics, *American Statistician* **14**, 17–21.

[2]   Hotelling, H. (1925). A general mathematical theory of depreciation, *Journal of the American Statistical Association* **20**, 340–353.

[3]   Hotelling, H. (1927). Differential equations subject to error, and population estimates, *Journal of the American Statistical Association* **20**, 340–353.

[4]   Hotelling, H. (1931). The generalization of Student's ratio, *Annals of Mathematical Statistics* **2**, 360–378.

[5]   Hotelling, H. (1932). Edgeworth's taxation paradox and the nature of demand and supply functions, *Journal of Political Economy* **40**, 577–616.

[6]   Hotelling, H. (1933). Analysis of complex of statistical variables into principal components, *Journal of Educational Psychology* **24**, 417–441, 498–520.

[7]   Hotelling, H. (1936). Relations between two sets of variates, *Biometrika* **28**, 321–377.

[8]   Hotelling, H. (1938). The general welfare in relation to problems of taxation and of railway and utility rates, *Econometrica* **6**, 242–269. (Presidential address to the Econometric Society at the meeting in Atlantic City, N.J., December 28, 1937).

[9]   Hotelling, H. (1940). The teaching of statistics, *Annals of Mathematical Statistics* **11**, 457–470.

[10]   Hotelling, H. (1941). Experimental determination of the maximum of a function, *Annals of Mathematical Statistics* **12**, 20–45.

[11]   Hotelling, H. & Pabst, M.R. (1936). Rank correlation and tests of significance involving no assumption of normality, *Annals of Mathematical Statistics* **7**, 29–43.

[12]   Levene, H. (1974). In memoriam: Harold Hotelling, 1895–1973, *American Statistician* **28**, 71–73.

[13]   Madow, W.G. (1960). Harold Hotelling, in *Contributions to Probability and Statistics: Essays in Honor of Harold Hotelling*, I. Olkin, S.G. Ghurye, W. Hoeffding, W.G. Madow & H.B. Mann, eds. Stanford University Press, Stanford, pp. 3–5.

[14]   Madow, W.G. (1960). Harold Hotelling as a teacher, *American Statistician* **14**, 15–17.

[15]   Neyman, J. (1960). Harold Hotelling: a leader in mathematical statistics, in *Contributions to Probability and Statistics: Essays in Honor of Harold Hotelling*, I. Olkin, S.G. Ghurye, W. Hoeffding, W.G. Madow & H.B. Mann, eds. Stanford University Press, Stanford, pp. 6–10.

[16]   Olkin, I., Ghurye, S.G., Hoeffding, W., Madow, W.G. & Mann, H.B., eds (1960). *Contributions to Probability and Statistics: Essays in Honor of Harold Hotelling*. Stanford University Press, Stanford.

[17]   Samuelson, P.A. (1960). Harold Hotelling as mathematical economist, *American Statistician* **14**, 21–25.

[18]   Working, H. & Hotelling, H. (1929). Applications of the theory of error to the interpretation of trends, *Journal of the American Statistical Association* **24**, Supplement, 73–85.

EDMUND A. GEHAN

Hotelling–Pabst Test *see* Spearman Rank Correlation

Household Epidemics *see* Chain Binomial Model

Human Genetics, Overview

Mendel's laws underlie the distribution of genetic traits observed in individuals. At each genetic locus, an individual receives one **gene** which is a copy of a randomly chosen one of the two genes of the father, and one which is a copy of a randomly chosen one of the two genes of the mother. Each individual passes on to each offspring a randomly chosen one of his two genes, independently to each offspring and independently of the gene contributed by his spouse. The different allelic forms of the genes at a locus, acting in combination with alleles at other loci and with environmental effects, give rise to different phenotypes, the observable characteristics of individuals. Alleles at loci on different chromosomes are inherited independently, but alleles at loci on the same chromosome are *linked*, or correlated, in their inheritance, owing to the process of meiosis which gives rise to the gamete cells.

At the population level, new alleles arise by mutation, and frequencies of alleles are influenced by the genetic forces of selection and the demographic forces of migration and population structure. Since populations are finite, allele frequencies will change over time under random genetic drift, even in the absence of directional genetic or demographic forces (*see* **Population Genetics**). Whereas genetic analysis of other species has been directed towards an understanding of evolution and population biology, or to the increase of crop yields and animal produce, human genetics has been primarily focused on an understanding of the genetic determinants of human disease.

The year 1900 saw the rediscovery of Mendel's work, 1901 the first discovery of a human **blood group** system, and 1902 the first application of Mendelian principles in medical genetics, setting the stage for the development of human medical and population genetics. With the analysis of data from human (as opposed to experimental) populations, came the need to address questions of **ascertainment** [11, 37]. With the discovery of blood group systems, came the first array of **genetic markers** that could be used both to assess human diversity and as markers in **linkage analysis**.

In the 1930s there was a rapid expansion in the development of approaches to the statistical analysis of human genetic data, with the work of Haldane, Hogben, and Fisher. Although Mendelian principles had been applied earlier in assessing the proportion of affected offspring in families ascertained for segregation of rare recessive diseases [1, 37], this period also saw the earliest formal **segregation analyses**,

comparing alternative models for the underlying basis of a genetic trait [12, 16], and consequently further development in a statistical framework and model for ascertainment [8]. Also at this time came the recognition that the methods of linkage analysis already used in experimental populations could be applied also to data collected from human families ascertained for a genetic disease [9, 13].

There is no strict separation between inferences of the genetic basis of traits from family data and from population data. One of the earliest applications of population genetic principles to human disease was Haldane's consideration of the expected frequencies of Mendelian genetic diseases in terms of mutation-selection balance [14]. One of the first statistical analyses of population data was that of Bernstein [2] leading to a resolution of the basis of the ABO blood types, while Fisher [10] regarded his analysis of the rhesus blood group system as a fine example of scientific inference. The resolution of human genetic blood groups and enzyme systems not only provided genetic markers for linkage analysis but also a source of extensive information on human diversity.

In fact, the discovery of many blood group systems in the first half of the century prompted many studies of the extent of human diversity, and a search for explanations of observed data on the basis of models of selection, and of the migration patterns of human history. Many of the population genetic ideas and models underlying such inferences were described by Cavalli-Sforza & Bodmer [5]. While **demography** may be the major factor influencing global patterns of human diversity, a gene need not itself be subject to differential selection in order for its selection to have an impact. The discovery of the many variants present in the human white blood cells (**HLA system**), and their multiple and complex associations with disease prompted renewed effort in understanding patterns of human variation. The phenomenon of "hitchhiking" [20], where the selective effects of genes at closely linked loci affect patterns of observed variation, has been used to explain unusually high frequencies of some human disease alleles in some human populations [35]. Thomson et al. [34] used human HLA data to examine the evolutionary interactions of selection, migration, and linkage. A more recent review of the statistical approaches to an understanding of associations of HLA and disease is given in [33]. Although current research in human genetics is often more focused towards individual data than to information at the population level, the data painstakingly compiled by Mourant et al. [23] remain a rich source of information, while the major work of Cavalli-Sforza et al. [6] shows how population allele frequencies reflect the imprint of human history.

While demography and genetic selection affect population allele frequencies, mutation is the source of new genetic variation. The estimation of mutation rates is therefore an important aspect of statistical genetics. It is hard to obtain precise estimates of human mutation rates by direct methods, since mutation rates are small. Indirect methods of estimation use current levels of genetic variation, and require assumptions about population size and structure. Over the 45 years since 1951 [25], the leader in study of human mutation rates by both direct [27] and indirect [26] methods has been J.V. Neel.

From 1935 to 1975 there were many developments in the statistical analysis of human genetic data observed on relatives, but the basic framework of segregation and linkage analysis, as developed by J.B.S. Haldane and R.A. Fisher, remained largely unchanged. For computational reasons, early analyses had been restricted to nuclear families or small pedigrees. With the widespread availability of digital computers, increasing interest in analysis of data on more extended pedigrees led to the development of new computational approaches [7]. With computational power permitting the analysis of larger data sets, and hence perhaps resolving more complex traits, came the necessity for more complex trait models such as the **mixed model in segregation analysis** [22]. In linkage analysis particularly, there were further developments, leading to a better understanding of how inferences could be drawn [15, 21] and to a better understanding of their properties of linkage likelihoods [31]. Ott [29] covers many of these developments.

Since 1980, with the development of molecular biology, there has been an explosion in the number of **polymorphisms** available for use as genetic markers in linkage analysis. Human genome maps at centimorgan density are now a reality [24], and the limitation in linkage analysis is no longer the availability of segregating markers, but the trait information. Simple Mendelian traits are rapidly being mapped, and the relevant genes identified. However, if a trait is exceedingly rare, or shows genetic heterogeneity, or

if its genetic basis is uncertain or complex involving alleles at several loci, then problems in linkage analysis remain.

The computation of a linkage likelihood over a pedigree requires a specific segregation analysis model for the trait to be assumed. For traits whose basis is uncertain, particularly of incomplete **penetrance** or delayed onset, linkage detection methods using only affected individuals have been developed. These are more robust to trait model assumptions; indeed, under the null hypothesis of no linkage, the distribution of the test statistic is often independent of trait model assumptions. Such methods date back to the 1930s, when Penrose [30] introduced sib pair methods, but more recently have been extended to other types of relationship [3, 19, 36]. In many cases, the use of only affected pedigree members can greatly increase robustness with little loss of power.

Once linkage has been detected, **multipoint linkage analysis** can help to localize the position of the gene more precisely. However, multipoint methods are computationally exceedingly intensive, particularly where there are many unobserved members of the pedigree. Moreover, there are limits to the resolution of linkage mapping (*see* **Genetic Map Functions**) [4]. The scale of resolution depends on the number of segregations that can be (explicitly or implicitly) observed. Where genetic homogeneity can be assumed, disequilibrium mapping [17] or **haplotype analysis** provides an alternative. Here the exact ancestry of current carriers of a disease allele is unknown, but their shared ancestry results in **linkage disequilibrium** with marker loci at small **genetic distance**. The large number of ancestral segregations provides for a finer mapping scale. Ultimately it may be possible to map at still finer scales by considering the matching and nonmatching segments of individual genomes [28].

Genetic heterogeneity is one of the major difficulties in resolving the genetic basis of any trait. Studies within a given population or of data on a single extended pedigree reduce the chance of heterogeneity within the data set, but such data sets are often limited in size, and results may not be relevant outside the particular population studied. Gradually, however, more complex traits are being resolved through advances both in the available genetic data and in methods of analysis and computation.

The classic text on human genetics is that of Stern [32]. The more recent text by Khoury et al.

[18] provides a thorough overview of approaches in modern genetic epidemiology, while Ott [29] is the best reference text on linkage analysis in human genetics.

References

[1]   Alpert, E. (1914). The laws of Naudin-Mendel, *Journal of Heredity* **5**, 492-497.

[2]   Bernstein, F. (1925). Zusammenfassende Betrachtungen über die erblichen Blutstrukturen des Menschen, *Zeitschrift für induktive Abstammungs- und VererbungsLehre* **37**, 237-270.

[3]   Bishop, D.T. & Williamson, J. (1990). The power of identity-by-state methods for linkage analysis, *American Journal of Human Genetics* **46**, 254-265.

[4]   Boehnke, M. (1994). Limits of resolution of genetic linkage studies: implications for positional cloning of human disease genes, *American Journal of Human Genetics* **55**, 379-390.

[5]   Cavalli-Sforza, L.L. & Bodmer W.F. (1971). *The Genetics of Human Populations*. Freeman, San Francisco.

[6]   Cavalli-Sforza, L.L., Menozzi, P. & Piazza, A. (1994). *The History and Geography of Human Genes*. Princeton University Press, Princeton.

[7]   Elston R.C. & Stewart, J. (1971). A general model for the genetic analysis of pedigree data, *Human Heredity* **21**, 523-542.

[8]   Fisher, R.A. (1934). The effects of methods of ascertainment on the estimation of frequencies, *Annals of Human Genetics* **6**, 13-25.

[9]   Fisher, R.A. (1934). The amount of information supplied by records of families as a function of the linkage in the population sampled, *Annals of Eugenics* **6**, 66-70.

[10]   Fisher, R.A. (1947). The *Rhesus* factor: a study in scientific method, *American Scientist* **35**, 95-102, 113.

[11]   Galton, F. (1904). Average number of kinfolk in each degree, *Nature* **70**, 529, 626.

[12]   Haldane, J.B.S. (1932). A method for investigating recessive characters in man, *Journal of Genetics* **25**, 251-255.

[13]   Haldane, J.B.S. (1934). Methods for the detection of autosomal linkage in man, *Annals of Eugenics* **6**, 26-65.

[14]   Haldane J.B.S. (1935). The rate of spontaneous mutation of a human gene, *Journal of Genetics* **31**, 317-326.

[15]   Haldane, J.B.S. & Smith, C.A.B. (1947). A new estimate of the linkage between the genes for colourblindness and haemophilia in man, *Annals of Eugenics* **14**, 10-31.

[16]   Hogben, L.T. (1931). The genetic analysis of familial traits. I. Single gene substitutions, *Journal of Genetics* **25**, 97-112.

[17]   Kaplan, N.L., Hill, W.G. & Weir, B.S. (1995). Likelihood methods for locating disease genes in nonequilibrium populations, *American Journal of Human Genetics* **56**, 18-32.

[18]   Khoury, M.J., Beaty, T.H. & Cohen, B.H. (1993). *Fundamentals of Genetic Epidemiology*. Oxford University Press, Oxford.

[19]   Lander, E.S. & Botstein, D. (1987). Homozygosity mapping: a way to map human recessive traits with the DNA of inbred children, *Science* **236**, 1567-1570.

[20]   Maynard Smith, J. & Haigh, J. (1974). The hitch-hiking effect of a favourable gene, *Genetical Research* **23**, 23-35.

[21]   Morton, N.E. (1955). Sequential tests for the detection of linkage, *American Journal of Human Genetics* **7**, 277-318.

[22]   Morton, N.E. & MacLean, C.J. (1974). Analysis of family resemblance. III. Complex segregation analysis of quantitative traits, *American Journal of Human Genetics* **26**, 489-503.

[23]   Mourant, A.E., Kopec, A.C. & Domaniewska-Sobczak, K. (1976). *The Distribution of Human Blood Groups and Other Polymorphisms*. Oxford University Press, Oxford.

[24]   Murray, J.C., Buetow, K.H., Weber, J.L. (and 24 others) (1994). A comprehensive human linkage map with centimorgan density, *Science* **265**, 2049-2064.

[25]   Neel, J.V. & Falls, H.F. (1951). The rate of mutation of the gene responsible for retinoblastoma in man, *Science* **114**, 419-422.

[26]   Neel, J.V. & Rothman, E.D. (1978) Indirect estimates of mutation rate in tribal Amerindians, *Proceedings of the National Academy of Sciences* **75**, 5585-5588.

[27]   Neel, J.V., Satoh, C., Goriki, K., Fujita, M., Takahashi, N., Asakawa, J. & Hazama, R. (1986). The rate with which spontaneous mutation alters the electrophoretic mobility of polypeptides, *Proceedings of the National Academy of Sciences* **83**, 389-393.

[28]   Nelson, S.F., McCusker, J.H., Sander, M.A., Kee, Y., Modrish, P. & Brown, P.O. (1993). Genomic mismatch scanning: a new approach to genetic linkage mapping, *Nature Genetics* **4**, 11-18.

[29]   Ott, J. (1991). *Analysis of Human Genetic Linkage*, 2nd Ed. Johns Hopkins University Press, Baltimore.

[30]   Penrose, L.S. (1935). The detection of autosomal linkage in data which consist of pairs of brothers and sisters of unspecified parentage, *Annals of Eugenics* **6**, 133-138.

[31]   Smith, C.A.B. (1953). Detection of linkage in human genetics, *Journal of the Royal Statistical Society, Series B* **15**, 153-192.

[32]   Stern, C. (1960). *Principles of Human Genetics*, 2nd Ed. Freeman, San Francisco.

[33]   Thomson, G. (1981). A review of theoretical aspects of HLA and disease associations, *Theoretical Population Biology* **20**, 168-208.

[34]   Thomson, G., Bodmer, W.F. & Bodmer J. (1976). The HL-A system as a model for studying the interaction between selection migration and linkage, in *Population Genetics and Ecology*, S. Karlin & E. Nevo, eds. Academic Press, New York, pp. 465-498.

[35] Wagener, D.K. & Cavalli-Sforza, L.L. (1975). Ethnic variation in genetic diseases: possible roles of hitch-hiking and epistasis, *American Journal of Human Genetics* **27**, 348–364.

[36] Weeks, D.E. & Lange, K. (1988). The affected-pedigree-member methods of linkage analysis, *American Journal of Human Genetics* **42**, 315–326.

[37] Weinberg, W. (1912). Zur Verebung der Anlage der Bluterkrankheit mit methodol. Erganzungen meiner Geschwistermethode, *Archiv für Rassen- und Gesellschaftsbiologie* **9**, 694–709.

E. THOMPSON

Huynh–Feldt Estimator *see* Analysis of Variance for Longitudinal Data

Hyper-Graeco–Latin Square *see* Orthogonal Designs

Hypergeometric Distribution

Consider a clinical study of five patients A, B, C, D, and E, two of whom are randomly assigned to a new therapy (surgery plus drug) and the remaining three to surgery alone. As healthy skeptics, we wish to test the statement that the patients' fates are unaffected by the new drug. Suppose that patients A and C respond. What is the probability distribution of the number of responders in the group assigned to the new therapy?

We can easily enumerate the possible outcomes (Table 1). There are 10 equally likely assignments of patients to the treatment groups, and under our assumption of predestined fate, the probability of two, one, or no responders in the new treatment group are 10%, 60%, and 30%, respectively.

Enumeration works well when the number of possibilities is small, such as the example in Table 1 of 10 possible assignments. However, as shown later, there is a rapid increase in the number of possible

Table 1   Assignments to new therapy (others to standard)

AC (two responders in new therapy):	1 way
AB, AD, AE, BC, CD, CE (one responder):	6 ways
BD, BE, DE (no responders):	3 ways

assignments with a modest increase in the scope of the number of patients.

The Hypergeometric Distribution

Consider a population of N patients, among whom A are "responders" and $B = N - A$ are "failures". Suppose we select a random sample of n patients. (That is, any subset of n patients has an equal chance of being the actual sample.) What is the probability distribution of the number of responders in the sample? The answer defines the *hypergeometric distribution*.

Combinatorial Considerations

Question: How many distinct n letter words can we make from an N letter alphabet, when no letter is repeated?

Answer:

$$\prod_{i=0}^{n-1}(N-i) = N(N-1)(N-2)\ldots(N-n+1).$$
(1)

The first letter can be selected N ways. For each of these, the second can be chosen in $(N-1)$ ways. Hence there are $N(N-1)$ two-letter words. For each of these two-letter words there are $(N-2)$ ways to select the third letter, or $N(N-1)(N-2)$ three-letter words. The general formula follows inductively.

Question: How many ways can we select n distinct letters from an N letter alphabet, if order is unimportant?

Answer:

$$\binom{N}{n} = \frac{N!}{n!(N-n)!} = \left[\prod_{i=0}^{n-1}(N-i)\right] \bigg/ n!, \quad (2)$$

where, by definition, $r! = r(r-1)(r-2)\ldots 1$ and $0! = 1$. [We define $\binom{N}{n}$ as zero if $n < 0$ or $n > N$.]

By applying (1) with $N = n$, there are $n!$ ways to arrange each collection of n distinct letters into words. Hence, the number of distinct selections of n letters from an N letter alphabet is the number of n letter words per (1) divided by $n!$ This gives us the right-most result in (2). By multiplying the numerator and denominator of the right-most part of (2) by $(N - n)!$, we obtain the middle expression of (2).

Hypergeometric Probability Function

The solution of the original question posed is defined as the probability of observing x responses in a random sample of n patients from a population containing A responders and $N - A$ nonresponders:

$$h(x; n, A, N) = \binom{A}{x} \binom{N-A}{n-x} \bigg/ \binom{N}{n} \quad (3)$$

$$= \binom{n}{x} \binom{N-n}{A-x} \bigg/ \binom{N}{A}. \quad (4)$$

Note that (4) tells us that the roles of n and A are interchangeable.

To derive (3), note that from (2), there are $\binom{N}{n}$ possible samples. Also from (2), we can select x responders from the population of A responders in $\binom{A}{x}$ ways and for each of those, we can complete the sample by selecting the nonresponders in $\binom{N-A}{n-x}$ ways. Hence, the numerator of (3) represents the number of possible samples with exactly x responders.

To obtain (4) from (3), one can simply replace the combinatorial terms by factorials [middle part of (2)].

In the example posed in the Introduction, $N = 5$ patients, $A = 2$ responders, and $n = 2$ sampled in the experimental treatment. From (3):

$$h(2; 2, 2, 5) = 1/10,$$

$$h(1; 2, 2, 5) = 6/10,$$

$$h(0; 2, 2, 5) = 3/10.$$

If $N = 20$ and $n = 10$, then there are $184\,756$ possible samples. Enumeration of the possible samples, as in the case where $N = 5$ and $n = 2$, would quickly become too time-consuming.

Properties of the Hypergeometric Distribution

Property 1. By straightforward algebra applied to (3):

$$h(x + 1; n, A, N)$$
$$= h(x; n, A, N) \left[\frac{(n - x)(A - x)}{(x + 1)(N - A - n + x + 1)} \right].$$
$$(5)$$

Property 2. Since from (5), the term in square brackets decreases with increasing x, the distribution is "unimodal" and has its mode at one (or both) of the integer values of x surrounding the x value where the term in square brackets is equal to unity. That is, the mode is adjacent to or equal to (if an integer):

$$x = \frac{(A + 1)(n + 1)}{N + 2} - 1. \quad (6)$$

A "unimodal" discrete distribution over a finite set of integers $0, 1, \ldots, K$ has probabilities that behave in one of the following ways: (i) increase to a peak and then decrease; (ii) have a peak at zero and decrease; or (iii) increase from zero to its peak at the highest possible x, K. Looking at increasing values of the random variable, it cannot show an increase in probability to the right of a decrease.

Property 3. The mean of the hypergeometric distribution, μ, is

$$\mu = nA/N. \quad (7)$$

Property 4. The variance of the hypergeometric distribution, σ^2, is

$$\sigma^2 = \frac{n(N - n)A(N - A)}{N^2(N - 1)}. \quad (8)$$

Property 5. Although the mean and mode do not seem to be related, it can be shown that the mean is always larger than the value defined by x in (6), and the mean is always within one unit of the value of x defined in (6). Thus, the mode must occur close to the mean.

Approximations

The approximations below can be "proven" by limit theory. The astute question, however, is: How large must the various quantities be before the approximation works to our satisfaction? Hence, rather than limit theory, we use exhaustive computer searches to explore the accuracy. The demonstrations are convincing in terms of closeness over a broad range of applications.

We approximate the cumulative distribution, which has exact value:

$$\Pr[X \leq x] = H(x; n, A, N)$$

$$= \sum_{j=0}^{x} h(j; n, A, N), \qquad (9)$$

where h is defined in (3).

Binomial Approximation

If the population, N, is "large", and the sample size, n, is a "small" fraction of the smaller of A (responders) and $(N - A)$ (failures), then the cumulative distribution satisfies the following approximation:

$$H(x; n, A, N) \cong \sum_{j=0}^{x} \binom{N}{j} p^j (1 - p)^{n-j}, \qquad (10)$$

where $p = A/N$.

The right-hand side of (10) is the cumulative **binomial distribution**.

Because of the "drop in the bucket" effect, successive trials are close to independent. Sampling without replacement (hypergeometric) is similar to sampling with replacement (binomial). (*see* **Sampling With and Without Replacement**).

Reality Check. We studied each of the 432.9 million binomial approximations where $100 \leq A \leq 1000$, $100 \leq N - A \leq 1000$, $n \leq 0.1A$ and $n \leq 0.1(N - A)$, and $x = 0, 1, \ldots, n$. The largest deviation between the cumulative distributions occurred where $A = 100$, $N - A = 100$, $n = 10$, and $x = 3$. Eq. (9) gave an exact value of 0.1656, while (10) gave an approximate value of 0.1719, for a difference of 0.0063.

Normal Approximation

Let us define the "smallest expected value" as

$$EC =$$
$$\min \left\{ \frac{An}{N}, \frac{(N - A)n}{N}, \frac{A(N - n)}{N}, \frac{(N - A)(N - n)}{N} \right\},$$
$$(11)$$

the smallest of the four expectations obtained per (7), interchanging the symmetric roles of n vs. $N - n$ and A vs. $N - A$.

If EC is "large", then

$$H(x; n, A, N) \cong \Phi((x - \mu)/\sigma), \qquad (12)$$

where Φ is the **standard normal** cumulative distribution. The values μ and σ are defined in (7) and (8).

Since the hypergeometric distribution is discrete, Yates [8] suggested that a better approximation might result by using the following, noting that all the probabilities occur at integer values:

$$\Pr[X \leq x + 0.5] = \Pr[X \leq x] \text{ for}$$

$$x = \text{integer in the hypergeometric}$$
$$\text{distribution.}$$

The basic idea is to approximate the discrete probability that the hypergeometric variable is equal to an integer, by the normal probability of falling within ± 0.5 of the integer (*see* **Yates's Continuity Correction**).

The "corrected approximation" is

$$H(x; n, A, N) \cong \Phi((x - \mu + 0.5)/\sigma). \qquad (13)$$

A rule of thumb, supposedly attributed to R.A. Fisher, claims that values of EC as low as 5 give satisfactory results.

Reality check of (13). We ran a computer check of all situations where $N \leq 250$ and $EC \geq 5$. The largest deviation between (13) and (9) occurred where $N = 250$, $A = 36$, $n = 37$, and $x = 5$. The exact probability from (9) is 0.5517, while the corrected normal approximation, (13), yielded 0.5347, for a deviation of 0.0170. The largest deviation in the "tail" (where the cumulative probability was small), occurred at $N = 245$, $A = 35$, $n = 35$, and $x = 1$. The exact probability is 0.0230, while the corrected normal approximation yields 0.0342 for a deviation of 0.0112. The computer routine compared over 19 million contingencies.

We also ran a computer check of all situations where $N \leq 250$, $EC \geq 7$, and the cumulative hypergeometric probability is below 20%. The largest deviation here was 0.0080, which occurred at $N = 250$, $A = 42$, $n = 42$, and $x = 3$. The exact value is

0.0462, while the corrected normal approximation is 0.0542.

The uncorrected normal approximation may be much more unreliable in the tails, where it is most important. For example, if $N = 50, A = 16, N = 17$, and $x = 3$ ($EC > 5$), then the exact hypergeometric cumulative probability (9), is 0.1056, while the uncorrected normal approximation, (12), is only 0.0611, a deviation of 0.0445.

For more information on other approximations, see [5] and [2].

Final Commentary

The reader may wonder why we introduced approximations in an era when exact calculations are routinely available on computers. Ironically, the very hardware and software that allowed us to investigate the adequacy of the approximations, in the most extensive study yet conducted, are the very same tools that allow us to use exact methods for every application. However, these approximations have been used in countless past research projects, and will continue to be employed by others. The investigation in this article indicates that the **P values** reported in these articles using binomial or corrected normal approximations are reasonably accurate, and that the inferences are qualitatively correct, provided that one is not an all-or-none type inference maker, based on a P value of 5% or 1%. Haber [2] shows that if the goodness criterion is a ratio of probabilities, then in the tails and with low expected numbers, the Yates correction was perceived to perform relatively poorly. This should not dissuade users.

In 1990, *Statistics in Medicine* devoted considerable coverage to the Yates correction (see [3] and the ensuing discussion). Shuster [6] used the binomial approximation for the analysis of **clinical trials** where the sample size is large but the events are rare. In effect, he interchanged the roles of A and n, as noted below (4).

Suissa & Shuster [7] relied heavily upon the hypergeometric distribution when they derived sample size requirements for clinical trials involving two independent samples. Their exact unconditional methods require fewer patients than a corresponding **Fisher's exact test**, when type I error and power are prespecified.

The term hypergeometric distribution [1] is based on the connection with the "hypergeometric series" defined by Euler in 1769. His series produced as special cases the geometric series which he was generalizing, and a polynomial whose coefficients are constant multipliers of the hypergeometric probabilities. For further details, see [4].

Generalization

The idea of the hypergeometric distribution can be extended to a multivariate setting as follows. Suppose a population contains N_j subjects of type j, $j = 1, 2, \ldots, J$. Suppose we wish to partition this population randomly into subgroups of size M_i, $i = 1, 2, \ldots, I$. Let X_{ij} be the number of subjects of type j in subgroup i. Then

$$\Pr\left[X_{ij} = x_{ij} : 1 \leq i \leq I, 1 \leq j \leq J\right]$$

$$= \prod_{i=1}^{I} M_i! \prod_{j=1}^{J} N_j! \left\{ N! \prod_{j=1}^{J} \prod_{i=1}^{I} x_{ij}! \right\}^{-1}, \quad (14)$$

where

$$N = \sum_{i=1}^{I} M_i = \sum_{j=1}^{J} N_j.$$

If $I = J = 2, N_1 = A, N_2 = N - A, M_1 = n$, and $M_2 = N - n$, then (14) reduces to (3), the hypergeometric. The marginal distribution of each X_{ij} is hypergeometric with $A = N_j$ and $n = M_i$.

Finally, note that for the fixed constants N_j and M_i, the probability given in (14) is inversely proportional to

$$\prod_{j=1}^{J} \prod_{i=1}^{I} x_{ij}!.$$

This fact drives computer programs dedicated to the exact analysis of two-dimensional **contingency tables** (*see* **Exact Inference for Categorical Data**).

The same concept can be extended to multidimensional situations with probabilities inversely proportional to the product of the factorials of the individual cell counts.

Acknowledgments

The author wishes to thank Professors James Kepner, P.V. Rao, Andrew Rosalsky, Andre Khuri, and Instructor Maria Ripol for helpful material.

References

[1] Guenther, W.C. (1983). Hypergeometric distributions, in *Encyclopedia of Statistical Sciences*, Vol. 3, S. Kotz & N.L. Johnson, eds. Wiley, New York, pp. 707–712.

[2] Haber, M. (1980). A comparison of some continuity corrections for the chi-squared test on 2 × 2 tables, *Journal of the American Statistical Association* **75**, 510–515.

[3] Haviland, M.G. (1990). Yates correction for continuity and the analysis of 2 × 2 contingency tables (with discussion), *Statistics in Medicine* **9**, 363–367.

[4] Larsen, R.J. & Marx, M.L. (1985). *An Introduction to Probability and its Applications*. Prentice-Hall, New York, Chapter 3.

[5] Patel, J.K. & Read, C.B. (1982). *Handbook of the Normal Distribution*. Marcel Dekker, New York, Chapter 7.

[6] Shuster, J.J. (1993). Fixing the number of events in large comparative trials with low event rates: a binomial approach, *Controlled Clinical Trials* **14**, 198–208.

[7] Suissa, S.S. & Shuster, J.J. (1985). Exact unconditional sample sizes, for the 2 × 2 binomial trial, *Journal of the Royal Statistical Society, Series A* **148**, 317–327.

[8] Yates, F. (1984). Tests of significance for 2 × 2 contingency tables, *Journal of the Royal Statistical Society, Series A* **147**, 426–463.

(*See also* **Logistic Regression, Conditional**)

JONATHAN J. SHUSTER

Hypergeometric Distribution, Multivariate *see* Multivariate Distributions, Overview

Hyperparameter *see* Prior Distribution

Hyperprior *see* Bayesian Methods

Hypothesis *see* Null Hypothesis

Hypothesis Testing

The global responses of patients with diabetic neuropathy who had been randomly assigned to one of two different treatments (*see* **Randomized Treatment Assignment**) are displayed in Table 1. If the treatments were equally efficacious, we would expect to see the same percentage of patients deteriorating or improving in both. Since the responses of individual patients will differ, even if given the same treatment, the resulting random variation means that we would not expect to see exactly the same percentage in each group. However, note that there are 14 patients with moderate or excellent response to treatment A and only three such patients on treatment B. Could this great a difference have happened "at random"? The basic idea behind hypothesis testing is to compute the **probability** of the pattern of data that we have observed, under the assumption that any differences are "purely random". If that probability is very low, then we would be tempted to reject the hypothesis that the differences between treatments is due to "random noise" alone. If the pattern that is seen also suggests a consistent difference in response between the treatments, we would be even more inclined to reject the hypothesis of equal effect.

In Table 1, around 30% of the patients on treatment A have a moderate or excellent response versus only 6% on treatment B. If we treat these two numbers as coming from independent **binomial** random variables with the same underlying probability of response, the probability of seeing as great or greater a difference is less than 0.001. Yet, the only excellent response was under treatment B. How can we claim that treatment A is better? What would have happened if we had compared only the percentage

Table 1 Responses of patients with diabetic neuropathy, to two randomly assigned treatments

| | Deterioration | | | Improvement | | |
	Severe	Slight	No change	Slight	Moderate	Excellent
Treatment A	1	2	20	9	14	0
Treatment B	3	2	26	15	2	1

of patients with an excellent response? Or the percentage of patients with any improvement? Or the percentage of patients who deteriorated? Of all parts of Table 1, the break between moderate improvement or better and all other responses is most favorable to treatment A. Is it acceptable to choose the most favorable part of the data before calculating the probability? What is the "right" way of applying hypothesis tests? Is there an "optimal" method of testing? Questions like this have generated a vast literature of books and articles, ranging from abstract mathematical dissertations, to philosophical discussions of the meaning of probability, to the interpretation of hypothesis tests run on medical, epidemiologic, and other biological data. There are at least two major schools of thought, and how one uses hypothesis tests or interprets them may differ, depending upon which school of thought is being invoked.

Historical Development

The basic idea behind hypothesis testing has been used in many branches of science for at least 200 years. One author [1] claims to have found the germ of the idea in a medical discussion from 1662. Other early references have included astronomical and sociological investigations (see [16]). However, the earliest clearly thought-out use of hypothesis testing probably belongs to **Karl Pearson**. Pearson was collecting biological data from all over the world and attempting to fit these data to specific probability distributions (see Galton et al. [12], for a formal statement of this program). The plan was to show the effects of natural selection and evolution on shifts in these distributions under the pressure of changes in the environment. To determine whether a given distribution fit the data, Pearson ordered the numbers and divided them into bins containing 5–20 adjacent numbers in a bin. He then computed the expected number of observations that he should have seen in each bin and compared the expected number to the observed number. If O_i = the observed number in bin i, and E_i = the expected number in bin i, then the sum

$$(O_1 - E_1)^2/E_1 + (O_2 - E_2)^2/E_2 + \cdots + (O_i - E_i)^2/E_i + \cdots$$

was used to determine if the fit was good. If this sum was too large, the proposed distribution was rejected. Pearson proved that, regardless of the underlying probability distribution being tested, if the sample size was large enough, this sum had a specific distribution, which he called a **chi-square(d) distribution**. Thus, he was able to test the hypothesis that the data followed a specific random pattern with an omnibus test.

Pearson's proof was not completely rigorous, and his exact calculations were in need of some minor adjustments (derived in [6]). However, his work contains the basic components of any modern hypothesis test:

1. a well defined probability distribution that describes the hypothesis that the differences in pattern are "purely random".
2. A test statistic that can be calculated from the data, which:
   (i) has a distribution that is the same regardless of the definition of "purely random"; and
   (ii) can be used to compute a probability that measures how well the observed data fit the distribution that defines "purely random".

R.A. Fisher, a younger contemporary of Pearson, derived most of the test statistics that we now use, in a series of papers and books during the 1920s and 1930s. Fisher also published a "cook book" of methods to popularize these tests [7], which went through 10 editions. **G.W. Snedecor**, who founded the first statistics department in the US at Iowa State University, published a textbook [20] that spread Fisher's methods and test statistics into even further use. In the 1970s, a review of the *Science Citation Index* showed that Snedecor's textbook was the single most frequently cited paper or book in the scientific literature of the time.

However, there were many questions about how to use these test statistics and which test statistics to use under which circumstances. In the late 1920s, Karl Pearson's son, **Egon Pearson**, approached the young Polish mathematician **Jerzy Neyman** with a question that was bothering him. If you test whether data fit a particular probability distribution, and the test statistic is not large enough to reject that distribution, how do you know that this is the "best" that could be done? How do you know that some other test statistic might not have rejected that probability distribution? The resulting collaboration between Egon Pearson and Neyman over the next few years produced a series of papers that revolutionized the nature of hypothesis testing and introduced some of the basic ideas that now govern this field.

Following on from this work by Neyman and Pearson, Eric Lehmann published a definitive textbook [15] that elaborated on the original Neyman–Pearson formulation. This version of the Neyman–Pearson formulation is the interpretation of hypothesis testing that is usually taught in elementary statistics courses, and it dominates much of the medical and epidemiologic literature, where hypothesis testing is used.

Fisher, the creator of most of our modern methods, was critical of the Neyman–Pearson formulation (see [9]; developed more fully in [11]). He felt that the formulation may have been very nice mathematics, but that it had nothing to do with the way in which hypothesis tests are actually used in scientific investigations. In addition, the statistical literature is filled with other objections to the validity of the Neyman–Pearson formulation in terms of its use of probability and its ability to interpret experimental results (for a survey of this work, see [2]). In general, these objections come from two schools of statistical reasoning. One school follows Fisher's approach and views hypothesis tests as rough tools of **inference** that should be used only in conjunction with other tools (for a full discussion, see [5]). The other school criticizes what they consider to be irrational components of hypothesis testing and proposes that inference should be based on the **likelihood** function. These critics, in turn, fall into two general categories, the Bayesians and those who would rest all inference on likelihood alone (*see* **Bayesian Methods; Likelihood**). Bayesian techniques do not make use of hypothesis tests but base their inference on credibility intervals that describe a highly probable range of values for a given parameter, based on prior knowledge and the data (*see* **Prior Distribution**). The likelihood approach to inference also rejects formal hypothesis testing and bases inference on ranges of the parameters that produce relatively high likelihoods for the observed data.

Since Lehmann's definitive text, hypothesis testing has been a fruitful area for statistical research. More recent developments include locally most powerful tests, restricted tests, investigations into the **robustness** of tests, and tests of nested (or **hierarchical**) and nonnested models (*see* **Separate Families of Hypotheses**). Some of these will be discussed briefly in what follows, but the reader should be aware that this continuing research means that the

nature of hypothesis testing and the applications of these techniques will continue to change.

The Neyman–Pearson Formulation

We shall start with a simple model and build on that. Consider two hypotheses about the nature of reality. In Table 1, the two hypotheses might be

H_0: the probability of moderate or better improvement is the same for patients on treatment A as it is on treatment B.

H_1: The probability of moderate or better improvement is twice as great on treatment A as it is on treatment B.

H_0 is called the **"null hypothesis"**. H_1 is called the **"alternative hypothesis"**. We are presented with data from a study and we are asked to make one of two decisions:

D_0: H_0 is true.
D_1: H_1 is true.

This situation can be displayed as a two-by-two table, as shown in Table 2. If the decision matches the true state of nature, there is no error. Otherwise, two types of error are possible. The probability of a type I error (deciding for the alternative hypothesis when the null hypothesis is true) is labeled α. The probability of a type II error (deciding for the null hypothesis when the alternative hypothesis is true) is labeled β.

One "solution" for this simple setup is to consider all possible patterns that the data might have and order them in terms of increasing evidence in favor of the alternative hypothesis. For instance, in comparing two treatments with respect to the frequency of improvements in Table 1, we have a total of 41 $(9 + 14 + 0 + 15 + 2 + 1)$ patients improving. A result that would be most favorable to the alternative hypothesis (that treatment A is better than treatment B) would be to assign all 41 to treatment A. The next most favorable would be to assign 40 to

Table 2 A decision table for choice between two hypotheses

Decision	True state of nature	
	H_0	H_1
D_0	No error	Type II error
D_1	Type I error	No error

treatment A and one to treatment B, etc. Once the possible outcomes are ordered, the analyst can pick a specific outcome (say, a break of 30A and 11B) and calculate the probability, based on the assumption of H_0, for each outcome that was as favorable or more favorable than that specific break point. Similarly, the analyst could compute the probability, based on the assumption of H_1, for each outcome that is less favorable than that specific break point. Let the decision be as follows:

D_1:   choose H_1 if the observed outcome is at that break or at one more favorable.

D_0:   choose H_0 if the observed outcome is one of the events less favorable than that break.

Then, the sum of the favorable probabilities at that break and beyond, under the null hypothesis, is the probability of a type I error, α. Similarly, the sum of the unfavorable probabilities less than that break, under the alternative hypothesis, is the probability of a type II error, β.

Another approach is to decide in advance what level of α (perhaps 0.05) error the analyst is willing to have (see **Level of a Test**). Then, each time the analyst is faced with a decision involving a simple null and a simple alternative hypothesis, the analyst can choose a break point that corresponds to that level of α. Then, in the long run, regardless of the exact problem at hand, the proportion of times the analyst will make a type I error will be α. However, for this to hold, the complete decision process (the choice of α, of the test statistic, and of the cut-point) must be set up in advance of seeing any data and independent of the outcome of a particular trial.

This situation of a simple null and simple alternative hypothesis seldom holds in real life. For instance, in Table 1 we can propose a simple null (that the probability of response is the same for both treatments), but a simple alternative would require that we pick a specific difference in probabilities for each type of response. If we want the alternative hypothesis to be more general, such as that the probability of improvement is greater for A and that the probability of deterioration is less for A, then we have to consider an infinitude of possible differences in probabilities of response. In such a case, the alternative hypothesis is called a composite hypothesis. However, although the comparison of a simple null and a simple alternative hypothesis seldom occurs in real-life problems, it is a useful first step in visualizing how one might proceed.

To be more realistic, let us consider a simple null hypothesis and a composite hypothesis of alternatives that are farther and farther away from the null. For instance, we might consider the null hypothesis that the probability of improvement is the same for both treatments and the composite alternative that the probability of improvement for A has the relationship

$$p_A = k p_B, \quad k > 1.$$

This includes the simple alternatives that $k = 2$ (probability of improvement for A is twice that of B), $k = 1.001$, $k = 10$, etc. As k increases, the "distance" between the simple null and the alternative increases. (There is a technical problem, here. If k gets large enough, then p_A will be greater than 1, but this can be taken care of by considering **odds** (see **Odds Ratio**) rather than probabilities.)

At this point, the Neyman–Pearson formulation has three parameters that govern the decision process: α, β, and δ the latter being the "distance" from the null to a specific simple alternative that is part of the composite alternative. Once they had reached this point in their development, Neyman and Pearson sought an optimum solution to the problem. Some of the critics of this formulation have attached on this attempt to find an optimum solution as one of the inherent problems. This is because one has to define what is meant by optimum, and the act of defining it often limits the nature of the solution. In this case, Neyman realized that there was no single definition of optimum when dealing with three freely ranging parameters. However, it was possible to define an optimum if the problem was constrained. Neyman's solution was the following:

1. fix α;
2. find a decision process that minimizes β for a range of δ-values.

They called $1 - \beta$, the probability of correctly deciding in favor of the alternative hypothesis, the **power** of the test procedure. Thus, in words, the optimum solution is one that fixes the probability of a type I error in advance (at, say, 0.05) and then has the greatest power for a specific range of alternative hypotheses. In this way, the analyst will make type I errors $100\alpha\%$ of the time across the entire spectrum of decisions that use this same α-level. At the same time, the analyst will be testing hypotheses is a way that is most favorable to the set of alternatives that have been chosen as important for each decision.

In such a model, the ideal decision process is one that is more powerful than any other for all possible alternatives. This is the uniformly **most powerful**, or UMP, test. If a UMP test exists, to follow the Neyman–Pearson formulation, the analyst should always use it. Unfortunately, as Neyman noted in the final paper that he wrote in this series [17], UMP tests seldom exist. In particular, they do not exist for the types of hypothesis tests most often used in medical and epidemiologic research.

There are two ways of overcoming this problem. The analyst can narrow the class of alternatives, or the analyst can seek the best decision process from a collection of decision processes that are constrained in some way. The first method (narrowing the class of alternatives) occurs with the use of restricted hypothesis tests and locally most powerful hypothesis tests (for a more complete discussion, see [18]). The second approach is done by requiring that the hypothesis tests have certain properties. Some of these properties are:

1. *unbiasedness* (the probability of a type II error is never less than α);
2. *symmetry* (the test statistic should produce the same value if the data are permuted – the nature of the permutation defining the type of symmetry);
3. *invariance* (the test statistic should produce the same value if all the data are subjected to a specific monotone transformation, such as multiplication by a constant, and an appropriate transformation is applied to the parameter value).

This has led to a plethora of terms to describe different types of optimum tests, such as UMP in the class of unbiased tests. Whether such tests are "optimum" for a given situation should depend upon whether the restriction of the alternative hypotheses or the properties defining the class of tests are appropriate to that situation. Just because a test has a nice name (such as "exact") does not mean that it is the "best" to use.

Criticisms of the Neyman–Pearson Formulation

The major criticisms of this formulation for hypothesis testing are three-fold: (i) the validity of the α-level depends upon the definition of probability as the long-run frequency of errors that might occur;

(ii) the computation of the significance level uses the probabilities of events that have not been observed; and (iii) the definition of optimum is purely arbitrary.

The Use of the Long-Run Frequency of Errors to Define α

Fisher [9] was one of the first to object on these grounds. Fisher pointed out that long-run frequency of error is a concept appropriate to quality control, where an inspector wants to be sure than no more than $100\alpha\%$ of defective products will pass. However, scientific investigation, said Fisher, is a process which involves a sequence of experiments, in which the conditions of each experiment are dependent upon the outcome of previous experiments. G.E.P. Box [3] added to this description by noting that the data from previous experiments are often reexamined in the light of later results. To Fisher, the fact that the analyst uses a cutoff significance level of 0.05 does not mean that the analyst will be wrong 5% of the time. For, according to Fisher, the analyst has no right to declare something is so until he can design a study that will invariably produce a significant result in favor of it.

There is a further problem with the Neyman–Pearson formulation whenever the observed P **value** is less than or equal to α. It does not allow the analyst to make any other decision. Thus, if α is set at 0.05, a P value of 0.04999 has the same interpretation as a P value of 0.00001. In Neyman–Pearson hypothesis testing, there is no such thing as "more significant", and the use of symbols such as * (for $P \leq 0.05$), ** (for $P \leq 0.01$), and *** (for $P \leq 0.001$) has no meaning. Attempts have been made to develop a theory of "evidence" that will allow for multiple decisions within this frequentist definition of probability. However, all have failed. (For a complete description of this problem, see [14].)

The Use of Events not Observed to Compute P Values

The power of an hypothesis test depends upon its ability to reject the null for events that are more favorable to the alternative. However logical the Neyman–Pearson development may seem, critics point out that it ends up with a counterintuitive procedure. Why should outcomes more extreme than the one observed play any role in the decision process?

These critics point out that the only reasonable computations involve the likelihood of the observations under the null hypothesis and the likelihood under the alternative hypothesis. The ratio of these likelihoods should be used to compare the hypotheses with respect to the data. This ratio is called the Bayes factor in the development of Bayesian statistical procedures (*see* **Bayesian Methods**).

The Definition of Optimum is Arbitrary

Neyman was faced with a three-parameter problem: α (the probability of a type I error), β (the probability of a type II error), and δ (the "distance" between the null and alternative hypotheses). His definition of optimum was to fix α and minimize β over a range of δ. Other definitions are possible. One could minimize the sum $\alpha + \beta$ or the odds of α over β. The major justification for Neyman's definition of optimum is that the resulting decision process mimics closely the way in which prior workers such as Fisher had used hypothesis tests. However, there is no reason why fixing α is appropriate for medical or epidemiologic problems. In fact, some critics have asked sarcastically why the analyst's long-run probability of error should have anything to do with whether treatment A is a life-saving procedure that should be used in medicine. One alternative, called sequential Bayes, proposes that there is a finite number of patients who will be treated (*see* **Adaptive and Dynamic Methods of Treatment Assignment**). Some of those will be treated in a controlled trial that compares treatment A to treatment B. Once the trial is over, all of the remaining patients will be given the treatment that has been declared better. The criterion proposed is to minimize the number of patients on the poorer treatment.

Cox's Formulation of Significance Testing

Many authors have agreed with Fisher's objections and proposed alternative approaches to hypothesis tests. Like Fisher, these authors would treat P values as rough tools for inspecting data. A full development of this idea is due to D.R. Cox [5]. To distinguish between his formulation and that of Neyman and Pearson, Cox called the informal use of P values "significance testing" (as opposed to hypothesis testing). Cox would have the analyst compute the P value of a test statistic but treat it as one of many descriptors of

the data. If the experiment was a difficult one to duplicate, or if the data from an epidemiologic study were difficult to accumulate, then the analyst should consider higher P values as "significant". If alternative experiments were easily and cheaply done, then the analyst should require lower P values before taking any decision in favor of an alternative hypothesis. In Cox's view, the cutoff P value is not set in advance, but is dependent upon the importance of the question, the ease of replication, and, to some extent, the data themselves. At all times, Cox warned, the evidence presented by a small P value should be part of a more general analysis of the data that pays attention to the estimated mean effects and to the plausibility of the results.

Cox claimed that there are two general ways in which significance tests and P values are used in scientific research. He called these "hypothesis dividing" and "hypothesis refining". In the hypothesis dividing mode, the scientist proposes two distinctly different hypotheses as explanations of reality. The scientist constructs an experiment or an observation that will lean one way for one hypothesis or the other way for the other hypothesis. The significance test is used to determine if there is enough information in the data to allow for a decision between the two hypotheses. The significance test is not necessarily used to decide in favor of one hypothesis or the other. That decision depends upon the design of the study and the nature of the data. The significance test is used only to discard certain studies as not providing enough information. (This echoes Fisher's view of significance tests.) In the hypothesis refining mode, the scientist has a complicated model of reality, involving many parameters, and he or she wishes to eliminate some of those parameters as having minor or negligible effects. Suppose, for instance, that we have been following a cohort of individuals for many years and wish to determine which baseline characteristics were predictive of some future event (such as a myocardial infarction). We might run a **logistic regression** using all the baseline variables that were collected and use significance tests to eliminate those that do not have a "significant" slope (*see* **Variable Selection**).

The Meaning of P Values

The P value of a test statistic is computed as the probability of a **critical region** of possible observations under the null hypothesis. However, it is difficult to define what that means in real life. In fact, the whole problem of linking the mathematical theory of probability to real life is a controversial one. Neyman finessed the problem by fixing the α-level and defining its meaning as the long-run proportion of times that an analyst will make a type I error. However, one cannot use this formulation to justify the statement that we are "$100(1 - \alpha)\%$ sure" that the null is false. Nor does this definition make sense if a hypothesis test is going to be applied to a nonreplicated event such as a definitive placebo controled clinical study of a potentially life-saving treatment (since, once the null hypothesis has been rejected, it is unethical to do another study).

In the mathematical theory of **probability**, we propose that there exists a space of "events". Probability is a measure (similar to length or area) on that space of events. The link between mathematical probability and real life is how we define that space of events. **W.S. Gossett** (who wrote under the pseudonym "Student") applied probability theory to the outcome of experiments and said that the space of events was the set of all possible outcomes of such an experiment. But, since only one outcome is seen, this is not a well-defined idea. In **sample survey** theory, the population is fixed and a sample of that population is chosen at random. The space of events is, then, the set of all possible **random samples** that might have been chosen. Since the **randomization** mechanism is known, this space is well defined. The uncertainty described by probability theory for sample surveys is not about the characteristics of the population (which are fixed) but about the estimates of those characteristics that are derived from the sample. In a **case–control study** the concept of a sample and population remains, but the calculated probabilities are the **conditional probabilities** that a person has a prior condition (e.g. a heavy coffee drinker), given that the person has the disease (for an excellent discussion of this, see [4]).

To justify the use of probability theory in controlled experiments, Fisher noted that the act of randomly assigning experimental units to treatments in a randomized controlled experiment generated a space that consisted of all possible random assignments. He was able to show that the classical distributions of test statistics that he had developed are approximations of the permutation probabilities that would result (*see* **Randomization Tests**). However, this meant that

hypothesis tests were valid only in the framework of a randomized controlled study (for a discussion of some of the consequences of this view, *see* **Intention-to-Treat Analysis**). Fisher objected to the observational studies connecting smoking with cardiovascular disease and cancer [10], because they used hypothesis tests to "prove" the case. Following the same logic, Fisher would have objected to the use of all hypothesis tests in epidemiology, in case–control studies, or in any type of clinical study that did not involve randomized assignment to treatment.

It is tempting to use probability statements to describe how "sure" one is about the results of the investigation. This would result in phrases such as "The probability that coffee is an important factor in the development of pancreatic tumors is less than 10%". However, the only way this can be done is to describe a space of events that is either related to the state of mind of the observer (personal or **subjective probability**; for a complete discussion, see [19]), or to a general opinion that one might expect in a community of knowledgeable scholars (an idea developed in [13]). All of these fall under the heading of Bayesian statistical methods (*see* **Bayesian Methods**).

Power and the Acceptance of the Null Hypothesis

An important element of the Neyman–Pearson formulation of hypothesis testing is the concept of power. The quality of a statistical test is determined by its power. One could construct a great many test statistics from the data in Table 1. A chi-square test for the independence of the rows and columns, for instance, can be computed based on the null hypothesis that the row (treatment) has nothing to do with the columns (responses) (*see* **Chi-Square Tests**). The P value for this test is greater than 0.50. On the other hand, one can use a Cochran–Armitage test (which is a restricted test) that concentrates on the class of alternatives where the probability of a patient's being in treatment A increases with the response (*see* **Trend Test for Counts and Proportions**). The P value for the Cochran–Armitage test is 0.04. The theory of restricted tests says that, if we believe that the only viable alternatives are that the better treatment is consistently better across all the possible responses, then the Cochran–Armitage test is more powerful and should be used rather than the chi-square test.

If we do not pay attention to power, then any test would be equally as "good". A *reductio ad absurdum* of this is to ignore the data from a study and pick a number from a table of **uniformly distributed** random numbers between zero and one. If the number is less than α, declare significance. Such a test is "exact". It also protects the α-level. But, the power is also exactly equal to α (since, regardless of the alternative hypothesis, it will reject the null $100\alpha\%$ of the time.)

In spite of the fact that the Neyman–Pearson formulation involves a decision to accept the null hypothesis, there is a general consensus among statisticians that hypothesis tests are not really designed for that. To quote Fisher [8],

> ... tests of significance (are) ... cogent for the rejection of hypotheses, but...by no means cogent for their acceptance...the logical fallacy of believing that a hypothesis has been proved to be true, merely because it is not contradicted by the available facts, has no more right to insinuate itself in statistical than in other kinds of scientific reasoning.

To deal with this problem, some have advocated that articles which describe the results of studies include information about the power of the study to detect a meaningful degree of effect. Alternatively, it has been urged that studies which result in a finding of no significant difference should include **confidence intervals** on the differences in effect that would be reasonable from the data. If the power of the study is inadequate to detect a meaningful effect or if the confidence interval contains meaningful differences in effect, then the study is inadequate to accept the null hypothesis (*see* **Clinical Significance vs. Statistical Significance**).

References

[1]   Armitage, P. (1983). Trials and errors: the emergence of clinical statistics, *Journal of the Royal Statistical Society, Series A* **146**, 321–334.

[2]   Berger, J. (1983). The frequentist viewpoint and conditioning, in *Proceedings of the Berkeley Conference in Honor of Jerzy Neyman and Jack Kiefer*, Vol. 1, L.M. LeCam & R.A. Olshen, eds. Wadsworth, Monterey.

[3]   Box, G.E.P. (1980). Sampling and Bayes' inference in scientific modeling and robustness, *Journal of the Royal Statistical Society, Series A* **143**, 383–340.

[4]   Cornfield, J. (1954). Statistical relationships and proof in medicine, *American Statistician* **8**, 19–23.

[5]   Cox, D.R. (1977). The role of significance tests, *Scandinavian Journal of Statistics* **4**, 49–70.

[6]   Cramér, H. (1946). *Mathematical Methods of Statistics*. Princeton University Press, Princeton, Chapter 30.

[7]   Fisher, R.A. (1925). *Statistical Methods for Research Workers*. Oliver & Boyd, Edinburgh.

[8]   Fisher, R.A. (1935). Statistical tests, *Nature* **136**, 474–475.

[9]   Fisher, R.A. (1955). Statistical methods and scientific inference, *Journal of the Royal Statistical Society, Series B* **17**, 69–78.

[10]   Fisher, R.A. (1958). Cigarettes, cancer, and statistics, *Centennial Review* **2**, 151–166.

[11]   Fisher, R.A. (1959). *Statistical Methods and Scientific Inference*. Oliver & Boyd, Edinburgh.

[12]   Galton, F., Pearson, K. & Weldon, R. (1898). Charge of this journal, *Biometrika* **1**, 1.

[13]   Keynes, J.M. (1921). *A Treatise on Probability*. Macmillan, London.

[14]   Kiefer, J. (1976). Admissibility of conditional confidence procedures, *Annals of Statistics* **4**, 836–865.

[15]   Lehmann, E. (1959). *Testing Statistical Hypotheses*. Wiley, New York.

[16]   Moroney, M.J. (1951). *Facts from Figures*. Penguin, Harmondsworth, Middlesex, Chapter 15.

[17]   Neyman, J. (1935). Sur la verification des hypotheses statistiques composées, *Bulletin de la Société Mathematique de France* **63**, 246–266; *Statistics* **4**, 49–70.

[18]   Salsburg, D.S. (1992). *The Use of Restricted Significance Tests in Clinical Trials*. Springer-Verlag, New York.

[19]   Savage, L.J. (1954). *The Foundations of Statistics*. Wiley, New York.

[20]   Snedecor, G.W. (1940). *Statistical Methods*. Iowa State University Press, Ames.

DAVID SALSBURG

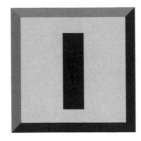

Ideal Point Model *see* **Multidimensional Scaling**

Idempotent Matrix *see* **Matrix Algebra**

Identifiability

Consider a vector $\mathbf{Y}$ of random variables having a distribution $F(\mathbf{y};\theta)$ that depends on an unknown parameter vector θ. θ is *identifiable* by observation of $\mathbf{Y}$ if distinct values for θ yield distinct distributions for $\mathbf{Y}$ [1]. A function $g(\theta)$ of the parameter vector is *identifiable* by observation of $\mathbf{Y}$ if $F(\mathbf{y};\theta_1) = F(\mathbf{y};\theta_2)$ for all $\mathbf{y}$ implies $g(\theta_1) = g(\theta_2)$. Note that θ is identifiable if and only if all functions of θ are identifiable.

There is some variation in the definition of identifiability, the preceding being the most general. Variants typically employ the density $f(\mathbf{y};\theta)$ or the expectation $E(\mathbf{Y};\theta)$ in place of the distribution; the latter variants may explicitly involve a design matrix X of regressors; for example, $E(\mathbf{Y};X,\theta)$. The basic concept, however, is that θ [or $g(\theta)$] is a function of the $\mathbf{Y}$ distribution, and hence observations of realizations of $\mathbf{Y}$ can be used to discriminate among distinct values of θ [or $g(\theta)$].

The term *estimable* is sometimes used as a synonym for identifiable, but is also used in more specific ways, especially in the context of linear models. For example, Scheffé [4] defines a linear function $\mathbf{c}'\theta$ of θ to be estimable if there exists an unbiased estimator of $\mathbf{c}'\theta$ that is a linear function of the observed realizations of $\mathbf{Y}$. This property has also been referred to as linear estimability. In epidemiology, estimability of $g(\theta)$ is sometimes used to mean that $g(\theta)$ can be consistently estimated from observed realizations of $\mathbf{Y}$. Several other definitions have been given; see, for example, [2], [3] and [5].

References

[1]   Bickel, P.J. & Doksum, K.A. (1977). *Mathematical Statistics*. Holden–Day, Oakland.
[2]   Lehmann, E.L. (1983). *Theory of Point Estimation*. Wiley, New York.
[3]   McCullagh, P. & Nelder, J.A. (1989). *Generalized Linear Models*. Chapman & Hall, New York.
[4]   Scheffé, H. (1959). *The Analysis of Variance*. Wiley, New York.
[5]   Seber, G.A.F. & Wild, C.J. (1989). *Nonlinear Regression*. Wiley, New York.

(*See also* **General Linear Model**)

SANDER GREENLAND

Identity Coefficients

Identity (k-, or kinship) coefficients were introduced by Cotterman [3], Malécot [10, 11], and Gillois [7] to answer questions of the following sort: if an individual X, is of **genotype** Aa, what is the probability that X's relative, Y, is aa? To answer a question of this kind efficiently, it is necessary to partition the problem into two parts: (i) a measure of the relationship connecting X and Y, and (ii) genotype probabilities conditioned on the relationship. The first part depends upon the concept of "identity by descent" (ibd); the second on assumptions about the mating system in the population.

The Concept of Identity by Descent

In Figure 1, Z is the offspring of X and Y, and X is the offspring of V and W. The transmitted gametes are labeled a, b, c, and d. It is clear from a consideration of Mendelism (*see* **Mendel's Laws**) that the **gene** a is an immediate replicate of either c or d, but not both. Let R denote the relation "is an immediate replicate of" and Pr denote probability, then

$$\mathrm{Pr}(a R c) + \mathrm{Pr}(a R d) = 1 \quad \text{and} \quad \mathrm{Pr}(a R c, a R d) = 0.$$

The following relations are defined in terms of the fundamental relation, R, where x, y, z, and z' are arbitrary genes at a single locus:

$R^0 =$ the identity relation

    (a gene is identical to itself),

$R^2 = [(x, y) : \exists\, z\ (x R z, z R y)],$

$R^3 = [(x, y) : \exists\, z\ \exists\, z'(x R z, z R z', z' R y)],$

$R^n = [(x, y) : \exists\, z\ \exists\, z'(x R z, z R^{n-2} z', z' R y)].$

These are the powers of the relation, R. For example, $z R^2 y$ means that x is the immediate replicate of a gene

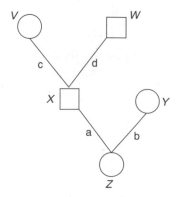

Figure 1   The concept of identity by descent

which is itself the immediate replicate of y. If we let $R^U = R^0 \cup R \cup R^2 \cup R^3 \cup \ldots \cup R^n$, the relation of identity by descent, I, is defined as

$$I = [(x, y) : \exists\, z\ ((x R^U y) \cup (y R^U x) \cup (x R^U z, y R^U z))].$$

In practice, instead of writing $x I y$, it is customary to write $x \equiv y$ to mean x is identical by descent (ibd) to y. This definition is simply a restatement in set-theoretic notation of Cotterman's original definition for which he used the term "derivative". Cotterman [3] states: "...derivative genes are genes which are relatively recently descended one from the other or both from some common gene". The qualification introduced by the phrase "relatively recently" is included in the definition presented above by restricting the size of n in the definition of R^U.

Arbitrary Relationships

Consider two related diploid individuals, X and Y. Label the genes of X a_1 and a_2, and the genes of Y a_3 and a_4. There are 15 "identity by descent" relations among the four genes, as shown in Figure 2. A line connecting two genes denotes that those genes are ibd, the lack of a line denotes that they are not ibd. Some of the events are combined; for example, $_{00}k_1$ is the probability of the union of two events. The notation is mnemonic: the first prescript is 0 if X is allozygous (i.e. has nonibd genes at the locus) and 1 if X is autozygous (i.e. has ibd genes at the locus), the second prescript refers to Y in the same way, and the postscript indicates the number of genes X and Y share in common, that is, the number that are ibd. An alternative notation [9] is: $_{11}k_2 = \Delta_1$, $_{11}k_0 = \Delta_2$, $_{2\,10}k_1 = \Delta_3$, $_{10}k_0 = \Delta_4$, $_{2\,01}k_1 = \Delta_5$, $_{01}k_0 = \Delta_6$, $_{00}k_2 = \Delta_7$, $_{2\,00}k_1 = \Delta_8$, $_{00}k_0 = \Delta_9$.

As an example, the k-coefficients for X and Y in Figure 3 are as shown. All coefficients with a leading prescript equal to one are zero because X is assumed to be allozygous. The probability that Y is autozygous and X and Y share no gene in common is $_{01}k_0 = 2/32$, because this can happen only if both gametes that form Y are derived from the gene in X's daughter that did not come from X; the probability of this is $(1/2)^4$. The probability that both X and Y are allozygous and they share no gene in common is $_{00}k_0 = (1/2)^3 + (1/2)^3 + (1/2)^4 = 10/32$, and so on. In this pedigree, the k-coefficients can be calculated from a simple application of basic Mendelism. In general,

$a_1\ a_3$ $a_1{-}a_3$ $a_1\ a_3$ $a_1\ a_3$ $a_1\ a_3$ $a_1{-}a_3$ $a_1\ a_3$

$a_2\ a_4$ $a_2\ a_4$ $a_2\ a_4$ $a_2{-}a_4$ $a_2\ a_4$ $a_2{-}a_4$ $a_2\ a_4$

$\Delta_9 = {}_{00}k_0$ $\Delta_8 = 2\,{}_{00}k_1$ $\Delta_7 = {}_{00}k_2$

$a_1\ a_3$ $a_1\ a_3$ $a_1\ a_3$ $a_1{-}a_3$ $a_1\ a_3$ $a_1{-}a_3$ $a_1\ a_3$

$a_2\ a_4$ $a_2\ a_4$ $a_2\ a_4$ $a_2\ a_4$ $a_2{-}a_4$ $a_2\ a_4$ $a_2{-}a_4$

$\Delta_4 = {}_{10}k_0$ $\Delta_6 = {}_{01}k_0$ $\Delta_2 = {}_{11}k_0$ $\Delta_3 = 2\,{}_{10}k_1$ $\Delta_5 = 2\,{}_{01}k_1$

$a_1{-}a_3$

$a_2{-}a_4$

$\Delta_1 = {}_{11}k_2$

Figure 2 The 15 ibd relationships between two individuals, X and Y, and their probabilities (k-coefficients). (The genes of X are labeled a_1 and a_2, those of Y, a_3 and a_4)

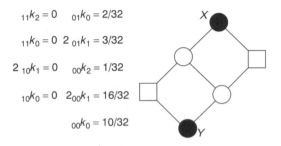

$_{11}k_2 = 0$ $_{01}k_0 = 2/32$

$_{11}k_0 = 0$ $2\,_{01}k_1 = 3/32$

$2\,_{10}k_1 = 0$ $_{00}k_2 = 1/32$

$_{10}k_0 = 0$ $2\,_{00}k_1 = 16/32$

$_{00}k_0 = 10/32$

Figure 3 A sample pedigree: calculating the k-coefficients

the nine k-coefficients are more difficult to calculate except in very simple pedigrees [5, 12, 14].

Genotype Pair Probabilities for Pairs of Relatives

The joint genotype distribution for a two-allelic locus in terms of the k-coefficients and the gene frequencies, p and q, of A and a, respectively, is shown in Table 1. For example, the probability that X and Y are both of genotype Aa is, according to the table, $\Pr(X = \text{Aa}, Y = \text{Aa}) = 2\,_{00}k_2\,pq + 2\,_{00}k_1\,pq + 4\,_{00}k_0\,p^2q^2$.

Noninbred Relatives

Often, one does not need the full set of k-coefficients because many relationships do not involve inbreeding. When neither X nor Y is inbred (when each has an **inbreeding** coefficient, $F = 0$), then all the k-coefficients are zero except for $_{00}k_2$, $2\,_{00}k_1$, and $_{00}k_0$.

The k-coefficients for a number of simple noninbred relationships are shown in Table 2. Bilineal relations are those for which $_{00}k_2 > 0$; unilineal relationships have $_{00}k_2 = 0$.

To calculate the k-coefficients for any noninbred relationship is straightforward. Let a and b be the gametes that form X and c and d those that form

Table 1 The joint genotype distribution of X and Y

X	Y	$_{11}k_2$	$2\,_{01}k_1$	$2\,_{10}k_1$	$_{11}k_0$	$_{10}k_0$	$_{01}k_0$	$_{00}k_2$	$2\,_{00}k_1$	$_{00}k_0$
AA	AA	p	p^2	p^2	p^2	p^3	p^3	p^2	p^3	p^4
AA	Aa	0	0	pq	0	$2p^2q$	0	0	p^2q	$2p^3q$
AA	Aa	0	0	0	pq	pq^2	p^2q	0	0	p^2q^2
Aa	AA	0	pq	0	0	0	$2p^2q$	0	p^2q	$2p^3q$
Aa	Aa	0	0	0	0	0	0	$2pq$	pq	$4p^2q^2$
Aa	aa	0	pq	0	0	0	$2pq^2$	0	pq^2	$2pq^3$
aa	AA	0	0	0	pq	p^2q	pq^2	0	0	p^2q^2
aa	Aa	0	0	pq	0	$2pq^2$	0	0	pq^2	$2pq^3$
aa	aa	q	q^2	q^2	q^2	q^3	q^3	q^2	q^3	q^4

Table 2 The k-coefficients for some simple relationships

Relationship	$_{00}k_2$	$_{200}k_1$	$_{00}k_0$
Unilineal			
Parent–offspring	0	1	0
Grandparent–grandchild	0	1/2	1/2
Half sibs	0	1/2	1/2
Avuncles	0	1/2	1/2
First cousins	0	1/4	3/4
Bilineal			
MZ twins	1	0	0
Full sibs	1/4	1/2	1/4
Double first cousins	1/16	6/16	9/16

Y. Let f_{ac} be the probability that a and c are ibd, f_{ad} be the probability that a and d are ibd, and so on. Let F_{XY} be the probability that a random gamete from X is identical to a random gamete from Y, i.e. the inbreeding coefficient of a, perhaps hypothetical, offspring of X and Y. Then

$$k_2 = f_{ac}f_{bd} + f_{ad}f_{bc}, \qquad 2k_1 = 4F_{XY} - 2k_2,$$

$$k_0 = 1 - 2k_1 - k_2$$

and the calculation is reduced to the methods used to calculate inbreeding coefficients. All of the k-coefficients in Table 2 can be calculated from these formulas.

Extensions

The k-coefficients described above apply to a single autosomal gene in a diploid organism. Several kinds of extensions are immediately apparent: to more than one autosomal locus [1, 2, 6], to more than two individuals [13], and to X-linked loci [4]. For a recent review and more extensive bibliography, see [8].

References

[1] Campbell, M.A. & Elston, R.C. (1971). Relatives of probands: models for preliminary genetic analysis, *Annals of Human Genetics* **35**, 225–236.

[2] Cockerham, C.C. & Weir, B.S. (1973). Descent measures for two loci with some applications, *Theoretical Population Biology* **4**, 300–330.

[3] Cotterman, C.W. (1940). A calculus for statistico-genetics, *Unpublished PhD thesis*. Ohio State University, Columbus, Ohio.

[4] Denniston, C. (1967). Probability and genetic relationship. *Unpublished thesis*, University of Wisconsin, Madison.

[5] Denniston, C. (1974). An extension of the probability approach to genetic relationships: one locus, *Theoretical Population Biology* **6**, 58–75.

[6] Denniston, C. (1975). Probability and genetic relationship: two loci, *Annals of Human Genetics* **39**, 89–104.

[7] Gillois, M. (1964). La relation d'identité en génétique. Thèse Faculté des Sciences de Paris.

[8] Gillois, M. (1988). Consanguinity, in *Proceedings of the Second International Conference on Quantitative Genetics*, B.S. Weir, E.J. Eisen, M.M. Goodman & G. Namkoong, eds. Sinauer, Sunderland, pp. 353–359.

[9] Jacquard, A. (1974). *The Genetic Structure of Populations*. Springer-Verlag, Berlin.

[10] Malécot, G. (1941). Etude mathématique des populations "mendéliennes", *Annales de l'Université de Lyon, Sciences, Section A* **2**, 25–37.

[11] Malécot, G. (1948). *Les mathématiques de l'hérédité*. Masson, Paris.

[12] Nadot, R. & Vaysseix, G. (1973). Apparentement et identité. Algorithme du calcul des coefficients d'identité, *Biometrics* **29**, 347–359.

[13] Thompson, E.A. (1974). Gene identities and multiple relationships, *Biometrics* **30**, 667–680.

[14] Vu Tien Khang, J., De Rochambeau, H., Chevalet, C. & Gillois, M. (1979). Analyse des pedigrees et calcul des coefficients d'identité par les arbres géniques, *Biometrical Journal* **21**, 367–387.

C. DENNISTON

Identity-by-Descent (ibd) *see* Linkage Analysis, Model-Free

Ignorable Dropout *see* Nonignorable Dropout in Longitudinal Studies

Illness–Death Process *see* Aalen–Johansen Estimator

Image Analysis and Tomography

Seeing is believing: sight is fundamental to our understanding of the world. This is as true in science as in everyday life. The collection of much statistical data is dependent upon human vision. For example, the examination of samples under a microscope, observing animal behavior, and the identification and counting of plant species in a field are all forms of image analysis. We are superb at analyzing the images projected onto our retinas, using one-third of our brains for vision. However, computers are being used more and more to automate and extend the potential of image analysis. Computers are better at extracting quantitative information from images than human observers: they can be more accurate and more consistent from day to day. Furthermore, computers may spare us from much tedious image interpretation.

We see effortlessly, most of the time. Progress was expected to be rapid when research commenced in the 1960s on computer-based image analysis. The task, however, has proved to be far more difficult. At least in part, this is because we are not conscious of the processes we go through in seeing. Biological objects present an even greater challenge to computer interpretation than man-made ones, because they tend to be more irregular and variable in shape.

Application Areas

Images to be analyzed in biostatistics may come from microscopy, medical scanning systems, electrophoresis, or simply from photographing illuminated objects. Figure 1 shows several such examples.

Figure 1(a) is a back-illuminated optical *microscope image* of cashmere goat fibers whose diameters were to be measured [38]. Measurement is made more difficult because the microscope has a shallow depth of focus and some fibers are out of focus, producing either dark or light edges to the fibers, so-called "Becke lines". There is a danger of misinterpretion if the optics that produced a particular image are not correctly understood. For example, the bas-relief type of images typical of differential interference contrast microscopy may be mistaken for three-dimensional features. However, tailoring image processing **algorithms** to particular forms of microscopy poses a considerable challenge. There are many optical microscope systems, including brightfield, darkfield, phase contrast, interference contrast, fluorescence, and confocal systems (see, for example [91]). There are also many other types of microscope systems such as scanning electron microscopes and confocal microscopes. Also, the theory of microscopy is complicated and agreement with data is less than perfect.

Figure 1(b) shows an example of an image produced by a *medical imaging system*, in this case a reconstructed slice (tomogram) from positron emission tomography (PET). It shows a transverse cross-section through a woman's thorax, with a tumor circled. There are many other medical imaging systems, such as conventional radiology, angiography, X-ray transmission computed tomography (CT), ultrasound imaging, magnetic resonance imaging (MRI), and single photon emission (computed) tomography (SPET or SPECT), each with its own characteristics requiring attention in analysis (for example, [16] and [72]). Tomographic methods, including CT, SPET, and PET, seek to reconstruct slices *within* the body from observations *outside*.

Figure 1(c) shows a type of *electrophoresis gel*, a DNA sequencing gel autoradiograph, produced as one stage in the **DNA sequencing** of gene fragments. About 50 mixtures of radioactively labeled fragments are positioned as distinct spots along one side of the gel. Each mixture then migrates down the gel, and DNA fragments produce separate, approximately horizontal bands. Finally, a photographic plate is placed over the gel. This blackens in response to radioactive emissions, thus producing an autoradiograph. Electrophoresis has many variants, including two-dimensional (2D) electrophoresis, electrofocusing, isotachophoresis, and several forms of immunoelectrophoresis [45]. Various forms of chromatography and chemical assays also produce pictorial information which can be interpreted by image analysis.

Finally, Figure 1(d) is an image of *illuminated objects*, in this case of 50 wheat grains, obtained using a video camera. This was part of an experiment to see if it was possible to estimate flour yield by digital image analysis [8]. Opportunities are almost limitless for digitally analyzing images of objects illuminated in many different ways. See, for example, the review by Price & Osborne [77] of imaging applications in agriculture and plant science, and by Sapirstein [85] of cereal variety identification from grains.

Types of Image

Digital images are obtained via an appropriate image capture device, such as a video camera or scanner.

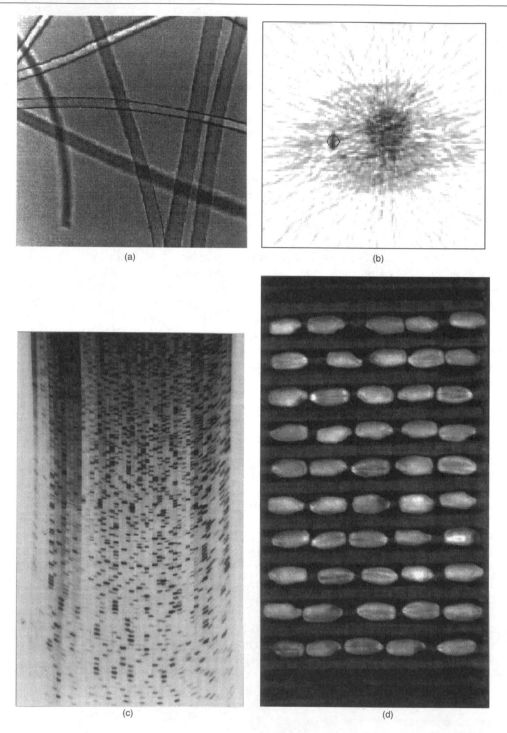

Figure 1   Examples of images: (a) microscope image of cashmere fibers; (b) positron emission tomogram (PET) of a transverse cross-section through a woman's thorax, with a tumor circled, reconstructed using the filtered-backprojection (FBP) algorithm (by courtesy of Max Lonneux and C. Michel, Positron Tomography Laboratory, UCL Belgium); (c) DNA sequencing gel autoradiograph; (d) wheat grains

A 2D digital image usually consists of a rectangular array of tiny squares called "picture elements", or *pixels* for short. Associated with each pixel is a number, representing the average *brightness* of that part of the original picture covered by the pixel. Usually, the brightness will be discretized to 8-bit resolution, i.e. there are $256 = 2^8$ shades of grey, with 0 representing black and 255 representing white.

The pixel brightness may represent *any* variate which has been measured on a 2D grid. Typically it is a measure of the intensity of reflected light, as in the wheat grains example [Figure 1(d)], or of transmitted light, as with the cashmere fibers [Figure 1(a)]. However, it could alternatively depend upon reflected or transmitted radiation in another part of the electromagnetic spectrum [such as gamma rays, Figures 1(b) and (c)].

The object being imaged may be essentially 2D, as with the DNA sequencing gel [Figure 1(c)], or three dimensional (3D). In the latter case, the *sampling procedure* may involve taking a cross-section, either physically or by a computer reconstruction [e.g. Figure 1(b) is a cross-section of a 3D tomography reconstruction: *tomography* techniques are, literally, those creating pictures of a slice, free of the effects of layers outside the focused plane]. Alternatively, a 3D object with either an opaque [wheat grains, Figure 1(d)] or a semi-transparent surface [cashmere fibers, Figure 1(a)], could be imaged simply by viewing it from a particular direction. Some sensors, such as confocal microscopes and magnetic resonance images, can collect *3D arrays* of data. These can be analyzed using similar methods to those for 2D images.

Although we only consider univariate, so-called *grayscale*, images in this article, it is worth pointing out the increasing use of *color* and *multispectral* image analysis. A color image actually consists of three grayscale images, representing light at red, green, and blue wavelengths, respectively. The wheat grains image [Figure 1(d)] is in fact the green component of a color image.

Methodologies

The ultimate aim of image analysis is usually to extract quantitative information, which may be in the form of binary presence/absence categories, or of measures of object location, length or area, shape statistics, etc. In some applications it may only be

possible or desirable to automate some stages in an analysis, leaving the rest to human interpretation. For example, in medical diagnosis the radiologist will want to look at the SPET image. Image analysis methods constitute an eclectic collection of techniques derived from many different theoretical standpoints:

1. The first, and probably most widely used, approach arose in the 1960s from the engineering discipline of *signal processing*, as typified by the books of Rosenfeld & Kak [83] and Jain [55]. Methods include histogram transformations, linear and nonlinear filters (*see* **Spectral Analysis**) and thresholding – techniques that we illustrate later.

2. An elegant approach, termed *mathematical morphology*, emerged from the Ecole des Mines in Fontainebleau, France, in the 1970s (*see* **Stereology**). It is based on the assumption that an image consists of structures which may be handled by set theory, leading to such highly effective methods as openings, closings, skeletonization, and watershed segmentation. The seminal works are Serra [86, 87]. Soille & Rivest [93] provide a useful introduction to the subject from an applications perspective.

3. From **artificial intelligence** have arisen approaches such as *syntactic* **pattern recognition** [28] and *computer vision* [6], but these methods have not often been applied in biostatistical contexts.

4. The 1980s saw the development of **Bayesian** *image analysis* [9, 31]. **Prior** *information* on an appropriate model for an image is combined with *data*, imperfect information about the image (such as pixel values affected by noise), in order to derive the *posterior distribution* for the image.

5. Yet another aspect of image analysis, namely that of extracting *measurements* such as lengths, areas, histograms, etc. from images, is identified as a distinct approach by Serra [87, p. 10]. These descriptors are subsequently interpreted using **stereology**, shape statistics, or classification methods.

Serra [87, p. 11] acknowledges that, although the different approaches to image analysis are somewhat contradictory, they each have their place. He suggests that an analysis might first require linear methods, then morphological ones, and finally either measurements or syntactic methods.

In the rest of this article we consider first the tomographic reconstruction of images, then the three major components of image analysis: enhancement, segmentation, and taking measurements, drawing on techniques from each of the above approaches and illustrating them using some of the images in Figure 1. We are concerned with the application of image analysis. Therefore, in this article we emphasize methods that we have found useful in practice. We are also conscious of only having space to present a subset from a very large field.

Tomography

In tomography the measured data are *projections*, from which the spatial distribution within a body is reconstructed. For example, Figure 2(a) shows PET recordings similar to those used to reconstruct the cross-section shown in Figure 1(b): these are data from only one of many planes collected in a single study. (The cross indicates the position of the cursor used as an aid to navigate through the 3D data set.) In PET, a radionuclide is introduced into the patient's bloodstream and then distributes throughout the body. Radionuclide decays are recorded on a PET scanner. The *distribution* and *intensity* of activity is recorded by the PET scanner, but the accumulated distribution of radionuclide in the body can only be inferred indirectly (by mathematical analysis) from the scanner projection data.

Projection measurements may be modeled as known linear functionals of an unknown spatial distribution (or image). The goal of reconstruction is to infer from the data the distribution within the specimen. Rosenfeld & Kak [83, Chapter 8] and Jain [55, Chapter 10] present the filtered-backprojection (FBP) algorithm [as used in Figure 1(b)] for reconstruction from data given by the Radon-transform (ray sums) of an image. See also Girard [34] and Bickel & Ritov [11], who study estimation of linear functionals and asymptotic convergence of FBP in PET.

Statistical interest has centered on PET and SPET, which exhibit significant statistical variability in camera recordings. A recent introduction to PET and SPET is given by Kay [58]. McColl et al. [68] describe statistical methods in neuroimaging, with special reference to these imaging modalities. However, many of the methods described apply more widely. We consider further: reconstruction

methodologies, use of prior information in fusing reconstructions from different modalities, and parametric mapping based on **pharmacokinetic modeling**. Reconstructions are used not only for clinical studies, providing a basis for individual patient diagnosis, but they also provide data for research studies.

Statistical Reconstruction

In pioneering work, Shepp & Vardi [88] and Lange & Carson [63] applied the **EM algorithm** for **maximum likelihood** (ML) estimation of **Poisson** count data in tomography. Both transmission and emission tomography are well modeled by a description [92] based on a spatially inhomogeneous **Poisson point process**. If $f(s)$ is the (unknown) distribution, then the distribution of recorded activity [in projections such as Figure 2(a)] is expressible as

$$g(t) = \int_{s \in \mathcal{X}} a(t|s) f(s) \mathrm{d}s,$$

or, in suitably discretized form, $g = Af$, with $A = (a_{ts})$. Conditional probabilities $a(t|s)$ are determined by the resolution and geometry of the acquisition camera and by the physics of photon transport through the body, and may be regarded as known. There is great generality in this specification, whether in radiology, CT, SPET, or PET, for precise modeling of physical effects (attenuation, scattering) including the ability to incorporate information from other modes. See, for example, Aykroyd & Green [3], Fulton et al. [29], Hutton et al. [54], Vardi & Lee [98], and Weir & Green [100]. This model flexibility and resulting gains in restoration quality have led to a growing interest in statistical reconstruction in clinical use.

Reconstruction (i.e. estimating f from observations on g) constitutes an *inverse problem*. Many reconstruction methods apply corrections using *back-projection* (*see* **Back-Calculation**), redistributing residual projection errors ($z = g - \hat{g}$) to provide the correction $\hat{f} + \hat{\delta f}$ to an initial estimate $\hat{f}$ by

$$\hat{\delta f}(s) \propto \int_{t \in y} a(t|s) z(t) \mathrm{d}t.$$

For example, ML–EM computations provide iterative improvements on a starting image, which is typically taken to be a **uniform distribution** within the body. ML–EM requires repetition of two steps:

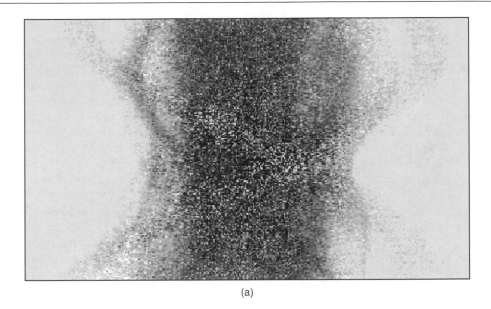

(a)

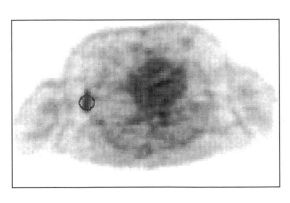

(b)

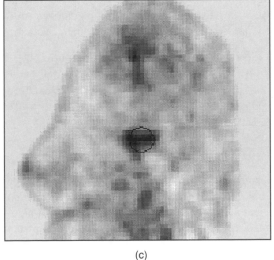

(c)

Figure 2 PET clinical study of a woman's thorax: (a) one plane of the projection data (with the cross indicating the position of the cursor used as an aid to navigate through the 3D data set); (b) a transverse cross-section, as in Figure 1(b), but reconstructed using four iterations of the OSEM algorithm; (c) a sagital cross-section, with a tumor circled (by courtesy of Max Lonneux and C. Michel, Positron Tomography Laboratory, UCL Belgium)

(i) project the current source estimate to produce fitted projection data, and (ii) backproject the ratio between observed and fitted projections to determine multiplicative corrections to be applied to the current source distribution. The usual convergence theory for EM algorithms shows that each iteration increases the likelihood and ML–EM converges from any starting image to an ML solution. There is a heavy computational burden, with arrays typically of size 128^3, but this can be eased by exploiting the sparse structure of the matrix A.

Figure 2(b) shows a 2D slice of a reconstruction, based on the EM algorithm, of the same projection data used with the FBP algorithm in Figure 1(b). In addition, Figure 2(c) shows a sagital slice through the 3D reconstruction. The gain in restoration quality of the statistical reconstruction is evident, with Figure 1(b) exhibiting streaking artifacts typical of FBP. The reconstruction was produced using the ordered subsets EM (OSEM) algorithm described in Hudson & Larkin [52], which is an adaption of Shepp & Vardi's iterative ML–EM algorithm. OSEM accelerates EM in its ML and Bayesian forms. Here four OSEM iterations were employed, each requiring similar computational effort to that required for the full FBP reconstruction, but far fewer than would be required in ML–EM for the same result.

Related Issues and Approaches

While the resolution of ML–EM images continues to improve with further iterations, they also exhibit an undesirable increase in noise. The effect is similar to bias–variance tradeoffs in nonparametric **density estimation**, and is attributable to the ill-posed inverse problem formulation. A choice of a regularized solution is therefore required. Approaches here include:

1. early stopping of iterations [as in Figure 2(b)];
2. a Bayesian specification of prior information or penalized likelihood criterion (*see* **Penalized Maximum Likelihood**) (see Green & Silverman [42]);
3. post-reconstruction smoothing (see Beekman & Viergever [7]).

Silverman et al. [89] propose an approach to reduce the buildup in noise within iterative reconstruction by local smoothing. The Shepp–Vardi ML–EM algorithm is readily modified to accomplish reconstruction by adopting prior information in a Bayesian formulation (e.g. [32], [41], and [48]) as required for regularization. Multiscale reconstruction may also be advantageous, and there are obvious applications of **wavelet** methodology with body organs creating discontinuities within the imaged region. Efficient convergence is also a critical factor.

Dynamics

Parametric mapping involves modeling functional parameters (e.g. metabolism or blood flow) on the basis of the time-varying distribution of activity of a tracer introduced into the bloodstream in a controlled manner. Time sequences of images result, with the aim of reconstruction being to provide maps of parameters of the model specifying dynamics, not the activity distribution itself.

Cunningham & Jones [22] propose a semiparametric spectral decomposition useful in compartmental models of **pharmacokinetic** studies. In this approach the total activity within prespecified regions of interest (or pixels) are collected over consecutive time intervals. The methodology is nonparametric. No specific compartmental model is assumed, but the time activity curves are expressed in terms of a dense set of basis functions. Cunningham & Jones provide a number of illustrations of the interpretability of such models; the review of O'Sullivan [73] extends this methodology. The method can be applied to time activity curves of indirect observations (projection data) equally well to determine significant modes. With indirect data a staged approach separating the spatial and temporal stages of the reconstruction may be adopted, as provided in the EMPIRA algorithm of Carson & Lange [17].

Enhancement

All images are subject to some degradation from their ideal forms, whether this is the presence of noise, blurring, or a warping/distortion of the image frame. Image enhancement is a set of methods for modifying images to reduce these effects, both to aid human interpretation and as a precursor to segmentation or other digital methods of analysis. In some images the degradation is relatively minor, and image enhancement is unnecessary for the particular application. However, in many cases this will not be so. We look at methods for correcting for warping, at filters, and at deconvolution, using the DNA sequencing gel in Figure 1(c) for illustration.

Registration and Unwarping

Unwarping of images is an important stage in many applications of image analysis. It may be needed to remove optical distortions introduced by a camera or viewing perspective [96], or to register an image with a reference grid such as a map, or to align two or more images. For example, matching is important in reconstructing a 3D shape from either a series of 2D sections or stereoscopic pairs of images. There is considerable interest in registering images produced by medical sensing systems with body atlas information [18, Section 3; 30] and in image fusion [2]. In tomography studies, MRI or CT provide accurate maps of *anatomy* while PET or SPET provide much lower resolution maps of *function*. Linking function to the anatomy is of interest. Image registration and segmentation techniques are required here.

There have been many approaches to finding an appropriate warp, but a common theme is the compromise between insisting that the distortion be *smooth* and achieving a *good match*. In some recently published cases the warp seems unnecessarily rough [19, Figure 8b; 44, Figure 7f]. Smoothness can be ensured by assuming a parametric form for the warp, such as the affine transformation, or by insisting that the warp satisfies partial differential equations such as Navier's equilibrium equations for elastic bodies [5]. Depending on the application, matching might be specified by points which must be brought into alignment [12], by local measures of **correlation** between images, or by the coincidence of edges [15].

In the DNA sequencing gel, shown in Figure 1(c), it is clear that bands are not aligned, because of a relative lengthening of the tracks near the center of the gel, known colloquially as a "smile" on the gel. Interpretation of electrophoretic gels often involves making comparisons between tracks, or between spot positions on different gels. Distortions are common. Figure 3(a) shows the result of an unwarping operation proposed by Glasbey & Wright [37]. Horgan et al. [51] show how affine and thin-plate spline transformations can be used to align two or more 2D electrophoretograms.

Filters

Filters have two roles in image analysis, either to *reduce noise* by smoothing or to *emphasize edges*, i.e. boundaries between objects or parts of objects. Filters are *linear* if the output values are linear combinations of the pixels in the original image, otherwise they are *nonlinear*.

Linear filters are well understood and fast to compute. They can be studied and implemented in either spatial or frequency domains. Linear filters can be categorized as *low-pass* or *high-pass*, according to whether they smooth by removing high-frequency components in images, or emphasize edges by removing low-frequency components. A third category, *band-pass* filters, remove both the lowest

and highest frequencies from images. Use of the **Fast Fourier Transform** leads to efficient computation for filters larger than 5×5. Further details can be found in Glasbey & Horgan [36, Chapter 3]. Note that smoothing filters are a form of kernel regression (*see* **Nonparametric Regression**). See, for example, Hastie & Tibshirani [47, Chapter 2] for a review of this and alternative statistical approaches to smoothing.

In filtering to reduce noise levels, linear smoothing filters inevitably blur edges, because both edges and noise are high-frequency components of images. Nonlinear filters are able to simultaneously reduce noise and preserve edges, but they have less secure theoretical foundations and can be slow to compute. The simplest, most studied, and most widely used nonlinear filter is the moving median. However, many other *robust estimators* of location have also been used [27]. Multiresolution methods based on wavelets are a new approach to smoothing images [25], which also offer great potential in other areas of image analysis.

Morphological filters are a subclass of nonlinear filters, the simplest of which are based on "max" and "min" operations. Substantial improvements in images can often be achieved using sequences of such filters. For example, another problem with Figure 1(c) is that the brightness in the background varies. This is a common problem in image analysis, and makes comparison of similar features in different parts of the image difficult. A morphological *closing* of the image can be used to estimate the background trend. The simplest closings are obtained by first replacing each pixel by the maximum local intensity in a region (e.g. using a *structuring element* which is a disc of radius R centered on each pixel), and then performing a similar operation on the resulting image, using the local minimum. Mathematically, the pixels, z_{ij}, in the closed image will be given by

$$z_{ij} = \min_{k,l} x_{i+k, j+l} \quad \text{and} \quad x_{ij} = \max_{k,l} y_{i+k, j+l},$$

where $(k^2 + l^2)^{1/2} \le R$ and $y_{i,j}$ denotes the original pixel value in row i, column j. If this filter is applied to Figure 3(a), then only the small groups of pixels which are darker than their surroundings will be substantially changed from y_{ij} to z_{ij}. These are the bands. By subtracting z from y, these bands will be made more distinct. Figure 3(b) shows the result using a disc of radius 10 pixels. This is known

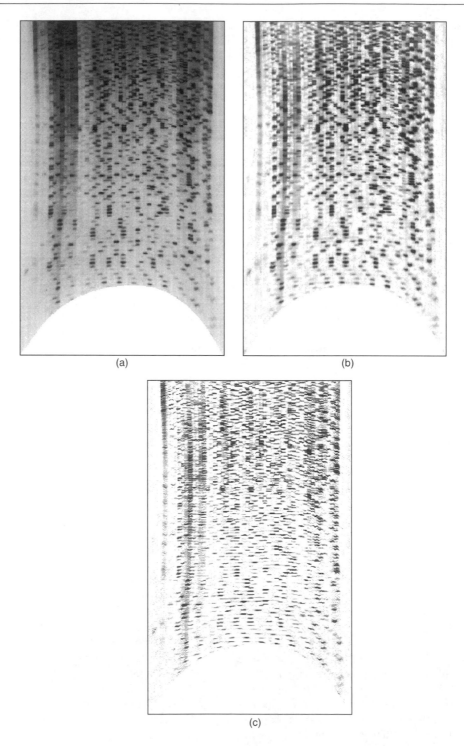

Figure 3 Enhancement of image of DNA sequencing gel autoradiograph: (a) after unwarping of Figure 1(c); (b) after application of top-hat transform to Figure 3(a) to remove background trend; (c) after constrained least squares deconvolution of Figure 3(b)

as a *top-hat filter*. Further morphological filters are discussed in [86], and [93].

Deconvolution

If an image has been contaminated by noise and blurring of forms which are either known or can be estimated, then filters can be constructed which optimally restore the original image. There are both linear and nonlinear deconvolution methods (see, for example [83, Chapter 7]). The fundamental linear method is the *Wiener filter*. Nonlinear restoration algorithms can do better than linear ones, but require substantially more computation. For example, *maximum entropy restoration* [90] is one method which exploits the constraint that the restored image is non-negative. However, as Donoho et al. [24] point out, there are many alternate methods which are equally good. Nonparametric methods for deconvolution generally require the selection of hyperparameters that control smoothing. Rice [80] evaluates generalized **cross validation** (GCV) in this context. See also Thompson et al. [97]. O'Sullivan & Pawitan [74] describe methods for indirect estimation problems and apply them in tomography.

Examination of the pixel values in Figure 3(b) shows the blurring to be well approximated by a Gaussian distribution with variance $\sigma^2 = 2$. This suggests the following model, in which we only consider blur down columns:

$$y_{ij} = \sum_{k=-m}^{m} w_k \, x_{i+k,j} + e_{ij},$$

$$\text{for } i = 1, \ldots, M, \; j = 1, \ldots, N,$$

where

$$w_k = \frac{1}{(2\pi\sigma^2)^{1/2}} \exp\left(\frac{-k^2}{2\sigma^2}\right),$$

$$\text{for } k = -m, \ldots, m,$$

M and N are the image dimensions, m is the integer part of 3σ, x_{ij} is an ideal unblurred version of the image, which is constrained to be nonnegative, and e_{ij} is uncorrelated noise. For a more general approach to blur estimation, see, for example, [79].

We can use information about the nature of the degradations to design a filter that will smooth y and enhance the edges, so as to get as close as

possible to restoring x. Deconvolution can be posed as a constrained **optimization** problem:

$$\text{minimize } S = \sum_{i=1}^{M} \sum_{j=1}^{N} \left(y_{ij} - \sum_{k=-m}^{m} w_k x_{i+k,j} \right)^2$$

with respect to x_{ij},

$$\text{for } i = 1, \ldots, M, \; j = 1, \ldots, N,$$

subject to $x_{ij} \geq 0$.

In the absence of the inequality constraint, and provided that we can consider x to be the realization of a random process, the optimal solution is the Wiener filter:

$$\hat{x}_{kl}^* = \frac{y_{kl}^*}{w_{kl}^*} \frac{|w_{kl}^*|^2}{|w_{kl}^*|^2 + S_{kl}^e / S_{kl}^x},$$

where y^* denotes the Fourier transform of y, and S_{kl}^x denotes the spectrum of x at frequency (k, l). For a derivation, see, for example, [83, Section 7.3]. The constrained problem can be solved iteratively by gradient descent. Further details are given in Horgan & Glasbey [50]. Figure 3(c) shows the result of deconvolving Figure 3(b). It can be seen that bands which are very close together have been separated in Figure 3(c), although they are indistinguishable in Figure 3(b).

Segmentation

Image segmentation is the division of an image into *regions* or *objects*. This is often a necessary step before the desired quantitative analysis can be carried out. As an example, we wish to segment the wheat grains image [Figure 1(d)], which was one of 38 such images. Each image consisted of 50 grains of the same type, and different images represented grains of different varieties or sites. The aim of the experiment was to see how well flour yield could be predicted from summary size and shape statistics obtained from each image. It is therefore natural to segment the images into individual grains before measuring and accumulating relevant summary statistics.

In some instances, of course, it is possible to estimate the parameters of interest without first resorting to segmentation. However, typically this requires strong model assumptions, upon which indirect inference can be based. Unfortunately, images are large data sets, e.g. a 512×512 image consists of more than 250 000 pixels. Therefore, there is considerable scope (as in other large data sets) for model assumptions to be violated. Often this has the consequence that the optimal solution for the theoretical model is a poor solution to the real problem! Consequently, in most problems it is necessary to segment an image first before measuring and analyzing the result. In this section we will briefly examine four classes of segmentation: thresholding, edge-based segmentation, region-based segmentation, and Bayesian approaches. The wheat grains image will illustrate some of the techniques discussed.

Thresholding

The simplest method of segmentation is thresholding, i.e. whenever a pixel's value is less than or equal to a certain number, t say, its value is replaced by 1, and otherwise given the value 2.

An obvious question is: How does one choose the threshold(s)? The simplest way is by applying some classification technique to the *histogram* of the pixel values. Glasbey [35] reviewed 11 histogram-based methods for choosing the thresholds automatically, most of which are fairly naive. Perhaps the most sophisticated is the minimum error thresholding technique of Kittler & Illingworth [61], which models the histogram as a mixture of Gaussian distributions. The parameters are estimated iteratively in such a way that the observed and estimated means and variances are equated.

Figure 4(a) shows the histogram of the wheat grains image. Clearly, there are two identifiable groups of pixels: light ones largely belonging to wheat grains, with a mean a little above 100, and dark ones, predominantly associated with the background. Note the non-Gaussian shape of the part of the histogram representing dark pixels, and especially the spike at zero due to the camera setting. Despite the fact that the histogram is not a mixture of Gaussians, we nevertheless applied the minimum error thresholding technique. It gave a value of $t = 66$. (Many other algorithms give a similar value.) Figure 4(b) shows the original wheat grains image, but with pixels whose values exceed 66 overlaid in black. This figure demonstrates a number of relevant issues. First, around each region overlaid in black is a grey halo. For the most part, these halos are 1 or 2 pixels wide. Mostly these represent "mixed" pixels, which are not definitively grain or background, but a mixture of both, caused by camera blur and shadows. In any event, where these halos are narrow, the boundaries of the overlaid regions are close enough to the true grain boundaries for most practical purposes. However, note that the darker parts of some of the grains have not been properly classified. This is perhaps not surprising, because histogram-based thresholding takes no account of spatial context. The remaining classes of segmentation discussed in this section attempt to account for spatial context in various ways. It is also possible to define an *adaptive threshold* which varies across an image (see, for example, [14]).

Edge-Based Segmentation

As the name implies, in edge-based segmentation an attempt is made to find edges in images, often by estimating a "derivative"; see [36, Chapter 3] for a description of some of the more popular edge detectors. One of the simplest edge detectors is *Prewitt's gradient filter*, which implicitly assumes a planar surface in a 3×3 window centered on each pixel, estimates the surface by least squares, and computes its maximal gradient. Figure 4(c) shows this gradient for the wheat grains image. Most of the grain boundaries are apparent, although there are some obvious gaps. Figure 4(d) is the result of thresholding Figure 4(c) at $t = 10$. Less obvious gaps are now apparent, as are some spurious features. This highlights the fundamental problem of edge-based segmentation, namely the absence of parts of boundaries and the presence of spurious edges. Edge tracking methods have been proposed by Hueckel [53], Martelli [67] and Breen & Peden [14], among others, but success is often only partial, especially in images that are more complex than the one analyzed here.

Region Growing and Merging

The basic idea behind region growing is the following. Suppose that one can find distinct points, or clusters of points, such that each distinct cluster belongs to a distinct object in the image, and the number of clusters equals the number of objects. Such points are typically called *seeds* or *markers*. Now grow out spatially from each cluster of seeds according to

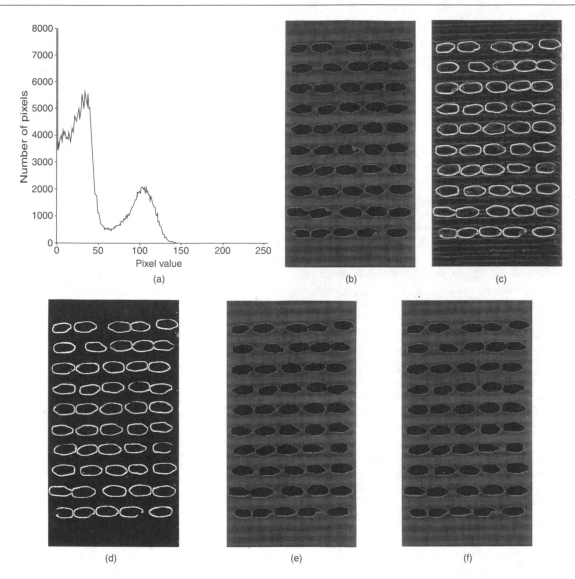

Figure 4 Approaches to segmenting the wheat grains image: (a) histogram of Figure 1(d); (b) after thresholding Figure 1(d) at $t = 66$ (pixels greater than the threshold are overlaid in black); (c) after applying Prewitt's gradient filter to Figure 1(d); (d) after thresholding Figure 4(c) at $t = 10$; (e) after applying seeded region-growing to Figure 1(d); (f) after applying a modified watershed transform to Figure 4(e)

some mechanism, allocating pixels to objects as they grow in a way that preserves the connectedness of the objects. This process will produce objects with complete boundaries, thereby overcoming a problem with edge-based segmentation mentioned above. Fast algorithms for a number of important region-growing algorithms have been developed in recent years by using data structures that come under the collective name of *priority queues* [13]. In this subsection we

apply two important region-growing algorithms to the wheat grains image.

Seeded region growing [1] first computes the mean grayscale of each cluster. Next, all neighboring pixels of clusters are examined, and the one whose grayscale value is closest to the mean of its neighboring cluster is assigned to that cluster, and the mean value of the cluster is updated. This process continues, one pixel at a time, until all pixels are assigned to a cluster (which by the end of the process is a complete object or region). For the wheat grains image we have chosen our seeds for the grains to be all pixels with a grayscale greater than 80, and our seeds for the background to be all pixels with a grayscale less than 40 [see Figure 4(a)]. Some of the pixels greater than 80 form small (spurious) islands near the bottom of the image [see Figure 4(b)]. Any connected region of pixels less than 100 pixels in area is therefore removed as a seed for the grains. The result of applying seeded region growing using these seeds is shown in Figure 4(e). Apart from the halos mentioned above, the segmentation appears to have found the grains very well. Seeded region growing appears to be quite robust to the choice of parameters; the important thing is to obtain a reasonable number of "representative" seeds for each distinct connected region in an image.

A point to notice in Figure 4(e) is that some of the grains are touching. It is important to separate these grains for subsequent measurements relevant to size, and particularly shape. To do this we employ a variant of a widely used region-growing technique called *watershedding* [69, 99]. The result, shown in Figure 4(f), is a reliable segmentation of the wheat grains. The remaining 37 images were mostly segmented as well and required very little manual intervention.

There are many other split-and-merge algorithms in the literature, most of them more complex than the one presented above. Haralick & Shapiro [46, Chapter 10] discuss a variety of such algorithms and Gordon [40] surveyed methods for constrained classification. The *Hough transform* (see, for example, [64]) can also be used for segmentation by identifying the linear or curved features in images.

Bayesian Approaches

The Bayesian approach to image segmentation received its initial impetus from the pioneering papers of Geman & Geman [31] and Besag [9]. Since then there has been a large number of papers on the subject. However, in the authors' opinion, these techniques are still only applicable for a specialized class of images, in which the models used are good representations of the data. As pointed out earlier, there is plenty of scope for the relatively simple model assumptions used in the Bayesian literature to be violated, because images are such large data sets.

However, because of its importance in the statistical literature, we give a brief survey of the area.

Many of the Bayesian approaches to image segmentation rest on variants of the following model as described in Besag [9]. Let S denote the set of all pixels in an image, and let $n = MN$ be the number of pixels in S. Assume that all pixels in the image belong to one of c classes, labeled $1, 2, \ldots, c$, respectively; we do not allow for mixed pixels. Let X_i denote the class to which pixel i belongs (double indexing of subscripts is unnecessary for the present discussion), and let $\mathbf{X} = (X_1, \ldots, X_n)$. Let y_i denote the value recorded at pixel i, and let $\mathbf{Y} = (y_1, \ldots, y_n)$.

Let $f(\mathbf{Y}|\mathbf{X}, \theta)$ denote the conditional density function of $\mathbf{Y}$ given $\mathbf{X}$, with parameter θ. Often (but not always, e.g. [59]) it is assumed that the observations are conditionally independent, i.e. $f(\mathbf{Y}|\mathbf{X}, \theta) = \prod f(y_i|X_i, \theta)$. Let $g(\mathbf{X}, \beta)$ denote the prior distribution of $\mathbf{X}$, with parameter β. In what follows we drop reference to θ and β. It is common to model g as a *locally dependent Markov Random Field* (MRF) [60]. Often, but not always, the local dependence is on the immediate eight neighbors of each pixel. MRFs usually produce a relatively simple structure for g (apart from a normalizing factor); they are also appealing because they can be modeled as limits to (possibly inhomogeneous) **Markov chains**. This means that they can be approximately simulated via **Markov chain Monte Carlo** (MCMC) techniques [10], and are therefore amenable to (computationally intensive) inference (*see* **Computer-Intensive Methods**).

The maximum a posteriori (MAP) estimator chooses $\mathbf{X}$ to maximize the posterior likelihood, which is proportional to $f(\mathbf{Y}|\mathbf{X})g(\mathbf{X})$. Unfortunately, this maximization is usually difficult because of the normalization factor mentioned above. In special cases, exact maximization (e.g. [43]) or approximate maximization [26] is possible. However, to circumvent this, Geman & Geman [31] used *simulated annealing* (an inhomogeneous MCMC technique) to find the global maximum of the posterior likelihood. Apart from being computationally intensive, this method sometimes produces gross mislabeling in certain classification problems and "oversmoothing" in related surface reconstruction and image restoration problems [9, 23, 66]. This phenomenon is most probably due to the method's strong dependence on the particular model chosen.

Partly as a consequence of these apparent limitations, Besag [9] introduced the *iterated conditional modes* (ICM) algorithm. Let $h(X_i|X_{S\setminus i})$ denote the distribution of X_i conditional on the other X_js; this will usually have a simple structure for an MRF. Let $\hat{\mathbf{X}}$ denote a provisional estimate of $\mathbf{X}$. ICM *iteratively* chooses $\hat{X}_i$ to maximize

$$p(X_i|\mathbf{Y}, \hat{X}_{S\setminus i}) \propto f(\mathbf{Y}|X_i, \hat{X}_{S\setminus i})h(X_i|\hat{X}_{S\setminus i}).$$

This simplifies in an obvious way when the y_is are independent conditional on $\mathbf{X}$. Besag shows that ICM never decreases the posterior likelihood and so will usually converge to a *local* maximum.

Variants of the above model include those of Geman et al. [33], who imposed constraints on the shapes of class boundaries, and Helterbrand et al. [49], who used boundary closure constraints. A somewhat different and interesting approach is adopted by Baddeley & van Lieshout [4]. They used prior distributions on $\mathbf{X}$ more appropriate for objects of a given shape and size; for instance, in the wheat grains example, these might be ellipses with given radii. The centers of these objects were modeled as nearest-neighbor Markov **point processes**. An algorithm similar to ICM was used to find a local maximum of the posterior distribution. One of Baddeley & van Lieshout's two examples involved fitting circles to an image of (roughly) circular pellets. Their segmentation fitted reasonably well in most places, but not everywhere, in part because the circularity assumptions were not quite right. Similar discrepancies might occur if the wheat grains were modeled as ellipses. Rather than assuming a fixed size and shape, Grenander and coworkers (see Grenander & Miller [44] and references therein) used *deformable templates* to define the boundaries of objects. This requires knowledge of the mean shape of objects, and variability about the mean. They also used jump-diffusion processes to model and simulate the process of interaction between objects. The associated segmentation process appears to be extremely computationally intensive. A related method is where segment boundaries are constrained to be smooth by including roughness penalties such as bending energies in an optimization criterion [71]. This is referred to as the fitting of "snakes" [57]. For further work in this area and a range of applications, see [3], [20], [76], [78], and [81].

We applied a form of ICM [9, Eq. (7)] to the wheat grains image, but the results were only slightly better than those produced by thresholding [Figure 4(b)]. It would seem that stronger prior constraints need to be incorporated. An appropriate Bayesian model and associated estimation procedure would almost certainly segment the wheat grains image as well as the region-based methods. However, it would require a lot of research (and probably data) to find the appropriate model and the estimation procedure is likely to be computationally intensive.

Measurement

The extraction of quantitative information is the end-point of most image analysis in biostatistics. The aim may simply be to count the number of objects in a scene, or measure their areas, or it may be more complex, such as describing the shapes of objects to discriminate between them.

It is straightforward to count the number of objects in an image provided that the segmentation has successfully associated one, and only one, component with each object. If this is not the case, then manual intervention may be necessary to complete the segmentation. However, short-cuts can sometimes be taken. For example, if the mean size of objects is known, then the number of objects in an image can be estimated, even when they are touching, through dividing the total area covered by all the objects by this average size. It is even possible to make allowance for objects overlapping each other provided that this process can be modeled, for instance by assuming that objects are positioned at random over the image and making use of the properties of Boolean models [21, pp. 753–759]. For example, Jeulin [56] has estimated the size distribution of a powder in such a way. Rudemo et al. [84] used a marked point process model to obtain estimates of plant densities in images of field crops.

Moments offer one method for summarizing segmented objects. If the object we are interested in is represented by all pixels $(i, j) \in A$, then the *(k, l)th moment* is

$$\mu_{kl} = \sum_{(i,j)\in A}\sum i^k j^l, \quad \text{for } k, l = 0, 1, 2, \dots.$$

In particular, the zeroth-order moment, μ_{00}, specifies the area of the object. First-order moments specify the location of an object. Higher-order moments are also mainly determined by an object's location. *Central moments*, defined by

$$\mu'_{kl} = \sum\sum_{(i,j)\in A} \left(i - \frac{\mu_{10}}{\mu_{00}}\right)^k \left(j - \frac{\mu_{01}}{\mu_{00}}\right)^l,$$

$$\text{for } k + l > 1,$$

are *locationally* – but not *rotationally* – invariant. If orientation is an important feature of an object, as it will be in some applications, then it is probably desirable for the moments to be sensitive to it. However, in other cases orientation is irrelevant and moment statistics are more useful if they are invariant to rotation as well as to location. One such method is based on first specifying the direction in which the object has the maximum value for its second-order moment. This direction is

$$\phi = \frac{1}{2}\tan^{-1}\left(\frac{2\mu'_{11}}{\mu'_{02} - \mu'_{20}}\right), \quad \text{if } \mu'_{02} > \mu'_{20},$$

and is otherwise this expression plus $\pi/2$. Direction ϕ, the *major axis* of the object, has second-order moment:

$$\lambda_1 = \mu'_{20}\sin^2\phi + \mu'_{02}\cos^2\phi + 2\mu'_{11}\sin\phi\cos\phi.$$

The direction perpendicular to ϕ, i.e. the *minor axis*, has the smallest second-order moment of

$$\lambda_2 = \mu'_{20}\cos^2\phi + \mu'_{02}\sin^2\phi - 2\mu'_{11}\sin\phi\cos\phi.$$

For a derivation, see Rosenfeld and Kak [83, Volume 2, pp. 288–290].

Perimeters of objects are also useful summary statistics. Let P denote the number of pixels on the boundary of object A, specified as follows. Pixel (i, j) is on the boundary if $(i, j) \in A$, but one of its four horizontal or vertical neighbors is outside the object, i.e.

$$(i + 1, j) \notin A \quad \text{or} \quad (i - 1, j) \notin A \quad \text{or}$$

$$(i, j + 1) \notin A \quad \text{or} \quad (i, j - 1) \notin A.$$

This gives an *8-connected* boundary, with pixels linked either horizontally, vertically, or diagonally. An unbiased estimator of the perimeter is given by

$$\frac{4}{\pi}\frac{P}{\sqrt{2}}$$

provided that either all orientations in the boundary occur equally often or the sampling grid is positioned

randomly on the object. This, and more complicated methods for estimating perimeters, are considered by Koplowitz & Bruckstein [62]. The use of scaling factors is part of stereology, a field which has traditionally been concerned with inference about objects using information from lower-dimensional samples, such as estimating volumes of objects from the areas of intersection with randomly positioned cutting planes (see, for example, [95, Chapter 11]). In particular, the scaling factor of $\pi/4$ arises in two of the so-called "six fundamental formulae" of classical stereology. However, the last 10 years have seen a revolution in stereology, with the discovery of the *disector* [*sic*] and other 3D sampling strategies [94]. Note, furthermore, that mathematical morphology can be used to study size distributions of objects in images. By performing openings, using structuring elements at a range of different sizes, a *granulometry* can be obtained [86, Chapter 10].

Shape information is what remains once location, orientation, and size features of an object have been dealt with. One commonly used shape statistic is a measure of *compactness*, which is defined to be the ratio of the area of an object to the area of a circle with the same perimeter. Another statistic often used to describe shape is a measure of *elongation*. This can be defined in many ways, one of which is as the ratio of the second-order moments of the object along its major and minor axes.

Summary statistics of area, perimeter, and major- and minor-axis lengths were obtained for the 50 wheat grains given by segmented regions in Figure 4(f). To illustrate these results, a **principal components analysis** was performed on the log transformed data. Table 1 gives the principal component coefficients. Figure 5 is a scatterplot of the first two principal components, which account for 99.1% of the variation in the correlation matrix. Each point is represented by that grain's outline.

Table 1 Principal component coefficients and percentages of correlation matrix explained for log-transformed summary statistics from 50 wheat grains given by segmented regions in Figure 4(f)

Component:	1	2	3	4
Percent variability:	80.1	18.9	0.9	0.003
Area	0.55	−0.21	0.34	0.74
Perimeter	0.53	0.32	−0.78	0.06
λ_1	0.49	0.54	0.52	−0.45
λ_2	0.42	−0.75	−0.06	−0.50

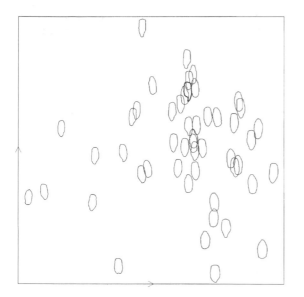

Figure 5 A scatterplot of the first two principal components of summary statistics from the segmented wheat grains [Figure 4(f)], with the first principal component along the horizontal axis. Each point is represented by that grain's outline, and the outline displayed in bold is an outlier in the third principal component

Examination of Table 1 and Figure 5 reveals that the first principal component is an indicator of grain size, while the second is a composite measure of compactness and elongation. The third principal component discriminates between one unusual grain outline, that shown in bold in Figure 5, and the rest. Comparison with Figure 1(d) shows that this grain is not particularly unusual, but rather that the segmentation has failed to recognize a particularly dark part of the grain. Berman et al. [8] used these summary statistics, together with those from a further 37 images, to predict flour yield. They found that the average area of grains in each image, together with averages of λ_1, λ_2, an estimate of volume of a prolate ellipsoid proportional to $\lambda_1\lambda_2^2$, and grain weight explained 65% of the variation in flour yield.

The description of shape is an open-ended task, because there are potentially so many aspects to an object even after location, orientation, and size effects have been removed. Other approaches include the use of *landmarks* [39] and warpings such as *thin-plate splines* and other *morphometric methods* [12], which consider image plane distortions needed to move landmarks to designated locations. Rohlf & Archie [82] and Mou & Stoermer [70] compared

alternate forms of *Fourier descriptors* to approximate object boundaries, and applied Zahn & Roskies' [101] method to describe the outlines of mosquito wings and diatoms, respectively. Further methods are discussed in the reviews of shape analysis by Pavlidis [75] and Mardia et al. [65].

References

[1]   Adams, R. & Bischof, L. (1994). Seeded region growing, *IEEE Transactions on Pattern Analysis and Machine Intelligence* **16**, 641–647.

[2]   Ardekani, B.A., Braun, M., Hutton, B. & Kanno, I. (1996). Minimum cross-entropy reconstruction of PET images using prior anatomical information obtained from MR, in *Quantification of Brain Function Using PET*, R. Myers, V. Cunningham, D. Bailey & T. Jones, eds. Academic Press, London, pp. 113–117.

[3]   Aykroyd, R.G. & Green, P.J. (1991). Global and local priors, and the location of lesions using gamma-camera imagery, *Philosophical Transactions of the Royal Society, London, Series A* **337**, 323–342.

[4]   Baddeley, A.J. & van Lieshout, M.J.M. (1993). Stochastic geometry models in high-level vision, *Advances in Applied Statistics* **20**, Supplement, 233–258.

[5]   Bajcsy, R. & Kovacic, S. (1989). Multiresolution elastic matching, *Computer Vision, Graphics and Image Processing* **46**, 1–21.

[6]   Ballard, D.H. & Brown, C.M. (1982). *Computer Vision*. Prentice-Hall, Englewood Cliffs.

[7]   Beekman, F.J. & Viergever, M.A. (1996). Evaluation of fully 3D iterative scatter correction and post-reconstruction filtering in SPECT, in *Three Dimensional Image Reconstruction in Radiology and Nuclear Medicine*, P. Greangeat & J.-L. Amans, eds. Kluwer, Dordrecht, pp. 163–175.

[8]   Berman, M., Bason, M.L., Ellison, F., Peden, G. & Wrigley, C.W. (1996). Image analysis of whole grains to screen for flour-milling yield in wheat breeding, *Cereal Chemistry* **73**, 323–327.

[9]   Besag, J. (1986). On the statistical analysis of dirty pictures (with discussion), *Journal of the Royal Statistical Society, Series B* **48**, 259–302.

[10]   Besag, J. & Green, P.J. (1993). Spatial statistics and Bayesian computation, *Journal of the Royal Statistical Society, Series B* **55**, 25–38.

[11]   Bickel, P.J. & Ritov, Y. (1995). Estimating linear functionals of a PET image, *IEEE Transactions on Medical Imaging* **14**, 81–87.

[12]   Bookstein, F.L. (1991). *Morphometric Tools for Landmark Data: Geometry and Biology*. Cambridge University Press, Cambridge.

[13]   Breen, E.J. & Munro, D.H. (1994). An evaluation of priority queues for mathematical morphology, in *Mathematical Morphology and its Applications to Image Processing*, J. Serra & P. Soille, eds. Kluwer, Dordrecht, pp. 249–256.

[14]   Breen, E.J. & Peden, G.M. (1994). Automatic thresholding and edge linking of ferritic steel weld images, *Journal of Computer-Assisted Microscopy* **6**, 167–179.

[15]   Burr, D.J. (1981). A dynamic model for image registration, *Computer Graphics and Image Processing* **15**, 102–112.

[16]   Bushberg, J.T., Seibert, J.A., Leidholdt, E.M. & Boone, J.M. (1994). *The Essential Physics of Medical Imaging.* Williams & Wilkin, Baltimore.

[17]   Carson, R.E. & Lange, K. (1985). The EM parametric image reconstruction algorithm, *Journal of the American Statistical Association* **80**, 20–22.

[18]   Colchester, A.C.F. & Hawkes, D.J., eds (1991). Information processing in medical imaging, in *Proceedings of the Twelfth International Conference on Information Processing in Medical Imaging.* Springer-Verlag, Berlin.

[19]   Conradsen, K. & Pedersen, J. (1992). Analysis of 2-dimensional electrophoretic gels, *Biometrics* **48**, 1273–1287.

[20]   Cootes, T.F., Taylor, C.J., Cooper, D.H. & Graham, J. (1995). Active shape models – their training and application, *Computer Vision and Image Understanding* **61**, 38–59.

[21]   Cressie, N.A.C. (1991). *Statistics for Spatial Data.* Wiley, New York.

[22]   Cunningham, V.J. & Jones, T. (1993). Spectral analysis of dynamic PET studies, *Journal of Cerebral Blood Flow and Metabolism* **13**, 15–23.

[23]   Devijver, P.A. & Dekesel, M.M. (1987). Learning the parameters of a hidden Markov random field model: a simple example, in *Pattern Recognition Theory and Applications*, P.A. Devijver & J. Kittler, eds. Springer-Verlag, Heidelberg, pp. 141–163.

[24]   Donoho, D.L., Johnstone, I.M., Hoch, J.C. & Stern, A.S. (1992). Maximum entropy and the nearly black object (with discussion), *Journal of the Royal Statistical Society, Series B* **54**, 41–81.

[25]   Donoho, D.L., Johnstone, I.M., Kerkyacharian, G. & Picard, D. (1995). Wavelet shrinkage: asymptopia? (with discussion), *Journal of the Royal Statistical Society, Series B* **57**, 301–369.

[26]   Ferrari, P.A., Frigessi, A. & Gonzaga de Sa, P. (1995). Fast approximate maximum *a posteriori* restoration of multicolour images, *Journal of the Royal Statistical Society, Series B* **57**, 485–500.

[27]   Fong, Y., Pomalaza-Raez, C.A. & Wang, X. (1989). Comparison study of nonlinear filters in image processing applications, *Optical Engineering* **28**, 749–760.

[28]   Fu, K.S. (1982). *Syntactic Pattern Recognition and Applications.* Prentice-Hall, Englewood Cliffs.

[29]   Fulton, R., Hutton, B., Braun, M., Ardekani, B. & Larkin, R. (1994). Use of 3D reconstruction to correct for patient motion in SPECT, *Physics in Medicine & Biology* **39**, 563–574.

[30]   Gee J.C., Reivich, M. & Bajcsy, R. (1993). Elastically deforming 3D atlas to match anatomical brain images, *Journal of Computer Assisted Tomography* **17**, 225–236.

[31]   Geman, S. & Geman, D. (1984). Stochastic relaxation, Gibbs distributions and the Bayesian restoration of images, *IEEE Transactions on Pattern Analysis and Machine Intelligence* **6**, 721–735.

[32]   Geman, S. & McClure, D. (1987). Statistical methods for tomographic image reconstruction, *Bulletin of the International Statistical Institute* **52**, 5–21.

[33]   Geman, D., Geman, S., Graffigne, C. & Dong, P. (1990). Boundary detection by constrained optimization, *IEEE Transactions on Pattern Analysis and Machine Intelligence* **12**, 609–628.

[34]   Girard, D.A. (1987). Optimal regularized reconstruction in computerized tomography, *SIAM Journal on Scientific and Statistical Computing* **8**, 934–950.

[35]   Glasbey, C.A. (1993). An analysis of histogram-based thresholding algorithms, *CVGIP: Graphical Models and Image Processing* **55**, 532–537.

[36]   Glasbey, C.A. & Horgan, G.W. (1995). *Image Analysis for the Biological Sciences.* Wiley, Chichester.

[37]   Glasbey, C.A. & Wright, F.G. (1994). An algorithm for unwarping multitrack electrophoretic gels, *Electrophoresis* **15**, 143–148.

[38]   Glasbey, C.A., Hitchcock, D., Russel, A.J.F. & Redden, H. (1994). Towards the automatic measurement of cashmere-fibre diameter by image analysis, *Journal of the Textile Institute* **85**, 301–307.

[39]   Goodall, C. (1991). Procrustes methods in the statistical analysis of shape (with discussion), *Journal of the Royal Statistical Society, Series B* **53**, 285–339.

[40]   Gordon, A.D. (1996). A survey of constrained classification, *Computational Statistics and Data Analysis* **21**, 17–29.

[41]   Green, P. (1990). Bayesian reconstruction from emission tomography data using a modified EM algorithm, *IEEE Transactions on Medical Imaging* **9**, 84–93.

[42]   Green, P. & Silverman, B. (1994). *Nonparametric Regression and Generalized Linear Models.* Chapman & Hall, London.

[43]   Greig, D.M., Porteous, B.T. & Seheult, A.H. (1989). Exact maximum *a posteriori* estimation for binary images, *Journal of the Royal Statistical Society, Series B* **51**, 271–279.

[44]   Grenander, U. & Miller, M.I. (1994). Representations of knowledge in complex systems (with discussion), *Journal of the Royal Statistical Society, Series B* **56**, 549–603.

[45]   Hames, B.D. & Rickwood, D. eds (1981). *Gel Electrophoresis of Proteins: A Practical Approach.* IRL Press, London.

[46]   Haralick, R.M. & Shapiro, L.G. (1992). *Computer and Robot Vision*, Vol. 1. Addison-Wesley, Reading.

[47]   Hastie, T.J. & Tibshirani, R.J. (1990). *Generalized Additive Models.* Chapman & Hall, London.

[48]   Hebert, T. & Leahy, R. (1992). Statistic-based MAP image reconstruction from Poisson data using Gibbs priors, *IEEE Transactions on Signal Processing* **40**, 2290–2302.

[49] Helterbrand, J.D., Cressie, N. & Davidson, J.L. (1994). A statistical approach to identifying closed object boundaries in images, *Advances in Applied Probability* **26**, 831–854.

[50] Horgan, G.W. & Glasbey, C.A. (1995). Uses of digital image analysis in electrophoresis, *Electrophoresis* **16**, 298–305.

[51] Horgan, G.W., Creasey, A.M. & Fenton, B. (1992). Superimposing two-dimensional gels to study genetic variation in malaria parasites, *Electrophoresis* **13**, 871–875.

[52] Hudson, H.M. & Larkin, R.S. (1994). Accelerated image reconstruction using ordered subsets of projection data, *IEEE Transactions on Medical Imaging* **13**, 601–609.

[53] Hueckel, M.H. (1971). An operator which locates edges in digitized pictures, *Journal of the Association for Computing Machinery* **18**, 113–125.

[54] Hutton, B.F., Hudson, H.M. & Beekman, F.J. (1997). A clinical perspective of accelerated statistical reconstruction, *European Journal of Nuclear Medicine* **24**, to appear.

[55] Jain, A.K. (1989). *Fundamentals of Digital Image Processing*. Prentice-Hall, Englewood Cliffs.

[56] Jeulin, D. (1993). Random models for morphological analysis of powders, *Journal of Microscopy* **172**, 13–21.

[57] Kass, M., Witkin, A. & Terzopoulos, D. (1988). Snakes: active contour models, *International Journal of Computer Vision* **1**, 321–331.

[58] Kay, J.W. (1994). Statistical models for PET and SPECT data, *Statistical Methods in Medical Research* **3**, 5–21.

[59] Kiiveri, H.T. & Campbell, N.A. (1992). Allocation of remotely sensed data using Markov models for image data and pixel labels, *Australian Journal of Statistics* **34**, 361–374.

[60] Kinderman, R. & Snell, J.L. (1980). *Markov Random Fields and Their Applications, Contemporary Mathematics*, Vol. 1. American Mathematical Society, Providence.

[61] Kittler, J. & Illingworth, J. (1986). Minimum error thresholding, *Pattern Recognition* **19**, 41–47.

[62] Koplowitz, J. & Bruckstein, A.M. (1989). Design of perimeter estimators for digitized planar shapes, *IEEE Transactions on Pattern Analysis and Machine Intelligence* **11**, 611–622.

[63] Lange, K. & Carson, R. (1984). EM reconstruction algorithms for emission and transmission tomography, *Journal of Computer Assisted Tomography* **8**, 306–316.

[64] Leavers, V.F. (1992). *Shape Detection in Computer Vision Using the Hough Transform*. Springer-Verlag, London.

[65] Mardia, K.V., Kent, J.T. & Walder, A.N. (1991). Statistical shape models in image analysis, in *Proceedings of the 23rd Symposium on the Interface: Computer Science and Statistics*, E.M. Keramidas, ed. Interface Foundation of North America, Fairfax Station, pp. 550–557.

[66] Marroquin, J., Mitter, S. & Poggio, T. (1987). Probabilistic solution of ill-posed problems in computational vision, *Journal of the American Statistical Association* **82**, 76–89.

[67] Martelli, A. (1976). An application of heuristic search methods to edge and contour detection, *Communications of the Association for Computing Machinery* **19**, 73–83.

[68] McColl, J.H., Holmes, A.P. & Ford, I. (1994). Statistical methods in neuroimaging with particular application to emission tomography, *Statistical Methods in Medical Research* **3**, 63–86.

[69] Meyer, F. & Beucher, S. (1990). Morphological segmentation, *Journal of Visual Communication and Image Representation* **1**, 21–46.

[70] Mou, D. & Stoermer, E.F. (1992). Separating *Tabellaria* (Bacillariophyceae) shape groups based on Fourier descriptors, *Journal of Phycology* **28**, 386–395.

[71] Mumford, D. & Shah, J. (1989). Optimal approximations by piecewise smooth functions and associated variational problems, *Communications on Pure and Applied Mathematics* **42**, 577–685.

[72] National Academy of Science, USA, Committee on the Mathematics and Physics of Emerging Dynamic Biomedical Imaging (1996). *Mathematics and Physics of Emerging Biomedical Imaging*. National Academy Press, Washington.

[73] O'Sullivan, F. (1994). Metabolic images from dynamics positron emission tomography studies, *Statistical Methods in Medical Research* **3**, 87–101.

[74] O'Sullivan, F. & Pawitan, Y. (1996). Bandwidth selection for indirect density estimation based on corrupted histogram data, *Journal of the American Statistical Association* **91**, 610–626.

[75] Pavlidis, T. (1978). A review of algorithms for shape analysis, *Computer Graphics and Image Processing* **7**, 243–258.

[76] Phillips, D.B. & Smith, A.F.M. (1994). Bayesian faces via hierarchical template modelling, *Journal of the American Statistical Association* **89**, 1151–1163.

[77] Price, T.V. & Osborne, C.F. (1990). Computer imaging and its application to some problems in agriculture and plant science, *Critical Reviews in Plant Science* **9**, 235–266.

[78] Qian, W. & Titterington, D.M. (1991). Pixel labelling for 3-dimensional scenes based on Markov mesh models, *Signal Processing* **22**, 313–328.

[79] Reeves, S.J. & Mersereau, R.M. (1992). Blur identification by the method of generalized cross-validation, *IEEE Transactions on Image Processing* **1**, 301–311.

[80] Rice, J. (1986). Choice of smoothing parameter in deconvolution problems, *Contemporary Mathematics* **59**, 137–151.

[81] Ripley, B.D. & Sutherland, A.I. (1990). Finding spiral structures in images of galaxies, *Philosophical Transactions of the Royal Society of London, Series A* **332**, 477–485.

[82] Rohlf, F.J. & Archie, J.W. (1984). A comparison of Fourier methods for the description of wing shape

in mosquitoes (Diptera: Culicidae), *Systematic Zoology* **33**, 302–317.

[83]   Rosenfeld, A. & Kak, A.C. (1982). *Digital Picture Processing*, 2nd Ed. Academic Press, San Diego.

[84]   Rudemo, M., Sevestre, S. & Andreasen, C. (1995). Marked point process models for cropweed images, *Scandinavian Image Analysis Conference - 95SCIA*. Swedish Society for Automated Image Analysis, Uppsala, pp. 23–31.

[85]   Sapirstein, H.D. (1995). Variety identification by digital image analysis, in *Identification of Food-Grain Varieties*, C.W. Wrigley, ed. American Association of Cereal Chemists, St Paul, pp. 91–130.

[86]   Serra, J. (1982). *Image Analysis and Mathematical Morphology*. Academic Press, London.

[87]   Serra, J. ed. (1988). *Image Analysis and Mathematical Morphology, Vol. 2: Theoretical Advances*. Academic Press, London.

[88]   Shepp, L. & Vardi, Y. (1982). Maximum likelihood reconstruction for emission tomography, *IEEE Transactions on Medical Imaging* **2**, 113–122.

[89]   Silverman, B.W., Jones, M.C., Wilson, J.D. & Nychka, D.W. (1990). A smoothed EM approach to indirect estimation problems, with particular reference to stereology and emission tomography (with discussion), *Journal of the Royal Statistical Society, Series B* **52**, 271–324.

[90]   Skilling, J. & Bryan, R.K. (1984). Maximum entropy image reconstruction: general algorithm, *Monthly Notices of the Royal Astronomical Society* **211**, 111–124.

[91]   Slayter, E.M. & Slayter, H.S. (1992). *Light and Electron Microscopy*. Cambridge University Press, Cambridge.

[92]   Snyder, D. & Miller, M. (1985). The use of sieves to stabilize images produced with the EM algorithm for emission tomography, *IEEE Transactions on Nuclear Science* **32**, 3864–3872.

[93]   Soille, P. & Rivest, J.-F. (1992). Principles and applications of morphological image analysis. Workshop Lecture Notes from 11th IAPR International Conference on Pattern Recognition.

[94]   Stoyan, D. (1990). Stereology and stochastic geometry, *International Statistical Review* **58**, 227–242.

[95]   Stoyan, D., Kendall, W.S. & Mecke, J. (1987). *Stochastic Geometry and Its Applications*. Wiley, Chichester.

[96]   Tang, Y.T. & Suen, C.Y. (1993). Image transformation approach to nonlinear shape restoration, *IEEE Transactions on Systems, Man and Cybernetics* **23**, 155–171.

[97]   Thompson, A.M., Brown, J.C., Kay, J.W. & Titterington, D.M. (1991). A study of methods of choosing the smoothing parameter in image restoration by regularization, *IEEE Transactions on Pattern Analysis and Machine Intelligence* **13**, 326–339.

[98]   Vardi, Y. & Lee, D. (1993). From image deblurring to optimal investments: maximum likelihood solutions for positive linear inverse problems, *Journal of the Royal Statistical Society, Series B* **55**, 569–612.

[99]   Vincent, L. & Soille, P. (1991). Watersheds in digital spaces: an efficient algorithm based on immersion simulations, *IEEE Transactions on Pattern Analysis and Machine Intelligence* **13**, 583–598.

[100]   Weir, I.S. & Green, P.J. (1994). Modelling data from single photon emission computed tomography, in *Statistics and Images*, Vol. 2, K.V. Mardia, ed. Carfax, Abingdon, pp. 313–338.

[101]   Zahn, C.T. & Roskies, R.Z. (1972). Fourier descriptors for plane closed curves, *IEEE Transactions on Computers* **21**, 269–281.

C.A. GLASBEY, M. BERMAN & H.M. HUDSON

Immunotoxicology

Immunotoxicology is a speciality of toxicology aimed at the detection, quantification, and interpretation of xenobiotic-induced direct and indirect alterations (stimulatory and/or suppressive) in the immune system and the resulting effects on morbidity (incidence of infection, duration of infection, incidence of tumors, etc.) and mortality. The immune system is a highly complicated network of lymphoid cells, nonlymphoid cells, soluble factors and regulatory molecules which protect humans from foreign substances and disease. The assays used in immunotoxicology (*see* **Bioassay**) can be divided into *in vivo* assays (in living animals) and *in vitro* assays (in cultured cells), and these can be further divided into immune function assays (measuring the responsiveness of the immune system to stimulation) and host resistance assays (measuring the ability of the immune system to protect the host from infectious agents and neoplasia) [4]. All host resistance and some immune function assays are done *in vivo*, with the remaining assays being done *in vitro* or through a combination of *in vitro* and *in vivo* methods [6]. In some cases, the same or similar immune function assays can be done in both *in vivo* and *in vitro* settings.

Host Resistance Assays

The most obvious endpoint for a host resistance assay is survival. These assays tend to be short-term and are performed in a two-step process [1, 8, 9]. In the first step, animals are exposed to a xenobiotic, generally using three dose groups and a control group. After a brief waiting period, the animals are then exposed to a carefully titrated concentration of some infectious agent (e.g. influenza virus), resulting in some known degree of mortality in the population (usually targeted for 20% in 4 days). The resulting data (the number dead out of the number exposed) are generally analyzed using pairwise comparisons (**Fisher's exact test** or its equivalent), sometimes accounting for multiple comparisons, and, when the study supports it, trend analysis (the Cochran–Armitage linear trend test). Seldom does the analysis include an analysis of the impact of titration variability in administering the infectious agent, a common problem.

More recent work utilizing infectious agents has moved away from mortality as an endpoint and has focused on body burden or tissue load of the infectious agent. Analysis of these assays is generally through the use of normality based statistical methods (e.g. **analysis of variance** (ANOVA)).

Other host resistance assays are similar to the infectious agent assays described above in that the endpoint can be viewed as a survival endpoint. An example would be administration of live tumor cells into the animal (PYB6 or B16F10 assays) with counts of the number of animals with and without tumors after a prescribed period. This type of assay is conducted in the same manner as the infectious agent survival assay described above, with administration of the xenobiotic followed by administration of the live tumor cells.

Another way in which this assay is examined is to count the number of tumors appearing in the animals. Here, the usual analysis is a comparison of the mean numbers of tumors in each dose group via a t test or a similar method. Seldom are these data analyzed by more complicated methods useful for count data such as **Poisson regression**, although there is some use of the Freeman–Tukey transformation method (*see* **Multinomial Distribution**). This is an area for further statistical development.

Immune Function Assays

Immune function assays are generally used to measure the functional competency of the immune system for dealing with antigenic response. In animals, these assays can be conducted *in vivo* by exposing animals to a xenobiotic followed by an antigen and then, following sacrifice, studying key components of the immune system (e.g. the numbers of antibodies producing B-cells in the

spleen [2]). In addition, for some species it is possible to perform immune function tests in peripheral blood lymphocytes, either through exposing the host to the xenobiotic and then removing blood and performing the assay or by removing blood and doing the entire assay *in vitro*. These types of studies can also be carried out in exposed and control human populations. In most cases, the data derived from these assays are count data with very high numbers (e.g. the number of plague-forming cells in a Petri dish following stimulation of lymphocytes with sheep red blood cell antigen) and they are analyzed under the basic assumption of normality (t tests and ANOVA) or through the use of similar **nonparametric** analyses. In some cases, the counts are converted to ratios (B-cells per million spleen cells) to control for fluctuations in physiology. Finally, some immune system markers are simple organ sizes (e.g. thymus weight, spleen weight, and cell counts) which are analyzed via assumptions of normality or **lognormality**.

In most of the analyses of immune function assays, care is taken to control for **multiple comparisons** (usually using Dunnett's' method) and, as with the analysis of host resistance assays, when data on dose–response are available, analyses for trend are common (e.g. **linear regression** and/or Jonkheere's test; *see* **Nonparametric Methods**).

Immunotoxicity and Risk Assessment

There have been considerable efforts in the past few years to develop methods to apply findings from immunotoxicity to the assessment of risks from exposure to xenobiotics (*see* **Risk Assessment**). The major challenge here is to synthesize a large array of assays into a single standard. There has been some work in this area, focusing on the relationship between immune function assays and host resistance assays [3, 5, 7], in which formal regression methods have been used. However, as general area of research, the utility of immunotoxicology for setting exposure standards is still emerging. One area of keen interest is the use of mechanistic models of immune function and response as a tool for understanding alterations due to xenobiotics.

References

[1]   Luster, M.I., Germolec, D.R., Bruccoleri, A. & Simeonova, P.P. (1997). Immunotoxicological methods and

applications: animal models, in *Comprehensive Toxicology*, I.A. Sipes, C.A. McQueen & A.J. Gandolfi, eds. Elsevier Science, Oxford.

[2]   Luster, M.I., Germolec, D.R., Kayama, F., Rosenthal, G.J., Comment, C.E. & Wilmer, J.L. (1995). Approaches and concepts in immunotoxicology, in *Experimental Immunotoxicology*, R. Smialowicz & M. Holsapple, eds. CRC Press, Boca Raton, pp. 103-123.

[3]   Luster, M.I., Portier, C., Pait, D.G., White, K.L., Gennings, C., Munson, A.E. & Rosenthal, G.J. (1992). Risk assessment in immunotoxicology. I. Sensitivity and predictability of immune tests, *Fundamental and Applied Toxicology* **18**, 200-210.

[4]   Luster, M.I., Munson, A.E., Thomas, P., Holsapple, M.P., Fenters, J., White, K., Lauer, L.D., Germolec, D.R., Rosenthal, G.J. & Dean, J.H. (1988). Development of a testing battery to assess chemical-induced immunotoxicity: National Toxicology Program's guidelines for immunotoxicity evaluation in mice, *Fundamental and Applied Toxicology* **10**, 2-19.

[5]   Luster, M.I., Portier, C., Pait, D.G., Rosenthal, G.J., Germolec, D.R., Corsini, E., Blaylock, B.L., Pollock, P., Kouchi, Y., Craig, W., White, K.L., Munson, A.E. & Comment, C.C. (1993). Risk assessment in immunotoxicology. II. Relationships between immune and host resistance tests, *Fundamental and Applied Toxicology* **21**, 71-82.

[6]   Munson, A.E. & LeVier, D. (1995). Experimental design in immunotoxicology, in *Methods in Immunotoxicology*, G. Burleson, J.H. Dean & A.E. Munson, eds. Wiley-Liss, New York, pp. 11-24.

[7]   Selgrade, M.K., Daniels, M.J. & Dean, J.H. (1992). Correlation between chemical suppression of natural killer cell activity in mice and susceptibility to cytomegalovirus: rationale for applying murine cytomegalovirus as a host resistance model and for interpreting immunotoxicity testing in terms of risk of disease, *Journal of Toxicology and Environmental Health* **37**, 123-137.

[8]   Thomas, P.T. & Sherwood, R. (1995). Host resistance models in immunotoxicology, in *Experimental Immunotoxicology*, R. Smialowicz & M. Holsapple, eds. CRC Press, Boca Raton, pp. 29-46.

[9]   Vos, J.G., Smialowicz, R.J. & van Loveren, H. (1994). Animal models for assessment, in *Immunotoxicology and Immunopharmacology*, 2nd Ed. J. Dean, M. Luster, I. Kimber & A. Munson, eds. Raven Press, New York, pp. 19-30.

(*See also* **Animal Screening Systems; Dose-Response Models in Risk Analysis**)

CHRISTOPHER J. PORTIER & DORI GERMOLEC

Impact Evaluation *see* Program Evaluation

Imperfect Use Pregnancy Rate *see* Reproduction

Implicit Stratification *see* Sampling in Developing Countries

Importance Sampling *see* Numerical Integration

Imputation *see* Missing Data in Clinical Trials

IMSL Mathematics and Statistics Libraries *see* Numerical Analysis

Inbreeding

Individuals with common ancestors are said to be related, and their offspring are inbred. If no further qualifications are made, then all humans are both inbred and related to everyone else simply because the population is finite. Each of us has two parents, and if we had four grandparents, eight grandparents, 16 great-grandparents, and so on, it would take only a few hundred years back in time before we would have more ancestors than there were people living on the planet at that time. Obviously our parents have some ancestors in common, but conventional definitions of inbreeding refer only to children whose parents are related through people in the past few generations.

Inbreeding in Pedigrees

The genetic consequences of inbreeding follow directly from basic Mendelian principles (*see*

Mendel's Laws). For each **gene**, an individual receives two alleles, one from each parent, and is generally equally likely to transmit either of these two alleles to a child. The random element in such transmission means that statements about inbreeding are usually expressed as probabilities. Because related people share ancestors, there is a chance that they receive copies of the same allele from those ancestors. Half-sibs, for example, may each receive copies of the same allele from their one common parent. Because this common parent has two alleles, there is a probability of one-half that the half-sibs receive alleles that are identical by descent (ibd). There is a further one-half probability that they would each transmit these ibd alleles to an offspring. A child of half-sibs, therefore, would have an inbreeding coefficient, F, of one-eighth.

A general approach is to specify some initial or reference population, in which all members are assumed to be unrelated, and inbreeding is then measured relative to that generation. It is generally accepted, for example, that Finland was settled by a relatively small group of people about 4000 years ago. It would be convenient to quantify inbreeding, for a random member of the presently living descendants of those founders, as the probability that the person receives two alleles that trace back to a single allele among the founders. Alleles that trace to distinct founding alleles will be considered not ibd.

If the common parent in the half-sib example itself had related parents, and had an inbreeding coefficient of F, then one-half the time it would transmit copies of the same allele to two offspring and the other half of the time it would transmit alleles that had probability F of being ibd. Such arguments lead to "path-counting" equations for inbreeding coefficients. If the parents of individual I have common ancestors A, with inbreeding coefficients F_A, and if there are n_A people in the loop from one parent through A and back to the other parent, then the inbreeding coefficient of I is

$$F_I = \sum_A \left(\frac{1}{2}\right)^{n_A} (1 + F_A).$$

In the half-sib case, the common parent A is the only common ancestor and $n_A = 3$ so that $F_I = 1/8$ as before. Full sibs have two parents in common, so the inbreeding coefficient of their children would be $1/8 + 1/8 = 1/4$. First cousins have four distinct parents, two of whom are full sibs, so they have two grandparents in common ($n = 5$ for each). The inbreeding coefficient of the children of first cousins is therefore 1/16, and this is the maximum amount of inbreeding tolerated by most marriage laws.

Just as the concepts of inbreeding and relatedness are closely connected, so are the probabilities of these events. The usual measure of relatedness for individuals X and Y, the coancestry coefficient (also called the coefficient of kinship) θ_{XY}, is defined as the probability that two alleles, one taken at random from the same locus of each of X and Y, are ibd. This definition provides a value of 1/4 for full sibs, 1/8 for half sibs and 1/16 for first cousins. If individuals X and Y have a child I, then

$$F_I = \theta_{XY}.$$

Although there is not complete independence among different genes, an inbreeding coefficient of F can be interpreted as meaning that a fraction F of the genes in such an individual has two alleles that are ibd. For alleles that are both harmful and recessive, such as the ΔF508 allele responsible for most cases of cystic fibrosis, inbreeding increases the proportion of people with the harmful trait by virtue of having two copies of the deleterious allele, not masked by a normal allele. The ΔF508 allele in Caucasian populations has a (relative) frequency of about $p = 0.05$. Among individuals whose parents are unrelated, the probability of having two copies of the allele, and therefore having cystic fibrosis, is about $p^2 = 0.0025$. Among people whose parents are cousins, however, $(1 - F) = 15/16$ of the time the probability is p^2, but $F = 1/16$ of the time it is the higher value of p. The total probability is more than doubled, to 0.0063. In general, the probability that an individual with an inbreeding coefficient of F is homozygous aa for allele a that has a frequency of p_a is

$$P_{aa} = p_a^2 + F p_a(1 - p_a). \tag{1}$$

The increased homozygosity brought about by inbreeding must be accompanied by an equivalent decrease in **heterozygosity**. If $\bar{a}$ indicates an allele different from a, then for inbred individuals

$$P_{a\bar{a}} = 2 p_a p_{\bar{a}}(1 - F). \tag{2}$$

Homozygotes have two alleles that have the same chemical composition, and so are identical in state. Such alleles may or may not be ibd. Heterozygotes have alleles that are not identical in state, and these alleles cannot be ibd.

There is often interest in the joint probability $P_{a,a}$ with which two individuals carry a specific allele a. It may be that one person, X, is alleged to be the father of a child but some other person Y is actually the father, and a is the allele known to have been received by the child from its father. The probability with which an allele chosen at random from one individual is ibd to one from the other is just the coancestry, so

$$P_{a,a} = p_a^2 + \theta p_a (1 - p_a) \tag{3}$$

when the two individuals have coancestry θ. There is a more complicated expression if the individuals are also inbred.

Inbreeding in Populations

Eqs (1) and (2) have been derived for inbred individuals, where F is necessarily positive. Alternatively, they could be used to relate **genotypic** frequencies P_{aa} and $P_{a\bar{a}}$ in some population to allele frequencies p_a and $p_{\bar{a}}$ in the same population, although it is then conventional to use the symbol f in place of F. A general treatment allows for variation among fs for different loci, and for different genotypes at a locus. Writing the frequency of allele a_i as p_i, the frequency of $a_i a_i$ homozygotes as P_{ii} and the frequency of $a_i a_j$ heterozygotes as P_{ij}:

$$P_{ii_k} = p_{i_k}^2 + \sum_{j \neq i} f_{ij} p_{i_k} p_{j_k},$$
$$P_{ij_k} = 2 p_{i_k} p_{j_k} (1 - f_{ij}), \quad i \neq j,$$

where the subscript k emphasizes that the equations hold for some particular population k.

Inferences about the f parameters are based on a model of repeated sampling from the population, and if this statistical sampling is random, the **multinomial distribution** is appropriate for large populations. Population data provide direct estimates of the genotypic frequencies, and **maximum likelihood** estimates for the p_as and fs, based on sample

genotype frequencies $\tilde{P}_{ijk}$ are

$$\hat{p}_{i_k} = \tilde{P}_{ii_k} + \tfrac{1}{2} \sum_{j \neq i} \tilde{P}_{ij_k},$$

$$\hat{f}_{ij_k} = 1 - \frac{\tilde{P}_{ij_k}}{2 \hat{p}_{i_k} \hat{p}_{j_k}}.$$

If a common value f, the "within-population inbreeding coefficient" is assigned to all the f_{ij}s, then iterative procedures are needed for maximum likelihood estimation. These procedures typically produce estimates of the order of 0.001 for human populations. The quantity f was written as F_{IS} by Wright [2], referring to the relation of alleles within individuals (I) relative to a subpopulation (S).

For a specific population, the within-population inbreeding coefficient f quantifies the excess homozygosity over that expected for random mating populations. **Population-genetic** analyses are likely to be concerned with the evolutionary processes that lead to extant populations, and therefore recognize that the present population itself results from genetic sampling. Because of the random processes involved in the choice of alleles transmitted between generations, as well as in other evolutionary forces such as selection and mutation, the genetic composition of a population cannot be specified with certainty over time. Instead, probabilistic models are needed.

Taking expectations $\mathcal{E}$ over populations (or over the evolutionary process) the frequency of allele a_i is written as p_i, and of genotype $a_i a_j$ is written as P_{ij}:

$$\mathcal{E} p_{i_k} = P_i,$$
$$\mathcal{E} P_{ij_k} = P_{ij}.$$

At this total-expectation level,

$$P_{ii} = p_i^2 + F p_i (1 - p_i),$$
$$P_{ij} = 2 p_i p_j (1 - F), \quad i \neq j, \tag{4}$$

where F is the "total inbreeding coefficient." Evidently, then (1) and (2) refer in expectation to all individuals with the pedigree leading to a specific F value – even though any particular individual is either inbred or not – and invoke the expected allele frequency rather than the frequency for a specific population.

The usual interpretation of (4) is that they apply as an average over populations. One application concerns a large population considered to consist of a number of subpopulations indexed by k. Eqs (1) and (2) hold for the subpopulations, but (4) holds for the total. Any variation in p_{i_k} over subpopulations causes $\mathcal{E}p_{i_k}^2$ to exceed p_i^2, so that $P_{ii} > p_i^2$ even if $P_{ii_k} = p_{i_k}^2$. This result is known as the "Wahlund principle." Wright [2] wrote F as F_{IT}, referring to the relation of alleles within individuals (I) relative to the total population (T).

The quantity $p_{i_k}^2$ can be regarded as the probability of two alleles in population k both being of type a_i:

$$P_{i,i_k} = p_{i_k}^2.$$

Taking expectations over populations:

$$P_{i,i} = p_i^2 + \theta p_i(1 - p_i),$$

illustrating why Wright wrote θ as F_{ST}, for the relationship between alleles within subpopulations (S) relative to the total population (T). The three measures of inbreeding are related by

$$f = \frac{F - \theta}{1 - \theta}.$$

It needs to be stressed that $P_{i,i}$ is the joint probability of two alleles in the same subpopulation being ibd, averaged over all subpopulations. Estimation of the inbreeding and coancestry coefficients F and θ requires data from more than one population. Otherwise there is no knowledge of the variation in allele frequencies among populations. If there is random mating within populations, then two alleles have the same relationship whether they are in the same or different individuals, $F = \theta$, and $f = 0$.

One method of estimation, under the random mating assumption, is to compare allelic variation within and among populations. The two means squares are MSW for within and MSA for among. For allele a_i and samples of size n alleles from each of r populations:

$$\text{MSW} = \frac{n}{r(n-1)} \sum_k p_{i_k}(1 - p_{i_k}),$$

$$\text{MSA} = \frac{n}{r-1} \sum_k (p_{i_k} - \overline{p}_i)^2,$$

where

$$\overline{p}_i = \frac{1}{r} \sum_k p_{i_k}.$$

The **variance components** for allele frequencies within and between populations are

$$\sigma_w^2 = p_i(1 - p_i)(1 - \theta),$$
$$\sigma_b^2 = p_i(1 - p_i)\theta,$$

and θ can be estimated [1] as

$$\hat{\theta} = \frac{\text{MSA} - \text{MSW}}{\text{MSA} + (n-1)\text{MSW}}.$$

Conditional Probabilities

It is now possible to return to the disputed **paternity** example. If the alleged father has been typed and found to carry the obligate paternal allele a, then the quantity of interest is the conditional probability $P_{a|a}$ with which some other man also carries the allele. If this unknown and untested other man belongs to the same population as the alleged father,

$$P_{a|a} = \frac{P_{a,a}}{p_a}$$
$$= p_a + \theta(1 - p_a),$$

which applies as an average over all populations. The allele frequency could be estimated from a sample from the total population, as opposed to the particular population to which the two men belong. Data from several populations would be needed if θ is to be estimated. If the two men belong to different populations, then

$$P_{a|a} = p_a.$$

Other Measures of Inbreeding

Identity coefficients describe other measures of inbreeding. These coefficients are the probabilities that sets of more than two alleles are ibd, and they are needed to express joint and conditional probabilities of genotypes, as opposed to alleles. They find use in questions of disputed identity where one person is found to have a particular genotype and is alleged to be the donor of some biological sample. This use is described in **statistical forensics**.

References

[1]   Weir, B.S. & Cockerham, C.C. (1984). Estimating *F*-statistics for the analysis of population structure, *Evolution* **38**, 1358–1370.
[2]   Wright, S. (1951). The genetical structure of populations, *Annals of Eugenics* **15**, 323–354.

B.S. WEIR

Incidence Density

An incidence density is an **incidence rate** and can be used to estimate a **hazard rate**.

M.H. GAIL

Incidence Density Ratio

The incidence density ratio is the ratio of the **incidence density** in one group to that in another group. The incidence density ratio approximates the **hazard ratio** if time intervals are small and can be estimated both from **cohort studies** and from **case–control studies** in which controls are selected by **density sampling**.

M.H. GAIL

Incidence Rate

The incidence rate is the number of persons who develop a disease of interest over a defined interval of time or age divided by the corresponding **person-years at risk** among members of the source population. Subjects are only "at risk" before they develop the disease of interest if, as is common, the incidence rate describes the rate of first occurrence of a disease. Usually, relatively short time intervals are used, compared with the timescale for development of disease, such as five-year intervals for a cancer incidence study. When individual follow-up data are not available to compute person-years at risk, the person-years are often estimated as the interval width times the population size at the midpoint of the interval. Synonyms for incidence rate include **incidence density** and person-years incidence rate. Incidence rate sometimes denotes a population **hazard rate**, rather than the estimate defined above. Sometimes the term incidence rate is used instead of **cumulative incidence rate**, but the concepts are distinct.

M.H. GAIL

Incidence–Prevalence Relationships

This article attempts a statistical view on the classical epidemiologic concepts of (age-specific) incidence and **prevalence**. Each individual's dynamics in the **Lexis diagram** is modeled by a simple three-state illness–death **stochastic process** in the age direction and individuals are recruited from a **Poisson process** in the time direction. Observable quantities are regarded as *estimators* of the *parameters* (incidence, prevalence, mortality, **mean** duration, etc.) of the statistical model.

The next section discusses increasingly complex versions of the classical epidemiologic relation

$$\text{prevalence} = \text{incidence} \times \text{duration},$$

and its generalization to age- and duration-specific incidence and mortality. Then some comments are provided on statistical techniques for estimating **incidence rates** from prevalence surveys, while the following section considers, conversely, the feasibility of estimating prevalence from information on incidence and mortality. The material is also relevant in the theory of **screening**, as briefly pointed out later.

A related topic *not* touched in this article is **inference** on mortality (or further morbidity) from follow-up of a **cross-sectional** sample, the so-called *prevalent cohort study*. This topic is treated in the articles **Delayed Entry** and **Biased Sampling of Cohorts in Epidemiology**.

Prevalence, Incidence, and Duration

Most – even rather elementary – textbooks in epidemiology contain versions of the statement

$$\text{prevalence} = \text{incidence} \times \text{duration}, \qquad (1)$$

see, for example, [15, pp. 65–66] or [10, pp. 64–66]. In broad generality, (1) is a conservation equation called Little's equation in queuing theory:

time-average number of units in the system
= arrival rule × average delay time per unit.

See Little [13] for the first general proof in the context of strictly stationary processes in steady state conditions and Ramalhoto et al. [20] for a comprehensive discussion.

In epidemiology, the archetypical situation concerns irreversible transitions between a healthy state H, a diseased state I, and the dead state D, simplest in the time- and age-homogeneous **Markov illness–death process** specified by intensities as follows:

$$H \xrightarrow{\ \alpha\ } I$$
$$\mu \searrow \quad \swarrow \nu$$
$$D$$

and fed by a stationary homogeneous **Poisson process** with (birth) intensity β. Here α is disease intensity for a healthy individual (the connection to the epidemiologic concept of disease incidence to be discussed below) and μ and ν are death intensities for healthy and diseased, respectively. Sometimes ν is called the **case fatality** rate or just lethality.

In this stochastic process our approach to prevalence is to imagine a **cross-sectional** sample taken at a particular time t, say $t = 0$. We may then calculate the expected number of healthy at $t = 0$ as

$$\int_0^\infty \beta \exp[-(\alpha + \mu)a]\,\mathrm{d}a = \frac{\beta}{\alpha + \mu}$$

since a person born at time $-a$ has probability $\exp[-(\alpha + \mu)a]$ of remaining alive and healthy until time 0; similarly the expected number of diseased at $t = 0$ is

$$\int_0^\infty \int_0^a \beta \exp[-(\alpha + \mu)y]\alpha \exp[-\alpha(a - y)]\,\mathrm{d}y\,\mathrm{d}a$$
$$= \frac{\alpha\beta}{(\alpha + \mu)\nu}.$$

Under the present assumptions, disease duration is **exponentially** distributed with mean ν^{-1}. Definition of disease incidence requires more care. The intensity α refers to the healthy only, while *disease incidence in the population* may be defined as the rate of occurrence of new disease in the whole population. This is

$$\beta \int_0^\infty \exp[-(\alpha + \mu)\alpha]\,\mathrm{d}a = \frac{\beta\alpha}{\alpha + \mu}$$

and we see that

$$E(\text{diseased}) = \frac{\beta\alpha}{\alpha + \mu}\nu^{-1}$$
$$= \text{disease incidence} \times \text{mean duration},$$

yielding (1) in the present interpretation of units of individuals (rather than the often used prevalence proportion in relative units).

Note, furthermore, that what we shall often term prevalence odds satisfies

$$\frac{E(\text{diseased})}{E(\text{healthy})} = \frac{\alpha\beta/[(\alpha + \mu)\nu]}{\beta/(\alpha + \mu)} = \frac{\alpha}{\nu},$$

that is,

prevalence odds = incidence × mean duration,

where incidence is now understood as *intensity of getting diseased for a healthy individual*.

Alho [5] viewed the above relations between prevalence, incidence, and duration in the macrodemographic context of stable population theory.

The above discussion may be generalized to *time-*, *age-* and disease *duration*-dependent intensities $\beta(t), \alpha(t, a), \mu(t, a)$, and $\nu(t, a, d)$, as documented by Keiding [11]. We may then also discuss such concepts as *age-specific prevalence*, expressing the probability of having the disease for a person at age a alive at time t. The general formulas become complicated and are not reproduced here, although some applications will be indicated below.

In the particular case of *time homogeneity*, which, though not very realistic nevertheless underlies most epidemiologic folklore, similar relations between prevalence, incidence, and duration result as above. In particular, the rate of occurrence of new cases in the population becomes

$$\beta \int_0^\infty \exp\{-[\alpha(a) + \mu(a)]\}\alpha(a)\,\mathrm{d}a,$$

and the expected number of diseased at $t = 0$ (prevalence on the population scale, "absolute" prevalence) becomes

$$\beta \int_0^\infty \int_0^a \exp\{-[\alpha(y) + \mu(y)]\}\alpha(y)$$
$$\times \exp[-\nu(a, a - y)]\mathrm{d}y\mathrm{d}a.$$

In the simple case where the case fatality rate $\nu(a, d)$ depends only on duration d but not age a, a change of order of integration yields

$$\int_0^\infty \beta \exp\{-[\alpha(y) + \mu(y)]\}\alpha(y)\mathrm{d}y$$
$$\times \int_0^\infty \exp[-\nu(v)]\mathrm{d}v,$$

where the first factor is incidence as just specified, while since $\exp[-\nu(v)]$ is the survival function of a diseased, the second factor is mean survival. This provides an interpretation of

$$\text{prevalence} = \text{incidence} \times \text{duration}$$

in the age-dependent case, and Keiding [11] specified how to obtain a similar interpretation when $\nu(a, d)$ depends also on a.

The relation *prevalence odds = disease intensity × mean duration* discussed in the time/age/duration homogeneous special case above, also generalizes to the age/duration inhomogeneous case, see again Keiding [11] and O'Neill et al. [18].

Inference on Incidence from Prevalence Data

As has been known in population statistics (**demography**) for hundreds of years, it is true under very restrictive stationarity assumptions (no dependence of birth and death rates on calendar time, no migration) that the age distribution of the living has density proportional to the survival function $(= 1 -$ distribution function) of the mortality. Inference on mortality rates is therefore in principle available from the age distribution of the living.

The simplest generalization of this to morbidity (disease incidence) is analysis of *current status data* where age-specific incidence rates are estimated from the age distributions of diseased and healthy in a cross-sectional sample. Diamond & McDonald

[8] gave a survey based on **parametric models** in discrete and continuous time while Keiding [11] and Keiding et al. [12] focused on variants of current **nonparametric survival analysis** techniques. Ades & Nokes [2] gave a useful practical discussion of the range and limitations of these ideas in modeling infectivity rates from seroprevalence studies; and Marschner [16] gave **sample size** calculations.

As emphasized by Preston [19], the crucial **stationarity** assumption may only be verified from at least two successive cross-sectional samples, which however might then be directly used for inference without the stationarity assumption. Recent work in this direction is due particularly to Marschner (for example [17]) and Ades [1] as well as a series of papers by Brunet & Struchiner (for example [6]), in the pseudo-stochastic mathematical biology tradition.

Inference on Prevalence from Incidence and Mortality Data

It is not uncommon that disease incidence and mortality are more directly estimable (e.g. from a historically prospective incidence study with follow-up) than prevalence. In that case the relations between prevalence, incidence and duration may be used to estimate prevalence, possibly calendar time-and/or age-specifically, see Keiding [11]. Such calculations will often be variations of the nonparametric **Aalen–Johansen estimator** of a transition probability in a nonhomogeneous Markov illness–death process, and this link provides a methodology for derivation of **standard errors**.

Application of such ideas has been primarily in the context of cancer [7, 9, 22], although there are also examples from neuroepidemiology [21, 23], reference [21] containing counterfactual and predictive "what if" calculations under specified past or future structures in incidence and mortality.

Screening

There are strong relations between the above material and the mathematical theory of **screening** for chronic disease [24, 25], in the simplest but also most important case by having the three states *Healthy, Preclinical* (where the patient feels healthy but screening can identify the disease), and *Clinical*(ly manifest) diseased. The same relations are valid, properly interpreted, and Zelen & Feinleib [25] actually also obtained a *prevalence = incidence × mean duration* result. O'Neill et al. [18] formalized a concept of *initiation*, equivalent to subclinical disease onset. The comprehensive exposition of the theory of screening by Albert et al. [3, 4] and Louis et al. [14] is based on probability densities rather than intensities as in this article and most of the other references.

References

[1] Ades, A.E. (1995). Serial HIV seroprevalence surveys: interpretation, design and role in HIV/AIDS prediction, *Journal of Acquired Immunodeficiency Syndrome* **9**, 490–499.

[2] Ades, A.E. & Nokes, D.J. (1993). Modeling age- and time specific incidence from seroprevalence: toxoplasmosis, *American Journal of Epidemiology* **137**, 1022–1034.

[3] Albert, A., Gertman, P.M. & Louis, T.A. (1978). Screening for the early detection of cancer – the temporal natural history of a progressive disease state, *Mathematical Biosciences* **40**, 1–59.

[4] Albert, A., Gertman, P.M., Louis, T.A. & Liu, S.-I. (1978). Screening for the early detection of cancer – II. The impact of screening on the natural history of the disease, *Mathematical Biosciences* **40**, 61–109.

[5] Alho, J.M. (1992). On prevalence, incidence and duration in general stable populations, *Biometrics* **48**, 587–592.

[6] Brunet, R.C. & Struchiner, C.J. (1996). Rate estimation from prevalence information on a simple epidemiologic model for health interventions, *Theoretical Population Biology* **50**, 209–226.

[7] Capocaccia, R. & de Angelis, R. (1997). Estimating the completeness of prevalence based on cancer registry data, *Statistics in Medicine* **16**, 425–440.

[8] Diamond, I.D. & McDonald, J.W. (1992). Analysis of current status data, in *Demographic Applications of Event History Analysis*, J. Trussel, R. Ilankinson & J. Tilton, eds. Clarendon Press, Oxford, pp. 231–252.

[9] Feldman, A.R., Kessler, L., Myers, M.H. & Naughton, M.D. (1986). The prevalence of cancer. Estimates based on the Connecticut Tumor Registry, *New England Journal of Medicine* **315**, 1394–1397.

[10] Ilennekens, C.H. & Buring, J.E. (1987). *Epidemiology in Medicine*. Little, Brown & Company, Boston.

[11] Keiding, N. (1991). Age specific incidence and prevalence: a statistical perspective (with discussion), *Journal of the Royal Statistical Society, Series A* **154**, 371–412.

[12] Keiding, N., Begtrup, K., Scheike, T.H. & Hasibeder, G. (1996). Estimation from current-status data in continuous time, *Lifetime Data Analysis* **2**, 119–129.

[13] Little, J.D.C. (1961). A proof for the queuing formula: $L = \lambda W$, *Operations Research* **9**, 383–387.

[14] Louis, T.A., Albert, A. & Heghinian, S. (1978). Screening for the early detection of cancer. III. Estimation of disease natural history, *Mathematical Biosciences* **40**, 111–144.

[15] MacMahon, B. & Pugh, T.F. (1970). *Epidemiology: Principles and Methods*. Little, Brown & Company, Boston.

[16] Marschner, I.C. (1994). Determining the size of a cross-sectional sample to estimate the age-specific incidence of an irreversible disease, *Statistics in Medicine* **13**, 2369–2381.

[17] Marschner, I.C. (1996). Fitting a multiplicative incidence model to age- and time-specific prevalence data, *Biometrics* **52**, 492–499.

[18] O'Neill, T.J., Tallis, C.M. & Leppard, P. (1985). The epidemiology of a disease using hazard functions, *Australian Journal of Statistics* **27**, 283–297.

[19] Preston, S.H. (1987). Relations among standard epidemiologic measures in a population, *American Journal of Epidemiology* **126**, 336–345.

[20] Ramalhoto, M.F., Amaral, J.A. & Cochito, M.T. (1983). A survey of J. Little's formula, *International Statistical Review* **51**, 255–278.

[21] Somnier, F.E., Keiding, N. & Paulson, O.B. (1991). Epidemiology of Myasthenia Gravis in Denmark: a longitudinal and comprehensive population survey, *Archives of Neurology* **48**, 733–739.

[22] Verdecchia, A., Capocaccia, R., Egidi, V. & Colini, A. (1989). A method for the estimation of chronic disease morbidity and trends from mortality data, *Statistics in Medicine* **8**, 201–216.

[23] Werdelin, L. & Keiding, N. (1990). Hereditary ataxias and associated disorders. Epidemiological aspects, *Neuroepidemiology* **9**, 321–331.

[24] Zelen, M. (1986). A review of the theory of screening for chronic diseases: single exam and the scheduling of examinations, in *Statistical Design: Theory and Practice*. Cornell University Press, Ithaca, pp. 27–41.

[25] Zelen, M. & Feinleib, M. (1969). On the theory of screening for chronic diseases, *Biometrika* **56**, 601–614.

NIELS KEIDING

Incident Case

An incident case is a subject who has just developed the disease or condition of interest for the first time. Incident cases of chronic diseases are particularly valuable for etiologic investigations because disease incidence, unlike disease **prevalence**, is determined by etiologic factors only and not by factors that influence survival following disease onset. To contrast incident with prevalent cases, *see* **Biased Sampling of Cohorts in Epidemiology; Case–Control Study, Prevalent; Cross-Sectional Study; Incidence–Prevalence Relationships; Prevalent Case**.

M.H. GAIL

Incidental Tumor *see* Tumor Incidence Experiments

Incomplete Block Designs

Experimental designs with fixed block size k in which the number of treatments (or levels of a single factor) v to be compared exceeds the available block size are called *incomplete block designs*. Such designs first arose in agricultural experiments and were studied by, among others, **Fisher, Yates**, and Bose. Incomplete block designs are currently used in a wide variety of subject areas, including agricultural field and animal experiments, food-tasting experiments, industrial processes, toxicology, educational psychology, and, occasionally, in **clinical trials**. For example, in animal experiments it may be desirable to compare the test treatments within a litter, but the number of treatments may exceed the available litter sizes. In food and beverage tasting experiments, the number of items to be tasted is often greater than the number of items a judge can taste within a reasonable time period. In an experiment to compare the tread wear on different kinds of automobile tires, each car can have, at most, four distinct tires and so, if the number of treatments to be tested is greater than four, the blocks (cars) are necessarily incomplete.

Most graduate and advanced undergraduate text books on experimental design contain some material on incomplete block designs, particularly **balanced incomplete block designs** (BIBDs) and **Youden squares**. Two such books, with an applied flavor, are by Lentner & Bishop [9], and John & Quenouille [6]. Das & Giri [3] contains a full account of all the major types of incomplete block designs, their analyses, and some selected construction results. John [5]

is a more theoretical discussion of the mathematical structure and analysis of incomplete block designs, and of the construction of such designs by the cyclic development of one or more initial blocks. This article describes briefly the different kinds of incomplete designs, their relationships to each other and to other well-known kinds of complete block designs (*see* **Randomized Complete Block Designs**), and general methods of analysis of such designs.

The incomplete block design problem is one of arranging the test treatments. Two technical concepts needed in a discussion of incomplete block designs are *binary* designs and *connected* designs.

An incomplete block design is said to be *binary* if no test treatment occurs more than once in any block. It can be shown that a design that is not binary may always be improved (in the sense of average or total **variance** of the treatment contrasts) by replacing all duplicates of test treatments in a given block with treatments not already in that block. Hence, we may restrict our attention to binary designs.

A design is said to be *disconnected* if the blocks of the design may be split into two groups in such a way that none of the test treatments that occurs in one group of blocks occurs in the other group of blocks. Treatments that occur in the different groups of blocks may not be compared due to **confounding** with the block effects. As a consequence, we also restrict our attention to designs that are not disconnected; that is, to designs that are *connected*.

There are many different types of incomplete block designs that are both binary and connected. *Balanced incomplete block designs* (BIBDs) have the property that all treatments occur in the same number of blocks, say r, and all pairs of treatments occur in the same number of blocks together, say λ. In BIBDs, all **paired comparisons** of treatments are estimated with equal precision. Kiefer [7, 8] has shown that BIBDs are optimal in the sense of having smallest average or total variance for the paired treatment comparisons.

A standard assumption in the analysis of block designs is that measurements on different experimental units are statistically independent. There are situations in which this is not a reasonable assumption. For example, in agricultural field experiments, fertilizer or irrigation may spill over from an experimental plot to its neighboring experimental plots. A family of experimental designs that is useful in such a situation is the *equineighbored* BIBDs in which each pair of test treatments occurs adjacent to each other in the same number of blocks.

One shortcoming of BIBDs is that for a given number of treatments and a given block size, the number of blocks required to construct a balanced incomplete block design may be too large to be of practical use. Yates [10] addressed this problem with a series of designs that he called **lattice designs**. Lattice designs exist only when $v = s^2$ and $k = s$, for some positive integer s, and are constructed using sets of mutually orthogonal **Latin squares**. Of course, the requirements that $v = s^2$ and $k = s$ are quite restrictive, so the application of lattice designs is somewhat limited.

Bose & Nair [1] discovered a more general alternative to BIBDs. In **partially balanced incomplete block designs**, all treatments occur in the same number of blocks and pairs of treatments occur together in λ_1 or λ_2 or λ_3 or ... or λ_m blocks together. (Two treatments that occur in the same block λ_l times are said to be in the *lth associate class*). BIBDs are special cases of partially balanced incomplete block designs for which $\lambda_1 = \lambda_2 = \cdots = \lambda_m = \lambda$. Lattice designs are also special kinds of partially balanced incomplete block designs.

Partially balanced incomplete block designs exist for more combinations of parameters than do BIBDs. Das [2] and Giri [4] showed how to construct incomplete block designs for still more combinations of parameters. Their **algorithm** starts with a partially balanced incomplete block design for v treatments in b blocks of size k. Augment each block in this design with α treatments that are not among the original v treatments. The result is a design for $v + \alpha$ treatments in b blocks of size $k + \alpha$. Such designs are called *reinforced designs*.

Youden squares [11] are incomplete block designs in which two sources of variation (**blocking**) may be eliminated. First used by Youden in greenhouse studies, these designs are related to Latin square designs. Indeed, removing any row and any column from a Latin square always yields a Youden square, but Youden squares may also be constructed from certain kinds of BIBDs.

Analysis of Incomplete Block Designs

Youden squares are distinct from the other types of incomplete block designs in that they involve two blocking factors rather than one.

In the analysis of incomplete block designs with a single treatment factor and a single blocking factor, the following linear model (*see* **General Linear Model**) is usually assumed:

$$Y_{ij} = \mu + \tau_i + \beta_j + \varepsilon_{ij}, \quad \text{for } i = 1, 2, \ldots v \text{ and}$$
$$j = 1, 2, \ldots, b,$$

where the τ_is denote the treatment effects and the β_js denote the block effects. No **interaction** among block and treatment effects is assumed. Indeed, because not all treatments occur in every block, not all block-treatment interactions are even estimable. The validity of the assumption of no interactions may be evaluated graphically by plotting the **residuals** from the fitted model against, for example, the predicted values. Degrees of freedom for the different factors are summarized in Table 1.

Computation of appropriate sums of squares is complicated in incomplete block designs due to the lack of **orthogonality** of block and treatment effects. Simple formulae for sums of squares do exist for BIBDs but for other incomplete block designs, even for a partially balanced incomplete block design with just two associate classes, the formulae become extremely complicated. For this reason, it is recommended that analyses be carried out using a computer package. If algebraic formulae are required, the reader is referred to the books by Das & Giri [3] and Lentner & Bishop [9].

The most common analysis of incomplete block designs is often called the *intrablock* analysis, because block differences are eliminated and all treatment **contrasts** may be expressed as differences among observations in the same blocks. This is essentially a **least squares** analysis, assuming that the block effects are fixed. Usually, the block effects are not of intrinsic interest and so the block sum of squares is computed *without* adjusting for treatment effects. Then, the treatment sum of squares is

Table 1 Degrees of freedom for the different factors

Source of variation	Degrees of freedom
Blocks	$b - 1$
Treatments	$v - 1$
Error	$bk - b - v + 1$
Corrected total	$bk - 1$

computed after adjusting for block effects. In linear models jargon, this is a *type I* **analysis of variance**, and is standard in most statistical packages, including SAS (*see* **Software, Biostatistical**). If the block effects *are* of intrinsic interest, a block sum of squares adjusted for treatment effects may be computed. This is commonly called a *type II* analysis of variance.

Yates [10] proposed an alternative analysis, which he called the *interblock* analysis, in which additional information about the treatment effects might be obtained by comparing experimental units in different blocks. In modern linear models terminology, the interblock analysis is a mixed effects analysis of variance in which the treatment effects are regarded as **fixed effects**, while the block effects are viewed as independent **random variables** with **mean** zero and variance σ_β^2. Modeling block effects by random variables is particularly appropriate when the blocks may be viewed as a sample from some population of blocks. For example, in **multicenter clinical trials** the centers at which the study takes place may be viewed as a representative sample of all possible centers (*see* **Random Effects**).

The interblock (mixed effects) analysis may be carried out using, for example, PROC GLM and PROC MIXED in the SAS computer package. Although the intrablock analysis has been the standard analysis for many years, the interblock analysis seems to be gaining in popularity as researchers are more inclined to view their block effects as random quantities.

References

[1]   Bose, R.C. & Nair, K.R. (1939). Partially balanced incomplete block designs, *Sankhyā* **4**, 337–372.

[2]   Das, M.N. (1958). Reinforced incomplete block designs, *Journal of the Indian Society of Agricultural Statistics* **10**, 73–77.

[3]   Das, M.N. & Giri, N.C. (1979). *Design and Analysis of Experiments*. Halstead Press, New York.

[4]   Giri, N.C. (1958). On reinforced P.B.I.B. designs, *Journal of the Indian Society of Agricultural Statistics* **12**, 45–56.

[5]   John, P.W.M. (1980). *Incomplete Block Designs. Lecture Notes in Statistics*, Vol. 1. Marcel Dekker, New York.

[6]   John, J.A. & Quenouille, M.H. (1977). *Experiments: Design & Analysis*, 2nd Ed. Macmillan, London.

[7]   Kiefer, J. (1958). On the nonrandomized optimality and randomized non-optimality of symmetrical designs, *Annals of Mathematics and Statistics* **29**, 675–699.

[8]   Kiefer, J. (1959). Optimum experimental designs, *Journal of the Royal Statistical Society, Series B* **21**, 272–319.

[9]   Lentner, M. & Bishop, T. (1986). *Experimental Design and Analysis*. Valley Book Co., Blacksburg.

[10]   Yates, F. (1940). The recovery of interblock information in balanced incomplete block designs, *Annals of Eugenics* **10**, 317–325.

[11]   Youden, W.J. (1940). Experimental designs to increase accuracy of greenhouse studies, *Contributions from Boyce Thompson Institute* **11**, 219–228.

D.R. CUTLER

Incomplete Contingency Table *see* Quasi-Independence

Incomplete Factorial Designs *see* Factorial Designs in Clinical Trials

Incomplete Follow-Up

Longitudinal (or follow-up) study data analysis is complicated by the diversity of possible outcomes and the different lengths of observation time. Some subjects die or relapse ("failures"), some remain alive or in remission ("survivors"), and some are *lost to follow-up* (e.g. drop out or withdraw from treatment) (Colton [2, pp. 299–302]). Even if one had the time to wait until all subjects met the outcome failure criterion, the problem of accounting for those who were lost to follow-up would remain. Thus, because of their *incompleteness*, longitudinal studies often are subject to selective influences (Hill & Hill [4, p. 27]).

Substantial **bias** in longitudinal studies can result from not considering the duration of the study and from inappropriate handling of incomplete data, even when only a small proportion of the observations is missing (Andersen [1, p. 80], Colton [2, pp. 237–250], Hill & Hill [4, pp. 188–203], Murray & Findlay [6].) Average duration of survival may be a convenient way to summarize "mean observation time" for the "failures" (Colton [2, pp. 299–302]). However, it is a meaningful term *vis-à-vis* mortality or relapse only when all study subjects have had the outcome; it has no meaningful interpretation in terms of survival or prognosis (Colton [2, pp. 237–250, 299–302]). Averaging survival time only among the failures, while ignoring those who have not lived long enough to experience the outcome within the period of observation, selects for early failure and overemphasizes negative outcomes (Colton [2, pp. 299–302]; Hill & Hill [4, pp. 188–203]).

Furthermore, conclusions based solely upon individuals with complete follow-up data presume that results recorded for the failure subgroup would not be affected by including those with incomplete data, i.e. both the survivor and lost-to-follow-up subgroups. In other words, this assumption presumes that the characteristic of "being followed up" does not correlate with the characteristic being measured, for example, survival (Hill & Hill [4, pp. 23–33]). However, the characteristic of being "lost to follow-up" may correlate with being either more or less likely to be alive or dead, so that the ratio of alive/dead may differ in traced versus untraced (i.e. lost) cases (Hill & Hill [4, pp. 188–203]). For example, in a study of treatment for alcoholism, treatment drop-outs may be more likely to relapse to heavy drinking than subjects who remain in treatment.

The magnitude of the incomplete follow-up problem increases as larger numbers of individuals drop out or are withdrawn. Consequently, conclusions drawn from the analysis of outcomes from follow-up data can be considerably biased by incomplete data. Between group differences in mean survival times can be attributed to the incomplete follow-up fallacy.

In all cases, the obvious data management solution is to conduct a comprehensive follow-up or, in the case of **clinical trials**, to emphasize study retention so that concerns regarding **missing data** due to incomplete follow-up do not arise. However, this can be a lengthy, not to mention costly, undertaking. Various statistical techniques have been developed to try to deal with this problem (Gibbons et al. [3], Little & Rubin [5], Rubin [7]).

References

[1] Andersen, B. (1990). Bias I, in *Methodological Errors in Medical Research: An Incomplete Catalogue*. Blackwell Scientific, Oxford, pp. 72–83.

[2] Colton, T. (1974). Fallacies in numerical reasoning, in *Statistics in Medicine*. Little, Brown & Company, Boston, pp. 299–302.

[3] Gibbons, RD, Hedeker, D., Elkin, I., Waternaux, C., Kraemer, H.C., Greenhouse, J.B., Shea, T., Imber, S.D., Sotsky, S.M. & Watkins, J.T. (1993). Some conceptual and statistical issues in analysis of longitudinal psychiatric data: application to the NIMH Treatment of Depression Collaborative Research Program dataset, *Archives of General Psychiatry* **50**, 739–750.

[4] Hill, A.B. & Hill, I.D. (1991). Collection of statistics: bias, in *Bradford Hill's Principles of Medical Statistics*, 12th Ed. Edward Arnold, London, pp. 23–33.

[5] Little, R. & Rubin, D. (1987). *Statistical Analysis With Missing Data*. Wiley, New York.

[6] Murray, G.D. & Findlay, J.G. (1988). Correcting for the bias caused by drop-outs in hypertension trials, *Statistics in Medicine* **7**, 941–946.

[7] Rubin, D.B. (1987). *Multiple Imputation for Nonresponse in Surveys*. Wiley, New York.

(*See also* **Nonignorable Dropout in Longitudinal Studies**)

HOWARD M. KRAVITZ

Incremental Lifetime Cancer Risk (ILCR) *see* Risk Assessment for Environmental Chemicals

Incubation Period *see* Latent Period

Incubation Period of Infectious Diseases

The incubation period is the time interval between exposure to a disease-causing agent and the onset of symptomatic disease. For example, the incubation period of an infectious disease refers to the time interval between infection or exposure to a viral or bacterial agent and the onset of symptomatic (clinical) disease. The incubation period is also called the clinical latency period (*see* **Latent Period**). The focus of this article is on modeling and estimating the incubation period of infectious diseases. However, some of the ideas may also be applicable to the incubation period of noninfectious disease, for example the incubation period of radiation-induced cancer that refers to the time interval from **radiation** exposure to cancer diagnosis.

The length of the incubation period depends on the disease and the infectious agent. It can be very short, perhaps only several days in the case of a streptococcal sore throat, or perhaps several weeks in the case of smallpox, or perhaps a decade in the case of the acquired immune deficiency syndrome (**AIDS**). After an individual is exposed to an infectious agent, the agent multiplies, and the host defenses are weakened. Eventually, the individual may experience the onset of clinical disease. Individuals may or may not be infectious (that is, capable of transmitting the infection to others) during the incubation period or subsequently.

The incubation period of a disease can be very variable among individuals [2, 21]. A single number, such as the **mean** or **median** incubation period, does not reveal the significant heterogeneity in incubation periods in a population for a given infectious diseases. The incubation period distribution, $F(t)$, is the probability that the incubation period is less than or equal to t time units. The probability density function of incubation periods usually is asymmetric and is **skewed** to the right. Sartwell [23, 24] suggested that the **lognormal distribution** adequately describes the incubation period distribution of a number of diseases. However, other **parametric models for survival** data may also adequately describe incubation period distributions, including the **Weibull, gamma**, log-logistic (*see* **Logistic Distribution**), and piecewise **exponential** models [9]. There is no requirement that all infected individuals eventually develop clinical disease. Thus, the distribution function, F, may not be proper. For example, one may postulate that a proportion, p, of infected individuals eventually develop clinical disease with incubation distribution, F_1, and the remaining proportion of infected individuals, $1 - p$, never develop disease; then we have the mixture model $F(t) = pF_1(t)$.

Studies of the incubation period distribution are important for several reasons. First, the incubation period distribution is important for forecasting the course of epidemics, and is used with either transmission models [1] or **back-calculation** approaches [9]. If the incubation period is long,

then infected individuals may be silently and unknowingly spreading the infection to others. Secondly, identification of **covariates** or cofactors that may lengthen the incubation period may lead to the development of effective therapeutic interventions. Thirdly, knowledge of the incubation period is useful in counseling infected patients about their prognosis. Finally, the incubation period is a critical parameter in designing **clinical trials** of early interventions and vaccines (*see* **Communicable Diseases; Infectious Disease Models; Vaccine Studies**).

The ideal study for estimating the incubation period is to monitor a **cohort** of uninfected individuals, determine the dates of infection, and then to follow the infected patients to determine the dates of the onset of clinical disease. The data for estimating the incubation period distribution would consist of the time interval between infection and disease for those patients who became infected. If an infected individual did not develop clinical disease at the time of last follow-up, then the data would be right **censored** at that time. Classical **survival analysis** techniques could be used to estimate the incubation period distribution from right-censored *data* [12]. **Kaplan–Meier** survival curves could be used to estimate $F(t)$ nonparametrically, the cumulative distribution function of incubation periods. Parametric models could also be fit to the right-censored incubation period data (*see* **Parametric Models in Survival Analysis**). A simple example is the case of a single point source epidemic, as might occur with salmonellosis where infection is transmitted from contaminated food or water [21]. In this example a cohort may be defined as all individuals who were exposed (e.g. individuals who are in a restaurant on the given day that contaminated food was served), in which case the date of exposure is known precisely. Another example of a point source epidemic for a noninfectious disease is the onset of leukemia associated with radiation exposure following the 1945 atomic bomb explosion in Hiroshima [11]. The incidence of leukemia appeared to peak about six years after exposure. Survival analyses could be performed on the time intervals from exposure to clinical disease, and of course some of these intervals may be right censored at the times of last follow-up (*see* **Epidemic Curve**).

Unfortunately, the ideal study of incubation periods can seldom be performed because of a number of important complications. First, it may not be possible to identify a cohort of initially uninfected individuals, and to follow them over time. Instead, we may only have available a sample of cases who already have clinical disease (see the section "Retrospective ascertainment" below). Even if a cohort is assembled and followed over time, it may not be possible to ascertain either the exact dates of infection (exposure) or the onset of clinical disease (see the section "Cohort studies" below). For example, an individual may already be infected at the time of enrollment in a cohort study, but the time that incident infection occurred is unknown. Many of these problems have surfaced in studies of the incubation period of AIDS, and have been the subject of active methodologic research among statisticians in recent years. In the next sections we discuss more fully these complexities and the methodologic approaches to address them. The issues are illustrated with studies of AIDS, although the methods are applicable more generally to other infectious diseases.

Retrospective Ascertainment

The first data on the incubation period of AIDS (time from HIV infection to AIDS diagnosis) were based on transfusion-associated AIDS cases [22]. In that study, AIDS cases were identified who had become infected by receiving a transfusion of infected blood. The date of infection was estimated retrospectively as the date of blood transfusion. There was an important selection criterion to get into the study, namely that subjects had to have AIDS. Early in an epidemic of a new disease the only data about incubation periods that may be gathered rapidly may come from symptomatic cases of disease who have already been identified. These cases of disease are then retrospectively studied to determine dates of exposure to the infectious agent. Such studies have been referred to as having "retrospective ascertainment" because only individuals with symptomatic disease are included and then they are retrospectively studied. A naive analysis of this type of data, which did not account for the selection criteria, could lead to serious underestimation of the incubation period. This is because the data are right **truncated**. Individuals with long incubation periods may not yet have symptomatic disease, and thus could not possibly be included in the data set. To analyze such data properly, the analysis must condition properly on the selection criteria [18, 19].

There are other **biases** with studies based on retrospective ascertainment. For instance in the transfusion example, patients who receive blood transfusion are often elderly and sick with chronic diseases, and thus they may die from other causes of death before developing AIDS. This leads to length-biased sampling: we are more likely to observe patients with shorter incubation periods, because patients with long incubation periods may die first from another disease and thus are never included in the data set. In a series of papers, statisticians have developed methods to correct for these and other biases (see, for example, [18], [19], and [25]). However, none of these methods can correct for the fundamental limitation of this sort of data: they are retrospective and involve only cases of disease and so without strong parametric assumptions they provide essentially no information about the prospective probability of getting a disease once one is infected.

Cohort Studies

A second type of study involves identifying a cohort of uninfected individuals, ascertaining as best one can the subsequent dates of infection, and following the infected individuals to ascertain the date of onset of clinical disease. The first issue concerns the difficulty in identifying the date of infection. The usual method is to test individuals serially with a laboratory assay such as the test for antibodies to the infectious agent. In the case of AIDS, individuals may be serially tested with ELISA or Western Blot assays to identify the dates of seroconversion to HIV antibodies [16]. A complication is that the date of seroconversion does not correspond to the date of infection. Infected individuals will be seronegative for antibodies to the virus until they develop detectable antibodies, usually within several months. Although we define the incubation period as the time from infection to the clinical diagnosis of disease, many studies cannot identify the actual dates of infection but only the time of antibody seroconversion. However, in the case of AIDS, the time from infection to antibody seroconversion is relatively short (approximate median is two months) compared with the much longer period from seroconversion to the onset of disease. Accordingly, many studies define the incubation period to be the time interval from antibody seroconversion (becoming antibody positive) to the onset of clinical disease. Nevertheless, this points out that the results of studies of incubation periods may depend on the choices of the assays that are used to ascertain infection or exposure to the infectious agent. PCR (polymerase chain reaction) testing may identify evidence of infection considerably earlier than antibody testing [17].

If individuals are periodically screened by laboratory tests for evidence of infection, then the date of infection can at best be determined up to an interval (i.e. interval censored). This interval is defined by the time of the latest screening test that was negative for infection, L, and the earliest screening test that was positive for infection, R. The term *doubly censored data* refers to time to event data for which both the time origin and failure time are censored. In cohort studies of the incubation period the data are frequently doubly censored because the date of infection is interval censored and the date of onset of clinical disease is right censored for those individuals who have not developed clinical disease by the time of the last follow-up.

A popular *ad hoc* approach for analyzing doubly censored data on incubation periods is to estimate (impute) the calendar date of infection by the midpoint of the interval. The imputed midpoint calendar date of infection is $S = (L + R)/2$. Then, standard survival analysis techniques for right-censored data are used on the incubation periods with imputed dates of infection. However, such approaches will typically be biased and give incorrect **variance** estimates. The bias of the estimated incubation resulting from midpoint imputation depends critically on the width of the intervals, $R - L$, the incubation distribution, and the density of infection times. For example, in the exponential growth phase of simple epidemics, midpoint imputation will tend to underestimate the time of infection and thus overestimates the incubation period. Law & Brookmeyer [20] studied the impact of midpoint imputation, and concluded that with a median incubation period of 10 years in the case of AIDS, the bias resulting from midpoint imputation associated with intervals even as large as two years is relatively small.

A more formal parametric approach for analyzing the doubly censored data in studies of the incubation period involves specifying parametric models and joint estimation of both the probability densities of infection times and of incubation times. The **likelihood** function is maximized to obtain the

maximum likelihood estimators. This approach was used by Brookmeyer & Goedert [10] to estimate the incubation period of HIV infection among hemophiliacs. Bacchetti & Jewell [4] used a weakly **semiparametric** approach. A discrete time scale was used with a separate parameter to represent the discrete **hazard** for each month. To avoid irregularities that result from trying to estimate a large number of parameters (e.g. wildly varying hazards from one month to the next with large variances), a **penalized likelihood** function was used that penalized for "roughness" in the estimated hazard function. A completely **nonparametric** approach to the problem has been given by De Gruttola & Lagakos [14]. However, the completely nonparametric estimate of the incubation period distribution, $F(t)$, is often numerically unstable, and it is not defined for all values of t.

Deconvolution Methods

Occasionally, population data may be available both about the incidence of clinical disease and infection rates in the population. The expected **cumulative incidence** of clinical disease up to calendar time $t, D(t)$, is related to infection rates $g(s)$ at calendar time s (numbers of new infections per unit time) and the incubation period distribution, by the convolution equation

$$D(t) = \int_0^t g(s)F(t - s)\,ds.$$

The basic idea is to use data on $D(t)$ and an estimate of $g(s)$ to glean information about F. This method was pioneered by Bacchetti & Moss [5] and Bacchetti [3] in connection with estimating the incubation period of HIV infection. The usefulness of the method depends on the availability of accurate information on the infection rates in the population, $g(s)$, and accurate disease **surveillance** data over time. For example, detailed information about historical infection rates was available in San Francisco on the basis of several epidemiologic surveys and cohort studies [5, 26]. The statistical framework is as follows. Let y_j represent the number of cases of disease in calendar interval I_j. Suppose that N, the cumulative number of infections that have occurred, is known. Then the vector of counts of cases of disease, **y**, has a **multinomial distribution** with sample size

N and cell probabilities that involve the incubation distribution and the known infection rates. Maximum likelihood estimation methods are used to estimate the parameters of the incubation period distribution. The method is closely related to the back-calculation methodology which uses data on $D(t)$ and an estimate of F to estimate historical infection rates $g(s)$. Back-calculation is a method for estimating past infection rates from disease surveillance data. The method requires reliable counts of numbers of cases of disease diagnosed over time and a reliable estimate of the incubation period distribution. The method has been used to obtain short-term projects of disease incidence and to estimate **prevalence** of infection [6, 9]. Early references on back-calculation are [7] and [8]

Synthesis of Studies of the Incubation Period

The main complications in the analysis and interpretation of studies of the incubation period include uncertainty in the dates of infection and the sampling criteria by which individuals are included in the data set. Accordingly, it is important to synthesize and compare estimates across studies because the estimates may be used on different methodologies with different underlying assumptions.

In the case of AIDS, many different methodologies outlined in this article have been used to study the incubation period distribution. The results from several different methodologies have been compared [15] and a general picture emerges [9]. The probability of developing AIDS within the first two years of HIV antibody seroconversion is very small, less than 0.03. Then the hazard of progression to AIDS begins to rise rapidly so that the cumulative probability of developing AIDS within seven years of seroconversion is approximately 0.25 and the median incubation period is nearly 10 years. When comparing incubation period estimates from different studies, an important consideration is whether treatments were available to delay progression and thus alter the incubation period distribution. Treatments such as AZT became available beginning in 1987 which may lengthen the incubation period. In the case of AIDS, the one covariate that has been shown to influence the length of the incubation period in multiple studies is the age at infection [13].

References

[1] Anderson, R.M. & May, R.M. (1992). *Infectious Diseases of Humans: Dynamics and Control*. Oxford University Press, Oxford.

[2] Armenian, H.K. & Lilienfeld, A.M. (1974). The distribution of incubations periods of neoplastic diseases, *American Journal of Epidemiology* **99**, 92–100.

[3] Bacchetti, P. (1990). Estimating the incubation period of AIDS by comparing population infection and diagnostic patterns, *Journal of the American Statistical Association* **85**, 1002–1008.

[4] Bacchetti, P. & Jewell, N.P. (1991). Nonparametric estimation of the incubation period of AIDS based on a prevalent cohort with unknown infection times, *Biometrics* **47**, 947–960.

[5] Bacchetti, P. & Moss, A.R. (1989). Incubation period of AIDS in San Francisco, *Nature* **338**, 251–253.

[6] Bacchetti, P., Segal, M. & Jewell, N.P. (1993). Back-calculation of HIV infection rates (with discussion), *Statistical Science* **8**, 82–119.

[7] Brookmeyer, R. & Gail, M.H. (1986). Minimum size of the acquired immunodeficiency syndrome (AIDS) epidemic in the United States, *Lancet* **2**, 1320–1322.

[8] Brookmeyer, R. & Gail, M.H. (1988). A method for obtaining short-term projections and lower bounds on the size of the AIDS epidemic, *Journal of the American Statistical Association* **83**, 301–308.

[9] Brookmeyer, R. & Gail, M.H. (1994). *AIDS Epidemiology: A Quantitative Approach*. Oxford University Press, New York.

[10] Brookmeyer, R. & Goedert, J. (1989). Censoring in an epidemic with an application to hemophilia-associated AIDS, *Biometrics* **45** 325–335.

[11] Cobb, S., Miller, M. & Wald, N. (1959). On the estimation of the incubation period in malignant disease, *Journal of Chronic Disease* **9**, 385–393.

[12] Cox, D.R. & Oakes, D. (1984). *Analysis of Survival Data*. Chapman & Hall, London.

[13] Darby, S.C., Doll, R. & Thakrar, R., Rizza, C. & Cox, D.R. (1990). Time from infection with HIV to onset of AIDS in patients with hemophilia in the United Kingdom, *Statistics in Medicine* **9**, 681–689.

[14] De Gruttola, V. & Lagakos, S.W. (1989). Analysis of doubly-censored survival data with applications to AIDS, *Biometrics* **45**, 1–11.

[15] Gail, M.H. & Rosenberg, P.S. (1992). in *AIDS Epidemiology: Methodologic Issues*, N. Jewell, K. Keietz, & V. Farewell, eds. Birkhauser, Boston, pp. 1–38.

[16] Haseltine, W.A. (1989). Silent HIV infections, *New England Journal of Medicine* **320**, 1487–1489.

[17] Horsborgh, C.R., Qu, C.Y., Jason, I.M., Holmberg, S., Longini, I., Schable, C., Mayer, K., Lifson, A., Schochetman, G., Ward, J., Rutherford, G., Evatt, B., Seage, G. & Jaffe, H. (1989). Duration of human immunodeficiency virus infection before detection of antibody, *Lancet* **2**, 637–640.

[18] Kalfbleisch, J.D. & Lawless, J.F. (1989). Inference based on retrospective ascertainment: an analysis of the data on transfusion related AIDS, *Journal of the American Statistical Association* **84**, 360–372.

[19] Lagakos, S., Barraj, L. & De Gruttola, V. (1988). Nonparametric analysis of truncated survival data with application to AIDS, *Biometrika* **75**, 515–523.

[20] Law, C.G. & Brookmeyer, R. (1992). Effects of midpoint imputation on the analysis of doubly censored data, *Statistics in Medicine* **11**, 1569–1578.

[21] Lilienfeld, A.M. & Lilienfeld, D.E. (1980). *Foundations of Epidemiology*, 2nd Ed. Oxford University Press, Oxford.

[22] Lui, K.J., Lawrence, D.N., Morgan, W.M., Peterman, T., Haverkos, H. & Bregman, D. (1986). A model based approach for estimating the mean incubation period of transfusion-associated acquired immunodeficiency syndrome, *Proceedings of the National Academy of Sciences* **83**, 3051–3055.

[23] Sartwell, P.E. (1950). The distribution of incubation periods of infectious disease, *American Journal of Hygiene* **51**, 310–318.

[24] Sartwell, P.E. (1966). The incubation period and the dynamics of infectious of disease, *American Journal of Epidemiology* **83**, 204–216.

[25] Wang, M.-C. (1992). The analysis of retrospectively ascertained data in the presence of reporting delays, *Journal of the American Statistical Association* **87**, 397–406.

[26] Winkelstein, W., Samuel, M., Padian, N.S., Wiley, J., Lang, W., Anderson, R. & Levy, J. (1987). The San Francisco Men's Health Study III. Reduction in human immunodeficiency virus transmission among homosexual/bisexual men, 1982–1986, *American Journal of Public Health* **77**, 685–689.

(*See also* **Sojourn Time in Disease Screening**)

RON BROOKMEYER

Independence *see* Statistical Dependence and Independence

Independence of a Set of Variables, Tests of

Suppose that p variables have been measured on each of n sample individuals. Denote the value of the jth variable for the ith individual by x_{ij}, and collect together the p values observed on the ith individual into the vector $\mathbf{x}_i' = (x_{i1}, \ldots, x_{ip})$. Then

$$\bar{\mathbf{x}} = \frac{1}{n}\sum_{i=1}^{n}\mathbf{x}_i = (\bar{x}_1, \ldots, \bar{x}_p)'$$

is the sample mean vector,

$$\mathbf{A} = (a_{ij}) = \sum_{i=1}^{n}(\mathbf{x}_i - \bar{\mathbf{x}})(\mathbf{x}_i - \bar{\mathbf{x}})'$$

is the corrected sum of squares and products matrix,

$$\mathbf{S} = (s_{ij}) = \frac{1}{n-1}\mathbf{A}$$

is the sample **covariance matrix,** and

$$\mathbf{R} = \mathbf{DSD}$$

is the sample **correlation** matrix, where

$$\mathbf{D} = \mathrm{diag}(s_{11}^{-1/2}, \ldots, s_{pp}^{-1/2}).$$

The two sample matrices $\mathbf{S}$ and $\mathbf{R}$ can be viewed as estimates of the corresponding population quantities $\boldsymbol{\Sigma}$ and $\boldsymbol{\Upsilon}$, respectively.

Situations often arise in which the p variables can be divided a priori into k distinct sets with p_i variables in the ith set ($i = 1, 2, \ldots, k$). For example, each child in a school class may have to sit an examination that comprises p separate tests, on each of which a mark of between 0 and 100 is awarded. However, these tests may be identifiably of four types: p_1 of them examine verbal ability, p_2 of them examine arithmetic ability, p_3 of them examine general knowledge, and p_4 of them examine logical reasoning. Clearly, *within* each set the individual tests are likely to be (highly) correlated, but a question of interest would then be whether the variables in different sets can be treated as independent. In this section, we consider testing independence of such sets of variables.

Without loss of generality, we can assume the variables to be arranged so that the first p_1 of them fall in the first set, the next p_2 in the second set, and so on. Denote by $\mathbf{S}_{ii}$ the sample covariance matrix of the variables in the ith set and by $\mathbf{S}_{ij}$ the matrix of sample covariances between those pairs of variables in which one variable comes from the ith set and the other from the jth set. Apply the same notation to the matrices $\mathbf{A}$, $\mathbf{R}$, $\boldsymbol{\Sigma}$, and $\boldsymbol{\Upsilon}$. Then the overall sample covariance matrix $\mathbf{S}$ can be expressed in partitioned form as

$$\mathbf{S} = \begin{pmatrix} \mathbf{S}_{11} & \mathbf{S}_{12} & \cdots & \mathbf{S}_{1k} \\ \mathbf{S}_{21} & \mathbf{S}_{22} & \cdots & \mathbf{S}_{2k} \\ \vdots & \vdots & & \vdots \\ \mathbf{S}_{k1} & \mathbf{S}_{k2} & \cdots & \mathbf{S}_{kk} \end{pmatrix},$$

and each of the matrices $\mathbf{A}, \mathbf{R}, \boldsymbol{\Sigma}$, and $\boldsymbol{\Upsilon}$ can be partitioned similarly. The null hypothesis that we are concerned with is

$$H_0: \boldsymbol{\Sigma}_{ij} = \mathbf{0}$$

for all $i \neq j$, the only requirement on the remaining unspecified matrices $\boldsymbol{\Sigma}_{ii}$ being that they are positive definite for all i. The alternative hypothesis is the general one, i.e. that $\boldsymbol{\Sigma}_{ij} \neq \mathbf{0}$ for at least one $i \neq j$.

Assuming **multivariate normality** of the data, the **likelihood ratio test** for this situation is obtained by maximizing the likelihood of the sample under the null hypothesis and dividing the result by the unconditional maximum of the likelihood. After some algebraic simplification the test statistic can be written

$$\Lambda = \frac{|\mathbf{A}|}{|\mathbf{A}_{11}| \cdots |\mathbf{A}_{kk}|},$$

and elementary properties of determinants establish that equivalent expressions for this statistic are

$$\Lambda = \frac{|\mathbf{S}|}{|\mathbf{S}_{11}| \cdots |\mathbf{S}_{kk}|}$$

or

$$\Lambda = \frac{|\mathbf{R}|}{|\mathbf{R}_{11}| \cdots |\mathbf{R}_{kk}|}.$$

Unfortunately, the exact sampling distribution of Λ is complicated and difficult to handle, so large-sample approximations are generally employed in practice. Standard likelihood-ratio theory provides the basic result that $-n \log \Lambda$ asymptotically follows the **chi-square distribution** with $\nu = \frac{1}{2}(p^2 - \sum_i p_i^2)$ **degrees of freedom** when H_0 is true, so this distribution can be used to find an approximate significance **level** for the test. However, a more accurate large-sample approximation was obtained by Box [2], who showed that when H_0 is true, then

$$\Pr(-a \log \Lambda \leq z) = \Pr(\chi_\nu^2 \leq z) + ba^{-2}[\Pr(\chi_{\nu+4}^2 \leq z)$$
$$- \Pr(\chi_\nu^2 \leq z)] + O(a^{-3}),$$

where

$$a = n - \frac{3}{2} - \frac{1}{3}\left(p^3 - \sum_i p_i^3\right)\left(p^2 - \sum_i p_i^2\right)^{-1}$$

and

$$b = \frac{1}{48}\left(p^4 - \sum_i p_i^4\right) - \frac{5}{96}\left(p^2 - \sum_i p_i^2\right)$$
$$- \frac{1}{72}\left(p^3 - \sum_i p_i^3\right)^2\left(p^2 - \sum_i p_i^2\right)^{-1}$$

(see also [1, p. 385], [6, p. 534], or [8, p. 90]). Alternatively, Muirhead [6, p. 537] reproduces tables from Davis & Field [3] that contain correction factors to make the percentage points of $-a \log \Lambda$ exactly those of χ_ν^2.

Two special cases of the above test are commonly of interest. The first is when $k = p$, in which case the null hypothesis becomes the hypothesis that all the variables are mutually uncorrelated (independent if normality of data is assumed); in other words, that $\boldsymbol{\Sigma}$ is a diagonal matrix. In this case the likelihood ratio statistic becomes

$$\Lambda = \frac{|\mathbf{S}|}{s_{11}s_{22}\cdots s_{pp}} = \frac{|\mathbf{A}|}{a_{11}a_{22}\cdots a_{pp}} = |\mathbf{R}|,$$

where $a_{jj} = \sum_{i=1}^n (x_{ij} - \bar{x}_j)^2$ and $s_{jj} = a_{jj}/(n-1)$ for $j = 1, \ldots, p$. Exact percentage points of $-(n - [2p+11]/6)\log \Lambda$ are given by Mathai & Katiyar [5] and reproduced by Seber [8, p. 612]. Alternatively, any of the above approximations can be used with $p_i = 1$ for all i.

The second special case is when there are just two a priori groups of variables; that is, $k = 2$ with p_1 and p_2 variables in the two groups respectively. In this case the sample covariance matrix $\mathbf{S}$ has the partitioning

$$\mathbf{S} = \begin{pmatrix} \mathbf{S}_{11} & \mathbf{S}_{12} \\ \mathbf{S}_{21} & \mathbf{S}_{22} \end{pmatrix},$$

with a corresponding form for each of the matrices $\mathbf{A}, \mathbf{R}, \boldsymbol{\Sigma}$, and $\boldsymbol{\Upsilon}$. The null hypothesis is now simply

$$H_0: \boldsymbol{\Sigma}_{12} = \mathbf{0},$$

and the likelihood ratio test statistic becomes

$$\Lambda = \frac{|\mathbf{A}|}{|\mathbf{A}_{11}||\mathbf{A}_{22}|} = \frac{|\mathbf{S}|}{|\mathbf{S}_{11}||\mathbf{S}_{22}|} = \frac{|\mathbf{R}|}{|\mathbf{R}_{11}||\mathbf{R}_{22}|}.$$

When the null hypothesis is true this statistic has Wilks's lambda distribution $\Lambda_{p_2,p_1,n-p_1-1}$, which has been tabulated extensively (see, for example, Seber [8, p. 565]), so that exact significance levels are easily found.

Note also that in this case we have $|\mathbf{S}| = |\mathbf{S}_{11}||\mathbf{S}_{22} - \mathbf{S}_{21}\mathbf{S}_{11}^{-1}\mathbf{S}_{12}|$ (using results for patterned matrices given, for example, by Seber [8, p. 519]), and equivalent expressions exist for $\mathbf{A}$ and $\mathbf{R}$. The likelihood ratio statistic can thus be reduced to the form

$$\Lambda = \prod_{i=1}^{q}(1 - r_i^2),$$

where $q = \min(p_1, p_2)$ and the r_i^2s are the nonzero **eigenvalues** of $\mathbf{S}_{22}^{-1}\mathbf{S}_{21}\mathbf{S}_{11}^{-1}\mathbf{S}_{12}$ (or, equivalently, of $\mathbf{S}_{11}^{-1}\mathbf{S}_{12}\mathbf{S}_{22}^{-1}\mathbf{S}_{21}$, or of either of these expressions with $\mathbf{A}_{ij}$ or $\mathbf{R}_{ij}$ replacing $\mathbf{S}_{ij}$ for $i, j = 1, 2$). These are the squared **canonical correlations** between the two sets of variables, which are important multivariate descriptors of the inter-set associations.

In this particular special case, it is possible also to derive a **union–intersection test** of the null hypothesis (which has not been found possible to date for the general case of k sets). To derive this test, we consider the univariate hypothesis

$$\rho_{ab}^2 = (\mathbf{a}'\mathbf{\Sigma}_{12}\mathbf{b})^2/[(\mathbf{a}'\mathbf{\Sigma}_{11}\mathbf{a})(\mathbf{b}'\mathbf{\Sigma}_{22}\mathbf{b})] = 0,$$

where ρ_{ab} is the correlation between two arbitrary linear combinations, one from each of the two sets of variables. A suitable test statistic for this univariate hypothesis is $(\mathbf{a}'\mathbf{S}_{12}\mathbf{b})/[(\mathbf{a}'\mathbf{S}_{11}\mathbf{a})(\mathbf{b}'\mathbf{S}_{22}\mathbf{b})]^{1/2}$ and, on maximization with respect to both $\mathbf{a}$ and $\mathbf{b}$, the union–intersection test statistic is found to be $\max_i r_i^2$. Critical values of this statistic have also been tabulated extensively; see, for example Pearson & Hartley [7, Tables 48 and 49] or Seber [8, p. 593].

Various other test statistics have been proposed for this last situation. Invariance arguments lead to statistics which are functions of the **eigenvalues** r_i^2, and the most popular variants are $\sum_{i=1}^{s} r_i^2$ or $\sum_{i=1}^{s}[r_i^2/(1 - r_i^2)]$. Muirhead [6, p. 548] discusses some power comparisons among the various statistics.

A final point concerns the behavior of all these test statistics when the data are not normal. Relatively few systematic studies have been conducted, although both Muirhead [6, p. 546] and Fang & Zhang [4, p. 170] give some results relevant to samples from elliptic distributions. Fang & Zhang derive forms of the likelihood ratio statistic appropriate for such samples, while Muirhead considers asymptotic null distributions of normal-based likelihood ratio test statistics when the data are actually from elliptic distributions. He quotes some **Monte Carlo** studies which indicate that the normal likelihood ratio test statistics should only be used with care if the data come from elliptic distributions.

References

[1]   Anderson, T.W. (1984). *An Introduction to Multivariate Statistical Analysis*, 2nd Ed. Wiley, New York.
[2]   Box, G.E.P. (1949). A general distribution theory for a class of likelihood criteria, *Biometrika* **36**, 317–346.
[3]   Davis, A.W. & Field, J.B.F. (1971). Tables of some multivariate test criteria, *Division of Mathematical Statistics Technical Paper No. 32*. CSIRO, Melbourne, Australia.
[4]   Fang, K.-T. & Zhang, Y.-T. (1990). *Generalized Multivariate Analysis*. Science Press, Beijing/Springer-Verlag, Berlin.
[5]   Mathai, A.M. & Katiyar, R.S. (1979). Exact percentage points for testing independence, *Biometrika* **66**, 353–356.
[6]   Muirhead, R.J. (1982). *Aspects of Multivariate Statistical Theory*. Wiley, New York.
[7]   Pearson, E.S. & Hartley, H.O. (1972). *Biometrika Tables for Statisticians*, Vol. 2. Cambridge University Press, Cambridge.
[8]   Seber, G.A.F. (1984). *Multivariate Observations*. Wiley, New York.

(*See also* **Multivariate Analysis, Overview; Multivariate Bartlett Test; Sphericity Test**)

W.J. KRZANOWSKI

Independent Pathway Model *see* Twin Analysis

Independent Samples *t*-Test *see* Student's *t* Distribution

Independent Variable *see* Explanatory Variables

Indian Statistical Institute

Research in the theory and applications of statistics as a new scientific discipline began in India in the early 1920s through the poineering initiative and efforts of **Prasanta Chandra Mahalanobis**. Soon after his return from England, Mahalanobis began to carry out statistical studies with the help of some part-time assistants. A chance meeting with Nelson Annandale (the then Director of the Zoological and Anthropological Survey of India) and subsequent interactions with him led to the first scientific paper by Mahalanobis on the statistical analysis of stature of Anglo-Indian males of Calcutta. This was followed by further research in **anthropometry**, in meteorology and in problems of flood control in North Bengal and Orissa. Gradually, a small group of young scientists was picked up by him in the Department of Physics, Presidency College, Calcutta, where he was a professor. This group formed the nucleus of a laboratory which later came to be known as the Statistical Laboratory.

In the early 1930s, realizing the necessity for a concerted effort for the advancement of theoretical and applied statistics in India, Mahalanobis, together with P.N. Banerjee and N.R. Sen, both professors of Calcutta University, convened a meeting on December 17, 1931, to consider various steps to be undertaken for the establishment of an association for the advancement of statistics in the country. As a result of this meeting, the Indian Statistical Institute (ISI) was registered as a non-Government and nonprofit-distributing learned society on April 28, 1932, with Sir R.N. Mookerjee as President and Professor P.C. Mahalanobis as (Honorary) Secretary. The total staff strength then was only two or three. From such a modest beginning, the Institute grew, under the remarkable leadership of Mahalanobis into an all-India organization which now has a staff strength of about 1600, including about 500 scientific staff. The Institute has its headquarters in Calcutta and centers at Bangalore and Delhi and a branch at Giridih. In addition, it has a network of service units of the Statistical Quality Control and Operations Research Division at Bangalore, Baroda, Calcutta, Chennai (formerly Madras), Coimbatore, Delhi, Hyderabad, Mumbai (formerly Bombay), Pune, and Tiruvananthapuram.

From the very beginning, Mahalanobis and his associates, who included S.S. Bose, R.C. Bose, S.N. Roy, K.R. Nair, K. Kishen, and H.C. Sinha, worked with zeal and enthusiasm for the development of statistical theory and methods, and in promoting research and practical applications in different areas of the natural and social sciences. *Sankhyā*, the Indian Journal of Statistics, was started in 1933 with Mahalanobis as its Editor, and received instant international recognition, which continues till today. Pioneering research activities were carried out in many areas of statistical theory, especially in the core areas of **multivariate analysis, sample surveys** and **experimental design**. Such activities were strengthened and new directions were opened up by Professor C.R. Rao and many others who joined the Institute in the 1940s and the tradition continues. The Institute pioneered the development of statistical methods in agricultural research and in the conduct of large-scale agricultural enquiries. This led to a large number of research publications and to the introduction of training activities offering short-term courses in statistics for officers in government departments and scientific institutions. The scientists of ISI, led by Mahalanobis, helped in introducing the first post-graduate degree course in Statistics in India at the Calcutta University in 1941, and in securing a separate section for Statistics in the Indian Science Congress.

Activities of the Institute gained further momentum from 1938. Mahalanobis started sample surveys to estimate the area under the jute crop in Bengal in 1937 as an exploratory project, which later grew to a full-scale survey of the entire province in 1941. Gradually, sample surveys of agricultural crops, and other socioeconomic surveys, became some of the most important activities of the Institute, and earned the Institute and Mahalanobis international reputation. Mahalanobis was appointed Honorary Statistical Advisor to the Cabinet, Government of India, and in 1950, through his initiative, the National Sample Survey (NSS) was started for conducting socioeconomic surveys of all-India coverage on a continuing basis. This was the first ever attempt in India to have a database for various developmental programs and the five year plans.

The ISI played a pioneering role in starting the Statistical Quality Control (SQC) movement in India by organizing a visit of W.A. Shewhart, the father of SQC, to India in 1948 and later by inviting other experts like W.E. Deming. SQC promotional work was gradually spread all over the industrial centers in India under a comprehensive program covering education and training, applied research, and consultancy services.

Research in economics was greatly stimulated when in 1954 Prime Minister Jawaharlal Nehru entrusted the preparation of the draft Second Five-Year Plan of the country to Mahalanobis and the Institute. The "draft" submitted by Mahalanobis and the plan models formulated by him in that connection have since been regarded as major contributions to economic planning in India. Since then many economists of the Institute have continued to work on various aspects of national planning and, until 1970, were directly helping the Planning Commission of the Government of India in the preparation of the long-term prospective plans for the country. Research in other disciplines of social sciences was also started in the Institute in the late 1950s. Mahalanobis's participation in 1946 in the annual scientific conferences of the Milbank Foundation led to the initiation of systematic studies in India on population growth. Earlier, the well-known Y-sample estimates for the 1941 census population were also derived by the ISI. Theoretical and empirical research in sociology using statistical techniques was started in the Institute for the first time in South-East Asia. Similarly, the development and introduction of psychometric tests for selection processes in different organizations was first made by the ISI in India besides carrying out basic research in psychometry (*see* **Psychometrics, Overview**). Studies of the phonetic structure of some major Indian languages have been made on a continuing basis in the Institute under the guidance and collaboration of the famous linguist Djordje Kostic.

The Institute, since its inception, recognized the need for development and use of accurate and fast computing equipment for the processing and analysis of data. Mahalanobis strongly believed that to be a good theoretical statistician one must also compute and must therefore have the best computing aids. The Institute has lived up to this tradition from the very beginning. In 1953 a small analog computer was designed and built in the Institute. In 1956 the Institute acquired a HEC-2M machine from the UK which was the first digital computer in India. In 1958 a digital computer URAL was received as a gift from the then USSR. From 1956 to the mid-1960s the Institute had been serving as a *de facto* national computer center for the country. In the early 1960s the Institute, in collaboration with Jadavpur

University, undertook the design, development, and fabrication of a fully transistorized digital computer, called ISIJU-1, which was commissioned in 1966 by Mr M.C. Chagla, the then Minister of Education, Government of India.

Quantitative analysis in the physical and earth sciences was one of the novel ideas that Mahalanobis pursued in the true spirit of the Institute. In addition to evolving some interesting techniques and obtaining some very interesting results from the analysis of directional geological data, the Institute also made a significant contribution by discovering the bones of a 16 m (+) long sauropod dinosaur named *Barapasaurus tagoreii*, from the lower Jurassic Kota rocks near Sironcha, Gadchiroli district, Maharashtra, in the 1960s. The discovery has helped in understanding the interesting problem about the origin and evolution of sauropod dinosaurs. It represents the only intermediate form between the prosauropods and the sauropods, and is called a "missing link" in the evolution of the sauropod dinosaur.

The Institute expanded its research, teaching, training, and project activities and earned national and international recognition over time. The substantial contributions of the Institute to theoretical and applied statistical work have culminated in the recognition of the Institute by the Government of India enacting *The Indian Statistical Institute Act, 1959 (No. 57)* which declared the Institute as an "Institution of National Importance" and empowered it to award degrees and diplomas. None other than Pandit Jawaharlal Nehru, the then Prime Minister of India, piloted the bill in Parliament. With this recognition, the already existing teaching and training programs were consolidated and expanded and courses for the degrees of Bachelor of Statistics (B.Stat. (Honors)) and Master of Statistics (M.Stat.) were started in June 1960. The Institute was also empowered to award Ph.D./D.Sc. degrees from the same time. Later on, courses leading to Master of Technology degrees were started in Computer Science and in Quality, Reliability and Operations Research. Recently, the Institute has also been empowered to grant degrees and diplomas in mathematics, quantitative economics, computer science and subjects related to statistics as well as statistics itself. A master's degree programme in quantitative economics has just been initiated.

The role and importance of ISI in conducting and promoting teaching of statistics has been appreciated by international bodies as well. In 1950 the **International Statistical Institute** initiated the International Statistical Education Centre (ISEC), Calcutta, jointly with ISI, to impart training in theoretical and applied statistics to participants selected from developing countries. The center is run by ISI under the auspices of UNESCO, the International Statistical Institute and the Government of India.

Recognition of the Institute by the Act of Parliament provided greater encouragement to research activities not only in statistics and mathematics but also in various branches of the natural and **social sciences**, without whose live contact, it was believed, the methodology of statistics could not grow. It is also due to this fact that "Unity in Diversity" has been adopted as the motto of the Institute.

The objectives of the Institute are:

1. to promote the study and dissemination of knowledge of statistics, to develop statistical theory and methods, and their use in research and practical applications generally, with special reference to problems of planning for national development and social welfare;
2. to undertake research in various fields of natural and social sciences with a view to the mutual development of statistics and these sciences; and
3. to provide for, and undertake, the collection of information, investigations, projects, and operational research for purposes of planning and the improvement of efficiency of management and production.

From the early days, the Institute has been in touch with many internationally famous scientists in different disciplines from all over the world. Some of these scientists have worked in the Institute for several months or even longer. **R.A. Fisher**, a pioneer of modern statistics, was a regular visitor to the Institute and lent it considerable support. J.B.S. Haldane, a geneticist of international repute, was a member of the faculty for several years beginning 1957. At the inspiration of these stalwarts and other renowned scientists, the Institute began to expand and/or undertake research activities in several areas of the natural and social sciences with the hope that collaboration under the same roof would foster the mutual development of statistics and other disciplines. In fact, the Institute stood up to

R.A. Fisher who called statistics a "key technology" of the century, in view of its intimate relevance to all scientific endeavors which involve experimentation, measurement and **inference** from sample to aggregate.

Coming to more recent times, the Institute has continued to pursue its goal of attainment of excellence in various fields of science. Fundamental research in statistics with its roots in applications has been the bottom line ever since the inception of the Institute. The contributions from the Institute in multivariate analysis, design and analysis of experiments, sample surveys, statistical methods of data analysis and statistical inference have found their places in textbooks and monographs, and the tradition continues. In addition, **probability theory** and **stochastic processes** have also been major areas of research in the Institute. The mathematicians of the Institute, in addition to collaborating with the statisticians, are also making fundamental contributions in several fields – topology, functional analysis, harmonic analysis, algebra, combinatorics, quantum mechanics, game theory, to name a few. The current trend of research in statistics not only carries forward the traditions set up in the Institute, but is also setting new directions, both in theory and applications, in different disciplines.

The Institute has been maintaining its tradition of high-quality research and development in the field of computer science. In 1979, a microprogrammed signal processing system using the **Fast Fourier Transform (FFT)** was designed and developed. Keeping pace with the global advances in computer technology, the activities of the Institute in the field of computer science gathered a tremendous momentum in the late 1970s, resulting in diversification of research in different areas including **algorithms** and complexity, parallel and distributed processing, fault-tolerant computing, VLSI, computational geometry, fuzzy sets and systems, wave propagation, atmospheric remote sensing, speech signal processing, cybernetics, **pattern recognition, neural networks, artificial intelligence**, image processing (*see* **Image Analysis and Tomography**), computer vision, document analysis, natural language processing, particle physics, fluid dynamics, plasma physics, etc. In recognition of its contributions in the field of computer science, the Government of India established, in collaboration with the United Nations Development Program (UNDP), one of the five national nodal centers for knowledge-based computing systems (NCKBCS) in ISI in the year 1988.

The different disciplines under the social sciences also continued to develop and flourish over time by carrying out basic research as well as inter- and multi-disciplinary programs. In economics, the Institute has come to be known as a specialized center for its significant contributions in different branches of theory and also for studies on such areas as demand analysis, poverty and levels of living, measurement of inequalities, production and prices, national income and allied topics, development and planning, etc. In **demography,** sociology, psychometry and linguistics also, the Institute maintained its distinctive feature for the focus and emphasis on quantitative aspects. Mention may be made, in this context, of the pioneering theory for teaching and training for hearing-impaired children, developed by D. Kostic. Based on this theory the Electronics Unit of the Institute, in collaboration with the Linguistic Research Unit and the Government of Tripura, designed, developed and fabricated a set of instruments for hard-of-hearing children of the Institute of Speech Rehabilitation, Government of Tripura, Agartala. This has come to be regarded as having significant impact on social welfare. Recently, the Institute has established a Policy Planning Research Unit at its Delhi Center and a Survey Research and Data Analysis Center in Calcutta.

Plant and human biology have been major areas of research in biological sciences in the Institute. Both basic and applied research are conducted, with emphasis on quantification, statistical design and analysis, and modeling. In the area of plant biology, research has included quantification of natural variability and modeling animal behavior, effect of interaction of rice varieties on yield, use of protein extracted from leaves to supplement human food, mathematical modeling of ecological and embryological phenomena, etc. In the area of human biology, researches have included anthropometric, genetic and biochemical studies on population affinities, micro-evolution, studies on utilizing data on anthropometric variability in designing car seats, human adaptation to differing environments, human ecology and growth, (*see* **Growth and Development**), and **genetic epidemiology**.

Over the years, the SQC & OR Division has grown to the size of having ten operating units all over the country and has uniquely served for promotion, education and training and technical guidance in total quality management methodology and quality assurance systems for the benefit of the manufacturing and service industry. It has thus, as was intended, played a leading role in the dissemination of new concepts, methods and techniques in the areas of quality and productivity.

The central library of the Institute is located at Calcutta with a network extending to other locations of the Institute. Over the years, the library of the Institute has attained the distinction of being one of the richest libraries in the country, particularly in the fields of statistics and related disciplines. The library has developed a well-equipped reprography and photography unit. The library's gift collections include the personal libraries of Mahalanobis and Shewhart. The library has been recognized as the depository library for World Bank Publications. A separate collection of books and journals in mathematics, statistics, etc. known as the Eastern Regional Center of the National Board of Higher Mathematics (NBHM), has been developed out of the grants from the NBHM.

The Documentation Research and Training Centre (DRTC) established at Bangalore in 1962 by the late S.R. Ranganathan, a doyen in the field of library and information science, is engaged in research, teaching and training in documentation and information science. The Institute awards post-graduate diplomas in documentation sciences.

The continual publication of many books and monographs and a large number of scientific papers in national and international journals by the scientific staff of the Institute give a good idea of the nature and extent of the contributions of the Institute to statistics and related fields. Scientists of the Institute have also received recognition from many national and international organizations by way of awards, titles, and fellowships. With a dynamic group pursuing and guiding research work in some of the most modern topics and frontier areas of statistics, mathematics, and in various fields of the natural and social sciences, there is close interaction with scientists from all over the world.

S.B. RAO

Indicator Variable *see* Dummy Variables

Indirect Assay *see* Biological Assay, Overview

Indirect Standardization *see* Standardization Methods

Individual(ized) Risk *see* Absolute Risk

Infant and Perinatal Mortality

An infant death is defined as the death of a live-born baby before a completed year after birth [24]. The concept of infant mortality did not emerge until the latter half of the nineteenth century, although data for much earlier periods have subsequently been used to construct infant mortality rates [3, 11]. Similarly, the idea that stillbirths and deaths in the first week of life could be grouped together and described as perinatal deaths was not put forward until 1948 [16], but perinatal mortality rates have been constructed retrospectively for earlier years.

The Emergence of the Concept of "Infantile Mortality"

In 1858, Sir John Simon, Medical Officer to the General Board of Health used the term "infantine death rate" for mortality among children under the age of five. In his introduction to *Papers Relating to the Sanitary State of the People of England* [18], he expressed the view that this rate was a proxy measure of the health of the population. Drawing attention to the wide differences between districts, he commented that these infantine death rates

> ... furnish a very sensitive test of sanitary circumstances; so that differences of infantine death-rate are, under certain circumstances, the best proof of differences of household condition in any number of compared districts. And, secondly, those places where infants are most apt to die are necessarily the places where survivors are most apt to be sickly ... [18].

He went on to suggest that, "Deaths which occur in excess within five years of birth are mainly due to two sets of causes; first to the common infectious diseases of childhood prevailing with unusual fatality; and secondly to the endemic prevalence of convulsive disorders, diarrhoea and pulmonary inflammation". A factor that he did not mention was differences in the completeness of registration of births. It was likely that some babies who died shortly after birth were not registered; in particular, babies born outside marriage in big cities.

William Farr first used the current definition of infant mortality indirectly when reporting deaths in 1875, although he did not explicitly use the term "infant", nor the word "infantile", which was more commonly used in the succeeding decades. He wrote, "I show that in 1000 infants born in 1875 no less than 158 died in the first year of life ..." [5].

Infantile Mortality and Stillbirth Registration

In the same report, William Farr commented on the implications of changes in the law that had made the registration of live births compulsory in 1875. He pointed out that, "In the case of children born alive – or who breathe – both the birth and death are registered, but still-born children are not registered in England" but "Under the provisions of the new Registration Act, no still-born children, however, should be buried without a certificate stating that they were still-born" [5]. There is good evidence that these certificates were also used to bury victims of infanticide [11].

An international survey undertaken for the Select Committee on Stillbirth Registration and published in 1893 showed that Britain and Ireland lagged behind many other countries in not having stillbirth registration [10]. Nearly 20 years later, a second and fuller survey was done by the "Special Committee on Infantile Mortality" set up by the **Royal Statistical Society** [17].

These surveys covered European countries, New Zealand, states of Australia and the US and provinces of Canada. The Royal Statistical Society's survey also covered other British colonies and some Latin American countries. It found that stillbirth registration was compulsory in most countries, but that, "The large majority of the countries where registration is not required are under the British Crown, and it may be concluded that the Registration Laws in force in such countries have been based on the English model." In contrast, Sweden had introduced registration of both live and still births and deaths as early as 1749, followed by Denmark and Norway in 1801.

The surveys found wide differences between the countries in their criteria for birth registration and for distinguishing between infant deaths and stillbirths. As William Farr had already pointed out, "In France, under the provisions of the Code Napoleon, children who die (either before or after birth) before registration, are recorded as still-born. Dr **Bertillon** estimates that twenty-two in 100 of the children registered in France as still-born breathed, and such children in England would be registered among the births and deaths" [5].

It was this problem that prompted the Royal Statistical Society's enquiry. When presenting the Committee's report to the Society, Reginald Dudfield focused his attention on the need for a definition of stillbirth, as none of the countries with stillbirth registration appeared to have one in their legislation [4]. He considered two sets of issues. The first was the question of "viability". This was linked to the **gestational age** after which the fetus should be considered a child capable of independent life. The second was how to establish whether the fetus or child was, or had been, alive at birth.

After asking the Obstetrical Section of the Royal Society of Medicine for a definition of stillbirth, he recommended the following slightly amended version:

A "still-born child" means a child whose body at birth measures not less than 13 inches (32 centimetres) in length from the crown of the head to the sole of the heel and who, when completely born (the head, body and limbs of the child, but not necessarily the afterbirth being extruded from the body of the mother), exhibits no sign of life – that is to say whose heart has ceased to function, as demonstrated by the absence of pulsation in the cord at its attachment to the body of the child and the absence of any heart-sounds or impulses.
NOTE: Crying and/or breathing – being secondary signs of life, manifested only when the heart is acting – can be relied upon as signs of life, but in the absence of either or both is not to be held to be proof of absence of life in the child [4].

When stillbirth registration was eventually introduced in England and Wales in 1927, a shorter definition based on gestational age was used:

"Stillborn" and "stillbirth" shall apply to any child who has issued forth from its mother after the twenty-eighth week of pregnancy and which did not at any time after being completely expelled from its mother breathe or show any other signs of life [6].

Public Concern About Infantile Mortality and Developments in Analysis

The Royal Statistical Society's enquiry came at a time when there had been a growing concern about infant mortality in a number of countries. In Britain, this had been prompted by the discovery that many potential recruits for the Boer War were unfit and by the campaign by the Women's Co-operative Guild for maternity services.

The Royal Statistical Society Committee also discussed the way in which the infantile mortality rate was calculated. It had defined this as the ratio of the deaths during the first year of life to births. Its enquiries had revealed, however, that some countries had used the estimated numbers alive under the age of one year instead. Given the relative inaccuracy of population estimates, the Committee recommended using births instead.

Having pointed out that some countries compiled their birth statistics by year of registration and others by year of occurrence, it recommended using occurrences. It also recommended that stillbirths should be tabulated separately and that in countries where live-born babies who died before registration were registered as stillbirths, they should actually be counted as infant deaths [17].

As a result of public concern about infant mortality, analyses of infant mortality by age at death in the Annual Reports of the Registrar General from 1904 were more detailed than in earlier years. In addition, a series of four reports on infant mortality was published by the Local Government Board, the government department responsible for public health. In the first of these, the Board's Chief Medical Officer, Arthur Newsholme reiterated John Simon's view in stating that, "Infant mortality is the most sensitive index we possess of social welfare and of sanitary administration, especially under urban conditions" [14]. These reports compared the infant mortality rates for different parts of England and Wales and discussed the comparisons and local data in relation to factors such as sex, legitimacy, family size, the quality of help available in childbirth, the ages of mothers, poverty, overcrowding and defective sanitation.

A similar concern about infant mortality in the US at the same period has been attributed to its emergence as a world power.

> The problem of infant mortality is one of the great social and economic problems of our day ... A nation may waste its forests, its water power, its mines, and to some degree, even its lands, but if it is to hold its own in the struggle for supremacy, its children must be conserved at any cost. On the physical, intellectual and moral strength of the children of today the future depends [9].

One response to this was the setting up of the Children's Bureau and its enquiry in 1913 into infant mortality in eight cities. This enquiry took a cohort approach, following up children born in a given year, and was analyzed by a statistician, Robert Morse Woodbury (*see* **Birth Cohort Studies**). Having considered the same broad range of factors as Arthur Newsholme, he concluded that the level of the father's earnings was the strongest "causal" factor associated with infant mortality [21].

These conclusions underpinned calls for political action to improve the conditions for young children and their parents, but these were not the only views held at the time. Followers of the **eugenics** movement took the view that heredity was the prime factor in infant mortality and that attempts to reduce it hindered natural selection by delaying or preventing the death of children who would survive as "weaklings" [15].

The introduction of new technology in the form of punched card equipment increased the extent to which infant mortality could be analyzed by cause, age at death, and other factors [3]. Peter McKinlay's analysis of the decline in infant mortality in England and Wales in the first quarter of the twentieth century showed that, "... all ages have not shared in this amelioration to the same extent ... as a general rule, the nearer to birth the less has the mortality been affected" [12].

In his analysis, he subdivided infant mortality into two categories, "(a) the death rate from 'congenital debility, malformation and premature birth' (number 28 of causes of death given for each separate district in the Annual Reports of the Registrar General), and (b) the remainder of the infant deaths under one year". He labeled these as "neo-natal"

and "post-natal", respectively, and called stillbirths "ante-natal" deaths.

He concluded from his analysis of differences between areas of England and Wales that

> only the provision of skilled assistance to mothers in childbed is of importance in connection with ante-natal mortality. ... The neo-natal death rate is related both to variations in external environment and in the obstetrical assistance available to mothers in childbed. ... The postnatal death rate seems to offer the greatest scope for administrative measures. In this case the health of the mother would appear to come first in order of appearance, environment also is of some importance, whereas the effects of variations in obstetrical services have now ceased to be reflected on the mortality of infancy [12].

The term "neonatal" was also used a few years later in an international analysis for the League of Nations [19]. This had a demographic focus and started by looking at trends in countries' infant mortality in relation to their birth rates, population changes and overall death rates. It brought together the two streams of opinion on infant mortality in stating that, "It is evident that the causes of infant mortality may be divided into two distinct categories: (a) those depending on the fitness of the infant to live at all, and (b) those arising from the unfitness of the surroundings to support infant life" [19].

In comparing the death rates for different countries, the author grouped together deaths of live-born babies under the age of one month with stillbirths, partly to get over the differences in stillbirth registration referred to earlier. The term "birth mortality" was suggested for this combined rate. This rate varied far less between countries than that for older babies. The author commented that, "Infant mortality has repeatedly been stated to be the best measure of the sanitary state of a country ... if the infant mortality rate is employed for this purpose, it should clearly be only the part relating to infants over 1 month" [19].

The Establishment of Current Definitions

In the latter half of the twentieth century, the current definitions of fetal death, stillbirth, and the components of the infant mortality rate have become established. They are shown in Figure 1. Introducing these definitions, the Registrar General's Statistical Review for England and Wales for 1951 commented

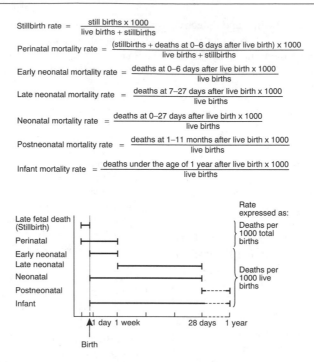

$$\text{Stillbirth rate} = \frac{\text{still births} \times 1000}{\text{live births} + \text{stillbirths}}$$

$$\text{Perinatal mortality rate} = \frac{(\text{stillbirths} + \text{deaths at 0–6 days after live birth}) \times 1000}{\text{live births} + \text{stillbirths}}$$

$$\text{Early neonatal mortality rate} = \frac{\text{deaths at 0–6 days after live birth} \times 1000}{\text{live births}}$$

$$\text{Late neonatal mortality rate} = \frac{\text{deaths at 7–27 days after live birth} \times 1000}{\text{live births}}$$

$$\text{Neonatal mortality rate} = \frac{\text{deaths at 0–27 days after live birth} \times 1000}{\text{live births}}$$

$$\text{Postneonatal mortality rate} = \frac{\text{deaths at 1–11 months after live birth} \times 1000}{\text{live births}}$$

$$\text{Infant mortality rate} = \frac{\text{deaths under the age of 1 year after live birth} \times 1000}{\text{live births}}$$

Figure 1 Definitions of stillbirth and infant morality rates. Reproduced from Macfarlane & Mugford [11] by permission of the office for National Statistics. © Crown copyright 1984

that the use of the term "neonatal period" was "now traditional among obstetricians and compilers of vital statistics" and its first use by writers of Annual Reviews had been in 1936 [7]. It also pointed out the term "perinatal mortality" had first been used in 1950. The term had been coined by a demographer Sigismund Peller, who took the view that time trends in early neonatal deaths had more in common with those in stillbirths than with those in the rest of the first year of life. [16]

In most developed countries, infant mortality rates have fallen persistently and dramatically in the latter half of the twentieth century to well below 10 infant deaths per 1000 live births. As the survival rates of preterm and immature babies have risen, the definitions used have been extended to include ever smaller babies and fetuses and countries still differ considerably in their criteria for registering live and still births. [8, 13].

The **World Health Organization**'s Expert Committee on Vital Statistics recommended in 1950 that, as a minimum, all countries register and tabulate all fetal deaths after the 28th completed week of gestation [22]. This was endorsed in the seventh revision of

the **International Classification of Diseases (ICD)**. This was the first to incorporate a definition of stillbirth that separates the definition of a dead-born fetus from the criteria for registration.

A quarter of a century later, a different approach was used in the ninth revision of the ICD. This recommended that *national* perinatal statistics should include all fetuses and babies delivered "weighing at least 500 g or, where birthweight is unavailable, the corresponding gestational age (22 weeks) or body length (25 cm crown–heel), whether alive or dead" [23]. It went on to acknowledge that countries' legal requirements might have different criteria for registration purposes and that international comparisons should be restricted to fetuses and babies "weighing 1000 g or more (or, where birthweight is unavailable, the corresponding gestational age (28 weeks) or body length (35 cm crown–heel)" [23].

The tenth revision of the ICD took yet another approach and defined the perinatal period "which commences at 22 completed weeks (154 days) of gestation (the time when birthweight is normally 500 g) and ends seven completed days after live birth" [24]. Although the ICD no longer uses the term stillbirth, the term still appears in the legislation of individual countries, such as the countries of the UK.

The relevance of the upper cutoff point for the perinatal period has often been questioned in recent years. Increasingly, the use of intensive care is enabling very immature babies to survive, but there is also a tendency for those that die to do so later after birth. One response to this is to redefine perinatal deaths as the sum of all stillbirths and neonatal deaths, as is done in Australia. Another, which takes into account the view that there are increasing differences between stillbirths and neonatal deaths, is to tabulate stillbirths, neonatal and postneonatal deaths separately and drop the use of the perinatal mortality rate.

The ninth revision of the ICD recommended using a special form of certificate for perinatal deaths, with the cause section subdivided into "main and other diseases or conditions in the fetus or infant," "main and other maternal conditions affecting the fetus or infant" and "other relevant circumstances" [23]. It did not indicate how these data should be analyzed. In response to this problem, the Office of Population Censuses and Surveys, now known as the **Office for National Statistics**, has devised a hierarchical classification to group causes of stillbirth and neonatal death from the forms of certificate it introduced in 1986 [1, 2]. This classification uses categories first proposed by Jonathan Wigglesworth for use with information derived from case notes [20] and also builds on the extensive research done over many years in Aberdeen, Scotland.

References

[1] Alberman, A., Botting, B., Blatchley, N. & Twidell, A. (1994). A new hierarchical classification of causes of infant deaths in England and Wales, *Archives of Disease in Childhood* **70**, 403–409.

[2] Alberman, A., Blatchley, N., Botting, B., Schuman, J. & Dunn A. (1997). Medical causes on stillbirth certificates in England and Wales; distribution and results of hierarchical classifications tested for the Office for National Statistics, *British Journal of Obstetrics and Gynaecology* **104**, 1043–1049.

[3] Armstrong, D. (1986). The invention of infant mortality, *Sociology of Health and Illness* **8**, 211–232.

[4] Dudfield, R. (1912). Still-births in relation to infant mortality, *Journal of the Royal Statistical Society* **76**, 1–26.

[5] Farr, W. (1877). Letter to the Registrar General, in *Thirty-eighth Annual Report of the Registrar General of Births, Deaths and Marriages in England*. Abstracts of 1875. Cd 1786. HMSO, London.

[6] General Register Office (1929). *The Registrar General's Statistical Review of England and Wales for the Year 1927*. HMSO, London.

[7] General Register Office (1954). *The Registrar General's Statistical Review of England and Wales for the Year 1951*. HMSO, London.

[8] Gourbin, C. & Masuy-Stroobant, G. (1995). Registration of vital data: are live and stillbirths comparable all over Europe?, *Bulletin of the World Health Organization* **73**, 449–460.

[9] Holt, L.E. (1913). Infant mortality, ancient and modern. An historical sketch, *Archives of Pediatrics* **30**, 885–915.

[10] House of Commons(1893). *Still-births in England and Other Countries*. Return to House of Commons. No 279. HMSO, London.

[11] Macfarlane, A.J. & Mugford, M. (1984). *Birth Counts: Statistics of Pregnancy and Childbirth*. HMSO, London.

[12] McKinlay, P.L. (1929). Some statistical aspects of infant mortality, *Journal of Hygiene* **28**, 394–417.

[13] Mugford, M. (1983). A comparison of reported differences of vital events and statistics, *WHO Statistics Quarterly* **26**, 201–212.

[14] Newsholme, A. (1910). *Report by the Medical Officer on Infant and Child Mortality*, Supplement to the Thirty-Ninth Annual Report of the Local Government Board for 1909-10. Cd 5263. HMSO, London.

[15] Pearson, K. (1912). The intensity of natural selection in man, *Proceedings of the Royal Society of London, Series B* **85**, 469–476.

[16] Peller, S. (1948). Mortality past and future, *Population Studies* **1**, 405–456.

[17] Royal Statistical Society (1912). Report of Special Committee on Infantile Mortality, *Journal of the Royal Statistical Society* **76**, 27–87.

[18] Simon, J. (1858). Introductory report, in *Papers Relating to the Sanitary State of the People of England*. HMSO, London.

[19] Stouman, K. (1934). The perilous threshold of life. League of Nations, *Quarterly Bulletin of the Health Organisation* **3**, 531–612.

[20] Wigglesworth, J.S. (1980). Monitoring perinatal mortality - a patho-physiological approach, *Lancet* **ii**, 684–686.

[21] Woodbury, R.M. (1925). *Causal Factors in Infant Mortality. A Statistical Study Based on Investigation in Eight Cities*, Children's Bureau Publication No 25. Government Printing Office, Washington.

[22] World Health Organization (1957). *Manual of the International Statistical Classification of Diseases, Injuries and Causes of Death*, 7th Rev., Vol. 1. WHO, Geneva.

[23] World Health Organization (1977). *Manual of the International Statistical Classification of Diseases, Injuries and Causes of Death*, 9th Rev., Vol. 1. WHO, Geneva.

[24]   World Health Organization (1992). *International Classi-
        fication of Diseases and Related Health Problems*, 10th
        Rev., Vol. 1. WHO, Geneva.

(*See also* **Birthweight; Cause of Death, Underlying
and Multiple; Death Certification; Midwifery,
Obstetrics, and Neonatology; Vital Statistics,
Overview**)

ALISON J. MACFARLANE

Infectious Disease Models

There are two major roles for stochastic infectious
disease models. Their study provides insights into
the spead of disease in a community, and they are
an essential component in the analysis of data from
empirical studies of infectious disease (*see* **Epidemic
Models, Stochastic**).

The Epidemic Threshold Theorem

A major insight provided by epidemic models is
that major epidemics can be prevented in a large
community by immunizing only a fraction of the
individuals. This property is sometimes referred to
as herd immunity, and is quantified by the **epidemic
threshold** theorem. Deterministic models for infectious diseases (*see* **Epidemic Models, Deterministic**)
indicate this result, but these models assume that both
the group of susceptible individuals and the group
of infective individuals are large throughout the epidemic. The stochastic version of the threshold theorem also requires a large susceptible group, but the
infection process may start with only one infective
individual. The stochastic threshold theorem is also
richer in that it quantifies the probability of a major
epidemic when a small number of infective individuals enter a large community that is currently free
from the disease.

In the overly simple setting of a large community
of homogeneous individuals, who mix uniformly (*see*
Random Mixing), the threshold theorem indicates
that the probability of a major epidemic is zero when
the proportion of individuals who are susceptible to
infection is less than $1/\theta$. The parameter θ, known

as the basic **reproduction number**, is the mean
number of individuals infected by the direct contacts
of an infective entering the community when all other
individuals are susceptible.

The epidemic threshold theorem holds under quite
general conditions, but the bound $1/\theta$ then depends
on the community structure and the heterogeneity
among individuals (see [7] and [8]).

Data on Outbreaks in Households

Infectious disease data have three features that distinguish them from other data. There is usually some
knowledge about the mechanism that generates the
data, the data are dependent, and the infection process
is only partially observable. A consequence of these
features is that the analysis of data is usually most
effective when it is based on a model that describes
aspects of the infection process. The level of detail
that should be incorporated into the model depends
on the objective of the study.

Disease transmission and the natural history of
diseases evolve in continuous time, but discrete time
models are often appropriate for data analysis. It may
be that events are only recorded to the nearest day,
say, or only the eventual outcomes of outbreaks are
observed. Data on the eventual number of cases in
households are often collected, because households
are a manageable unit size and data on eventual
infection can be verified by laboratory tests, which
makes them relatively reliable.

Chain Binomial Models

In a household having initially s susceptible individuals, there will be $1, 2, \ldots,$ or s eventual cases.
The probability of a specified number of eventual
cases in an infected household is computed in terms
of disease transmission probabilities by considering
the likelihood of the various chains of infection. To
illustrate, suppose that one of a total of five susceptible individuals of a household is infected and starts
an outbreak in the household. Assume that the outbreak evolves without further infection from outside.
Four eventual cases in the household could result via
a number of different chains of infection. One such
chain is $1 \rightarrow 2 \rightarrow 1 \rightarrow 0$, which means that the single initial infective infected exactly two household
members, who in turn infected exactly one member,

and the last remaining susceptible member escaped infection throughout.

A simple **chain binomial model** would compute the probability for this chain, given one introductory case, as

$$\binom{4}{2} p_1^2 q_1^2 \binom{2}{1} p_2 q_2 \binom{1}{0} p_1^0 q_1 = 12 p_1^2 q_1^3 p_2 q_2,$$

where q_i is the probability that a susceptible escapes infection when exposed to i infectives for the duration of their infectious periods and $p_i = 1 - q_i$. The probability that the number of eventual cases in a household is x is the sum of chain probabilities over all chains with x eventual cases.

The **EM algorithm** is a convenient tool for finding maximum likelihood estimates when fitting chain binomial models to size of household outbreak data. This is pointed out with reference to **partner studies** for HIV infection in [11] and is discussed more fully in the review paper [6] (*see* **AIDS and HIV**).

Models that capture the infection mechanism of the data generally contain parameters with clear interpretations and are well suited for testing epidemiologically important hypotheses. For example, with a chain binomial model for the size of household outbreaks, we can test the Reed–Frost hypothesis $q_2 = q_1^2$, or the Greenwood hypothesis $q_2 = q_1$. The Reed–Frost assumption is appropriate for diseases that spread primarily by direct person-to-person contact.

Many methods of analysis of household data assume that each household outbreak evolves essentially independently after the initial infection of the household. This assumption is often of concern. Longini & Koopman [10] propose an analysis based on a pragmatic chain binomial model that also allows infection from outside the household.

Epidemic Chain Models with Random Effects

It is instructive to think about disease transmission in terms of a continuous infectivity function $\lambda(t)$ that indicates how infectious an infective is t time units after being infected. The infectivity function reflects both the level of infectious agent emitted by the infective and his or her rate of making contacts with others. Often, the infectivity function is zero for a period immediately after infection, because the infectious organism is developing within the body and no infectious agent is emitted.

When disease transmission is person-to-person, the probability that a given susceptible individual escapes infection when exposed to a given infective is $q_1 = \exp[-\int_0^T \lambda(t)\,dt]$, where T is the duration of time from infection until the end of the infectious period.

Epidemic chain binomial models assume that infectives are homogeneous, in the sense that they all have the same infectivity function. When infectives have different infectivity functions, we still use chain binomial models if the infectives can be partitioned into homogeneous groups. Otherwise, we proceed by considering the q_1 for each infective to be a realization from a probability distribution. In these **random effects** models, see [4, Chapter 3], the probabilities of the epidemic chains are expressed in terms of the **moments** of q_1. This allows for heterogeneity in the infectivity of infected individuals. Heterogeneity in susceptibility or among households can be allowed for in a similar way. An application of random effects models to data on *Shigella sonnei* in households is given by Baker & Stevens [3].

A comprehensive analysis of infectious disease data on household outbreaks, allowing infection from outside the household, variation in the duration of the infectious period, and **covariates**, is described by Addy et al. [1].

Continuous Time Data for Households

Sometimes, when daily data are available on symptoms shown by infected individuals, the analysis is based on a continuous time model. The standard model used is a compartmental model for the irreversible compartments Susceptible $\rightarrow$ Exposed $\rightarrow$ Infective $\rightarrow$ Removed, referred to as the SEIR model. An individual in the exposed category is infected, but not yet infectious, and said to be in the **latent period**. The final category is called removed, because these individuals play no further part in the infection process. These individuals may simply have recovered and have acquired immunity from further infection for the duration of the epidemic. It is of interest to estimate characteristics, such as the mean and variance, of the latent and infectious periods. This can be done by assuming a parametric model for the distribution of the latent and infectious periods, as described in [2, Chapter 15] and [4, Chapter 4]. It is also of interest to make inferences about the functional form of the infectivity function, which is considered in the context of transmission of the human immunodeficiency virus (HIV) by Shiboski & Jewell [12] on the basis of data on partners of individuals infected with HIV.

Data on an Epidemic in a Community

Regression Analysis

When data are available on the days on which individuals show symptoms of disease, and these can be used to deduce the date of infection, with reasonable accuracy, then a comprehensive regression analysis is possible. The response variable is the indicator of infection for each susceptible individual on each day. The **Mantel–Haenszel** test statistic has been suggested as a way of reducing the number of covariates, see [4, Chapter 5]; however, a **logistic regression** model is also convenient for determining which covariates are needed in the model. When a final set of covariates is arrived at it is useful to fit a **loglinear** regression model in these covariates to the binary data. The preference for the loglinear model stems from the more direct epidemiologic interpretation of its parameters in the infectious disease context. More specifically, if Y is the indicator of escaping infection for a given susceptible on a given day, then fitting the model $Y \simeq \text{binomial}[1, \exp(-\beta'\mathbf{x})]$ is useful, because with this model $\beta'\mathbf{x}$ can be interpreted as the force of infection acting on the susceptible on that day. The covariate $\mathbf{x}$ might include the number of infectives in the community and the number of infectives in the susceptible's household, for example. An illustration of such a regression analysis is given in [4, Chapter 6].

Martingale Methods

The fact that the infection process is observed only partially causes the likelihood function based on continuous time data to be very complicated. This has encouraged the development of pragmatic methods based on simplifying assumptions and approximations. In contrast, methods of analysis derived from martingales for **counting processes** have proved successful for developing simple methods of statistical inference for some crucial parameters, such as the basic reproduction number, for quite general models. Tutorial accounts of these methods are given in [5] and [4, Chapter 7].

Vaccine Efficacy

A major motivation for the study of infectious diseases is to gain insight into ways in which they can be controlled and to determine requirements for their control. The most successful method of intervention continues to be vaccination (*see* **Vaccine Studies**). The epidemic threshold theorem plays a key role here, but it can only be applied if parameter estimates are available. A crucial parameter is the vaccine efficacy. Traditionally, vaccine efficacy has been estimated by $1 - (AR_V/AR_U)$, where AR_V is the attack rate among vaccinated individuals and AR_U is the attack rate among unvaccinated individuals. The attack rate is the proportion of individuals infected in the specified risk group over a nominated period of time. As a measure of the protective effect that the vaccine provides, this concept of vaccine efficacy suffers from depending on both the community from which the data come and on the time period over which the data are collected. Recently, there has been a more careful study of the interpretation and estimation of vaccine efficacy, see [9]. Typically, as a concept of protection against infection, vaccine efficacy might be interpreted as α, where the force of infection acting on vaccinated individuals is $\alpha g(t)$ at chronological time t when the force of infection exerted on an unvaccinated susceptible is $g(t)$. Depending on the vaccine, α may be a constant in $[0, 1]$ or a separate realization on a random variable for each vaccinated individual.

The HIV/AIDS Epidemic

The appearance of AIDS stimulated new interest in the problems of modeling and data analysis for infectious disease studies. A distinguishing feature of infection with HIV is the very long time between infection and diagnosis with AIDS. This has made it feasible, and of interest, to assess the size of the epidemic, forecast its progress, and study characteristics of disease progression during the course of the epidemic (*see* **AIDS and HIV**).

References

[1]   Addy, C.L., Longini, I.M. & Haber, M. (1991). A generalized stochastic model for the analysis of infectious disease final size data, *Biometrics* **47**, 961–974.

[2]   Bailey, N.T.J. (1975). *The Mathematical Theory of Infectious Diseases and its Applications*. Griffin, London.

[3]   Baker, R.D. & Stevens, R.H. (1995). A random effects model for analysis of infectious disease final-state data, *Biometrics* **51**, 956–968.

[4]   Becker, N.G. (1989). *Analysis of Infectious Disease Data*. Chapman & Hall, London.

[5]   Becker, N.G. (1993). Martingale methods for the analysis of epidemic data, *Statistical Methods in Medical Research* **2**, 93–112.

[6]   Becker, N.G. (1997). Uses of the EM algorithm in the analysis of data on HIV/AIDS and other infectious diseases, *Statistical Methods in Medical Research* **6**, to appear.

[7]   Becker, N.G. & Dietz, K. (1995). The effect of household distribution on transmission and control of highly infectious diseases, *Mathematical Biosciences* **127**, 207–219.

[8]   Becker, N.G. & Hall, R. (1996). Immunization levels for preventing epidemics in a community of households made up of individuals of different types, *Mathematical Biosciences* **132**, 205–216.

[9]   Halloran, M.E., Haber, M. & Longini, I.M. (1992). Interpretation and estimation of vaccine efficacy under heterogeneity, *American Journal of Epidemiology* **136**, 328–343.

[10] Longini, I.M. & Koopman, J.S. (1982). Household and community transmission parameters from final distributions of infections in households, *Biometrics* **38**, 115–126.

[11] Madger, L. & Brookmeyer, R. (1993). Analysis of infectious disease data from partner studies with unknown source of infection, *Biometrics* **49**, 1110–1116.

[12] Shiboski, S.C. & Jewell, N.P. (1992). Statistical analysis of the time dependence of HIV infectivity based on partner study data, *Journal of the American Statistical Association* **87**, 360–372.

(*See also* **Communicable Diseases; Incubation Period of Infectious Diseases**)

NIELS G. BECKER

Infectious Diseases *see* Communicable Diseases

Infectivity Titration

In an experiment to assay the virulence of a suspension of living, self-reproducing organisms

(which we refer to here as "particles"), doses derived by successive dilution of the original suspension are administered to groups of host organisms, and the proportion of hosts infected at each dilution is recorded. The "independent action" or "one-hit" theory [13–15] assumes that infection can be initiated by one particle, which, for some reason or other, is "effective". Particles act independently, any one particle having a probability, p, of being effective on a particular occasion. The biological interpretation of p depends on the host–pathogen system. It may be the probability of a particle being retained in the host, or reaching a totally susceptible site; or, on a stochastic model, it may depend on the relative rates at which particles divide and die within a host [4] (*see* **Stochastic Processes**).

Situations for which this model has been proposed include the infection of plants by viruses [6], the titration of viruses in egg membranes [16] or portions of membrane [10], the infection of animals by bacteria [20, 21], and the initiation of tumors in animals by viruses [7].

Suppose that at the ith dilution, the mean number of particles per inoculum is λ_i, and that n_i hosts are inoculated, of which r_i are infected. If the probability of infection, p, is the same for all hosts, the probability that a host receiving this inoculum will not be infected is the first term in the **Poisson distribution**,

$$P_i = \exp(-\lambda_i p). \tag{1}$$

If this dose has a concentration equal to a fraction x_i of the original preparation, we can define $\gamma_i = \lambda_i p = \gamma x_i$, say, where γ is the mean number of effective particles per inoculum in the undiluted preparation. From a set of results at a series of different dilutions one could estimate γ as in the **dilution method for bacterial density estimation**, or the "most probable number" method (*see* **Serial Dilution Assay**).

Note, first, that the parameter to be estimated here depends both on the density of the particles in the original preparation and on the probability of infection, p. In the dilution method for counting viable bacteria it is assumed that a particle present in the inoculum will be detected without fail, so that $p = 1$ for all hosts. The absolute density of particles in a preparation can then be estimated. In the more general situation considered here, the absolute density of particles cannot be estimated without some further assumption about the probability of infection. Nevertheless, an infectivity titration can be used to compare two or more microbial populations, inoculated into randomly assigned hosts (*see* **Biological Assay, Overview**).

Note, secondly, that if p is not equal to unity universally, it may vary between hosts, and this feature leads to a number of important modifications of the model described above. However, variation in infectivity between individual particles does not invalidate the simple model, provided the hosts are identical in their susceptibility.

Host Variability

Suppose that p varies from host to host with a distribution function $F(p)$. (We avoid the use of a capital letter for the **random variable** p, as P is customarily used in the different sense of (1) above.) Then, the probability of noninfection is

$$P_i = \int_0^1 \exp(-\lambda_i p) \mathrm{d}F(p). \tag{2}$$

Expression (2) is a **moment generating function** for the distribution $F(p)$, and may be expanded in terms of the moments. Since p is restricted to the range (0,1), the terms involving the higher moments are, in practice, negligible for all except very large values of λ_i, and a good approximation is

$$P_i \cong \exp(-\lambda_i \mu)[1 + (\lambda_i^2 \mu_2)/2], \tag{3}$$

where μ and μ_2 are, respectively, the mean and variance of p. Expression (3) shows that the effect of host variability is to flatten the dose–response curve relating P_i to λ_i or to the known concentration factor x_i, the proportionate effect being greater at the higher concentrations.

The general effect of host variability was noted in [21]. The precise effect has been studied for a number of specific distributional forms, including the **gamma distribution** [1, 16], truncated **exponential** [1, 5], **beta** [5] and two-point [2, 7] distributions. For the gamma (or type III) distribution with density function

$$f(p) = \exp(-p/\mu k)(p/\mu k)^{(1/k)-1}/(\mu k)\Gamma(1/k), \tag{4}$$

with mean μ and variance $\mu_2 = k\mu^2$, (2) gives

$$P_i = (1 + \lambda_i \mu k)^{-(1/k)}, \tag{5}$$

which is equivalent to (3) to $O(k)$ and tends to (1) as $k \to 0$. The gamma distribution, having infinite range, is strictly inappropriate as a distribution for p, but may be regarded as an adequate model for small values of μ, when truncation at $p = 1$ would have little effect.

The two-point distribution places probability masses α_i at values $p = \pi_i, i = 1, 2$, with $\pi_1 < \pi_2$. If $\pi_2 \gg \pi_1$, the effect on the dose–response curve relating the probability of infection, $Q_i = 1 - P_i$, to x_i or $\log x_i$, is to suggest a "shelf" at approximately $Q = \alpha_2$, since only the hosts with the higher level of susceptibility will be infected at the lower concentrations.

Further insight into the flattening effect [5] follows by regarding the response curve as the distribution function of a tolerance distribution (*see* **Quantal Response Models**). Let V denote the variance of the tolerance distribution of $\log x$ from (2), V_0 the corresponding value from (1) for homogeneous hosts, and $V_{\log p}$ the variance of $\log p$. Then, as noted in [5],

$$V = V_0 + V_{\log p}. \tag{6}$$

This increase in variance caused by host variability corresponds to the flattening of the dose–response curve. Many authors [8, 10, 20] have used probit analysis to analyze dose–response curves in infectivity titrations (*see* **Quantal Response Models**). It is known [11] that the exponential model (1) leads to a tolerance distribution for the log dose closely similar to a normal distribution, and that, with logs taken to base 10, the expected slope of a probit line is about 1.8–2.0. The expression (6) shows that, in general, probit slopes against log dose for infectivity experiments will usually be less than 1.8. Systematic values below 1.8 would indicate host variability, whilst values above 2.0 would suggest departure from independent action.

Detection and Estimation of Host Variability

Probit analysis provides a rough way of checking the evidence for host variability and of estimating its magnitude through the parameter $V_{\log p}$. A better approach is based on the more correct models (1) and (2).

For a test of the null hypothesis of zero variability in a titration experiment with n hosts at each dilution,

Moran [16, 17] proposed the statistic

$$T = \sum r_i(n - r_i), \qquad (7)$$

and evaluated its null distribution for series with various dilution ratios. Moran's statistic is symmetric as between infected and noninfected hosts, and thus does not use the fact, shown by (3), that departures from the null model (1) will tend to be associated with excessive numbers of noninfections at high doses.

Armitage [1] proposes a score test (see **Likelihood**), based on the likelihood function derived from (3). The test statistic is

$$\phi = \sum \left[\frac{n_i \hat{Q}_i - r_i}{\hat{Q}_i} \right] \frac{(\hat{\gamma}_0 x_i)^2}{2}. \qquad (8)$$

Here, $\hat{\gamma}_0$ is the maximum likelihood estimate of γ under the null model (1), and $\hat{Q}_i$ is the corresponding estimate of Q_i. Note that in (8) the discrepancies between observed and expected frequencies are more heavily weighted at the higher doses. A modified statistic ϕ' is available when γ is estimated by a consistent but inefficient estimator, such as that suggested by Fisher [9] based on $\sum r_i$.

Moran's T is identically zero for series with $n = 1$, and is therefore inappropriate in that situation. Experiments are likely to require larger values of n, but may sometimes be designed in blocks, each with $n = 1$.

Stevens [22] proposes the statistic R, equivalent to Moran's [18] $D + 1$, defined as the number of dilutions between (and including) the first at which not all hosts are infected, and the last at which at least one is infected. As an example, in the following series of increasing dilutions with single observations (+ representing infection),

$$\ldots + + 0 + 0 + + 0 0 \ldots,$$

the value of R is 5. As with T, there is no differential weighting of the two extremes of the response curve. An alternative simple statistic [3] is J, defined as the number of infected hosts at dilutions beyond that at which the first noninfection occurs. In the example, $J = 3$. The statistic J has been shown [3] to be highly correlated with the efficient statistic ϕ and to be more powerful than R in the detection of small departures from the null model.

All tests of host variability must be one-sided, since the null hypothesis lies at one end of the parameter range. It might be argued that such tests are pointless, since some degree of host variability must exist except in the extreme case where $p = 1$ for all hosts. However, one situation leading to a mean μ less than unity might arise if a proportion, μ, of hosts were invariably susceptible, the remaining proportion, $1 - \mu$, being totally resistant. In that case, there would be no variability. Contradiction of the null hypothesis in a test for variability, then, at least rules out that possible scenario. In general, though, it will be more useful to estimate the degree of variability than to test for evidence of its existence.

Maximum likelihood estimation of k follows from the likelihood equations based on (3) [1], and less efficient estimates may be based on the simple test statistics such as T.

Dependent Action Models

Most log dose–response curves encountered in infectivity experiments are sufficiently flat to support the independent action or "one-hit" theory, for which other evidence exists [13, 15]. If infection depended on cooperation between more than one particle, the resulting "multi-hit" log dose–response curve would be steeper than that given by (1). Iwaszkiewicz & Neyman [12] discuss the estimation of the critical number of effective particles required for infection, and introduce the concept of host variability by allowing the critical number to vary between hosts, the effect again being to flatten the log dose–response curve. Independent action could conceivably also give rise to a steeper curve. In the production of tumors by viruses, for example, tumors might be too faint to be detected unless several occurred close together [19]. In the absence of host variability, the response curve would then be steeper than the exponential form (1).

References

[1]   Armitage, P. (1959). Host variability in dilution experiments, *Biometrics* **15**, 1–9.

[2]   Armitage, P. (1959). An examination of some experimental cancer data in the light of the one-hit theory of infectivity titrations, *Journal of the National Cancer Institute* **23**, 1313–1330.

[3]   Armitage, P. & Bartsch, G.E. (1960). The detection of host variability in a dilution series with single observations, *Biometrics* **16**, 582–592.

[4]   Armitage, P., Meynell G.G. & Williams, T. (1965). Birth–death and other models for microbial infection, *Nature* **207**, 570–572.

[5]   Armitage, P. & Spicer, C.C. (1956). The detection of variation in host susceptibility in dilution counting experiments, *Journal of Hygiene* **54**, 401–414.

[6]   Bald, J.G. (1937). The use of numbers of infections for comparing the concentration of plant virus suspensions. I. Dilution experiments with purified suspensions, *Annals of Applied Biology* **24**, 33–35.

[7]   Bryan, W.R. (1956). Biological studies on the Rous sarcoma virus. IV. Interpretation of tumor–response data involving one inoculation site per chicken, *Journal of the National Cancer Institute* **16**, 843–863.

[8]   Finter, N.B. & Armitage, P. (1957). The membrane piece technique for *in vitro* infectivity titrations of influenza virus, *Journal of Hygiene* **55**, 434–456.

[9]   Fisher, R.A. (1922). On the mathematical foundations of theoretical statistics, *Philosophical Transactions of the Royal Society of London, Series A* **222**, 309–368.

[10] Fulton, F. & Armitage, P. (1951). Surviving tissue suspensions for influenza virus titration, *Journal of Hygiene* **49**, 247–262.

[11] Irwin, J.O. (1942). The distribution of the logarithm of survival times when the true law is exponential, *Journal of Hygiene* **42**, 328–333.

[12] Iwaszkiewicz, K. & Neyman, J. (1931). Counting virulent bacteria and particles of virus, *Acta Biologiae Experimentalis, Varsovie* **6**, 101–142. Reprinted in Neyman, J. (1967). *A Selection of Early Statistical Papers of J. Neyman.* Cambridge University Press, Cambridge.

[13] Meynell, G.G. (1957). The applicability of the hypothesis of independent action to fatal infections in mice given *Salmonella typhimurium* by mouth, *Journal of General Microbiology* **16**, 396–404.

[14] Meynell, G.G. (1957). Inherently low precision of infectivity titrations using a quantal response, *Biometrics* **13**, 149–163.

[15] Meynell, G.G. & Meynell, E.W. (1958). The growth of micro-organisms *in vivo* with particular reference to the relation between dose and latent period, *Journal of Hygiene* **56**, 323–346.

[16] Moran, P.A.P. (1954). The dilution assay of viruses. I, *Journal of Hygiene* **52**, 189–193.

[17] Moran, P.A.P. (1954). The dilution assay of viruses. II, *Journal of Hygiene* **52**, 444–446.

[18] Moran, P.A.P. (1958). Another test for heterogeneity of host resistance in dilution assays, *Journal of Hygiene* **56**, 319–322.

[19] Parker, R.F., Bronson, L.H. & Green, R.H. (1941). Further studies of the infectious unit of vaccinia, *Journal of Experimental Medicine* **74**, 263–281.

[20] Peto, S. (1953). A dose–response equation for the invasion of micro-organisms, *Biometrics* **9**, 320–335.

[21] Reid, D.B.W. & MacLeod, D.R.E. (1954). The relation between dose and mortality for *Salmonella dublin*, *Journal of Hygiene* **52**, 18–23.

[22] Stevens, W.L. (1958). Dilution series: a statistical test of technique, *Journal of the Royal Statistical Society, Series B* **20**, 205–214.

P. ARMITAGE

Inference

Inference is usually defined as the process of drawing conclusions from facts, available evidence, and premises. *Statistical inference* is the term associated with the process of making conclusions on the basis of data that are governed by probability laws. More generally conclusions are made that are uncertain. The objective measurement of the uncertainty is one of the principal goals of statistical inference. In practical applications of statistical inference data are available and the aim of the inference is to draw conclusions about models which potentially may have generated the data. *Data analysis* is the colloquial expression which is often used to describe the statistical inferential process.

Examples of such situations are: a randomized **clinical trial** is being carried out to determine which of two therapy programs is superior for the treatment of **AIDS**; a **sample survey** is taken in a community having a contaminated public water supply to determine if families having higher concentrations of contaminated water also have higher rates of congenital abnormalities; data are available from individuals diagnosed as having an acute myocardial infarct – how is the infarct incidence related to age and gender?

Implicit in the inferential process is a defined population and an experimental plan which describes how data is generated from the population. The experimental plan for data collection may be very well laid out, as in a clinical trial, or may be quite informal, such as data collected from a hospital to carry out an **observational study**. The less formal the experimental plan for data collection, the greater the opportunities for blunders and systematic biases. Furthermore, any conclusions drawn from the data, strictly speaking, apply only to the population from which the data have been generated. Populations that are not well defined also create opportunities for the injection of systematic errors in the inferential process. In what follows it will always be assumed that there is both a well-defined population and a data collection plan which does not create opportunities for systematic error.

There is a general lack of agreement on the best ways to carry out statistical inferences. These differences have led to different "schools of statistical inference". These "schools" are often referred to as the frequentist, likelihood, Bayesian, and fiducial schools of inference. Major articles appear in this Encyclopedia reflecting the different schools of inference. Important criticisms have been made against some of the ideas in each of these schools of inference. Even within a school there may be sharp disagreements. In this article the major views of different schools of inference will be compared, with special emphasis on the frequency school of inference.

The problem may be formulated by considering that data represent realizations of a **random variable** X having a family of **probability** distributions $\{P_\theta(x)\}$ which is indexed by θ. The random variable X and parameter θ may be vector valued. Realizations of X are denoted by x. To concentrate on ideas, we will assume that all operations described below are defined and any required regularity conditions are satisfied. We define $f_\theta(x)$ to be a probability density function (pdf) or frequency function of X. The main goal of the inference is to draw conclusions about θ. More generally, if θ is vector valued, then the inference may be concerned with drawing inferences on a subset of values of θ. The remaining parameters are referred to as **nuisance parameters**.

The most important class of inference problems is when the vector X is composed of independent identically distributed (iid) random variables having the joint distribution $\prod_i f_\theta(x_i)$. The **likelihood** is central to nearly all schools of inference and is defined by being proportional to the joint distribution, i.e. $L(\theta|x) \propto \prod_i f(x_i|\theta)$. Usually the likelihood is defined as equal to the joint distribution except for the omission of a multiplicative constant which does not depend on θ.

In some cases the likelihood function can be written as

$$L(\theta|x) = L_1(\theta|t(x))L_2(x),$$

where $t(x)$ is a function of the observations and may be a vector. In this case $t(x)$ is called a **sufficient statistic**. Hence the probability distribution of X, conditional on $t(x)$, is not a function of θ. As a result, $t(x)$ contains all the relevant data for making inferences about θ. A minimal sufficient statistic corresponds to the smallest dimension of $t(x)$ for which the distribution of X, conditional on $t(x)$, is not a function of θ. Note that the likelihood function is a sufficient statistic. Using only the sufficient statistic to make inferences on θ leads to a data reduction method in which the sample x is replaced by $t(x)$. This data reduction does not lose any information on θ.

Frequentist School of Inference

The frequentist school of inference is the most widely used method of inference in practice. Much of the foundations were laid by Fisher [12–18], Neyman [23], and Neyman & Pearson [24–28]. However, Fisher and Neyman & Pearson have serious disagreements about basic issues. Articles describing aspects of the frequency school of inference are scattered throughout this Encyclopedia. Major articles are: **Hypothesis Testing, Estimation**, and **Maximum Likelihood**. Other articles discussing aspects of estimation are: **Confidence Intervals and Sets, Consistent Estimator, Cramér–Rao Inequality, Efficiency and Efficient Estimators, Generalized Maximum Likelihood, Minimum Variance Unbiased (MVU) Estimator, Sufficient Statistic**, and **Unbiasedness**. Articles discussing the frequentist theory of hypothesis testing and related topics are: **Alternative Hypothesis, Critical Region, Likelihood Ratio Tests, Most Powerful Test, Neyman–Pearson Lemma, Null Hypothesis** and **Level of a Test**. Two basic texts on frequentist inference are Lehmann [21, 22].

The basic idea underlying the frequentist school of inference is to evaluate the inferential process by assuming that an "experiment" is repeated an infinite number of times. Procedures having "better properties", as judged by long-term behavior, are deemed superior. Throughout the frequentist formulation of inference there is an attempt to derive statistical methods that have "optimal" properties in the context of an infinite number of repetitions of the experiment.

In general, all probability statements generated by the frequency theory of inference are based on the frequentist interpretation of probability. Yet the conclusions are targeted at specific data sets or specific experiments. Critics dismiss the concept of using methods based on properties associated with an infinite repetition of experiments. Outcomes that did not happen should not be used to evaluate observed outcomes. They point out that the goal of a data analysis is to make an inference from the particular experiment which has generated the data, not from a hypothetical infinite repetition of experiments. Widely used methods such as tests of significance and confidence procedures are subject to these criticisms. The critics agree that frequentist ideas may be relevant prior to carrying out an experiment, but are irrelevant after the experiment is carried out. Nevertheless, these frequentist-based methods have proven to be very useful in practice. Their applicability is continuing to expand despite the presence of sharp criticisms.

For example, suppose $X_1, X_2, \ldots, X_n$ represent iid random variables following a $N(\theta, \sigma^2)$ distribution with θ unknown and σ^2 known. The $100(1 - 2\alpha)\%$ **confidence interval** is $\bar{x} \pm z_\alpha \sigma \sqrt{n}$, where $\bar{x}$ is the sample mean and z_α is the normal deviate which cuts off probability α in the tail of the normal distribution. The formal probability statement is $\Pr\{\bar{X} - z_\alpha \sigma / \sqrt{n} < \theta < \bar{X} + z_\alpha \sigma / \sqrt{n}\} = 1 - 2\alpha$. For any fixed $\bar{x}$, the population mean is either within the interval or is outside the interval. Hence, this statement only assigns a probability 0 or 1 that the population mean θ is included within the interval. The probability $(1 - 2\alpha)$ refers to the process of calculating such intervals over infinite repetitions of the experiment. Operationally, confidence coefficients are usually chosen to be high (95% or 99%) and individuals "act" as if the statement is correct that the population mean is included within the interval. An additional criticism of confidence intervals is that no distinction is made as to whether the population parameter is likely to have a higher probability of being in the neighborhood of $\bar{x}$ compared with being at the ends of the interval. Intuitively, most individuals would agree that the value of the parameter is more likely to be in a neighborhood of $\bar{x}$ compared with being located in a neighborhood around the boundary of the confidence interval.

The operational use of confidence regions is essentially associating a "degree of belief" with the statement that the parameter θ is located within the calculated confidence region on the basis of specific data. The high values chosen for confidence coefficients are so close to unity, that practitioners behave as if the statement is "certain". However, this same idea of using a degree of belief to measure

the uncertainty of an inference can also be used to ascribe different degrees of belief for comparing values within a confidence region. To illustrate ideas, consider the calculation of confidence intervals for a mean as described earlier. Suppose a spectrum of confidence intervals is calculated by choosing different confidence coefficients. The point $\bar{x}$ is a degenerate confidence interval with confidence zero. Then for any potential value of the population parameter θ', there corresponds a confidence interval for which θ' is the end-point, i.e., the normal deviate corresponding to $z_{\alpha'} = \sqrt{n}(\theta' - \bar{x})/\sigma$ (if $\theta' > \bar{x}$) or $z_{\alpha'} = \sqrt{n}(\bar{x} - \theta')/\sigma$ (if $\theta' < \bar{x}$). Then the ratio of degrees of belief comparing the value θ' relative to $\bar{x}$ is α' for the population mean. Hence each end-point of a 95% two-sided confidence interval has a degree of belief of 0.025 of being the population mean compared with the sample average, whereas each end-point of a 10% two-sided confidence interval ($z_{0.45} = 0.12$) has a degree of belief of 0.45 (collectively 0.90) of being the population mean relative to $\bar{x}$.

Among the most widely used techniques in the frequentist theory of inference is the test of significance (*see* **Hypothesis Testing**). Central to a test of significance are the **null** and **alternative hypotheses**, i.e. $H_0: \theta = \theta_0$ and $H_1: \theta \neq \theta_0$. The alternative hypothesis can also be one-sided, $H_1: \theta > \theta_0$ or $H_1: \theta < \theta_0$. The test of significance consists of calculating evidence which is "unfavorable" to the null hypothesis. The test of significance consists of using a statistic $T(x)$ so that large values of $T(x)$ indicate departures from the null hypothesis $H_0: \theta = \theta_0$. If $T_0(x)$ represents the value of the statistic from an experiment, then the test of significance calculates $P = \Pr\{T(X) \geq T_0(x) | \theta = \theta_0\}$. This so-called **P value** is interpreted as discrediting the null hypothesis if P is small (usually $P \leq 0.05$) and in favor of the null hypothesis if P is large. The role of the alternative hypothesis is to specify the statistic $T(x)$.

The P value is widely interpreted as summarizing the statistical evidence of an experiment. If a small value is calculated ($P \leq 0.05$), then either one has observed a rare event if H_0 is true, or if H_0 is not true, then the model for carrying out the calculation (assuming $\theta = \theta_0$), is wrong. Ordinarily the conclusion is made that the model is incorrect and H_0 is rejected.

The logic of the significance test is that if the observed $T_0(x)$ is evidence against the null hypothesis, then larger values of $T(x)$ would constitute even stronger evidence against H_0. The logic of significance tests is questioned, in that a hypothesis may be rejected on the basis of experimental outcomes which were not observed.

The test of significance does not recognize that there may be different interpretations on the P value which are dependent on both the sample size and the magnitude of the deviation from H_0. An experiment in which there is a negligible deviation from the null hypothesis, but having a very large sample size, will result in a small P value, whereas an experiment in which there is a large deviation from H_0, but with a small sample size, may not result in small P value. The uncritical use of tests of significance may result in misleading conclusions. It is often recommended that: (i) if P is small, then information should be presented on the magnitude of the deviation from the null hypothesis, and (ii) if P is large, then evidence should be presented on the power of the test.

Randomization and Permutation Tests

One of the important applications of significance tests is when the sample space is generated by the investigator. This has no analogy with any of the other methods of inference. It occurs whenever an experimental design makes use of randomization. We shall refer to these tests as **randomization tests**.

To illustrate ideas, consider an experiment where the location parameters of two treatment groups are to be compared by a significance test. The most widely used example is a randomized clinical trial in which patients are assigned to each of two treatment groups such that each patient has the same probability of being assigned to each group. If there are $2n$ patients available for the experiment and each group is assigned n patients, then there will be

$$N = \binom{2n}{n}$$

possible assignments. Hence there will be N points in the sample space. Suppose the null hypothesis is that there is no difference in outcome among the two groups. If $\bar{x}_1$ and $\bar{x}_2$ represent the sample average for each group, then $\bar{x} = (\bar{x}_1 + \bar{x}_2)/2$ will always be constant for the experiment. Hence, to show a difference in the location parameters the differences between the two sample averages $\bar{x}_1 - \bar{x}_2 = (\bar{x}_1 - \bar{x})$ will be considered. The sample space will consist of N possible values of the differences between the

two sample averages, each having probability equal to $1/N$ of arising due to the randomization. Hence, if $D_0 = |\bar{x}_1 - \bar{x}_2|$ represents the absolute value of the observed difference between the group sample averages, then the test of significance calculates $P = $ (number of absolute differences $\geq D_0$)/N. No further assumptions need to be made about the probability distributions of the outcomes. Essentially the randomization tests are distribution-free. The validity of the procedure is justified by the randomization which injected probability into the experiment. Of course, the inference only applies to patients who are in the clinical trial, i.e. the inference procedure concludes which is the best treatment for the population of patients that have been entered in the trial. To have a broader inference of making the conclusions apply to the population of patients having disease, it would be necessary to have a random sample of patients entered on the clinical trial.

A closely related set of procedures are *permutation tests*. We distinguish between randomization and permutation tests. Randomization tests are characterized by the investigator purposely introducing probability into the experimental design, whereas in permutation tests it is *assumed* that the sample space consists of equally likely outcomes. Consider the following example of a permutation test. Suppose the water supply in a community was a blend coming from several sources. Depending on the location of the residence, there would be different amounts of water from each source in the blend of water available to each residence. One of the water sources was found to be contaminated. From the time the contaminated source was put into service until the discovery of contamination there were 20 live births in the community. Two babies were born with congenital abnormalities. The amount of water going to each mother's residence during her pregnancy was known during this period of time. Is there an association between the contaminated water and birth defects? A permutation test would assume that each baby has the same risk of having a congenital abnormality. Hence there will be

$$\binom{20}{2} = 190$$

different ways in which two birth defect infants can be distributed among the 20 infants. If the residences with the two highest amounts of contaminated water also had the two birth defects, then this could happen with probability $P = 1/190 = 0.005$ if

2038   Inference

there is no relationship between birth defects and
the contaminated water supply. This probability is so
low that the frequentist would conclude a relationship
between contaminated water and birth defects. Most
people would intuitively agree there may be a relationship. A P value of 0.05 would arise if the two
birth defect babies came from residences in which
the amount of contaminated water delivered to the
households during pregnancy ranked fourth and fifth
highest. There are nine other more extreme outcomes
than the observed fourth and fifth. If pairs of numbers represent the rankings then these outcomes are:
(1, 2), (1, 3), (1, 4), (1, 5), (2, 3), (2, 4), (2, 5), (3, 4)
and (3, 5). Since under the permutation test assumption any one of the possible 190 outcomes has the
same chance of occurring, the number of outcomes
equal to or more extreme than the one observed is
$10/190 = 0.053$.

The randomization and permutation tests have
generated the field of distribution-free or **nonparametric** methods. These methods do not require knowledge of the probability distribution of the observed
outcome, as our two examples illustrate. To ease
computations the observations are often replaced by
ranks or **scores**. Very little statistical efficiency is
lost by these substitutions.

Conditioning

An important modification of frequentist inference is
the possibility of using information (data) to consider
only a subset of the sample space. This may be done
by conditioning on some aspect of the observed data
which will result in a reduced sample space (*see*
Conditionality Principle). The conditioning can only
be done after the experiment has been completed
and the data are available. Fisher [17] has advocated
conditioning on the relevant subset of the sample
space. The conditional sample space is also referred
to as *recognizable subsets* or *reference sets*.

Cox [10] presented a very interesting example
which leads one to make a conditional inference on
a recognizable subset. His example is as follows.
Suppose there are two normal populations, $N(\theta, \sigma_1^2)$
and $N(\theta, \sigma_2^2)$, having the same mean, but different
variances. The mean is unknown, but the variances
are known with $\sigma_1^2 \gg \sigma_2^2$. The experiment consists
of choosing a population with probability 1/2 and
drawing one observation, x. The population is known
which is sampled. Consider a test of $H_0: \theta = 0$ vs.

$H_1: \theta = \theta' \simeq \sigma_1$. Consider two tests – a conditional
and an unconditional test to be made at an $\alpha =
0.05$ level of significance. The conditional test is
made on the population from which the sample was
drawn. This leads to rejection regions $x > 1.64\sigma_1$
or $x > 1.64\sigma_2$ depending on which population has
been sampled. However, this is not the most powerful test over the entire sample space. Application of
the Neyman–Pearson theory results in a test which
approximately has rejection regions $x > 1.28\sigma_1$ or
$> 5\sigma_2$ depending on which population has been sampled. If the sample is from the second population,
then almost complete discrimination is made between
$\theta = 0$ against a much larger value of θ. As a result we
can have a significance level of 10% if one is sampling from the first population. The power of the first
test is 0.26 if population one is sampled and nearly
unity if population 2 is sampled. Alternatively, the
unconditional test has a power of 0.80. Thus, considering the overall sample space the first test has an
average power of 0.63. Cox states

> if the object of the analysis is to make statements by
> a rule with certain specified long-run properties, the
> unconditional test just given is in order . . . . If, how-
> ever, our object is to say "what can we learn from
> the data we have", the unconditional test is surely
> no good. The unconditional test says that we can
> assign a higher level of significance than we ordinar-
> ily do, because if we were to repeat the experiment,
> we might sample some other distributions. But this
> fact seems irrelevant to the interpretation of an obser-
> vation which we know may come from a distribution
> with variance σ_1^2. That is, our calculations of power,
> etc. should be made conditionally within the distri-
> bution known to have been sampled.

Cox's example shows that the inference procedure
should not be determined solely by considerations
of power when one is considering repetitions of
the experiment. In this example the indicator of the
population sampled is called an **ancillary statistic**
because it contains no information about θ. In general
an ancillary statistic is defined as a function of the
observations whose distribution is not a function of
the parameter. In Cox's example, if δ is an indicator
variable indicating which experiment is chosen, then
the data are (δ, x) and δ is an ancillary statistic. The
recognizable subset conditions on δ, i.e. $f(x|\delta)$.

Another illuminating example is provided by
Berger & Wolpert [5]. Assume $X_1, X_2 \ldots, X_n$
are iid having a **uniform distribution** over the

interval $\left(\theta - \frac{1}{2}, \theta + \frac{1}{2}\right)$. The sufficient statistics are $U = \min(X_i)$, $V = \max(X_i)$. Their joint distribution is $f(\mu, v) = n(n-1)(v-u)^{n-2}$, $\theta - \frac{1}{2} < \mu \le v < \theta + \frac{1}{2}$. However, $R = V - U$ is an ancillary statistic because its distribution is independent of θ. The distribution of (U, V) conditional on $R = r$ is uniform over the interval $\theta - \frac{1}{2} \le \mu < \theta + \frac{1}{2} - r$ and should be the starting point for the statistical inference. In particular, a $100(1 - \alpha)\%$ confidence interval is $(u + v)/2 \pm (1 - r)(1 - \alpha)/2$. In this example it is clear that the range is an ancillary statistic. However, in other situations the proper ancillary statistic may not be obvious and there may be competitive ancillary statistics.

The problem becomes more complex when $\theta = (\theta_1, \theta_2)$ and the inference is to be made on θ_1 with θ_2 being regarded as a vector of nuisance parameters. If the likelihood factors into

$$L(x|\theta_1, \theta_2) = L_1(\theta_1|x, a(x))L_2(\theta_2|a(x)),$$

then the distribution of $a(x)$ is independent of θ_1 and $a(x)$ is ancillary for θ_1. An example of this likelihood decomposition is when the data consists of pairs (Y_i, X_i), $i = 1, 2, \ldots, n$, which are iid following a bivariate normal distribution with $E(Y_i) = \mu_y$, $\text{var}(Y_i) = \sigma_y^2$, $E(X_i) = \mu_x$, $\text{var}(X_i) = \sigma_x^2$, and $\text{cov}(X_i, Y_i) = \rho\sigma_x\sigma_y$. The object of the inference is on the parameters $\alpha = \mu_y - \beta\mu_x$ and $\beta = \rho\sigma_y/\sigma_x$ as $E(Y_i|X_i) = \alpha + \beta X_i$. The likelihood can be written

$$L(\mu_x, \mu_y, \sigma_x^2, \sigma_y^2, \rho | x, y)$$
$$= L_1(\mu_y, \tau^2, \alpha, \beta | x, y)L_2(\mu_x, \sigma_x^2 | x),$$

where $\tau^2 = \text{var}(Y_i|X_i) = \sigma_y^2(1 - \rho^2)$ and

$$L_1(\mu_y, \tau^2, \alpha, \beta | x, y)$$
$$= \tau^{-n} \exp\left\{-\sum_{i=1}^{n}[y_i - (\alpha + \beta x_i)]^2/2\tau^2\right\}$$

$$L_2(\mu_x, \sigma_x^2 | x)$$
$$= \sigma_x^{-n} \exp\left\{-\sum_{i=1}^{n}(x_i - \mu_x)^2/2\sigma_x^2\right\}.$$

Thus the regression analysis is conditional on the observed values of x_i which are treated as fixed constants.

When the likelihood factors can be written in terms of minimal sufficient statistics which factor into $L(\theta_1, \theta_2 | t_1, t_2) = L_1(\psi | t_1, t_2), L_2(\theta_1, \theta_2 | t_2)$, then it is possible to consider the distribution of t_1 conditional on t_2 in order to make inferences on $\psi = \psi(\theta_1, \theta_2)$. This is the case for the **two by two contingency table** for comparing two **binomial distributions**. Conditioning on the total number of successes allows an inference to be made on the ratio of two **odds** in which one of the success probabilities is regarded as a nuisance parameter. Similarly, for comparing two **Poisson distributions**, with rate parameters (θ_1, θ_2), the likelihood can be written

$$L(\theta_1, \theta_2 | s_1, s_2) = (\theta_1/\theta_2)^{s_1}\theta_2^t \exp[-(\theta_1 + \theta_2)]$$
$$= L_1(\psi = \theta_1/\theta_2 | s_1)$$
$$\times L_2(\theta_1, \theta_2 | t = s_1 + s_2),$$

which admit of an inference on ψ by conditioning on the sum of the observed events. In both of these examples t contains "no information" about the parameter of interest, ψ. Cox [10] proposed a criterion for determining if t gives no information about ψ when nuisance parameters are present.

An important use of invoking a conditional inference arises in some censoring situations. To illustrate ideas suppose an investigator is testing a drug on patients in which the outcome is success or failure. The experiment is carried out until one observes a single failure. Hence the number of observations is a random variable following a **geometric distribution**. However, the investigator has only enough drug to treat 10 patients. The experiment could then have a maximum of 10 patients and the truncated distribution for the sample size would be

$$\Pr\{N = n | N \le 10\} = \theta^{n-1}(1 - \theta)/(1 - \theta^{10}),$$
$$\text{for } n = 1, 2, \ldots, 10,$$
$$\Pr\{N = 10\} = \theta^9.$$

The experiment is carried out and the fifth patient had a failure. Should the statistician use the likelihood $\theta^4(1 - \theta)$ in making the inference, or the truncated likelihood? To continue the story, the investigator tells the statistician afterwards that just before the experiment started the drug manufacturer had agreed to make available as much drug as needed. Hence there would be no need for the truncated distribution. In a final development, the drug manufacturer changed its offer to only make available the amount of drug for a maximum of 20 patients. This would change the truncated distribution. What should the statistician do? The actual experiment did not need the extra drugs, but an unconditional inference would have required taking account of the limited supply. The change of mind of the drug manufacturer would change the truncated probability distribution. Yet the manufacturer's decision had nothing to do with the actual experiment that was carried out with the available drug supply. Common sense dictates that the inference should be made conditional on what happened, not what could have happened. There was enough drug to carry out the experiment as planned. The likelihood should be conditional on the actual drug supply expended.

Estimation

The most widely used methods of **estimation** among frequentists are **minimum variance unbiased (MVU) estimation** and the method of **maximum likelihood**. Other methods in use are the **method of moments** and **generalized estimating equations**. The principle of having **unbiased** estimates sometimes leads to problems. For example, suppose $\overline{X}$ is the sample average of a sequence of n iid random variables having a $N(\theta, \sigma^2)$ distribution with σ^2 known. Then the minimum variance unbiased estimate of θ is the sample average. However, if it is desired to estimate θ^2, then we note that $E(\overline{X}^2) = \theta^2 + \sigma^2/n$. Therefore, if $T = \overline{X}^2 - \sigma^2/n$, $E(T) = \theta^2$ and T is an unbiased estimate of θ^2. However, θ^2 is always nonnegative, but there is a positive probability that $T = \overline{X}^2 - \sigma^2/n$ will be negative giving a nonsensical estimate. In general, if $g(\theta)$ is some function of θ, and T is an unbiased estimate of θ, then $g(T)$ is ordinarily not an unbiased estimate of $g(\theta)$. Despite some anomalies with the concept of unbiased estimation, the applications of the minimum variance unbiased criteria to estimation problems is very useful in applications – especially for models linear in the parameters.

Another widely used estimation procedure is the method of maximum likelihood. Estimates of θ, denoted by $\hat{\theta}$, are formed by maximizing the likelihood function, i.e. $L(\theta|x) = \max_\theta L(\theta|x)$. The properties of the maximum likelihood estimates are that they are: consistent, asymptotic minimum variance unbiased, and asymptotically normal. In addition, the

maximum likelihood estimate has the property that the estimate of $g(\theta)$ is $g(\hat{\theta})$.

Both minimum variance unbiased estimation and maximum likelihood estimation supply both point and confidence region estimates. Their justification is based on properties associated with infinite repetitions of sampling. However, Bayesian ideas have been used to justify maximum likelihood estimation.

Likelihood School of Inference

The use of the likelihood function is basic to many of the methods associated with frequentist inference. It was introduced by Fisher [12–16] as an information summary. It is essentially a minimal sufficient statistic for θ. Edwards [11] discusses the history of the likelihood function, and Berger & Wolpert [5] contains a thorough development of the statistical implications when the likelihood function is used as a basis for inference. Many of the ideas building on Fisher's early work are attributed to Barnard [1–4] and Birnbaum [6, 7].

Fisher initially introduced the likelihood function to obtain maximum likelihood estimates of parameters. The justification for maximum likelihood estimation has been made in terms of its large-sample properties relying on the frequency concepts of probability. Furthermore, ratios of likelihoods form the basis of likelihood ratio tests and the general Neyman–Pearson theory of hypothesis tests. However, all properties of these methods are judged by their behavior over the entire sample space of possible observations. This is at odds with the likelihood school of inference who regard the sample space as irrelevant after the experiment has been done. The only relevant quantities are the sample data, x, and its incorporation into the likelihood function, $L(\theta|x)$.

The basis of all **Bayesian inference** is the likelihood function. If $p(\theta)$ is the **prior distribution** on θ and $\pi(\theta|x)$ is the posterior distribution, then we have the well-known relationship $\pi(\theta|x) \propto L(\theta|x)p(\theta)$. Hence, whatever implications for inference arise from the likelihood function also apply to Bayesian inference methods.

The basis for the use of the likelihood in statistical inference is contained in the likelihood principle (*see* **Foundations of Probability**). It states that all information about θ from an experiment is contained in the likelihood function. Furthermore, two likelihood functions (from the same or different experiments) contain the same information about θ if they are proportional to one another.

The importance of the likelihood function in inference arises from its justification based on the widely accepted ideas of sufficiency and conditionality. Conversely, the likelihood function has been shown to lead to sufficiency and conditionality. These proofs were originally made by Birnbaum [6] and are correct for discrete observations. Others have modified his arguments for the continuous case. We summarize the main ideas borrowing from the development of Berger & Wolpert [5]. The ideas of conditionality and sufficiency have been discussed earlier in this article. There are two versions of each which are modified by the adjectives "weak" and "strong". We informally state the weak versions, which are all that is necessary in the proofs found in the literature.

Weak Conditionality Principle (WCP). Suppose there are two or more possible experiments, each having possibly different probability distributions, and each giving rise to different experimental outcomes. However, they all have in common the same parameter, θ. Consider the mixed experiment in which experiment i is chosen to be carried out with probability p_i. Then the WCP states that the evidence about θ from the mixed experiment is the experiment actually performed.

Weak Sufficiency Principle (WSP). Consider an experiment in which $t(X)$ is a sufficient statistic for θ. Then if x_1 and x_2 represent two different outcomes, but $t(x_1) = t(x_2)$, then the evidence about θ is the same for each outcome.

It has been proved that the WCP and the WSP imply the likelihood principle and conversely the likelihood principle implies both the WCP and WSP. The proof for the continuous case can be found in Berger & Wolpert [5].

The proponents of inference based on the likelihood principle view the rejection of the likelihood principle as also logically rejecting the WSP or WCP. However, the WSP is one of the basic ideas in frequency inference. The WCP is regarded as simply "common sense".

The likelihood principle is incompatible with many of the methods used in the frequency theory of inference. For example, **randomization**, significance tests, hypothesis testing, confidence intervals, and randomization tests are all contraindicated by the likelihood principle. It is of interest that although randomization is rejected by the WCP, there has been no effort to negate randomized clinical trials. The idea of randomized clinical trials and the general idea of randomization appear to have been accepted by the likelihood and Bayesian schools of inference, notwithstanding the variance with the likelihood principle. One reason for accepting randomization is that it is regarded as a way to obtain "balance" among different groups being compared with respect to unknown factors affecting the outcomes.

Censoring which did not occur is considered irrelevant. For example, suppose in a clinical trial patients are only followed for a maximum period of time (say 10 years). If one had data from such a trial where the end-point was death and all patients died within the 10-year period, then the censoring at 10 years is of no consequence. Yet in calculating the behavior of a frequentist statistical procedure, it is necessary to consider infinite repetitions of the trial in which some patients may have survived 10 years and would be censored.

Stopping rules are deemed irrelevant. Hence, **sequential** methods are treated as if data arose from fixed-size experiments. For example, if X is N(θ, σ^2) then one may sample from this population until the sample average exceeds a fixed constant, i.e. $\bar{x} > k\sigma/\sqrt{n}$. By the law of the iterated logarithm (*see* **Limit Theorems**), there is a finite probability that the event will happen. However, for (say) $\theta = 0$ and large k, the necessary number of observations may be very large. If a frequentist desires to exclude $\theta = 0$ from a 95% confidence limit, then it is only necessary to choose $k = 1.96$. Of course, this entire procedure would be misleading from a frequentist point of view. The likelihood argument is that the inference should not interpret the usual confidence interval in the frequency sense. A frequentist would also take account of the ultimate sample size in placing confidence intervals on θ. Alternatively, the Bayesian approach to this problem is to incorporate the possibility of $\theta = 0$ in a prior distribution.

Suppose one observed four successes in 10 trials from sampling a binomial distribution. This gives rise to the likelihood function $L(\theta|x) = \theta^4(1-\theta)^6$, where θ is the probability of success in a single trial. Alternatively, suppose one samples from this population until four successes are observed. If this experiment took 10 observations to observe four successes, then it will give rise to the same likelihood as observing four successes in 10 trials. The likelihood principal would treat both experiments as generating the same information even though the sampling distributions associated with each experiment are different.

One of the principal criticisms of the use of the likelihood function for inference is the need to specify the model generating the data. Furthermore, it does not encompass any nonparametric methods.

Methods for solely using the likelihood function for inference are not well developed. We cite a few examples of the use of a likelihood function for making inferences.

The ratio of likelihoods can measure the relative support of two values of θ, e.g. $L(\theta_1|x)/L(\theta_2|x)$. Since the maximum likelihood estimate $\hat{\theta}$ maximizes the likelihood, it can serve as a normalization factor and one may consider $L(\theta|x)/L(\hat{\theta}|x)$ to measure the relative support of any θ to $\hat{\theta}$. Likelihood contours may be calculated by setting $L(\theta|x)/L(\hat{\theta}|x) = k$ for a range of values of k. If we consider values of the parameter satisfying

$$L(\theta|x)/L(\hat{\theta}|x) \leq k,$$

then, we can obtain an expression analogous to a confidence region for θ.

Using the likelihood when nuisance parameters are present raises complications. Suppose $\theta = (\theta_1, \theta_2)$ and θ_2 is a nuisance parameter. One approach is to substitute the maximum likelihood estimate of $\hat{\theta}_2(\theta_1)$ in the ratio $L(\theta_1, \hat{\theta}_2(\theta_1)|x)L(\hat{\theta}_1, \hat{\theta}_2|x)$. For example, consider the likelihood function of a sample of n observations from a N(m, σ^2) distribution, i.e.

$$L(m, \sigma^2|x) = \sigma^{-n} \exp\left\{-\frac{1}{2}\sum_{i=1}^{n}(x_i - m)^2/\sigma^2\right\}.$$

The maximum likelihood estimate of σ^2, as a function of m, is $\hat{\sigma}^2(m) = \sum_{i=1}^{n}(x_i - m)^2/n$. Then one has

$$L(m, \hat{\sigma}^2(m)|x)/L(\hat{m}, \hat{\sigma}^2|x) = \left\{1 + \frac{(\hat{x} - m)^2}{s^2}\right\}^{-n/2}$$

$$\cong \{1 + t^2/n\}^{-n/2},$$

where $ns^2 = \sum_{i=1}^{n}(x_i - \bar{x})^2$ and $t^2 = n(\hat{x} - m)^2/s^2$. This is the **Student t distribution** (except for the

normalizing constant), but with n in place of $(n - 1)$. If we desired bounds on m, then we could set $L(m, \hat{\sigma}^2(m)|x)/L(\hat{m}, \hat{\sigma}^2|x) \leq k$. Then for large n we have the interval $\hat{x} \pm s(-2\log k)^{1/2}/\sqrt{n}$.

The general application of likelihood methods may be extended by noting that for large samples

$$L(\theta|x)/L(\hat{\theta}|x) \simeq \exp\{-(\theta - \hat{\theta})^2/2\sigma^2(\hat{\theta})\},$$

where

$$\sigma^2(\hat{\theta}) = -\left(\frac{\partial^2 \log \theta}{\partial \theta^2}\right)^{-1}_{\theta=\hat{\theta}}$$

Hence, the maximum likelihood estimate and the estimate of its asymptotic variance can be used to make likelihood-type inferences for large samples. The result extends to the multivariate situation.

Bayesian School of Inference

In this section we illustrate and contrast Bayesian methods of inference with frequency methods. The application of Bayesian methods to problems of medicine and biology is growing. In large measure the expansion in applications is due to the development of new computing **algorithms** which allow the calculations of posterior distributions having large numbers of parameters. This class of computer algorithms are called **Markov chain Monte Carlo** methods. Two widely used algorithms for this purpose are the Gibbs sampler and the Metropolis-Hastings algorithms: cf. Tanner & Wong [34], Smith [31], Tierney [35], Smith & Gelfand [32], and Smith & Roberts [33]. Breslow [8], in a review paper, cites many applications of Bayesian methods to biostatistics, i.e. **longitudinal data** models, **small area estimation**, **risk assessment** based on species to species **extrapolation**, **bioequivalence** and sequential clinical trials (*see* **Data and Safety Monitoring**).

The Bayes paradigm is that all inferences are based on calculating the posterior distribution of θ. The difficulty in utilizing Bayesian methods is due to both the dependence on model specification, and the meaning of Bayesian probability statements. To utilize Bayesian methods it is necessary to specify both the likelihood function and a prior distribution. Prior distributions may be chosen by subjective opinion or may reflect previous data or knowledge. Issues arise when informationless prior distributions are chosen which contain no information or parameters. The interpretation of a Bayesian probability is that it measures a degree of belief. It allows attaching a posterior probability (degree of belief) associated with hypotheses. This is in contrast to frequentist inference which attaches a value of 0 or 1 to the truth of a hypothesis. Bayesian methods are often judged in practice by their behavior over infinite repetitions. The book by Savage [30] still remains as a cogent treatise advocating the use of Bayesian methods.

Elements

The basis of all Bayesian inference is that, "Any inferential process that does not follow from some likelihood function and some set of priors has objectively verifiable deficiencies", cf. [9]. Bayesian inference places probability distributions on parameters. The elements of Bayesian inference are: that a prior distribution $p(\theta)$ summarizes information about θ prior to experimentation; the likelihood $L(\theta|x)$ incorporates information utilizing data; and the posterior distribution $\pi(\theta|x)$ depicts the probability distribution of θ after incorporating the data. More formally, the relationship between these quantities is

$$\pi(\theta|x) \propto L(\theta|x)p(\theta).$$

This expression is a direct consequence of Bayes' theorem and shows how prior beliefs are changed with the availability of data.

The interpretation of $\pi(\theta|x)$ is that it is a degree of belief, taking on values within the unit interval. In what follows it will be assumed for simplicity that θ has a prior distribution having a probability density function. This assumption is not necessary, but it eases the formalism.

Ratios of posterior distributions are often used to indicate "support" for comparing two different values of θ, i.e. $\pi(\theta_1|x)/\pi(\theta_2|x)$. If one of the θs is the mode of $\pi(\theta|x)$ (denoted by θ_m), then $\pi(\theta|x)/\pi(\theta_m|x)$ compares the degree of belief of an arbitrary θ with the modal value. If θ is one dimensional, then a graph of the ratio vs. θ is particularly useful.

Although there is a great deal of debate on the choice of the prior distribution, the importance of the prior distribution diminishes when the sample size is large. This is easily seen by noting that if we write

$L(\theta|x) = \prod_{i=1}^{n} L(\theta|x_i)$, then

$$\log[\pi(\theta|x)] = \log[L(\theta|x)p(\theta)]$$
$$= \sum_{i=1}^{n} \left[\log L(\theta|x_i) + \frac{1}{n} p(\theta) \right],$$

and noting that the second term in brackets goes to zero as $n \to \infty$.

The normalizing constant $P(x)$ is $P(x) = \int_{\Omega} L(\theta|x) p(\theta) \mathrm{d}\theta$ and is the expected value of the likelihood averaged over the prior distribution. The integral is over the parameter space of θ. Hence, the posterior distribution can be written

$$\pi(\theta|x) = L(\theta|x)p(\theta)/P(x).$$

Note that $P(x)$ is proportional to the posterior probability of observing the data x.

An important aspect of Bayesian inference is predicting a future observation (*see* **Prediction**). If y represents a future observation and x represents data already observed, then the predictive likelihood of y is

$$L(y|x) = \int_{\Omega} L_1(\theta|y)\pi(\theta|x)\mathrm{d}\theta,$$

where $L_1(\theta|y)$ is the likelihood of a single new observation. The quantity $L(y|x)$ is the likelihood of observing a future observation given the data represented by x. If $L(y|x)$ is normalized, then

$$f(y|x) = L(y|x) \bigg/ \int_{-\infty}^{\infty} L(y|x)\mathrm{d}y$$

is the predictive distribution of y. It is clear that the predictive distribution is not necessarily restricted to predicting a single observation, but can predict an arbitrary number of observations. The book by Geisser [19] is a principal reference for predictive distributions.

A fundamental problem in statistical inference is to carry out an inference when nuisance parameters are present. The methods of Bayesian inference can deal with the problem in a relatively straightforward way. Suppose $\boldsymbol{\theta} = (\boldsymbol{\theta}_1, \boldsymbol{\theta}_2)$ and inference is to be made on $\boldsymbol{\theta}_1$ with $\boldsymbol{\theta}_2$ regarded as a vector of nuisance parameters. The methods of Bayesian inference deal with this problem by considering the marginal posterior distribution of $\boldsymbol{\theta}_1$, i.e.

$$\pi(\boldsymbol{\theta}_1|x) = \int_{\Omega_2} \pi(\boldsymbol{\theta}_1, \boldsymbol{\theta}_2|x)\mathrm{d}\boldsymbol{\theta}_2.$$

The comparable problem in the frequency theory of inference can be carried out only in special cases when minimal sufficient statistics exist.

Example

To illustrate ideas we shall consider the Bayesian analysis for comparing two binomial distributions. If (p_i, s_i, n_i) represent the success probabilities, number of successes, and sample sizes, respectively, for $i = 1, 2$, then the likelihood is

$$L(p_1, p_2|s_1, s_2)$$
$$= p_1^{s_1}(1 - p_1)^{n_1-s_1} p_2^{s_2}(1 - p_2)^{n_2-s_2}.$$

Define the new parameters (α, β) by the logit transformations (*see* **Logistic Regression**), i.e.

$$\log[p_1/(1 - p_1)] = \alpha, \quad \log[p_2/(1 - p_2)] = \alpha + \beta.$$

Note that $e^\beta = p_2(1 - p_1)/p_1(1 - p_2)$. The reparameterized likelihood can be written

$$L(\alpha, \beta|s, t) = e^{\alpha t + \beta s}/(1 + e^\alpha)^{n_1}(1 + e^{\alpha+\beta})^{n_2},$$

where $t = s_1 + s_2$ and $s = s_2$. The reparameterization allows one to test $H_0 : p_1 = p_2$ by considering β only. The parameter α is a nuisance parameter.

The sampling theory of inference considers the distribution of s conditional on t, which results in α being dropped. This is the basis of the analysis of 2×2 tables with all marginal totals fixed. The explicit conditional distribution is

$$f(s|t, \beta) = C(s, t)e^{\beta s} \bigg/ \sum_{z=0}^{r} C(z, t)e^{\beta z},$$
$$s = 0, \dots, r,$$

when $r = \min(t, n_2)$ and

$$C(s, t) = \binom{n_1}{t - s}\binom{n_2}{s}.$$

The Bayesian analysis finds the posterior distribution of (α, β) from which the marginal distribution of β can be calculated. Let the prior distributions of (α, β) be taken as

$$p(\alpha, \beta) \propto e^{\alpha t' + \beta s'}/(1 + e^\alpha)^{n_1'}(1 + e^{\alpha+\beta})^{n_2'},$$

where the prime quantities are parameters of the prior distribution, but subject to the condition $0 \leq s' \leq t' \leq$

$n_1' + n_2'$. Then the posterior distribution is

$$\pi(\alpha, \beta|s, t) \propto e^{\alpha t'' + \beta s''}/(1 + e^\alpha)^{n_1''}(1 + e^{\alpha+\beta})^{n_2''},$$

where $s'' = s + s'$, $t'' = t + t'$, $n_1'' = n_1 + n_1'$, and $n_2'' = n_2 + n_2'$. Since the form of the posterior is the same as the likelihood, the prior distribution is called a *natural conjugate* or *conjugate distribution*. Finally, the marginal posterior distribution is

$$\pi(\beta|s'', t'') \propto e^{\beta s''} \int_0^1 \frac{v^{t''-1}(1 - v)^{n''-t''-1}dv}{[1 - v + ve^\beta]^{n_2''}},$$

where $n'' = n_1'' + n_2''$. The integral can be found using numerical methods (*see* **Numerical Integration**).

Prior Distributions

The choice of a prior distribution is an important first step in implementing a Bayesian analysis. Prior distributions may be chosen on the basis of other similar experiments, subjective opinion, or the acknowledgment that nothing is known about the parameters, and the prior is informationless.

There is a great deal of debate when the prior distribution is informationless. Jeffreys [20] proposed that if a parameter takes on values over the real line, that the prior distribution be uniform, whereas if θ takes on values over the positive real line, that $\log \theta$ have a uniform distribution. Therefore the informationless prior for location and scale parameters, as suggested by Jeffreys, are $p(m) = 1$ $(-\infty < m < \infty)$ for a location parameter and $p(\sigma) = 1/\sigma$ $(0 < \sigma < \infty)$ for a scale parameter. Both are improper distributions in that their integrals over the parameter space do not exist. Another view of the improper prior distribution for the scale parameter is that it is flat over the range of the parameters of the likelihood functions. Therefore the posterior distribution is essentially the likelihood function.

Nevertheless the posterior distributions do satisfy all conditions for distribution functions. For example, suppose $X_1, \dots, X_n$ are iid $N(m, \sigma^2)$ with m and σ^2 both unknown. The likelihood function is

$$L(m, \sigma^2|\mathbf{x}) = \sigma^{-n} \exp\left\{-\frac{1}{2}\sum_{i=1}^{n}(x_i - m)^2/2\sigma^2\right\},$$

resulting in the posterior distribution

$$\pi(m, \sigma^2|\mathbf{x}) \propto L(m, \sigma)/\sigma.$$

If the marginal distribution of m is obtained by integrating over σ, then we obtain

$$\int_0^\infty \pi(m, \sigma^2|\mathbf{x}) \mathrm{d}\sigma \propto [1 + t^2/(n-1)]^{-(n-1)/2},$$

with $t^2 = n(\bar{x} - m)^2/s^2$, $s^2 = \sum_{1=1}^n (x_i - \bar{x})^2/(n - 1)$, which is Student's t with $n - 1$ degrees of freedom. Finally, integrating our Student's t results in unity, i.e.

$$\int_{-\infty}^\infty \int_0^\infty \pi(m, \sigma^2|\mathbf{x}) \mathrm{d}\sigma \mathrm{d}m = 1.$$

Jeffreys has also suggested an algorithm for constructing informationless priors on the basis of the Fisher information. If $X_1, X_2, \ldots, X_n$ are iid with likelihood function $L(\sigma|\mathbf{x}) = \prod_{i-1}^n f(x_i|\theta)$, then the Fisher **information** in the sample is

$$I_n(\theta) = \mathrm{E}\left(\frac{\partial \log L(\theta|x)}{\partial \theta}\right)^2$$

$$= n\mathrm{E}\left(\frac{\partial \log f(x|\theta)}{\partial \theta}\right)^2 = nI(\theta).$$

Jeffreys' algorithm for an informationless prior is $p(\theta) \propto I(\theta)^{1/2}$. Since the Fisher information is invariant under transformations, the Jeffreys algorithm is also invariant with respect to transformations. The Jeffreys alogrithm for many parameters is to take $p(\theta) \propto |I(\theta)|^{1/2}$, where $|I(\theta)|$ is the determinant of the matrix of partial cross derivatives.

An important class of prior distributions is when the posterior distribution belongs to the same family of distributions as the prior distributions. These are called *conjugate* or *normal conjugate* prior distributions. For example, consider the distribution of the sample mean arising from n iid observations arising from a N(m, σ^2) with σ^2 known. The likelihood is $L(m|x) = \exp[-n(\bar{x} - m)^2/2\sigma^2]$. The conjugate prior distribution is $p(m) \propto \exp[-n'(m - m')^2/2\sigma^2]$, where (n', m') are parameters of the prior distribution. Then the posterior distribution of m is

$$\pi(m|x) \propto L(m|x)p(m) \propto \exp[-n''(m - m'')/2\sigma^2],$$

where $n'' = n + n'$ and $m'' = (n\bar{x} + n'm')/n''$. Although the quantity n in the likelihood is an integer, the parameter n' is not restricted to be an integer but only to be nonnegative. Note that as $n' \to 0$, $p(m) \propto 1$, which results in an improper prior in the limit. The form of the posterior distribution shows that the prior distribution contributed n' observations having a mean of m' to the likelihood. The informationless prior corresponding to $n' \to 0$ contributes no information to the likelihood.

There exist conjugate prior distributions for all of the distributions having minimal sufficient statistics. The book by Raiffa & Schlaifer [29] contains a compendium and an extensive discussion of conjugate prior distributions. In all of these conjugate prior distributions it is possible to interpret the parameters of the prior as adding additional information to the data.

To cite another example, in addition to the normal distribution, consider the likelihood arising from observing s successes out of n trials from a binomial distribution. The likelihood is $L(\theta|s) = \theta^s(1 - \theta)^{n-s}$ and the conjugate prior is $p(\theta) \propto \theta^{s'}(1 - \theta)^{n'-s'}(0 \leq s' \leq n')$ resulting in the beta posterior distribution. $\pi(\theta|s) \propto \theta^{s''}(1 - \theta)^{n''-s''}$, with $s'' = s + s'$ and $n'' = n + n'$. The prior distribution has contributed s' successes from n' trials. Jeffreys [10] proposed that the informationless prior for this situation take $s' = 1/2$ and $n' = 1$, i.e. $p(\theta) \propto [\theta(1 - \theta)]^{-1/2}$. The prior contributes a "half" a success from a single trial to the likelihood.

In any event, there is a determination of the information for every conjugate prior distribution. As a result, if the prior is based on past information, than it can lead to the fitting of the parameters of the conjugate prior distributions. The same remark holds for choosing priors by a subjective assessment. Any subjective assessment that is incorporated into a conjugate prior can be interpreted with regard to its information content.

Over the past several decades much of the debate concerning Bayesian inference has been concentrated on the use of prior distributions. It is unlikely that there will be closure on this topic. However, when the prior distribution can be interpreted with respect to information content, priors having information equivalent or less than one unit of information and which are smooth over the parameter space are unlikely to have a major effect on the likelihood function.

References

[1] Barnard, G.A. (1947). The meaning of significance level, *Biometrika* **34**, 179–182.

[2] Barnard, G.A. (1949). Statistical inference (with discussion), *Journal of the Royal Statistical Society, Series B* **11**, 115–139.

[3] Barnard, G.A. (1967). The use of the likelihood function in statistical inference, in *Proceedings of the Fifth Berkeley Symposium on Mathematical Statistics and Probability*. University of California Press, Berkeley.

[4] Barnard, G.A. (1974). On likelihood, in *Proceedings of the Conference on Foundational Questions in Statistical Inference*, O. Barndorff-Nielsen, P. Blaesild, & G. Schou, eds. Department of Theoretical Statistics, University of Aarhus.

[5] Berger, J.O. & Wolpert, R.L. (1984). *The Likelihood Principle*. Institute of Mathematical Statistics, Hayard.

[6] Birnbaum, A. (1962). On the foundations of statistical inference, *Journal of the American Statistical Association* **57**, 269–306.

[7] Birnbaum, A. (1972). More on concepts of statistical evidence, *Journal of the American Statistical Association* **67**, 858–861.

[8] Breslow, N. (1990). Biostatistics and Bayes, *Statistical Science* **5**, 269–298.

[9] Cornfield, J. (1969). The Bayesian outlook and its application (with discussion), *Biometrics* **25**, 617–657.

[10] Cox, D.R. (1958). Some problems connected with statistical inference, *Annals of Mathematical Statistics* **29**, 357–371.

[11] Edwards, A.W.F. (1972). *Likelihood*. Cambridge University Press, Cambridge.

[12] Fisher, R.A. (1921). On the mathematical foundations of theoretical statistics, *Philosophical Transactions of the Royal Society of London, Series A* **222**, 309–368.

[13] Fisher, R.A. (1970). *Statistical Methods for Research Workers*. Oliver & Boyd, Edinburgh.

[14] Fisher, R.A. (1925). Theory of statistical estimation, *Proceedings of the Cambridge Philosophical Society* **22**, 700–725.

[15] Fisher, R.A. (1934). Two new properties of mathematical likelihood, *Proceedings of the Royal Society of London, Series A* **144**, 285–307.

[16] Fisher, R.A. (1935). The fiducial argument in statistical inference, *Annals of Eugenics* **6**, 391–398.

[17] Fisher, R.A. (1956). *Statistical Methods and Scientific Inference*. Oliver & Boyd, Edinburgh.

[18] Fisher, R.A. (1966). *The Design of Experiments*, 8th Ed. Oliver & Boyd, Edinburgh.

[19] Geisser, S. (1993). *Predictive Inference: An Introduction*. Chapman & Hall, New York.

[20] Jeffreys, H. (1961). *Theory of Probability*, 3rd Ed. Oxford University Press, Oxford.

[21] Lehmann, E.L. (1983). *Theory of Point Estimation*. Wiley, New York.

[22] Lehmann, E.L. (1986). *Testing Statistical Hypotheses*, 2nd Ed. Wiley, New York.

[23] Neyman, J. (1937). Outline of a theory of statistical estimation based on the classical theory of probability, *Philosophical Transactions of the Royal Society of London, Series A* **236**, 333–380.

[24] Neyman, J. & Pearson, E.S. (1933). On the testing of statistical hypotheses in relation to probabilities a priori, *Proceedings of the Cambridge Philosophical Society* **29**, 492–510.

[25] Neyman, J. & Pearson, E.S. (1933). On the problem of the most efficient tests of statistical hypotheses, *Philosophical Transactions of the Royal Society of London, Series A* **231**, 289–337.

[26] Neyman, J. & Pearson, E.S. (1936). Sufficient statistics and uniformly most powerful tests of statistical hypotheses, *Statistical Research Memoirs* **1**, 113–137.

[27] Neyman, J. & Pearson, E.S. (1936). Unbiased critical regions of Type A and Type A_1, *Statistical Research Memoirs* **1**, 1–37.

[28] Neyman, J. & Pearson, E.S. (1938). Contributions to the theory of testing statistical hypotheses, *Statistical Research Memoirs* **2**, 25–57.

[29] Raiffa, H. & Schlaifer, R. (1961). *Applied Statistical Decision Theory*. Graduate School of Business Administration, Harvard University, Cambridge, Mass.

[30] Savage, L.J. (1954). *The Foundations of Statistics*. Methuen, London.

[31] Smith, A.F.M. (1991). Bayesian computational methods, *Philosophical Transactions of the Royal Society of London, Series A* **337**, 369–386.

[32] Smith, A.F.M. & Gelfand, A.F. (1992). Bayesian statistics without tears: a sampling–resampling perspective, *American Statistician* **46**, 84–88.

[33] Smith, A.F.M. & Roberts, G.O. (1993). Bayesian computation via the Gibbs sampler and related Markov chain Monte Carlo methods, *Journal of the Royal Statistical Society, Series B* **55**, 3–23.

[34] Tanner, M. & Wong, W. (1987). The calculation of posterior distributions by data augmentation (with discussion), *Journal of the American Statistical Association* **82**, 528–550.

[35] Tierney, L. (1994). Markov chains for exploring posterior distributions (with discussion), *Annals of Statistics* **22**, 1701–1762.

(*See also* **Inference, Foundations of**)

M. ZELEN

Inference, Foundations of

Humans learn considerable information (and misinformation) from birth and throughout their lives. This ability arises through some combination of genetic influences, direct experience in the surrounding environment, and input from others, both through interpersonal interaction (i.e. parents, friends, teachers, etc.) and stored and supplied societal information (i.e.

media, books, paintings, digital information, analog information, etc.). Some learning is relatively direct and easy to assimilate (e.g. falling off a bicycle can be painful and lead to injury), but much other learning is more difficult, because of both variability in observed relationships and the complex and sophisticated underlying models and concepts that "explain" observations (e.g. the currently accepted models of particle physics or molecular biology). Multiple distinct intellectual pathways have contributed to the current methods of biostatistical inference. These pathways include randomness, **probability**, regular variability, statistical modeling, and observational vs. experimental data collection.

The ideas of randomness go back at least to biblical times where the casting of lots was used. However, the modern ideas of probability were initially developed with respect to games of chance [8]. **Jacob Bernoulli's** proof of the strong **law of large numbers** [12] set the scene for interpreting probabilities as the limit of the proportion of times that an event would occur in a long sequence of repeated identical trials. In this context it was natural that probability was thought of in a frequentist sense: "fair" games could be repeated with equal probabilities of differing outcomes in cards or dice.

A second intellectual thread was the observation that in repeatable situations with variable outcomes there was a regularity or **pattern** to the variability observed. Repeated measurements taken in the (presumed) same or similar situation clustered around some (presumed) true value. It was natural to consider ways of dealing with this variation in outcome, and natural that at some point the mathematical theory of probability theory would be used as one possible way of assessing the variability.

Probability as a concept becomes more difficult as one thinks about it. Einstein, for example, did not believe that probability was an inherent property of the universe: his view is often quoted as "God does not play dice with the universe" [3]. However, most physicists believe that probability is basic to the quantum mechanical structure of the universe. Regular variability that could "mimic" probability theory could also result from the mathematics of **chaos theory** that make it clear that very small changes in initial conditions, for even relatively simple nonlinear systems, can lead to dramatic changes in outcome over time. If for no other reason than an inability to delineate precisely the initial conditions,

variability in biological systems can be expected to be the commonly observed situation. As an example of possible chaos theory, multiple card shuffling could be expected (with a number of shuffles) to approximate the usual mathematical model that all permutations are equally likely; yet there are skilled individuals who can shuffle cards with perfect knowledge of how the cards will interleave.

At the same time there are (seemingly) unique situations where only one event will be observed. For example, one presidential election, one football game, or the treatment of an individual patient may be at issue. Yet individuals evaluate such situations and at least implicitly attach **odds** or probabilities to these situations; some consistently do an excellent job, while others do not do so well. This suggests that the evaluation of probabilities or the **likelihood** of outcomes also can be related to the personal or individual beliefs of humans. This **subjective** version of probability, or **Bayesian** probability, has become another contributor to current thinking about statistical inference. Of course, thinking Bayesians also believe in an external frequentist probability (otherwise one could not talk about the data swamping the prior probability, or a state of nature). Savage [11] argues that unless one follows a Bayesian behavior system one will be in a position to lose, *no matter what the true state of nature*, if forced to bet. Note, however, that in this formulation the state of nature has an external (frequentist?) probability associated with it. Modern philosophers of science have discussed extensively the concepts of probability and **causality** when the relationships are statistical rather than deterministic. Such considerations are expected, given the current physical models of the universe. Probabilities in deterministic situations, where maximal information is not available, that have some frequency distribution of the outcome, lead to frequency-based probabilities. Because one may wish to use probabilities in a setting where an experimental set-up with inherent indeterminism may not be repeated, there is also a need for probability that is not personal or subjective but that also is not justified by appeal to the strong law of large numbers. However, here the probability is inherent in the laws governing certain situations (e.g. quantum mechanics in physics); such probabilities are sometimes called propensity-based probabilities (e.g. [6]). In most statistical settings these latter two concepts of probability are combined and called *frequentist*.

Inference in the statistical sense has been used to describe procedures that analyze data that come from (at least conceptually) some underlying set of probability distributions. When this is the case statements can often be made that only make sense in the context of the underlying distributions. For example, one constructs an interval in such a way that 95% of the time the mean of the underlying probability distribution for repeated samples from the distribution will lie in the interval; that is, one constructs a 95% **confidence interval**. Or one compares the change in sitting diastolic blood pressure from a baseline measurement to 12 weeks in two groups: one that is **randomized** to a placebo treatment and another group randomized to a new presumed antihypertensive drug. The *P* **value** for a treatment difference is used to summarize the strength of evidence for a treatment difference. Or, in the same experiment, a Bayesian **prior distribution** about the treatment differences is updated given the data from the experiment, and the probability that the change in blood pressure is more in the new drug group is used as a summary to show the new drug is effective. In each case the inference (in the every-day use of the word) is summarized by *statements that depend upon an underlying probability model combined with the observed data*. Such inference is *statistical inference*. Statisticians often perform other activities that are not statistical inference *per se*, but when combined with further processing of the data are associated with statistical inference in many situations. Descriptive statistics, including summary statistics (e.g. sample **mean, median, standard deviation**, minimum, and maximum), **graphic** plots (e.g. scatter diagrams, histograms, line graphs of mean or median values), computer visualization of multiple variables at a time, or two-dimensional projections of higher dimensional space, etc., are not statistical inference *per se*. However, plots with confidence sets or intervals would directly involve statistical inference.

The concepts of probability theory were integrated into one formal theory of statistical inference by **Jerzy Neyman** and **Egon Pearson** (e.g. [10]). They developed their formal framework for **hypothesis testing** introducing the familiar concepts of the **null hypothesis**, the **alternative hypothesis**, type I and II errors (*see* **Level of a Test**), **power**, etc. Some philosophers of science conclude that scientific paradigms can never be essentially (i.e. up to statistical variability) proven to be true. They can

only be shown to be consistent with the facts at hand; however, further data or theory combined with data may show them to be inconsistent. While this is true for complex theories, particularly in physics, for other situations (e.g. a drug lowers blood pressure on the average in some population), "theories" or "facts" could be more clearly established conceptually. Hypothesis testing, combined with Occam's razor (the simplest possible explanation is to be preferred; *see* **Parsimony**), gives a paradigm for scientific endeavor. Hypothesis testing fits nicely into this paradigm as "null hypotheses" (usually straw men shown to be false) are to be rejected. The new theory had many other benefits: by selecting conventional levels for the significance level it led to an acceptable level of scientific proof that is largely used today both by scientific journals and regulatory authorities; it allowed experiments to be designed and sample sizes to be computed using the concept of statistical power, or equivalently type I and type II errors. Hypothesis testing about the parameters of a state of nature leads naturally to the concept of confidence regions and intervals because of the duality between hypothesis testing and confidence intervals (e.g. [2]).

Hypothesis testing was not without its problems. Cornfield [4, 5] lists problems with the formal hypothesis testing paradigm. For example, if the significance level is formally set at 0.05 and one performs an experiment and fails to reject a null hypothesis, then no amount of additional evidence should ever be allowed to lead to rejection of the null hypothesis! Furthermore, in a complex situation hypothesis testing can be used to plan experiments, but if one wants formally to take into account already known, but very complex, facts and/or beliefs, then this is difficult to incorporate rationally into the formal scientific inference. Bayesian statistics would appear to be the solution to the incorporation of complex facts already known. The Bayesian prior estimate of the state of nature (or the distribution of a parameter(s) of interest) seems ideal for such situations. However, there are also problems with using Bayesian statistical methods [7]: (i) different individuals will have (often drastically) different prior beliefs – whose prior distribution should be used; (ii) humans are at best very imperfect Bayesians and cannot process data as probability models suggest we should [9]; and (iii) like the frequentist models, in practice difficulties and new data can arrive that would not have been adequately addressed in the elicitation of prior beliefs.

(For example, new animal data suggest a toxicity problem with the long-term use of a drug or biologic; another drug with the same molecular mechanism of action reports findings.) There is no known method of statistical inference that can withstand all rational criticism. Thus, the actual application of statistics to important biostatistical problems necessarily is far from **algorithmic**; scientific judgment and reasoning, as well as intuition, often enter into important decision making in addition to formal statistical inference – as embodied, say, by hypothesis testing, confidence regions, model building, or Bayesian analysis. That is to say, while statistical inference is based upon the mathematical theory of probability, the decisions and understandings that result from the statistical inference have many arbitrary aspects, both technical (e.g. the significance level to be used in a test) and judgmental (e.g. an experiment has so much **missing data** that one decides to disregard it altogether). This results in important decisions using both statistical inference and other human decision making capacities in many instances. There is good reason to believe that humans are at best very imperfect Bayesian or frequentist statisticians [9].

The rapid continuing increase in computing power has led to innovations in statistical inference methodology. For example, the ability to resample from samples of distributions (e.g. **bootstrap** techniques), to implement **Markov chain Monte Carlo** methods, and to simulate from permutation distributions (especially the randomization distribution; *see* **Randomization Tests**) allow approaches to inference that use the same underlying ideas of the last 60 years but are new techniques that were not feasible a generation ago.

Another important path to understanding modern concepts of inference – especially in biostatistics – is to understand the important difference between observationally collected data and experimental data where the observer can intervene in the system to establish stronger scientific inference. For example, the history of medicine is replete with harmful treatments given for hundreds of years [1]. The **scientific method** and appropriate experimentation has led to rapid progress in science in general, and biology and medicine in particular. Until the advent of the scientific method (or, more realistically, a growing appreciation of the scientific method) plausible, but incorrect, systems of understanding human and animal biology were seemingly accepted if they were internally self-consistent and advocated by authority. Selected subject-matter application areas of biostatistics, besides medical biostatistics, may have other difficulties. For example, epidemiologic studies, ecologic, and wild animal studies are often necessarily restricted to observational data collection and/or mathematical modeling. The inability to experiment gives less cogent scientific inference and potentially a larger probability of mistaken "knowledge" due to potential underlying **biases**. No matter how firm the basis of statistical inference, the possibility of bias from unknown sources cannot be discounted. Other areas, such as plants for food and animal breeding, are more amenable to more classic experimentation; yet even here the heterogeneity is a large issue (say compared with electrons which are all assumed to be the same in particle physics). The idea of randomization, as introduced by **R.A. Fisher**, allows much more cogent experimentation, especially in human populations, than observational data or even less controlled experimental data that may be subject to unknown important biases.

In the previous paragraph the term *the scientific method* was used. There appears to be no entirely satisfactory definition that encompasses all the situations where one might use this term. Often books on the philosophy of science introduce it by implication. One definition is: "a method of research in which a problem is identified, relevant data are gathered, a hypothesis is formulated from these data, and the hypothesis is empirically tested" [13]. Such a definition is in accord with the statistical theory of hypothesis testing.

Statistical inference in the medical biological sciences has difficulties that do not arise in the physical sciences, at least to the same degree. One of the cornerstones of modern science is the ability to replicate results. If one group reports a simple method of cold fusion, then other experimenters around the world may try to replicate the results. In experiments with animals, and especially humans, the sanctity of life introduces ethical concerns. In certain situations there may be a strong **ethical** and practical prohibition against replicating a result. If a therapy has been "shown" to prolong life as compared with a placebo, then further placebo-controlled experimentation may be considered unethical and/or impracticable. The lack of the ability to replicate can lead to the unchecked propagation of a false "fact". Furthermore, because of the need to monitor for patient benefit and/or safety, a minimal amount of information adequate for showing benefit or harm is the rule not the exception. That is to say, if a society decides that proof consists of rejecting a null hypothesis at the 0.05 significance level, then a randomized **clinical trial** with mortality as an endpoint might be argued to be unethical if the trial does not stop when reaching this level of significance, taking into account the **multiple comparison** issues of sequential monitoring. All experimentation seems beset with difficulties, and without a doubt Murphy was an optimist (*cf*. Murphy's Law: Anything that can go wrong will). However, human experimentation may have even deeper difficulties. Subjects may deliberately unblind therapy in a randomized trial (*see* **Blinding or Masking**). Subjects may exercise the right to withdraw, go on vacation, and miss a crucial follow-up visit, etc. The combination of these and other factors leads to more dispute *that is unresolved by convincing data* than in the more "hard" sciences. Statistical inference may investigate the **sensitivity** to such experimental deviations, but the cogency of the results is usually lessened in ways difficult to quantify.

Statistical inference and associated experimental design for drugs, biologics, and devices for human use is further complicated by very important practical matters. The rewards and development costs of new therapies and diagnostic tests for human use are both extremely large in many situations. Also, the competitive nature of the market-place plays a large role in the development of new modalities of treatment or diagnosis. The first sponsor of an approved modality is in a very favorable position. This, plus possible humanitarian reasons, puts a premium on the speed of development. The large stakes place intense pressures on both industry and regulatory agencies. This can result in a very strict adherence to statistical inference guidelines for such research. However, treatments – for example a drug – are rarely all good or bad. An appropriate dose needs to be found; furthermore, the appropriate amount and/or method of delivery may differ for important human subgroups (e.g. race, older individuals and children, individuals with impaired organ function, and genetically distinct subsets). The best designs and development programs from a statistical inference point of view may not be used because of other considerations.

In summary, statistical inference in biostatistics is formally the same as in other applied areas. However, practical and ethical issues can introduce limitations not seen in many other areas of applied statistics.

References

[1]   Ackerknecht, E.H. (1973). *Therapeutics from the Primatives to the 20th Century*. Hafner, New York (translated from the German).

[2]   Bickel, P.J. & Doksum, K.A. (1977). *Mathematical Statistics: Basic Ideas and Selected Topics*. Holden-Day, San Francisco, p. 178.

[3]   Clark, R.W. (1973). *The Life and Times of Einstein. An Illustrated Biography*. Wings Books, New York, p. 216.

[4]   Cornfield, J. (1966). Sequential trials, sequential analysis and the likelihood principle, *American Statistician* **20**, 18–22.

[5]   Cornfield, J. (1969). The Bayesian outlook and its application (with discussion), *Biometrics* **25**, 617–657.

[6]   Fetzer, J.H. (1993). *Philosophy of Science*. Paragon House, New York, p. 97.

[7]   Fisher, L.D. (1996). Commentary: comments on Bayesian and frequentist analysis and interpretation of clinical trials, *Controlled Clinical Trials* **17**, 423–434.

[8]   Hald, A. (1990) *A History of Probability and Statistics and Their Applications before 1750*. Wiley, New York, Chapters 3–5.

[9]   Kahneman, D., Slovic, P. & Tversky, A., eds (1982). *Judgment Under Uncertainty: Heuristics and Biases*. Cambridge University Press, New York.

[10]   Neyman, J. & Pearson, E.S. (1967). *Joint Statistical Papers of J. Neyman and E.S. Pearson*. University of California Press, Berkeley.

[11]   Savage, L.J. (1972). *The Foundations of Statistics*. Dover Publications, New York.

[12]   Stigler, S.M. (1986). *The History of Statistics: The Measurement of Uncertainty before 1900*. The Belknap Press of Harvard University, Cambridge, Mass., Chapter 2.

[13]   *The Random House Dictionary of the English Language*. The Unabridged Edition (1967). Random House, New York, p. 1279.

(*See also* **Foundations of Probability; Inference**)

L. FISHER

Infinitely Divisible Distributions
see Central Limit Theory

Influence *see* Diagnostics

Influence Function in Survival Analysis

The influence function of an estimator was introduced by Hampel [5] in the context of robust estimation (*see* **Robustness**). Broadly speaking, the influence function evaluated at a possible data point x indicates how the estimator is changed by the addition of a data point with value x. As an example, the influence function for the sample mean is identically equal to x, showing that a single data point has an influence on the mean directly proportional to its value. This reflects the fact that the sample mean is very sensitive to **outliers**. However, the influence function for the sample **median** is a step function. The median is the simplest example of an estimator with bounded influence function. Several more **efficient** estimators with bounded influence functions have been proposed as more robust estimators [5]. An introduction to the influence function is given in [9].

The influence function of an estimator is computed by first writing the estimator as a functional of a distribution function. For an estimator that is a function of independent, identically distributed observations, this distribution function will be the empirical distribution function, $F_n(x)$ (*see* **Goodness of Fit**). For example, the sample mean $\overline{X} = n^{-1} \sum X_i$ can be expressed as $\int x dF_n(x)$. This estimates the same functional of the true distribution function $\int x dF(x)$: estimators with this property are called Fisher **consistent**. We can write the sample median as $F_n^{-1}\left(\frac{1}{2}\right)$, (with a suitable definition of inverse for a noncontinuous function), and this estimates $F^{-1}\left(\frac{1}{2}\right)$.

We use the general notation $T(F)$ for a functional of a distribution function. Then we define the influence function for $T(F)$ by

$$IC(x; T, F) = \lim_{t \to 0} t^{-1}\{T[(1-t)F + t\delta_x] - T(F)\},$$
$$(1)$$

if this limit exists. In (1) δ_x is the distribution function that puts mass 1 at the point x. For $T(F) = \int x dF(x)$, we have $IC(x; T, F) = x$, and for $T(F) = F^{-1}\left(\frac{1}{2}\right)$, we have

$$IC(x; T, F) = \begin{cases} \dfrac{1}{f[F^{-1}(1/2)]}, & \text{if } x < 0, \\ 0, & \text{otherwise.} \end{cases}$$

The influence function defined in (1) is constructed from the so-called Gâteaux derivative of the functional T. The definition can be extended by computing the Gâteaux derivative of more complex functionals, such as functionals $T(F, u)$ that depend on an additional real parameter, or bivariate functionals $T(F, G)$, say.

In survival data analysis, the estimators of interest are typically more complex than simple functions of independent and identically distributed observations, and the definition of the influence function needs these more complex functionals. Consider the case of a single sample of independent, possibly **censored**, observations $(X_1, \delta_1), \ldots, (X_n, \delta_n)$, where X_i is the observed failure or censoring time, and δ_i is 1 if X_i is uncensored, and 0, otherwise. Assuming the random censorship model, we write $X = \min(X^0, Y)$, where X^0 has distribution $F(\cdot)$, the failure time distribution of interest, and Y has distribution G.

The influence function of the **Kaplan–Meier** estimate of the survival distribution F was introduced in [8, Eqs. (2.1),(2.2)]. This used a representation, due to Peterson [6], of the cumulative hazard function as a functional of two subsurvival functions: $S_u(\cdot)$, and $S_c(\cdot)$, where $S_u(t) = \Pr(X > t, \delta = 1)$, and $S_c(t) = \Pr(X > t, \delta = 0)$. This gives a pair of influence functions for the Kaplan–Meier estimator of $S(t) = 1 - F(t)$:

$$IC_1(s; T, S_u, S_c)(t)$$
$$= S(t)\left\{\int_0^{\min(s,t)} \frac{dS_u(x)}{(S_u + S_c)^2(x)} + \frac{1(x \leq t)}{(S_u + S_c)(s)}\right\},$$
$$IC_2(s; T, S_u, S_c)(t)$$
$$= S(t)\left\{\int_0^{\min(s,t)} \frac{dS_u(x)}{(S_u + S_c)^2(x)}\right\}.$$

The first term in IC_1 is the effect a new observation at time s has on the estimate of $S(t)$ by increasing the size of the risk set, if $s \leq t$. This is the only effect of a new censored observation, as is seen from the expression for IC_2. The second contribution to IC_1 corresponds to the additional jump point in the Kaplan–Meier estimate of $S(t)$ when a new, uncensored, observation at time s is added.

In addition to providing a descriptive summary of how sensitive an estimator can be to outliers, the influence function can be used to compute the asymptotic variance of an estimator. We assume for notational convenience that we have a simple functional of one distribution function $T(F)$. If this functional is differentiable, then we can write

$$T(G) = T(F) + \mathrm{d}T_F(G - F) + R, \qquad (2)$$

where G is some distribution function, $\mathrm{d}T_F$ is the differential of $T(F)$ and is a linear functional, and R is a remainder term. For many statistical functionals, $\mathrm{d}T_F(G - F)$ will take the form

$$\mathrm{d}T_F(G - F) = \int IC(x; T, F)\mathrm{d}G(x),$$

where IC is defined in (1), but has been standardized so that $\int IC(x)\mathrm{d}F(x) = 0$. If we now let $G = F_n$, then we have an expression for the estimator $T(F_n)$ as the true value $T(F)$, plus a linear combination $n^{-1}\sum IC(X_i; T, F)$ and a random remainder term. Under some conditions that, in particular, ensure that the remainder goes to 0 in a suitable sense as $n \to \infty$, we may conclude that $\sqrt{n}[T(F_n) - T(F)]$ is asymptotically normally distributed with mean 0 and variance $\int IC^2(x; T, F)\mathrm{d}F(x)$.

The argument sketched above is an example of the *functional delta method*, described in [1, II.8], and [4]. The ordinary **delta method** uses an approximate linearization of a nonlinear function to find the limiting distribution of an estimator. The functional delta method uses the same argument with the functional derivative $\mathrm{d}T$ defined by (2). In fact, the functional derivative is not well defined by (2): we need to specify in what sense R converges to 0, as G becomes arbitrarily close to F. There are three main notions of convergence, leading to Gâteaux, compact, and Fréchet differentiability. While the definition of the influence function in (1) uses the weak notion of Gâteaux differentiability, the asymptotic argument requires that T be either compact or Fréchet differentiable. For a fuller discussion of this, see [1, II.8]. Since functional derivatives also obey a chain rule, the functional delta method can be used to find the asymptotic distribution for functions of estimators as well. The asymptotic variance of the cumulative hazard estimator was computed using this method in [8]. The functional delta method is applied to the Kaplan–Meier estimator and several functions of it in [1, IV.3] and to more complex product limit estimators in [1, IV.4].

Another important use of the influence function in survival analysis is to suggest influence **diagnostics**, or case-deletion diagnostics, for use in the **proportional hazards** regression model, analogously to the way regression diagnostics are computed routinely for linear regression models. It is shown in [3] and [10] that a sample estimate of the influence function can be used to approximate $\hat{\beta} - \hat{\beta}_{-i}$, where $\hat{\beta}$ is the usual estimate of the regression parameter in Cox's proportional hazards regression model and $\hat{\beta}_{-i}$ is the estimate obtained when the ith observation is deleted. Storer & Crowley [11] consider various other ways to estimate $\hat{\beta} - \hat{\beta}_i$. Barlow & Prentice [2], in a discussion of various definitions of **residuals** for proportional hazards regression, relate the estimated influence function to a particular type of residual, and thereby also extend the definitions of [3] and [10] to **time-dependent covariates**. Further development, with emphasis on applications, is given in [7]. There is also a helpful summary in [1, VII.3].

References

[1]   Andersen, P.K., Borgan, Ø., Gill, R.D. & Keiding, N. (1993). *Statistical Models Based on Counting Processes*. Springer-Verlag, New York.

[2]   Barlow, W.E. & Prentice, R.L. (1988). Residuals for relative risk regression, *Biometrika* **75**, 65–74.

[3]   Cain, K.C. & Lange, N.T. (1984). Approximate case influence for the proportional hazards regression model with censored data, *Biometrics* **40**, 493–500.

[4]   Gill, R.D. (1989). Non- and semi-parametric maximum likelihood estimators and the von Mises method (Part 1), *Scandinavian Journal of Statistics* **16**, 97–128.

[5]   Hampel, F.R. (1974). The influence curve and its role in robust estimation, *Journal of the American Statistical Association* **69**, 383–394.

[6]   Peterson, A.V. (1977). Expressing the Kaplan–Meier estimator as a function of empirical sub-survival functions, *Journal of the American Statistical Association* **72**, 854–858.

[7]   Pettitt, A.N. & Bin Daud, I. (1989). Case-weighted measures of influence for proportional hazards regression, *Applied Statistics* **38**, 51–68.

[8]   Reid, N. (1981). Influence functions for censored data, *Annals of Statistics* **9**, 78–92.

[9]   Reid, N. (1983). Influence functions, in *Encyclopedia of Statistical Sciences*, Vol. 4, S. Kotz & N.L. Johnson, eds. Wiley, New York, pp. 117–120.

[10] Reid, N. & Crépeau, H. (1985). Influence functions for proportional hazards regression, *Biometrika* **72**, 1–9.

[11] Storer, B.E. & Crowley, J. (1985). A diagnostic for Cox regression and general conditional likelihoods, *Journal of the American Statistical Association* **80**, 139–147.

(*See also* **Residuals for Survival Analysis; Survival Distributions and Their Characteristics**)

N. REID

Information

It is natural to try to quantify the amount of information provided by a set of data concerning an unknown quantity of interest. R.A. Fisher, in a classic 1925 work [1], proposed that the statistical information provided by a set of data on a parameter θ be defined as the inverse of the variance of an **efficient** estimator of θ. This quantity is equal to the Fisher information $I(\theta)$ defined in the article, **Information Matrix**. More broadly, one may define the information provided by a given estimator $\tilde{\theta}$, not necessarily an efficient one, to be the inverse of its variance. Intuitively, the lower the variance of an estimator, the more precisely it estimates the underlying parameter. Thus, the definition just given says simply that information equals precision.

The above concept of information arises in various contexts; here, we give two examples of interest in biostatistics.

The first example is the situation of combining several independent (asymptotically) **unbiased** estimates of the same parameter θ. This situation arises in a number of settings in biostatistics; for example, **stratified** analysis and **meta-analysis**. Typically, estimates are combined by weighted averaging. It is a classical result that the optimal method of weighting, in terms of minimizing the variance of the combined estimator, is to weight each individual estimate, $\tilde{\theta}_i$, according to the inverse of its variance, v_i. This result, which is an easy consequence of the Cauchy–Schwarz inequality, is the most basic version of the weighted **least squares** schemes that abound in applied statistics.

Intuitively, the weight assigned to a given estimate is in proportion to the amount of information contributed by that estimate. The variance of the combined estimator is easily derived, and by reciprocation the information content of the combined estimate is found to be the sum of v_i^{-1}. Thus, it is seen that the information content of an optimally weighted average of several independent estimates is equal to the sum of the information contents of the individual estimates.

The second example is the situation of sequential monitoring in clinical trials (*see* **Data and Safety Monitoring**). With certain popular monitoring schemes, particularly that of Lan & DeMets [3], it is necessary at each interim analysis to have some measure of how far the trial has progressed. A simple measure of trial progress is elapsed calendar time from the date the trial began. Some workers, however, argue that a more appropriate measure of trial progress is the proportion of statistical information accumulated by the time of the interim analysis, relative to the total amount of information that is expected to be accumulated by the planned end of the trial.

This measure of trial progress is often referred to as *information time*. The proportion of information accumulated is reflected fully by the sample size in certain special cases, but not in general. For instance, in a study monitored sequentially using the **logrank test**, the information is reflected by the number of events, while in a longitudinal study analyzed using a mixed linear model with a random slope and intercept for each subject (*see* **Mixed Effects Models for Longitudinal Data**), the information content is a function of the ratio of within-subject to between-subject variance and the observation pattern of the various individuals. See [4] for a more detailed discussion.

The foregoing conceptualizations of information are related, as will be indicated below, to S. Kullback's notion of discrimination information. Kullback's information measure, also known as relative entropy and by various other names, is in turn related to the entropy-based definition of information used in the Shannon–Weaver theory of information and coding. Consider a data vector $\mathbf{X}$ relating to the parameter θ. Let $f(\mathbf{X}|\theta)$ denote the joint density (or mass function) of $\mathbf{X}$ under θ, which, viewed as a function of θ, is the **likelihood** function. In addition, define

$$Z(\theta_1 : \theta_0) = \log \frac{f(\mathbf{X}|\theta_1)}{f(\mathbf{X}|\theta_0)},$$

which is the **likelihood ratio test** statistic for testing $H_0: \theta = \theta_0$ vs. $H_1: \theta = \theta_1$. Kullback defines the mean information for discriminating between these two hypotheses when the true θ value is θ_1 to be

$$\mathrm{Inf}(\theta_1 : \theta_0) = \mathrm{E}_{\theta_1}[Z(\theta_1 : \theta_0)]$$
$$= \int f(\mathbf{X}|\theta_1) \log \frac{f(\mathbf{X}|\theta_1)}{f(\mathbf{X}|\theta_0)} \, d\mathbf{X},$$

where the integral is replaced by a sum when $\mathbf{X}$ is discrete. Kullback demonstrates that this information measure possesses a number of basic properties that one would intuitively expect from an information measure. For example, the information provided by two random vectors $\mathbf{X}$ and $\mathbf{Y}$ is equal to the sum of the information provided by $\mathbf{X}$ and the information associated with the conditional distribution of $\mathbf{Y}$ given $\mathbf{X}$. For more detailed discussion, see [2].

Kullback shows, furthermore, by a Taylor expansion of the likelihood ratio, that if θ_0 and θ_1 are close and suitable regularity conditions hold, then

$$\mathrm{Inf}(\theta_1 : \theta_0) \doteq \tfrac{1}{2} I(\theta_1)(\theta_1 - \theta_0)^2;$$

in the case of a vector parameter, the right-hand side becomes $\tfrac{1}{2}(\theta_1 - \theta_0)^\mathrm{T} \mathbf{I}(\theta)(\theta_1 - \theta_0)$, where $\mathbf{I}(\theta)$ here is the Fisher information matrix. Thus, there is a direct connection between Kullback's notion of information and Fisher's.

If the data are reduced down to some (not necessarily efficient) estimator $\tilde{\theta}$ of θ that is approximately normally distributed with mean θ, then the Fisher information of the reduced data is approximately equal to the inverse of $\mathrm{var}_\theta(\tilde{\theta})$. This observation provides a further way of viewing inverse variance as information.

In particular, considering the **maximum likelihood** estimator (MLE) $\hat{\theta}$ of θ, assuming suitable conditions, it is known that when the sample size is large, the estimator $\hat{\theta}$ is approximately normal. Thus, if the data were reduced down to the MLE $\hat{\theta}$, then the Fisher information for the reduced data would be approximately equal to the inverse of $\mathrm{var}_\theta(\hat{\theta})$. Now this quantity is equal precisely to the Fisher information for the unreduced data. In other words, the information contained in the MLE is approximately equal to the information in the entire data, reflecting the efficiency of the MLE.

This finding may be arrived at also by a route starting from the Kullback definition of information. Suppose that θ_0 and θ_1 are close and the sample size is large. Then, assuming suitable conditions, it is known that the likelihood ratio statistic $Z(\theta_1 : \theta_0)$ is approximately equivalent to the Wald statistic $Z_\mathrm{Wald} = (\hat{\theta} - \theta_0)/\mathrm{var}_\theta(\hat{\theta})^{1/2}$ [in practice $\mathrm{var}_\theta(\hat{\theta})$ has to be estimated on the basis of $\hat{\theta}$] (*see* **Likelihood**). This statistic depends on the data only through $\hat{\theta}$, so that we see again that the information in $\hat{\theta}$ alone is approximately equal to the information in the entire data.

References

[1]   Fisher, R.A. (1925). Theory of statistical estimation, *Proceedings of the Cambridge Philosophical Society* **22**, 700–725.

[2]   Kullback, S. (1959). *Information Theory and Statistics*. Wiley, New York (Dover, New York, 1968; Peter Smith Publisher, Magnolia, Mass., 1978).

[3]   Lan, K.K.G. & DeMets, D.L. (1983). Discrete sequential boundaries for clinical trials, *Biometrika* **70**, 659–663.

[4]   Lan, K.K.G. & Zucker, D.M. (1993). Sequential monitoring of clinical trials: the role of information and Brownian motion, *Statistics in Medicine* **12**, 753–765.

(*See also* **Large-Sample Theory**)

D.M. ZUCKER

Information Bias *see* Bias in Case–Control Studies

Information Matrix

Let $\mathbf{X}$ be an n-vector of observations relating to a vector parameter $\boldsymbol{\theta}$. In addition, let $f(\mathbf{X}|\boldsymbol{\theta})$ denote the joint density (or mass function) of $\mathbf{X}$ under $\boldsymbol{\theta}$, which, viewed as a function of $\boldsymbol{\theta}$, is the **likelihood** function. A key role in statistics is played by the matrices $\mathbf{I}^{(\mathrm{o})}$ and $\mathbf{I}$ defined as follows, where the expectation below is taken under $\boldsymbol{\theta}$:

$$\mathbf{I}_{pq}^{(\mathrm{o})}(\boldsymbol{\theta}) = \frac{\partial^2}{\partial \theta_p \partial \theta_q} \log f(\mathbf{X}|\boldsymbol{\theta}),$$

$$\mathbf{I}_{pq}(\boldsymbol{\theta}) = \mathrm{E}\left[\mathbf{I}_{pq}^{(\mathrm{o})}(\boldsymbol{\theta})\right].$$

The matrix $\mathbf{I}(\boldsymbol{\theta})$ is called the Fisher information matrix, or sometimes, for emphasis, the expected information matrix. For a scalar parameter θ, the term used is simply Fisher information (*see* **Information**). The matrix $\mathbf{I}^{(\mathrm{o})}(\boldsymbol{\theta})$ is called the observed information matrix. Generally, the elements of the matrices $\mathbf{I}(\boldsymbol{\theta})$ and $\mathbf{I}^{(\mathrm{o})}(\boldsymbol{\theta})$ will have magnitude of order n.

The basic classic results concerning the information matrix are stated below. The most familiar setting for these results is that of independent, identically distributed (iid) observations, but they extend to more general settings. For the results to hold, certain technical conditions are required (see, for example, [4, Chapter 5]); such conditions generally hold in typical applied statistics settings. Below we denote the inverse of the information matrix $I(\theta)$ by V^*.

Cramér–Rao Inequality

Let $\tilde{\theta}$ be any unbiased estimate of θ, and denote by V its **covariance matrix**. Then the matrix $V - V^*$ is nonnegative definite. In particular, in the case of a scalar parameter θ, this result says that the variance of any unbiased estimator of θ cannot be less than V^*. There also exists an asymptotic version of this result in which unbiasedness is replaced by asymptotic unbiasedness and covariance is replaced by asymptotic covariance.

Behavior of MLEs

The **maximum likelihood** estimate (MLE) $\hat{\theta}$ of the true θ is defined as the maximizer for given data X of the function $f(X|\theta)$ over all θ. The estimator $\hat{\theta}$ is approximately distributed according to the **multivariate normal distribution** with mean vector θ and covariance matrix V^*. In light of what was said above, this indicates an asymptotic optimality property of the MLEs.

Estimation of V^*

The matrix $I^{(o)}(\hat{\theta})$ is a **consistent** estimator of $I(\theta)$ in the sense that $I(\theta)^{-1}I^{(o)}(\hat{\theta})$ **converges** to the identity matrix in large samples. Correspondingly, $I^{(o)}(\theta)^{-1}$ consistently estimates V^*.

The above results extend to more general forms of likelihood often encountered in biostatistics, including **quasi-likelihood** [3, Chapter 9] and **partial likelihood** [2]. Asymptotic optimality properties of MLEs in these more general settings also have been developed; see, respectively, [3, Section 9.5] and [1].

References

[1] Begun, J.M., Hall, W.J., Huang, W.-M. & Wellner, J.A. (1983). Information and asymptotic efficiency in parametric–nonparametric models, *Annals of Statistics* **11**, 432–452.

[2] Cox, D.R. (1975). Partial likelihood, *Biometrika* **62**, 269–276.

[3] McCullagh, P. & Nelder, J.A. (1989). *Generalized Linear Models*, 2nd Ed. Chapman & Hall, London.

[4] Rao, C.R. (1973). *Linear Statistical Inference and Its Applications*, 2nd Ed. Wiley, New York.

(*See also* **Large-Sample Theory**)

D.M. ZUCKER

Information Sandwich *see* Likelihood

Informative Dropout *see* Nonignorable Dropout in Longitudinal Studies

Informed Consent *see* Ethics of Randomized Trials

Initiation of Disease *see* Incidence–Prevalence Relationships

Inliers *see* Fraud, Detection of

Inner Product *see* Matrix Algebra

Instantaneous Incidence Rate *see* Hazard Rate

Instrumental Data *see* Measurement Error in Epidemiologic Studies

Instrumental Variable

The **errors-in-variables** model differs from the classical **linear regression** model in that the "true" explanatory variables are not observed directly, but are masked by measurement error. For such models, additional information is required to obtain consistent estimators of the parameters. A variable that is correlated with the true explanatory variable but uncorrelated with the measurement errors is one type of additional information. Variables meeting these two requirements are called *instrumental variables*.

B.S. EVERITT

Integrated Health Systems *see* Health Services Organization in the US

Integrated Risk Information System *see* Risk Assessment for Environmental Chemicals

Intelligence Quotient (IQ) *see* Eugenics

Intention-to-Treat Analysis

Intention-to-treat (ITT) analysis (also referred to as "as-randomized" or "method effectiveness" analysis [20]) is defined in the context of a randomized clinical trial (RCT). In a RCT design for the comparison of treatments, subjects are randomly assigned to different treatments. Once this randomized assignment to treatment is made, the ITT principle requires that any comparison of the treatments is based upon comparison of the outcome results of all patients in the treatment groups to which they were randomly assigned. This approach is recommended to maintain the benefits of randomization.

Randomization provides two important features. First, the treatment assignment is based on chance

alone. The characteristics of the group of patients receiving the different treatments should be roughly equivalent at the onset of the trial, with the only difference being their treatment assignment. If, during the implementation of the trial, the groups continue to be distinguished only by their treatment assignment, then any differences in the outcomes of the groups at the end of the study (*see* Outcome Measures in Clinical Trials) can be attributed solely to difference in treatment. Secondly, randomization provides the theoretical foundation for the statistical tests of significance that are used to test for observed differences (*see* Randomization Tests) [2, 7]. These two benefits of randomization are the foundations of the science of comparative clinical trials.

Unfortunately, once a clinical trial begins, several predictable, as well as unforeseen, conditions can (and usually do) influence the actual vs. the intended protocol under which individual subjects in each group are studied (*see* Clinical Trials Protocols). Thus, the groups, as treated, may no longer be comparable at the end of the trial. These circumstances may include: subjects who do not adhere to the assigned treatment regimen (*see* Compliance Assessment in Clinical Trials); subjects whose eligibility for trial participation has changed or was incorrect at the start of the trial (*see* Eligibility and Exclusion Criteria); subjects whose treatment assignment was incorrect; or subjects who terminate participation in the trial prior to the measurement of the main clinical outcome.

Partial or complete noncompliance with the regimen of the assigned treatment is fairly common in medical treatment trials. Patients may not be able to tolerate the side effects of their randomly assigned treatment and may request the termination of all medication or switch to another of the study treatments. Less common is a clerical or computer error that results in a patient being given medication other than that randomly assigned. Although such patients may take their medication faithfully, they will be noncompliant with their assigned treatment. In the extreme, widespread failure to comply with the assigned regimen can destroy a study. For example, in a trial comparing an active treatment with a control, if nearly all of the subjects randomly assigned to the active treatment do not take the drug, then a comparison of efficacy between the two groups will be meaningless. Less extreme, but very common, are instances where patients do not take the prescribed dosage of a treatment, or take the drug intermittently or for a limited duration [9, 20].

It is expected that, in general, there will be reasonable adherence to protocol in a substantial proportion of patients within each of the treatment groups. For those subjects not adhering to the protocol, the question may be raised as to whether they should be excluded from the analysis, the concern being that they do not provide information relevant to the efficacy of treatment taken as prescribed. By definition, ITT analysis does not allow treatment comparisons using only those subjects compliant with the therapies under test. Use of ITT analysis requires, with very few exceptions, that all subjects with valid outcomes be (i) included in the analysis and (ii) analyzed according to their randomly assigned treatment. Subjects who comply with their randomly assigned treatment for only a short time after its initiation, or switch to a competing treatment, are still considered, for analysis purposes, in their randomly assigned treatment group. This ensures that the randomization is protected; that is, the treatment groups can be assumed to include patients equivalent prior to the onset of therapy, and the possibility that the analysis could have been inadvertently biased by "selective" exclusion or inclusion of subjects into treatment groups is eliminated (*see* **Selection Bias**).

Contrary to the strict interpretation of the ITT principle, investigators may attempt to compare groups defined not solely by the original randomization but by factors that might be influenced by the treatments under test. In the face of substantial noncompliance, the comparison of only those patients in the trial that actually complied with the prescribed treatment is intuitively appealing. However, in addition to the difficulty of defining compliance in an objective manner, it has been seen that subjects who comply tend to fare differently and in a sometimes unpredictable way from those who do not comply [1, 3, 12, 22]. Thus, any observed differences among treatment groups constructed in this manner may be due not to treatment, but to factors associated with compliance.

The ITT analysis approach often provides a conservative estimate of the effect of a treatment administered as prescribed. The inclusion of noncompliant patients in the assessment of efficacy, barring some peculiar **dose–response** relationship, dilutes the difference between outcomes in the treatment and control groups. For the same reasons, ITT analysis may underestimate the risk of adverse side effects.

The ITT approach may be viewed as evaluating a *treatment strategy,* as contrasted to evaluating the efficacy of a treatment taken as prescribed [12]. The effectiveness of a treatment strategy is a reasonable approximation to the effectiveness of a prescribed regimen in the community [15]. Patients prescribed a treatment outside of a clinical trial often exhibit the same or an increased level of noncompliance, without the extra encouragement to comply that is provided in most clinical trials.

In contrast to the issue of noncompliance with the study treatment regimen, the determination of a subject's eligibility for trial participation after initiation of randomized treatment is a circumstance where many clinical trialists feel that a strict interpretation of the ITT principle can produce study results that are simply not credible [9, 13]. For example, in a comparative study of treatments for sepsis in newborns, treatment must usually be started as soon as there is a presumptive diagnosis of sepsis. Sepsis is too dangerous to be left untreated, and definitive laboratory tests are not immediately available, so treatment is usually started at the first sign of infection. If subjects with a presumptive diagnosis are assigned treatment by randomization, then a portion in each of the treatment groups will be later proven not to have had sepsis. Strict application of the ITT principle requires that the subjects proved not to have had sepsis nevertheless be included in the analysis in the treatment group to which they were assigned. A more relaxed application acknowledges that sepsis was or was not present *prior to randomization* and that its presence *was not known* due to the absence of confirmatory laboratory information. Thus, the exclusion from analysis of those patients without sepsis, and thus ineligible for the trial, would be appropriate since there is no conceivable way in which the treatment assignment could have influenced which subjects previously had sepsis. The choice of analysis in this example affects not only the credibility of the study report, which might have included in the analysis patients without sepsis, but also the measure of the effect of treatment. Including the subjects without sepsis in the treated groups would provide biased estimates of efficacy, since those without the disease would be counted as cured. In contrast, for the assessment of safety, inclusion of all subjects with and without a definitive diagnosis of sepsis is reasonable. The larger sample size will allow for the detection of differences in rarer side effects.

There is a concern that if exceptions to ITT analysis, as in the sepsis example above, are routinely allowed, then analysts will inevitably be tempted to adopt exceptions or exclusions that do **bias** the results of a study. An example, not as clear as the sepsis trial, is the administration of a study drug other than that actually assigned. This can happen on rare occasions because of a clerical error at the start of treatment, or, more commonly, because a subject decides to change medication early in the course of their assigned treatment. The first example seems simple enough; an unintentional clerical mistake resulted in an incorrect drug being dispensed. It might, therefore, be reasonable to include the subject in the analysis as having taken the received treatment. The second example, however, raises severe problems, since the drug itself may have caused the switch, possibly due to a perceived lack of efficacy or unpalatable side effects [17]. Most analysts would consider the latter example to constitute crossing the ITT "line in the sand".

Patients dropping out of a clinical trial before their endpoint can be measured can bias a study severely regardless of the analysis approach utilized. If, for example, one of the tested treatments has unpleasant side effects, patients with mild disease might view the side effects as a hardship when contrasted to their mild affliction, and discontinue participation. This would create an imbalance among the treatment groups with regard to severity of disease. Information on some clinical outcomes such as mortality might be obtainable given enough time, even if a subject drops out from a study. Other outcomes, such as laboratory evaluations at a specific time point after baseline, will not be available from alternative sources. Clinical trials should be designed and organized with the resources available and directed so that dropouts will be minimal and hopefully at random [8]. Several authors have proposed methods for imputing data for patient endpoints on the basis of previous data obtained in the study [4, 10, 11, 14] (*see* **Missing Data in Clinical Trials**).

The above discussion has centered around comparative trials of efficacy, with the primary example the comparison of an active treatment with a placebo, and the inherently conservative nature of an ITT analysis has been mentioned. A large number of clinical trials, known as **equivalence trials**, seek to show that a new treatment is equal to an established treatment with regard to efficacy, while being less toxic or less expensive. Suppose that the new drug, however, is

less efficacious than the established drug. If subjects who fail to comply with their assignment to the new treatment, or who switch to the standard treatment, are, for analysis purposes, considered in the group to which they were originally assigned, the difference between outcomes in the two groups is brought closer together. The established treatment group will include subjects taking the less effective treatment or taking no treatment, and the new treatment group will include subjects taking the more effective treatment and/or no treatment. Thus, the ITT approach for equivalence trials may tend to mask true differences, making it easier to conclude that treatments are equivalent when they are, in fact, not [13].

Statisticians and clinical trialists generally agree that some form of the ITT principle is appropriate for most efficacy trials. The strictness of application of the principle still raises considerable discussion.

Alternative Analysis Strategies

Alternatives to ITT analysis generally attempt either to restrict analysis to those subjects who have adhered to a treatment protocol, or to incorporate measures of compliance to treatment in comparative analyses. Many titles have been given to the first of these approaches including "as-treated analysis" [6], "treatment received" [16], "explanatory approach" [19], "method effectiveness" [20], "per-protocol" [20], "efficacy analyzable patients" [9], and "biologic efficacy" [21]. The phrase "as-treated" (AT) analysis will be used in this article.

In AT analysis (i) only patients considered compliant with one of the study treatments are included in the analysis, and (ii) outcomes of subjects are attributed to the treatment groups on the basis of the treatment actually taken, regardless of their randomly assigned treatment. It is argued that the primary interest of a comparative clinical trial is in testing whether a treatment, taken as prescribed, is effective. In contrast, the ITT approach dictates that all subjects be included in the analysis, even those who have not taken the prescribed treatment; and that subjects who have complied with a study treatment other than that assigned by randomization nevertheless be counted as having taken the assigned treatment. The ITT approach is counterintuitive to many clinicians and other scientists. It is considered by AT proponents as incorrect, and it is understood by those arguing for either ITT or AT analysis that ITT analysis will, in the face of noncompliance, provide a diluted estimate of efficacy.

The primary argument against the AT approach is that it can lead to biased comparisons of treatment groups, in contrast to the ITT approach as outlined above. That is, it can lead to claims of efficacy even when a treatment is nonefficacious. There are also some difficult practical problems with AT analysis, including difficulty in defining compliance [12, 18], difficulty in determining which subjects are compliant, and loss of sample size when analysis is limited to compliant subjects.

Another alternative to ITT analysis has been developed in recent work [5, 20], which attempts to incorporate measures of compliance into the statistical analysis. This approach focuses on the information that compliance has to offer, rather than on considering compliance as a defining characteristic for the inclusion of patients in, or the exclusion of patients from, analysis. The goal of the new work is to use compliance data to provide better estimates of, or understanding of, the clinical response to treatment. These model-based approaches currently require assumptions about compliance, either its relation to treatment or to outcome, that may be difficult to accept or verify. Nonetheless, this work may help to breach the gap between the current ITT and AT positions, and may be particularly useful for analyzing equivalence trials (*see* **Noncompliance, Adjustment for**).

Current Status

ITT analysis is a widely used strategy for the analysis of comparative clinical trials in the definitive comparison of treatments for both regulatory and nonregulatory assessments. "AT analysis" is used frequently as a secondary and confirmatory analysis to the ITT analysis, or for explanatory or exploratory assessment of efficacy in subgroups defined by characteristics or factors that could have differential response rates, such as compliance, gender or ethnic groups.

References

[1]   Azurin, J.C. & Alvero, M. (1971). Cholera incidence in a population offered cholera vaccination: comparison of cooperative and uncooperative groups, *Bulletin of the World Health Organization* **44**, 815–819.

[2]   Byar, D.P., Simon, R.M., Friedewald, W.T., Schlesselman, J.J., DeMets, D.L., Ellenberg, J.H., Gail, M.H. & Ware, J.H. (1976). Randomized clinical trials: perspectives on some recent ideas, *New England Journal of Medicine* **295**, 74–80.

[3]   Canner, P.L., Forman, S.A., Prud'homme, G.J., Berge, K.G. & Stamler, J. (1980). Influence of adherence to treatment and response of cholesterol on mortality in the Coronary Drug Project, *New England Journal of Medicine* **303**, 1038–1041.

[4]   Efron, B. (1994). Missing data and the bootstrap (Abstract), *Journal of the American Statistical Association* **89**, 463–474.

[5]   Efron, B. & Feldman, D. (1991). Compliance as an explanatory variable in clinical trials, *Journal of the American Statistical Association* **86**, 9–26.

[6]   Ellenberg, J.H. (1996). Intent-to-treat analysis versus as-treated analysis, *Drug Information Journal* **30**, 535–544.

[7]   Fisher, L., Dixon, D.O., Herson, J., Frankowski, R., Hearron, M.S. & Peace, K.E. (1990). Intention to treat in clinical trials, in *Statistical Issues in Drug Research and Development*, K.E. Peace, ed. Marcel Dekker, New York.

[8]   Freidman, L.M., Furberg, C.D. & DeMets, D.L. (1996). *Fundamentals of Clinical Trials*, 3rd Ed. Mosby-Year Book, St. Louis.

[9]   Gillings, D. & Koch, G. (1991). The application of the principle of intention-to-treat to the analysis of clinical trials, *Drug Information Journal* **25**, 411–424.

[10]   Greenless, J.S., Reece, W.S. & Zieschang, K.D. (1982). Imputation of missing values when the probability of response depends on the variable being imputed (Abstract), *Journal of the American Statistical Association* **77**, 251–261.

[11]   Laird, N.M. (1988). Missing data in longitudinal studies (Abstract), *Statistics in Medicine* **7**, 305–315.

[12]   Lee, Y.J., Ellenberg, J.H., Hirtz, D.G. & Nelson, K.B. (1991). Analysis of clinical trials by treatment actually received: is it really an option?, *Statistics in Medicine* **10**, 1595–1605.

[13]   Lewis, J.A. & Machin, D. (1993). Intention-to-treat–who should use ITT?, *British Journal of Cancer* **68**, 647–650.

[14]   Little, R.J.A. & Rubin, D.B. (1987). *Statistical Analysis with Missing Data*. Wiley, New York.

[15]   Newell, D.J. (1992). Intention-to-treat analysis: implications for quantitative and qualitative research, *International Journal of Epidemiology* **21**, 837–841.

[16]   Peduzzi, P., Wittes, J. & Detre, K. (1993). Analysis as-randomized and the problem of non-adherence: an example from the veterans affairs randomized trial of coronary artery bypass surgery, *Statistics in Medicine* **12**, 1185–1195.

[17]   Peduzzi, P., Detre, K., Wittes, J. & Holford, T. (1991). Intent-to-treat analysis and the problem of crossovers, *Journal of Thoracic and Cardiovascular Surgery* **101**, 481–487.

[18] Redmond, C., Fisher, B. & Wieand, H.D. (1983). The methodologic dilemma in retrospectively correlating the amount of chemotherapy received in adjuvant therapy protocols with disease-free survival, *Cancer Treatment Reports* **67**, 519–526.

[19] Schwartz, D. & Lellouch, J. (1967). Explanatory and pragmatic attitudes in therapeutical trials, *Journal of Chronic Diseases* **20**, 637–648.

[20] Sheiner, L.B. & Rubin, D.B. (1995). Intention-to-treat analysis and the goals of clinical trials, *Clinical Pharmacology and Therapeutics* **57**, 6–15.

[21] Sommer, A. & Zeger, S.L. (1991). On estimating efficacy from clinical trials, *Statistics in Medicine* **10**, 45–52.

[22] Tarwotjo, I., Sommer, A., West, K.P., Djunaedi, E., Loedin, A.A., Mele, L. & Hawkins, B. (1987). Influence of participation on mortality in a randomized trial of vitamin A prophylaxis, *American Journal of Clinical Nutrition* **45**, 1466–1471.

JONAS H. ELLENBERG

Inter-Rater Reliability *see* Agreement, Measurement of

Interaction

Interaction is most often considered in the context of regression models, including the special case of models underlying the **analysis of variance** (ANOVA). In these models, the response variable is linked in some manner to a linear predictor of the form

$$\alpha + \beta_1 X_1 + \beta_2 X_2 + \cdots + \beta_k X_k,$$

where the X_is represent **explanatory variables**, and α and the β_is represent parameters to be estimated. Here, for exposition purposes, the X_is will be regarded as representing separate factors of interest, or perhaps functions of a measurement or coding of a single factor. In this case, the linear predictor reflects an additive relationship such that a change in X_i induces the same change in the linear predictor whatever the values of the other explanatory variables.

In this framework, an interaction term is defined by the product of two or more X_is. Consider the special case of two explanatory variables. Then the linear

predictor can be expanded and be represented by

$$v(X_1, X_2) = \alpha + \beta_1 X_1 + \beta_2 X_2 + \beta_{12} X_1 X_2.$$

The coefficient β_{12} then represents a departure from an **additive model** for the simultaneous effect of X_1 and X_2 on the response. A test of the hypothesis $\beta_{12} = 0$ is used to examine whether there is evidence for such a departure. Technically, such a test is undertaken as a standard test for a nonzero regression coefficient in the **regression** model being considered.

If X_1 is continuous, then plots of v against X_1, with X_2 fixed, provide an illustration of interaction effects. In the absence of interaction, the curves are parallel for different values of X_2. If X_2 is also continuous, then parallel curves also arise when v is plotted against X_2 with X_1 fixed. The nature of the variables may determine the most natural means of presentation. For example, if X_1 represents an experimental treatment level and X_2 a covariate that specifies some intrinsic characteristic of a subject, then it is natural to plot v against X_1 with X_2 fixed. If X_1 and X_2 are *categorical*, then interaction effects are often displayed by the presentation of values of v for different values of X_1 and X_2 in a two-way table.

The absence of interaction, when there is particular interest in the effect of both X_1 and X_2 on the response variable, indicates that the separate effects of the two variables are additive. If interest primarily focuses only on X_1, and X_2 is regarded as a covariate, then the lack of interaction indicates that the effect of X_1 is independent of X_2. Particularly in analysis of variance procedures, the interaction of a treatment variable X_1, with a covariate X_2 which varies in a haphazard or largely uncharacterizable way, may be regarded as random variation that may be used in the estimation of the error of treatment contrasts (*see* **Random Effects**).

When the term $\beta_{12} X_1 X_2$ is referred to as an interaction term, terms of the form $\beta_i X_i$ are often referred to as main-effect terms. This derives predominantly from the ANOVA literature, and is particularly relevant to the orthogonal effects that derive from the coding of explanatory variables commonly used there (*see* **Analysis of Variance**). More generally, the interpretation of main-effect terms may depend very critically on the particular representation of the explanatory variables used to define X_i, particularly in the presence of interaction terms.

A distinction is sometimes made between qualitative and quantitative interactions. A qualitative interaction is one in which the direction of the effect of X_1, say, differs depending on the value of X_2. A quantitative interaction would reflect changes in the magnitude of the X_1 effect with X_2, which do not induce a change in the direction of the effect.

Another distinction is between synergistic (*see* **Synergy of Exposure Effects**) and antagonistic interactions. Assume that a change in X_1 induces a change δ_1 in the linear predictor through the term $\beta_1 X_1$, and a change in X_2 similarly induces a change δ_2. If δ_1 and δ_2 have the same sign, say "+", then a synergistic interaction is one which causes the change in the linear predictor due to changes in both X_1 and X_2 to be greater than $\delta_1 + \delta_2$. In contrast, an antagonistic interaction will result in a change less than the sum of the individual effects.

Interactions are always defined in terms of a specific model. Another model which is defined with a transformation of the response variable or a different relationship between the response variable and the linear predictor will not necessarily manifest the same interactions. Some formal attention has been paid to defining "removable interactions", but it is probably best to consider alternative models for this purpose on a case by case basis.

For models with more than two factors, products of all pairs of variables can be considered, and would be termed second-order or two-way interactions. In the obvious way, interactions of order m can be defined by introducing a product of m variables. When factors are defined with a set of binary **dummy variables**, interactions between factors involve products of these dummy variables, and the set of cross products corresponding to a pair of factors can be regarded as a single interaction term with **degrees of freedom** corresponding to the number of nonlinearly dependent cross products that can be defined. For factors with I and J levels, the degrees of freedom would be $(I - 1)(J - 1)$.

It has been argued that any model with an interaction term must have all main effects corresponding to terms in the interaction in the model. Such an approach produces what are called **hierarchical models**. While there are examples in which this requirement is viewed as too strong, it is in almost all situations sensible formally to test for nonzero interaction effects in the presence of the main effects.

A comprehensive review of interaction has been given by Cox [1]. In epidemiology, interaction is closely linked with the term **effect modification**.

Reference

[1]   Cox, D.R. (1984). Interaction, *International Statistical Review* **52**, 1–31.

(*See also* **Experimental Design in Biostatistics; Multiple Linear Regression**)

V.T. FAREWELL

Interaction Contrast *see* Contrasts

Interaction in Factorial Experiments

An important benefit obtained by using **factorial experiments** is the ability to determine whether **interactions** are present. In this context, interaction may be defined as the modification of the effect of a factor on a response, due to the influence of another factor. Put another way, the presence of an interaction means that the relationship between one factor and a response is different for different levels of another factor.

A typical factorial model which includes the interaction between factors A and B can be written as

$$\mu_{ij} = \mu_{..} + \alpha_i + \beta_j + \gamma_{ij}, \quad \text{for all } i, j,$$

where μ_{ij} represents the mean response across all observations when factor A is at level i and factor B is at level j, $\mu_{..}$ represents the overall mean, α_i represents the main effect for the ith level of factor A, β_j represents the main effect for the jth level of factor B, and γ_{ij} represents the interaction effect of the ith level of factor A and the jth level of factor B. This model clearly indicates that the effects of the factors are not simply additive, as would be the case if the interaction term were deleted (*see* **Additive Model**). Note that since the present discussion is concerned with understanding the meaning and utility of the interaction term, no constraints are imposed on the model parameters, and so models given will generally be overparameterized models.

By manipulation of the model given above, and defining the main effects as $\alpha_i = \mu_{i.} - \mu_{..}$ and $\beta_j = \mu_{.j} - \mu_{..}$, the interaction term can be expressed as a difference of differences; namely

$$\gamma_{ij} = (\mu_{ij} - \mu_{i.}) - (\mu_{.j} - \mu_{..})$$
$$= (\mu_{ij} - \mu_{.j}) - (\mu_{i.} - \mu_{..}),$$

where the "." in the subscript indicates summation over all levels of that subscript. Some authors refer to functions like $\mu_{ij} - \mu_{aj} - \mu_{ib} + \mu_{ab}$, i.e. differences of differences of cell means, as interaction effects. While such quantities are readily evaluated and interpreted from tables or graphs of treatment combination means, they are not equal to the interaction effects defined above. Such functions are actually the corresponding functions of the interaction effects, namely, $\gamma_{ij} - \gamma_{aj} - \gamma_{ib} + \gamma_{ab}$. Hence, it is true that if any of the functions $\mu_{ij} - \mu_{aj} - \mu_{ib} + \mu_{ab}$ are nonzero, then interactions are present.

Traditionally, the presence of interactions in a model has been viewed as something to be avoided, if possible. Didactic presentations of factorial models often emphasize testing for the significance of the interaction terms (*see* **Hypothesis Testing**), with the hope that the test statistics would be nonsignificant. If this no-interaction model is tenable, the relationship between the two factors and the response is easy to explain. However, in many real-life situations, interactions are appropriately included in the statistical model, since the relationship between a set of factors and the response goes beyond the simple additive (i.e. no-interaction) model.

Indeed, in certain situations the presence of interactions is viewed as desirable. For example, consider a randomized **clinical trial** where repeated measurements are taken through the course of a study comparing the effects of two different treatments on a disease of interest. The researcher anticipates that at the time of **randomization**, the average response will be the same in both treatment groups, but will eventually become different as the treatments have their desired effect. It is this divergence of response that is appropriately reflected by the treatment–time interaction effect in the analysis model.

The number of two-factor interaction terms in the model, corresponding to the **degrees of freedom** associated with that interaction effect, is the product of the numbers of levels of the two main effects in the models. By extension, the number

of degrees of freedom associated with higher-order interaction terms increases multiplicatively with the number of effects included in the interaction term. This is especially noticeable when the number of levels of one or more of the factors increases beyond a simple dichotomy. In this situation, estimates of interaction effects may become unstable if the number of such terms increases but the sample size remains fixed. This instability is partly due to the loss of degrees of freedom associated with the estimated residual **variance**, since the number of observations at the combinations of the factor levels may become too small. Furthermore, computational problems can occur because the model specification may have included some interaction terms in the model which involve unobserved treatment combinations. Strong computational **algorithms** will build in methods for recognizing and dealing appropriately with such possibilities.

As indicated in the graph (Figure 1), the interaction of two classification factors, or of a classification and a continuous factor, is straightforward to graph, and hence to interpret. However, comparable interpretation of interaction effects containing two or more continuous factors is considerably more complex. Practical experience suggests that it is next to impossible to explain and/or interpret interaction effects containing more than three terms in a straightforward verbal manner. While graphs may be useful in this regard, if the graphs involve more than one, or possibly two, continuous factors, the dimensionality of the required graph may be unreasonable.

In some situations, clarity of interpretation of interaction effects can be obtained by modeling these

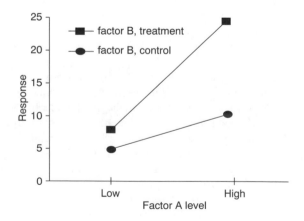

Figure 1   Graph of A–B interaction effect

effects with nested effects (*see* **Multilevel Models**) rather than as true interaction effects. That is, instead of using the terms α_i, β_j, and γ_{ij} in the model that deals with factors A and B and the A $*$ B interaction, we use α_i and terms for effect B that are different for each level of A. This may be more useful as one attempts to understand the underlying relationships among the variables.

When constructing a model with the possible inclusion of interactions, the investigator should be attentive to the convention of using the hierarchy principle for determining which interactions should be included in a model. For a model to be hierarchical, the inclusion of any interaction term mandates that all lower-order effects which include the effects in the interaction must also be included in the model (*see* **Hierarchical Models**). That is, if the AB interaction effect is in the model, then the A and B main effects must also be included. By extension, if the ABC interaction effect is used in a model, then the interaction effects AB, AC, and BC, as well as the A, B, and C main effects, must be included.

Interaction is something different from what epidemiologists refer to as **confounding**. In that literature, confounding refers to the change found in the relationship between a factor (often called an effect in epidemiology) and a response when another effect (the confounding effect) is added to the model. Interaction effects need not be included in a model for confounding to be present. Rather, confounding refers to the presence of significant **correlation** among the effects.

The use of interaction effects can be especially useful, and perhaps difficult to implement, when **time-dependent covariates** are used in the model. For example, in the analysis of growth of infants in the first year of life (*see* **Growth and Development**), it would be useful to utilize information about whether the child is being breast-fed at each measurement time. Inclusion of an indicator variable about the breast-feeding condition will simply yield a linear shift of the growth curve. However, if the interaction term involving feeding condition and age is included in the model, the rate of growth can be modeled differently under the two feeding conditions.

References

[1] Fisher, L.D. & van Belle, G. (1993). *Biostatistics: A Methodology for the Health Sciences*. Wiley, New York, pp. 435–443.

[2] Forthofer, R.N. & Lee, E.S. (1995). *Introduction to Biostatistics: A Guide to Design, Analysis, and Discovery*. Academic Press, San Diego, pp. 395–404.

[3] Neter, J., Kutner, M.H., Nachtsheim, C.J. & Wasserman, W. (1996). *Applied Linear Statistical Models*. Richard D. Irwin, Chicago, pp. 805–812.

ROBERT ANDERSON

Interaction Model

Interaction models for **categorical data** are **loglinear models** describing association among categorical variables. They are called interaction models because of the analytic equivalence of loglinear **Poisson regression** models describing the dependence of a count variable on a set of categorical explanatory variables and loglinear models for **contingency tables** based on **multinomial** or product multinomial sampling. The term is, however, somewhat misleading, because the interpretation of parameters from the two types of models are very different. *Association models* would probably be a better name.

Instead of simply referring the discussion of interaction and association models to the section on loglinear models, we will consider these models from the types of problems that one could address in connection with analysis of **association**. The first problem is a straightforward question of whether or not variables are associated. To answer this question, one must first define association and dissociation in multivariate frameworks and, secondly, define multivariate models in which these definitions are embedded. This eventually leads to a family of so-called graphical models that can be regarded as the basic type of interaction or association. The second problem concerns the properties of the identified associations. Are associations homogeneous or heterogeneous across levels of other variables? Can the strength of association be measured and in which way? To solve these problems, one must first decide upon a natural measure of association among categorical variables and, secondly, define a parametric structure for the interaction models that encapsulates this measure. Considerations along these lines eventually lead to the family of hierarchical loglinear models for nominal data and models simplifying the basic loglinear terms for **ordered categorical data**.

Graphical Interaction Models

What is meant by association between two variables? The most general response to this question is indirect. Two variables are dissociated if they are *conditionally* independent given the rest of the variables in the multivariate framework in which the two variables are embedded. Association then simply means that the two variables are not dissociated.

Association in this sense is, of course, not a very precise statement. It simply means that conditions exist under which the two variables are not independent. Analysis of association will typically have to go beyond the crude question of whether or not association is present, to find out what characterizes the conditional relationship – for instance, whether it exists only under certain conditions, whether it is homogeneous, or whether it is modified by outcomes on some or all the conditioning variables. Despite the inherent vagueness of statements in terms of unqualified association and dissociation, these statements nevertheless define elegant and useful models that may serve as the natural first step for analyses of association in multivariate frames of inference. These so-called *graphical* models are defined and described in the subsections that follow.

Definition

A graphical model is defined by a set of assumptions concerning pairwise conditional independence given the rest of the variables of the model.

Consider, for instance, a model containing six variables, A to F. The following set of assumptions concerning pairwise conditional independence defines four constraints for the joint distribution $\Pr(A, B, C, D, E, F)$. The family of probability distributions satisfying these constraints is a graphical model:

$$A \perp C|BDEF \Leftrightarrow \Pr(A, C|BDEF)$$
$$= \Pr(A|BDEF)\Pr(C|BDEF),$$
$$A \perp D|BCEF \Leftrightarrow \Pr(A, D|BCEF)$$
$$= \Pr(A|BCEF)\Pr(D|BCEF),$$
$$B \perp E|ACDF \Leftrightarrow \Pr(B, E|ACDF)$$
$$= \Pr(B|ACDF)\Pr(E|ACDF),$$
$$C \perp E|ABDF \Leftrightarrow \Pr(C, E|ABDF)$$
$$= \Pr(C|ABDF)\Pr(E|ABDF).$$

Interaction models defined by conditional independence constraints are called "graphical interaction models", because the structure of these models can be characterized by so-called interaction graphs, where variables are represented by nodes connected by undirected edges if and only if association is permitted between the variables. The graph shown in Figure 1 corresponds to the set of conditional independence constraints above, because there are no edges connecting A to C, A to D, B to E, and C to E.

Interaction graphs are visual representations of complex probabilistic structures. They are, however, also mathematical models of these structures, in the sense that one can describe and analyze the interaction graphs by concepts and **algorithms** from mathematical graph theory and thereby infer properties of the probabilistic model. This connection between probability theory and mathematical graph theory is special to the graphical models.

The key notion here is conditional independence, as discussed by Dawid [5]. While the above definition requires that the set of conditioning variables always includes all the other variables of the model, the results described below imply that conditional independence may sometimes be obtained if one conditions with certain subsets of variables.

Graphical models for multidimensional tables were first discussed by Darroch et al. [5]. Since then, the models have been extended both to continuous and mixed categorical and continuous data and to regression and block recursive models. Whittaker [9], Edwards [7], Cox & Wermuth [4], and Lauritzen [8] present different accounts of the theory of graphical models. The sections below summarize some of the main results from this theory.

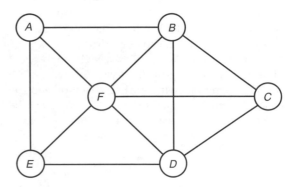

Figure 1   An interaction graph

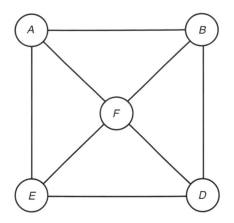

Figure 2 An interaction graph obtained by collapsing the model defined by Figure 1 over variable C

The Separation Theorem

The first result connects the concept of graph separation to conditional independence.

First, we present a definition: a subset of nodes in an undirected graph separate two specific nodes, A and B, if all paths connecting A and B intersect the subset. In Figure 1, (B, D, F) separate A and B, as does (B, E, F). E and C are separated by both (A, D, F) and (B, D, F).

The connection between graph separation and conditional independence is given by the following result, sometimes referred to as the separation theorem.

Separation Theorem.   If variables A and B are conditionally independent given the rest of the variables of a multivariate model, A and B will be conditionally independent given any subset of variables separating A and B in the interaction graph of the model.

The four assumptions on pairwise conditional independence defining the model shown in Figure 1 generate six minimal separation hypotheses:

$$A \perp C|BDF, \quad A \perp C|BEF, \quad A \perp D|BEF,$$
$$B \perp E|ADF, \quad C \perp E|ADF, \quad C \perp E|BDF.$$

Closure and Marginal Models

It follows from the separation theorem that graphical models are closed under marginalization, in the sense

that some of the independence assumptions defining the model transfer to marginal models.

Collapsing, for instance, over variable C of the model shown in Figure 1 leads to a graphical model defined by conditional independence of A and D and B and E, respectively, because the marginal model contains separators for both AD and BE (Figure 2).

Loglinear Representation of Graphical Models for Categorical Data

No assumptions have been made so far requiring variables to be categorical. If all variables are categorical, however, the results may be considerably strengthened both with respect to the type of model defined by the independence assumptions of graphical models and in terms of the available information on the marginal models.

The first published results on graphical models [5] linked graphical models for categorical data to loglinear models:

> A graphical model for a multidimensional contingency table without **structural zeros** is loglinear with generators defined by the cliques of the interaction graph.

The result is an immediate result of the fact that any model for a multidimensional contingency table has a loglinear expansion. Starting with the saturated model, one removes all loglinear terms containing two variables assumed to be conditional independent. The loglinear terms remaining after all the terms relating to one or more of the independence assumptions of the model have been deleted define a hierarchial loglinear model with parameters corresponding to each of the completely connected subsets of nodes in the graph.

The interaction graph for the model shown in Figure 1 has four cliques, $BCDF, ABF, AEF$, and DEF, corresponding to a loglinear model defined by one four-factor interaction and three three-factor interactions.

Separation and Parametric Collapsibility

While conceptually very simple, graphical models are usually complex in terms of loglinear structure. The problems arising from the complicated parametric structure are, however, to some degree to be compensated for by the properties relating to collapsibility of the models.

Parametric collapsibility refers to the situation in which model terms of a complete model are unchanged when the model is collapsed over one or more variables. Necessary conditions implying parametric collapsibility of loglinear models are described by Agresti [1, p. 151] in terms which translate into the language of graphical models:

> Suppose variables of a graphical model of a multi-dimensional contingency table are divided into three groups. If there are no edges connecting variables the first group with connected components of the subgraph of variables from the third group, then model terms among variables of the first group are unchanged when the model is collapsed over the third group of variables.

Parametric **collapsibility** is connected to separation in two different ways. First, parametric collapsibility gives a simple proof of the separation theorem, because a vanishing two-factor term in the complete model also vanishes in the collapsed model if the second group discussed above contains the separators for the two variables. Secondly, separation properties of the interaction graph may be used to identify marginal models permitting analysis of the relationship between two variables. If one first removes the edge between the two variables, A and B, and secondly identifies separators for A and B in the graph, then the model is seen to be parametric collapsible on to the model containing A and B and the separators with respect to all model terms relating to A and B.

The results are illustrated in Figure 3, where the model shown in Figure 3(a) is collapsed on to marginal models for $ABCD$ and $CDEF$. The separation theorem is illustrated in Figure 3(b). All terms relating to A and B vanish in the complete model. The model satisfies the condition for parametric collapsibility, implying that these parameters also vanish in the collapsed model. The second property for the association between E and F is illustrated in Figure 3(c). C and D separate E and F in the graph from which the EF edge has been removed. It follows, therefore, that E and F cannot be linked to one and the same connected component of the subgraph for the variables over which the table has been collapsed. The model is therefore parametric collapsible on to CDEF with respect to all terms pertaining to E and F.

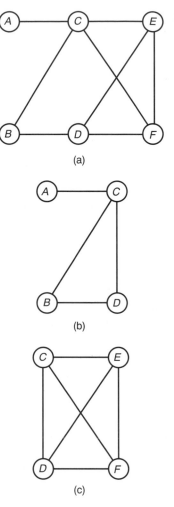

Figure 3 Collapsing the model given in (a) illustrates the separation theorem for A and B (b), and parametric collapsibility with respect to E and F (c)

Decomposition and Reducibility

Parametric collapsibility defines situations in which inference on certain loglinear terms may be performed in marginal tables because these parameters are unchanged in the marginal tables. Estimates of, and test statistics for, these parameters calculated in the marginal tables will, however, in many cases differ from those obtained from the complete table. Conditions under which calculations give the same results may, however, also be stated in terms of the interaction graphs.

An undirected graph is said to be *reducible* if it partitions into three sets of nodes – X, Y, and Z – if

Y separates the nodes of X from those of Z and if the nodes of Y are completely connected. If the interaction graph meets the condition of reducibility, it is said to decompose into two components, $X + Y$ and $Y + Z$. The situation is illustrated in Figure 4, which decomposes into two components, $ABCD$ and $CDEF$.

It is easily seen that reducibility above implies parametric collapsibility with respect to the parameters of X and Z, respectively. It can also be shown, however, that likelihood-based estimates and test statistics obtained by analysis of the collapsed tables are exactly the same as those obtained from the complete table.

Regression Models and Recursive Models

So far, the discussion has focused on models for the joint distribution of variables. The models can, however, without any problems, be extended first to multidimensional regression models describing the conditional distribution of a vector of dependent variables given another vector of **explanatory variables** and, secondly, to block recursive systems of variables. In the first case, the model will be based on independence assumptions relating to either two dependent variables or one dependent and one independent variable. In the second case, recursive models have to be formulated as a product of separate regression models for each recursive block conditionally given variables in all prior blocks. To distinguish between symmetric and asymmetric relationships edges between variables in different recursive blocks, interaction graphs are replaced by arrows.

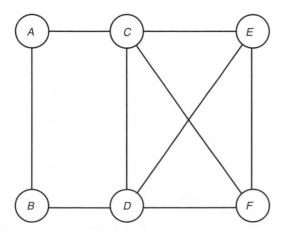

Figure 4 An interaction graph of a reducible model

Parametric Structure: Homogeneous or Heterogeneous Association

The limitations of graphical models for contingency tables lie in the way in which they deal with higher-order interactions. The definition of the graphical models implies that higher-order interactions *may* exist if more than two variables are completely connected.

It is therefore obvious that an analysis of association by graphical models can never be anything but the first step of an analysis of association. The graphical model will be useful in identifying associated variables and marginal models where associations may be studied, but sooner or later one will have to address the question of whether or not these associations are homogeneous across levels defined by other variables and, if not, which variables modify the association. The answer to the question of homogeneity of associations depends on the type of measure that one uses to describe or measure associations. For categorical data, the natural measures of association are measures based on the so-called cross product ratios [2] (*see* **Odds Ratio**). The question therefore reduces to a question of whether or not cross product ratios are constant across different levels of other variables, thus identifying loglinear models as the natural framework within which these problems should be studied.

Ordinal Categorical Variables

In the not unusual case of association between ordinal categorical variables, the same types of argument apply against the hierarchical loglinear models as against the graphical models. Loglinear models are basically interaction models for nominal data; and, as such, they will give results that are too crude and too imprecise for ordinal categorical data. The question of whether or not the association between two variables is homogeneous across levels of conditioning variables can, for ordinal variables, be extended to a question of whether or not the association is homogeneous across the different levels of the associated variables. While not abandoning the basic loglinear association structure, the answer to this question depends on the further parameterization of the loglinear terms of the models. We refer to a recent discussion of these problems by Clogg & Shihadeh [3].

Discussion

The viewpoint taken here on the formulation of inter-action models for categorical data first defines the family of graphical models as the basic type of models for association and interaction structure. Loglinear models are, from this viewpoint, regarded as parametric graphical models, meeting certain assumptions on the nature of associations not directly captured by the basic graphical models. Finally, different types of models for ordinal categorical data represent yet further attempts to meet assumptions relating specifically to the ordinal nature of the variables.

References

[1]   Agresti, A. (1990). *Categorical Data Analysis*. Wiley, New York.
[2]   Altham, P.M.E. (1970). The measurement of association of rows and columns for an $r \times s$ contingency table, *Journal of the Royal Statistical Society, Series B* **32**, 63–73.
[3]   Clogg, C. & Shihadeh, E.S. (1994). *Statistical Models for Ordinal Variables*. Sage, Thousand Oaks.
[4]   Cox, D.R. & Wermuth, N. (1996). *Multivariate Dependencies. Models, Analysis and Interpretation*. Chapman & Hall, London.
[5]   Darroch, J.N., Lauritzen, S.L. & Speed, T.P. (1980). Markov fields and log-linear models for contingency tables, *Annals of Statistics* **8**, 522–539.
[6]   Dawid, A.P. (1979). Conditional independence in statistical theory, *Journal of the Royal Statistical Society, Series B* **41**, 1–15.
[7]   Edwards, D. (1995). *Introduction to Graphical Modelling*. Springer-Verlag, New York.
[8]   Lauritzen, S.L. (1996). *Graphical Models*. Oxford University Press, Oxford.
[9]   Whittaker, J. (1990). *Graphical Models in Applied Multivariate Statistics*. Wiley, Chichester.

SVEND KREINER

Interblock Analysis *see* Incomplete Block Designs

Interim Analyses *see* Data and Safety Monitoring

Interim Analysis of Censored Data

In many chronic disease **clinical trials**, the major endpoint of interest is time to an event, such as time to disease progression or time to death. Often, the focus of the clinical trial is the comparison of time to event among different treatment groups. In such trials, patients enter the study during some **staggered entry** accrual period, and the final analysis is planned after a predetermined follow-up period. Usually, at the final analysis, not all events are observed, giving rise to **censored** survival data.

For ethical as well as practical reasons, these trials are monitored periodically and interim analyses are performed (*see* **Data and Safety Monitoring**). It is now common practice for all large-scale clinical trials to be monitored formally. Independent data-monitoring boards have been established for most large-scale government-sponsored clinical trials, and, increasingly, such monitoring boards are being established for pivotal clinical trials conducted by private industry such as pharmaceutical companies. The role of the data-monitoring board is to serve as an external oversight committee that reviews periodically the data from the trial as they accrue and to advise on the early termination of the trial or modification of the protocol on the basis of the emerging results (*see* **Clinical Trials Protocols**). Reasons for the termination of a trial are complex, and include serious toxicity, unexpected adverse events, design and/or logistical issues too serious to address, such as very low accrual or event rates, external information, established benefit, or no trend of interest. The board also considers carefully issues of data quality and the consistency of results across various endpoints and over time before making their recommendation.

There has been a great deal of statistical research devoted to early termination of a trial, if, during an interim analysis, a sufficiently large or small treatment difference is observed in the primary endpoint. The major question is: How large or small must the treatment difference be during the interim analysis to warrant terminating the trial? To this end, a test statistic is computed at each interim analysis and compared with a stopping boundary. If the test statistic crosses the boundary at an interim analysis, then the trial is terminated; otherwise, the trial continues until the next interim analysis. This process is continued, if necessary, until the time of a planned final analysis, and is referred to as **sequential** testing. We focus our discussion on upper boundaries only; that is, we allow the possibility of stopping the trial only if a sufficiently large treatment difference is observed during an interim analysis. In some settings, both upper and lower boundaries, allowing termination if either a sufficiently large or small treatment difference is observed, may be implemented (*see* **Data and Safety Monitoring**).

Statistical methods for sequential testing have been available for a long time, but only since the early 1980s have they been used routinely in monitoring clinical trials. One reason is that standard sequential methods require that the trial be monitored continually. Although there are many experimental conditions where this is feasible, it is generally not flexible enough to accommodate the needs of most large-scale clinical trials, where, administratively, it is too difficult for the data to be maintained for continual monitoring. Moreover, continual review is not feasible in a system where the data are monitored by an independent board that, of necessity, can meet only, at most, several times a year. The flexible method proposed by Lan & DeMets [10] has proven to be a useful way of monitoring trials that allow the number and timing of interim analyses to be left unspecified. Their method depends on specifying an alpha-spending function that may be translated into stopping boundaries. We discuss this strategy for sequential monitoring in more detail later in the article. Other strategies for monitoring clinical trials that include the use of the triangular test, the truncated sequential probability ratio test, and the restricted procedure are discussed in [25] (*see* **Sequential Analysis**).

To derive sequential tests, we must be able to characterize the joint distribution of the sequentially computed test statistics used with censored survival data. The difficulty is that there are two time axes that must be considered in evaluating the distribution of sequentially computed test statistics. Time to event for individuals is measured from the time they enter the trial, and it is the distribution of these patient times that are compared among treatments. However, sequential monitoring occurs over calendar time, which is measured as time from the start of the study. These issues are considered in more detail below. Later, we describe how the results for

the joint distribution of sequentially computed test statistics for right censored data may be used in conjunction with the flexible methods of Lan & DeMets to construct stopping rules.

Formalization of the Problem

We assume that n individuals enter the trial at calendar times $E_1, \ldots, E_n$. Each individual i has a potential survival time T_i, possibly unobserved, measured from the time of entry (*see* **Survival Analysis, Overview**). The distribution of T_i may depend on a vector of **covariates**, which includes a treatment indicator, denoted by Z_{0i}, and possible additional covariates $\mathbf{Z}_{1i}$. The relationship between survival time and the covariates is often modeled through the hazard function given by

$$\lambda(u|Z_0, \mathbf{Z}_1, \boldsymbol{\beta})$$
$$= \lim_{h \to 0} h^{-1} \times \Pr(u \le T < u + h | T \ge u, Z_0, \mathbf{Z}_1),$$

where $\boldsymbol{\beta}$ denotes a vector of parameters that may be finite dimensional (parametric model) or infinite dimensional (**semiparametric** or **nonparametric** models). The main objective is testing the null hypothesis of no treatment effect on the survival distribution (*see* **Hypothesis Testing**). For example, if we consider only treatment indicator Z_0, then the nonparametric null hypothesis may be posed as

$$H_0: \lambda(u|Z_0 = 1) = \lambda(u|Z_0 = 0), \quad u \ge 0. \quad (1)$$

Parametric or semiparametric models may also be used for this purpose; for example, we may assume the hazard function follows a **proportional hazards** model:

$$\lambda(u|Z_0, \mathbf{Z}_1) = \lambda_0(u) \exp(\beta_0 Z_0 + \boldsymbol{\beta}_1^{\mathrm{T}} \mathbf{Z}_1), \quad (2)$$

where $\lambda_0(u)$ is some unknown baseline hazard function, $\mathbf{Z}_1$ is a vector of additional covariates, and the null hypothesis is $H_0: \beta_0 = 0$.

If an interim analysis is conducted at calendar time t (measured from the start of the study), then individual i will have censored survival data if $T_i > t - E_i$. Censoring may also occur from other random loss-to-follow-up causes. We define V_i to be the potential censoring time due to causes unrelated to the time of an interim analysis. Thus, assume that for individual i there exists a vector of random variables $(E_i, T_i, V_i, \mathbf{Z}_i)$, $i = 1, \ldots, n$, some of which are possibly unobserved. At analysis time t, the observable random variables are $\{X_i(t), \delta_i(t), \mathbf{Z}_i\}$, for all $i = 1, \ldots, n$, such that $E_i \leq t$. Here, $X_i(t) = \min(T_i, V_i, t - E_i)$ is the observed time-on-study at analysis time t, and $\Delta_i(t) = 1$ if $T_i \leq \min(t - E_i, V_i)$, 0 otherwise, denotes the failure indicator at time t. It is important to note that the data available for an individual at different interim analysis times may vary. For example, an individual with censored time-to-event data at time $t[\Delta_i(t) = 0]$ may at some later time t' be uncensored $[\Delta_i(t') = 1]$.

Typically, a test statistic is computed using all the available data at time t. This statistic, which we denote by $W(t)$, is used to test the null hypothesis H_0 of no treatment difference; that is, the null hypothesis is rejected when $W(t)$ or $|W(t)|$ is sufficiently large, depending on whether we are considering one-sided or two-sided alternatives. The most widely used methods for testing the nonparametric null hypothesis given by (1) are the class of *weighted logrank tests*. Special cases of this general class include the **logrank test**. [12, 14], Prentice's [16] generalization of the Wilcoxon test (*see* **Wilcoxon–Mann–Whitney Test**), and the G^ρ tests of Harrington & Fleming [8]. If, instead, the null hypothesis is stated using a parametric or semiparametric model such as (2), then $W(t)$ may be a standard Wald or score test statistic derived from the **likelihood** for a parametric model or from Cox's [4] **partial likelihood** for the semiparametric model (2).

In a sequential time-to-event trial, the study is monitored at interim times $t_1, \ldots, t_K$. At each analysis time, t_j, we compute the test statistic $W(t_j)$, which incorporates all of the information up to the analysis time. If this statistic exceeds the stopping boundary value b_j, i.e.

$$|W(t_j)| \geq b_j,$$

then we may terminate the study and reject the null hypothesis. The boundary values b_j must be chosen in such a way as to preserve the **level of the test**. For example, if we wish to test at level of significance α, then the b_j must satisfy

$$\mathrm{Pr}_{H_0} \left\{ \bigcup_{j=1}^{K} [|W(t_j)| \geq b_j] \right\} = \alpha, \qquad (3)$$

where Pr_{H_0} denotes probability computed under the null hypothesis. To evaluate probabilities such as those in (3), we require the joint distribution of $[W(t_1), \ldots, W(t_K)]$. The particular challenge in deriving this joint distribution arises from the fact that the data for any individual contributing to the test statistic at different interim times may vary. A **Lexis diagram** is very helpful in explaining the interrelationship of these two time-scales. For an excellent example that illustrates the use of a Lexis diagram, we refer the reader to [9]. Careful consideration of patient time vs. calendar time has allowed derivation of the joint sequential distribution for most test statistics commonly used with right censored data. Some of the main results are as follows.

A random vector has normal independent increments if its joint distribution is the same as a vector of partial sums or independent normal random variables. Tsiatis [20, 21], Slud [18], and Gu & Lai [6] show that a general class of time sequential nonparametric statistics (i.e. weighted logrank statistics) are asymptotically distributed with an independent increments normal structure. The independent increments structure is the basis for most sequential designs and analyses, enabling the immediate application of standard group sequential methods and software to compute probabilities such as those given by (3). Assuming the proportional hazards model of Cox [3] (*see* **Cox Regression Model**), Gu & Ying [7], generalizing the work of Tsiatis [21], Sellke & Siegmund [17], and Tsiatis, et al. [23], showed that the test statistic based on maximizing the partial likelihood [4] also has this independent increment structure.

Recently, Tsiatis et al. [22], under the assumption of a parametric model with a single test parameter of interest (usually corresponding to a treatment difference) and a finite number of **nuisance parameters**, proved that the joint distribution of sequentially computed maximum likelihood estimators, and the joint distribution of sequentially computed score tests, have this independent increments structure.

In summary, most test statistics for right censored data, properly normalized, have a joint asymptotic distribution corresponding to an independent increments multivariate normal random vector with variance proportional to statistical **information**. Here, information refers to the usual notion of Fisher information for parametric models. An extended definition of information for semiparametric and nonparametric models is given by Bickel et al. [2]; this is beyond the scope of this article. One important example worth mentioning is the logrank test. In a randomized trial, the information for the logrank test is proportional to the number of events.

Flexible Sequential Boundaries

We now describe how sequential boundaries $b_1, \ldots, b_K$ may be constructed satisfying (3), using the flexible method proposed by Lan & DeMets [10]. The key to this method is to note that the rejection region given in (3) may be partitioned as follows:

$$|W(t_1)| \geq b_1, \text{ or}$$

$$|W(t_1)| < b_1, |W(t_2)| \geq b_2, \text{ or}$$

$$\ldots$$

$$|W(t_1)| < b_1, \ldots, |W(t_{K-1})|$$
$$< b_{K-1}, |W(t_K)| \geq b_K.$$

Denote these mutually exclusive rejection regions as $R_1, \ldots, R_K$. If we define the rejection probabilities γ_j such that $\Pr_{H_0}(R_j) = \gamma_j, j = 1, \ldots, K$, then (3) will be satisfied when

$$\sum_{j=1}^{K} \gamma_j = \alpha. \tag{4}$$

If we know the joint distribution of $[W(t_1), \ldots, W(t_K)]$, then for any set of $\gamma_j, j = 1, \ldots, K$, satisfying (4), we may recursively derive the boundary values $b_j, j = 1, \ldots, K$, so that $\Pr_{H_0}(R_j) = \gamma_j$. This is the method proposed by Slud & Wei [19] to be used with the sequentially computed Gehan–Wilcoxon test, [5] (*see* **Nonparametric Methods**).

Lan & DeMets suggest that the rejection probabilities be linked directly to the information available at the different interim analyses through the use of an "α-spending function". The use of information-based methods is discussed by Lan & Zucker [11]. Specifically, define a monotone increasing function $\alpha(\pi)$ for $0 \leq \pi \leq 1$ such that $\alpha(0) = 0$ and $\alpha(1) = \alpha$, where $\pi = \pi(t)$ denotes the proportion of statistical information at an interim analysis time t, with 100% information at the time of a final analysis. If we define MI as the maximum information and $I(t)$ as information at interim analysis time t, then the proportion of information at t would be $\pi(t) =$ $I(t)/MI$. The rejection probabilities, γ_j, are set equal to $\{\alpha[\pi(t_j)] - \alpha[\pi(t_{j-1})]\}$, where $t_0 = 0$ and $\pi(0) = 0$. By definition, these satisfy (4) and may be used to define stopping boundaries $b_j, j = 1, \ldots, K$. The term α-spending function refers to the fact that the probability of rejecting the null hypothesis using this strategy, by time t_j, if the null hypothesis is true, is $\alpha[\pi(t_j)]$, or, "we have spent $\alpha[\pi(t_j)]$ of the significance level by time t_j". The procedure guarantees that the level of significance will be equal to some prespecified α regardless of the number of interim analyses or the timing of these analyses.

As an example of the application of this method, consider the use of the logrank test in a randomized trial to test for the equality of the survival distribution between two treatments. In this case, the information is proportional to the number of deaths. Let $D(t)$ denote the number of deaths observed until time t and D^* denote the maximum number of deaths that determines the end of the trial. At the first analysis time, t_1, we compute the proportion of information $\pi(t_1) = D(t_1)/D^*$. The first boundary value, b_1, is the solution to

$$\Pr_{H_0}[|W(t_1)| \geq b_1] = \alpha[\pi(t_1)].$$

After this is determined, we compute the observed value of the test statistic. If it exceeds b_1, then we stop and reject H$_0$; otherwise, we continue to the next monitoring time.

Consider the jth $(j = 2, \ldots, K-1)$ analysis time t_j, and suppose that the boundary values $b_1, \ldots, b_{j-1}$ have been computed. At t_j, the proportion of information $\pi(t_j)$ is equal to $D(t_j)/D^*$, and the boundary value b_j solves the following equation:

$$\Pr_{H_0}[|W(t_1)| \leq b_1, \ldots, |W(t_{j-1})| \leq b_{j-1},$$
$$|W(t_j)| \geq b_j] = \alpha[\pi(t_j)] - \alpha[\pi(t_{j-1})].$$

The solution is easily computed using the independent increments property of the logrank statistic and the recursive numerical integration **algorithm** of Armitage, et al. [1]. The computations may be carried out using available statistical software such as EAST (Early Stopping, Cytel Corporation). Again, the observed value of the test statistic is determined and compared with the cutoff. If it exceeds b_j, then we stop and reject H$_0$; otherwise, we continue to the next monitoring time.

If we continue until the final analysis time, then we "use up" the remaining significance level; that is, we compute b_K, where

$$\text{Pr}_{H_0}[|W(t_1)| \leq b_1, \ldots, |W(t_{K-1})| \leq b_{K-1},$$

$$|W(t_K)| \geq b_K = \alpha - \alpha[\pi(t_{K-1})].$$

To implement these methods for sequential stopping, we must specify the maximum information and the α-spending function prior to the initiation of the trial. The choice of group sequential stopping rules has received a great deal of attention by many authors, including Pocock [15], O'Brien & Fleming [13], and Wang & Tsiatis [24]. The expected stopping times at various alternatives is the criterion that is most often used for comparing competing group sequential tests with the same significance level and **power**. Because α-spending functions and stopping boundaries have a one-to-one relationship, results on the choice of stopping boundaries may be used to determine the choice of the α-spending functions. Space limitations preclude detailed discussion of these issues; we note that two common α-spending functions have received considerable attention in the literature. These functions correspond to what are referred to as the O'Brien–Fleming boundary and the Pocock boundary, respectively, [10]. The former function tends to be very conservative at the early stages of the study, while the latter is more liberal. For an O'Brien–Fleming boundary, we take $\alpha(\pi) = \alpha_1(\pi)$, where

$$\alpha_1(\pi) = 4 - 4\Phi \left(\frac{z_{\alpha/4}}{\sqrt{\pi}} \right),$$

and for a Pocock boundary, we take $\alpha(\pi) = \alpha_2(\pi)$, where

$$\alpha_2(\pi) = \alpha \log[1 + (e - 1)\pi].$$

In these formulas, e is a constant whose natural logarithm is equal to one, and $\Phi(\cdot)$ and z_x are the cumulative density function and $1 - x$ **quantile** of a **standard normal** random variable, respectively.

The choice of maximum information (MI) is closely related to the power necessary to detect a clinically important alternative. When designing a clinical trial, the information necessary to detect a clinically important difference, with some predetermined power, when using a test at a specified level of significance, is computed. For example, if we test the null hypothesis (1) using the logrank test with significance level α for a clinical trial where patients are randomized with probability 0.5 to each of two treatments, then the number of events necessary to detect a treatment difference corresponding to a log hazard ratio of β_0, with power $1 - \eta$, is given by

$$4 \left(\frac{z_{\alpha/2} + z_\eta}{\beta_0} \right)^2.$$

However, when the data are monitored at several interim analysis times with the possibility of early stopping, there is a loss of power. Hence, the maximum information must be inflated by a factor that depends on the spending function, the significance level, power, and the number of interim analyses. For example, if we use the O'Brien–Fleming-type spending function with five interim analyses at the 0.05 level and 90% power, then the information must be increased by 3%. In contrast, an increase of 21% would be necessary with a Pocock-type spending function. The results of Wang & Tsiatis [24] may be used to determine the inflation factor as a function of K, α, η, and the type of spending function.

In summary, we have described a class of flexible and comprehensive methods for developing stopping rules for clinical trials with censored data, which may be used with parametric, semiparametric, and nonparametric models. These methods are used commonly by **data and safety monitoring boards**, as they guarantee the preservation of the significance level and power of the test while still allowing for early termination at interim times that do not have to be specified in advance.

References

[1]   Armitage, P., McPherson, C.K. & Rowe, B.C. (1969). Repeated significance tests on accumulating data, *Journal of the Royal Statistical Society, Series A* **132**, 235–244.

[2]   Bickel, P.J., Klaassen, C.A., Ritov, Y. & Wellner, J.A. (1993). *Efficient and Adaptive Estimation for Semiparametric Models*. Johns Hopkins University Press, Baltimore.

[3]   Cox, D.R. (1972). Regression models and life tables, *Journal of the Royal Statistical Society, Series B* **34**, 187–220.

[4]   Cox, D.R. (1975). Partial likelihood, *Biometrika* **62**, 269–276.

[5]   Gehan, E.A. (1965). A generalized Wilcoxon test for comparing arbitrarily singly censored samples, *Biometrika* **52**, 203–223.

[6]   Gu, M. & Lai, T. (1991). Weak convergence of time-sequential censored rank statistics with applications to

sequential testing in clinical trials, *Annals of Statistics* **19**, 1403–1433.

[7] Gu, M. & Ying, Z. (1995). Group sequential methods for survival data using partial score processes with covariate adjustment, *Statistica Sinica* **5**, 793–804.

[8] Harrington, D.P. & Fleming, T.R. (1982). A class of rank test procedures for censored survival data, *Biometrika* **69**, 553–566.

[9] Keiding, N., Bayer, T. & Watt-Boolsen, S. (1987). Confirmatory analysis of survival data using left truncation of the life times of primary survivors, *Statistics in Medicine* **6**, 939–944.

[10] Lan, G.K.K. & DeMets, D.L. (1983). Discrete sequential boundaries for clinical trials, *Biometrika* **70**, 659–663.

[11] Lan, G.K.K. & Zucker, D.M. (1993). Sequential monitoring of clinical trials: The role of information and Brownian motion, *Statistics in Medicine* **12**, 753–765.

[12] Mantel, N. (1966). Evaluation of survival data and two new rank order statistics arising in its consideration, *Cancer Chemotherapy Reports* **50**, 163–170.

[13] O'Brien, P.C. & Fleming, T.R. (1979). A multiple testing procedure for clinical trials, *Biometrics* **35**, 549–556.

[14] Peto, R. & Peto, J. (1972). Asymptotically efficient rank invariant test procedures, *Journal of the Royal Statistical Society, Series A* **135**, 185–206.

[15] Pocock, S.J. (1977). Group sequential methods in the design and analysis of clinical trials, *Biometrika* **64**, 191–199.

[16] Prentice, R.L. (1978). Linear rank tests with right censored data, *Biometrika* **65**, 167–179.

[17] Sellke, T. & Siegmund, D. (1983). Sequential analysis of the proportional hazards model, *Biometrika* **70**, 315–326.

[18] Slud, E. (1984). Sequential linear rank statistics for two sample censored survival data, *Annals of Statistics* **12**, 551–571.

[19] Slud, E. & Wei, L.J. (1982). Two-sample repeated significance tests based on the modified Wilcoxon statistic, *Journal of the American Statistical Association* **77**, 862–868.

[20] Tsiatis, A.A. (1981). The asymptotic joint distribution of the efficient scores test for the proportional hazards model calculated over time, *Biometrika* **68**, 311–315.

[21] Tsiatis, A.A. (1982). Repeated significance testing for a general class of statistics used in censored survival analysis, *Journal of the American Statistical Association* **77**, 855–861.

[22] Tsiatis, A.A., Boucher, H. & Kim, K. (1995). Sequential methods for parametric survival models, *Biometrika* **82**, 165–173.

[23] Tsiatis, A.A., Rosner, G.L. & Tritchler, D.L. (1985). Group sequential tests with censored survival data adjusting for covariates, *Biometrika* **72**, 365–373.

[24] Wang, S.K. & Tsiatis, A.A. (1987). Approximately optimal one-parameter boundaries for group sequential trials, *Biometrics* **43**, 193–199.

[25] Whitehead, J. (1992). *The Design and Analysis of Sequential Clinical Trials*, 2nd Ed. Ellis Horwood, New York.

(*See also* **Sample Size Determination in Survival Analysis**)

A.A. TSIATIS

Interim Sacrifice *see* Preclinical Treatment Evaluation

Interior Point Method *see* Linear Programming

Interlaboratory Study

It is useful to distinguish between *efficiency* or *proficiency tests*, which monitor laboratories participating in studies of the performance of specific tests, and studies to determine the *precision* and *accuracy* of test methods. The distinction between these two objectives is not made clearly in the extensive literature dealing with interlaboratory testing, also known as *collaborative testing*. Even Youden & Steiner [2] are not clear on this dual situation. Indeed, they introduce a new technique, known as the "two-sample chart", which is an appropriate procedure for proficiency tests, but recommend it also for the study of a test method for which it is less appropriate. For the sake of clarity, we deal separately with these two types.

Proficiency Tests

Suppose that a test method has been proposed, say for the determination of a certain constituent of human blood. A fairly large number of laboratories are interested in the test, and are willing to participate in a study designed to determine how well the test is carried out in laboratories using the test. Samples from two materials, A and B, are prepared and distributed to 30 laboratories. Each laboratory agrees to repeat the test 10 times on each sample. A simple tabulation will list, for each laboratory, the average and the standard deviation of the 10 replicates for A and for B.

h and k Charts

It is important to obtain an overall, yet detailed, overview of the data before proceeding to further analysis. This is accomplished by two charts, denoted h and k. The statistic h is calculated for each participant laboratory, for each material. It is defined by

$$h_{ij} = \frac{y_{ij} - \overline{y}_j}{s_j}, \qquad (1)$$

where y_{ij} is the average of the replicate measurements made by participant i for material j; $\overline{y}_j$ is the average of all y_{ij} over all participants (all i) for a given value of j; and s_j is the standard deviation of all y_{ij} over i for a given value of j.

Note that h is *positive* when the participant in question obtains, on the average, a value *higher* than the average of all participants; and that h is *negative* if the value obtained for the participant is *below* the average. The denominator s_j standardizes the difference $y_{ij} - \overline{y}_j$. A plot is made for of all the h_{ij}-values for both materials A and B, arranged by participants.

The statistic k measures the relative variability between the replicate measurements of any participant for a given material. It is defined by

$$k_{ij} = \frac{s_{ij}}{(s_r)_j},$$

where s_{ij} is the standard deviation among the replicates for participant i and material j and $(s_r)_j$ a *pooled* standard deviation, is the square root of the average of s_{ij}^2 over all participants for material j.

A value of k greater than 1 indicates a participant whose replicates vary more than the average. A k-value less than one indicates that the laboratory has lower than average inter-replicate variability. The k_{ij}-values are plotted in a similar way to h_{ij}.

The Two-Sample Ellipse

Youden & Steiner [2] suggested that a plot be made in which points represent the participants (laboratories). The abscissa for each point is the average value obtained by the laboratory in question for material A; the ordinate is the average value it obtained for material B. Their graph, and their interpretation of it, are based, however, on assumptions that are not always true. We therefore present a modification of their method, a modification that is less dependent on unverified assumptions.

We plot, for each laboratory, the average result it gets for material B against its average result for material A. If the laboratory is subject to systematic error – for example, a tendency to get high (or low) values – then this is likely to show up in both A and B. For high values, the point (A,B) will tend to be in the first quadrant (north-east); for low values, the point will be in the third quadrant (south-west). If this is true for many laboratories, then the points will tend to lie along a positive slope (south-west to north-east). Thus, the appearance of the graph will tell us something about possible systematic errors in the laboratories.

An ellipse is then drawn, based on contours of the **bivariate normal distribution**, containing approximately 95% of the points. Copies of the ellipse, with the experimental points, are sent to all participating laboratories. The copy sent to any laboratory whose point fell outside the ellipse should identify its position, but this should not be done on the copies sent to other laboratories.

The procedure should allow nonconforming laboratories to study their laboratory technique in order to find causes for their discrepancy. This should lead to an improvement in the technique employed by the laboratory.

Study of a Test Method

An interlaboratory study of a test method must be conducted in accordance with a number of general principles.

The test method should be described, and identical copies of the protocol should be given to all participating laboratories. This should be unambiguous, so that all participants carry it out in essentially the same way.

The materials to be analyzed in accordance with the test method should cover as wide a range as necessary. For example, if the test method is one for the determination of glucose in serum, then the materials (serum with glucose) should cover the range from low glucose content to high glucose content, the extremes being determined by the range over which the test method is applicable. Each of the materials should be as homogeneous as possible so that all participants receive the same set of materials. There should be at least four, and preferably six or more, materials.

The laboratories should all be competent in carrying out the test, and equipped with the necessary instrumentation. In each laboratory there should be an individual to whom the data analyst can turn for information. This person should be able to produce the data provided by the experimenters, and answer questions about the participants in the laboratory, about the test method, about the manner in which the measurements were made, and about anything unusual that may have happened. A minimum of six laboratories is desirable.

If the method is new or not totally known to all of the participants, then it is advisable to carry out a preliminary pilot study to familiarize the participants with the test method. This preliminary study does not have to include *all* of the materials.

If the interlaboratory study fails to satisfy the above requirements, then the entire test may well be a waste of time and money.

Repeatability and Reproducibility

Repeatability characterizes variability among replicates obtained in the same laboratory on the same material. We have seen that the standard deviation $(s_r)_j$ is an average measure of this property for material j.

If we consider two replicates from the same laboratory, from the same material, their difference, which is zero on the average, has a standard deviation of $\sqrt{2}(s_r)_j$, and we expect the absolute value of this difference to lie (with 95% confidence) between $0 - 1.96\sqrt{2}(s_r)_j$ and $0 + 1.96\sqrt{2}(s_r)_j$.

Thus, the critical difference, in absolute value is $1.96\sqrt{2}(s_r)_j$ or $2.77(s_r)_j$. This is called the repeatability of the method for material j.

Reproducibility refers to variability *among* laboratories. The s_j in (1) is a measure of the variability. However s_j contains also a part of the variability among replicates, reduced by n, where n is the number of replicates. We have

$$s_j^2 = s_L^2 + \frac{(s_r)_j^2}{n},$$

where s_L^2 is the variability among laboratories only (*see* **Variance Components**). Thus,

$$s_L^2 = s_j^2 - \frac{(s_r)_j^2}{n}.$$

If this difference turns out to be negative (as it sometimes does), then s_L^2 is considered to be zero.

The total variability among single measurements obtained in different laboratories is characterized by a standard deviation equal to

$$s_R = \left[s_L^2 + (s_r)^2 \right]^{1/2}.$$

The quantity s_R is called the "standard deviation of reproducibility", and for reasons similar to those explained for repeatability, the quantity

$$1.96\sqrt{2}(s_R)_j, \quad \text{or } 2.77(s_R)_j,$$

is called the "reproducibility" for material j.

Transformations of Scale

Transformations of the scales of data by nonlinear functions are widely used. In our experience, transformations of scale are unnecessary in most cases, and even harmful in some cases. A simple 'row-additive' model, on the original scale of the data, is entirely appropriate for most interlaboratory data [1]. This model incorporates a constant for the participant laboratory, and a participant-specific scale factor multiplying constants for materials. A nonlinear transformation of scale results in a distorted error term and is, for that reason, to be avoided.

Certain features of the data may show up in one test and fail to show up in another test. It is necessary, in analyzing data, to look at them from many perspectives. The widespread idea that a single mathematical model must be "fitted" to the data is simply erroneous: in most cases, a single mathematical model cannot represent all of the data. The practice, also widespread, of *rejecting* the values that do not fit the preconceived mathematical model is equally erroneous, as discussed below.

Tests for Outliers

The statistics for interlaboratory studies is discussed in a fairly large number of "standard procedures". Most of these devote a large proportion of their instructions and recommendations to a discussion of **"outliers"**. Statistical tables appear in many of them to allow the person responsible for the analysis of the data to "reject" nonconforming portions of the data. The rejection is based on the probability that a value as discrepant as the suspected outlier can occur. This entire course of action is based on a misunderstanding of interlaboratory testing.

In proficiency testing, the isolation of laboratories that disagree with the majority of participants is a major objective. But this is no longer the case in the evaluation of a test method. Here, a discrepant value should be considered as an indication that something went wrong. This could have happened for a number of different reasons. One of these is that the laboratory that obtained the discrepant value made a mistake. Another is that the laboratory did not follow the procedure stipulated by the organizers of the study. In that case, the question arises whether the stipulation was sufficiently precise to eliminate other experimental procedures. If it was not, then the details need to be rewritten in greater detail.

The "rejection" of values without examining these possibilities sweeps nonconforming values under the rug and ends up with an overly optimistic picture of the experimental test.

Apart from these considerations, the probability rationale underlying the treatment of outliers is faulty. A particular laboratory may be seen to be giving generally low readings. However, if we apply the common rejection criteria, we will reject some values and retain the others. This is clearly illogical: rigid application of a single rejection criterion will give a false picture, not only of the performance of this laboratory, but of the entire study.

One more outlier test should be discussed: Youden's ranking test. This test rejects laboratories that are consistently low or consistently high. It does this by ranking the materials within each laboratory and then summing the ranks. A laboratory that exhibits a very low or very high sum of **ranks** is considered an outlier.

This test is based on a false mathematical assumption, namely that the ranks are distributed at random among the laboratories. In accordance with this view, for a laboratory that obtains, say, a low rank for material A, the ranks it obtains for any other material are *totally independent* of the one it had for material A. This means that laboratories do not differ *systematically* from each other. This assumption is false for literally hundreds of data sets published in a variety of journals. Unfortunately, the ranking test is quite popular. It is used extensively in publications by the Association of Official Analytical Chemistry (AOAC), mostly because it is recommended in [2]. If used, this test, like other outlier tests, will result in overly optimistic evaluations of test methods.

Conclusion

The many procedures published for the purpose of providing statistical analyses of interlaboratory data are, by and large, faulty. Some are based on invalid assumptions, and some use poor logic. Many are based on mathematical considerations and are therefore popular. Mathematical models constitute a useful tool, but in order to lead to valid treatments, they must accord with the assumptions, as well as with the objectives, of the studies. Unfortunately, this is not generally the case with the mathematical treatment of interlaboratory data. The methods summarized in this article are designed to reveal useful information about the test methods. They look at the data in great detail, rather than presenting merely summary parameters.

References

[1] Mandel, J. (1961). Non-additivity in two-way analysis of variance, *Journal of the American Statistical Association* **56**, 878–888.
[2] Youden, W.J. & Steiner, E.H. (1975). *Statistical Manual of the Association of Official Analytical Chemists.* AOAC, Washington.

(*See also* **Laboratory Quality Control**)

J. MANDEL

Internal Control Group *see* Biased Sampling of Cohorts in Epidemiology

Internal Pilot Study *see* Cooperative Heart Disease Trials

Internal Validation Sample *see* Misclassification Error

Internal Validity *see* Validity and Generalizability in Epidemiologic Studies

International Agency for Research Against Cancer (IARC)

The International Agency for Research on Cancer (IARC) was established in May 1965, through a resolution of the XVIIth World Health Assembly as an extension of the **World Health Organization** after a French initiative. IARCs founding members were the Federal Republic of Germany, France, Italy, the UK, and the US. The Agency's headquarters' building was provided by its host, and is located in Lyon, France. Today, IARC's membership has grown to 16 countries (founding states plus Australia, Belgium, Canada, Denmark, the Russian Federation, Finland, Japan, Norway, the Netherlands, Sweden, and Switzerland). IARC activities are mainly funded by the regular budgetary contributions paid by its participating states. Each contribution is according to a formula which shares the first 70% equally amongst all participating states and apportions the remaining 30% depending upon the individual country's GNP.

A major goal of the IARC is the identification of causes of cancer, so that preventive measures may be adopted against them. The Governing Council has repeatedly stated that research dealing with treatment and other aspects of cancer patient care should not be a part of IARC's mission, nor should the Agency be directly involved in the implementation of control measures, except in cases where it is necessary in order to assess the effectiveness of the mechanisms of carcinogenicity, or when the experimental intervention is needed to permit identification of causes. Nor does IARC deal in the formulation of policies or legislation aimed at controlling carcinogens.

The main emphasis of research is on epidemiology, environmental carcinogenesis, and research training. This emphasis reflects: (i) the generally accepted notion that 80% of all cancers are, directly or indirectly, linked to environmental factors, and thus are preventable; (ii) the recent recognition of the fact that epidemiology may play an important part in cancer prevention and in the evaluation of prevention measures; and (iii) the fact that geographic variations in cancer incidence almost certainly reflect differences in the environment and are therefore particularly well suited for international research efforts.

Epidemiologic research is in two main areas: **descriptive epidemiologic** studies show the trends of cancer incidence and mortality in different populations and geographic areas, and **analytic epidemiologic** studies focus on the **associations** between incidence and mortality and specific risk factors (diet, some professional exposures, etc.).

Recent years have seen renewed interest for the study of genetic factors (*see* **Genetic Epidemiology, Overview**) and other host factors contributing to cancer. This trend came about after an increasing body of evidence showing that genetic mutations play a critical part in carcinogenesis, because of the potential importance of host factors in the modification of the carcinogenic effect of environmental agents (*see* **Environmental Epidemiology**), and because of the potential usefulness of genetic methods in the identification of people at high cancer risk who could benefit from a specific intervention.

Throughout its existence, IARC has had an active programme in biostatistics, involving several professional biostatisticians. Emphasis has been given not only to the optimal utilization of methods, but also to the development of new methodology in response to the needs of cancer research. Contribution to **case–control** and **cohort study** methodology, evaluation of **screening** programs, long-term animal experiments and descriptive epidemiology are among the fields in which IARC has made notable methodologic contributions.

IARC publishes several series: the *Scientific Publications* series (145 volumes), the *IARC Monographs on the Evaluation of Carcinogenic Risks to Humans* (67 titles and eight supplements), the *Technical Reports* series, the *Directory of Agents being Tested for Carcinogenicity* (29 volumes) and a few other nonserial publications. Of particular importance to statisticians are the volumes on statistical methods in cancer research [1–4].

IARC has around 150 staff members at the Agency's Headquarters in Lyon, and welcomes every year an average of over 600 visiting scientists and trainees from over 30 countries.

References

[1]   Breslow, N.E. & Day, N.E. (1980). *Statistical Methods in Cancer Research*, Vol. 1: *The Analysis of Case-Control Studies*. IARC, Lyon.

[2]   Breslow, N.E. & Day, N.E. (1986). *Statistical Methods in Cancer Research*, Vol. 2: *The Design and Analysis of Cohort Studies*. IARC, Lyon.

[3]   Estève, J., Benhamou, E. & Raymond, L. (1994). *Statistical Methods in Cancer Research*, Vol. 4: *Descriptive Epidemiology*. IARC, Lyon.

[4]   Gart, J.J., Krewski, D., Lee, P.N., Tarone, R.E. & Wahrendorf, J. (1986). *Statistical Methods in Cancer Research*, Vol. 3: *The Design and Analysis of Long-Term Animal Experiments*. IARC, Lyon.

International Biometric Society

The International Biometric Society is an

international society for the advancement of biological science through the development of quantitative theories and the application, development, and dissemination of effective mathematical and statistical techniques. To this end the Society welcomes to membership biologists, mathematicians, and others interested in applying similar techniques.

The Society was founded on September 6, 1947, at the First International Biometric Conference at Woods Hole, Massachusetts, in the US. The first President of the Society was **R.A. Fisher** from Britain and the first Secretary was **Chester I. Bliss**, from the US. The founders of the Society were motivated by the need for an organization that would foster international cooperation in the methodology and applications of statistics to biology. Biological research was defined broadly and included medicine, agronomy, public health, epidemiology, psychometrics, crop forecasting, paleontology, plant and animal husbandry, design of experiments, etc.

Structure of the Society

The Society is comprised of geographically delimited Regions or Groups that operate both independently and in consort with the international parent organization. Each Region or Group has its own set of officers and operates scientific and educational programs within its own geographic areas as well as maintaining an active role in the activities of the parent organization. The Governing Body of the Society is its Council, with members of Council elected by the membership at large. The election procedures ensure that all geographic areas have appropriate representation on the Council. The Society had seven Regions in 1948 and in 1995 had 18 Regions and 17 Groups covering virtually the entire world. The total membership in 1995 was approximately 6300.

Publications of the Society

The Society publishes **Biometrics** (Founding Editor **Gertrude M. Cox,** US) a peer-reviewed journal with the general purpose "to promote and extend the use of mathematical and statistical methods in pure and applied biological sciences". Potential authors do not need to be members of the Society to submit articles for publication. *Biometrics* was first published in 1945 as the *Biometrics Bulletin* and is currently published quarterly with special issues from time to time. The *Biometric Bulletin*, first published in 1983 (Founding Editor, Robert O. Kuehl, US) also published quarterly by the Society provides information on Society activities, Regional and Group activities, scientific abstracts from Biometric Society Regional meetings, as well as expository papers on biometric applications in various areas of the world. The Society, in collaboration with the **American Statistical Association** publishes quarterly the *Journal of Agricultural, Biological and Environmental Statistics* (Founding Editor, Dallas E. Johnson, US), which focuses on the methodology and applications of statistics to the named fields. The first issue appeared in 1996.

Society Networks

The Society supports a series of Regional biostatistical networks. The networks provide a linkage between countries with established biostatistical centers and those with little or no expertise. Joint conferences, short courses, individual training and provision of journals and computer **software** are components of the activities that make available biometric design and analysis to the scientists in developing countries.

International Biometric Society Conferences

Since the first International Biometric Conference (IBC) in 1947 there have been 17 IBCs in countries around the world. The conferences provide a forum for the presentation of scientific papers, discussion of these papers and interactions with biostatistical colleagues with different types of problems and perspectives. The Regions apply to host the biannual meetings and the conferences attract a large number of attendees from many different countries. The Society celebrated the fiftieth anniversary of its founding at the eighteenth IBC in Amsterdam in 1996. Over 700 people attended from more than 60 countries. The nineteenth IBC will be held in 1998 in Cape Town, South Africa.

For additional information about the International Biometric Society, contact the IBS Business Office, 808 17th Street, NW, Suite 200, Washington, DC, 20006-3910, USA. Tel: 1-202-223-9669; Fax: 1-202-223-9569.

J.H. ELLENBERG

International Classification of Diseases (ICD)

The International Classification of Diseases (commonly known as the ICD) is a classification system designed to group together similar diseases, injuries, and related health problems to facilitate statistical analysis of these conditions. The classification is designed to have a finite number of categories encompassing the entire range of morbid conditions. A specific disease or condition is given its own separate category title in the classification only when separate identification is warranted because of its frequency of occurrence or importance as a medical or public health concern. However, many category titles in the classification contain groups of separate but usually related morbid conditions. There is a unique place for inclusion into one of the categories for every disease or morbid condition; therefore, a number of residual categories are reserved throughout the classification for those conditions which do not belong under one of the more specific titles. The International Classification of Diseases is a statistical classification, not a nomenclature or extensive list of approved names for morbid conditions; however, the concepts of classification and nomenclature are closely related. Some classifications are so detailed (e.g. in zoology and botany) that they in fact become nomenclatures, but these very detailed classifications often lose their value for statistical purposes.

History and Development of the International Classification of Diseases

Interest in classifying diseases and studying disease patterns is usually traced back to the work of **John Graunt** and his tabulations of causes of death based on the London Bills of Mortality in the seventeenth century. During the eighteenth and early nineteenth centuries, several classifications of diseases were prepared. The first to approach classification of diseases systematically was François Bossier de Lacroix (1706–1777), writing under the name Sauvages, in his treatise, *Nosologia Methodica*. During the same period, the naturalist and physician Carolus Linnaeus (1707–1778) prepared, in addition to his seminal classification of botany, a treatise entitled *Genera Morborum*. By the beginning of the nineteenth century, the disease classification in general use was *Synopsis Nosologiae Methodicae*, prepared by William Cullen (1710–1790) and published in 1785 [1].

When the General Register Office of England and Wales was established in 1837, **William Farr** (1807–1883) was named as its first medical statistician. Farr found the Cullen classification, still in use, to be outdated and not sufficiently useful for statistical summarization. In his annual "Letters", published in the Annual Reports of the Registrar General, Farr urged the adoption of a new, uniform, statistical classification of diseases. He noted that many diseases were denoted by more than one term, some terms were used to describe more than one disease, vague terms were used, and complications were recorded instead of primary diseases [2].

The importance of a uniform statistical classification was recognized at the first International Statistical Congress meeting in Brussels in 1853. The Congress asked Farr and Marc d'Espine of Geneva to prepare an internationally acceptable uniform classification of causes of death. At the next meeting of the Congress in 1855 in Paris, Farr and d'Espine each submitted his own classification and the Congress adopted a compromise list of 139 rubrics; the compromise list reflected Farr's arrangement into five groups: epidemic diseases, constitutional (general) diseases, local diseases arranged according to anatomical site, developmental diseases, and diseases directly resulting from violence. Over the next 30 years, this classification was revised four times but it maintained the general structure proposed by Farr.

In 1891, the **International Statistical Institute**, successor to the International Statistical Congress, charged a committee to prepare a new classification of causes of death. The committee, chaired by Jacques **Bertillon** (1851–1922), submitted its classification to the Institute in 1893, and it was adopted. This Bertillon Classification, as it was called, consisted of 161 rubrics as well as an abridged classification of 44 titles and another of 99 titles. These were based on Farr's principle of distinguishing between general diseases and those localized to a particular organ or anatomical site. The Bertillon Classification received general approval and was put into use by several countries and a number of cities. The 1899 meeting of the Institute passed a resolution acknowledging the use of this "system of cause of death nomenclature" in all the statistical offices in North America, and some in South America and Europe. The resolution further "insists vigorously that this system of nomenclature be adopted in principle and without revision, by all the statistical institutions of Europe" and "approves...the system of decennial revision proposed by the American Public Health Association ...".

The French Government, as a response to the International Statistical Institute's 1899 resolution, convened in Paris, in 1900, the first International Conference for the Revision of the Bertillon or International List of Causes of Death. This conference adopted a classification consisting of 179 groups and an abridged list of 35 groups, and it reaffirmed the desirability of decennial revisions. Accordingly, the International List of Causes of Death, and its successor classifications, has been revised approximately every 10 years thereafter.

Bertillon continued his leadership in classification matters, and the revisions of 1900, 1910, and 1920 were carried out under his guidance. During the decade following his death in 1922, there was an increasing interest in expanding the classification to accommodate morbidity and other **vital statistics** interests. At the same time, there was recognition of the need to involve other international agencies, particularly the Health Organization of the League of Nations, in future revision activity. To coordinate efforts, an international commission, known as the Mixed Commission, was created with equal representation from the International Statistical Institute and the Health Organization of the League of Nations. This Commission drafted the proposals for the fourth (1929) and fifth (1938) revisions of the International List of Causes of Death.

In 1946, the newly established **World Health Organization** was given the responsibility for the next (sixth) revision of the International List of Causes of Death and to develop an International List of Causes of Morbidity. In 1948, the International Conference for the Sixth Revision of the International Lists of Diseases and Causes of Death met in Paris. The Conference secretariat was the joint responsibility of competent French authorities and the World Health Organization. The Sixth Decennial Revision Conference introduced a new era in international vital and health statistics. In addition to recommending a comprehensive list of conditions for both morbidity and mortality, the *Manual of the International Statistical Classification of Diseases, Injuries, and Causes of Death*, the Conference agreed on rules for selecting the underlying **cause of death**, a Medical Certificate of Cause of Death form (*see* **Death Certification**), and special lists and guidelines for tabulation. These recommendations were endorsed by the first World Health Assembly in 1948, resulting in World Health Organization Nomenclature Regulations which member countries have agreed to follow.

The International Conference for the Seventh Revision of the International Classification of Diseases was held under WHO auspices in 1955; the Eighth Revision Conference took place in 1965. The seventh revision was limited to a few essential changes and amendments or corrections. The eighth revision, while more extensive than the seventh, still maintained the basic structure of the classification and the general concept of classifying diseases according to etiology rather than manifestation.

The International Conference for the Ninth Revision of the International Classification of Diseases, again convened by WHO, took place in 1975. During the period when the seventh and eighth revisions were in force, there was a growing use of the International Classification of Diseases for indexing hospital records and for other morbidity applications. These expanding uses were recognized in the ninth revision, which added considerable detail and specificity to the classification. Also introduced was an optional method of classifying selected conditions according to their manifestation in a particular organ or site as well as by the underlying general disease. In addition, based on recommendations of the Ninth Revision Conference, the World Health Assembly approved the publication by WHO of two supplementary classifications on a trial basis: one for Impairments, Disabilities, and Handicaps [4] and one for Procedures in Medicine [3] (*see* **Classifications of Medical and Surgical Procedures**). These were to be adjuncts to the International Classification of Diseases, not integral parts of the basic classification.

Planning for the preparation of the tenth revision began even before the publication of the ninth revision. Early on, it was apparent that the expanded uses of the classification and the resultant complexities and additional detail required more than the usual 10-year cycle for this revision. The longer time period would not only allow broad solicitation of input from users and producers of the data but would also permit trials of some of the major changes being proposed. Therefore, WHO, with the concurrence of member states, postponed the Tenth Revision Conference from 1985 to 1989, with the planned implementation of the tenth revision consequently also delayed.

Characteristics of the Tenth Revision

The formal title of the tenth revision of the International Classification of Diseases (usually refered to as ICD-10) is *International Statistical Classification of Diseases and Related Health Problems, Tenth Revision* [6]. It comprises three volumes: Vol. 1 contains the main classifications; Vol. 2 contains guidance and rules for use of the ICD; and Vol. 3 is the alphabetic index.

ICD-10 is a variable-axis classification evolved from the original principles of organization proposed by Farr. It is designed as a three-character code with fourth-character subdivisions where appropriate. A letter is used in the first position and a numerical digit in the second, third, and fourth positions. The fourth character is preceded by a decimal point. Therefore, individual alphanumeric codes range from A$nn.n$ to Z$nn.n$, where n represents any of the ten digits from 0 to 9. The letter U is not used. The alphanumeric characteristic of ICD-10 codes is an innovation designed to permit more flexibility in maintaining a hierarchical sequence of diseases while adding more detail to the classification; previous revision code numbers were completely numeric. Vol. 1 contains the list of three-character categories and the tabular list of inclusions and four-character subdivisions. The "core" classification is the list of three-character categories representing the level of reporting required for the WHO mortality database and for routine international comparisons. Many countries use the ICD only at this level of detail; further subdivision of disease categories may not be possible given the quality of the original diagnostic data. Both the core classification and the fully detailed tabular list with its fourth-character detail are arranged into 21 main chapters, and chapters into blocks of related conditions headed by an appropriate block title. In the tabular list, but not in the list of three-character categories, inclusion terms are provided under each code number as examples or guides to the intended content of the category. However, the inclusion terms so listed are not intended to be exhaustive for any given category, and the Alphabetic Index (Vol. 3) serves as a much more detailed guide to the correct placement of conditions into ICD categories.

Vol. 1 also contains a separate classification of morphology of neoplasms which may be used in addition to the main ICD codes which usually classify neoplasms only by behavior and site. These morphology codes are the same as those appearing in the adaptation of the International Classification of Diseases called the *International Classification of Diseases for Oncology* (ICD-O) [5]. In addition, Vol. 1 contains key definitions adopted by the World Health Assembly to facilitate international comparisons of data, and special tabulation lists recommended for the uniform statistical summarization and presentation of both morbidity and mortality data based on the International Classification of Diseases.

ICD-10 came into force on January 1, 1993; however, the actual implementation of this revision of the classification in countries around the world did not begin in earnest until 1995 and the next several years thereafter.

References

[1]   Knibbs, G.H. (1929). The International Classification of Disease and Causes of Death and its Revision, *Medical Journal of Australia* **1**, 2–12.

[2]   Registrar General of England and Wales (1839). *First Annual Report*. Registrar General of England and Wales, London.

[3]   World Health Organization (1978). *International Classification of Procedures in Medicine*, Vols 1 and 2. World Health Organization, Geneva.

[4]   World Health Organization (1980). *International Classification of Impairments, Disabilities and Handicaps. A Manual of Classification Relating to the Consequences of Disease*. World Health Organization, Geneva.

[5]   World Health Organization (1990). *International Classification of Diseases for Oncology*, 2nd Ed. World Health Organization, Geneva.

[6]   World Health Organization (1992). *International Statistical Classification of Diseases and Related Health Problems*, 10th Rev., 3 Vols. World Health Organization, Geneva.

(*See also* **Cause of Death, Automatic Coding; Mortality, International Comparisons**)

Robert A. Israel

International Society for Clinical Biostatistics

The International Society for Clinical Biostatistics (ISCB) was founded in May 1979 with the aim to stimulate research on the principles and methodology used in the design and analysis of clinical research, to increase the relevance of statistical theory to clinical practice, and to further the communication between statisticians and clinicians. The Society also seeks to promote high and harmonized standards of statistical practice as well as to promote better understanding of the use and interpretation of biostatistics by the general public, and by national and international organizations and agencies in the public and commercial domains with an interest in, and/or responsibilities for, public health. The Society also has a policy of furthering training in the area of biostatistics.

The ISCB is constituted by an executive committee and led by a President. The Executive Committee consists, in addition to the President, of a Vice-President, a Treasurer, a Secretary and up to eight members including the Past President and the Newsletter Editor. The Society's Permanent Office is located in Denmark at the following address: ISCB Permanent Office, PO Box 25, DK-3480 Fredensborg, Denmark (tel.: +45 48 484 100; fax: +45 48 484 200).

Scientific Meetings, Courses, and Publications

The ISCB organizes an annual scientific meeting open to anybody with an interest in statistical applications in the field of medicine, including statisticians, clinicians, epidemiologists, and pharmacologists.

Between its foundation in 1979 and 1997, 18 annual meetings have been held (there was no annual meeting in 1981), all but one of them in Europe – the 1997 meeting was in Boston, US. Three of these meetings have been joint meetings with other societies; in 1985 with the German Gesellschaft für Medizinische Dokumentation, Informatik und Statistik (GMDS), and in 1991 and 1997 with the Society for Clinical Trials (SCT). The planned locations for the next few annual meetings are Dundee, Scotland, in 1998, Heidelberg, Germany (joint meeting with GMDS), in 1999, and Trento, Italy, in 2000.

A special feature of the meeting is a mini-symposium devoted to a particular (pseudo-) medical field. In recent years these have included health care assessment and pharmacoeconomics, methodologic issues of **prevention trials**, and organ transplantation.

The Society does not publish its own journal, but by an arrangement with the publishers, John Wiley & Sons Ltd, reviewed papers from the annual meetings are published in issues of *Statistics in Medicine*. In addition, a twice/thrice yearly newsletter, *ISCB News*, is published.

The Society also performs an educational role in the sense of organizing courses on particular statistical topics relevant to the application of statistics in medicine (*see* **Teaching Medical Statistics to Statisticians**). These have generally been run in conjunction with annual meetings, either as pre- or postconference activities, with faculties of foremost researchers in their field.

The Society recognizes the political and economic difficulties of some countries and actively promotes and supports the establishment of national groups.

Special Working/Interest Groups

In recent years the Society has developed a number of working groups. With the development of European and ICH (International Conference on Harmonization) biostatistics guidelines in the 1990s, the ISCB established two groups with interests in drug development statistical regulatory issues: "Statistics in European Drug Regulation", concerned with the lack of statistical expertise within the European regulatory authorities, and "Statistics in Regulatory Affairs", whose remit is to consider and influence the development of regulatory requirements, guidelines, and other documents concerning the scientific aspects of data collection, management, analysis, and reporting (*see* **Drug Approval and Regulation**).

Other working parties have been established (by the year 1997) – one on **fraud** and one on Education.

Membership

The membership during the mid-1990s has been fairly stable and numbering around 800 members from some 30 countries from around the world, with the majority coming from the European Union. Nonmembers attending an annual meeting automatically become members for that year. The annual membership fee in 1997 is 15 pounds Sterling, with a student fee of half this amount. The Society has a running agreement with John Wiley & Sons Ltd whereby ISCB members may subscribe to *Statistics in Medicine* at a favorable rate.

JORGEN SELDRUP

International Statistical Institute

The International Statistical Institute (ISI) was established in 1885 in London, closely following an exploratory contact of statisticians in Paris. Its predecessor organization, the International Statistical Congress (ISC), was started in 1853 in Brussels under the leadership of the famous Belgian statistician **Adolphe Quetelet**. The ISC remained in existence until 1876 when the German–French rivalries of the time, apparently through an intervention of Chancellor Bismarck, led to the dissolution of this intergovernmental statistical cooperation. The ISI, under the circumstances, was started as a non-governmental instrument of international statistical cooperation, with heavy reliance on its elected membership, which consists of outstanding statisticians of the world in their personal professional capacity. ISI is considered today the world academy of statisticians.

At the beginning of 1997 ISI had 1991 elected members, distinguished statisticians active in academia, government, and the private sector of about 100 countries. At the same time, 161 persons who are the heads of national and international statistical offices participate as ex officio members in ISI. In addition to its elected and ex officio members, ISI involves in its Associations (Sections) a substantial number of statisticians who are active in specialized areas of statistics. These Associations are: the Bernoulli Society for Mathematical Statistics and Probability (1670 members); the International Association for Official Statistics (480 members); the International Association for Statistical Computing (750 members); the International Association of Survey Statisticians (1160 members); and the International Association for Statistical Education (332 members). The Sections of ISI maintain open membership for all interested statisticians; many elected or ex officio ISI members also hold membership in one or more of these specialized Associations. The total of about 4400 Association members include those ISI members who hold membership both in these Sections and in the ISI. ISI is incorporated as a not-for-profit institution in The Netherlands (with its Permanent Office, established in 1913, located in Voorburg, a town adjacent to The Hague).

The goal of ISI is the development and improvement of statistical methods, and their application throughout the world, all in the widest sense of the word. While in the nineteenth century ISI was the only international statistical organization, by the end of the twentieth century the international statistical system has numerous other components, which are parts of the United Nations (UN), the regional commissions of the UN, the specialized agencies of the UN (such as UNESCO, WHO, or FAO), and the regional organizations formally outside the UN system such as the European Union (with its statistical office EUROSTAT) and the Organization for Economic Cooperation and Development (OECD). The role played by ISI has changed since its inception accordingly. In the nineteenth century, for example, the promotion of standardization of statistical methodology in the official statistics of countries was a key task: the acceptance of the first **International Classification of Diseases** at the 1893 Chicago Session of the ISI was an historic step in this regard. Today the intergovernmental organizations such as the UN, its specialized agencies, the European Union, and the OECD are the main forums for these types of endeavor.

It is convenient to group present-day ISI activities into five areas: (i) conference services, (ii) publications, (iii) research activities, (iv) membership services, and (v) other functions.

In respect of *conferences*, the biennial ISI Sessions are the most outstanding. The 1997 Session in Istanbul is the fifty-first such undertaking (during World Wars I and II no Sessions were held). Recent Sessions were held in Tokyo (1987), Paris (1989), Cairo (1991), Florence (1993), and Beijing (1995). The number of participants in recent Sessions has reached about 1500 with nearly 500 invited and contributed papers presented on a wide array of statistical, theoretical, methodological, and application questions. Smaller, and more specialized conferences were held in Dublin (1992), Voorburg (1994), and Washington (1996), in cooperation with other national and international statistical organizations.

The *publications* of ISI include scientific journals, such as the *International Statistical Review*, the *Statistical Theory and Method Abstracts*, books such as the Kendall–Buckland–Marriott *Dictionary of Statistical Terms*, which came out in several editions (between 1957 and 1990), the volume *The Future of Statistics. An International Perspective* (1994), as well as the *Newsletter of the ISI*, etc. [1–5]. In addition, there are numerous journals and publications by the five ISI Associations dealing with areas of their specialization.

ISI has been a promoter of *research activities* since its inception. The *Bulletins of the ISI* go back to the nineteenth century: these volumes have been issued after each of the ISI Sessions and printed in the host country where the Sessions were held. These "Bulletins" are a repository of and testimonial to the manifold research efforts undertaken by statisticians in numerous countries over the last 110 years or so. Later, in connection with the "World Fertility Survey" in the 1970s and 1980s, ISI has set up an internal research facility regarding population issues, albeit budgetary restrictions by the end of the 1980s made this venture financially unsustainable. The research function of ISI, however, has been maintained. Today, it involves holding Cutting Edge Conferences on acute methodological, theoretical or topical matters such as the statistical issues of derivatives trading, the index numbers of stock markets, or the demographic crisis of the transition countries. It also involves projects at the ISI Permanent Office such as the multilingual glossary of statistical terms, the ISI life expectancy program, and historical statistical investigations and commemorations. Moreover, the five ISI Associations are involved in a wide range of similar activities.

The *membership services* of ISI are primarily administrative in nature and result in the publication of the *Directory of ISI* which lists all ISI members as well as containing a listing of national and international statistical organizations and societies. The five ISI Associations also have directories of their members.

Among the *other functions* of ISI mention should be made of the site (home page) maintained on the **internet** (http://www.cbs.nl/isi). Also, every second year (at the time of the world-wide Session) ISI awards the "Jan Tinbergen Prize" to the three most deserving statistical studies submitted by young statisticians from developing countries. Each winner receives 5000 Dutch Guilders, transportation to and free stay at the Session, and an opportunity to present the winning study. Still another endeavor of ISI is its "World Numeracy Program", which aims at spreading quantitative literacy on a world-wide basis, primarily via the involvement of national statistical societies, the UNESCO, and other bodies.

ISI also attempts to promote cooperation with statisticians active in other, primarily nonstatistical, organizations dealing with biometrics, econometrics, psychometrics, astronomy, classification science, linguistics, etc. It is believed that in addition to the studies emanating from specialized and subspecialized areas within statistics identified as such, there are significant intellectual and practical gains to be made by fostering more integration with the rather dispersed statistical professionals active in all other fields. The Sessions of ISI, therefore, are being opened up for meetings with the "sister organizations" active in statistics.

References

[1]   *International Statistical Review*, V. Nair & W. de Vries, eds. Published three times per year in April, August, and December. ISI, P.O. Box 950, 2270 AZ Voorburg, The Netherlands.

[2]   Marriott, F.H.C., ed. (1990). *A Dictionary of Statistical Terms*, 5th Ed. Longman, Harlow, 232 pp.

[3]   *Newsletter of the International Statistical Institute*, Z.E. Kenessey, ed. Published every four months. ISI, P.O. Box 950, 2270 AZ Voorburg, The Netherlands.

[4]   *Statistical Theory and Method Abstracts*, C. van Eeden & J. Mijnheer, eds. Published four times a year in January, April, July, and October. ISI, P.O. Box 950, 2270 AZ Voorburg, The Netherlands.

[5]   *The Future of Statistics: An International Perspective*, Z.E. Kenessey, ed. Proceedings of the "Long Term Perspectives of International Statistics" conference, held in Voorburg, 1994. ISI, P.O. Box 950, 2270 AZ Voorburg, The Netherlands.

Z. KENESSY

Internet

The internet (lower case i) is the world's largest computer network, connecting millions of machines worldwide. It offers exciting new ways for people to communicate with each other and new ways to disseminate and access information. The Internet (upper case I), which is a term used to describe what can be done over the internet, has been described as potentially the most exciting and revolutionary development in information since Caxton's printing press. It opens up whole new vistas for academics, the business community, and the general public, providing easier access to information, faster means of communication and exchange of ideas, and new ways of using leisure time.

The internet began with the military, in the late 1960s. The Advanced Research Projects Agency, a branch of the US Department of Defense, sought a way of exchanging military research information between sites. One essential criterion was that the network had to be able to survive a nuclear war. If one computer in the network was destroyed, then the information would simply take another route. This led to a computer network known as ARPANET. From its military origins, it grew considerably as more US government departments and agencies gained access to the network. In 1983, the military network moved to a separate, more secure system and in 1984, the US National Science Foundation created the NSFNET, which linked supercomputers together to allow access by any US educational establishment, irrespective of location.

The ARPANET and NSFNET networks laid the foundations for the wide area network of computers that spans the globe and which is now known as the internet. Essentially, it is a network of networks. Each country has many networks for educational, government, and commercial purposes. Each of these separate networks, such as AARNET in Australia, NSFNET in the USA, and JANET in the UK, is an entity in itself. There are also networks operated by commercial Internet Service Providers, who provide access to homes and businesses throughout the world. Each of these networks is made up of smaller, local networks. This whole collection of networks interconnects across the world, allowing each site access to every other site, irrespective of the starting point. This vast interconnecting network forms what is referred to as the internet.

The interconnection of computers to form the internet is based on TCP/IP protocols which allow computers of different types, running different operating systems, to communicate with each other. Each computer on the internet is identified by its IP number, which is an hierarchical number similar in nature to a telephone number with country, area, and district codes. However, there are also names for the machines, which are easier to remember, and when a name is known it can be looked up in a Domain Name Service (DNS).

In the same way that ARPANET passed its information through any available route, depending on which machines were available, information can be routed across the internet by any available route. This makes the whole system extremely robust to failures of individual machines or subnetworks. The machines and networks that make up the internet change from day to day and year to year, but that is not important, as it was designed from its earliest beginnings to be robust to such evolution.

Types of Use

Running over the physical structure of the internet are many different types of service, in the same way that telephone companies supply many types of service over telephone lines. This array of services is generally termed the Internet (upper case I). The Internet can be used in a variety of ways, which see exciting new developments every few months. The principal types of activity are communication between individual people or within a group, gaining access to information, and operating software held on a remote computer. These main areas are outlined below.

Communication

Electronic mail (often referred to as "e-mail") is a form of communication in which text entered by an individual into one computer system is then sent in electronic form to another, where it can be read by the intended recipient. This type of communication can take place between any systems which are connected to the internet and which have software installed for sending and receiving e-mail. The messages are not transferred around the world instantaneously, but are delivered in minutes rather than days. This has made e-mail a popular form of communication. The e-mail address of an individual can often be found in the WhoWhere database [6].

In addition to messages between individuals, it is also possible for one person to send a single message to a group of others. Messages sent to a particular Internet address are then automatically broadcast to a list of participants of a "discussion group". Discussion groups of this kind exist for an enormous number of different interests.

Transfer of messages to the individual mailboxes of people interested in a particular subject can be avoided by conducting the discussion through UseNet news groups or conferencing, where all the messages are brought together on electronic bulletin boards and accessed by interested parties at their convenience.

Again using text exchanges, technologies such as Internet Relay Chat (IRC) and Talker services enable people to conduct discussions where the text typed by each individual is seen by all the others involved, in real time. Each day there are many people holding discussions, limited only by the speed at which they can type.

As the bandwidth of the internet increases, so the possibility of conducting real-time audio conversations becomes a reality, with full motion video an additional option. This is currently not possible everywhere, but it is spreading rapidly. Again, this need not be confined to one-to-one exchanges. Linking many people together allows computer video conferencing to take place, with the consequent reduction in the need for people to travel the world to meet face to face for discussion.

File Transfer

When information is transferred in message form it is usually also possible to attach other files to the main message. However, computer files of any type, such as programs, word processor files, data, or text, can also be transferred from one system to another over the internet. This method of transfer uses the File Transfer Protocol (FTP). This facility is very convenient for a variety of purposes, and it is particularly effective for large files. It also forms the backbone of many of the systems for gaining access to information.

Information Searching and Browsing

The Internet has provided a means by which a vast amount of information can be made available in electronic form and accessed by an enormous number of people. The variety and extent of the information now available is staggering. Methods of access to the information are independent of the type of computer a user has, which takes us closer to Universal Access to information. One of the difficulties faced by users is locating the information of particular interest to them. Early information systems were based on a hierarchical file structure and used a "gopher" system of access. More recent developments have been based on "hypertext" links, where a keyword in one document is linked to another related document. This is a less structured, but more flexible, system of organization. This has also led to a greater need for searching mechanisms to locate material of interest.

A great deal of attention has been focused on the richer form of presentation of information within a framework called the World Wide Web. The Web, as it is often called, started at CERN (the European

Laboratory for Particle Physics in Geneva) in 1989, as a system to allow researchers in high-energy physics to exchange papers and information about their experiments. Its use grew exponentially and it is now a major part of the Internet. The Web is accessed by a "browser" which can be used to navigate through this information in a convenient manner, simply by clicking on words or images (called hyperlinks) which transfer the reader to another, related, document or resource. Resources are identified by their Uniform Resource Locator (URL), which identifies the machine containing the resource and where the resource is in the machine's filestore. Hyperlinks may point to resources on the same machine, or on another system anywhere else in the world. Navigation between systems is handled by the browser and is invisible to the user, who is free to appreciate the information available without concern for the technicalities of its retrieval. The most commonly used browsers are Netscape Navigator^{TM}, Internet Explorer^{TM}, and Mosaic^{TM}. The Web allows close integration of text, graphics, sound, animation, and "virtual reality" 3-D worlds. Recent developments may be found at the World Wide Web consortium site [8].

Remote Software

One feature of the Internet is that a user in one geographic location can access a computer system in another place. This allows software or processing power available on one machine to be operated from a remote location. However, recent developments have allowed the reverse to happen, so that software can be downloaded from a remote site on to a local machine and then run automatically, without further expertise required on the part of the user. This makes computing much more accessible to the general public, as very little knowledge about the technology is required before using it. Currently, the most popular computer language for such developments is Java. Code written in Java will run on many types of machine without modification. Information on recent developments may be found at [4].

Intranets

Many organizations have seen the potential that the Internet has for the free distribution of information and have applied the Internet principles to their own organizations. They have set up what are called Intranets, which are freely accessible by everyone within the organization but are inaccessible from outside. It is easy to see the benefits that may be gained by running such a private Internet world.

Internet Uses in Biostatistics

In the world of biostatistics, the potential benefits of using the Internet outlined above are all available. In particular, the use of e-mail has had a large effect on the working lives of many people, and the Web is having an increasing effect on the way in which information is made available in biostatistics (and, indeed, on the construction of this Encyclopedia [9]). One of the great benefits of this revolution is that it allows biostatisticians who are geographically isolated from colleagues to maintain contact in a convenient way, and so to feel part of a wider community. In addition to individual contacts, e-mail discussion lists provide a particularly helpful forum for this. There are many lists and information sources relevant to the interests of biostatisticians. Some Internet sites provide helpful listings of other sites of interest in a particular subject area. An example for statistics is at [2].

For the provision of information, many organizations have now created Web sites. This includes professional societies, and Web sites now exist for most of the major societies, the interests of which include biostatistics. These sites provide valuable, up-to-date information on professional activities. In particular, it is becoming increasingly common for conference information and registration facilities to be provided on the Web. Research organizations of all types are also making use of the Internet. In addition to general information on their activities, research papers are often made available. This provides a very fast means of disseminating research ideas and results. A useful list of organizations in the general statistics area which have Web sites is provided at [3]. In addition, information about statistical software, and sometimes also the software itself, is readily accessible. A useful starting point for exploring this area is [5].

A significant area of interest in biostatistics is the availability of data and information from application areas in medicine and the health sciences. From this perspective, the Internet can be thought of as providing access to a vast library of information held at a large number of sites throughout the world.

Where the data themselves are not made available, for copyright or other reasons, the Internet can still be extremely useful in identifying and contacting the site at which information may be held. In addition to the lists of professional and research organizations mentioned above, a useful starting point for information is the World Health Organization (WHO) site at [7], which also provides links to a large number of organizations with medical and health interests.

The huge amount of information available over the Internet, and the vast number of sites that now exist, can sometimes lead to difficulties in locating the particular site or information that may be of interest. A number of different automatic search facilities are available, and these can be extremely helpful in locating relevant items. These facilities are generally based on keywords provided by the user. However, some care is generally required in the selection of these keywords. For example, providing the simple keyword "biostatistics" is likely to lead to a huge number of relevant sites being identified. An example of a general search facility is at [1].

The development and use of the Internet has taken place at such a phenomenal rate that it is difficult to predict what further changes will take place in the future. One likely area is commercial electronic publishing. Some journals are already available over the Internet and others are likely to follow. Another is conferences, where a "virtual conference" over the Internet can provide a cheaper and more accessible alternative to the traditional physical event. While particular developments are difficult to predict, it is certain that the Internet will continue to have an increasingly large effect on the way in which biostatistics is conducted.

References

[1]   The AltaVista search facility: http://www.altavista.com/

[2]   The CTI Centre for Statistics, a useful starting point in finding information or discussion lists of interest in the general area of statistics: http://www.stats.gla.ac.uk/cti/

[3]   The International Association for Statistical Computing, where lists of organizations relevant to statistics and some of its application areas are held: http://www.stat.unipg.it/iasc/

[4]   The Java language, information on: http://www.sun.com/java/

[5]   The Statlib archive, which is particularly useful for locating information about software in statistics: http://lib.stat.cmu.edu/

[6]   The WhoWhere database of Email addresses: http://www.whowhere.com/

[7]   The World Health Organization: http://www.who.ch/

[8]   The World Wide Web consortium site: http://www.w3.org/pub/WWW/

[9]   *The Encyclopedia of Biostatistics* web site: http://www.wiley.co.uk/eob/

ADRIAN W. BOWMAN, JAMES CURRALL &
STUART G. YOUNG

Interpenetrating Samples

Interpenetrating sampling (IPS), also known as interpenetrating subsampling and replicated sampling, was introduced in the pioneering contribution of **P.C. Mahalanobis** [17, 18]. Mahalanobis used IPS for the jute and rice acreage surveys in Bengal and Bihar, eastern states of India, as early as 1937. Since then, many countries of different continents have started using IPS in their large-scale **sample surveys**. The United Nations Subcommission on Statistical Sampling strongly recommended the use of IPS in 1949 [26]. IPS was originally proposed in assessing the **nonsampling errors** as the so-called "interviewer errors". Interviewer effects in the measurements from IPS are compared in the **fixed-effects** setup, and the **variance component** due to interviewers is measured in the **random-effects** setup. IPS has also turned out to be an effective method of estimating the **variance** of the **estimator** of a parameter of interest in complex surveys (see Deming [3, 4], Lahiri [14], and Yates [27]). In fact, IPS is the foundation of modern **resampling** methods like **jackknife** [24] and **bootstrap** [5], and also replication methods [20, 21].

IPS consists of selecting a sample in the form of $k(k \geq 2)$ samples using the identical sampling design from the same population. Sample sizes in k samples may or may not be equal. If k interviewers are assigned to collect information from k samples, then the interviewer effects can be studied and compared. Samples may or may not be drawn independently. The sampling design can be a complex design, that is, **multistage, stratified**, with equal or unequal probabilities. Let θ be the parameter of interest and $t_1, \ldots, t_k$ be the k estimators of θ based on k IPS. First, assume that

$$\mathrm{E}(t_j) = \theta, \qquad \mathrm{var}(t_j) = \sigma^2,$$

$$\mathrm{cov}(t_j, t_{j'}) = \rho\sigma^2, \quad j \neq j'.$$

Consider the following estimator $\hat{\theta}$ of θ

$$\hat{\theta} = \sum_{j=1}^{k} w_j t_j,$$

where the w_js are fixed constant (known or unknown), with $\sum_{j=1}^{k} w_j = 1$. It can be seen that

$$\mathrm{var}(\hat{\theta}) = \sigma^2 (1 - \rho) \sum_{j=1}^{k} w_j^2 + \rho\sigma^2.$$

An estimator of $\mathrm{var}(\hat{\theta})$ is

$$\widehat{\mathrm{var}}(\hat{\theta}) = \frac{\displaystyle\sum_{j=1}^{k} w_j^2}{1 - \displaystyle\sum_{j=1}^{k} w_j^2} \sum_{j=1}^{k} w_j(t_j - \hat{\theta})^2.$$

It can be checked that

$$\mathrm{E}[\widehat{\mathrm{var}}(\hat{\theta})] = \mathrm{var}(\hat{\theta}) - \rho\sigma^2.$$

As a result, $\widehat{\mathrm{var}}(\hat{\theta})$ is an **unbiased** estimator of $\mathrm{var}(\hat{\theta})$ when $\rho = 0$, $\widehat{\mathrm{var}}(\hat{\theta})$ overestimates $\mathrm{var}(\hat{\theta})$ when $\rho < 0$, and $\widehat{\mathrm{var}}(\hat{\theta})$ underestimates $\mathrm{var}(\hat{\theta})$ when $\rho > 0$. If $w_1 = \cdots = w_k = 1/k$, then $\hat{\theta} = [(t_1 + \cdots + t_k)/k] = \bar{t}$ and

$$\widehat{\mathrm{var}}(\hat{\theta}) = \frac{1}{k(k-1)} \sum_{j=1}^{k} (t_j - \bar{t})^2.$$

In the case where k samples are drawn independently, $\widehat{\mathrm{var}}(\hat{\theta})$ is an unbiased estimator of $\mathrm{var}(\hat{\theta})$. Thus, IPS provides a quick, simple, and effective way of estimating the variance of the estimator even in a complex survey. The case $\mathrm{var}(t_j) = \sigma_j^2, j = 1, \ldots, k$, is considered in Murthy [22], Koop [12] and others. Suppose that $t(j)$ is the value of $\bar{t}$ when

the jth estimator of θ from the jth investigator is omitted. Then

$$t(j) = \frac{t_1 + \cdots + t_{j-1} + t_{j+1} + \cdots + t_k}{k-1},$$

$$j = 1, \ldots, k.$$

Let

$$t(\cdot) = \frac{t(1) + t(2) + \cdots + t(k)}{k}.$$

The jackknife version of $\bar{t}$ is given by

$$\hat{\theta}^J = k\bar{t} - (k-1)t(\cdot).$$

It can now be seen that $\hat{\theta}^J = \bar{t}$, and, consequently, the expression of $\mathrm{var}(\hat{\theta}^J)$ in Efron & Stein [6]

$$\widehat{\mathrm{var}}(\hat{\theta}^J) = \frac{k-1}{k} \sum_{j=1}^{k} [t(j) - t(\cdot)]^2,$$

is exactly the same as $\widehat{\mathrm{var}}(\hat{\theta}) = \widehat{\mathrm{var}}(\bar{t})$ given above. For comparison of several **ratio and regression estimators** based on IPS with or without jackknife, see Ghosh & Gomez [9, 10].

In IPS, k samples are drawn from the same population using the identical sampling design. If k samples are selected with replacement so that they are independent, then one can see its similarity in principle with the modern Bootstrap Sampling (BSS) (see Efron & Tibshirani [7]). In BSS, the observed data are a **random sample** of size n from an unknown probability distribution F. Bootstrap samples are random samples of size n drawn with replacement from the observed data or the empirical distribution $\hat{F}$. If we treat the observed data as a finite population of size n, then BSS are, in fact, IPS with $k = n$. Of course, there is no interviewer effect for bootstrap samples.

In IPS, three basic principles of **experimental designs**; namely, **randomization**, replication, and local control, are used. The main purpose of IPS is to identify, reduce, and control errors due to interviewers. IPS is used extensively not only in agriculture but also in **social sciences, demography**, and many other fields (see Hansen et al. [11], Lahiri [15], Som [25], Fellegi [8], Bailey et al. [1], Levy & Lemeshow [16]). Fractile graphical analysis developed in [19], based on IPS, is used in comparing, analyzing, and testing the separation between two populations when a concomitant variable (*see* **Covariate**) is measured in addition to the response variable. Details on the theory of IPS are available in [2], [13], and [23].

References

[1]   Bailey, L., Moore, T.F. & Bailer, B.A. (1978). An inter-
      viewer variance study for the eight impact cities of
      the national crime survey cities sample, *Journal of the
      American Statistical Association* **73**, 16–23.
[2]   Cochran, W.G. (1977). *Sampling Techniques*, 3rd Ed.
      Wiley, New York.
[3]   Deming, W.E. (1960). *Sample Design in Business
      Research*. Wiley, New York.
[4]   Deming, W.E. (1963). On some of the contributions of
      interpenetrating network of samples, in *Contribution to
      Statistics*, C.R. Rao, ed. Statistical Publishing Society,
      Calcutta, pp. 57–66.
[5]   Efron, B. (1979). Bootstrap methods: another look at
      the jackknife, *Annals of Statistics* **7**, 1–26.
[6]   Efron, B. & Stein, C. (1981). The jackknife estimate of
      variance, *Annals of Statistics* **9**, 586–596.
[7]   Efron, B. & Tibshirani (1993). *An Introduction to the
      Bootstrap*. Chapman & Hall, New York.
[8]   Fellegi, I. (1964). Response variance and its estima-
      tion, *Journal of the American Statistical Association* **59**,
      1016–1041.
[9]   Ghosh, S. & Gomez, R. (1986). Comparison of ratio
      estimators based on interpenetrating sub-samples with
      or without jackknifing, *Journal of the Indian Society of
      Agricultural Statistics* **38**, 200–210.
[10] Ghosh, S. & Gomez, R. (1987). Interpenetrating sub-
      sampling regression estimation with or without jack-
      knifing, *Communications in Statistics – Simulation and
      Computation* **16**, 1105–1116.
[11] Hansen, M.H., Hurwitz, W.N. & Madow, W.G. (1953).
      Sample Survey Methods and Theory. Wiley, New York.
[12] Koop, J.C. (1967). Replicated (or interpenetrating) sam-
      ples of unequal sizes, *Annals of Mathematical Statistics*
      38, 1142–1147.
[13] Koop, J.C. (1988). The technique of replicated or inter-
      penetrating samples, in *Handbook of Statistics*, Vol. 6,
      P.R. Krishnaiah & C.R. Rao, eds. Elsevier, Amsterdam,
      pp. 336–368.
[14] Lahiri, D.B. (1954). Technical paper on some aspects of
      the development of the sample design: National Sample
      Survey Report No. 5, *Sankhyā* **14**, 264–316.
[15] Lahiri, D.B. (1957). Observations on the use of inter-
      penetrating samples in India, *Bulletin of the Interna-
      tional Statistical Institute* **36**, Part 3, 144–152.
[16] Levy, P.S. & Lemeshow (1991). *Sampling of Popula-
      tions: Methods and Applications*. Wiley, New York.
[17] Mahalanobis, P.C. (1944). On large-scale sample sur-
      veys, *Philosophical Transactions of the Royal Society
      of London, Series B* **231**, 329–451.
[18] Mahalanobis, P.C. (1946). Recent experiments in statis-
      tical sampling in the Indian Statistical Institute, *Journal
      of the Royal Statistical Society* **109**, 325–378.
[19] Mahalanobis, P.C. (1960). A method of fractile graph-
      ical analysis, *Econometrica* **28**, 325–351.
[20] McCarthy, P.C. (1966). Replication: an approach to the
      analysis of data from complex surveys, *PHS Publication

No. 1000, Series E, No. 14*. US Government Printing
      Office, Washington.
[21] McCarthy, P.C. (1969). Pseudo-replication: half-sam-
      ples, *International Statistical Review* **37**, 239–264.
[22] Murthy, M.N. (1964). On Mahalanobis' contributions to
      the development of sample survey theory and methods,
      in *Contribution to Statistics*, C.R. Rao, ed. Statistical
      Publishing Society, Calcutta, pp. 282–316.
[23] Murthy, M.N. (1967). *Sampling Theory and Methods*.
      Statistical Publishing Society, Calcutta.
[24] Quenouille, M. (1949). Approximate tests of correlation
      in time series, *Journal of the Royal Statistical Society,
      Series B* **11**, 18–44.
[25] Som, R.K. (1965). Use of interpenetrating samples in
      demographic studies, *Sankhyā, Series B* **27**, 329–342.
[26] United Nations (1949). *Recommendations for the Prepa-
      ration of Sample Survey Reports, Series C, No. 1*. United
      Nations, New York.
[27] Yates, F. (1981). *Sampling Methods for Censuses and
      Surveys*, 4th Ed. Oxford University Press, London.

SUBIR GHOSH

Interquartile Range *see* Order Statistics

Interval Censoring

Interval censoring is commonly used to denote a type of sampling scheme or to describe a type of observed incomplete data. By interval-censored data we mean that a random variable of interest is known only to lie in an interval, instead of being observed exactly. In most applications of **survival analysis**, the random variable is the time until some event such as death or a disease. A common example of interval-censored survival data occurs in medical or health studies that entail periodic follow-up. Many **clinical trials** and longitudinal studies (*see* **Cohort Study**) fall into this category [16, 41]. In this situation an individual due for the scheduled observations for a clinically observed change in disease status may miss some observations and may return with a changed status, thus contributing an interval-censored time of the occurrence of the change. Another example arises in the acquired immune deficiency syndrome (**AIDS**) studies [25] that concern the human immunodeficiency virus (HIV) infection and the AIDS **incubation period** (the time from HIV infection to AIDS diagnosis). In this case, if a subject is HIV positive at the beginning of the study, then his or her HIV infection time is usually determined by a retrospective study of the subject's history. Thus only an interval given by the last HIV negative test and the first HIV positive test is known for the HIV infection time.

An important special case of interval-censored data is current status data [11, 26, 29]. In this situation each subject is observed only once for the occurrence of the event of interest and the only information available is the status of the occurrence of the event at the observation time. In other words, the observation of the time until the event is either left-censored (the survival time is known only to be less than the observation time) or right-censored (the survival time is known only to be greater than the observation time), depending on whether the event is or is not seen. One example of current status data is **cross-sectional** data [28, 35]. Another example is given by no-lethal tumors when the time to tumor onset is of interest, but not directly observable [12] (*see* **Tumor Incidence Experiments**). Note that for the first example the current status data occur usually due to study designs, while for the second case the current status data occur due to the inability to measure the variable. In the literature, current status data are also referred to as Case I interval-censored data, while the more general case is referred to as Case II interval-censored data [21].

Another special case of interval-censored data is left-censored data, in which the observation of the time until the event of interest is either left-censored or exactly known. One reason behind the occurrence of the left-censored data is the inability to measure the variable of interest when it is below a certain level. An example is the severity of an adverse event related to a drug, which sometimes can be determined only when it is over a certain degree.

To this point, survival time has been defined in a way that starts from time zero, or a known time point. A more general framework is to define survival time as the time between two related events. This illustrates another more complicated type of interval-censored data, namely doubly interval-censored data [19, 45], in which the times of the occurrences of both events defining the survival time are interval censored. A common example of such data is given by the AIDS studies discussed above

when the variable of interest is AIDS incubation time [4, 9, 17].

Interval censoring can also occur on **covariates** that are related to the survival time of interest. Such an example occurs in the AIDS study on an antiviral drug when the effect of the anti-viral resistance related to the drug on the survival time of the subjects under study is of interest. In this situation it is often the case that the occurrence of the resistance can be known only to belong to an interval. In what follows we concentrate on the interval censoring that occurs on the survival time of interest.

For the analysis of interval-censored data, one way is to use parametric methods [13, 36], which are relatively straightforward. For example, the log **spline** methods can be used to estimate the distribution function [31]. Another way, which we focus on below, is to apply semiparametric or nonparametric methods. First, we discuss the **nonparametric maximum likelihood estimate** (NPMLE) of a distribution function for survival time. We then move to regression analysis of interval-censored data and the comparison of different distribution functions. Unless specifically mentioned, the discussion will be confined to interval-censored data, although some methods discussed may also apply to doubly interval-censored data.

Nonparametric Maximum Likelihood Estimates

In medical and health studies, the estimation of a cumulative distribution function (cdf) of survival time (the survival function) is perhaps the most important and common task (*see* **Survival Distributions and Their Characteristics**). Let T denote the survival time of interest in a survival study and let F denote its cdf. Suppose that the observed data can be represented by $\{I_i\}_{i=1}^n$, where $I_i = (L_i, R_i]$ is the interval known to contain the unobserved survival time associated with the ith subject. If $L_i = 0$, then we have a left-censored observation, and if $R_i = \infty$, then we have a right-censored observation. Let $\{s_j\}_{j=0}^{m+1}$ denote the unique ordered elements of $\{0, \{L_i\}_{i=1}^n, \{R_i\}_{i=1}^n, \infty\}$, α_{ij} be the indicator (*see* **Dummy Variables**) of the event $(s_{j-1}, s_j] \subseteq I_i$, and $p_j = F(s_j) - F(s_{j-1})$. Assume that the censoring mechanism is independent of the survival time, that is, the censoring is noninformative (*see* **Censored Data**). Then the log **likelihood** can be written as

$$l(p) = \sum_{i=1}^{n} \log[F(R_i) - F(L_i)]$$

$$= \sum_{i=1}^{n} \log \left(\sum_{j=1}^{m+1} \alpha_{ij} p_j \right)$$

and the problem of finding the NPMLE of F becomes that of maximizing $l(p)$ with respect to $p = (p_1, \ldots, p_{m+1})$ subject to the constraints $\sum_{j=1}^{m+1} p_j = 1$ and $p_j \geq 0$, $j = 1, \ldots, m+1$ [18, 37]. Note that a more general way to express an interval-censored observation is to use the finite union of disjoint intervals [50], and in this case the discussion here equally applies.

To maximize $l(p)$ with respect to p, a simple and common way is to use the self-consistency **algorithm** proposed by Turnbull [50] (*see* **Turnbull Estimator**), which can be seen as an application of the EM algorithm [10] and iterates the equation $p_j^{\text{new}} = n^{-1} \sum_{i=1}^{n} [\alpha_{ij} p_j^{\text{old}} / (\sum_{l=1}^{m+1} \alpha_{il} p_l^{\text{old}})]$ until convergence. This approach is easy to implement, but is known to have a slow convergence rate. An alternative is to apply the convex minorant algorithm presented by Groeneboom [20], which promises to converge faster than the self-consistency algorithm. A third approach is to use the vertex-exchange or other algorithms proposed for the mixture model problem based on the fact that the maximization problem here is essentially similar to that arising in the fitting of mixture models (see [6]). The advantage of this approach is the availability of the statistical package C.A.MAN [7], which includes the EM and the vertex-exchange algorithms. All the above algorithms are iterative, and in fact there is no closed form for the NPMLE of F.

For current status data, however, a closed form of the NPMLE can be found [3, 48]. In this case, the NPMLE of F can be shown to be equal to the **isotonic regression** of $\{d_1/n_1, \ldots, d_m/n_m\}$ with weights $\{n_1, \ldots, n_m\}$, where $d_j = \sum_{i \in S_j} I(T_i \leq s_j)$, $n_j = |S_j|$, and S_j denotes the set of subjects who are observed at s_j, $j = 1, \ldots, m$. Thus by using the max–min formula for an isotonic regression [5], the NPMLE of F can be written as

$$\hat{F}_n(s_j) = \max_{u \leq j} \min_{v \geq j} \left(\sum_{l=u}^{v} d_j \Big/ \sum_{l=u}^{v} n_j \right).$$

For doubly interval-censored data it should be noted that the likelihood involves not only the

distribution of the survival time, but also the distribution of the originating event that defines the survival time. In this situation, one method of finding the NPMLE is to use the self-consistency algorithm proposed by DeGruttola & Lagakos [9]. This algorithm, however, is notoriously slow and can suffer starting value problems. An alternative is to apply the algorithm given by Gomez & Lagakos [19], which is very fast and stable, but could be less efficient. Some of other self-consistency algorithms that can be used in this situation could be found in Leung & Elashoff [32], Sun [45], and Tu [49].

A self-consistent estimate of F may not be an NPMLE. To verify this, one approach is to use the so-called Kuhn–Tucker conditions (see [18]). Note that at the NPMLE, p_j can be nonzero only if s_{j-1} is a left endpoint L_i for some subject i, and s_j is a right endpoint R_k for some possibly different subject k. Some of the p_js that satisfy this criterion may also be zero. The Kuhn–Tucker conditions can also be applied to identify these zero p_js, thus speeding up the self-consistency algorithm. Another approach is to use the fact that an estimate $\hat{p}$ is an NPMLE if and only if $\sup_{1 \leq j \leq m+1} \sum_{i=1}^{n} (\alpha_{ij} / \sum_{l=1}^{m+1} \alpha_{il} \hat{p}_l) = n$ [6]. For the conditions for the uniqueness of NPMLEs, see Gentleman & Geyer [18].

It can be shown that the NPMLE is **consistent** [21]. Furthermore, in the case of current status data, Groeneboom & Wellner [21] showed that $\hat{F}_n$ has a limiting, nonnormal distribution at $n^{1/3}$ **convergence** rate as $n \to \infty$. Note that this is different from the usual $n^{1/2}$ convergence rate. However, the integral of $\hat{F}_n$ and its linear functionals can be shown to have asymptotic normal distributions with $n^{1/2}$ convergence [21, 24]. For the case of general interval-censored data, no equivalent results are available, although some results can be found in Groeneboom & Wellner [21]. Also, in this case no simple variance estimate for $\hat{F}_n$ exists, except using observed Fisher **information** or **bootstrap** estimates. Other areas that remain unexplored include the estimation of F when the censoring mechanism depends on the survival time and the study of the asymptotic properties of $\hat{F}_n$ from doubly interval-censored data.

Regression Analysis

Regression analysis of survival data is commonly performed to study the effect of various covariate factors such as treatment, sex, and age on survival time. In the case of interval-censored data the methods available for the regression analysis are mainly two types: the full likelihood-based method and the marginal likelihood-based method. Let X_i denote the covariate vector associated with the ith subject and assume that the censoring mechanism is independent of both the survival time and the covariates. By using the notation given above, the log likelihood has the form:

$$l(p) = \sum_{i=1}^{n} \log[F(R_i|X_i) - F(L_i|X_i)]$$

$$= \sum_{i=1}^{n} \log \left\{ \sum_{j=1}^{m+1} \alpha_{ij}[F(s_j|X_i) - F(s_{j-1}|X_i)] \right\},$$

where $F(T|X)$ denotes the cdf of T given covariates X.

The regression model that is discussed most in the literature for the analysis of interval-censored data is perhaps the **Cox regression**, or **proportional hazards** (PH), model [8] given by [1, 15, 23, 44]

$$\lambda(t|X) = \lambda_0(t) \exp(\boldsymbol{\beta}'\mathbf{X}),$$

where $\lambda_0(t)$ denotes the unknown baseline hazard function and $\boldsymbol{\beta}$ the regression coefficients. For inference about $\boldsymbol{\beta}$ and the cumulative hazard function $\Lambda_0(t) = \int_0^t \lambda_0(s)\mathrm{d}s$, a natural method is the full likelihood approach, which maximizes $l(p)$ over $\boldsymbol{\beta}$ and $\Lambda_0(t)$ simultaneously. For example, Huang [22] studied this approach for current status data and showed that the maximum likelihood estimate (mle) of the regression coefficients is consistent and **efficient**. Moreover, he showed that the mle has an asymptotic normal distribution with an $n^{1/2}$ convergence rate. In contrast, the mle of the cumulative hazard function is consistent with an $n^{1/3}$ convergence rate and its asymptotic distribution remains unknown. The full likelihood approach can also be used for the regression analysis of doubly interval-censored data [30].

Under the PH model, an alternative to the above full likelihood approach is the marginal likelihood approach [42]. This approach defines a marginal likelihood as the summation of the probabilities of the ranking of the T_is over the set of all possible rankings of the T_is that are consistent with the observed interval-censored data. This approach is the direct generalization of the corresponding approach commonly used for right-censored data [27] and has the advantage of not involving $\lambda_0(t)$. The disadvantage is that it does not have a simple and easily manageable form, resulting in computational problems. Also, little is known about its properties.

Although the PH model yields sound results in many cases, there are situations where other models may provide a better fit to interval-censored data. For example, the **proportional odds** regression model, given by

$$\log\{[F(t|X)/[1 - F(t|X)]\} = \alpha(t) + \boldsymbol{\beta}'\mathbf{X},$$

is commonly used for environmental health data and its application to current status data has been discussed by Rossini & Tsiatis [40], where $\alpha(t)$ is a monotone-increasing function. Lin & Ying [33] discussed the **additive hazards** regression model $\lambda(t|X) = \lambda_0(t) + \boldsymbol{\beta}'\mathbf{X}$ and Rabinowitz et al. [39] studied the accelerated regression model $\log(T) = \boldsymbol{\beta}'X + \varepsilon$ for the regression analysis of interval-censored data. Sun [47] considered a **logistic regression** model for interval-censored discrete survival data.

Although a great deal of research for the regression analysis of interval-censored data has been done, there is no approach as simple as the **partial likelihood** method [8] for right-censored data. Also, there are no methods available for model checking for any of the previously mentioned models.

Comparison of Distribution Functions

A comparison of different distribution functions is often the primary goal of clinical trials and longitudinal studies. In the case of interval-censored data, one way of performing the comparison is to use the above described regression techniques by defining X as group or treatment indicators, and to base the comparison on the score tests for the regression coefficients equal to zero [15, 39] (*see* **Likelihood**). Another method, which is similar to the score test method and has received great attention in the literature, is to base the comparison on a rank test [14, 43]. For example, Self & Grossman [43] considered the linear regression model $T = \alpha + \boldsymbol{\beta}'X + \varepsilon$, where α is a constant and ε denotes the error term. Under the model, they derived the **linear rank tests** defined as the score tests for $\beta = 0$ from the marginal likelihood of the ranking of the Ts. In Sun [46], a nonparametric test, a generalization of the **logrank test** for the right-censored data [27], is proposed. For more references on rank tests, see Petroni & Wolfe [38].

A third approach to the comparison of distribution functions is to form a test by a direct comparison of the estimates of the different distribution functions [2, 38]. Permutation tests (*see* **Randomization Tests**) can also be formed for a comparison [34]. Note that most of the above comparison tests require the same censoring distribution.

Concluding Remarks

There remain many problems in the analysis of interval-censored data. One is that the properties of many of the proposed methods remain unknown, and this is especially the case for doubly interval-censored data. Another general problem is the censoring mechanism behind interval censoring. Most of the methods discussed above assume that censoring is noninformative and do not apply to informatively censored data, for which methods that take into account the censoring mechanism need to be developed.

Acknowledgments

The author is grateful to Drs Steve Lagakos, Qiming Liao, Jane Lindsey, and Ilsoon Yang for reading the article and making many helpful comments and suggestions. He also wishes to thank Drs Dianne Finkelstein, Mei-Ling Lee, and Marcello Pagano for their comments.

References

[1]   Alioum, A. & Commenges, D. (1996). A proportional hazards model for arbitrarily censored and truncated data, *Biometrics* **52**, 512–524.

[2]   Andersen, P.K. and Ronn, B.B. (1995). A nonparametric test for comparing two samples where all observations are either left- or right-censored, *Biometrics* **51**, 323–329.

[3]   Ayer, M., Brunk, H., Ewing, G., Reid, W. & Silverman, E. (1955). An empirical distribution function for sampling with incomplete information, *Annals of Mathematical Statistics* **26**, 641–647.

[4]   Bacchetti, P. & Jewell, N.P. (1991). Nonparametric estimation of the incubation distribution of AIDS based on a prevalent cohort with unknown infection times, *Biometrics* **47**, 947–960.

[5]   Barlow, R.E., Bartholomew, D.J., Bremner, J.M. & Brunk, H.D. (1972). *Statistical Inference under Order Restrictions*. Wiley, New York.

[6]   Böhning, D., Schlattmann, P. & Dietz, E. (1996). Interval censored data: a note on the nonparametric maximum likelihood estimator of the distribution function, *Biometrika* **83**, 462–466.

[7]   Böhning, D., Schlattmann, P. & Lindsay, B.G. (1992). Computer assisted analysis of mixtures (C.A.MAN): statistical algorithms, *Biometrics* **48**, 283–303.

[8]   Cox, D.R. (1972). Regression models and life-tables (with discussion), *Journal of the Royal Statistical Society, Series B* **34**, 187–220.

[9]   DeGruttola, V.G. & Lagakos, S.W. (1989). Analysis of doubly-censored survival data, with application to AIDS, *Biometrics* **45**, 1–11.

[10] Dempster, A.P., Laird, N.M. & Rubin, D.B. (1977). Maximum likelihood from incomplete data via the EM algorithm (with discussion), *Journal of the Royal Statistical Society, Series B* **39**, 1–38.

[11] Diamond, I.D. & McDonald, J.W. (1992). Analysis of current status data, in *Demographic Applications of Event History Analysis*, J. Trussell, R. Hankinson & J. Tilton, eds. Clarendon Press, Oxford, pp. 231–252.

[12] Dinse, G.E. & Lagakos, S.W. (1983). Regression analysis of tumour prevalence data, *Applied Statistics* **32**, 236–248.

[13] Farrington, C.P. (1996). Interval-censored data: a generalized linear modeling approach, *Statistics in Medicine* **15**, 283–292.

[14] Fay, M.P. (1996). Rank invariant tests for interval censored data under the grouped continuous model, *Biometrics* **52**, 811–822.

[15] Finkelstein, D.M. (1986). A proportional hazards model for interval-censored failure time data, *Biometrics* **42**, 845–854.

[16] Finkelstein, D.M. & Wolfe, R.A. (1985). A semiparametric model for regression analysis of interval-censored failure time data, *Biometrics* **41**, 933–945.

[17] Frydman, H. (1995). Semiparametric estimation in a three-state duration-dependent Markov model from interval-censored observations with application to AIDS data, *Biometrics* **51**, 502–511.

[18] Gentleman, R. & Geyer, C.J. (1994). Maximum likelihood for interval censored data: consistency and computation, *Biometrika* **81**, 618–623.

[19] Gomez, G. & Lagakos, S.W. (1994). Estimation of the infection time and latency distribution of AIDS with doubly censored data, *Biometrics* **50**, 204–212.

[20] Groeneboom, P. (1990). Nonparametric likelihood estimators for interval censoring and deconvolution, *Technical Report* 378, Statistics Department, Stanford University.

[21] Groeneboom, P. & Wellner, J.A. (1992). *Information Bounds and Nonparametric Maximum Likelihood Estimation*, DMV Seminar, Band 19. Birkhauser, New York.

[22] Huang, J. (1996). Efficient estimation for the proportional hazards model with interval censoring, *Annals of Statistics* **24**, 540–568.

[23] Huang, J. & Wellner, J.A. (1994). Regression models with interval censoring, in *Proceedings of the Kolmogorov Semester*. Euler Institute, St Petersburg.

[24] Huang, J. & Wellner, J.A. (1995). Asymptotic normality of the NPMLE of linear functionals for interval censored data, case I, *Statistica Neerlandica* **49**, 153–163.

[25] Jewell, N.P. (1994). Non-parametric estimation and doubly-censored data: general ideas and applications to AIDS, *Statistics in Medicine* **13**, 2081–2095.

[26] Jewell, N.P. & Laan, M. van der (1995). Generalizations of current status data with applications, *Lifetime Data Analysis* **1**, 101–110.

[27] Kalbfleisch, J.D. & Prentice, R.L. (1980). *The Statistical Analysis of Failure Time Data*. Wiley, New York.

[28] Keiding, N. (1991). Age-specific incidence and prevalence: a statistical perspective (with discussion), *Journal of the Royal Statistical Society, Series A* **154**, 371–412.

[29] Keiding, N., Begtrup, K., Scheike, T.H. & Hasibeder, G. (1996). Estimation from current status data in continuous time, *Lifetime Data Analysis* **2**, 119–129.

[30] Kim, M.Y., DeGruttola, V.G. & Lagakos, S.W. (1993). Analyzing doubly censored data with covariates, with application to AIDS, *Biometrics* **49**, 13–22.

[31] Kooperberg, C. & Stone, C.J. (1992). Logspline density estimation for censored data, *Journal of Computational and Graphical Statistics* **1**, 301–328.

[32] Leung, K.M. & Elashoff, R.M. (1996). A three-state disease model with interval-censored data: estimation and applications to AIDS and cancer, *Lifetime Data Analysis* **2**, 175–194.

[33] Lin, D.Y. & Ying, Z. (1996). Additive hazards regression models for survival data, in *Proceedings of the 1st Seattle Symposium in Biostatistics: Survival Analysis*. Seattle, Washington.

[34] Mantel, N. (1967). Ranking procedures for arbitrarily restricted observation, *Biometrics* **23**, 65–78.

[35] Marschner, I.C. (1994). Determining the size of a cross-sectional sample to estimate the age-specific incidence of an irreversible disease, *Statistics in Medicine* **13**, 2369–2381.

[36] Odell, P.M., Anderson, K.M. & D'Agostino, R.B. (1992). Maximum likelihood estimation for interval-censored data using a Weibull-based accelerated failure time model, *Biometrics* **48**, 951–959.

[37] Peto, R. (1973). Experimental survival curves for interval-censored data, *Applied Statistics* **22**, 86–91.

[38] Petroni, G.R. & Wolfe, R.A. (1994). A two-sample test for stochastic ordering with interval-censored data, *Biometrics* **50**, 77–87.

[39] Rabinowitz, D., Tsiatis, A. & Aragon, J. (1995). Regression with interval-censored data, *Biometrika* **82**, 501–513.

[40] Rossini, A. & Tsiatis, A. (1996). A semiparametric proportional odds regression model for the analysis of current status data, *Journal of the American Statistical Association* **91**, 713–721.

[41] Samuelsen, S.O. & Kongerud, J. (1994). Interval censoring in longitudinal data of respiratory symptoms in aluminium potroom workers: a comparison of methods, *Statistics in Medicine* **13**, 1771–1780.

[42] Satten, G.A. (1996). Rank-based inference in the proportional hazards model for interval censored data, *Biometrika* **83**, 355–370.

[43] Self, S.G. & Grossman, E.A. (1986). Linear rank tests for interval-censored data with application to PCB levels in adipose tissue of transformer repair workers, *Biometrics* **42**, 521–530.

[44] Shiboski, S. & Jewell, N. (1992). Statistical analysis of the time dependence of HIV infectivity based on partner study data, *Journal of the American Statistical Association* **87**, 360–372.

[45] Sun, J. (1995). Empirical estimation of a distribution function with truncated and doubly interval-censored data and its application to AIDS studies, *Biometrics* **51**, 1096–1104.

[46] Sun, J. (1996). A nonparametric test for interval-censored failure time data with application to AIDS studies, *Statistics in Medicine* **15**, 1387–1395.

[47] Sun, J. (1997). Regression analysis of interval-censored failure time data, *Statistics in Medicine* **16**, 497–504.

[48] Sun, J. & Kalbfleisch, J.D. (1993). The analysis of current status data on point processes, *Journal of the American Statistical Association* **88**, 1449–1454.

[49] Tu, X.M. (1995). Nonparametric estimation of survival distributions with censored initiating time, and censored and truncated terminating time: application to transfusion data for acquired immune deficiency syndrome, *Applied Statistics* **44**, 3–16.

[50] Turnbull, B.W. (1976). The empirical distribution with arbitrarily grouped censored and truncated data, *Journal of the Royal Statistical Society, Series B* **38**, 290–295.

JIANGUO SUN

Interval Scale *see* Measurement Scale

Intervention Analysis in Time Series

When data are collected in the form of time series there are important questions concerning "changes" in the series. Changes may be "man-made" or they may arise "naturally". How efficient was a preventive program to decrease the monthly number of accidents? How did the frequency of traditional neurological diagnostic methods change after the introduction of computer tomography? How did the pattern of morbidity in a population change after an environmental accident? Notifications of diseases, entries in a hospital, injuries due to accidents, etc. are usually collected in fixed equally spaced intervals. Such time series observations are likely to be dependent. ARIMA models [autoregressive integrated moving average models (*see* **ARMA and ARIMA Models**) and Box–Jenkins models [1]] allow the stochastic dependence of consecutive data to be modeled. Intervention analysis proposed by Box & Tiao [2] is an extension of ARIMA modeling allowing study of the magnitude and structure of changes of ARIMA processes.

The well-known two-sample t test for a change in level after an intervention may not be appropriate in this situation due to the possible dependency of the observations. In addition, this test allows only an assessment of the magnitude of a change and not of its structure. Since the series may be nonstationary, large changes of the series could occur even when no intervention takes place (*see* **Stationarity**). Intervention analysis may allow an investigator to distinguish between what can be expected due to nonstationarity alone and what cannot.

Analogous questions of "change" may arise when studying time series data recorded in an individual patient; changes of time series, for example, may occur after the intervention "treatment". Dependence of consecutive observations may be important when data such as blood glucose are recorded within a single patient over time. Such studies on individual subjects may be interesting and relevant in basic medical research and in clinical applications. In clinical research they may allow physicians the assessment of individual treatment effects. Decisions on treatment strategy may be based on knowledge of the stochastic processes representing the observed time series, thus allowing full use to be made of the recorded data [4].

Intervention Models

Let $y_{t-1}, y_t, y_{t+1}, \dots$ denote the observations (number of entries in a hospital, etc.) at equally spaced times, $t - 1, t, t + 1, \dots$ (e.g. yesterday, today, tomorrow, etc.). The intervention model states that y_t (or a suitably transformed version of the series) may be decomposed into two parts, an "explained"

part u_t and an "unexplained" or "noise" part n_t,

$$y_t = u_t + n_t. \tag{1}$$

The Noise Series n_t

The noise series (*see* **Noise and White Noise**) or unexplained part n_t is an autoregressive integrated moving average ARIMA(p, d, q) process given by

$$w_t = \nabla^d n_t, \tag{2}$$

$$w_t = \phi_1 w_{t-1} + \dots + \phi_p w_{t-p}$$
$$+ a_t - \theta_1 a_{t-1} - \dots - \theta_q a_{t-q} \quad \text{or}$$

$$\phi(B) w_t = \theta(B) a_t. \tag{3}$$

∇ is the differencing operator such that $\nabla n_t = n_t - n_{t-1}$ and the integer d is the number of times n_t has to be differenced to obtain a stationary series w_t. B is the backward shift operator (*see* **Backward and Forward Shift Operators**) such that $Bw_t = w_{t-1}, B^k w_t = w_{t-k}, \phi(B)$ and $\theta(B)$ are polynomials in B:

$$\phi(B) = 1 - \phi_1 B - \dots - \phi_p B^p \quad \text{and}$$
$$\theta(B) = 1 - \theta_1 B - \dots - \theta_q B^q. \tag{4}$$

$\phi(B)$ is called the autoregressive operator of order p and $\theta(B)$ the moving average operator of order q. The parameters of the noise process $\phi_1, \dots, \phi_p$ and $\theta_1, \dots, \theta_q$ are constrained such that the roots of $\phi(z)$ and $\theta(z)$ in the complex z-plane lie outside the unit circle. a_t is a *white noise* series consisting of independent identically distributed normal random variables with mean zero and variance σ_a^2. The ARIMA model for the noise n_t may be extended to the seasonal ARIMA model by including seasonal autoregressive and moving average operators. In the absence of u_t, the observed series y_t is just the ARIMA process n_t.

The Explained Part u_t

The explained part u_t is the "response" of a system to a dummy input variable I_t:

$$u_t = f(I_t). \tag{5}$$

The input I_t is usually taken as the unit pulse function p_t,

$$p_t = \begin{cases} 1, & \text{for } t = T, \\ 0, & \text{otherwise,} \end{cases} \tag{6}$$

or the unit step function s_t,

$$s_t = \begin{cases} 1, & \text{for } t \geq T, \\ 0, & \text{otherwise.} \end{cases} \qquad (7)$$

The pulse function p_t may represent, for example, an unusual event which acts only at time T. The step function s_t represents, for example, a preventive measure starting at time T. Since the "noise process" n_t may be nonstationary, large changes of the series could occur even when no intervention takes place.

Basic Patterns of Response

Figure 1 shows basic intervention models. In the first line the two dummy input variables s_t and p_t are depicted. The lines (a), (b), and (c) below show "responses" corresponding to the following three models:

1. Figure 1(a): *the simplest, case*

$$f(I_t) = \omega_0 I_t. \qquad (8)$$

The response is just the pulse- or step-input I_t multiplied by ω_0. The parameter ω_0 measures the "strength" of the effect. In this model, and

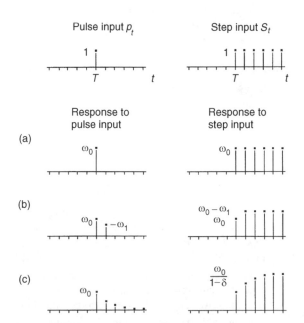

Figure 1   Responses to a unit pulse and step input: (a), (b), and (c) basic patterns of response

with the step function as input, the new level is reached immediately.

2. Figure 1(b): *a refined model*:

$$f(I_t) = \omega_0 I_t - \omega_1 I_{t-1}, \quad \text{or}$$
$$f(I_t) = (\omega_0 - \omega_1 B)I_t, \quad \text{or}$$
$$f(I_t) = \omega(B)I_t, \qquad (9)$$

where $\omega(B) = \omega_0 - \omega_1 B$ is a polynomial of first order in B.

In this refined model, and with the step function as input, the final level is reached in two steps. If $\omega_0 = 0$ the response is as in (a) but 1 time unit delayed.

3. Figure 1(c): *gradual approach to equilibrium*:

$$f(I_t) = \omega_0(I_t + \delta I_{t-1} + \delta^2 I_{t-2} + \cdots)$$
$$= \omega_0(I_t + \delta B I_t + \delta^2 B^2 I_t + \cdots)$$
$$= \omega_0(1 + \delta B + \delta^2 B^2 + \cdots)I_t$$
$$= [\omega_0/(1 - \delta B)]I_t. \qquad (10)$$

In this basic type of response the final level is reached only gradually.

The above three types of response are special cases of the *general response*

$$f(I_t) = v(B)I_t$$
$$= [\omega(B)/\delta(B)]I_t, \qquad (11)$$

where $\omega(B) = \omega_0 - \omega_1 B - \cdots - \omega_s B^s$ and $\delta(B) = 1 - \delta_1 B - \cdots - \delta_r B^r$ are polynomials in B. The corresponding model,

$$y_t = f(I_t) + n_t, \qquad (12)$$

is called an intervention model of order r. $v(B)$ is the transfer function containing infinitely many parameters in general. $\omega(B)/\delta(B)$ is a parsimonious "rational lag representation" of the transfer function $v(B)$ containing only $s + r + 1$ parameters [2].

The noise part of the model is usually obtained from the preintervention period in the same way as the ordinary ARIMA model. Standard software such as SAS or BMDP (*see* **Software, Biostatistical**) allows maximum likelihood estimation of ARIMA models and intervention models. Inspection of the data may suggest a pattern by which the known event has changed the series. Additional help may be obtained by inspection of the residuals from the corresponding model. A different way to obtain a model for the response consists in postulating one or several expected "types of change" and studying if the data provide evidence for a particular type of change.

Example

During an investigation concerned with the relationship between air pollution and respiratory diseases the environmental accident of "Schweizerhalle" occurred. In that investigation a series of medical data had been collected during about one year: the daily number of respiratory symptoms per child in a randomly selected group of preschool children (called "SYMPTOMS"). On November 1, 1986, a Sandoz storehouse containing chemical substances burned down in Schweizerhalle, located near Basle. After many people experienced symptoms and, additionally, when dead fish appeared in the Rhine, public pressure demanded investigation of possible health effects. In addition to studies specially set up for this purpose, it seemed recommendable to analyze the ongoing study with regard to the question of whether health effects could be discovered on the date of the accident.

For the preaccident period of the series SYMPTOMS an *AR(1) model* was identified. Figure 2 illustrates the process of intervention model building. Three intervention models of increasing complexity are fitted to the series SYMPTOMS in a way that each additional parameter allows for a refined explanation of the data. The simplest model is as follows:

1. Intervention model of *order zero*,

$$y_t = \omega_0 s_t + n_t, \qquad (13)$$

where s_t is the unit step function. The estimated parameters of this model are shown in Table 1 below the univariate model. Figure 2(a) shows, in the second row, the estimated function $\omega_0 s_t$ (the point labeled 370 corresponds to the date of the accident). This model gives a better fit to the data ($\sigma_a^2 = 0.00454$) than the univariate model ($\sigma_a^2 = 0.00476$). However, this simplified model does not fully represent all characteristic properties of the series: it predicts, for example, that the final level is reached immediately. It is

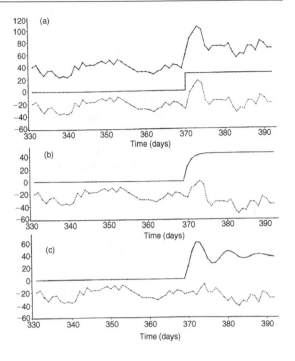

Figure 2 Three intervention models of increasing complexity. (a) Model of order zero. Upper curve: series y_t (SYMPTOMS). Second curve: "explained" part u_t. Third curve: noise series $n_t = y_t - u_t$ (shifted downwards). (b) Model of order one. Upper curve: "explained" part u_t. Lower curve: noise series $n_t = y_t - u_t$ (shifted downwards). (c) Model of order two. Same arrangement as in (b). Curves are shown multiplied by 100. Explanation in the text

therefore natural to consider the following more elaborate model.

2. Intervention model of *order one*,

$$y_t = \omega_0 (1 - \delta_1 B)^{-1} s_t + n_t. \qquad (14)$$

The parameters are given in Table 1 and the corresponding curves are presented in Figure 2(b). The residual variance decreases to $\sigma_a^2 = 0.00441$. This model allows for gradually reaching the final level [upper curve of Figure 2(b)]. However, the additional parameter δ_1 has a relatively large standard error. In addition, one recognizes from the lower curve of Figure 2(b) that the noise series n_t still has an unexplained "bump". This suggests introducing an additional refinement of the model.

Table 1   Summary of intervention models

Model type	Estimated parameters $\pm$ se	Residual variance
Univariate	$\phi_1 = 0.91 \pm 0.02$ $\mu = 0.368 \pm 0.039$	0.00476
Intervention (order 0)	$\phi_1 = 0.87 \pm 0.03$ $\mu = 0.343 \pm 0.026$ $\omega_0 = 0.274 \pm 0.058$	0.00454
Intervention (order 1)	$\phi_1 = 0.87 \pm 0.03$ $\mu = 0.331 \pm 0.027$ $\omega_0 = 0.239 \pm 0.065$ $\delta_1 = 0.46 \pm 0.16$	0.00441
Intervention (order 2)	$\phi_1 = 0.87 \pm 0.03$ $\mu = 0.334 \pm 0.026$ $\omega_0 = 0.203 \pm 0.033$ $\delta_1 = 1.21 \pm 0.07$ $\delta_2 = 0.75 \pm 0.07$	0.00420

3. Intervention model of *order two*,

$$y_t = \omega_0 (1 - \delta_1 B - \delta_2 B^2)^{-1} s_t + n_t. \quad (15)$$

The "explained" part of the model $u_t = \omega_0 (1 - \delta_1 B - \delta_2 B^2)^{-1} s_t$ may be rewritten

$$(1 - \delta_1 B - \delta_2 B^2) u_t = \omega_0 s_t, \quad \text{or}$$

$$u_t - \delta_1 u_{t-1} - \delta_2 u_{t-2} = \omega_0 s_t \quad \text{or}$$

$$u_t = \delta_1 u_{t-1} + \delta_2 u_{t-2} + \omega_0 s_t. \quad (16)$$

This second-order difference equation may represent vibrations of discrete systems (in analogy to the differential equations of order two in continuous physical systems). The lowest part of Table 1 shows the estimated parameters of this model. The parameters ω_0, δ_1 and δ_2 have small standard errors and the residual variance drops to $\sigma_a^2 = 0.00420$. The "bump" in the noise series n_t [lower curve of Figure 2(c)] has disappeared.

The upper curve of Figure 2(c), u_t, shows the characteristic behavior of a "damped vibration". The final increase of the series over the level of the preaccident period is estimated by the gain $g = \omega_0 (1 - \delta_1 - \delta_2)^{-1} = 0.376$, i.e. an increase of approximately 0.38 respiratory symptoms per child per day. The introduction of additional parameters into the model did not reduce the residual variance any further. Thus, identification of a sequence of models of increasing complexity showed that the response of the series SYMPTOMS after the accident of Schweizerhalle may be parsimoniously represented by an intervention model of second order. The model corresponds to what is known in continuous physical systems as a "damped vibration". After an initial overshoot, the series settles down to a new equilibrium at a higher level.

The results obtained support the hypothesis that the number of symptoms per child increased after the accident. The identified intervention model states that after an initial overshoot following the accident the series settles down to a new level. Unfortunately, data were not available for a longer period after the accident; thus, there is a possibility that "return to normal" could have been missed. The question of whether under the impression of the accident more symptoms were recorded (than were actually present) cannot be answered entirely satisfactorily. However, other studies conducted in this context point toward an increase in respiratory symptoms in the general population. A more detailed presentation of this study may be found in [6].

Remarks

Extensions of models as described and illustrated above are possible: intervention analysis with input consisting of multiple pulses, for example, may be used to analyze questions such as "Are there more deaths due to infarction in years with influenza A than in years without?" The sequence of pulses then represents years with influenza A.

Responses to an intervention need not to occur instantaneously; a preventive program may show an effect eventually after a delay. In addition, effects of preventive programs need not show a "permanent" effect. Decomposing the dummy input into a short-term and a long-term component may help to decide if an effect is only transient. Outliers in ARIMA time series may be detected and removed by introducing corresponding pulse inputs.

A complementary method to intervention analysis is **forecasting**: a forecast obtained from data before the intervention may be compared with actual data obtained after the intervention [3].

Literature

A nontechnical introduction to intervention analysis is given by McCleary & Hay [8]. The classical reference to ARIMA models by Box & Jenkins [1] does not include intervention analysis. The authorative presentation of intervention analysis is that of Box & Tiao [2]. Jenkins [7] provides instructive case studies in the fields of business, industry, and economics. A review, examples, and references of studies concerned with intervention analysis in medicine may be found in [5]. Applications and references of studies concerned with intervention modeling of *single patient* time series are presented in [4].

References

[1]   Box, G.E.P. & Jenkins, G.M. (1976). *Time Series Analysis: Forecasting and Control*, Rev. Ed. Holden-Day, San Francisco.

[2]   Box, G.E.P. & Tiao, G.C. (1975). Intervention analysis with applications to economic and environmental problems, *Journal of the American Statistical Association* **70**, 70–79.

[3]   Box, G.E.P. & Tiao, G.C. (1976). Comparison of forecast and actuality, *Applied Statistics* **25**, 195–200.

[4]   Crabtree, B.F., Ray, S.C., Schmidt, P.M., O'Connor, P.J. & Schmidt, D.D. (1990). The individual over time: Time series applications in health care research, *Journal of Clinical Epidemiology* **43**, 241–260.

[5]   Helfenstein, U. (1996). Box–Jenkins modelling in medical research, *Statistical Methods in Medical Research* **5**, 3–22.

[6]   Helfenstein, U., Ackermann-Liebrich U., Braun-Fahrländer, Ch. & Wanner, H.U. (1991). The environmental accident of "Schweizerhalle" and respiratory diseases: a time series analysis, *Statistics in Medicine* **10**, 1481–1492.

[7]   Jenkins, G.M. (1979). *Practical Experiences with Modelling and Forecasting Time Series*. Gwilym Jenkins & Partners (Overseas) Ltd, St. Helier.

[8]   McCleary, R. & Hay, R.A. (1980). *Applied Time Series Analysis for the Social Sciences*. Sage, Beverly Hills.

ULRICH HELFENSTEIN

Interviewer Bias

Interviewer bias is a type of information **bias** (*see* **Bias in Observational Studies; Bias, Overview**) that arises when an interviewer consciously or unconsciously elicits inaccurate information from study subjects. Interviewer bias can result in **differential error**, which can seriously distort disease–exposure **associations**, if the interviewer is aware of the disease status and exposure hypothesis in a **case–control study**, or if the interviewer is aware of the exposure status and outcome hypothesis in a **cohort study**. In the former case, the interviewer may probe more deeply for evidence of exposure among cases than among **controls**. In the latter case, the interviewer may try to elicit evidence of health effects more assiduously in exposed than in unexposed cohort members. Methods used to minimize interviewer bias include providing structured questionnaires (*see* **Questionnaire Design**), training interviewers to follow a fixed pattern of questioning, and, where possible, keeping interviewers unaware of the disease status and exposure hypotheses of greatest interest in case–control studies, and unaware of exposure status and health outcome hypotheses of greatest interest in cohort studies (*see* **Blinding or Masking**).

(*See also* **Bias in Case–Control Studies; Bias in Cohort Studies; Interviewing Techniques**).

M.H. GAIL

Interviewing Techniques

Interviewers have a variety of roles and responsibilities in conducting a **survey**. Primarily, they are responsible for the collection of data by administering a data collection instrument (*see* **Questionnaire Design**). Other roles include conducting screening interviews to ensure the respondent selected meets the requirements of the survey design plan, gaining respondent cooperation, accurately coding and editing data, and representing the survey sponsor to the public. Twenty years ago, interviewer techniques were almost exclusively designed for household, face-to-face interviews. In recent years, the advent of **computer-assisted interviewing** (CAI), which includes computer-assisted telephone interviewing (CATI) and computer-assisted personal interviewing (CAPI), have had a marked effect on the techniques used by survey interviewers. The following standard techniques, as well as techniques used specifically for CAI, are based on contemporary interviewer training manuals [1, 2].

Introducing the Survey and Gaining Cooperation

An interviewer's first contact with the respondent is crucial for several reasons. First, the purpose and importance of the survey is communicated. Secondly, rapport between the interviewer and respondent is established. Thirdly, and perhaps most important, cooperation of the respondent to participate is usually received.

The interviewer must convey the purpose and importance of the study in a simple and direct manner. This is sometimes awkward if the interviewer must read verbatim a long and complex script. After reading the introduction, the interviewer must be able to paraphrase effectively what was read so that the respondent begins to feel and understand that it is important to participate. Discussing participation in a confident, friendly, empathetic tone can help to eliminate hesitancy on the respondent's part. Interviewers can allay concerns by suggesting that they start the interview and reiterating that the respondent does not have to answer any question that may be too personal. This is an effective way to coach a reluctant respondent to participate and allows the respondent to feel that he/she has some control over the interview situation.

Typically, respondents are given assurances of **confidentiality** and, if under the auspices of an official agency, authorization for the survey during the first contact. While this may seem like a technical requirement, respondents often feel more at ease and are more willing to respond once they know the purpose of the survey, and they understand that the information they are providing will be held strictly confidential. Reluctant respondents often are concerned about how they were selected. Virtually every interviewer has had a respondent ask: "How did you get my name?" If the survey is a **random sample**, then interviewers need to explain the process in a clear and concise manner. Interviewers should listen carefully to all questions and comments from the respondent and should answer only what is asked.

Handling respondents who refuse to participate (*see* **Nonresponse**) is probably the most challenging component of an interviewer's job. In any survey, there are respondents who simply do not want to be interviewed. Some respondents refuse outright and others indicate refusal indirectly by avoiding the interview or constantly rescheduling. While a relatively high number of initial interview contacts result in rescheduling, few refusals actually do occur in a well-planned survey. The interviewer is the major influence on the motivation of the respondent and on the quality of the responses received. Interviewers can subtly communicate their interest in the study, their enthusiasm about their work, and even their positive feelings about the respondent, all of which increase survey cooperation.

Interviewers are trained to convert a potential refusal into cooperation. A good interviewer will use techniques that reduce covert negative issues likely to cause refusals. Respondents may be mistrustful of the interviewer, may see participating in a survey as an invasion of their privacy, or may not understand or believe assurances of confidentiality and anonymity. Respondents may also feel threatened about the survey's topic, especially if it is sensitive. Interviewers can discuss the respondent's concerns in an open, relaxed manner and usually can convince them to start the interview.

Interviewing a Survey Respondent

Ask Each Question Exactly as Worded. This is a standard long held in survey design. If questions are not read exactly as worded, they may not yield comparable results. Research has shown that even minor changes in wording can change response distributions. It is true, however, that interviewers are allowed to depart from the standard wording, but that is only after they have first asked the standard form of the question and attempted to get an answer.

Ask Every Question.   Although the answer to a given question may seem obvious, interviewers must ask the question and obtain a response. Occasionally, the respondent provides an answer which applies to a question asked later in the interview. In this case, the interviewer should verify the answer to the question.

Maintain Positive Rapport.   Offering the respondents some assurance that they are doing well and that their responses are valuable can increase their willingness to participate. Comments such as "Yes, I see" show the respondents that their answers are important and interesting to the interviewer. This can stimulate a respondent to talk further and to engage more actively in the survey process.

Use Effective Probing Techniques.   When the respondent's answer does not meet the question's objective, or when a respondent seems to have misunderstood the question, interviewers need to probe for clarification or correction. One of the most common probes is to ask the respondent to repeat the answer – this often prompts the respondents to expand on the answer, offer more information, or correct an answer. Another common probe technique is to reread the question. This often results in the respondent paying closer attention to the question and revising the answer.

In general, interviewers should not probe by paraphrasing a question, offering additional explanations (unless this is provided for in the interviewer's manual), or assuming responses that may seem obvious from prior answers. Rather, probing should take the form of more general questions ("What do you mean?") or should be an attempt to improve the specificity of a response ("Could you put your answer in terms of days?").

The danger of probing is that the interviewer can influence the respondent's answer and approach to other questions. Also, it can unnecessarily prolong the interview and convey a more conversational, informal tone. It is important for the interviewer to probe only when necessary and then return to asking survey questions. Probes should be neutral and not convey a right or wrong answer. For example, if the respondent

says she had between five and eight visits to the doctor, a **biased** probe would be "So, would you say five is about right?" and a neutral probe would be "Would you say the number of visits was closer to five or closer to eight?" Interviewers can also probe using statements and questions that indicate their uncertainty, such as "I don't know quite what you mean," or "Which figure would you say comes closer?" It is important when using these sorts of probes to keep the tone positive, and not intimate that the respondent gave a wrong answer. In fact, some interviewers find it useful to probe with a suggestion that it is the interviewer who is misunderstanding (e.g. "I'm not sure what you mean by that; could you tell me a little more?").

One exception to the probing guidelines above is when an interviewer is conducting a cognitive interview. Cognitive interviews are typically used in pretests to identify flawed questions prior to fielding the survey. Cognitive interviewers specialize in applying cognitive psychology principles to understanding the survey response process. These interviewers depart freely from the questionnaire to probe intensively. Probes are not used to help record or code information given by the respondent; rather, they are qualitative in nature and used to determine whether the respondent is having difficulty comprehending the question, recalling the information asked, or using an inappropriate response strategy (like estimating or guessing). Examples of typical probes used in cognitive interviews include "Can you paraphrase for me what you think this question is asking?", "Tell me how you arrived at your answer?", and "How sure are you that your answer is correct?"

Interviewer's Manner and Nonverbal Communication

Whether in person or on the telephone, interviewers must uniquely combine a friendly approach with an official, businesslike manner. Respondents often begin to talk about the subject matter of a questionnaire, and if the interviewer becomes distracted or becomes too engaged in social conversation with the respondent, it is often difficult to return to asking survey questions.

It is important that interviewers maintain an objective attitude. They should never indicate a personal opinion about a reply or a survey topic.

Furthermore, they need to be acutely aware of facial expressions, mannerisms, tone of voice, and other spontaneous reactions to respondent answers. Expressions of surprise, amusement, disapproval, or even sympathy may cause respondents to give untrue answers or to withhold information. Objectivity is the most effective method for putting respondents at ease and making them feel free to answer questions honestly.

For telephone interviews, it is essential that the interviewer's tone be pleasant and friendly, that they speak clearly, and that they are familiar enough with the instrument to avoid long pauses or delays. Pauses on the telephone are awkward, and may give the impression that the interviewer is waiting for an explanation from the respondent. Hesitation and expressed uncertainty about what to ask may create a negative impression in a telephone contact that would not have necessarily occurred in a face-to-face interview.

Telephone surveys, in general, are administered more quickly than a face-to-face interview because interviewers tend to read the questions faster and respondents tend to answer quicker and are less inclined to engage in social discourse. However, rushing can also give the appearance of lacking confidence and may cause the listener to misunderstand. Telephone interviewing should be confined to shorter data-collection instruments (*see* **Telephone Sampling**).

Computer-Assisted Interviewing (CAI)

Field data collection using computers is a new approach in many surveys. Clear benefits of CAI are that it eliminates editing responsibilities of the interviewer and keying of questionnaire data, resulting in quicker availability of results. Using a computer to collect interview data offers some important advantages to actual interviewer techniques as well.

First, the computer presents the correct sequence of questions based on the information and the responses already entered. This relieves the interviewer of a burden as they do not need to follow skip instructions, check items, and so forth. The computer also checks responses to ensure that all applicable items are answered appropriately. For example, where possible answers to a question are

1 (Yes) or 2 (No), the computer will reject other answers, and prompt the interviewer either to reask the question or to check the entry they made. Clearly, the use of computers is expected to help interviewers do their job more efficiently by eliminating tedious paperwork and freeing them to concentrate on actual data collection and building rapport with respondents.

One advantage of CAI interviews is that the program can easily provide on-screen instructions or other helpful information. For example, the screen may display previously provided names of family members so that the interviewer can refer to them by name in follow-up questions. This helps the interviewer administer the questions in a more friendly, casual manner. During the interview, the disadvantage to a lot of on-screen instructions and information is that the interviewer must not devote much time to reading the screen and trying to familiarize her/himself with instructions and other screen entries. This can hurt the interviewer's credibility as a well-trained professional, and can serve to distract and/or disengage the respondent. The interviewer's training must thoroughly familiarize the interviewer with the screens and instrument flow.

Another advantage of CAI is that each displayed screen can have an accompanying HELP screen, readily providing interviewers with screen-specific information, definitions, and explanations. This preserves the interviewer's sense of confidence, and improves data quality.

In CAPI surveys, interviewers have to be sensitive to the respondents' perception of the use of a computer to enter data. Some respondents perceive the computer as a means of entering their data into some sort of an open "information highway", and need to be assured that computers actually go further to protect confidential data. The computer may also serve as a barrier to good eye contact between the interviewer and respondent. In addition, if the interviewer is not comfortable with the computer program, they may spend too much time attending to the computer to the exclusion of the respondent. One point that interviewers should remember is that the respondent usually cannot see the screen that the interviewer is looking at, in contrast to being able to see a paper and pencil questionnaire. Also, because the interviewing program will perform internal consistency edits based on information previously and subsequently provided, the programs often identify inconsistent answers that the interviewer has to probe about. If this is not done in a sensitive manner (e.g. "I must have entered something wrong – let me ask that question again."), respondents may begin to feel defensive about their answers and disengage from the survey process.

Last, interviewers may have more difficulty showing cards, life history calendars, or other tools that they need to give to the respondent during the interview. Depending on where the computer is set up, if it is sitting on the interviewer's lap and the respondent is not close by, too much distance may be created which will make these survey aides awkward to use. Also, if interviewers are forced to stand while conducting CAPI interviews, they lose the mobility to use ancillary interviewing tools smoothly.

Conclusion

Good interviewing techniques apply to all modes of interviewing: face-to-face, telephone, CATI, and CAPI. Each interviewing mode also makes unique demands on the interviewer. The current trend towards increasing use of CAI requires interviewers to fortify themselves with all the standards of good interviewing techniques, and develop automation skills as an additional requirement. Interviewers are also being required to administer a survey for an increasingly resistant respondent pool, and to manipulate the dynamics of the interviewing situation to maintain respondent cooperation and interest. Newer and more effective training strategies need to be developed to equip interviewers with all the skills demanded by a fast-paced, changing survey environment.

References

[1]   US Bureau of the Census (1996). HIS-100C CAPI Manual for HIS Field Representatives, *National Health Interview Study*. US Bureau of the Census, Washington.

[2]   Westat, Inc. (1996). *Interviewer Training Manual, Race/Ethnicity Study*. Westat Inc., Rockville.

(*See also* **Interviewer Bias**)

SUSAN SCHECHTER &
ADRIENNE ONETO QUASNEY

Intrablock Analysis *see* Incomplete Block Designs

Intraclass Correlation *see* Correlation

Intracluster Correlation *see* Sample Surveys

Invariance *see* Sufficient Statistic

Invariance Principle *see* Limit Theorems

Inverse Chi-Square Distribution *see* Fiducial Probability

Inverse Cumulative Distribution Function (cdf) Transformation *see* Uniform Distribution

Inverse Gaussian Distribution

In 1828 the English botanist Robert Brown described observations made on the motion of plant pollen immersed in water. He found a swimming, dancing motion from pollen from many different plants and he extended his research to include particles of fossilized plants and mineral specimens. Apparently, he believed that he had discovered a new type of particle. His work led to the realization that the motion was a physical phenomenon rather than biologic.

Bachelier (1900) and Einstein (1905) derived the normal distribution as the model for **Brownian motion**. Wiener (1923) gave the theory of a measure on the path space. Schrodinger (1915) considered Brownian motion with a positive drift, and obtained the distribution of the first passage time to describe the position of a particle performing Brownian motion. Tweedie [5] noticed the inverse relationship between cumulant **generating functions**, and proposed the name inverse Gaussian distribution. Wald [6] obtained the distribution as an approximation of the sample size distribution in a **sequential** probability ratio test. The distribution is sometimes known as Wald's distribution.

The probability density function of the inverse Gaussian distribution, denoted by IG(μ, λ), is

$$f_X(x : \mu, \lambda) = \left(\frac{\lambda}{2\pi x^3}\right)^{1/2} \exp\left[\frac{-\lambda(x-\mu)^2}{2\mu^2 x}\right],$$

with $\mu > 0$, $\lambda > 0$, and $x > 0$. The mean is μ and the variance is μ^3/λ. The unimodal density function, a member of the **exponential family**, is skewed to the right (*see* **Skewness**). Its shape resembles other skewed density functions such as the **lognormal, Weibull**, and **gamma**. It can be obtained from the Wiener process $X(t)$ with positive drift ν and variance parameter σ^2 (*see* **Brownian Motion and Diffusion Processes**). Starting at zero, the time, T, for $X(t)$ to reach the barrier $a(a > 0)$ for the first time is called the *first passage time* and has an inverse Gaussian distribution with $\mu = a/\nu$ and $\lambda = a^2/\sigma^2$.

Unlike the Weibull or gamma distributions, the inverse Gaussian distribution allows exact sampling distributions. The **sufficient statistics** $\overline{X}$ and $T = \sum(1/X - 1/\overline{X})$, or a one-to-one function of $\overline{X}$ and T, are the basic quantities which are used in all of the **hypothesis tests, confidence intervals**, etc. $\overline{X}$ is also inverse Gaussian and λT is independently distributed as a **chi-square distributed** variable with $n - 1$ **degrees of freedom**.

Statistical methods based on the distribution have been developed to include the point and interval **estimation** of parameters, prediction intervals, estimation of the cumulative distribution function (cdf), analysis of **residuals** (one-way and two-way), **regression** analysis, and reliability analysis (*see* **Survival Analysis, Overview**).

The distribution has been used to describe phenomena in many of the sciences. In the biosciences, Sheppard & Savage [4] made use of the distribution to describe the length of time a particle remains in the blood. Since then it has been used in modeling maternity data, crop field size, shelf life, and many other types of data. Eaton & Whitmore [2] modeled the length of stay in a hospital as an inverse Gaussian variable.

For additional information, see [1] and [3].

References

[1] Chhikara, R.S. & Folks, J.L. (1989). *The Inverse Gaussian Distribution*. Marcel Dekker, New York.
[2] Eaton, W.W. & Whitmore, G.A. (1977). Length of stay as a stochastic process: a general approach and application to hospitalization for schizophrenia, *Journal of Mathematical Sociology* **5**, 273–292.
[3] Johnson, N.L. & Kotz, S. (1970). *Distributions in Statistics: Continuous Univariate Distributions*, Vol. 1. Wiley, New York.
[4] Sheppard, C.W. & Savage, L.J. (1951). The random walk problem in relation to the physiology of circulatory mixing, *Physical Review* **83**, 489–490.
[5] Tweedie, M.C.K. (1957). Statistical properties of inverse Gaussian distributions I, *Annals of Mathematical Statistics* **28**, 362–377.
[6] Wald, A. (1944). On cumulative sums of random variables, *Annals of Mathematical Statistics* **15**, 283–296.

J. LEROY FOLKS

Inverse Regression *see* Calibration

Inversion Formula *see* Characteristic Function

Inversion Method *see* Simulation

Irreducible Chain *see* Markov Chains

Irwin, Joseph Oscar

Born: December 17, 1898, in London, UK.
Died: July 27, 1982, in Schaffhausen, Switzerland.

As the leading theoretician amongst British medical statisticians in the 1930s and in subsequent decades,

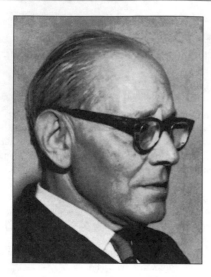

Reproduced by permission of the Royal Statisical Society

Oscar Irwin played an important role in linking developments in statistical theory to applications in medical research.

At school, Irwin had specialized in classics before he took up mathematics. In 1917 his entry to Cambridge on a scholarship was delayed first by illness, and then by a crucial period working under **Karl Pearson** on anti-aircraft trajectories. On achieving his degree in 1921, he joined Pearson's staff at University College. Renewed illness led to a period of recuperation in Switzerland which initiated a life-long love of that country and, in later life, to his marriage to a Swiss wife.

In 1928, Irwin joined **R.A. Fisher's** department at Rothamsted, and thus became one of the few statisticians to work both with Karl Pearson and Fisher. A decade later, when Fisher and **Egon Pearson** occupied adjacent floors at University College, Irwin was said to be one of the few people to be *persona grata* in both departments. During his period with Fisher, ending in 1931, Irwin came to grips with the mathematical theory published during the 1920s by Fisher, who always retained a high opinion of Irwin's mathematical ability.

In 1931, Irwin joined the staff of the **Medical Research Council (MRC)**, housed at the London School of Hygiene and Tropical Medicine, where he was to stay for most of the next 30 years. As an MRC worker, Irwin had only a part-time university appointment. However, for about 25 years he taught a course in statistical methods, introducing many relatively recent developments in the subject. During the war years (1940–1945) he worked in Cambridge, teaching statistics to mathematicians, many of whom followed a subsequent career in statistics.

Irwin retired in 1965, after which he worked for a short time at the Galton Laboratory, University College London, before moving to Switzerland. He was a Visiting Professor at the University of North Carolina, Chapel Hill during three sabbatical periods.

Irwin's early papers reveal great mathematical fluency, which he retained throughout his life. In a paper of 1927 [1] he derived the distribution of the **mean** (*see* **Sampling Distribution**) from various distributions using the **characteristic function**. At Rothamsted he wrote on the influence of climatic factors on crop yield, but was perhaps more intrigued by theoretic work on topics such as the **analysis of variance**. In 1931, he started a series of expository papers on 'Recent advances in mathematical statistics', with bibliographies, which were particularly influential at a time at which few books on statistical theory existed.

His move to the MRC enlarged his research interests. He wrote several papers on **factor analysis**, but during the 1930s, while his colleague and close contemporary **Austin Bradford Hill** devoted himself largely to epidemiologic and (later) clinical research, Irwin's interests focused on laboratory experimentation. There were papers with H. Barkwith on the **dilution method** of estimating bacterial densities, and a developing interest in the methodology of **biological assay**, stimulated by his membership of a committee of the British Pharmacopoeia Commission. There was a major paper in the 1937 *Journal of the Royal Statistical Society*, *Supplement* [3], and papers with E.A. Cheeseman clarifying the **maximum likelihood** solution in probit analysis (*see* **Quantal Response Models**).

His 1935 paper in *Metron* [2] described the "exact" test for **two-by-two tables**, derived and published independently from **Yates'** 1934 paper and Fisher's insertion in the 1934 edition of *Statistical Methods for Research Workers* (*see* **Fisher's Exact Test**). He also wrote extensively on theories of **accident proneness**.

After the war he embarked on many long-term collaborative research programs, often for official committees. These included collaborative assays, especially for the standardization of vitamins, nutritional studies, work on physiologic responses to hot climates, laboratory tests for pertussis vaccines, and tests for the carcinogenicity of tars and mineral oils (*see* **Tumor Incidence Experiments**). The latter work led to papers on the analysis of animal carcinogenicity tests by **actuarial methods**. His earlier work on accident proneness stimulated a revived interest in long-tailed discrete distributions, with some pioneering studies of the Waring distributions.

Irwin played a very active role in the affairs of the **Royal Statistical Society**, as President in 1962–1964, Editor of the *Journal, Series B* from 1949 to 1959, Chairman of the Study Section in 1934–1935 and of the Research Section in 1947–1949, and recipient of the Guy Medal in Silver. He was President of the British Region of the **International Biometric Society** during 1958 and 1959.

Oscar Irwin was a man of wide cultural interests and fine sensitivity. In some ways he was ill-adapted to the more robust features of professional life, and preferred quiet and intimate conversation to public forum and debate. He exhibited great kindness to visiting scientists and students; several young medical visitors to the London School of Hygiene were given tutorials on Fisher's *Statistical Methods for Research Workers*, a book for which Irwin retained undying respect throughout his life.

References

[1]   Irwin, J.O. (1927). On the frequency distribution of the means of samples from a population having any law of frequency with finite moments with special reference to Pearson's Type II, *Biometrika* **19**, 225–239.

[2]   Irwin, J.O. (1935). Tests of significance for differences between percentages based on small numbers, *Metron* **12**, 83–94.

[3]   Irwin, J.O. (1937). Statistical method applied to biological assays, *Journal of the Royal Statistical Society, Supplement* **4**, 1–60.

P. ARMITAGE

Isodemographic Base Map *see* Mapping Disease Patterns

Isometry *see* Allometry

Isoquant *see* Linear Programming

Isotonic Inference

Isotonic inference concerns situations in which a set of parameters is assumed, a priori, to satisfy certain order restrictions. In the most common case, where data are arranged in ordered groups, the **mean** value of a **random variable** is assumed to change monotonically with the ordering of the groups. It is then reasonable to take account of the order restrictions in making inferences about the group means, such as point or interval estimations or significance tests. Isotonic inference extends more generally to situations where there are various shape constraints on response curves, such as convexity, concavity, or sigmoidicity.

One approach to such problems is to assume a parametric model that incorporates those order or shape constraints such as a **linear regression** equation or a particular **dose–response** function. The inference based on the parametric model can, however, be considerably **biased** and variable when the specified model is incorrect. It has been pointed out in environmental toxicology applications, for example, that no parametric dose–response model can be assumed to hold generally at very low doses of interest, and yet a monotone and convex relationship might reasonably, and more reliably, be assumed. We are therefore concerned in this article mainly with methods of inference that avoid the need to specify a rigid parametric model, but nevertheless allow for those order restrictions.

There is a large literature on **estimation** and testing (*see* **Hypothesis Testing**) in the areas of isotonic and order-restricted inferences, and comprehensive surveys of these areas include [3] and [37].

One general approach to the isotonic inference is **maximum likelihood** estimation. The problem of finding order-restricted maximum likelihood estimates is often solved by using **isotonic regression**. In its simplest case an explicit solution is obtained by the pool-adjacent-violators method, but in more general cases it is solved only by some nonlinear programming, see [40] and [9], for example, or by the aid of a formal **Bayesian** approach, as in [36]. For a restricted **likelihood ratio test** the usual asymptotic chi-square distribution theory does not apply. In some cases, the resulting distributions are known to be a mixture of χ^2 distributions, but in other cases some **computer-intensive methods** such as parametric **bootstrap** tests [9], or an asymptotic conservative approximation method [40] may be used. The maximum likelihood approach is outlined in another article (*see* **Isotonic Regression**). Here we are concerned mainly with other approaches to isotonic inference. As a natural method of incorporating prior knowledge in particular applications, a Bayesian approach is also briefly mentioned.

The Case for Isotonic Inference

The data in Table 1 are measurements of the half-life of an antibiotic drug in relation to the dose administered. The usual **analysis of variance** (ANOVA) is obviously inappropriate, because of the ordering of the doses, and one possible approach is to assume a parametric model. The simplest model for the monotone relationship is linear regression. However, it is generally difficult to assume that a linear relationship holds over a wide range of an **explanatory variable**. For the dose–response relationship there are of course more natural response curves, such as a sigmoid function, but it is still often difficult to assume a particular model for the given set of data. Furthermore, it also sometimes suffices to show an overall upward trend or to detect a steep **change-point** in the responses. It is then unnecessary to assume a rigid parametric model, and a nonparametric trend test or some

multiple comparisons procedure is more appropriate (*see* **Simultaneous Inference**). We need assume only a monotone relationship in the mean half-life,

$$H_1: \mu_1 \leq \cdots \leq \mu_a, \tag{1}$$

where at least one inequality is strong, so that the null model $H_0: \mu_1 = \cdots = \mu_a$ is excluded.

The data in Table 2 show ordinal (i.e. **ordered**) **categorical data** typical of a Phase III comparative **clinical trial**. Assuming a **multinomial** model with cell probabilities p_{ij}, the **null hypothesis** that the two treatments are equal can be expressed as $p_{1j} = p_{2j}$, $j = 1, \ldots, 4$, or equivalently as

$$p_{ij} = p_{i\cdot}p_{\cdot j}. \tag{2}$$

Eq. (2) is the familiar independence hypothesis for a two-way **contingency table**. However, the usual **goodness-of-fit chi-square test** is inappropriate, since we are interested in a more restricted alternative

$$p_{11}/p_{21} \leq \cdots \leq p_{14}/p_{24}$$
$$H_2 : \text{or}$$
$$p_{11}/p_{21} \geq \cdots \geq p_{14}/p_{24},$$

where at least one inequality is strong, implying that treatment 1 is superior to treatment 2 in efficacy or vice versa. **Ordered categorical data** are a special case of rank data with many ties, and any method for rank data can be applied to ordered categorical data, and vice versa.

If ordered categorical data are obtained at several doses, as in Table 3, then we are interested in testing

Table 1   Half life of an antibiotic in rats

Dose (mg/kg)	Data (h)					Average
5	1.17	1.12	1.07	0.98	1.04	1.076
10	1.00	1.21	1.24	1.14	1.34	1.186
25	1.55	1.63	1.49	1.53		1.550
50	1.21	1.63	1.37	1.50	1.81	1.504
200	1.78	1.93	1.80	2.07	1.70	1.856

Table 2   Efficacy in a phase III trial of antibiotics

Drug	Not effective	Slightly effective	Effective	Excellent
AMPC	3	8	30	22
S6472	8	9	29	11

Table 3   Usefulness in a dose-finding clinical trial

Drug	Undesirable	Slightly undesirable	Not useful	Slightly useful	Useful	Excellent
Placebo	3	6	37	9	15	1
AF 3 (mg/kg)	7	5	33	21	10	1
AF 6 (mg/kg)	5	6	21	16	23	6

the two-way **ordered alternative**:

$$H_3 : p_{i+1,j}/p_{i,j} \le p_{i+1,j+1}/p_{i,j+1},$$
$$i = 1, \ldots, a-1;$$
$$j = 1, \ldots, b-1,$$

which implies that higher doses are superior to lower doses in efficacy.

A similar hypothesis

$$H_4 : \mu_{i+1,j+1} - \mu_{i+1,j} - \mu_{i,j+1} + \mu_{i,j} \ge 0,$$
$$i = 1, \ldots, a-1; j = 1, \ldots, b-1,$$

has been considered for normal means from a two-way layout experiment, which implies that the differences, $\mu_{ij} - \mu_{i'j}$, tend upwards as the level j increases for any $i > i'$; see [13].

Various Extensions of the Monotone Relationship

A monotone dose–response relationship may be disturbed by toxicity at higher doses, and a **nonparametric** testing procedure for the downturn (or "umbrella") hypothesis,

$$H_5 : \mu_1 \le \cdots \le \mu_{\tau+1} \ge \mu_{\tau+2} \ge \cdots \ge \mu_a,$$
$$\tau = 1, \ldots, a-1,$$

has been proposed in [44]; here τ is an unknown turning point.

Some other extensions arise when responses show monotone relationships with the passage of time. Frequently encountered examples include the monotonic change of occurrence probabilities of some events, increasing treatment effects, and increasing **hazard rates** with time. For instance, the hypothesis

$$H_6 : \mu_2 - \mu_1 \le \mu_3 - \mu_2 \le \cdots \le \mu_a - \mu_{a-1}$$

arises from the analysis of the age–period–cohort effects model (*see* **Age–Period–Cohort Analysis**) where only the second-order differences are estimable in each effect along with the time axis; see [19]. Hypothesis H_6 is equivalent to H_6': $\mu_i - 2\mu_{i+1} + \mu_{i+2} \ge 0$, and may be called the "convexity hypothesis". Hypothesis H_6 is of course mathematically different from hypothesis H_5, but there are some similarities in their shapes, and

with a slight modification the test for H_6 performs well also as a test for H_5. Convexity, concavity and sigmoidicity constraints are commonly employed also in the field of bioassay as reasonable shape constraints on a dose–response relationship (*see* **Biological Assay, Overview; Quantal Response Models**).

As seen from the above examples, isotonic inference is closely related to **change-point** analysis. Actually, a one-sided change-point model may be formulated as a set of particular monotone relationships,

$$H_7 : \mu_1 = \cdots = \mu_\tau < \mu_{\tau+1} = \cdots = \mu_a,$$
$$\tau = 1, \ldots, a-1, \tag{3}$$

with τ an unknown change-point parameter, so that a useful statistic for change-point analysis is useful also for isotonic inference. Interestingly, (3) defines $a-1$ edges of the convex cone defined by the simple ordered alternative (1).

For other extensions, including **tree-structured**, star-shaped, unimodality, and symmetry models, the reader is referred to [3] and [37].

Testing a Simple Ordered Alternative in Normal Means

We wish to test a simple ordered alternative H_1 in the one-way layout model

$$y_{ij} = \mu_i + \varepsilon_{ij}, \quad i = 1, \ldots, a; j = 1, \ldots, n_i,$$

where the ε_{ij} are assumed to be independently distributed as **normal** $N(0, \sigma^2)$ with known **variance** σ^2. Then there are two major streams of overall trend tests and multiple contrast type tests. Most cases of unknown variance can be dealt with similarly, if an **unbiased** variance estimator distributed as a multiple of χ^2 is available.

Overall Trend Tests

One possible approach is the restricted likelihood ratio test developed extensively in [3] (*see* **Isotonic Regression**). The approach does not, however, possess any obvious optimal property for such restricted alternatives, and is rather difficult to extend to higher-way problems.

Abelson & Tukey [1] proposed a linear score statistic which maximizes the minimum **power** in the region defined by H_1 within the class of linear tests. This has been extended to the most stringent and somewhat most powerful (MSSP) test for a more general restricted alternative by Schaafsma [38, 39]. In the balanced case, Abelson & Tukey's score is determined by equalizing powers at all the $a - 1$ edges of H_1 and is given by

$$c_i \propto -[i(1 - i/a)]^{1/2} + \left[(i-1)\left(1 - \frac{i-1}{a}\right)\right]^{1/2},$$
$$i = 1, \ldots, a.$$

Extending Taguchi's idea [46], the cumulative χ^2 test was introduced in [14], and its power has been compared with that of the previous two approaches. The test statistic χ^{*2} is the sum of squares of the standardized accumulated statistics

$$y_i^* = \frac{1}{\sigma}\left(\frac{1}{N_i} + \frac{1}{N_i^*}\right)^{-1/2}(\overline{Y}_i^* - \overline{Y}_i),$$
$$i = 1, \ldots, a - 1, \qquad (4)$$

where $N_i = n_1 + \cdots + n_i$, $N_i^* = n_{i+1} + \cdots + n_a$, and $\overline{Y}_i = (y_1. + \cdots + y_i.)/N_i$, $\overline{Y}_i^* = (y_{i+1}. + \cdots + y_a.)/N_i^*$ with $y_i. = (y_{i1} + \cdots + y_{in_i})$, $i = 1, \ldots, a$. The χ^{*2} statistic is characterized by the strong positive **correlations** between the serial components y_i^*, and in particular by the expansion for the balanced case in a series of independent χ^2 variables,

$$\chi^{*2} = \frac{1}{1 \cdot 2}\chi_{(1)}^2 + \frac{a}{2 \cdot 3}\chi_{(2)}^2 + \cdots + \frac{a}{(a-1) \cdot a}\chi_{(a-1)}^2,$$

where $\chi_{(l)}^2$ is the 1 df χ^2 statistic for detecting the departure from the null model in the direction of Chebyshev's lth order orthogonal polynomial. Hence χ^{*2} tests mainly, but not exclusively, a linear trend; see [18] and [31] for details.

Multiple Contrast Type Tests

Several multiple comparison procedures have been proposed for ordered parameters. Williams [49] proposed a closed testing procedure based on the maximum likelihood estimator for defining the maximal noneffective dose level. Marcus [26] modified the method by changing the estimator at the control level from $\overline{y}_1.$ to $\hat{\mu}_1$, the maximum likelihood estimator of μ_1, so that his statistic is the maximal component of Bartholomew's $\overline{\chi}^2$. The limiting

distribution of the latter statistic is obtained in [50], where upper percentiles are tabulated, including the case of unknown variance. The maximal component of χ^{*2} has been proposed also for this purpose, and is called the "max t" method, where t stands for the y_i^* of (4). The statistic is characterized as the likelihood ratio test for the change-point hypothesis H_7, and an exact and very efficient algorithm for calculating the **P value** has been obtained by Hawkins [11] (*see* **Change-Point Problem**). The power functions of these closed multiple testing procedures have been compared in [26], [43], and [25]. More general multiple tests for ordered parameters are obtained in [28].

Confidence Interval

A **confidence interval** taking advantage of order restrictions can be obtained by inverting an appropriate test for order restricted alternatives. For example, Marcus & Peritz [27] and Schoenfeld [41] obtain confidence intervals for normal means by inverting a multiple contrast type test and the restricted likelihood ratio test, respectively. Wynn [53] gives a general methodology for obtaining one-sided confidence intervals, and Hayter [12] obtains confidence intervals based on the one-sided **studentized range** test. In particular, in the bioassay problem, Schmoyer [40] obtains improved upper confidence bounds for the responses at very low doses by assuming sigmoidicity in the dose–response curve.

There is no extensive work on the design of experiments on the ordered parameters, although optimal allocation has been discussed in [24] (*see* **Optimal Design**).

Applications

A test of Abelson & Tukey, the cumulative χ^2 test, and some of the multiple comparison procedures, are now applied to the data in Table 1. Since the variance σ^2 is unknown, it is replaced by the usual unbiased estimate of variance, $\hat{\sigma}^2 = \sum\sum(y_{ij} - \overline{y}_i.)^2/(24 - 5) = 0.020741$.

The linear score statistic of Abelson & Tukey is calculated as

$$(-c_1\overline{y}_1. - c_2\overline{y}_2. + c_3\overline{y}_3. + c_4\overline{y}_4. + c_5\overline{y}_5.)/\hat{\sigma}$$
$$= 9.1206,$$

with scores $c_1 = c_5 = (\sqrt{6}+1)/\sqrt{5} = 1.543$, $c_2 = c_4 = (4 - \sqrt{6})/\sqrt{20} = 0.3467$, and $c_3 = 0$, giving a

P value of 2.2×10^{-8} as evaluated by the t distribution with 19 df.

The null distribution of cumulative χ^2 statistic $\sum y_i^{*2}$ is well approximated by $d\chi_f^2$, a multiple of the χ^2 variable with df f, where the constants d and f are given by

$$d = 1 + \frac{2}{a-1}$$
$$\times \left(\frac{\lambda_1}{\lambda_2} + \frac{\lambda_1 + \lambda_2}{\lambda_3} + \cdots + \frac{\lambda_1 + \cdots + \lambda_{a-2}}{\lambda_{a-1}} \right),$$
$$f = (a-1)/d, \qquad (5)$$

with $\lambda_i = N_i / N_i^*$. An even better approximation based on the expansions by Laguerres' orthogonal polynomials, and also the approximation under the alternative hypothesis, are given in [15]. Then the P value of the statistic

$$F^* = (a-1)^{-1} \chi^{*2}|_{\sigma^2=\hat{\sigma}^2} = 54.739$$

can be evaluated as 1.1×10^{-8} by the **F distribution** with df $(f, \sum n_i - a)$, where $f = 2.067$ from (5).

The maximal component of the $\chi^{*2}|_{\sigma^2=\hat{\sigma}^2}$ is obtained at the partition between levels 2 and 3:

$$\max t = \left[\left(\frac{1}{10} + \frac{1}{14} \right) (0.02741) \right]^{-1/2}$$
$$\times \left(\frac{23.00}{14} - \frac{11.31}{10} \right) = 8.584,$$

the one-sided P value of which is evaluated as 1.1×10^{-7} by the recurrence formula based on the Markov property of $y_i^* s$. According to the closed testing procedure of [28], the process proceeds to the final step where the t statistic between levels 1 and 2 shows a nonsignificant result at the one-sided significance level 0.10, thus suggesting finally the difference between the dose levels (1,2) and (3,4,5).

In applying the Williams [49] procedure and the modified Williams procedure of [26], we need the maximum likelihood estimaters of the μ_i, which are

$$\hat{\mu}_1 = 1.076, \qquad \hat{\mu}_2 = 1.186,$$
$$\hat{\mu}_3 = \hat{\mu}_4 = 1.524, \qquad \hat{\mu}_5 = 1.856,$$

by the pool-adjacent-violators method. Since $\hat{\mu}_1 = \bar{y}_{1.}$, both statistics coincide and equal

$$w = \max \sqrt{m}(\hat{\mu}_i - \bar{y}_{1.})/\hat{\sigma}$$
$$= \sqrt{m}(\bar{y}_{5.} - \bar{y}_{1.})/\hat{\sigma} = 8.357,$$

where we take the repetition number m as the harmonic mean of the n_is for referring approximately to the tables for upper percentiles in the balanced case by [49] and [50], respectively. In any case, the statistic w is highly significant and the closed testing procedure stops with the nonsignificant result between levels 1 and 2, thus again suggesting a difference between the dose levels (1, 2) and (3, 4, 5).

For a more general likelihood $L(\mathbf{y}, \boldsymbol{\theta}, \mathbf{v})$ with the ordered parameter $\boldsymbol{\theta}$, and possibly with the **nuisance parameter** $\mathbf{v}$, arguments similar to those used above apply if the asymptotic normality of the likelihood estimators is assured. In particular, the cumulative χ^2 and the max t statistics can be based on the cumulative efficient scores evaluated at the null hypothesis and extended easily to two-way problems; see [16], [17], and [7] for details.

Testing Ordered Alternatives in Binomial Probabilities

The data in Table 4 are from a dose–response **clinical trial**. Assuming that the y_i are independently distributed as **binomial** $B_{in}(n_i, p_i)$ we are interested in testing the simple **ordered alternative**

$$H_1: p_1 \leq \cdots \leq p_a.$$

If the quantitative measures $d_1 < \cdots < d_a$ are attached to the y_i, then the locally most powerful test against a wide range of monotone relationships of p_i to d_i is obtained by Cochran [6] and Armitage [2] (*see* **Trend Test for Counts and Proportions**). For the case where there is no information on d_i, the likelihood ratio test has been developed by Chacko [5]. The tests based on the cumulative χ^2 and its maximal component have also been extended as follows:

the cumulative $\chi^2 : \chi^{*2} = \sum y_i^{*2}$,

the maximal component of $\chi^{*2} : \max t = \max y_i^*$,
$$(6)$$

Table 4 Dose finding trial for a heart disease drug

Dose (mg/day)	Improved	Not improved
100	20	16
150	23	18
200	27	9
225	26	9
300	9	5

where y_i^* is given by (4) with σ replaced by $[\bar{Y}(1-\bar{Y})]^{1/2}$, $\bar{Y} = \sum y_i / \sum n_i$, and y_i. replaced by y_i in defining Y_i. Formula (5) is also valid for the χ^{*2} to give a two-sided P value of 0.113 when applied to Table 4. For max t, another exact algorithm is available based on the Markov property of the y_i^* to give a one-sided P value of 0.044 for Table 2 at the partition between levels (1, 2) and (3, 4, 5); see [51], [52], and [25] for the algorithm. The Cochran–Armitage test gives a slightly larger one-sided P value of 0.049 since there is a slight downturn tendency in this example.

Analyzing the Two-Way Contingency Table with Ordered Column Categories

Two-Sample Problem

First consider the two-sample problem presented by Table 2. A popular approach to the analysis is to use a nonparametric test based on a linear score statistic such as Wilcoxon's (*see* **Wilcoxon–Mann–Whitney Test**). Now, for the two-sided alternative H_2 the two statistics,

the cumulative χ^2 : $\chi^{*2} = \chi_1^2 + \cdots + \chi_{b-1}^{*2}$,   (7)

the maximal component of χ^{*2} :

$$\max \chi^2 = \max \chi_j^2, \qquad (8)$$

can be defined in terms of the accumulated efficient scores, where χ_j^2 is the goodness-of-fit χ^2 statistic for the 2×2 **table** formed by accumulating the first j and the remaining $b - j$ columns. The χ_j^2 is, however, identical to the y_i^{*2} of (6) if the binomial data are arranged in a $2 \times b$ table in an obvious way and exactly the same distribution theory applies also to this case. The two-sided P values are 0.039 for χ^{*2} and 0.154 for max χ^2, whereas it is 0.025 for the Wilcoxon test. In this case the Wilcoxon test shows the smallest P value, since approximately a linear trend is observed in p_{1j}/p_{2j}, $j = 1, \ldots, 4$. If these tests are applied to the last two rows of Table 3 for comparing AF 3 mg and AF 6 mg, then the two-sided P values are 0.0128, 0.0096, and 0.0033 for the Wilcoxon, the χ^{*2}, and max χ^2 methods, respectively. It has been verified by **simulation** that, when evaluated as two-sample nonparametric tests, the Wilcoxon method is useful for the location shift

of the underlying symmetrical and light-tailed distributions such as the **logistic** or normal, the max χ^2 method is useful for skewed or heavy-tailed distributions, and the cumulative χ^2 method is characterized by its **robustness**, having relatively high **power** over a wide range of underlying distributions – normal, heavy-tailed, or skewed.

Another important approach to the problem is to assume an underlying continuous distribution for each treatment and to compare the parameters describing those distributions. The **proportional-odds** and **proportional-hazards** models are important examples; see [30] for details.

General a-Sample Problem

For a general a-sample problem the Wilcoxon test is extended to the Kruskal–Wallis test. The same type extensions are available for the χ^{*2} and its maximal component by defining the χ_j^2 in (7) and (8) as the goodness-of-fit χ^2 statistic for the accumulated $a \times 2$ table for the partition between columns j and $j + 1$. The constants for the χ^2 approximation of χ^{*2} are obtained by

$$d = 1 + \frac{2}{b-1}$$
$$\times \left(\frac{\gamma_1}{\gamma_2} + \frac{\gamma_1 + \gamma_2}{\gamma_3} + \cdots + \frac{\gamma_1 + \cdots + \gamma_{b-2}}{\gamma_{b-1}} \right),$$
$$f = (a-1)(b-1)/d,$$

with $\gamma_j = C_j / C_j^*$, $C_j = y_{\cdot 1} + \cdots + y_{\cdot j}$, and $C_j^* = y_{\cdot j+1} + \cdots + y_{\cdot b}$. The max χ^2 can be evaluated by the calculation **algorithm** based on the Markov property of the subsequent χ_j^2s [25].

For the row-wise multiple comparisons based on the cumulative χ^2, the statistic

$$S = \max ||(\mathbf{a}' \otimes \mathbf{C}^{*'})\mathbf{z}||^2$$

is defined where $\otimes$ is a Kronecker product, $\mathbf{z}$ a vector of $\sqrt{y_{\cdot\cdot}} y_{ij}/(y_{i\cdot} y_{\cdot j})^{1/2}$ arranged in dictionary order, $\mathbf{C}^{*'}$ a $b - 1 \times b$ matrix defined so that the (j, j')th element of $\mathbf{C}^{*'}\mathbf{C}^*$ is $(\gamma_j/\gamma_{j'})^{1/2}$ for $j \le j'$ and the maximum is taken over all $\mathbf{a}$ that satisfy $\mathbf{a}'\mathbf{a} = 1$, and $(\sqrt{y_{1\cdot}}, \ldots, \sqrt{y_{a\cdot}})\mathbf{a} = 0$. When $a \ge b$ and under the null model, the statistic S is asymptotically distributed as the largest root of the Wishart matrix $W(\mathbf{C}^{*'}\mathbf{C}^*, a - 1)$, which is well approximated by $\gamma_{(1)}\chi^2(a - 1)$ with $\gamma_{(1)}$ the largest root of $\mathbf{C}^{*'}\mathbf{C}^*$.

The statistic S gives the Scheffé-type multiple comparison test, and has been applied to taste-testing data of five foods in five ordered categorical responses of [4] to obtain the significant classification of rows (foods) (1, 2), (3, 4) and (5). The max χ^2 is also applied to the data for multiple comparisons of the columns to obtain a highly significant classification (1, 2, 3) and (4, 5). The resulting block interaction model is expressed as

$$p_{ij} = p_{i\cdot}p_{\cdot j}q_{\mu\nu}, \quad \mu = 1, 2, 3, \nu = 1, 2,$$

if i belongs to the μth subgroup of rows and j to the νth subgroup of columns. The goodness-of-fit χ^2 has been compared with the fitting of the proportional-odds model [45] and its extension [29]; see [20] and [22] for details. The Scheffé-type multiple comparison method is applied to the normal distribution model in [21], for classifying subjects based on the similarity of the time series profiles defined by repeated measurements.

Two-Way Contingency Table with Natural Orderings in Both Rows and Columns

Assuming a multinomial model $M(y_{\cdot\cdot}, p_{ij})$ for the data y_{ij} in Table 3 the cumulative χ^2 statistic and its maximal component are defined for testing H$_3$ using the cumulative efficient scores evaluated at the null hypothesis. These are

the doubly cumulative $\chi^2 : \chi^{**2} = \sum\sum \chi_{ij}^2,$

the maximal component of χ^{**2} : max max $\chi_{ij}^2,$

with the χ_{ij}^2 being the goodness-of-fit χ^2 for the 2×2 tables obtained from partitioning and accumulating rows and columns at $i = 1, \ldots, a-1$, and $j = 1, \ldots, b-1$, respectively. The χ^{**2} is for the two-sided version of H$_3$, and max max χ^2 is applicable to both one- and two-sided problems. When applied to Table 3 the two-sided P values are approximately 0.0065 for the χ^{**2} and exactly 0.0142 for max max χ^2. The details of the P value calculations and other variations of the test statistics are given in [22] and [23]. As a semiparametric model for the ordered two-way table the constant-**odds ratio** model has been proposed by Wahrendorf [48] based on Plackett's [32] coefficient of association for **bivariate distributions** (*see* **Association, Measures of**).

As an example of the higher-way layouts, a three-way contingency table with age at four levels, existence of the metastasis into the lymph node at two levels, and the soaking grade at three levels, is analyzed in [22]. An example of highly fractional factorial experiments with ordered categorical responses is given in [10]; see also the discussion following that article (*see* **Factorial Experiments**).

Bayesian Approach to Isotonic Inference

Since the purpose of an isotonic inference is to make use of the prior knowledge to enhance the efficiency of test and estimation, it is natural to consider a Bayesian approach. For example, an essentially complete class of tests for orderly constrained hypothesis is obtained as the whole set of Bayes tests with a **prior distribution** defined on those constrained supports. The cumulative χ^2 and max t methods are derived from this idea; see [47], [16], and [7]. More specifically, in bioassay problems, the Dirichlet prior has been introduced for the successive differences of the responses for doses d_i, $p(d_i) - p(d_{i-1})$, $i = 1, \ldots, a+1$; $p(d_0) = 0$, $p(d_{a+1}) = 1$, reflecting the nondecreasing nature of the dose–response relationship, see [34] and [35], for example. Shaked & Singpurwalla [42] discuss the defect of the Dirichlet prior, and introduce concavity constraints on the shape of a dose–response curve, reflecting a situation encountered in practice. Because of computational difficulties, however, they are unable to compute posteriors beyond modal estimates. The computational problem was overcome only recently by Gelfand & Kuo [8], who showed how a sampling-based approach could be used to develop the desired marginal posterior distributions and their features, for Dirichlet and product–beta priors. Ramgopal et al. [33] consider convex, concave, and ogive constraints to specify the shape of dose–response curves, and extend the sampling-based approach to calculating any posterior feature of interest in these generalized constrained problems.

References

[1] Abelson, R.P. & Tukey, J.W. (1963). Efficient utilization of non-numerical information in quantitative analysis: general theory and the case of the simple order, *Annals of Mathematical Statistics* **34**, 1347–1369.

[2] Armitage, P. (1955). Test for linear trends in proportions and frequencies, *Biometrics* **11**, 375–386.

[3] Barlow, R.E., Bartholomew, D.J., Bremner, J.M. & Brunk, H.D. (1972). *Statistical Inference Under Order Restrictions*. Wiley, Chichester.

[4] Bradley, R.A., Katti, S.K. & Coons, I.J. (1962). Optimal scaling for ordered categories, *Psychometrika* **27**, 355–374.

[5] Chacko, Y.C. (1966). Modified chi-square test for ordered alternatives, *Sankhyā, Series B* **28**, 185–190.

[6] Cochran, W.G. (1954). Some methods for strengthening the common χ^2 test, *Biometrics* **10**, 417–451.

[7] Cohen, A. & Sackrowitz, H.B. (1991). Tests for independence in contingency tables with ordered categories, *Journal of Multivariate Analysis* **36**, 56–67.

[8] Gelfand A.E. & Kuo, L. (1991). Nonparametric Bayesian bioassay including ordered polytomous response, *Biometrika* **78**, 657–666.

[9] Geyer, C.J. (1991). Constrained maximum likelihood exemplified by isotonic convex logistic regression, *Journal of the American Statistical Association* **86**, 717–724.

[10] Hamada, M. & Wu, C.F.J. (1990). A critical look at accumulation analysis and related methods (with discussion), *Technometrics* **32**, 119–130.

[11] Hawkins, D.M. (1977). Testing a sequence of observations for a shift in location, *Journal of the American Statistical Association* **72**, 180–186.

[12] Hayter, A.J. (1990). A one-sided Studentized range test for testing against a simple ordered alternative, *Journal of the American Statistical Association* **85**, 778–785.

[13] Hirotsu, C. (1978). Ordered alternatives for interaction effects, *Biometrika* **65**, 561–570.

[14] Hirotsu, C. (1979). The cumulative chi-squares method and Studentized maximal contrast method for testing an ordered alternative in a one-way analysis of variance model, *Reports of Statistical Application Research, Union of Japanese Scientists and Engineers* **26**, 12–21.

[15] Hirotsu, C. (1979). An *F*-approximation and its application, *Biometrika* **66**, 577–584.

[16] Hirotsu, C. (1982). Use of cumulative efficient scores for testing ordered alternatives in discrete models, *Biometrika* **69**, 567–577.

[17] Hirotsu, C. (1983). Defining the pattern of association in two-way contingency tables, *Biometrika* **70**, 579–589.

[18] Hirotsu, C. (1986). Cumulative chi-squared statistic as a tool for testing goodness of fit, *Biometrika* **73**, 165–173.

[19] Hirotsu, C. (1988). A class of estimable contrasts in an age-period-cohort model, *Annals of Institute of Statistical Mathematics* **40**, 451–465.

[20] Hirotsu, C. (1990). Discussion on Hamada and Wu's paper, *Technometrics* **32**, 133–136.

[21] Hirotsu, C. (1991). An approach to comparing treatments based on repeated measures, *Biometrika* **78**, 583–594.

[22] Hirotsu, C. (1992). *Analysis of Experimental Data, Beyond Analysis of Variance* (in Japanese). Kyoritsu-shuppan, Tokyo.

[23] Hirotsu, C. (1997). Two-way change-point model and its application, *Australian Journal of Statistics* **39**, 205–218.

[24] Hirotsu, C. & Herzberg, A.M. (1987). Optimal allocation of observations for inference on k ordered normal population means, *Australian Journal of Statistics* **29**, 151–165.

[25] Hirotsu, C., Kuriki, S. & Hayter, A.J. (1992). Multiple comparison procedure based on the maximal component of the cumulative chi-squared statistic, *Biometrika* **79**, 381–392.

[26] Marcus, R. (1976). The powers of some tests of the equality of normal means against an ordered alternative, *Biometrika* **63**, 177–183.

[27] Marcus, R. & Peritz, E. (1976). Some simultaneous confidence bounds in normal models with restricted alternatives, *Journal of the Royal Statistical Society, Series B* **38**, 157–165.

[28] Marcus, R., Peritz, E. & Gabriel, K.R. (1976). On closed testing procedure with special reference to ordered analysis of variance, *Biometrika* **63**, 655–660.

[29] McCullagh, P. (1980). Regression models for ordinal data, *Journal of the Royal Statistical Society, Series B* **42**, 109–142.

[30] McCullagh, P. & Nelder, J.A. (1989). *Generalized Linear Models*, 2nd Ed. Chapman & Hall, London.

[31] Nair, V.N. (1986). On testing against ordered alternatives in analysis of variance models, *Biometrika* **73**, 493–499.

[32] Plackett, R.L. (1965). A class of bivariate distributions, *Journal of the American Statistical Association* **60**, 516–522.

[33] Ramgopal, P., Laud, P.W. & Smith, A.F.M. (1993). Nonparametric Bayesian bioassay with prior constraints on the shape of the potency curve, *Biometrika* **80**, 489–498.

[34] Ramsey, F.L. (1972). A Bayesian approach to bioassay, *Biometrics* **28**, 841–858.

[35] Ramsey, F.L. (1973). Correction, *Biometrics* **29**, 830.

[36] Robert, C.P. & Hwang, J.T.G. (1996). Maximum likelihood estimation under order restrictions by the prior feedback method, *Journal of the American Statistical Association* **91**, 167–172.

[37] Robertson, T., Wright, F.T. & Dykstra, R.L. (1988). *Order Restricted Statistical Inference*. Wiley, New York.

[38] Schaafsma, W. (1966). Hypothesis testing problems with the alternative restricted by a number of inequalities, *Doctoral dissertation*. University of Groningen, Noordhoff, Groningen.

[39] Schaafsma, W. (1968). A comparison of the most stringent and the most stringent somewhere most powerful tests for certain problems with restricted alternatives, *Annals of Mathematical Statistics* **39**, 531–546.

[40] Schmoyer, R.L. (1984). Sigmoidally constrained maximum likelihood estimation in quantal bioassay, *Journal of the American Statistical Association* **79**, 448–453.

[41] Schoenfeld, D.A. (1986). Confidence bounds for normal means under order restrictions, with application to dose-response curves, toxicology experiments, and low-dose extrapolation, *Journal of the American Statistical Association* **81**, 186–195.

[42] Shaked M. & Singpurwalla, N.D. (1990). A Bayesian approach for quantile and response probability estimation with applications to reliability, *Annals of the Institute of Statistical Mathematics* **42**, 1–19.

[43] Shirley, E. (1979). The comparison of treatment with control group means in toxicological studies, *Applied Statistics* **28**, 144–151.

[44] Simpson, D.G. & Margolin, B.H. (1986). Recursive nonparametric testing for dose response relationships subject to downturn at high doses, *Biometrika* **73**, 589–596.

[45] Snell, E.J. (1964). A scaling procedure for ordered categorical data, *Biometrics* **20**, 592–607.

[46] Taguchi, G. (1966). *Statistical Analysis* (in Japanese). Maruzen, Tokyo.

[47] Takeuchi, K. (1979). Test and estimation problems under restricted null and alternative hypotheses (in Japanese), *Journal of Economics* **45**, 2–10.

[48] Wahrendolf, J. (1980). Inference in contingency tables with ordered categories using Plackett's coefficient of association for bivariate distributions, *Biometrika* **76**, 15–21.

[49] Willams, D.A. (1971). A test for differences between treatment means when several dose levels are compared with a zero dose control, *Biometrics* **27**, 103–117.

[50] Williams, D.A. (1977). Some inference procedures for monotonically ordered normal means, *Biometrika* **64**, 9–14.

[51] Worsley, K.J. (1983). The power of likelihood ratio and cumulative sum tests of a change in a bionomial probability, *Biometrika* **70**, 455–464.

[52] Worsley, K.J. (1986). Confidence regions and tests for a change point in a sequence of exponential family of random variables, *Biometrika* **73**, 91–104.

[53] Wynn, H.P. (1975). Integrals for one-sided confidence bounds: A general result, *Biometrika* **62**, 393–396.

C. HIROTSU

Isotonic Regression

Many regression problems involve minimizing a weighted sum of squares subject to the restriction that the solution must satisfy certain side conditions. A function $f(x)$ defined on a finite index set of numbers $\mathcal{X} = \{x_1, x_2, \ldots, x_k\}$ is isotonic or order preserving if x, y are in $\mathcal{X}$ and $x < y$ implies $f(x) \leq f(y)$. Isotonic regression minimizes a weighted sum of squares subject to the condition that the regression function is isotonic. A simple example is a one-way **analysis of variance** for ordered normal means, in which the variable $x_i = i$ indexes the groups. With each point x_i in $\mathcal{X}$ we associate a positive weight w_i, usually the number of observations on which it is based. Suppose that $g(x)$ is a given function defined on $\mathcal{X}$, then the isotonic regression of $g(x)$ with weights $w_1, w_2, \ldots, w_k$ is denoted by $g^*(x)$ and minimizes the weighted sum of squares,

$$\sum_{i=1}^{k} w_i[g(x_i) - f(x_i)]^2,$$

in the class of all isotonic functions $f(x)$ defined on $\mathcal{X}$. Note that $g^*(x)$ is the isotonic function closest to $g(x)$ as measured in weighted **least squares** distance. For a one-way analysis of variance for nondecreasing ordered normal means, $g(x_i)$ is the observed mean for group i, w_i is the number of observations on which the mean is based and $f(x_i) = \mu_i$ is the mean for group i and $\mu_1 \leq \mu_2 \leq \cdots \leq \mu_k$. For the simple case of ordinary **linear regression** with a single independent variable, $g(x_i)$ is the mean value of the independent **explanatory** variable at x_i, w_i is the number of observations on which it is based, and $f(x) = a + bx$ is a linear regression function. Isotonic regression allows $f(x)$ to be any isotonic function rather than restricting the regression function $f(x)$ to be linear. While isotonic regression can be viewed as a smoothing procedure, one disadvantage is that the isotonic estimates are essentially step functions and, hence, are not smooth everywhere. The degree of smoothness depends on the type of assumptions made; for example, that the function is nondecreasing or convex. Another disadvantage is that the isotonic estimators are biased. Isotonic regression is important because it provides **maximum likelihood** estimators for a large class of problems involving ordered parameters, as well as solving many more constrained statistical problems than the weighted least squares problem stated above. One simple example is unimodal simple regression, which consists of an up-phase in which $E(Y|X = x)$ is increasing with x and a down-phase in which $E(Y|X = x)$ is decreasing with x. If the turning point is known, then it is possible to use isotonic regression for each phase separately. If the turning point is unknown, a simple modification of this idea yields the solution (see [3] for details and examples).

A number of efficient **algorithms** for isotonic regression are available, especially for the case of a single independent variable (see [2] for details). The pooled-adjacent-violators algorithm is widely used, but is only applicable for the case of a simple order. A simple order is when $x_1 < x_2 < \cdots < x_k$, and this implies $f(x_1) \leq f(x_2) \leq \cdots \leq f(x_k)$. This algorithm basically involves, possibly repeated, weighted averages of the unconstrained estimates. For recent extensions of this algorithm, including the case of concave regression and additive isotonic models, see [5] and [1], respectively. Other types of ordering such as quasi- and partial ordering exist; for example, when we have more than one independent variable, partial orderings, which deal with situations such as noncomparable elements in $\mathcal{X}$, arise (see [4] for details on types of ordering).

References

[1]   Bacchetti, P. (1989). Additive isotonic models, *Journal of the American Statistical Association* **84**, 289–294.
[2]   Barlow, R.E., Bartholomew, D.J., Bremner, J.M. & Brunk, H.D. (1972). *Statistical Inference under Order Restrictions*. Wiley, New York.
[3]   Frisen, M. (1986). Unimodal regression, *Statistician* **35**, 479–485.
[4]   Robertson, T., Wright, F.T. & Dykstra, R.L. (1988). *Order Restricted Statistical Inference*. Wiley, New York.
[5]   Tang, D. & Lin, S.P. (1991). Extension of the pool-adjacent-violators algorithm, *Communications in Statistics – Theory and Methods* **20**, 2633–2643.

(*See also* **Isotonic Inference**)

J.W. McDonald

Item Response Theory *see* Rasch Models

Iterated Conditional Modes (ICM) Algorithm *see* Image Analysis and Tomography

Iterative Gene Counting *see* Gene Frequency Estimation

Iterative Proportional Fitting

Iterative proportional fitting (IPF), also known as iterative proportional scaling, is an **algorithm** for constructing tables of numbers satisfying certain constraints. In its simplest form, the algorithm enables one to construct two-way **contingency tables** with specified marginal totals and a prescribed degree of association; from a more general perspective, it may be viewed as a cyclic ascent algorithm which maximizes a specific objective function. The algorithm can also be used to construct **maximum likelihood** estimators for table entries based upon hierarchical **loglinear models** for **Poisson**, **multinomial**, or product multinomial models. We will illustrate these aspects of the algorithm and its applications by describing some simple cases.

Suppose that we are given two pairs $\mathbf{u} = (u_1, u_2)$ and $v = (v_1, v_2)$ of positive numbers satisfying $u_1 + u_2 = v_1 + v_2$, and a further positive number ψ. The IPF algorithm will enable us to construct the *unique* **two-by-two table** $\mathbf{b} = (b_{ij})$ such that, for all i and j,

$$b_{i+} = u_i, \qquad b_{+j} = v_j, \qquad \frac{b_{11}b_{22}}{b_{12}b_{21}} = \psi,$$

where the subscript $+$ denotes the result of summing over the subscript it replaces. The algorithm goes like this. Begin with the 2×2 table $\mathbf{a} = (a_{ij})$ defined by $a_{11} = \psi$, $a_{12} = a_{21} = a_{22} = 1$, noting that the cross-ratio $a_{11}a_{22}/a_{12}a_{21} = \psi$ (see **Odds Ratio**). Next, scale the rows of $\mathbf{a}$ to form the table $\mathbf{a}' = (a'_{ij})$:

$$a'_{ij} = a_{ij} \times \frac{u_i}{a_{i+}}, \qquad (1)$$

for $i = 1, 2$ and $j = 1, 2$. It is easy to check that $\mathbf{a}'$ has the desired row sums, as well as having cross-ratio ψ. We now scale the columns of $\mathbf{a}'$ to form the table $\mathbf{a}'' = (a''_{ij})$:

$$a''_{ij} = a'_{ij} \times \frac{v_j}{a'_{+j}}. \qquad (2)$$

One can check that $\mathbf{a}''$ has the desired column sums and cross-ratio, although the row sums are no longer (u_i). This completes one cycle of the IPF algorithm, beginning with the table $\mathbf{a}$.

The algorithm continues by repeatedly scaling the rows, as in (1), and then the columns, as in (2), to have the desired totals. After a number of cycles, the row totals are closer to (u_i) than they were initially, the column totals are exactly (v_j), and the cross-ratio is exactly ψ. The sequence of tables so defined converges pointwise to a 2×2 table **b** with all the desired properties; uniqueness also follows.

It is instructive to examine why these assertions are true, for in doing so we obtain further insights into the IPF algorithm. To do this, we introduce the notion of **information** (or I-) divergence between two tables $\mathbf{c} = (c_{ij})$ and $\mathbf{d} = (d_{ij})$, satisfying $c_{++} = d_{++}$, defined as follows:

$$I(\mathbf{c}|\mathbf{d}) = \sum_{ij} c_{ij} \log \left(\frac{c_{ij}}{d_{ij}} \right).$$

(A similar definition applies to singly indexed arrays.) It can be proved that $I(\mathbf{c}|\mathbf{d}) \geq 0$, and that $I(\mathbf{c}|\mathbf{d}) = 0$ if and only if $\mathbf{c} = \mathbf{d}$. Although not a symmetric function of its arguments, I behaves in many ways like a metric on tables, and it provides the basis of a proof of convergence of the IPF algorithm. We return to our construction of a table **b** having row totals **u**, column totals **v**, and cross-ratio ψ. First define the table $\mathbf{c} = (c_{ij})$ as follows:

$$c_{ij} = \frac{u_i v_j}{w},$$

where $w = u_+ = v_+$. The tables $\mathbf{a}, \mathbf{a}', \mathbf{a}'', \ldots$ become closer to **c** as the iterations continue, closeness here being in the sense of I-divergence. More precisely, we can check that

$$I(\mathbf{c}|\mathbf{a}) = I(\mathbf{c}|\mathbf{a}'') + I(\mathbf{v}|\mathbf{a}'_2) + I(\mathbf{u}|\mathbf{a}_1), \quad (3)$$

where $\mathbf{a}_1 = (a_{i+})$ and $\mathbf{a}'_2 = (a'_{+j})$. The convergence and uniqueness assertions above all follow from repeated use of this expansion and the stated properties of I. As long as there exists at least one table **c** with the desired marginal totals, we can begin the IPF algorithm with any table having the desired cross-ratio, and expect to converge to the stated limit. The repeated scaling gives tables closer and closer in the sense of I-divergence to the table **c**, all the while retaining the original cross-ratio, and the row and column totals converge to their desired values.

All of the discussion so far applies with minimal changes to $r \times s$ tables; in the more general case, there are further cross-ratios to take into account.

Whereas in a 2×2 table there is only one cross-ratio whose value can be fixed, in an $r \times s$ table, there are $(r-1)(s-1)$ multiplicatively independent cross-ratios. A convenient set (cf. [12]) is the following:

$$\psi_{ij} = \frac{b_{ij} b_{rs}}{b_{is} b_{rj}}, \quad i = 1, \ldots, r-1; j = 1, \ldots, s-1.$$

Here we constructed our cross-ratios in relation to the index values r and s. Other choices give equivalent results; indeed there are quite different ways of defining the quantities which are preserved. This issue is addressed in the theory of **loglinear models**; see [11], [2], and [12]. Given an arbitrary set of $(r-1)(s-1)$ positive numbers (ψ_{ij}), and positive numbers $\mathbf{u} = (u_i)$ and $\mathbf{v} = (v_j)$ satisfying $u_+ = v_+$, the IPF algorithm may be initiated with the table $\mathbf{a} = (a_{ij})$ given by $a_{ij} = \psi_{ij}, i = 1, \ldots, r-1; j = 1, \ldots, s-1$, and $a_{rj} = 1 = a_{is}, i = 1, \ldots, r; j = 1, \ldots, s$. With this initial table, the steps are just as before, and the resulting sequence of tables converges to the unique table having row totals (u_i), column totals (v_j), and cross-ratios (ψ_{ij}).

We turn now to reasons for constructing such tables. One is simply to demonstrate the fact that the row totals, column totals, and cross-ratios of two-way tables may be specified independently, and to show how to obtain tables with arbitrarily specified (but consistent) values of these quantities. Historically, the algorithm was first used to adjust sample frequencies to expected marginal totals. In the examples in Deming [5], we have a table $\mathbf{n} = (n_{ij})$ based upon a **sample survey**, and marginal totals (N_{i+}) and (N_{-j}), but *not* the individual cell frequencies $\mathbf{N} = (N_{ij})$, from a census of the population. The result of applying the IPF algorithm with initial table **n**, and desired marginal totals (N_{i+}) and (N_{+j}), can then be regarded as an estimate of what would have been obtained by cross-tabulating the entire population, instead of only a sample thereof. A modern treatment of these ideas can be found in [2], where the procedure is known as *raking* the table **n**. The third application of the algorithm we note is to the construction of maximum likelihood estimates of table entries under loglinear models. We simply describe the results here; the reader may consult standard references such as [11], [2], or [1] for fuller details. Suppose that $\mathbf{n} = (n_{ij})$ is a two-way table of independent Poisson counts with parameters $\lambda = (\lambda_{ij})$. Then the maximum likelihood estimate $\hat{\lambda}$ of λ under the *multiplicative model* for the (λ_{ij}), has the same row and column totals as **n**, and all cross-ratios equal to 1. In this case, the IPF algorithm begins with a table all of whose entries are 1, and scales the row and column totals to match those of the data **n**. The algorithm converges after a single cycle to the unique maximum likelihood estimator $\hat{\lambda}$.

Three- and Higher-Way Tables

There are a number of ways in which the IPF algorithm may be used with three-way tables. We illustrate two of these. Suppose that we have an $r \times s$ table $\mathbf{u} = (u_{ij})$ and an $s \times t$ table $\mathbf{v} = (v_{jk})$ of positive numbers satisfying $u_{+j} = v_{j+}$ for $j = 1, \ldots, s$. By analogy with our earlier construction, we might be interested in obtaining an $r \times s \times t$ table $\mathbf{b} = (b_{ijk})$ having

$$b_{ij+} = u_{ij}, \qquad b_{+jk} = v_{jk}.$$

This can be solved rather straightforwardly. For example, the table $\mathbf{c} = (c_{ijk})$ given by

$$c_{ijk} = \frac{u_{ij}v_{jk}}{w_j},$$

where $w_j = u_{+j} = v_{j+}, j = 1, \ldots, s$, is readily checked to have ij-margin **u** and jk-margin **v**.

Of course, this is not the end of the story. We may also be interested in any further structure concerning the table **b** which may be specified, in addition to these marginal totals. It turns out that we may also ask that the table has predetermined values of certain cross-ratios. In this example, and more generally, we need rules to tell us which marginal totals and which cross-ratios can be specified independently. The issue is best discussed in the language of **hierarchical** loglinear models for multiway tables, where these are commonly described in terms of the marginal subtables which constitute the **sufficient statistics** for the models (under either independent Poisson, multinomial, or independent multinomial sampling). We refer to [1], [2], and [11] for details concerning these models. In this language, the cross-ratios that we have been specifying are the antilogarithms of elements of subspaces **orthogonal** to those that define the hierarchical loglinear model corresponding to the specified marginal totals. For example, by specifying margins corresponding to the indices ij and jk, as we did in our example, we are also able to specify independently cross-ratios corresponding to the pair

ik and the triple ijk – that is, all interactions other than those involved in the loglinear model defined by the prescribed marginal totals.

Now let us suppose that, in addition to **u** and **v** as above, we are given a $t \times r$ table $\mathbf{w} = (w_{ki})$ of positive numbers satisfying $w_{k+} = v_{+k}$ and $w_{+i} = u_{i+}$ for all k and i. Can we use IPF to construct a table $\mathbf{b} = (b_{ijk})$ satisfying

$$b_{ij+} = u_{ij}, \quad b_{+jk} = v_{jk}, \quad b_{i+k} = w_{ki},$$

and having prescribed values for the ijk cross-ratios? One might think that this would be quite straightforward. Begin with a suitable initial table **a**. Then scale to achieve the ij, jk, and ki marginal totals **u**, **v**, and **w**, respectively. One cycle of the algorithm would be three such scalings, and after a few cycles, we might expect to have a table with the specified cross-ratios, and essentially the desired marginal totals.

How can this version of IPF go wrong? A clue is provided by our indication of the method used to prove that IPF converges. We made use of the existence of a table **c** satisfying the marginal constraints, and then everything followed. However, in the case of three-way tables, it is not hard to specify three consistent, positive two-way tables, for which *no* three-way table exists having positive entries, and the three specified tables as two-way marginal totals. A simple example is given by three 2×2 tables each having 1 in the diagonal cells and 2 in the off-diagonal cells. Although they are clearly consistent, it is easy to check that no $2 \times 2 \times 2$ table can exist with positive entries and these margins. Use of the IPF algorithm with an initial table whose entries are all 1, and these three marginal tables, results in a cycle through the same three tables. The tables constructed do not converge. Summarizing this discussion, we can say that only if there exists a three-way table with the given two-way tables as marginal totals is the IPF algorithm guaranteed to converge to a limiting table with the desired marginal totals and three-way cross-ratios. When it does, this table is uniquely specified by these properties.

We note that in the application of this result to maximum likelihood estimation with loglinear models, the assumption of the existence of *some* table with the given marginal totals is trivially satisfied as long as the observed table $\mathbf{n} = (n_{ijk})$ has positive entries, for in this case **n** itself suffices. If the observed table has some zero entries, but positive two-way marginal totals, the IPF algorithm still converges, but to a table with some zero entries. In a sense, this is an extended maximum likelihood estimator: one on the boundary of the natural parameter space.

The foregoing discussion applies without change to higher-way tables. For example, suppose that we have an initial four-way table $\mathbf{a} = (a_{ijkl})$, and we wish to scale it to have prescribed ij, jk, kl, and li marginal totals. What cross-ratios (equivalently, what loglinear structure) of this initial table will be preserved throughout the iterations, and could therefore be specified independently of the marginal totals? The answer is: all interactions other than those involved in the loglinear model defined by the prescribed marginal totals, that is, the ik, jl, ijk, ijl, ikl, jkl, and $ijkl$ interactions. Note that we still need to know that there exists a table with the specified marginal totals before the algorithm is guaranteed to converge to a limiting table with all the desired properties.

Finite Termination: Decomposable Models

Decomposable models are a class of loglinear models for complete multiway tables which possess closed-form expressions for their MLEs under the standard sampling models; see [11] and [2]. It turns out that the IPF algorithm behaves rather well for this class of models. Suppose that a set of marginal totals to be fitted via IPF defines a decomposable loglinear model. If the initial table is constant, and the margins to be fitted are taken in a suitable order, the algorithm converges after just one cycle. Furthermore, there *always* exists a table with the given set of tables as marginal subtables, when the corresponding model is decomposable. Finally, as long as the specified tables are all positive, the table whose existence has just been described has positive entries.

History

Fienberg [7] presents a discussion of the history of the IPF algorithm. Some additional references can be found in [8]. The most important early papers are [6] and [13].

Numerical Aspects

Haberman [11] proves that tables constructed by the IPF algorithm converge to their limit at a geometric (also called first-order) rate. This means that, asymptotically, the difference between the nth iterate and the limit is bounded above by ρ^n for some ρ between zero and unity. (This compares unfavorably with the behavior of Newton or modified Newton algorithms, which typically exhibit what is known as quadratic convergence.) In many cases, ρ may be quite close to unity, and so convergence may be rather slow, giving rise to a literature concerning speeding up of the algorithm. However, at that point, the algorithm ceases to be the one we are discussing.

The great advantage of the IPF algorithm is its simplicity, stability, and economy of space. When a table is large, and the number of iterations is not a limiting factor, it is the method of choice for the problems we have discussed. For other problems, such as the calculation of MLEs under loglinear models, Newton-type methods are preferred, because of their speed of convergence and the fact that variance–**covariance matrices** are an automatic byproduct. FORTRAN IV versions of the IPF algorithm can be found in [9] and [10].

Variants and Generalizations

It is implicit in the foregoing discussion that the tables being considered are all *complete*, that is, are fully rectangular, or rectangular parallelepipeds, etc., and have no so-called **structural zeros**. This was because the algorithm is mostly used, and its properties are most easily discussed, in that context. However, variant forms of the algorithm are used successfully with tables having a variety of other structures, and preserving features corresponding to models other than hierarchical loglinear models; see [11].

For generalizations of a different kind, see [4] and [3]. In these papers, applications of the algorithm beyond contingency tables are given, and its connections to the information measure I and entropy are more fully explored.

References

[1]   Agresti, A. (1990). *Categorical Data Analysis*. Wiley, New York.

[2]   Bishop, Y.M.M., Fienberg, S.E. & Holland, P.W. (1975). *Discrete Multivariate Analysis*. MIT Press, Cambridge, Mass.

[3]   Csiszar, I. (1975). *I*-divergence geometry of probability distributions and minimization problems, *Annals of Probability* **3**, 146–158.

[4]   Darroch, J.N. & Ratcliff, D. (1972). Generalized iterative scaling for loglinear models, *Annals of Mathematical Statistics* **43**, 1470–1480.

[5]   Deming, W.E. (1964). *Statistical Adjustment of Data*. Dover, New York.

[6]   Deming, W.E. & Stephan, F.F. (1940). On a least squares adjustment of a sampled frequency table when the expected marginal totals are known, *Annals of Mathematical Statistics* **11**, 427–444.

[7]   Fienberg, S.E. (1970). An iterative procedure for estimation in contingency tables, *Annals of Mathematical Statistics* **41**, 907–917.

[8]   Fienberg, S.E. & Meyer, M.M. (1983). *Encyclopedia of Statistical Sciences*, Vol. 4, S. Kotz & N.L. Johnson, eds. Wiley, New York, p. 2275.

[9]   Haberman, S.J. (1972). Loglinear fit for contingency tables, *Applied Statistics* **21**, 218–225.

[10] Haberman, S.J. (1973). Printing multidimensional tables, *Applied Statistics* **22**, 118–126.

[11] Haberman, S.J. (1974). *The Analysis of Frequency Data*. University of Chicago Press, Chicago.

[12] Plackett, R.L. (1981). *The Analysis of Categorical Data*, 2nd Ed. Griffin, London.

[13] Stephan, F.F. (1942). An iterative method of adjusting sample frequency tables when the expected marginal totals are known, *Annals of Mathematical Statistics* **13**, 166–178.

(*See also* **Categorical Data Analysis**)

T.P. SPEED

Iteratively Reweighted Least Squares *see* Generalized Linear Model

Itô Calculus *see* Computer Algebra

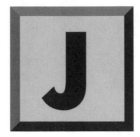

J-Shaped Distribution

As a sequel to Khinchin's definition of **unimodality**, a J-shaped distribution function is defined. A characterization for a related distribution is given using a well-known result of Khinchin on unimodality and a characterization theorem for a **U-shaped** probability density function by Ghosh and Shanbhag.

We define the following:

Definition 1. A distribution function $F(x)$ is said to be negative-tailed (positive-tailed) J-shaped if there exists a value $x = a$ such that $F(x)$ is convex (concave) for $x < a$ ($x > a$) and $F(a) = 1$ (0). The point $x = a$ is called a negative (positive) pivot of $F(x)$.

Definition 2. If a J-shaped distribution $F(x)$ is differentiable except at a countable subset of the set of reals, then the derivative $F'(x)$ is called a J-shaped probability density function.

We observe that for a negative-tailed J-shaped distribution function $F(x)$ with a negative pivot at $x = a$ we have $F(x) = 1$ at $x = a$ and for $x > a$. Since a constant function is both concave and convex, we conclude that a negative-tailed J-shaped distribution is unimodal with vertex at $x = a$. Hence, by Khinchin's theorem [3, p. 92] its **characteristic function** $p(t)$ has the following representation:

$$p(t) = [\exp(ita)/t] \int_0^t q(u)\mathrm{d}u, \quad \text{for a real } t.$$

Similarly, the characteristic function $r(t)$ of a positive-tailed J-shaped distribution has the following representation:

$$r(t) = [\exp(itc)/t] \int_0^t s(u)\mathrm{d}u, \quad \text{for a real } t,$$

where c is the positive pivot.

Examples

The following are two examples of J-shaped density functions:

1. Let a random variable X measure the level of nicotine intake by human beings. Then the frequency distribution of X amongst patients with lung cancer is likely to be negative-tailed J-shaped.
2. If a cohort of children is followed from birth to age 5 years, the distribution of age at death, amongst those who die, is likely to be positive-tailed J-shaped. Conversely, among those who die in a cohort of individuals followed from, say, age 65 to 70 years, the distribution of age at death is likely to be negative-tailed J-shaped.

Related Distributions

The concepts of a U-shaped probability density function and a bimodal distribution are related to J-shaped distribution. We define the following:

Definition 3.   Let X be an absolutely continuous random variable. Then the probability density function of X is said to be U-shaped if there exist real numbers a, b, and c such that $a < b < c$, $\Pr \{X < a\} = 0$, $\Pr \{X > c\} = 0$, $\Pr \{X < x\}$ is concave in (a, b) and convex in (b, c).

The following theorem [2] gives a characterization for a U-shaped density function.

Theorem.   Let X be an absolutely continuous random variable with probability density function $h(x)$. Then $h(x)$ is bounded and U-shaped if and only if the characteristic function of X is given by

$$f(t) = p[\exp(itb) - \exp(ita)]/it$$
$$- q\exp(itc)/t \int_0^t r(u)\mathrm{d}u, \quad \text{for a real } t,$$

where $r(u)$ is a characteristic function, a, b, c, and p are real numbers, and q is real and positive.

Definition 4.   A distribution function $F(x)$ is said to be bimodal if there exist real numbers a, b, and c with $a < b < c$ such that (i) $F(x)$ is convex for $x < a$; (ii) $F(x)$ is concave for $a < x < b$; (iii) $F(x)$ is convex for $b < x < c$; and (iv) $F(x)$ is concave for $x > c$. The points $x = a$ and $x = c$ are called two vertices of $F(x)$. The point $x = b$ is called an antimode of $F(x)$.

If $a = c$, then $F(x)$ is unimodal in Khinchin's sense.

The following theorem [1] characterizes a bimodal distribution.

Theorem.   The function $f(t)$ is the characteristic function of a bimodal distribution function $F(x)$ with vertices a and c, with $a < c$, if and only if

$$f(t) = F(a)h(t) + \{F(c) - F(a)\}g(t)$$
$$+ \{1 - F(c)\}k(t),$$

where $h(t)$ is the characteristic function of a negative-tailed J-shaped distribution with a negative pivot at $x = a$, $g(t)$ is the characteristic function of a U-shaped distribution over (a, c), and $k(t)$ is the characteristic function of a positive-tailed J-shaped distribution with a positive pivot at $x = c$.

References

[1]   Ghosh, P. (1978). A characterization of a bimodal distribution, *Communications in Statistics – Theory and Methods* **7**, 475–477.

[2]   Ghosh, P. & Shanbhag, D.N. (1972). A note on the characterization of a U-shaped probability density function, *Journal of Applied Probability* **9**, 684–685.

[3]   Lukacs, E. (1970) *Characteristic Function*. Griffin, London.

PANKAJ GHOSH

Jaccard Coefficient of Numerical Taxonomy *see* Agreement, Measurement of

Jackknife Method

The primary purpose of this technique is the estimation of the **standard errors** and the **bias** of estimators, $T(\mathbf{x})$. These Ts may be either too complicated to admit analytical derivation of the **sampling distributions**, or based on $\mathbf{x}$s from a probability model that is too difficult or impossible to specify. The essence of the computations for random samples of size n is the re-evaluation of the estimator on subsamples, which are typically produced by leaving out one observation at a time. For instance, the result of leaving out the ith datum may be denoted by $T_i = T[\mathbf{x}(i)]$, where $\mathbf{x}(i)$ is the particular subsample of size $n - 1$ without the observation x_i.

The idea of appropriately differencing to reduce biases of order n^{-1} is credited to Quenouille. The original (1949) article [5] involves a **serial correlation** context, where the two subsets are the first and second half of the series. The second [6] has a more general context. Tukey [11] named the tool in 1958 for its parallel with the rough-and-ready boy-scout implement. He also coined the term *pseudovalues* for the individual differences, $nT - (n - 1)T_i$. These are the simple ingredients for the standard error estimator. Tukey argued that in many instances these may be treated as approximately independent and their ordinary sample variance would be a reasonable estimator of var $[T(\mathbf{x})]$. This variance estimator was shown to be appropriate in large samples for the bias-corrected point estimator as well. Approximate **confidence intervals** and **hypothesis tests** are based on treating a standardized estimator as a normal or a **Student** t.

The methodology was extended to more general bias structures by Gray & Schucany [2]. Important early contributions to the theoretical foundations, by Rupert Miller, his students, and others were reviewed in 1974 [4]. There were early results on consistency of variance estimators for a broad classes of problems, including functions of **maximum likelihood** estimators (MLEs) and functions of **U-statistics**. A rigorous demonstration of the asymptotics for MLEs is given in [7]. The estimators that do not jackknife well have discontinuous *influence functions* (see [1, Section 11.6] or [8, Section 2.2.1]), of which the most notable example is the **median**. The approximate confidence intervals work better after symmetrizing **transformations**, for example, $\log s^2$ and $\tanh^{-1} r$.

The encyclopedia entry by Hinkley [3] contains the logical foundation, elementary notation, and some illustrative calculations. Efron & Tibshirani [1] give an excellent overview and the relationship of the jackknife to the **bootstrap**. These are distinct sample reuse approaches to getting information about the sampling distribution of $T(\mathbf{x})$. The bootstrap does this by simulating from the empirical distribution function, $F_n(x)$, the best estimate of $F(x)$ in a certain sense. The jackknife may be viewed as studying T in the neighborhood of F_n by quadrature (*see* **Numerical Integration**) rather than by **Monte Carlo**. For a more theoretical treatment of the jackknife and bootstrap, see [8].

Censored data are an important feature of some biostatistical problems. A recent examination of the suitability of jackknifing Kaplan–Meier integrals (*see* **Kaplan–Meier Estimator**) may be found in [10]. Stefanski & Cook [9] establish a relationship between the jackknife and SIMEX, which is a **simulation**-based method of inference for measurement error models.

References

[1] Efron, B. & Tibshirani, R. (1993). *An Introduction to the Bootstrap*. Chapman & Hall, New York.

[2] Gray, H.L. & Schucany, W.R. (1972). *The Generalized Jackknife Statistic*. Marcel Dekker, New York.

[3] Hinkley, D.V. (1983). Jackknife methods, in *Encyclopedia of Statistical Sciences*, Vol. 4, N.L. Johnson, S. Kotz, & C.B. Read, eds. Wiley, New York, pp. 280–287.

[4] Miller, R.G. (1974). The jackknife - a review, *Biometrika* **61**, 1–17.

[5] Quenouille, M. (1949). Approximate tests of correlation in time series, *Journal of the Royal Statistical Society, Series B* **11**, 18–44.

[6] Quenouille, M. (1956). Notes on bias in estimation, *Biometrika* **43**, 353–360.

[7] Reeds, J.A. (1978). Jackknifing maximum likelihood estimates, *Annals of Statistics* **6**, 727–739.

[8] Shao, J. & Tu, D. (1995). *The Jackknife and the Bootstrap*. Springer-Verlag, New York.

[9] Stefanski, L.A. & Cook, J.R. (1995). Simulation-extrapolation: the measurement error jackknife, *Journal of the American Statistical Association* **90**, 1247–1256.

[10] Stute, W. & Wang, J.-L. (1994). The jackknife estimate of a Kaplan-Meier integral, *Biometrika* **81**, 602–606.

[11] Tukey, J.W. (1958). Bias and confidence in not quite large samples (abstract), *Annals of Mathematical Statistics* **29**, 614.

(*See also* **Cross-Validation**)

WILLIAM R. SCHUCANY

Jackknife Repeated Replication *see* Resampling Procedures for Sample Surveys

James–Stein Estimator

The discovery of Stein [6] that the sample mean of a normal population is inadmissible in three or more dimensions was based on an argument using the estimator

$$\mathbf{d}^1(\mathbf{x}) = \left(1 - \frac{b}{a + |\mathbf{x}|^2}\right)\mathbf{x},$$

where we observe $\mathbf{X} = \mathbf{x}$, with $\mathbf{X} \sim \mathrm{N}(\boldsymbol{\theta}, \mathbf{I})$, a p-dimensional normal random variable (*see* **Multivariate Normal Distribution**). If $p \geq 3$, Stein showed that, for sufficiently small b and sufficiently large a,

$$E_\theta |\mathbf{d}^1(\mathbf{X}) - \theta|^2 < E_\theta |\mathbf{X} - \theta|^2, \quad \text{for all } \theta, \quad (1)$$

demonstrating the inadmissibility of $\mathbf{X}$ under squared error loss. This result only demonstrated the existence of a better estimator, as Stein did not give specific values of a and b that would satisfy (1). This was remedied in James & Stein [4], where it was shown that the estimator

$$\mathbf{d}^{JS}(\mathbf{x}) = \left(1 - \frac{c}{|\mathbf{x}|^2}\right)\mathbf{x} \quad (2)$$

dominates $\mathbf{X}$ as long as $0 \leq c \leq p - 2$. In fact, James & Stein [4] show that the optimal value of c is $c = p - 2$, and using this value (2) is usually referred to as the *James–Stein estimator*. Starting from (2), entire families of improved estimators of θ have been derived. Note, in particular, that since $\mathbf{X}$ is a **minimax** estimator of θ, any estimator that dominates it is also a minimax estimator. Thus, research began into finding better families of minimax estimators of a multivariate normal mean.

One of the most important developments was due to Baranchik [1], who proved that estimators of the form

$$\mathbf{d}^B(\mathbf{x}) = \left(1 - \frac{r(|\mathbf{x}|)}{|\mathbf{x}|^2}\right)\mathbf{x}$$

are minimax provided that (i) $0 \leq r(\cdot) \leq 2(p-2)$; and (ii) the function r is nondecreasing.

An immediate consequence of Baranchik's result was the minimaxity of (and the dominance of $\mathbf{X}$ by) the *positive-part Stein estimator*

$$\mathbf{d}^+(\mathbf{x}) = \left(1 - \frac{p-2}{|\mathbf{x}|^2}\right)^+ \mathbf{x}, \quad (3)$$

where $(\cdot)^+$ indicates that the quantity in parentheses is replaced by 0 whenever it is negative. This represents a great improvement over (2), as it does not suffer from aberrant behavior when $\mathbf{x}$ is near 0. (There, the James–Stein estimator can actually get infinitely large). In fact, the positive-part estimator (3) is so good that even though it is known to be inadmissible, it took over 25 years to exhibit an estimator that dominates it. (The inadmissibility of (3) follows from Brown [2], who showed that the admissible estimators must be generalized Bayes estimators. Because of the "point" at $|\mathbf{x}|^2 = p - 2$, (3) is not smooth enough to be generalized Bayes. The work of Efron & Morris

[3, Section 5] showed that (3) was close to being a Bayes rule, and hence close to admissible, so it was suspected that it would be difficult to dominate. Finally, Shao & Strawderman [5] exhibited a dominating estimator.)

References

[1]   Baranchik, A.J. (1970). A family of minimax estimators of the mean of a multivariate normal distribution, *Annals of Mathematical Statistics* **41**, 642–645.

[2]   Brown, L.D. (1971). Admissible estimators, recurrent diffusions, and insoluble boundary value problems, *Annals of Mathematical Statistics* **42**, 855–903. (Corrigenda: *Annals of Statistics* **1**, 594–596.)

[3]   Efron, B. & Morris, C.N. (1973). Stein's estimation rule and its competitors – an empirical Bayes approach, *Journal of the American Statistical Association* **68**, 117–130.

[4]   James, W. & Stein, C. (1961). Estimation with quadratic loss, in *Proceedings of the Fourth Berkeley Symposium on Mathematics Statistics and Probability*, Vol. 1. University of California Press, Berkeley, pp. 311–319.

[5]   Shao, P.Y.-S. & Strawderman, W.E. (1994). Improving on the James–Stein positive-part estimator. *Technical Report*, Department of Statistics, Rutgers University.

[6]   Stein, C. (1956). Inadmissibility of the usual estimator for the mean of a multivariate distribution, *Proceedings of the Third Berkeley Symposium on Mathematical Statistics and Probability*, Vol. 1. University of California Press, Berkeley, pp. 197–206.

(*See also* **Decision Theory; Shrinkage; Shrinkage Estimation**)

George Casella

Java *see* Internet

Jeffreys, Harold

Born: April 22, 1891, in Fatfield, Co. Durham, UK.
Died: March 18, 1989, in Cambridge, UK.

The career of Harold Jeffreys is easily described. From his local school he went up to Cambridge, where he stayed for the rest of his life. His continuous 75 years as a fellow of St John's College is a record for any Oxbridge college. He was Plumian Professor of Astronomy and Experimental Philosophy, received numerous scientific awards, and was knighted.

During most of his life, and certainly up until his retirement from the Chair in 1958, he was best known for his important work in geophysics and related fields. The data he studied therein, and the general interest in the philosophy of science present in Cambridge in the 1920s, combined and culminated in the publication in 1939 of his book, called simply *Theory of Probability*. The substantially revised, third edition appeared in 1961 [1]. It is still in print and considered by many statisticians to be essential reading, not just for historical reasons, but because of its modern manner of thought. He was a poor oral communicator but his writing is superb. He stands with literature's greatest in the effective use of the English language.

There are two major novelties in the Theory, as he liked to call his book. The first lies in the concept of probability: the second in the development, from this concept, of operational procedures for handling data. He addressed the problem of how one's uncertainty about quantities of scientific interest, like hypotheses or values of constants, should be described. In the first chapter he demonstrated, on the basis of some simple ideas, that this could only be done through probability; so that one could speak of the probability of a hypothesis being true. Furthermore, statements of these uncertainties had to combine according to the rules of probability. One of these rules is **Bayes' theorem** and because of its ubiquity, the subject, when treated from this viewpoint, has become known as Bayesian statistics (*see* **Bayesian Methods**). The Theory was the first modern book on Bayesian statistics. This attitude towards probability was quite different from that of his near-contemporary, **R.A. Fisher**, who was, in the 1930s, revolutionizing statistics. Fisher used only the probability of data, given the hypothesis, whereas Jeffreys was advocating and justifying the concept of the probability of the hypothesis, given the data. Fisher's ideas found general acceptance and Jeffreys was initially treated as a maverick.

Although, at the time, their results seemed in good numerical agreement, it is now appreciated that they typically differ. If data x on hypothesis H has density $p(x|H)$, then Fisher used the tail-area probability $\int_x^\infty p(t|H)dt$, or **P value**, to describe the status of H. Jeffreys used a direct probability $p(H|x) \propto p(x|H)p(H)$. In the use of the integral in the former but not in the latter, which satisfies the **likelihood** principle, the ideas contrast and the numerical values differ.

Jeffreys differed from **de Finetti** in regarding the numerical value of a probability as being shared by all rational persons, whereas de Finetti thought of it as subjective. If Jeffreys was right, then he had to have some way of producing the rational probability. The way he explored, and which later workers have followed, is first to describe a rational view of ignorance. This forms a reference point from which other states can be described, using Bayes' theorem. The invariance ideas he used have been extended into a modern development of reference priors.

Jeffreys' views have influenced the philosophy of science, and are in marked contrast to those of **Karl Popper**, who advocated the view that a hypothesis could only be disproved, whereas probability admitted values near one, effectively amounting to proof. Jeffreys was a great geophysicist who also created an original way of conducting the scientific method.

Reference

[1]   Jeffreys, H. (1961). *Theory of Probability*, 3rd Ed. Clarendon Press, Oxford.

DENNIS V. LINDLEY

Job-Exposure Matrices

Epidemiologic investigation of occupational hazards requires information on illness among workers and on their occupations or occupational exposures. Two families of epidemiologic investigations can be distinguished: industry-based studies and community-based studies. Each has unique advantages and disadvantages. Historically, community-based studies were based on analyses of job titles. With growing realization that there can be substantial variation in exposure profiles among workers who share the same job title, and that workers in different occupations can have common exposures, increasing attention has been paid to ascertaining subjects' occupational exposures (*see* **Occupational Epidemiology; Occupational Health and Medicine; Occupational Mortality**).

Since taking measurements in subjects' current workplaces is usually neither feasible nor useful for diseases of long latency, other approaches have been developed to ascertain subjects' past occupational exposures. If subjects can be interviewed, they can be asked about their exposure to various chemicals, but information thereby obtained is not sufficiently valid. Another approach is to obtain information about the jobs that subjects did and then have experts in industrial hygiene estimate the chemicals that may have been present in such workplaces. If the information collected about subjects' jobs is reasonably detailed, and the experts knowledgeable, then this can lead to quite valid exposure estimates. However, it is an expensive labor-intensive enterprise.

The job exposure matrix (JEM) approach was developed to provide a relatively inexpensive way of inferring exposures when the investigator has information on subjects' job histories. A JEM is simply a correspondence system for translating any occupation code into a list of exposures. The JEM provides the means for bringing together, for the purpose of statistical analysis, groups of subjects who share common exposures, irrespective of their occupations. A JEM consists of two primary axes, an exhaustive and mutually exclusive classification of occupations, and a list of substances. The occupation axis can be further subdivided by industries, by time periods, and conceivably by geographic areas. In the simplest form, the entry in the matrix could be a **binary** indicator of whether a worker in occupation i should be considered exposed to substance j. Applying each column in turn to a set of occupation histories allows the investigator to infer the exposure status of each study subject to each substance in the JEM. A more refined JEM could contain quantitative indicators of the probability of exposure to the substance in the job and estimates of the degree of exposure.

If the number of JEM substances is lengthy and the matrix entries are valid, this could generate useful data. While a handful of community-based JEMs have been developed in a few countries [1], they have not found wide applicability. The main limiting factor is the lack of valid and generalizable JEMs which are sufficiently broad in scope as to satisfy a wide range of research needs [3] (*see* **Validity and Generalizability in Epidemiologic Studies**). By contrast, a JEM can also be developed in the context of a **cohort study** and can be very useful if based on company records or expertise [2]. Such a JEM would not normally be applicable outside the cohort for which it was developed.

References

[1]   Coughlin, S.S. & Chiazze, L. (1990). Job-exposure matrices in epidemiologic research and medical surveillance, *State of the Art Reviews in Occupational Medicine* **5**, 633–646.

[2]   Goldberg, M., Kromhout, H., Guenel, P., Fletcher, A.C., Gerin, M., Glass, D.C., Heedrok, D., Kauppinen, T. & Ponti, A. (1993). Job-exposure matrices in industry, *International Journal of Epidemiology* **22**, Supplement 2, S10–S15.

[3]   Siemiatycki, J. (1996). Exposure assessment in community-based studies of occupational cancer, *Occupational Hygiene* **3**, 41–58.

JACK SIEMIATYCKI

Join-Count Statistics *see* Clustering

Joint Action *see* Synergy of Exposure Effects

Joint Probability Function *see* Random Variable

Jonkheere–Terpstra Test *see* Ordered Alternatives

Journal of Agricultural, Biological, and Environmental Statistics *see* American Statistical Association

Journal of Biopharmaceutical Statistics

The *Journal of Biopharmaceutical Statistics* (*JBS*) is an international, applied, biopharmaceutical statistical journal, published four times per year by Marcel Dekker, Inc., 270 Madison Avenue, New York, NY 10016. It was founded in 1988 by its Editor-in-Chief, Karl E. Peace, Ph.D., Chief Scientific Officer, Biopharmaceutical Research Consultants, Inc., P.O. Box 2506, Ann Arbor, MI 48106, in conjunction with Marcel Dekker, Inc. The first issue of the *JBS* appeared in 1991.

The *JBS* provides an information resource for applied statisticians working in biopharmaceutical areas through publication of (i) high quality applications of statistics in biopharmaceutical research and development (*see* **Pharmacoepidemiology, Overview**) and (ii) expositions of statistical methodology with clear and immediate applicability to such work. Although not exhaustive, biopharmaceutical areas include particularly those attendant to the drug, device, or biologic research development processes; drug screening; assessment of pharmacological activity; pharmaceutical formulation and scale-up; preclinical safety assessment; **bioavailability, bioequivalence,** and **pharmacokinetics; phase I, Phase II** and Phase III clinical development (*see* **Clinical Trials, Overview**); pre-market approval assessment of clinical safety (*see* **Drug Approval and Regulation**); **post-marketing surveillance**; manufacturing and quality control; technical operations; and regulatory issues (*see* **Drug Approval and Regulation**). Papers submitted to the *JBS* for publication consideration should emphasize the application of statistical methods, rather than the methods *per se* – whether new or established. Substantive aspects of the application should be presented. The process of problem formulation appropriate to the statistical method should be specifically addressed. Of particular importance is attention to statistical design (*see* **Experimental Design in Biostatistics**) and protocol development (*see* **Clinical Trials Protocols**). In reflecting applied statistics as a scientific discipline, the *JBS* aims to provide models in the biopharmaceutical areas of proper design, analysis, and interpretation of both experimental and **observational studies**.

Manuscripts submitted to the *JBS* for publication consideration are reviewed by the editor, a regional editor and two editorial board members or appropriate experts. Review below regional editors is blinded to author identity. Authors are blinded to reviewer identity. General criteria for acceptance include originality, quality, and significance of the application or methods as well as the quality of the presentation.

Publications in the *JBS* reflect the international nature of biopharmaceutical research, with contributions by authors from every continent and many countries, e.g. Australia, Canada, China, England, Finland, Germany, Japan, South Africa, Switzerland, and the US. As of October, 1997, the fourth issue of the seventh volume is in press, and all issues of the eighth volume are compiled.

KARL E. PEACE

Journal of Clinical Epidemiology

The *Journal of Clinical Epidemiology* represents a continuation, under a new name, of the *Journal of Chronic Diseases* (*JCD*), which was inaugurated in 1955. During that era, before the proliferation of specialty journals in such fields as **gastroenterology**, geriatrics (*see* **Gerontology and Geriatric Medicine**), and **rheumatology**, journals concerned specifically with medical research were oriented almost exclusively to studies of pathophysiology and biologic mechanisms. Clinical studies of chronic disease were seldom encouraged or accepted, because the care of chronic disease was seldom regarded as a scientific activity in the explicatory type of laboratory research usually conducted as "clinical investigation". The investigative methods needed to study patient care and to do **clinical trials**, however, were different from those of laboratory experiments; and reports using those methods would be either unappreciated by laboratory scientists, or regarded as too pragmatic for the often theoretical orientation of biostatistical and other journals concerned with methodology. Thoughtful reviews of clinical topics and appraisals of research methods would also usually take more space than most journals were willing to allocate. The *JCD* thus offered an orientation, appreciation, editorial policy, and space that had previously been unavailable.

The first volume of the journal immediately showed its new orientation, and its lively interest in methodology. The first paper in the first issue was **Merrell** & Shulman's "Determination of prognosis in chronic disease, illustrated by systemic lupus erythematosus". The paper described the medical use of **life-table** analyses for the course of clinical ailments, and was repeatedly cited thereafter for many years as the classic publication in that field. Another classic methodologic publication in the first volume was Louis Lasagna's discussion of an investigative method that was then in its infancy: "The controlled clinical trial: theory and practice". The discussion had a substantial influence on the planning and analyzing of cancer trials at the National Institutes of Health (NIH) during the late 1950s. A third methodologic classic in Volume 1 was **Harold Dorn's** essay, "Some applications of biometry in the collection and evaluation of medical data". The latter paper contains Dorn's often quoted remark that

> Reproducibility does not establish validity, since the same mistake can be made repeatedly; but without reproducibility an observed relationship becomes merely an isolated historical event and adds nothing to accumulated scientific knowledge.

During the next few early years, the journal's continuing focus on clinical issues in chronic disease was reflected by publications concerned with topics that today might be classified as **neurology**, metabolism, rheumatology, gastroenterology, **hepatology, psychiatry**, neonatology, congenital anomalies (*see* **Teratology**), atherosclerosis (*see* **Cardiology and Cardiovascular Disease**), hematology, **oncology**, and such chronic infections as tuberculosis and syphilis. Victor McKusick's pioneering work in clinical genetics first appeared in the *JCD* in a series of instalments under the general title of "Heritable disorders of connective tissue".

In addition to these clinical topics, the early volumes of the journal continued to offer a forum for methodology. The papers referred to classification of arthritis, evaluation of **screening** tests, discussions of epidemiologic principles, uses of interview data to assess **prevalence** of disease, the measurement of pain and pain relief, uses of nonmedical

interviewers to obtain data about specific symptoms, and variability of daily blood pressure measurements. The methodologic studies, then as now, revealed the frequent, but often unrecognized, problems of **bias** in research with human groups. **Donald Mainland**, after analyzing results of a questionnaire given to a class of 129 first-year medical students, concluded that "... more than one-half of them held opinions which, if allowed to influence the selection of subjects in a forward-going etiologic survey, would bias the results".

Sidney Cobb et al., reporting on "differences between respondents and nonrespondents in a morbidity survey involving clinical examination" demonstrated the type of bias that might arise from low response rates in studies for the estimation of prevalence. The authors recommended a procedure that (like many other recommendations about how to deal with bias) has often been subsequently neglected: "A study of the nonresponse problem (should) be built into each new field investigation as it is planned."

The journal also become involved in topics that were overtly controversial or that would later generate controversy. In a controlled trial reported elsewhere in 1952, anticoagulant therapy had been found unequivocally effective in reducing short-term deaths in patients with acute myocardial infarction. Many clinicians claimed, however, that the results of the trial were inconsistent with their own clinical experience, particularly for the predominance of "low risk" patients who had excellent prognoses without treatment. Only much later would it be realized that the anticoagulant trial, despite an untreated control group, was not randomized (*see* **Randomization**) or double-blind, and that the proanticoagulant results could easily be attributed to a **biased** assignment of patients. Nevertheless, anticoagulant therapy was being so vigorously advocated that physicians who failed to use it might be sued for malpractice if a patient with myocardial infarction died. In a pair of editorials in the journal in 1956, the virtues of anticoagulant therapy received a spirited denunciation by David Rytand and a vigorous defense by William Foley.

The *JCD*, in its early years, published several instalments of research, conducted by the US Public Health Service, as the Tuskegee study of "Untreated syphilis in the male Negro". The research was originally regarded as a splendid investigation of the **natural history** of a disease, but the work later became controversial and received many ethical rebukes for continuing to assess "natural history" at a time when presumably effective therapy (with penicillin) had become available. During subsequent debates about the moral and methodological issues, T.G. Benedek (in the 1978 *JCD*) pointed out that the rebukers had often overlooked the ethical context of the era in which the research was done.

The modern fervor (and dispute) about lowering cholesterol was just beginning. Several papers on how to reduce cholesterol with diet or medication had appeared in the *JCD* (and elsewhere), but an international group of experts, after a meeting in Geneva, stated in 1957 that

> There was no clear cut scientific evidence to show that any particular factor causes... coronary artery disease. Numerous public statements by scientific and other writers... give the impression that the atherosclerosis problem has been largely solved. The chief culprit is purported to be fat and diet. According to these opinions, all one has to do to mend the situation is to change one's eating habits so as to include a special kind of low-fat diet. Unfortunately, scientific proof of a causal relationship between fats in the diet (and) coronary artery disease is still lacking.

Forty years later, many experts would claim that the proof has now become convincing; but others would still argue that it is not.

In 1957, after the death of J. Earle Moore (the founding editor), the co-editors became Louis Lasagna and David Seegal. In 1966, David P. Earle became editor with Martin Branfonbrener added as co-editor a year later. In 1978, Earle again became sole editor, with Brandfonbrener and Walter O. Spitzer working as associate editors. When Earle retired, the journal resumed the geographically separated, dual-editor pattern that had originally been set by J.E. Moore in Baltimore and D. Seegal in New York. The co-editors after 1982 were Alvan R. Feinstein in New Haven and Walter O. Spitzer in Montreal.

Throughout its 33 years, the journal has published some outstanding, memorable papers. Some of them have already been mentioned, but several others can be noted as "golden oldies". They are: Seegal's 1962 editorial on the virtues of saying "I don't know"; E. Schimmel's 1963 editorial on "The physician as pathogen"; another 1963 editorial in which the author concluded that without better clinical "science at the bedside, modern medical research may yield an intricately designed, expensively produced, doubly-blind

controlled, statistically significant chaos"; a 1965 reprinting of J. Evelyn's treatise, originally published in 1961, on the hazards of air pollution in London; and a randomized double-blind trial, by C.R.B. Joyce and R.M.C. Welldon, in 1965, on "The objective efficacy of prayer".

With further passage of time, the contents of the journal gradually changed as other journals became available in subspecialty medical domains, and in new specialties such as rehabilitation and geriatrics. Many of the clinical reviews and symposia that formerly might have appeared in the journal became submitted and published elsewhere. The journal's symposia increasingly began to reflect its additional methodologic orientation, with topics that included the role of computers in medicine, quantitative principles in the design and analysis of long-term studies (*see* **Longitudinal Data Analysis, Overview**), and the development of indexes (or rating scales) to measure **health status** or to describe functional status and **quality of life**. The statistical philosophies that guided the US National Institutes of Health (NIH) in its approach to clinical-trial research were first described by several statisticians in a 1966 *JCD* "biometrics seminar" called "The role of hypothesis testing in clinical trials". The discussion included the often-quoted remark by **Jerome Cornfield** that, "I do not believe that anything that is good science can be bad statistics." The many unresolved controversies about retrospective **case–control studies** were discussed in a frequently cited 1979 symposium edited by Michel Ibrahim and W.O. Spitzer. Many other methodologic issues in epidemiology were considered in a memorial "festschrift", in 1986, for Abraham Lilienfeld.

The journal's clinical scope was still broad and the clinical topics still emphasized diagnosis, prognosis, course, and therapy, but most of the clinical publications began to include the kinds of group data and statistical analyses that today would make the work be classified as **clinical epidemiology**. The latter domain expanded the scope of "epidemiology" to include many topics in which the people under study were in clinical, rather than community, settings. The topics under study were also expanded to include behavioral, social, and familial factors – personality traits, emotional adjustment, urbanization, **social class**, social isolation, and familial structures and relationships – that could affect the development or management of human ailments such as heart disease, cancers, renal disease, schizophrenia, and disability.

Although all of these topics could today be included in the broad scope of contents for "clinical epidemiology", the journal's most striking expansion was in methodology. The *JCD* became the prime publication for creative scholarship in the analysis and development of methods for research in quantitative clinical epidemiology. The orientation required a special blend of thought: a sophisticated knowledge of clinical distinctions in human ailments; an intense awareness of epidemiologic subtleties in the way that groups of people are formed and collected; and mathematical attention to the statistical strategies with which results can be quantitatively summarized and interpreted.

Scholars who work in the multidisciplinary intersection produced by the manifold methodologic challenges of quantitative clinical epidemiology are also relatively homeless. Their interests are often too quantitative or epidemiologic to be appreciated by clinical journals, too clinical to be approved by journals of epidemiology or public health, and too clinically or epidemiologically "applied" to be welcomed by journals of mathematical or biologic statistics. By opening this multidisciplinary forum, the *JCD* became a leading outlet for methodologic advances in medical research concerned with groups of people.

The methodologic analyses and advances were sometimes presented within the text of publications on specific ailment-oriented topics, but often the methods themselves were the main focus of discussion. The methods included such clinical issues as the role of **co-morbidity** (a term and concept introduced in the *JCD* in 1970); the acquisition of cogent, high-quality data in interviews and questionnaires (*see* **Questionnaire Design**); the evaluation of diagnostic and technologic tests (*see* **Diagnostic Tests, Evaluation of**); decisions about what kind of data to assemble in describing personality, behavior, **quality of care**, or quality of life; defining the "range of normal" (*see* **Normal Clinical Values, Reference Intervals for**); and the role of necropsy research in revealing the fallacies of using "cause-specific" death certificate data for individual decisions or collective concepts about the distribution of disease.

The epidemiologic methods referred to problems that produce biased or inaccurate results in data for groups. The problems included diverse issues in life-table analysis, the first empirical demonstration of the distortion known as **Berkson's fallacy**, and attention to every aspect of the assembly, maintenance, and collection of data for the people investigated in randomized trials, **cohort studies**, case–control studies, community **cross-sections, ecologic studies**, and other architectural structures for research. The statistical concepts included problems in planning sample sizes for diverse investigative situations (*see* **Sample Size Determination**), estimating relative risks, assessing the role of repeated measures and **regression to the mean**, determining **prevalence** in longitudinal or cross-sectional studies, and understanding or evaluating the virtues and hazards of old multivariable analytic methods (such as **linear regression**) and newer **multivariate analysis** (such as binary regression, logistic **transformations, discriminant functions**, and the **proportional hazards** model).

To acknowledge its focus on the intimate interchange between qualitative challenges in clinical science and quantitative issues in statistics, the *Journal of Chronic Diseases* in 1988 changed its name to the *Journal of Clinical Epidemiology*. The fertile interchange has led to many useful collaborations among clinicians, epidemiologists, psychosocial scientists, and statisticians, while producing valuable interdisciplinary cross-fertilization and communication. It has made medical people aware of the need for satisfactory "numeracy" and "reliability" in communicating with their statistical and psychometric colleagues, while making statisticians and psychometricians aware of the need for satisfactory "literacy" and "sensibility" in communicating with medical people.

The satisfactory adjustment of interdisciplinary communication is not easy. Sometimes a statistical author may submit a paper that is aimed exclusively at statisticians, and that is incomprehensible to a medical reader. By 1979, the problem was happening often enough in the *JCD* to make David Earle publish an editorial urging "potential authors to write their manuscripts so that the clinical relevance is clearly apparent, and put as much of the derivation as possible in an appendix or to publish the mathematics elsewhere". The editors of the *JCE* have often made analogous requests.

Sometimes a reviewer who is a rigorous quantitative methodologist may make demands that are impossible for an investigator to attain. A psychometric reviewer may ask, almost as a matter of routine, that **Cronbach's alpha** be calculated for a five-category ordinal scale for which the calculation (which requires an inventory of individual items) cannot be done. A biostatistical reviewer may ask for analyses of data that cannot be obtained because the research project is completed, or may want the authors to use complex multivariable procedures (beyond those already employed) that may bring more smoke and heat to the results but little light.

From the medical-content side of the spectrum, an epidemiologist may insist that the research is worthless because it was a cohort study rather than a randomized trial, or vice versa; or the reviewer may dismiss the research as useless and beyond repair because the investigators should have chosen an entirely different control group. A clinical reviewer, unwilling to learn some basic principles of numeracy, may complain about the "obscurity" of statistical writing that contains nothing more esoteric than simple regression and **correlation** coefficients. These problems have not been common, however. In general, the journal seems to have had outstanding success in attracting suitable authors, getting capable, open-minded reviewers, and producing relatively clear interdisciplinary communications. The term "clinical epidemiology" covers many methods and orientations. They include causal elucidations by a classical epidemiologist, patient care decisions by a classical clinician, analytic improvements by a classical statistician, and diverse mixtures of some or all of these activities. (At some levels of definition – such as "disease", "chronic disease", "clinical", or "epidemiology" – an encompassing vagueness may be more satisfactory than an excluding precision.)

Under the new title, the *JCE* continued its basic policies, but added some new sections. Controversial topics were regularly published as trios containing a presentation, dissent, and response. Some of the more prominent controversies discussed in this variance-and-dissent format have been classification and directionality in epidemiologic research, the use of the **kappa** statistic, and the role of Popperian causality (*see* **Causation**) in scientific reasoning. This format, which allows direct airing for controversial topics, has been popular with readers, and has subsequently been emulated at other journals. A "Second Thoughts" section was made available for "lighter" essays that would be "fun" to read. James F. Jekel was invited to prepare periodic summaries, called "Rainbow Reviews", of the reports

(with multicolored covers) regularly issued by the US **National Center for Health Statistics**. With the continued application of clinical epidemiology to studies of pharmaceutical agents, a new section on **pharmacoepidemiology** was added in 1991.

In 1996, the *JCE* began publishing supplements containing the abstracts submitted to the annual meeting of the International Clinical Epidemiology Network (INCLEN). The *JCE* has also published supplements on the SUPPORT study of outcomes and risks of treatment, policy for management of asymptomatic hypercholesterolemia, pharmacoepidemiology in developing countries, ethics in epidemiology, long-term health effects of silicone breast implants, and postvasectomy sequelae. Special issues or sections of issues were devoted to a symposium on **meta-analysis** and to a memorial set of papers for Petr Skrabanek.

In 1995, after the absorption of Pergamon Press, Elsevier Science became the new publisher, while encouraging the maintenance of previous editorial policies and editorial freedom. When W.O. Spitzer "retired" in 1995, the journal moved its European office to Leiden, and Jan Vandenbroucke joined A.R. Feinstein as co-editor. The journal has been fortunate in having outstanding workers in the field – too many to be listed here – as members of its advisory and editorial consultant board, and as *ad hoc* reviewers. As noted in a 1997 editorial, the journal tries to "maintain both the appearance and reality of being open-minded about... controversy, dissent, and ferment (which) are the source of creative scientific growth and development". The journal has also continued its efforts to provide "high quality scientific papers" and "leadership... in methodologic issues that are the scientific basis and creative outlets of research in clinical epidemiology".

In an early "credo", the editors of the ancestor *JCD* described their "willingness to experiment, to be provocative... (and) to avoid stodginess and pomposity". The editors said they were willing to give a "day in court... (to) facts and opinions... which might otherwise not have been printed elsewhere" and were "never preoccupied (with) format and length of contribution so long as they seemed appropriate to the material at hand". This original credo has survived and prevailed, and it endures at the *JCE*.

ALVAN R. FEINSTEIN

Journal of Epidemiology and Biostatistics

The *Journal of Epidemiology and Biostatistics* was founded in November 1995, with the first issue published in June 1996, and three further issues published within the first year of operations. Peter Boyle and Carlo La Vecchia in the first issue set out the aims and scope [1]. They had perceived that there had been a rapid expansion in the need for, and the provision of, information on which decisions on public health issues could be made.

> Epidemiology is increasingly seen as providing the scientific basis for decision-making in Public Health which, in turn, is increasingly being recognized as a priority by governments, as witnessed by the growth of schools of Public Health in many countries. This expansion is not confined to any one particular area or topic but exists in a large number of areas of subject matter such as cancer, heart disease, acquired immune deficiency (AIDS), other chronic diseases, and congenital malformations, infectious diseases, health services research and economics, pharmacoepidemiology and nutritional disorders.

The scope of the Journal is such that it will be useful for practitioners, both clinical and scientific, research, and also for teaching. It is intended that published materials should be clear and understandable to a wide audience, thus increasing the bounds of knowledge of epidemiology and biostatistics to readers from other related disciplines.

The editorial office of the Journal, published in the UK, is in Milan at the European Institute of Oncology, and the Editorial Board spans a wide range of related disciplines, including epidemiological methodology, biostatistics, chronic disease, **nutrition, clinical trials** and drug surveillance (*see* **Pharmacoepidemiology, Overview**). It is also highly international with more that 60 members from Europe, North America, and the Pacific basin.

The Journal offers several novel characteristics, primarily the rapid lead time from submission to publication. There is no charge for submission to the Journal. Manuscripts will normally be reviewed and authors notified within 30 days of receipt of the decision to accept or reject the work. There is an express review process within five working days, although there is an administrative charge. All manuscripts will be reviewed by at least two internationally recognized experts on the subject. In addition to full-length manuscripts the journal also publishes review articles, novel hypotheses, short communications, book reviews and editorials.

The address for submissions is:

Professor Peter Boyle (Editor), *Journal of Epidemiology and Biostatistics*, Division of Epidemiology and Biostatistics, European Institute of Oncology, Via Ripamonti 435, 20141 Milan, Italy. Fax: +39 2 57 48 98 13.

The final distinctive feature of the Journal is the use of color print in both diagrams and script, where they enhance and complement the text. Color prints or preferably 35 mm transparencies are therefore welcomed with submissions.

Reference

[1] Boyle, P. & La Vecchia, C. (1996). Introducing the Journal of Epidemiology and Biostatistics (Editorial), *Journal of Epidemiology and Biostatistics* **1**, 1–2.

PETER BOYLE

Journal of the American Statistical Association: Its Organization and Purpose

The **American Statistical Association** (ASA) was founded in 1839 by men concerned about issues surrounding the nation's decennial **census** taking. Almost 50 years later, General Walker (ASA President 1883–1896), a towering figure who was impassioned in his desire and beliefs that all workers (most especially government workers and researchers throughout the land) should embrace the statistical method in their daily work, led the association beyond the then-local horizons of Boston with the adoption of a number of measures, the most fundamental one being the establishment in 1888 of a *New Series* of publications of the ASA. This title reflected the fact that previously there had been a *Collection* of the ASA (with the first and possibly only volume in

1847) plus other occasional papers, many of which had been destroyed in the Great Fire of Boston in 1872. An account of these earlier collections can be found in [4]. This *New Series* subsequently assumed the title *Quarterly Publications of the American Statistical Association* and in 1922 was renamed *Journal of the American Statistical Association (JASA)*. The header *New Series* however continued for 44 years, eventually being removed with the 1932 volume. Today, *JASA* still appears quarterly.

For its first 40 years with only two exceptions, ASA held four quarterly (or three quarterly and one annual) meetings per year; after 1894 the quarterly meetings were dropped but the annual meetings continued. Papers read at these meetings constituted a large proportion of the articles in *JASA* in its first 20 years or so. In 1928, read papers were assembled together as a Proceedings section of *JASA*, a practice continued until 1937 after which there was a return to the earlier custom whereby such read papers intermingled with general papers. This was finally discontinued with the publication of separate Proceedings of the Business and Economic Section in 1954 and of the Social Statistics Section in 1958.

Articles reflected the interests of ASA members who were primarily economists, accountants, social scientists, political scientists, historians, health professionals, and the like. That is, members were users of statistical science in their substantive field, and so articles were focused on advancing knowledge and new theories in those fields rather than in statistical methodology *per se*. Indeed, the first article of Volume 1, on water power [6] and the second one on parks and open spaces [3], illustrate amply the concerns of members with societal issues (in these cases people's basic well-being). In addition, there were numerous Reports, Miscellany, News and Notices, and Reviews entries. These articles typically included reports on **vital statistics** (of every imaginable stripe – deaths, births, divorces, diseases, suicides, etc. recorded for national, state and local municipalities, as well as international regions); they covered reviews of important papers from abroad (most often mathematical developments from British publications); and they included book reviews, among other topics. Starting in 1897, regular reports of the ASA Secretary as read at the annual meetings were included; see [1]. The Proceedings and Scientific Program of these meetings began to be published in 1910 [2]. Reports of various ASA committees would at

times also be published. In short, *JASA* was the vehicle to convey information – both scientific results and operational news – to the membership.

Today, the nature and content of *JASA* have changed, at least on the surface if not in its aims. In a formal sense, the general articles now appear within the Applications and Case Studies Section or the Theory and Methods Sections. The split into separate divisions was implemented in 1968 and visible in 1970 when papers in each section were assembled together. The Applications Section was expanded to the Applications and Case Studies Section in 1989. Book reviews had been collected together from the beginning. In 1989, this section was expanded to the (General) Review Section, though book reviews still constitute the bulk of the material in this section. The extensive Reports and much of the Miscellany articles have disappeared from *JASA*; the News and Notices articles also no longer appear in *JASA*. These were essentially moved to *The American Statistician* when it began in 1947 and later to the monthly *Amstat News* begun in 1974, with the exceptions that the Reports of the Annual Meetings continued to appear in *JASA* until the 1971 meeting and the Board of Directors and related Reports until the 1969 Report, when these reports shifted to *The American Statistician*. *The American Statistician* from its inception also included articles demonstrating the uses of statistics, articles that previously occupied many pages of *JASA*. As its founding editors said, *The American Statistician* would serve as an adjunct to the technical papers published in *JASA*.

From the content viewpoint, a reading of Information for Authors, which currently appears in each issue of *JASA*, reveals that the Applications and Case Studies Section seeks articles that contribute to a substantive field through the use of sound or innovative uses of statistical methods, present data useful to such fields, or discuss and evaluate such data and findings; methodological innovations are not requirements. This descriptor reflects very accurately and keeps intact the tenor and the goals of ASA as exemplified in the articles of the very early issues of *JASA*. Then and now the important new theoretical results were directed at the field of application with new statistical theory that may have emerged being incidental to the major thrust.

By the time of ASA's Seventy-fifth Anniversary in 1914, changes were looming on the horizon. The so-called mathematical method had appeared through

correlation, and has remained as an integral part of statistical science. Nevertheless, mathematical statistical articles still assumed a relatively small proportion of *JASA* articles until about the 1950s. By the 1960s, mathematically based articles had become more dominant. These articles now appear in the Theory and Methods Section. As defined in the Information for Authors, this Section "publishes articles that make original contributions to the foundations, theoretical development, and methodology of statistics and probability". This mandate is "interpreted broadly... and may include computational and graphical methods as well as more traditional mathematical methods". However, such articles should be, and are, motivated by a practical problem arising from a substantive application.

The General Section includes the traditional Book Review Section plus Review Papers covering an area of applied statistics or a review of some specific statistical theory. Special topic papers may also appear in this general section.

In addition, at its April 1907 meeting, it was decided to ask the ASA President to address the association at its annual meeting and that this Address be published as the lead article in the following March issues of *JASA*. Accordingly, the first Presidential Address was delivered by Wright on January 17, 1908 (see [7]). Interestingly, though the ASA had but five presidents for its first 70 years, each serving till death (Fletcher 1839–45, Shattuck 1846–51, Jarvis 1852–82, Walker 1883–96, and Wright 1897–1909), subsequent presidents were limited to one year terms; and further, today, the Address of the ninety-second president appears in Volume 92.

Today, in substance *JASA* is dominated by theoretical mathematically based statistical methodology, although its authors continue to be motivated by real world problems. The advances in the substantive field that totally dominated *JASA* prior to about 1950–60 are now found in other ASA journals, namely *Journal of Business and Economic Statistics* (begun in 1983), *Journal of Educational and Behavorial Statistics* (1976), *Journal of Computational and Graphical Statistics*, (1992), *Journal of Agricultural Biological and Environmental Statistics* (1996 and a joint venture with the International Biometric Society), and *Technometrics* (1959 and a joint venture with the American Society of Quality). In addition, the magazines *STATS* (1989) and *Chance* (1988) are targeted to the student and/or man-in-the-street nonstatistician

audience. Earlier, ***Biometrics*** (called *Biometrics Bulletin* 1945–46) was launched under **Gertrude Cox's** editorship by the Biometrics Section of ASA to publish articles on the use of mathematical and statistical methodology in biology (including agriculture); this journal was fully assumed by the **International Biometric Society** in 1951. This applications orientation of the membership is still vibrant today and has been a strong and persistent thread throughout. The strength of this view was reflected by the unsuccessful efforts of the ASA's mathematical members to have the *Annals of Mathematical Statistics* (begun in 1930, and first edited by Harry Carver) as an ASA publication.

The first *JASA* Editor was Davis Dewey, who served from 1888 to 1907. The division in 1969 brought with it a separate editor for each section: the Applications (predecessor of the Applications and Case Studies) Section, Theory and Methods Section, and Book Review (now the General Review) Section.

With the exception of the occasional invited paper and also Invited Discussants to selected articles typically addressing a major applied topic, articles are unsolicited. Potential authors submit manuscripts to the Editor(s). Papers deemed not to fit the overall aims of the journal would be returned to the authors without going through the formal reviewing process. That said, in a typical scenerio, the Editor disseminates the submissions to a cadre of Associate Editors, who take the responsibility for selecting and monitoring the refereeing process. Double-blind refereeing for the Applications and Case Studies and the Theory and Methods Sections was instituted in 1996.

The 1995 Editors (see [5]) reported that the Applications and Case Studies Section received 127 new manuscripts (140 in 1994) and that the acceptance rate (of new and resubmissions) was 22% for 1995 (25% for 1994). The Theory and Methods Section received 466 new submissions in 1995 (451 in 1994) with an acceptance rate of 30% (19% in 1994). In the General Section, in 1995, one-third of new books received were sent out for reviews, both new review manuscripts received in 1995 were rejected, while two of the three received in 1994 were accepted in 1995. Subsequently, there were 27 Applications and Case Studies papers, 132 Theory and Methods papers, five Review papers, 44 Book Reviews and 25 Telegraphic Review articles published in 1996, plus the Presidential Address and **Fisher Lecture**, and relevant editorially related information, occupying 1768 pages. In contrast, Volume 1 published 11 Leading Articles and 49 Reviews and Miscellany articles in 492 pages. Volume 1 spanned 2 years; it was not until Volume 19 in 1924 that one volume per year began.

Throughout its long history, *JASA* has continued to be a premier journal serving the entire international statistical community. It remains the flagship publication of the ASA.

References

[1]   Dewey, D.R. (1897). Report of the Secretary of the American Statistical Association, *Journal of the American Statistical Association* **5**, 234–235.

[2]   Doten, C.W. (1910). Proceedings of the Seventy-first Annual Meeting of the American Statistical Association, New York, December 27–30, 1909, *Journal of the American Statistical Association* **12**, 36–39.

[3]   Gould, E.R.L. (1888). Park areas and open spaces in American and European Cities, *Journal of the American Statistical Association* **1**, 49–61.

[4]   Green, S.A. (1889). An account of the collections of the American Statistical Association, *Journal of the American Statistical Association* **1**, 328–330.

[5]   Lambert, D., Hollander, M. & Agresti, A. (1996). Editors' Report for 1995, *Journal of the American Statistical Association* **91**, 443–443.

[6]   Swain, G.F. (1888). Statistics of water power employed in manufacturing in the United States, *Journal of the American Statistical Association* **1**, 1–44.

[7]   Wright, C.D. (1908). Address of Carroll D. Wright, President of the American Statistical Association, at its Annual Meeting in Boston, January 17, 1908, *Journal of the American Statistical Association* **11**, 1–16.

L. BILLARD

Journal of the American Statistical Association: Its Writings

From noble beginnings in 1888, the *Journal of the American Statistical Association (JASA)* quickly became firmly established as a premier journal in the dissemination of the statistical method. This article invites us to ride through that past as we glimpse delights and mysteries of the writings of the **American Statistical Association** (ASA) as preserved in the *Journal*.

The overriding characteristic of ASA's first century of writings was that, with few exceptions, articles were distinctly nonmathematical in nature. The ASA, as reflected in *JASA*, was primarily an association of economists, historians, political scientists, social scientists, census-takers, demographers, health professionals, and the like, who used the statistical method as a tool in the pursuit of truth and enlightenment in the context of the substantive discipline. Thus, articles frequently generated new theory and policies within those disciplines. Furthermore, they were often a repository of extensive data sets gathered in the course of the studies undertaken; indeed, there would be pages and pages of data at times, a perhaps tedious but nevertheless refreshing sharing of information. The central role played by the applied statistician (in today's parlance) was cemented when, on the occasion of ASA's 75th anniversary in 1914, a series of papers was prepared focusing on the service and importance of statistics in government, history, sociology, business, economics; and Pearl [39] wrote on the "new" field of biology for which the term "biometry" had been recently coined. Throughout these years, however, there was a recognition that the English school (especially **Galton, Karl Pearson**, and **Yule**) was producing important new ideas, with reviews of specific works from *Biometrika* and the **Royal Statistical Society** appearing in *JASA*. Nevertheless, there were initially serious doubts as to whether those ideas developed primarily in a purely biological setting could be transferred to the nonbiological settings that dominated *JASA*.

During the first 20–30 years there were essentially only two areas of statistical theory that received attention in *JASA* papers. The first area covered concepts relating to averages, variation, and distributions. Dewey's review [18] of Galton's work, *Natural Inheritance*, reflected the prevailing sentiments of the late 1800s and of what was coming over the horizon when he conveyed Galton's opinion that "statisticans are apt to be content with averages ... What is wanted is a method of calculating distribution, and a graphic scheme for reading the distribution".

Falkner [19] developed several basic principles on the theory and practice of statistics including concepts of enumeration, aggregation, **estimation**, variation, and consistency, in each case basing his arguments on logical reasoning and conclusions from what his numerical illustrations revealed. This paper was typical for the day in that the statistical theory emerged in response to the need to develop new theories in a substantive area, in this case price theory (with the Consumer Price Index concept emerging from this work). It also evoked great interest, generating considerable subsequent activity. Holmes [29] felt that an average alone was inadequate, and introduced the concept of mixtures of distributions. Holmes' article also elicited the first letter to the editor by none other than the "most eminent" Galton himself [21]. Swain [51] looked at the method of averages; and later a review paper by Mitchell [37] and Bailey's review [3] of Yule's book [63] established the basic "theoretical" foundations for **frequency distributions**. In the 1920s, there was a second wave of activity, this time mathematical in nature, starting with the fundamental papers of Carver [9, 10].

Motivated by the desire to provide visual representations of frequency distributions, concurrent work on the concepts of graphs and tables proceeded, albeit slowly (*see* **Graphical Displays**). Ripley [47] laid the groundwork for general graphical principles but consensus was hard to muster. Eventually, the ASA joined with 16 other national associations to establish guidelines for graphical presentations of data, with the preliminary report [7] outlining 17 basic principles, the most mundane of which was that the "arrangement of a diagram should proceed from left to right" (Principle 1). Likewise, tables had no systematic principles for construction until, following Watkins' article [54] on the theory of tabulation, Falkner [20] laid out several underlying principles (including the need to number tables for ease of identification).

Correlation and **regression** related concepts also emerged during these first 20–30 years. While it would be many years before these terms would be so identified, regression actually appeared early, primarily in forecasting **population growth** rates, in and of itself a topic that occupied many pages. Interestingly, Crum [15], in reviewing a population forecast (using a quadratic relation), stated that "to most statisticians the method of least squares must always form an almost insuperable obstacle". A scant 15 years later would see a major change in this perspective! In the early 1900s, there were many papers concerned with determining whether curves (or plots) for two or more response variables were similar. The crucial question

as to whether the important theoretical results being advanced in Britain carried over to the applications that dominated *JASA* was answered affirmatively in a major paper by Persons [41], in which he depended ultimately on numerical arguments, though he did provide some algebraic formulas as well. In general, *JASA* articles tended to report on these overseas developments with its own articles focusing more on explaining the uses and limitations of these new theories. For example, Reed [45] demonstrated how it was feasible to have perfect correlation and a correlation coefficient of zero, that is, the coefficient was a measure of a linear relationship; and Day [17] clarified some of the then-still confusions between seemingly related, but in actuality distinct, concepts. In contrast, when time (or space) as an index was a critical element to the plots, leading articles on correlation concepts, beginning with Magee [36], did grace the pages of *JASA*. Magee's work lead eventually to a major entry by Persons [42]. Persons' work is a tortuous journey through several numerical examples but eventually we were introduced to what would later be termed the **autocorrelation** coefficient for time-dependent series, among other new concepts. This paper served as a springboard for numerous major articles in **time series** theory in the 1920s and 1930s, with a subsequent decline until the 1960s when interest was renewed in *JASA* pages. However, regression related articles appeared consistently over the decades with **general linear models** and in the last 20 years **generalized linear models** and related topics making their appearance.

Despite the fact that tensions between the non-mathematical and mathematical statistician (defined as the use(r) of correlation related ideas) were clearly building by the mid-1900s, the pages of *JASA* in these early years were also clearly vibrating with an unmistakable excitement. The statistical community, by dint of pure intellectual strength and logical thinking, was reasoning its way through to clarity on such issues as the closeness of fit of two curves, of **causation** as opposed to **association**, of time as a dependent entity, of **goodness of fit** and the comparison of observed and expected frequencies, and of correlation as distinct from contingency. The first entry by Karl Pearson [40] involved an exchange of views with Harris et al. [25] on **contingency tables**. The 1930 date reflected the continued attention to the subject well beyond the first proposed use (to resolve questions surrounding women's suffrage and the legalized sale of alcoholic liquors) in Gehlke [22].

While distributions and correlation served as the two major areas of statistical theory developed prior to about 1920, other theory did filter through though almost always as an aid to wrestling with particular theories of central concern to a field of application. Thus, we saw the concept of probable error [44], adequate sample sizes [50] (*see* **Sample Size Determination**), **seasonal** effects [59], smoothing (*see* **Nonparametric Regression**) [14], **moving average** [31], and **hypothesis testing** [55]. We saw the beginnings of **sample surveys** and the survey instrument (*see* **Questionnaire Design**) with Holmes' [28] treatise on the importance of a survey being "representative" and "systematically" conducted, and on how, when, and what questions should be asked. However, it was not until 1915 [23] that the ASA formed a standing committee to establish standards and guidelines for survey instruments, and 1916 when Hobson [26] provided a theoretical structure for these instruments.

While these theoretical developments were unquestionably important to the emergence of statistics as a science, they were in reality largely incidental to *JASA* articles. A more accurate reflection overall was that articles provided a window into the prevailing societal issues of the day. In fact, they open pages on our (often long forgotten) history lessons of a century ago. We read, for example, about the opening of the West, especially through articles on crops (plantings and yields) and railways (freight, mileages, revenues and expenses). We can trace historical ideas pertaining to foods (what is consumed, how prepared, availability), women (their education, children, occupations), accidents (railway, and factory accidents), poverty, anthropology, immigration (countries of origin, where settled, and impact), divorces, suicides, and living conditions, to name but a few. These all received considerable attention.

Kopf [33], in his portrayal of **Florence Nightingale** as the "passionate statistician", reminded us that she used "the statistical method as a means of developing a basis of established fact for social reform", that she was a pioneer in graphical illustrations of statistics and issued "her original tabulation of the appalling morbidity and mortality statistics of the British Army ... [in] January, 1858", and that she "drew up a standard list of diseases ... and a set of

model hospital statistical forms". Most importantly, her study (with **William Farr**) of the results tabulated in these forms led to the radically new awakening that "a (large) field of qualified statistical inquiry had been opened by the introduction of her forms". Nightingale was surely one of the first biostatisticians. Certainly, the collection and tabulation of disease statistics as a concept was to grow unabated from this time forward.

Consequently, throughout *JASA* there was considerable attention devoted to the study of diseases, motivated primarily by a concern for living conditions, especially in the cities, and for working conditions, most notably in factories. For example, in a paper important both for its theory and its impact on typhoid, Winslow [59] ascertained that there was a seasonal component to the fatality rate. Furthermore, in trying to resolve the debates over this issue, he identified a "serious source of error ... introduced by the lapse of time between the reporting ... and fatality"; he then adjusted the apparent death rates in an attempt to obtain the true death rate. This reporting lag problem is still with us today most recently in connection with **AIDS** diagnosis. In fact, another difficulty with analysing AIDS data, that pertaining to the changing definitions of AIDS is also not new, the general problem of definition having been identified as early as 1892. Abbott [1], attempting to improve the collection and administration of **vital statistics**, called for standard medical nomenclature and classification of diseases. Thus was set in motion a series of papers leading to Wilbur's article in which the development of a classification system is traced through the debates surrounding the **Bertillon** classification scheme first reported to the **International Statistical Institute** in 1893 up to the adoption of the revised classifications that were to take effect in 1910 (*see* **International Classification of Diseases (ICD)**).

For the health professional, there are extensive data available for a very large number of diseases both from the US and from abroad. Thus, it is possible to trace the progress of cholera, pneumonia, diarrhea, typhoid fever, tuberculosis, influenza, dysentery, croup, diphtheria, measles, scarlet fever, whooping cough, and so on; all were pervasive and persistent and received considerable attention. The famous influenza epidemic of 1918 immediately drew attention and was quickly brought up for discussion at the March 1919 meeting of the ASA. There was a call that the ASA join with the **American Public**

Health Association to encourage a "thorough statistical study of the epidemic", and to recognize a need for "methods of higher analytic description of the disease". The session closed with endorsement of a resolution that addressed several critical and urgent aspects (see [53]). This action typified the central role played in responding to important societal issues of the day.

A new stage in health policy was reached when Winslow [60], in a study of smallpox, declared that "... statistical evidence of the protective effect of vaccination is absolutely conclusive". Preventive measures of a different ilk emerged following Chaddock's finding that the practice of calculating the death rate for an entire city obscured the fact that the rate was higher in some parts of the city than in others [11]. More specifically, it was higher in those parts of the city that had poor sanitation or poor housing conditions, or for workers plying their trade in dangerous occupations in unhealthy environments. It is sobering to ponder the expectation that tuberculosis would soon be extinct as expressed by Newsholme in 1903 that there was "more hope of the almost complete extermination of tuberculosis than of any of the acute infectious diseases, with the possible exception of typhus and small-pox" (see [2]). Woodward [61] pointed out the importance of death rates "to show where and how sanitary work (was) needed" and what measures should therefore be taken.

The health and welfare of the population was the strong thread that bound together and motivated so much of the work on diseases, working and living conditions, and related concerns. The first issue of *JASA* even had an article on park areas and open spaces in cities because of their positive impact on the citizens' health [24]. This thread threatened to unravel, however, when it came to cancer. There had been an observed rise in the number of cancer cases. Whether this was due to a real increase in incidence or to the way the data were grouped was hotly disputed. Indeed, King & Newsholme [32] and Willcox [58] framed the debate and its progress (or lack thereof) with their aptly titled articles "On the alleged increase in cancer". As far as the cancer question was concerned, how to group correctly by age was still a contentious issue, Young's theory on age grouping [62] notwithstanding. Willcox concluded (incorrectly, we now know) that there was no real increase in incidence and that the apparent increase was an artifact of an inappropriate use of age. In an unrelated study, we

note that it was not until 1923 that smoking attracted attention [30], while cancer itself did not receive further major attention until the **Berkson** & Gage article [4] on the five-year survival curve for cancer patients. Furthermore, **Cutler** [16], in his review of statistical evidence for an association between lung cancer and smoking, concluded that the "relative importance of smoking, air pollution, and occupational exposure to cancerigenic materials remains to be established", though unlike Willcox he did acknowledge as his starting point the great increase in deaths from lung cancer. Brownlee [8], in a review of the Surgeon-General's Report, felt that "the Committee has not established the case for causality in lung cancer" (*see* **Smoking and Health**).

Parallel to the work on diseases was a large body of work on birth and death rates. These ranged from tables of counts, often buried in the numerous municipal reports on vital statistics, to the mathematical equations that emerged in the 1920s. It should be remarked that recording these vital statistics accurately was still quite a task in the 1800s. Deaths, in particular, were especially difficult to track, with neither of the two solutions proposed by Price [43], namely searching newspapers for death notices or comparing census returns with death records, being workable. Earlier, the American Medical Association at its founding in 1847 joined with the ASA in its call for a standard **death certificate**, subsequently adopted in 1900. Also, at its first annual meeting in 1907 the American Public Health Association proposed resolutions regarding statements on causes of death (see [46]).

The first "study" of death rates came with Macauley's conclusion [35] that a person's age rather than weight served as a more accurate indication of future longevity. Later, Hoffman [27] studied death rates via improved health and sanitary conditions. The prolific Hoffman contributed significantly to this question, and was the first to propose that death rates should be calculated for various age, gender, race, occupation, and other categories. Willcox [57] observed that a decline in death rates over the 20 previous years compared with the previous 80–100 years coincided with a decrease in fluctuations, attributed by Willcox to successful efforts in controlling unhealthy environments. Then, in a marked departure from the past, beginning with Lotka [34], the 1920s and 1930s saw a series of papers by Lotka, **Pearl**, and Reed, developing mathematical formulations, typically logistic equations or variations thereof, to describe birth, death, or more generally, growth rates. This work is still fundamental today, albeit based on deterministic rather than the more accurate **stochastic** model approach. As an aside, Schultz [49], using the Lotka–Pearl–Reed **logistic** model, projected the maximum attainable population of the US, to occur by 2100 at 196 million! Schultz's paper is important for its calculation of the **standard error** of a forecast (for regression models), and the particular warning that this standard error increases as the predictor variable moves farther away from the mean of the observed values.

Who could quarrel with Newsholme's [38] assertion that "To die of old age is the most laudable ambition of all"? We may, however, argue today with his conclusion that "To die of old age is comparatively rare". To these, we add Sydenstricker & Brundage's warning that the available statistics of disease incidence were confined almost entirely to deaths [52]. These statements succinctly summarize and explain the motivation behind and intense interest in health and diseases, indeed the welfare of the populace, an interest unabated in biometry to this day. In the early years, most overtly biostatistical contributions appeared in the form of brief commentary on the large number of reports detailing various vital statistics, especially those related to health, diseases, birth, and death statistics. These regular reports covered local municipal figures, other data aggregated by regions, as well as figures from overseas. By the 1930s, the emphasis had shifted, with a decrease in the number of international reports, and with the relatively sterile lists that characterized the US reports being replaced by detailed articles containing analyses, theoretical developments, and interpretations supplementing the still plentiful data sets.

Given the founding origins of the ASA, it is not surprising that the association has played a role, to varying degrees of activity over the years, in resolving societal issues of concern. Often major initiatives were undertaken to address some of these issues. These can include technical issues such as those surrounding the graphical method or sampling surveys, or issues such as the influenza epidemic, the standardized death certificate, or the classification of diseases, as discussed above.

Reports, either as papers or committee reports, have appeared in *JASA* throughout its history. Some have served as a motivating force for new theoretical developments. An important example of the latter is the report of the committee established by the then ASA President S.S. Wilks in 1950 to examine the statistical methods used in the Kinsey report (see **Cochran** et al. [12]). An appendix to that committee's report is the exposition by Cochran et al. [13] on the principles of sampling, still well worth reading. Since then there have continued to be numerous important articles on sampling – what to sample, types of samples, problems with sampling, response and **nonresponse** issues, and so on. These issues of course are of special interest to those focused on census-taking. Indeed, the census has been a major and important thread throughout, ranging from the founders' concerns with the 1840 census, through the establishment of a permanent Census Bureau in 1902 as a direct result of ASA efforts, to the special issue of *JASA* devoted to the Undercount in the 1990 Census (edited by Schenker; see [48] and the papers therein), to the 1996 Census Blue Ribbon Panel appointed by the 1996 ASA President.

Finally, perhaps the most surprising aspect of ASA writings in its first century is the relatively few articles on **hypothesis testing** and **experimental design**, despite the fact that the 1920s and 1930s were an especially active time for these topics. These were clearly identified as mathematical theories and so their publication in other outlets (most often British sources) in part reflected the applied orientation of most ASA members. Those members committed to mathematical statistics started to look to the new journal *Annals of Mathematical Statistics*, launched in 1930, to publish their work. Later, in 1945, the Biometrics Section of the ASA founded the forerunner of *Biometrics*, which in its first 20 years was dominated by design of experiments (including regression) and agriculture with a few articles arising from a medical setting. In more recent years, that balance has been largely reversed (see [5] for a review). However, the 1960s saw a return to articles on basic statistical methodologies, most particularly in statistical **inference** broadly defined – **analysis of variance**, especially **optimal designs**, hypothesis testing, **sequential analysis, chi-square tests, estimation,** and a relatively large number of nonparametric tests (*see* **Nonparametric Methods**) that have continued to grow in number and impact into the 1990s. By and large, by 1990 the topics being covered in broad terms have not changed, though the level of their mathematical content increased substantially. Moving into the 1990s, however, has brought a shift in emphasis to methods that rely on both mathematical and computational tools, such as **imaging,** smoothing, and **Markov chain Monte Carlo** methods.

Our special interest herein has been ASA's writings variously described under the rubric of biostatistics or biometry. An expanded vision of some of what we saw on this journey can be found in Billard [6], whose perspective was to look at all of statistics in *JASA* up to 1939 as a prologue for projecting the future of statistics into the next century.

References

[1] Abbott, S.W. (1892). The necessity of a revision of the classification and nomenclature employed in the vital statistics of Massachusetts, *Journal of the American Statistical Association* **3**, 279–284.

[2] Abbott, S.W. (1904). The decrease of consumption in New England, *Journal of the American Statistical Association* **9**, 1–20.

[3] Bailey, W.B. (1911). Review of *"An Introduction to the Theory of Statistics"*, by G.U. Yule, *Journal of the American Statistical Association* **12**, 765.

[4] Berkson, J. & Gage, R.P. (1952). Survival curve for cancer patients following treatment, *Journal of the American Statistical Association* **47**, 501–575.

[5] Billard, L. (1995). The roads travelled, *Biometrics* **51**, 1–11.

[6] Billard, L. (1997). A voyage of discovery, *Journal of the American Statistical Association* **92**, 1–12.

[7] Brinton, W.C. (Chair) (1915). Joint Committee on Standards for Graphic Presentations, *Journal of the American Statistical Association* **14**, 790–797.

[8] Brownlee, K.A. (1965). A review of "smoking and health", *Journal of the American Statistical Association* **60**, 722–739.

[9] Carver, H.C. (1921). The mathematical representation of frequency distributions, *Journal of the American Statistical Association* **17**, 720–731.

[10] Carver, H.C. (1921). The mathematical representation of frequency distributions, *Journal of the American Statistical Association* **17**, 885–892.

[11] Chaddock, R.E. (1914). Records of health and sanitary progress, *Journal of the American Statistical Association* **14**, 319–334.

[12] Cochran, W.G., Mosteller, F. & Tukey, J.W. (1953). Statistical problems of the Kinsey Report, *Journal of the American Statistical Association* **48**, 673–716.

[13] Cochran, W.G., Mosteller, F. & Tukey, J.W. (1954). Principles of sampling, *Journal of the American Statistical Association* **49**, 13–35.

[14] Cross, I. (1908). Strike statistics, *Journal of the American Statistical Association* **11**, 168–194.

[15] Crum, F.S. (1901). A study of municipal growth, *Journal of the American Statistical Association* **7**, 464–466.

[16] Cutler, S.J. (1955). A review of the statistical evidence on the association between smoking and lung cancer, *Journal of the American Statistical Association* **50**, 267–282.

[17] Day, E.E. (1918). A note on "The correlation of historical economic variables and their misuse of coefficients in this connection", by W.I. King, *Journal of the American Statistical Association* **16**, 115–118.

[18] Dewey, J. (1889). Galton's statistical methods, *Journal of the American Statistical Association* **1**, 331–334.

[19] Falkner, R.P. (1892). The theory and practice of price statistics, *Journal of the American Statistical Association* **3**, 119–140.

[20] Falkner, R.P. (1916). Statistical tabulation and practice, *Journal of the American Statistical Association* **15**, 192–200.

[21] Galton, F. (1892). Note from Mr. Francis Galton to Mr. George K. Holmes on the subject of distribution, *Journal of the American Statistical Association* **3**, 271–273.

[22] Gehlke, C.E. (1917). On the correlation between the vote for suffrage and the vote on the liquor questions: a preliminary study, *Journal of the American Statistical Association* **15**, 524–532.

[23] Gillin, J.L. (1915). The social survey and its further developments, *Journal of the American Statistical Association* **14**, 603–610.

[24] Gould, E.R.L. (1888). Park areas and open spaces in cities, *Journal of the American Statistical Association* **1**, 49–61.

[25] Harris, J.A., Treloar, A.E. & Wilder, M. (1930). Professor Pearson's note on our papers on contingency, *Journal of the American Statistical Association* **25**, 323–327.

[26] Hobson, A. (1916). The use of the correspondence method in original research, *Journal of the American Statistical Association* **15**, 210–218.

[27] Hoffman, F.L. (1906). The general death-rate of large American cities, 1871–1904, *Journal of the American Statistical Association* **10**, 1–75.

[28] Holmes, G.K. (1890). Mortgage statistics, *Journal of the American Statistical Association* **2**, 1–21.

[29] Holmes, G.K. (1892). Measures of distribution, *Journal of the American Statistical Association* **3**, 141–157.

[30] Holt, W.L. (1923). A statistical study of smokers and non-smokers at the University of Tennessee, *Journal of the American Statistical Association* **18**, 766–772.

[31] King, W.I. (1915). New method for computing the moving average, *Journal of the American Statistical Association* **14**, 798–800.

[32] King, G. & Newsholme, A. (1893). On the alleged increase in cancer, *Proceedings of the Royal Society* **54**, 209–242.

[33] Kopf, E.W. (1916). Florence Nightingale as statistician, *Journal of the American Statistical Association* **15**, 388–404.

considered are comparisons, critical evaluations and new applications of existing methods, contributions to **probability theory** which have a clear practical bearing (including the formulation and analysis of **stochastic processes**), statistical computation or simulation where original methodology is involved and original contributions to the foundations of statistical science.

Series C (Applied Statistics) promotes papers that are driven by real-life problems and that make a novel contribution to the subject. Practical examples should be central to papers, to motivate the work and to justify any methodologic developments. Papers describing interdisciplinary work are especially welcome, as are those that give interesting novel applications of existing methodology or provide new insights into the practical application of techniques. Other types of papers considered are those on design issues [e.g. in relation to experiments (*see* **Experimental Design in Biostatistics**), surveys (*see* **Sample Surveys**; **Surveys, Health and Morbidity**) or **observational studies**], which should feature an adequate description of a substantial application and a justification for any new theory, and papers describing developments in statistical computing, provided that they are driven by practical examples.

Series D (The Statistician) encourages papers on the practice of statistics and the role of the professional statistician. In addition, *The Statistician* aims to further the study and understanding of statistical techniques, to promote the proper application of statistical methods in practice, and to provide an international focus of information exchange between statisticians in all fields. Papers on the **teaching** and communication of statistics, statistical computing, reviews and those of historical and biographical interest are of particular interest. All papers should be aimed at a general statistical audience, with an emphasis on exposition rather than the description of technical detail.

Looking ahead, although, in all the first 160 years of the *Journal of the Royal Statistical Society*, the journal has depended on the imprint of ink on paper in a printing press to record its history, this reliance will not continue exclusively in the future. As manuscripts are now almost always created in electronic form, the journal's production process and availability are adapting to reflect the instantaneousness of the new medium.

(*See also* **Royal Statistical Society**)

M.C. OWEN

[34] Lotka, A.J. (1918). The relation between the birth rate and death rate in a normal population and the rational basis of an empirical formula for the mean length of life given by William Farr, *Journal of the American Statistical Association* **16**, 121–130.

[35] Macaulay, T.B. (1891). Weight and longevity, *Journal of the American Statistical Association* **2**, 287–296.

[36] Magee, J.D. (1912). The degree of correspondence between two series of index numbers, *Journal of the American Statistical Association* **13**, 174–181.

[37] Mitchell, W.C. (1905). Methods of presenting statistics of wages, *Journal of the American Statistical Association* **9**, 325–343.

[38] Newsholme, A. (1921). National changes in health and longevity, *Journal of the American Statistical Association* **17**, 689–719.

[39] Pearl, R. (1914). The service and importance of statistics to biology, *Journal of the American Statistical Association* **14**, 40–48.

[40] Pearson, K. (1930). On the theory of contingency I. Note on Professor J. Arthur Harris' papers on the limitation in the applicability of the contingency coefficient, *Journal of the American Statistical Association* **25**, 320–323.

[41] Persons, W.M. (1910). The correlation of economic statistics, *Journal of the American Statistical Association* **12**, 287–322.

[42] Persons, W.M. (1917). On the variate difference correlation method and curve-fitting, *Journal of the American Statistical Association* **15**, 602–642.

[43] Price, M.L. (1907). A method of dealing with unregistered deaths, *Journal of the American Statistical Association* **10**, 491–492.

[44] Pritchett, H.S. (1891). A formula for predicting the population of the United States, *Journal of the American Statistical Association* **2**, 278–286.

[45] Reed, W.G. (1917). The coefficient of correlation, *Journal of the American Statistical Association* **15**, 670–684.

[46] Resolutions (1907). Rules of statistical practice, *Journal of the American Statistical Association* **10**, 523–532.

[47] Ripley, W.Z. (1899). Notes on map making and graphics representation, *Journal of the American Statistical Association* **6**, 313–326.

[48] Schenker, N. (1993). Undercount in the 1990 census, *Journal of the American Statistical Association* **88**, 1044–1046.

[49] Schultz, H. (1930). The standard error of a forecast from a curve, *Journal of the American Statistical Association* **25**, 139–185.

[50] Smith, M.R. (1895). Almshouse women, *Journal of the American Statistical Association* **4**, 219–262.

[51] Swain, H.H. (1898). Comparative statistics of railroad rates, *Journal of the American Statistical Association* **6**, 115–145.

[52] Sydenstricker, E. & Brundage, D.K. (1921). Industrial establishment disability records as a source of morbidity statistics, *Journal of the American Statistical Association* **17**, 584–598.

[53] Van Buren, G.H., Crum, F.S. & Kopf, E.W. (1919). Statistics of the influenza epidemic, *Journal of the American Statistical Association* **16**, 490–492.

[54] Watkins, G.P. (1915). Theory of statistical tabulation, *Journal of the American Statistical Association* **14**, 742–757.

[55] Westergaard, H. (1916). Scope and method of statistics, *Journal of the American Statistical Association* **15**, 225–291.

[56] Wilbur, C.L. (1909). A statistical pilgrimage, *Journal of the American Statistical Association* **11**, 624–635.

[57] Willcox, W.F. (1916). The nature and significance of the changes in the birth and death rates in recent years, *Journal of the American Statistical Association* **15**, 1–15.

[58] Willcox, W.F. (1917). On the alleged increase in cancer, *Journal of the American Statistical Association* **15**, 701–782.

[59] Winslow, C.-E.A. (1902). A statistical study of the fatality of typhoid fever at different seasons, *Journal of the American Statistical Association* **8**, 103–125.

[60] Winslow, C.-E.A. (1903). Statistics of smallpox and vaccination, *Journal of the American Statistical Association* **8**, 279–284.

[61] Woodward, W.C. (1907). The practical application of vital statistics, *Journal of the American Statistical Association* **10**, 485–488.

[62] Young, A.A. (1900). The comparative accuracy of different forms of quinquennial age groups, *Journal of the American Statistical Association* **7**, 27–39.

[63] Yule, G.U. (1911). *An Introduction to the Theory of Statistics*. Griffin, London.

L. BILLARD

Journal of the Royal Statistical Society

In May 1838, following the establishment of the Society during 1834, the Council launched the first volume of the *Journal of the Statistical Society of London*:

> The Council of the Statistical Society of London is of opinion that the time has arrived when the Fellows of the Society, and the public, will hail with satisfaction the appearance of a Journal devoted to the collection and comparison of Facts which illustrate the condition of mankind, and tend to develop the principles by which the progress of society is determined.

Since in the 1830s the "Science of Statistics" was in its infancy, in their introduction to the new journal the Council felt it necessary to add some explanation about the objects of the Society and its journal. Within the extensive scope of the subject the importance of medical statistics was already recognized:

> Mechanics discover the means of abridging human labour; Chemistry enters largely into the economy of Arts; Medicine practises on the bodies of men; all these sciences operate upon human interests and their powers and effects are susceptible of statistical exposition.

Reviewing the content of the journal in 1865, the Council divided the subject-matter into seven classes: "commercial", "industrial", "financial", "moral and social", "vital", and "miscellaneous", the last category comprising papers not presented for reading to the Society. **W.A. Guy** was an early presenter of papers, such as "Influence of the seasons and weather on sickness and mortality" and "Influence of employment and health". **William Farr**, of still greater authority, made his debut with the paper "Mortality of lunatics" and "The influence of elevation on the fatality of cholera". Other contributions included the reports of the Committee on Medical Statistics (1837) and of the Committee on Sickness among the Metropolitan Police Force (1839–40).

Although as long ago as 1863 the Society had been urged to publish discussions at its meetings, the proposal had been defeated. It was not until the June issue in 1873 that reports of the oral discussion and the authors' replies began to appear, and the practice of having both a formal proposing and seconding of a vote of thanks, as now, did not begin until 1909.

In January 1887, the Society was granted its Royal Charter, and the journal accordingly changed its name to the *Journal of the Royal Statistical Society*. Another important change at that time was the introduction of reviews of books on statistical and economic subjects in 1886, under the heading "Notes on some recent Additions to the Library".

Up to that point in the journal's history the papers published had been almost entirely of a descriptive nature, with large numbers of tables presenting data, but without detailed analysis. It was only around the turn of the century that the mathematical foundations began to be developed in the pages of the journal, with papers such as "On the theory of correlation" by **G. Udny Yule** (1897) and "On the representation of statistics

by mathematical formulae" by **F.Y. Edgeworth**, in four parts, concluded in the 1899 volume.

In June 1928, the Society formed its first "Study Group" for holding informal meetings. This was followed in 1933 by the formation of the first of its Sections, the Industrial and Agricultural Research Section. The papers presented at the first two meetings of the Section were published in a supplementary issue with part II of the main journal in the Society's centenary year. A second supplement was issued with part IV of the journal. The *Supplements*, two parts per volume, were initially designed to cater for the "considerable developments in the application of modern statistical methods to technical problems met with in industry and agriculture" during the previous two decades.

World War II caused the research activities of the Industrial and Agricultural Research Section to be abandoned. Only about four meetings could be held in each session during the early years. The 1940–41 volume of the *Supplement* was slim and the next volume did not appear until 1946. However, papers continued to be accepted and published as "read" papers even though they could not be presented. One effect was therefore that written, rather than oral contributions to the discussion appeared, and this practice persisted and grew after the war.

Some work, however, was carried out around the country under the Industrial Applications Group formed for the purpose. This prompted the Society to split the Section into two: the Industrial Applications Section and the Research Section.

The Industrial Applications Section was constituted as several Local Groups around the country whose purpose was primarily to organize meetings, whereas the *Supplement* was intended to be primarily the vehicle for publication of the proceedings of Research Section meetings and to fulfill the need "for a medium of publication for research work (not necessarily theoretical or mathematical) which is of general interest to statisticians". An editorial panel was set up for the journal under the editorship of **M.G. Kendall**, B.L. Welch and **F. Yates**. Research Section meetings did not have the status of the Ordinary Meetings of the Society until 1958 when the meetings were called Research Methods Meetings (later changed to the current "Ordinary Meetings organized by the Research Section" in 1969).

By 1947 the *Supplement* had grown into a scientific journal of high repute. The Council therefore

decided that from 1948 the Society's two publications would both be issued under the main title of the *Journal of the Royal Statistical Society*, the original journal being distinguished by the subtitle "Series A (General)" and the *Supplement* by the subtitle "Series B (Methodological)". Though the names had changed, the volume numbers ran on sequentially. Series A remained the organ of the Society as a whole, with publication of papers from Ordinary Meetings (other than the research type), the annual report of Council, book reviews, obituaries and other features from time to time.

Since the war, the Council had been aware of the absence of a publication devoted to the practical statistical problems that arise in the many fields of human activity. To fill this gap, *Applied Statistics* was launched in 1952. It officially became the *Journal of the Royal Statistical Society*, Series C, in 1964. The President, **Austin Bradford Hill**, defined its aims in the first issue as follows.

> *Applied Statistics* has been founded, therefore, to meet the needs of all workers concerned with statistics – not of professional statisticians only but also of those innumerable workers in industry, commerce, science, and other branches of daily work, who must handle and understand statistics as part of their tasks. Its aim, in short, is to present, in one way or another but always simply and clearly, the statistical approach and its value, and to illustrate in original articles modern statistical methods in their everyday applications.

The journal published three issues per volume and initially was designed more as a magazine than as a learned journal. It contained reports of the meetings of the various Groups, articles expounding statistical methods and illustrating their application, and features entitled "Questions and answers", "Notes and comments", "Letters to the Editors" and book reviews. Gradually, though, the journal became more technical in character.

In December 1966, J.A. Nelder and B.E. Cooper organized a meeting on "Statistical programming – the present situation and future prospects" at the Atlas Laboratory, Chilton, UK. The five papers presented and an account of the discussion were published in *Applied Statistics* in 1967. As a result of the meeting, the "Statistical algorithms" section of the journal was started in 1968. The main aims of the section were:

to ensure that published algorithms are clearly organized, well documented, and standardized in notation and terminology, so that they will be readily understandable to a large number of readers; ... also, that the algorithms are programmed as far as possible in languages which are widely available and clearly defined independently of individual implementations.

These aims only began to outlive their usefulness by the mid-1990s when the publication of statistical algorithms ceased. By this time over 300 had been published.

In 1968, Series A made a break with tradition when it ceased to publish the Sauerbeck index of wholesale prices, which it had published annually since 1886, latterly from material supplied by the editor of the *Statist*. Other changes arising from concern over overlap with Series C refocused its editorial policy and included a change in its subtitle to "Statistics in society" and a decrease from four issues per volume to three in 1988. In contrast, Series B and Series C increased from three issues to four in 1993.

The year 1993 also saw the addition of *The Statistician* to Series A, B, and C following the merger with the Institute of Statisticians. This has resulted in an integration and reorganization of the content of the four journals, with the intention that from 1998 *The Statistician* will contain book reviews, the annual report, obituaries, and the presidential address, instead of Series A.

The scope of each series can now be summarized as follows.

Series A (Statistics in Society) has a particular focus on statistics relevant to social issues interpreted broadly to include medical, educational, legal, demographic, and general social issues. Review papers and historical, biographical, or philosophical papers are also encouraged. Although analyses should be thorough and well presented, innovative statistical methods are not essential for publication. Methodological papers are also welcomed as long as the methods are relevant and illustrative applications involving appropriate data are provided.

Series B (Methodological) publishes papers that contribute to the understanding of statistical methodology and/or develop and improve statistical methods. The kinds of contribution considered include descriptions of new methods of collecting or analysing data, with the underlying theory, an indication of the scope of application and preferably a real example. Also

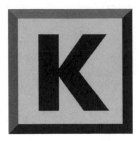

Kalman Filtering and Smoothing

Kalman filtering and smoothing algorithms are designed for **time series** models in state space form, as defined later in this article. Although the state space framework is introduced in the engineering literature, a substantial number of contributions in the statistical and econometric literature have emphasized the importance of the state space model for the statistical analysis of time series. This is primarily due to the Kalman filter and its relationship to the prediction error decomposition which allows the likelihood function of state space models to be evaluated in a simple and straightforward way. Another feature of the state space framework is its generality: most practical Gaussian time series models can be formulated as a state space model. More recent developments emphasize the importance of efficient smoothing algorithms for estimation, inference and diagnostic checking of state space models.

This article presents the most important algorithms for univariate state space models. Proofs are not given and technical details are avoided, but appropriate references are given to the literature for further reading. A number of applications will show the importance of Kalman filtering and smoothing for the statistical analysis of time series.

Local Level Model

The most elementary time series model in the state space framework is the local level model which combines a random walk component μ_t and a disturbance term ε_t as

$$y_t = \mu_t + \varepsilon_t, \quad \varepsilon_t \sim \text{NID}(0, \sigma_\varepsilon^2),$$
$$t = 1, \ldots, T, \quad (1)$$
$$\mu_{t+1} = \mu_t + \eta_t, \quad \eta_t \sim \text{NID}(0, \sigma_\eta^2),$$

where NID indicates that the disturbances are normally distributed and independent of each other. The disturbances are mutually uncorrelated. The specification of the local level model is completed by assuming that the initial value, μ_1, is random with an infinite variance, that is $\mu_1 \sim \text{N}(0, \kappa)$, where $\kappa \to \infty$. The diffuse initial condition is imposed because the **stochastic process** (1) is nonstationary (*see* **Stationarity**). The statistical properties of the local level model (1) are investigated in detail in [8] (*see* **Structural Time Series Models**).

Model (1) allows the level of the time series to vary over time depending on the signal to noise ratio, $q = \sigma_\eta^2/\sigma_\varepsilon^2$. When q is small, the level μ_t evolves very smoothly. In the extreme case of $q = 0$, the level is a constant. However, when q is large, the behavior of the time series is close to a random walk model because the influence of the measurement disturbance ε_t is small relative to η_t so that $y_t \approx \mu_t$.

The estimation of the unobservable level, μ_t, conditional on the variances σ_ε^2 and σ_η^2, is done recursively using the Kalman filter and smoother, for $t = 1, \ldots, T$. In general, the variances σ_ε^2 and σ_η^2 are unknown and they are treated as hyperparameters. The likelihood function can be evaluated by the Kalman filter via the prediction error decomposition. Maximizing the likelihood function with respect to

σ_ε^2 and σ_η^2 via a quasi-Newton optimization routine is referred to as hyperparameter estimation. The exact score vector is obtained via a very efficient smoother. The computation of diagnostic statistics and goodness of fit measures also rely on the Kalman filter and smoother.

Illustration

Figure 1 presents a time series of 150 daily observations on the level of blood glucose in a patient. The data were recorded by the patient himself each morning. The data are subject to measurement error and there are likely to be differences from day to day owing to variations in behavior. The doctor wishes to estimate the underlying level of blood glucose, in order to monitor the patient's state of health and to determine whether to change the amount of insulin taken. It will be shown that the local level model can be used to extract the required information using Kalman filtering and smoothing.

Kalman Filtering and Smoothing

Assuming that the variances σ_ε^2 and σ_η^2 are known, the one-step-ahead predictor of the level, i.e. the estimator of μ_{t+1} given the data set $Y_t = \{y_1 \ldots, y_t\}$ as denoted by $a_{t+1} = \mathrm{E}(\mu_{t\,|\,1}|Y_t)$, is evaluated recursively by the Kalman filter. It also evaluates the prediction error variance, denoted by $p_{t+1} = \mathrm{var}(\mu_{t+1}|Y_t) = \mathrm{var}(a_{t+1})$, recursively. The Kalman filter for the local level model (1) is given by

$$v_t = y_t - a_t, \qquad f_t = p_t + \sigma_\varepsilon^2,$$
$$a_{t+1} = a_t + k_t v_t, \quad p_{t+1} = p_t + \sigma_\eta^2 - k_t p_t, \tag{2}$$

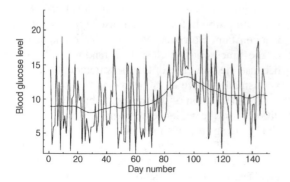

Figure 1   Daily records of blood glucose and estimated level

for $t = 1, \ldots, T$, with $k_t = p_t/f_t$ and the initializations $a_1 = 0$ and $p_1 = \kappa$, where κ is the large variance of μ_1. The Kalman filter is said to be in a "steady state" when the variance p_t has converged to a constant $\bar{p}$, for $t = \bar{t}, \ldots, T$, so that f_t and k_t are also constant.

The estimate of the level a_t is effectively constructed by putting exponentially declining weights on the past observations. This is seen directly by reformulating the update as $a_{t+1} = (1 - k_t)a_t + k_t y_t$. The rate of decline is determined by the "gain" k_t which depends on the variances σ_ε^2 and σ_η^2. The one-step-ahead prediction error of the observation is $v_t = y_t - \mathrm{E}(y_t|Y_{t-1})$ with variance $f_t = \mathrm{var}(v_t)$. The prediction errors are important from a statistical point of view because they are serially independent for a correctly specified model.

Estimators conditional on the set of all available observations, Y_T, are defined as smoothed estimators and they are evaluated by a backwards operating algorithm which requires the output of the Kalman filter. For example, the smoothed estimators of the disturbances and their corresponding variances are defined as

$$\mathrm{E}(\varepsilon_t|Y_T) = \hat{\varepsilon}_t = \sigma_\varepsilon^2 e_t,$$
$$\mathrm{var}(\varepsilon_t|Y_T) = \mathrm{var}(\hat{\varepsilon}_t) = \sigma_\varepsilon^4 d_t,$$
$$\mathrm{E}(\eta_t|Y_T) = \hat{\eta}_t = \sigma_\eta^2 r_t,$$
$$\mathrm{var}(\eta_t|Y_T) = \mathrm{var}(\hat{\eta}_t) = \sigma_\eta^4 n_t, \tag{3}$$

where

$$e_t = v_t/f_t - k_t r_t, \qquad d_t = 1/f_t + k_t^2 n_t,$$
$$r_{t-1} = r_t + e_t, \qquad n_{t-1} = n_t + d_t - 2k_t n_t, \tag{4}$$

for $t = T, \ldots, 1$, with initialization $r_T = 0$ and $n_T = 0$. The Kalman filter storage of the quantities v_t, f_t, and k_t is required for $t = 1, \ldots, T$. The quantity r_t is a weighted sum of future prediction errors, i.e. v_j for $j = t+1, \ldots, T$.

The smoothed estimator of the level μ_t, i.e. the estimator of μ_t given the data set Y_T as denoted by $\hat{\mu}_t = \mathrm{E}(\mu_t|Y_T)$, is evaluated by the simple forwards recursion

$$\hat{\mu}_{t+1} = \hat{\mu}_t + \hat{\eta}_t, \quad t = 1, \ldots, T, \tag{5}$$

where $\hat{\mu}_1 = p_1 r_0$ and $\hat{\eta}_t = \sigma_\eta^2 r_t$. The forwards recursion (5) follows implicitly from the model specification (1). The smoothed level can also be evaluated backwards together with the recursions (4), i.e.

$$\hat{\mu}_{t-1} = \hat{\mu}_t - \hat{\eta}_{t-1} = \hat{\mu}_t - \sigma_\eta^2 r_{t-1},$$

$$t = T + 1, \ldots 1,$$

where $\hat{\mu}_{T+1} = a_{T+1|T}$ is obtained from the Kalman filter.

When observation y_t is missing, the Kalman filter and smoother equations still apply but with $v_t = 0$ and $f_t \to \infty$ so that $1/f_t = 0$ and $k_t = 0$.

Hyperparameter Estimation

Kalman filtering and smoothing assume that the variances σ_ε^2 and σ_η^2 are known. In practice, they are not known and they need to be estimated. The variances are treated as hyperparameters and they are re-parameterized to enforce them to be nonnegative, i.e.

$$\sigma_\varepsilon^2 = \exp(2\psi_\varepsilon), \qquad \sigma_\eta^2 = \exp(2\psi_\eta),$$

and the hyperparameter vector is $\boldsymbol{\psi} = (\psi_\varepsilon, \psi_\eta)'$. Hyperparameter estimation of $\boldsymbol{\psi}$ involves numerical maximization of the likelihood function with respect to $\boldsymbol{\psi}$.

The likelihood function for Gaussian time-series models is obtained via the prediction error decomposition. For a given $\boldsymbol{\psi} = \boldsymbol{\psi}^*$, the Kalman filter computes the log-likelihood function as given by

$$l(\boldsymbol{\psi}^*) = -\frac{1}{2}\sum_{t=1}^{T}\log f_t - \frac{1}{2}\sum_{t=1}^{T}v_t^2/f_t,$$

apart from some constant. When the Kalman filter reaches a "steady state" quickly, so that most f_ts are constant, maximizing $l(\boldsymbol{\psi})$ is close to minimizing the

sum of squared one-step-ahead prediction errors, that is $\sum_{t=1}^{T} v_t^2$.

Numerical optimization routines based on quasi-Newton schemes require score information. The score vector for $\boldsymbol{\psi}$ at position $\boldsymbol{\psi}^*$ is evaluated by

$$s(\boldsymbol{\psi}^*) = \frac{\partial l(\boldsymbol{\psi})}{\partial \boldsymbol{\psi}}\bigg|_{\boldsymbol{\psi}=\boldsymbol{\psi}^*}$$

$$= \begin{bmatrix} \exp(2\psi_\varepsilon^*)\sum_{t=1}^{T}(e_t^2 - d_t) \\ \exp(2\psi_\eta^*)\sum_{t=1}^{T}(r_t^2 - n_t) \end{bmatrix}, \qquad (6)$$

where the scalars e_t, d_t, r_t, and n_t are obtained from the smoother (4). The score vector is zero for $\boldsymbol{\psi} = \tilde{\boldsymbol{\psi}}$, where $\tilde{\boldsymbol{\psi}}$ maximizes $l(\boldsymbol{\psi})$. Maximum likelihood estimation of $\boldsymbol{\psi}$ for the Gaussian local level model (1) is carried out by numerically maximizing $l(\boldsymbol{\psi})$ using a quasi-Newton optimization routine which requires the score vector $s(\boldsymbol{\psi})$.

The process of hyperparameter estimation for the local level model (1), with starting values $\psi_\varepsilon^* = 1$ and $\psi_\eta^* = 0$, using the blood glucose data is represented in Table 1. For each step in the numerical optimization procedure, $l(\boldsymbol{\psi})$ gets closer to its maximum and $s(\boldsymbol{\psi})$ gets closer to zero. The maximum likelihood estimates are $\hat{\sigma}_\varepsilon^2 = 17.89$ and $\hat{\sigma}_\eta^2 = 0.20$ so that the signal to noise ratio is $q = 0.0112$. The relatively small q value should produce a rather smooth curve for μ_t. Figure 1 includes the plot of the smoothed estimator $\hat{\mu}_t$ through the observations y_t.

Diagnostic Checking and Goodness of Fit

Once the maximum likelihood estimator for $\boldsymbol{\psi}$ is identified, the process of model evaluation can be

Table 1 Hyperparameter estimation local level

Iteration	ψ_η^*	$s(\psi_\eta^*)$	ψ_ε^*	$s(\psi_\varepsilon^*)$	$l(\boldsymbol{\psi}^*)$
0	0	4.3738	1	155.3585	−328.9512
1	0.0274	−7.5609	1.9460	−88.9225	−327.8231
2	−0.6805	−2.4358	1.9022	−85.9225	−320.6576
3	−0.7298	−0.5045	1.4410	−0.3900	−298.0500
4	−0.7628	−0.2798	1.4406	−0.0075	−298.0370
5	−0.7896	−0.1167	1.4418	−0.1155	−298.0318
6	−0.8029	−0.0318	1.4417	0.0188	−298.0308
7	−0.8076	−0.0050	1.4420	−0.016	−298.0307
8	−0.8032	−0.0002	1.4420	0.0051	−298.0307
9	−0.8032	0.0000	1.4420	−0.0000	−298.0307

started. The main tools for diagnostic checking rely on the standardized one-step-ahead prediction errors

$$\tilde{v}_t = v_t/\sqrt{f_t},$$

for $t = 1, \ldots, n$. The Kalman filter is required only for computing the prediction errors.

The purpose of diagnostic checking (*see* **Diagnostics**) is to validate the proposition that the prediction errors are standard NID deviates, that is $\tilde{v}_t \sim$ NID$(0, 1)$, for a correctly specified model. The following diagnostic test statistics and graphs are useful in this respect:

1. A graphical inspection for **serial correlation** is based on the correlogram with approximate standard error $1/(T-1)^{1/2}$ (*see* **Autocorrelation Function**). The portmanteau statistic for serial correlation is the Box–Ljung Q-statistic, i.e.

$$Q_P = T(T+2) \sum_{j=1}^{P} \hat{\rho}_j^2/T - j,$$

where $\hat{\rho}_j$ is the sample autocorrelation at lag j and P is a predetermined constant. The Q statistic is χ^2 distributed with $P - n + 1$ degrees of freedom, where n is the number of hyperparameters.

2. The normality χ^2 test, with two degrees of freedom, is based on measures for skewness and kurtosis, i.e.

$$N = \frac{T}{6}\left(\frac{m_3}{m_2^{3/2}}\right)^2 + \frac{T}{24}\left(\frac{m_4}{m_2^2} - 3\right)^2,$$

where m_i is the ith order sample cumulant of $\tilde{v}_t$.

3. Heteroscedasticity diagnostic H is based on a ratio of two sums of squared prediction errors where the sums are taken from two exclusive subsamples in Y_n of equal length h. The ratio is an F test with degrees of freedom (h, h).

Goodness-of-fit statistics are used for assessing the overall model fit. The basic measure of goodness of fit in time series models is the variance of the prediction errors in a steady state, i.e. $\overline{f}$. The standard coefficient of determination is

$$R^2 = 1 - \frac{(T-1)\overline{f}}{\sum_{t=1}^{T}(y_t - \overline{y})^2},$$

where $\overline{y}$ is the sample mean of the observations y_t. For the local level model it is better to compare the prediction error variance with the variance of first differences, i.e. $\Delta y_t = y_t - y_{t-1}$. This leads to

$$R_{\mathrm{D}}^2 = 1 - \frac{(T-1)\overline{f}}{\sum_{t=2}^{T}(\Delta y_t - \overline{\Delta y})^2},$$

where $\overline{\Delta y}$ is the sample mean of the observations Δy_t. It should be noted that R_{D}^2 can be negative, indicating a worse fit than a random walk. Comparisons of fit between different models should be based on an information criterion such as the one of **Akaike** which is given by AIC $= \log \overline{f} + 2(m-1)/T$, where m is the number of hyperparameters plus the number of nonstationary components. For a local level model, the AIC is $\log \overline{f} + 4/T$.

Figure 2 plots the prediction errors for the blood glucose data together with the corresponding correlogram and histogram. It shows that not all the serial correlation is removed and that the prediction errors are somewhat skewed distributed. However, the overall diagnostic statistics are satisfactory,

$$Q_{12} = 6.43_{(0.84)}, \qquad N = 4.08_{(0.13)},$$
$$H = 0.99_{(0.51)},$$

with the P values as subscripts. The goodness-of-fit statistics are

$$\overline{f} = 19.74, \qquad R^2 = 0.94,$$
$$R_{\mathrm{D}}^2 = 0.06, \qquad \mathrm{AIC} = 3.01,$$

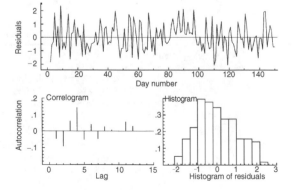

Figure 2   Prediction errors and diagnostic plots

which are all satisfactory. For example, the prediction error variance and the AIC for a model with a fixed level are given by 20.86 and 3.06, respectively.

Outliers and Breaks

The detection of **outliers** and structural breaks in the local level model (1) is based on the disturbances ε_t and η_t. Large absolute values of η_t may indicate the need for a step intervention (break) and large absolute values of ε_t may indicate a pulse intervention (outlier). Graphical inspection of the standardized smoothed disturbances (3), to be referred to as auxiliary residuals, has proved to be effective and efficient for detecting and identifying irregularities in time-series data. The auxiliary **residuals** are calculated directly via the smoother (4), that is

$$e_t^* = e_t/\sqrt{d_t}, \qquad r_t^* = T_t/\sqrt{n_t},$$

for $t = 1, \ldots, n$. The auxiliary residual e_t^* is associated with the disturbance ε_t and r_t^* is associated with the disturbance η_t; see (3). Auxiliary residuals are equal to t tests of the associated intervention. Thus, e_t^* is the t test of an impulse intervention at time t and r_t^* is the t test of a step intervention at time t. It should be stressed that the auxiliary residuals can be calculated even when the associated standard deviation of the disturbance (e.g. σ_ε) is zero.

The auxiliary residuals e_t^* and r_t^* for the blood glucose data are plotted in Figure 3. The level residual plot reveals that the level moves upwards dramatically after observation 80. The plot of the observations in Figure 1 confirms this feature clearly. Also, it is shown that r_t^* is highly serially correlated.

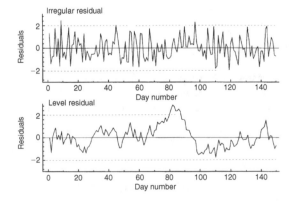

Figure 3   Auxiliary residuals

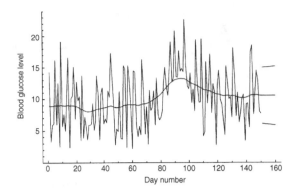

Figure 4   Blood glucose data, level, and forecasts

Forecasting

The model that fits the present data set satisfactorily may also be suitable to forecast future values (*see* **Forecasting**). The forecast function of the local level model is

$$\tilde{y}_{T+l|T} = a_{T+l}, \quad \text{var}(\tilde{y}_{T+l|T}) = p_{T+l} + \sigma_\varepsilon^2,$$
$$a_{T+l+1} = a_{T+1}, \qquad p_{T+l+1} = p_{T+l} + \sigma_\eta^2, \tag{7}$$

for $l = 1, 2, \ldots$. The forecast function of the local level model is a horizontal straight line. It projects the estimate of the level at time T into the future. The variance of the forecast reveals how the uncertainty of the forecasts increases with l.

Figure 4 displays the observations and estimated level together with forecasts $\tilde{y}_{T+l|T} = 10.609$, for $l = 1, \ldots, 10$, and the corresponding forecast error bounds which are based on $\pm[\text{var}(\tilde{y}_{T+l|T})]^{1/2}$. The forecast error for $l = 1$ is equal to 4.458 and for $l = 10$ it is equal to 4.654.

The State Space Model

The linear state space model for a univariate time series y_t is given by

$$y_t = \mathbf{Z}_t \boldsymbol{\alpha}_t + \mathbf{G}_t \mathbf{u}_t, \quad \mathbf{u}_t \sim \text{NID}(\mathbf{0}, \mathbf{I}),$$
$$t = 1, \ldots, T, \tag{8}$$
$$\boldsymbol{\alpha}_{t+1} = \mathbf{T}_t \boldsymbol{\alpha}_t + \mathbf{H}_t \mathbf{u}_t, \quad \boldsymbol{\alpha}_1 \sim \text{NID}(\mathbf{a}, \mathbf{P}),$$

where $\boldsymbol{\alpha}_t$ is the ($k \times 1$) state vector. The system vectors and matrices $\mathbf{Z}_t$, $\mathbf{G}_t$, $\mathbf{T}_t$ and $\mathbf{H}_t$ for $t = 1, \ldots, T$, are assumed to be deterministic and known. If specific elements of the system vectors and matrices are unknown, they will be treated as hyperparameters.

The local level model is transformed into state space by setting $\mathbf{Z}_t = \mathbf{T}_t = 1$, $\mathbf{G}_t = (\sigma_\varepsilon, 0)$, $\mathbf{H}_t = (0, \sigma_\eta)$, $\mathbf{a} = 0$ and $\mathbf{P} = \kappa$ so that $\boldsymbol{\alpha}_t$ is the level and $\mathbf{u}_t$ is the 2×1 vector of disturbances.

The first equation of (8) is the measurement equation and the second equation is the transition equation. The state vector $\boldsymbol{\alpha}_t$ is modeled as a multivariate autoregression of order 1. The appearance of the disturbance vector $\mathbf{u}_t$ in the measurement and transition equations is general rather than restrictive. The system vector and matrix, $\mathbf{G}_t$ and $\mathbf{H}_t$, can be interpreted as a selection vector and matrix, respectively. The restriction of mutual independence between the two sets of disturbances is the special case $\mathbf{H}_t \mathbf{G}_t' = 0$, for $t = 1, \ldots, T$. The state space model (8) is time invariant when the system matrices are constant over time. Most practical time series models, including the local level model, can be cast as time-invariant state space models.

Kalman Filter

The Kalman filter for the general univariate state space model is given by

$$
\begin{aligned}
v_t &= y_t - \mathbf{Z}_t \mathbf{a}_t, \\
F_t &= \mathbf{Z}_t \mathbf{P}_t \mathbf{Z}_t' + \mathbf{G}_t \mathbf{G}_t', \\
\mathbf{K}_t &= (\mathbf{T}_t \mathbf{P}_t \mathbf{Z}_t' + \mathbf{H}_t \mathbf{G}_t') F_t^{-1}, \\
\mathbf{a}_{t+1} &= \mathbf{T}_t \mathbf{a}_t + \mathbf{K}_t v_t, \\
\mathbf{P}_{t+1} &= \mathbf{T}_t \mathbf{P}_t \mathbf{T}_t' + \mathbf{H}_t \mathbf{H}_t' - \mathbf{K}_t F_t \mathbf{K}_t',
\end{aligned}
\tag{9}
$$

for $t = 1, \ldots, T$, with the initializations $\mathbf{a}_1 = \mathbf{a}$ and $\mathbf{P}_1 = \mathbf{P}$. The one-step-ahead prediction error is $v_t = y_t - \mathrm{E}(y_t | \mathbf{Y}_{t-1})$ and F_t is the variance of v_t. The $(k \times 1)$ vector $\mathbf{K}_t$ is called the Kalman gain. The proof of the Kalman filter can be found, for example, in [1] and [8].

The initialization of the Kalman filter (9) is easily derived as

$$
\begin{aligned}
\mathbf{a}_1 &= \mathrm{E}(\boldsymbol{\alpha}_1 | \mathbf{Y}_0) = \mathrm{E}(\boldsymbol{\alpha}_1) = \mathbf{a}, \\
\mathbf{P}_1 &= \mathrm{var}(\boldsymbol{\alpha}_1 | \mathbf{Y}_0) = \mathrm{var}(\boldsymbol{\alpha}_1) = \mathbf{P},
\end{aligned}
$$

where $\mathbf{a}$ and $\mathbf{P}$ are the unconditional mean and variance matrix of the initial state vector, respectively. The Kalman filter cannot be applied straightforwardly in nonstationary cases where some (diagonal) elements of $\mathbf{P}$ are set equal to κ, where $\kappa \to \infty$. It is

shown in Koopman [13] how to deal with these cases efficiently. Alternative solutions for dealing with diffuse initial conditions are in [2], [3], [6], and [16].

The Kalman filter provides a general tool for handling missing observations. When the observation y_t is missing, the prediction error v_t, the inverse F_t^{-1} and the Kalman gain $\mathbf{K}_t$ are set to zero. Therefore, the Kalman update equations become

$$
\mathbf{a}_{t+1} = \mathbf{T}_t \mathbf{a}_t, \qquad \mathbf{P}_{t+1} = \mathbf{T}_t \mathbf{P}_t \mathbf{T}_t' + \mathbf{H}_t \mathbf{H}_t',
$$

which are the so-called forecasting equations.

After the Kalman filter has processed all observations up to time $t = T$, we may wish to forecast future observations, i.e. $\tilde{y}_{T+l} = \mathrm{E}(y_{T+l} | \mathbf{Y}_T)$ with standard error $[\mathrm{var}(\tilde{y}_{T+l})]^{1/2}$. Forecasting may be interpreted as filtering future observations that are missing. The forecasting equations are therefore the same as the Kalman filter equations for a missing observation y_t. The prediction error v_t, the inverse F_t^{-1} and the Kalman gain $\mathbf{K}_t$ are set to zero and the forecasting equations reduce to

$$
\begin{aligned}
\tilde{y}_{T+l} &= \mathbf{Z}_{T+l} \mathbf{a}_{T+l}, \\
\mathrm{var}(\tilde{y}_{T+l}) &= \mathbf{Z}_{T+l} \mathbf{P}_{T+l} \mathbf{Z}_{T+l}' + \mathbf{G}_{T+l} \mathbf{G}_{T+l}', \\
\mathbf{a}_{T+l+1} &= \mathbf{T}_{T+l} \mathbf{a}_{T+l}, \\
\mathbf{P}_{T+l+1} &= \mathbf{T}_{T+l} \mathbf{P}_{T+l} \mathbf{T}_{T+l}' + \mathbf{H}_{T+l} \mathbf{H}_{T+l}',
\end{aligned}
\tag{10}
$$

for $l = 1, 2, \ldots$. The vector $\mathbf{a}_{T+l+1}$ contains the forecasts of each element of the state vector, and the square root of the corresponding diagonal element of $\mathbf{P}_{T+l+1}$ is the standard error of the forecast. For the unusual case of a time-variant state space model, the system matrices for time $t = T + l$, where $l = 1, 2, \ldots$, needs to be known.

Smoothing

The work of de Jong [4, 5], Kohn & Ansley [10] and Koopman [11] leads to a smoothing algorithm for the general univariate state space model (8) as given by

$$
\begin{aligned}
e_t &= F_t^{-1} v_t - \mathbf{K}_t' \mathbf{r}_t, \\
\mathrm{var}(e_t) &= D_t = F_t^{-1} + \mathbf{K}_t' \mathbf{N}_t \mathbf{K}_t, \\
\mathbf{r}_{t-1} &= \mathbf{Z}_t' F_t^{-1} v_t + \mathbf{L}_t' \mathbf{r}_t, \\
\mathrm{var}(\mathbf{r}_{t-1}) &= \mathbf{N}_{t-1} = \mathbf{Z}_t' F_t^{-1} \mathbf{Z}_t + \mathbf{L}_t' \mathbf{N}_t \mathbf{L}_t,
\end{aligned}
\tag{11}
$$

for $t = T, \ldots, 1$, where $\mathbf{L}_t = \mathbf{T}_t - \mathbf{K}_t \mathbf{Z}_t$. The backwards recursions are initialized by $\mathbf{r}_T = 0$ and $\mathbf{N}_T = 0$. The Kalman filter output of v_t, F_t^{-1} and $\mathbf{K}_t$, should be stored for $t = 1, \ldots, T$. The standardized smoothing quantities are given by

$$e_t^* = e_t / \sqrt{D_t}, \qquad r_{i,t}^* = r_{i,t} / \sqrt{N_{ii,t}}, \qquad (12)$$

for $i = 1, \ldots, k$ and $t = 1, \ldots, T$. The ith element of the vector $\mathbf{r}_t$ is denoted by $r_{i,t}$ and the ith diagonal element of $\mathbf{N}_t$ is denoted by $N_{ii,t}$. The adjustments for (11) are very minor when dealing with a diffuse initial state vector; see [13].

The smoothed state vector $\mathbf{a}_{t|T} = \mathrm{E}(\boldsymbol{\alpha}_t | \mathbf{Y}_T)$ with variance matrix $\mathbf{P}_{t|T} = \mathrm{var}(\boldsymbol{\alpha}_t | \mathbf{Y}_T)$ can be evaluated by

$$\mathbf{a}_{t|T} = \mathbf{a}_t + \mathbf{P}_t \mathbf{r}_{-1}, \qquad \mathbf{P}_{t|T} = \mathbf{P}_t - \mathbf{P}_t \mathbf{N}_{-1} \mathbf{P}_t, \qquad (13)$$

for $t = T, \ldots, 1$. A substantive amount of additional memory space is required for storing $\mathbf{a}_t$ and $\mathbf{P}_t$ of the Kalman filter. Self-contained proofs of (11) and (13) are given by de Jong [4, 5] and Kohn & Ansley [10]. The state smoother (11) and (13) can also be obtained by re-formulating the classical Anderson and Moore [1] fixed interval smoothing algorithm; see the Appendix.

The output of the smoother (11) can be used to construct the smoothed estimator of the disturbance vector $\mathbf{u}_t$ conditional on the full data set $\mathbf{Y}_T$, that is $\hat{\mathbf{u}}_t = \mathrm{E}(\mathbf{u}_t | \mathbf{Y}_T)$, and its variance matrix. For the usual case of $\mathbf{H}_t \mathbf{G}_t' = 0$, we obtain the smoothed disturbances for the measurement and transition equations by, respectively,

$$\mathbf{G}_t \hat{\mathbf{u}}_t = \mathbf{G}_t \mathbf{G}_t' e_t, \quad \mathrm{var}(\mathbf{G}_t \hat{\mathbf{u}}_t) = \mathbf{G}_t \mathbf{G}_t' D_t \mathbf{G}_t \mathbf{G}_t',$$

$$\mathbf{H}_t \hat{\mathbf{u}}_t = \mathbf{H}_t \mathbf{H}_t' \mathbf{r}_t, \quad \mathrm{var}(\mathbf{H}_t \hat{\mathbf{u}}_t) = \mathbf{H}_t \mathbf{H}_t' \mathbf{N}_t \mathbf{H}_t \mathbf{H}_t', \qquad (14)$$

for $t = 1, \ldots, T$. More general results and proofs for the smoothed disturbances are given by Koopman [11]. Note that when the variance $\mathbf{G}_t \mathbf{G}_t'$ is nonzero and the variance matrix $\mathbf{H}_t \mathbf{H}_t'$ is diagonal, the individual standardized smoothed disturbances are given by e_t^* and $r_{i,t}^*$ of (12), for $i = 1, \ldots, k$.

An efficient algorithm for calculating the smoothed estimator of the state vector, i.e. $\hat{\boldsymbol{\alpha}}_t = \mathbf{a}_{t|T} = \mathrm{E}(\boldsymbol{\alpha}_t | \mathbf{Y}_T)$, is given by

$$\hat{\boldsymbol{\alpha}}_{t+1} = \mathbf{T}_t \hat{\boldsymbol{\alpha}}_t + \mathbf{H}_t \hat{\mathbf{u}}_t, \quad t = 1, \ldots, T, \qquad (15)$$

where $\mathbf{H}_t \hat{\mathbf{u}}_t = \mathbf{H}_t \mathbf{H}_t' \mathbf{r}_t$ and $\hat{\boldsymbol{\alpha}}_1 = \mathbf{a} + \mathbf{Pr}_0$. The forwards recursion (15) can be applied after the smoothing algorithm (11) has stored the vector $\mathbf{r}_t$ using the storage space of the Kalman filter, for $t = 1, \ldots, T$. The additional storage space for the state smoother (13) is not required. Also, the recursion (15) is computationally much more efficient compared to the first equation of (13); see [11].

Missing observations are handled by the Kalman filter and smoother as follows. The Kalman filter sets to zero the prediction error v_t, the inverse F_t^{-1} and the Kalman gain K_t, associated with the missing observation y_t, so that the smoothing step at time t reduces to

$$\mathbf{t}_{t-1} = \mathbf{T}_t' \mathbf{r}_t, \qquad \mathbf{N}_{t-1} = \mathbf{T}_t' \mathbf{N}_t \mathbf{T}_t.$$

The missing value y_t does not affect (15). In fact, $\mathbf{Z}_t \hat{\boldsymbol{\alpha}}_t$ is the best linear unbiased estimator of the missing value y_t conditional on $\mathbf{Y}_T$. The exact signal smoother (15) applies to state space models with diffuse initial conditions as well, but it requires a minor adjustment; see [12].

Applications

Hyperparameter Estimation

The hyperparameter vector $\boldsymbol{\psi}$ contains all the unknown elements of the system matrices of the state space model. Maximum likelihood estimation of $\boldsymbol{\psi}$ is carried out by numerically maximizing the log-likelihood function $l(\boldsymbol{\psi})$ using search information contained in the score vector $s(\boldsymbol{\psi})$. The prediction error decomposition allows the log-likelihood function to be calculated for a specific value $\boldsymbol{\psi} = \boldsymbol{\psi}^*$ via

$$l(\boldsymbol{\psi}^*) = -\frac{T}{2} \log 2\pi - \frac{1}{2} \sum_{t=1}^{T} \log F_t - \frac{1}{2} \sum_{t=1}^{T} F_t^{-1} v_t^2, \qquad (16)$$

where v_t and F_t are obtained from the Kalman filter (9) for $t = 1, \ldots, T$; see [8]. Note that the Kalman filter quantities depend on the hyperparameter vector $\boldsymbol{\psi}$ in a highly nonlinear fashion. When the ith element of the hyperparameter vector $\boldsymbol{\psi}$ relates only to the system matrices $\mathbf{G}_t$ and $\mathbf{H}_t$, for $t = 1, \ldots, T$, its score value, evaluated at $\boldsymbol{\psi} = \boldsymbol{\psi}^*$, is given by

$$
s(\boldsymbol{\psi}^*)_i = \left. \frac{\partial l(\boldsymbol{\psi})}{\partial \psi_i} \right|_{\boldsymbol{\psi} = \boldsymbol{\psi}^*} = \sum_{t=1}^{T} \frac{\partial \mathbf{G}_t}{\partial \psi_i} \mathbf{G}_t'(e_t^2 - D_t)
$$

$$
+ \sum_{t=1}^{T} tr \frac{\partial \mathbf{H}_t}{\partial \psi_i} \mathbf{H}_t'(\mathbf{r}_t \mathbf{r}_t' - \mathbf{N}_t),
$$

$$
(17)
$$

which can be computed directly by the smoother (11); see [14]. So each step in the process of hyperparameter estimation requires only one Kalman filtering and smoothing pass to obtain the log likelihood and the exact score vector. When hyperparameters are related to the system matrices $\mathbf{Z}_t$ and $\mathbf{T}_t$, for $t = 1, \ldots, T$, the exact score vector can still be evaluated by smoothing, but with the inclusion of (13). It is argued by Koopman & Shephard [14] that it is computationally more efficient to calculate the numerical score in such situations. More details on hyperparameter estimation, including a discussion on the choice of starting values for $\boldsymbol{\psi}$, can be found in [15].

Diagnostic Checking, Outliers, and Breaks

The basic procedure of diagnostic checking and assessing goodness-of-fit criteria was discussed earlier. The same methodology applies to all time-series models in the state space framework. The detection of outliers and breaks in general is based on the vector of disturbances, $\mathbf{u}_t$. Harvey & Koopman [9] use auxiliary residuals for a general and efficient method of detecting and identifying irregularities in time series data. The auxiliary residuals are defined as standardized smoothed disturbances and they can be calculated using the smoothing algorithms (11) and (14). By a single Kalman filtering and smoothing pass, $k + 1$ sets of residuals are available for detecting and distinguishing between outliers in y_t and breaks in the state vector $\boldsymbol{\alpha}_{t+1}$.

De Jong & Penzer [7] point out that the auxiliary residuals are equivalent to the t tests of corresponding interventions and that they can be calculated via (11) for any $\mathbf{G}_t$ and $\mathbf{H}_t$, $t = 1, \ldots, T$. For example, the auxiliary residual $r_{i,\tau}^*$ of (12) is the t test of the estimated coefficient δ in the extended state equation

$$
\boldsymbol{\alpha}_{t+1} = \mathbf{T}_t \boldsymbol{\alpha}_t + \delta \mathbf{x}_{i,\tau} + \mathbf{H}_t \mathbf{u}_t,
$$

where the $k \times 1$ vector $\mathbf{x}_{i,\tau}$ is a zero vector, except that the ith element at time $t = \tau$ is unity. In a similar way, the auxiliary residual e_τ^* of (12) is the t test of the estimated coefficient δ in the extended measurement equation

$$
y_t = \mathbf{Z}_t \boldsymbol{\alpha}_t + \delta x_{0,\tau} + \mathbf{G}_t \mathbf{u}_t,
$$

where the scalar $x_{0,\tau}$ is zero except at time $t = \tau$ where it is unity.

It is important to stress that the auxiliary residuals are serially correlated. Harvey & Koopman [9] develop tests for skewness, kurtosis, and normality taking into account the implied ARMA correlation structure of the auxiliary residuals (*see* **ARMA and ARIMA Models**). The normality tests are useful statistics for detecting potential irregularities in time series such as outliers and breaks.

Signal Extraction and Weight Functions

The plot of the smoothed signal, i.e. $\mathbf{Z}_t \hat{\boldsymbol{\alpha}}_t$ for $t = 1, \ldots, T$, together with the observations y_t, is useful for checking whether the estimated model has captured the most important features of the data. Also, a plot of individual elements of $\hat{\boldsymbol{\alpha}}_t$ is of interest. The smoothed estimator of the state vector at time τ is a linear function of all data points $Y_T = \{y_1, \ldots, y_T\}$, i.e. $\hat{\boldsymbol{\alpha}}_\tau = \sum_{t=1}^{T} \mathbf{w}(\tau)_t y_t$, where $\mathbf{w}(\tau)_t$ is a sequence of weight vectors for $t = 1, \ldots, T$. In understanding the behavior of an element of the state vector, it can be informative to plot the pattern of weights associated with some smoothed estimator at time τ.

The weight vectors $\mathbf{w}(\tau)_t$ of $\hat{\boldsymbol{\alpha}}_\tau$ are obtained by applying Kalman filtering and smoothing, where the original observations y_t are replaced by zero values except at time τ where the observation y_τ is replaced by unity. The smoothed state vector of (15) contains the weights, i.e. $\hat{\boldsymbol{\alpha}}_t = \mathbf{w}(\tau)_t$.

Appendix

The Kalman filter evaluates the estimator of the state vector $\mathbf{a}_t = \mathbf{a}_{t|t-1} = \mathrm{E}(\boldsymbol{\alpha}_t | \mathbf{Y}_{t-1})$ and the variance matrix $\mathbf{P}_t = \mathbf{P}_{t|t-1} = \mathrm{var}(\boldsymbol{\alpha}_t | \mathbf{Y}_{t-1})$, where $\mathbf{Y}_{t-1} = \{y_1, \ldots, y_{t-1}\}$ for $t = 1, \ldots, T$. Corresponding estimators conditional on all observations Y_T are referred to as smoothed estimators and they are evaluated by a backwards operating smoothing algorithm.

A well known smoothing algorithm for the evaluation of $\mathbf{a}_{t|T} = E(\boldsymbol{\alpha}_t|\mathbf{Y}_T)$ and $\mathbf{P}_{t|T} = \mathrm{var}(\boldsymbol{\alpha}_t|\mathbf{Y}_T)$, for $t = 1, \ldots, T$, is the state smoother formulated by Anderson & Moore [1], hereafter referred to as the AM formulation, as given by

$$\mathbf{a}_{t|T} = \mathbf{a}_{t|t} + \mathbf{P}_{t|t}\mathbf{T}_t'\mathbf{P}_{t+1}^{-1}(\mathbf{a}_{t+1|T} - \mathbf{a}_{t+1}), \quad (18)$$

$$\mathbf{P}_{t|T} = \mathbf{P}_{t|t} + \mathbf{P}_{t|t}\mathbf{T}_t'\mathbf{P}_{t+1}^{-1}(\mathbf{P}_{t+1|T} - \mathbf{P}_{t+1})$$
$$\times \mathbf{P}_{t+1}^{-1}\mathbf{T}_t\mathbf{P}_{t|t}, \quad t = T, \ldots 1, \quad (19)$$

where

$$\mathbf{a}_{t|t} = \mathbf{a}_t + \mathbf{P}_t\mathbf{Z}_t'F_t^{-1}v_t, \quad (20)$$

$$\mathbf{P}_{t|t} = \mathbf{P}_t - \mathbf{P}_t\mathbf{Z}_t'F_t^{-1}\mathbf{Z}_t\mathbf{P}_t, \quad (21)$$

with $\mathbf{a}_{t|t} = E(\boldsymbol{\alpha}_t|\mathbf{Y}_t)$ and $\mathbf{P}_{t|t} = \mathrm{var}(\boldsymbol{\alpha}_t|\mathbf{Y}_t)$. The smoother requires the output of the Kalman filter (9). A similar formulation of the AM smoother can be found in [8]. The AM smoother is computationally not efficient owing to many matrix multiplications and the inversion of matrix $\mathbf{P}_t$. However, it can be re-formulated as follows.

Define

$$\mathbf{r}_{t-1} = \mathbf{P}_t^{-1}(\mathbf{a}_{t|T} - \mathbf{a}_t), \quad (22)$$

$$\mathbf{N}_{t-1} = \mathbf{P}_t^{-1}(\mathbf{P}_t - \mathbf{P}_{t|T})\mathbf{P}_t^{-1}, \quad (23)$$

for $t = 1, \ldots, T$. Consequently, substitute $\mathbf{a}_{t|t}$ of (18) using (20), substitute the first $\mathbf{P}_{t|t}$ of (19) using (21) and after rearranging (18) and (19), we obtain

$$\mathbf{P}_t^{-1}(\mathbf{a}_{t|T} - \mathbf{a}_t) = \mathbf{Z}_t'F_t^{-1}v_t + \mathbf{L}_t'\mathbf{P}_{t+1}^{-1}$$
$$\times (\mathbf{a}_{t+1|T} - \mathbf{a}_{t+1}), \quad (24)$$

$$\mathbf{P}_t^{-1}(\mathbf{P}_{t|T} - \mathbf{P}_t)\mathbf{P}_t^{-1} = -\mathbf{Z}_t'F_t^{-1}\mathbf{Z}_t + \mathbf{L}_t'\mathbf{P}_{t+1}^{-1}$$
$$\times (\mathbf{P}_{t+1|T} - \mathbf{P}_{t+1})\mathbf{P}_{t+1}^{-1}\mathbf{L}_t, \quad (25)$$

where $\mathbf{L}_t = \mathbf{T}_t\mathbf{P}_{t|t}\mathbf{P}_t^{-1} = \mathbf{T}_t(\mathbf{I} - \mathbf{P}_t\mathbf{Z}_t'F_t^{-1}\mathbf{Z}_t) = \mathbf{T}_t - \mathbf{K}_t\mathbf{Z}_t$. Given the definitions of $\mathbf{r}_{t-1}$ and $\mathbf{N}_{t-1}$, the smoothing recursions (24) and (25) become

$$\mathbf{r}_{t-1} = \mathbf{Z}_t'F_t^{-1}v_t + \mathbf{L}_t'\mathbf{r}_t,$$
$$\mathbf{N}_{t-1} = \mathbf{Z}_t'F_t^{-1}\mathbf{Z}_t + \mathbf{L}_t'\mathbf{N}_t\mathbf{L}_t, \quad (26)$$

and it follows from definitions (22) and (23) that $\mathbf{r}_T = 0, \mathbf{N}_T = 0$ and

$$\mathbf{a}_{t|T} = \mathbf{a}_t + \mathbf{P}_t\mathbf{r}_{t-1},$$
$$\mathbf{P}_{t|T} = \mathbf{P}_t - \mathbf{P}_t\mathbf{N}_{t-1}\mathbf{P}_t, \quad (27)$$

for $t = T, \ldots, 1$. A self-contained proof of the state smoothing algorithm (26) and (27) can be found in [4], [5], and [10].

References

[1]   Anderson, B.D.O. & Moore, J.B. (1979). *Optimal Filtering*. Prentice Hall, Englewood Cliffs.
[2]   Ansley, C.F. & Kohn, R. (1985). Estimation, filtering and smoothing in state space models with incompletely specified initial conditions, *Annals of Statistics* **13**, 1286–1316.
[3]   Ansley, C.F. & Kohn, R. (1990). Filtering and smoothing in state space models with partially diffuse initial conditions, *Journal of Time Series Analysis* **11**, 275–293.
[4]   De Jong, P. (1988). A cross-validation filter for time series models, *Biometrika* **75**, 594–600.
[5]   De Jong, P. (1989). Smoothing and interpolation with the state space model, *Journal of the American Statistical Association* **84**, 1085–1088.
[6]   De Jong, P. (1991), The diffuse Kalman filter, *Annals of Statistics* **19**, 1073–1083.
[7]   De Jong, P. & Penzer, J. (1996). Diagnosing shocks in time series, Discussion paper, LSE Statistics Dept.
[8]   Harvey, A.C. (1989). *Forecasting, Structural Time Series Models and the Kalman Filter*. Cambridge University Press, Cambridge.
[9]   Harvey, A.C. & Koopman, S.J. (1992). Diagnostic checking of unobserved components time series models, *Journal of Business and Economic Statistics* **10**, 377–389.
[10] Kohn, R. & Ansley, C.F. (1989). A fast algorithm for signal extraction, influence and cross-validation in state space models, *Biometrika* **76**, 65–79.
[11] Koopman, S.J. (1993). Disturbance smoother for state space models, *Biometrika* **80**, 117–126.
[12] Koopman, S.J. (1996). Analytic filtering and smoothing for state space models, Discussion paper, LSE Statistics Dept.
[13] Koopman, S.J. (1997). Exact initial Kalman filtering and smoothing for nonstationary time series models, *Journal of the American Statistical Association* **92**, 1630–1638.
[14] Koopman, S.J. & Shephard, N. (1992). Exact score for time series model in state space form, *Biometrika* **79**, 823–826.
[15] Koopman, S.J., Harvey, A.C., Doornik, J.A. & Shephard, N. (1995). *STAMP 5.0 Structural Time Series*

Analyser, Modeller and Predictor. Chapman & Hall, London.

[16]   Snyder, R.D. & Saligari, G.R. (1996). Initialization of the Kalman filter with partially diffuse initial conditions, *Journal of Time Series Analysis* **17**, 409–424.

(*See also* **Prediction**)

SIEM JAN KOOPMAN

Kaplan–Meier Estimator

The Kaplan–Meier estimator is a **nonparametric** estimator which may be used to estimate the **survival distribution** function from **censored data**. The estimator may be obtained as the limiting case of the classical actuarial (**life table**) estimator, and it seems to have been first proposed by Böhmer [2]. It was, however, lost sight of by later researchers and not investigated further until the important paper by Kaplan & Meier [12] appeared. Today the estimator is usually named after these two authors, although sometimes it is denoted the product–limit estimator (*see* **Aalen–Johansen Estimator**). Below we describe the Kaplan–Meier estimator, illustrate its use in one particular case, and discuss estimation of the median and mean survival times. Furthermore, we show how the Kaplan–Meier estimator can be given as the product–integral of the **Nelson–Aalen estimator**, and indicate how this may be used to study its statistical properties. For almost four decades the Kaplan–Meier estimator has been one of the key statistical methods for analyzing censored survival data, and it is discussed in most textbooks on survival analysis. Rigorous derivations of the statistical properties of the estimator are provided in the books by Fleming & Harrington [7] and Andersen et al. [1]. In particular the latter presents formal proofs of almost all the results reviewed below as well as an extensive bibliography.

The Estimator and Confidence Intervals

Consider the survival data situation where we want to study the time to death (or some other event) for a homogeneous population with survival distribution function $S(t)$ representing the probability that an individual will be alive at time t. Assume that we have a sample of n individuals from this population. Our observation of the survival times for these individuals will typically be subject to right-censoring, meaning that for some individuals we only know that their true survival times exceed certain censoring times. The censoring is assumed to be independent in the sense that the additional knowledge of censorings before any time t does not alter the risk of failure at t. We denote by $t_1 < t_2 < \cdots$ the times when deaths are observed and let d_j be the number of individuals who die at t_j.

The Kaplan–Meier estimator for the survival distribution function then takes the form

$$\hat{S}(t) = \prod_{t_j \le t} \left(1 - \frac{d_j}{r_j}\right), \qquad (1)$$

where r_j is the number of individuals at risk (i.e. alive and not censored: in the **risk set**) just prior to time t_j. If there are no censored observations, then (1) reduces to one minus the empirical distribution function. The variance of the Kaplan–Meier estimator is estimated by Greenwood's formula:

$$\hat{\sigma}^2(t) = \hat{S}(t)^2 \sum_{t_j \le t} \frac{d_j}{r_j(r_j - d_j)}. \qquad (2)$$

In the case of no censoring, (2) reduces to $\hat{S}(t)[1 - \hat{S}(t)]/n$, the standard **binomial** variance estimator.

In large samples the Kaplan–Meier estimator, evaluated at a given time t, is approximately normally distributed so that a standard $100(1 - \alpha)\%$ confidence interval for $S(t)$ takes the form

$$\hat{S}(t) \pm z_{1-\alpha/2}\hat{\sigma}(t), \qquad (3)$$

with $z_{1-\alpha/2}$ the $1 - \alpha/2$ fractile of the **standard normal** distribution. The approximation to the normal distribution is improved by using the log-minus-log transformation (*see* **Quantal Response Models**) giving the **confidence interval**

$$\hat{S}(t)^{\exp\{\pm z_{1-\alpha/2}\hat{\sigma}(t)/[\hat{S}(t)\ln\hat{S}(t)]\}}. \qquad (4)$$

This interval is satisfactory for quite small sample sizes [3]. Confidence intervals with small-sample properties which are comparable with (4), or even slightly better, may be obtained by using the arcsine-square-root transformation [3] or by basing the confidence interval on the **likelihood ratio test** [5,

Section 4.3; 16]. Note that all these confidence intervals should be given a pointwise interpretation. Simultaneous confidence bands for the survival distribution function are considered below.

Right-censoring is not the only kind of data incompleteness in survival analysis. Often, e.g. in epidemiologic applications, individuals are not followed from time zero (in the relevant time scale, typically age), but only from a later entry time (conditional on survival until this entry time). Thus, in addition to right-censoring, the survival data are subject to left truncation. For such data we may, in principle at least still use the Kaplan–Meier estimator (1) and estimate its variance by (2). The number at risk, r_j, is now the number of individuals who have entered the study before time t_j and are still in the study just prior to t_j. However, for left-truncated data the numbers at risk, r_j, will often be low for small values of t_j. This will result in estimates $\hat{S}(t)$ which have large sampling errors and which therefore may be of little practical use. What can be usefully estimated in such situations is the conditional survival distribution function, $S(t|t_0) = S(t)/S(t_0)$, representing the probability of survival to time t given that an individual is alive at time $t_0 < t$. It may be useful to estimate such conditional distribution functions for several values of t_0 (at which there are reasonable numbers at risk), there being nothing canonical about any particular value. The estimation is performed as described earlier, the only modification being that the product in (1) and the sum in (2) are restricted to those t_j for which $t_0 < t_j \leq t$.

An Illustration

As an illustration we use data from a randomized clinical trial for patients with histologically verified liver cirrhosis. Patients were recruited from several hospitals in Copenhagen between 1962 and 1969 and were followed until death, lost to follow-up, or until the closing date of the study, October 1, 1974. The time variable of interest is time since entry into the study. Patients are right censored if alive on October 1, 1974, or if lost to follow-up before that date.

We consider only the 138 placebo-treated male patients. Their median age at entry was 57 years, while the lower and upper quartiles were 51 and 66 years, respectively. Of the 138 patients, 88 died during the study. The Kaplan–Meier estimate of the survival distribution function for these patients is

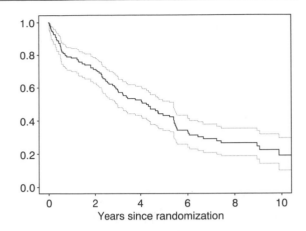

Figure 1 Kaplan–Meier estimate of the survival distribution function for 138 placebo-treated male patients with liver cirrhosis with 95% log-minus-log-transformed confidence intervals

shown in Figure 1 with 95% confidence intervals computed according to (4). From the figure we see, for example, that the five years survival probability is estimated as 43.0% with a 95% confidence interval from 34.0% to 51.9%, while the estimated 10 years survival probability is 18.4% with a confidence interval from 9.7% to 29.3%. We return to the liver cirrhosis example below in connection with median and mean survival times and simultaneous confidence bands. A further discussion and analysis of the data are given by Schlichting et al. [15]. The data were also used for illustrative purposes by Andersen et al. [1].

Median Survival Time and Related Quantities

The use of the Kaplan–Meier estimator is not restricted to estimating survival probabilities for given times t. It may also be used to estimate fractiles such as the **median survival time** and related quantities like the interquartile range (*see* **Quantiles**).

Consider the pth fractile, ξ_p, of the cumulative distribution function $F(t) = 1 - S(t)$, and assume that $F(t)$ has a positive density function $f(t) = F'(t) = -S'(t)$ in a neighborhood of ξ_p. Then ξ_p is uniquely determined by the relation $F(\xi_p) = p$, or equivalently, $S(\xi_p) = 1 - p$. The Kaplan–Meier estimator is a step function and hence does not necessarily attain the value $1 - p$. Therefore a similar relation cannot be used to define the estimator $\hat{\xi}_p$ of the pth fractile. Rather, we define $\hat{\xi}_p$ to be the smallest value of t for which $\hat{S}(t) \leq 1 - p$, i.e. the time t where $\hat{S}(t)$ jumps from a value greater than $1 - p$ to a value less than or equal to $1 - p$. In large samples $\hat{\xi}_p$ is approximately normally distributed with a variance that may be estimated by

$$\widehat{\text{var}}(\hat{\xi}_p) = \frac{(1 - p)^2 \hat{\sigma}^2(\hat{\xi}_p)}{[\hat{f}(\hat{\xi}_p)\hat{S}(\hat{\xi}_p)]^2}. \tag{5}$$

Here $\hat{f}(t)$ is an estimator for the density function $f(t) = -S'(t)$ (*see* **Density Estimation**). One may, for example, use

$$\hat{f}(t) = \frac{1}{2b}\left[\hat{S}(t - b) - \hat{S}(t + b)\right] \tag{6}$$

for a suitable bandwidth b (corresponding to a kernel function estimator with uniform kernel). Furthermore, for $p < q$, $\hat{\xi}_p$ and $\hat{\xi}_q$ are approximately binormally distributed, and their correlation may be estimated by

$$\widehat{\text{corr}}(\hat{\xi}_p, \hat{\xi}_q) = \frac{\hat{\sigma}(\hat{\xi}_p)\hat{S}(\hat{\xi}_q)}{\hat{\sigma}(\hat{\xi}_q)\hat{S}(\hat{\xi}_p)}. \tag{7}$$

Note that $\hat{S}(\hat{\xi}_p)$ in (5) and (7) is equal to or only slightly less than $1 - p$, and that (5) could have been simplified if we had used this approximate equality. We have chosen not to do so since then $\hat{S}(\hat{\xi}_p)$ in (5) and (7) cancels with the same factor in $\hat{\sigma}(\hat{\xi}_p)$; cf. (2).

The above results may be used in the usual way to determine approximate confidence intervals, e.g. for the median survival time $\xi_{0.50}$ and the interquartile range $\xi_{0.75} - \xi_{0.25}$, as illustrated below. For the purpose of determining a confidence interval for a quantile (fractile) like the median it is, however, better to apply the approach of Brookmeyer & Crowley [4]. For the pth fractile one then uses as a confidence interval all hypothesized values ξ_p^0 of ξ_p which are not rejected when testing the null hypothesis $\xi_p = \xi_p^0$ against the alternate hypothesis $\xi_p \neq \xi_p^0$ at the α level (*see* **Hypothesis Testing**). Such test-based confidence intervals can be read directly from the lower and upper confidence limits for the survival distribution function in exactly the same manner as $\hat{\xi}_p$ can be read from the Kaplan–Meier curve itself (*see* **Median Survival Time**).

For the liver cirrhosis data an estimate of the median survival time is 4.27 years (standard

error 0.66 years), while the lower and upper quartiles are estimated as 1.46 years (0.35 years) and 8.97 years (1.13 years), respectively, with an estimated correlation of 0.28. In these computations the bandwidth $b = 1$ year was used in (6). An estimate of the interquartile range of the survival distribution function is $8.97 - 1.46 = 7.51$ years, with standard error $(0.35^2 + 1.13^2 - 2 \times 0.35 \times 1.13 \times 0.28)^{1/2} = 1.09$ years. From this an approximate 95% confidence interval for the median survival time is $4.27 \pm 1.96 \times 0.66$, i.e. from 2.98 to 5.56 years, while 95% confidence limits for the interquartile range are from 5.37 to 9.65 years. For the median survival time it is, as mentioned earlier, better to read the confidence limits directly from the pointwise confidence intervals for the survival distribution function given in Figure 1. This gives 95% confidence limits for the median survival time from 3.02 years to 5.41 years. Note that no estimate of the density function is needed here.

Mean Survival Time

Owing to right-censoring, in most survival studies it will not be possible to obtain reliable estimates for the mean survival time $\mu = \int_0^\infty t f(t)\mathrm{d}t = \int_0^\infty S(t)\mathrm{d}t$ (*see* **Life Expectancy**). This is one important reason why, in survival analysis, the median is a more useful measure of location than the mean. What may be usefully estimated from right-censored survival data is the expected time lived in a given interval $[0, t]$, i.e. $\mu_t = \int_0^t S(u)\mathrm{d}u$. This is estimated by

$$\hat{\mu}_t = \int_0^t \hat{S}(u)\mathrm{d}u,$$

the area below the Kaplan–Meier curve between 0 and t. Such an estimate may be of interest in its own right, or it may be compared with a similar population-based estimate to assess the expected number of years lost up to time t for a group of patients. In large samples, $\hat{\mu}_t$ is approximately normally distributed with a variance that may be estimated by

$$\widehat{\text{var}}(\hat{\mu}_t) = \sum_{t_j \leq t} \frac{(\hat{\mu}_t - \hat{\mu}_{t_j})^2 d_j}{r_j(r_j - d_j)},$$

a result which may be used to give approximate confidence limits for μ_t. By letting t tend to infinity, the above results may be extended to the estimation of the mean μ itself [8]. However, the conditions (mainly on the censoring) needed for such an extension to be valid are usually not met in practice.

In the liver cirrhosis study no patient was followed for more than 13 years, making the estimation of the mean survival time impossible. We may, however, estimate the expected number of years lived up to a given time t. In particular, estimates for the expected number of years lived up to 5 years and 10 years after the start of the study are 3.29 years (standard error 0.17 years) and 4.73 years (0.33 years), respectively.

Redistribute-to-the-Right Algorithm and Self-Consistency

We mentioned earlier the relationship between the Kaplan–Meier estimator and the empirical distribution function in the case of no censoring. The redistribute-to-the-right algorithm and the concept of self-consistency, both due to Efron [6], further illustrate this relation.

For notational convenience we assume that there are no ties, and we denote by $t_1^0 < t_2^0 < \ldots < t_n^0$ the ordered times of deaths and censorings combined. The redistribute-to-the-right algorithm is as follows. First, we construct the ordinary empirical (survival) distribution function which places probability mass $1/n$ at each of the observed times t_j^0. If $t_{j_1}^0$ is the smallest t_j^0 that corresponds to a censored observation, then we remove its mass and redistribute it equally among the $n - j_1$ time-points to the right of it. Then, if $t_{j_2}^0$ is the second smallest censored observation, we remove its mass, which will be $1/n + 1/[n(n - j_1)]$, and redistribute it equally among the $n - j_2$ time-points to its right, etc. This algorithm will converge in a finite number of steps to the Kaplan–Meier estimator (1) (with the modification that it is set equal to zero after t_n^0 also when this last time-point corresponds to a censored observation).

A self-consistent estimator $\tilde{S}(t)$ for the survival distribution function equals $1/n$ times an estimate for the number of individuals who survive time t. More precisely,

$$\tilde{S}(t) = \frac{1}{n}\left[\#(t_j^0 > t) + \sum_{t_j^0 \leq t} a_j(t) \right], \qquad (8)$$

where $a_j(t) = \tilde{S}(t)/\tilde{S}(t_j^0)$ if the observation at t_j^0 corresponds to a censored observation, and $a_j(t) = 0$ if it corresponds to an observed death. It turns out that the Kaplan–Meier estimator (modified as just indicated) is the unique self-consistent estimator. Turnbull [17] (see **Turnbull Estimator**) used the idea of self-consistency to derive an iterative procedure (a version of the **EM algorithm**) for estimating the survival distribution function nonparametrically from arbitrarily grouped, censored, and truncated data, while Gill [9] showed that the self-consistency equation, (8), may be interpreted as a generalized score equation.

Product–Integral Representation and Relationship to the Nelson–Aalen Estimator

Usually one assumes that the survival distribution function $S(t)$ is absolute continuous with density function $f(t) = -S'(t)$, hazard rate function $\alpha(t) = f(t)/S(t)$, and cumulative hazard rate function $A(t) = \int_0^t \alpha(u)\mathrm{d}u$. However, the Kaplan–Meier estimator is discrete in nature, and the same applies to the Nelson–Aalen estimator for the cumulative hazard rate function. This makes it useful to be able to handle both discrete and continuous distributions within a unified framework. Let us therefore review how the survival distribution function $S(t)$ and the cumulative hazard rate function $A(t)$ are related for distributions which need neither to be continuous nor discrete. For such distributions

$$A(t) = -\int_0^t \frac{\mathrm{d}S(u)}{S(u-)}, \qquad (9)$$

where $S(t-)$ denotes the left-hand limit of the survival distribution function at t. For an absolute continuous distribution, (9) specializes to $A(t) = -\ln S(t) = \int_0^t \alpha(u)\mathrm{d}u$. For a discrete distribution it gives $A(t) = \sum_{u \leq t} \alpha_u$, where the discrete hazard, α_t, is the conditional probability of death exactly at time t given that death has not occurred earlier. To express the survival distribution function by the cumulative hazard rate function it is convenient to use the product–integral π, defined as the limit of approximating finite products in a similar manner as the ordinary integral $\int$ is defined as the limit of approximating finite sums (see **Product-Integration**). With the use of the product–integral we may write

$$S(t) = \prod_{u \le t} [1 - \mathrm{d}A(u)]. \qquad (10)$$

For a continuous distribution, (10) specializes to the well-known relation $S(t) = \exp[-A(t)]$, while for a discrete distribution it takes the form $S(t) = \prod_{u \le t} (1 - \alpha_u)$.

The Nelson–Aalen estimator for the cumulative hazard rate function is $\hat{A}(t) = \sum_{t_j \le t} d_j / r_j$. This corresponds to a distribution with all probability mass concentrated at the observed failure times and with discrete hazard $\hat{\alpha}_j = d_j / r_j$ at t_j. Using (10), the corresponding survival distribution function takes the form

$$\hat{S}(t) = \prod_{u \le t} [1 - \mathrm{d}\hat{A}(u)] = \prod_{t_j \le t} (1 - \hat{\alpha}_j), \qquad (11)$$

i.e. it is the Kaplan–Meier estimator (1). Thus the Kaplan–Meier and Nelson–Aalen estimators are related in exactly the same way as are the survival distribution function and the cumulative hazard rate function themselves. This fact is lost sight of when one considers the relations $A(t) = -\ln S(t)$ and $S(t) = \exp[-A(t)]$ which are only valid for the continuous case. In fact, the latter relations have led researchers to suggest the estimators $-\ln \hat{S}(t)$ and $\exp[-\hat{A}(t)]$ for the cumulative hazard rate function and the survival distribution function, respectively. The numerical differences between these two estimators and the Nelson–Aalen and Kaplan–Meier estimators will be of little importance in most cases. But the fact that the Nelson–Aalen and Kaplan–Meier estimators are related through (9) and (10) indicates that they are the canonical nonparametric estimators for the cumulative hazard rate function and the survival distribution function. This statement is supported by the fact that they may both be given a **nonparametric maximum likelihood** interpretation [11].

Martingale Representation and Statistical Properties

The product–integral formulation (11) of the Kaplan–Meier estimator shows its close relationship to the Nelson–Aalen estimator, and it is the key to the study of its statistical properties. In fact, these are closely related to those of the Nelson–Aalen estimator. We here indicate a few main steps and refer to Andersen et al. [1, Section IV.3] for a detailed account.

Let $J(t) = 1$ if there is at least one individual at risk just before time t; $J(t) = 0$ otherwise. Furthermore, introduce $A^*(t) = \int_0^t J(u)\mathrm{d}A(u)$, and let

$$S^*(t) = \prod_{u \le t} [1 - \mathrm{d}A^*(u)]. \qquad (12)$$

We note that (12) is almost the same as $S(t)$ [cf. (10)] when there is only a small probability that there is no one at risk at times $u \le t$. By a general result for product–integrals (Duhamel's equation), we may write

$$\frac{\hat{S}(t)}{S^*(t)} - 1 = -\int_0^t \frac{\hat{S}(u-)}{S^*(u)} \mathrm{d}(\hat{A} - A^*)(u). \qquad (13)$$

Here $\hat{A} - A^*$ is a square integrable martingale (*see* **Nelson–Aalen Estimator**). It follows that the right-hand side of (13) is a stochastic integral and hence itself a mean zero square integrable martingale. As a consequence of this, $\mathrm{E}[\hat{S}(t)/S^*(t)] = 1$ for any given t, so the Kaplan–Meier estimator is almost **unbiased**. Furthermore, the predictable variation process of the martingale on the right-hand side of (13) may be used to arrive at an estimator for the variance of $\hat{S}(t)/S^*(t)$. From this, Greenwood's formula (2) follows provided one adopts a general model, not necessarily continuous. Greenwood's formula may also be derived through a standard **information** calculation starting with a binomial-type likelihood for such a general model.

A further consequence of (13) is that $\sqrt{n}(\hat{S} - S)/S$ is asymptotically equivalent to $-\sqrt{n}(\hat{A} - A)$ and therefore converges weakly to a mean zero Gaussian martingale. In particular, for a fixed t, the Kaplan–Meier estimator (1) is asymptotically normally distributed, a fact that was used in connection with the confidence intervals (3) and (4). Also, the asymptotic distributional results of the estimators for the median and mean survival times reviewed earlier are consequences of this weak convergence result.

Confidence Bands

The weak convergence of $\sqrt{n}(\hat{S} - S)/S$ to a mean zero Gaussian martingale also makes it possible to derive confidence bands for the survival distribution function, i.e. limits that contain $S(t)$ for all t in an interval $[\tau_1, \tau_2]$ with a prespecified probability. Two important types of such confidence bands are the equal precision bands [14] and the Hall–Wellner bands [10]. Borgan & Liestøl [3] derived transformed versions of these confidence bands and compared them with the nontransformed ones.

The standard and log-minus-log transformed equal precision bands are obtained by replacing $z_{1-\alpha/2}$ in (3) and (4) by $d_{1-\alpha}(\hat{c}_1, \hat{c}_2)$, the $1 - \alpha$ fractile in the distribution of the supremum of the absolute value of a standardized Brownian bridge over the interval from $\hat{c}_1$ to $\hat{c}_2$ (*see* **Brownian Motion and Diffusion Processes**). Here

$$\hat{c}_i = \frac{n[\hat{\sigma}(\tau_i)/\hat{S}(\tau_i)]^2}{1 + n[\hat{\sigma}(\tau_i)/\hat{S}(\tau_i)]^2}, \quad i = 1, 2. \quad (14)$$

The fractile $d_{1-\alpha}(\hat{c}_1, \hat{c}_2)$ may be found (approximately) by solving (with respect to d) the following nonlinear equation:

$$\frac{4\phi(d)}{d} + \phi(d)\left(d - \frac{1}{d}\right)\ln\left[\frac{\hat{c}_2(1 - \hat{c}_1)}{\hat{c}_1(1 - \hat{c}_2)}\right] = \alpha,$$

with $\phi(d)$ the standard normal density. The equal precision bands require $0 < \hat{c}_1 < \hat{c}_2 < 1$, so they cannot be extended all the way down to $t = 0$. Typically, one will also omit the largest values of t.

The nontransformed Hall–Wellner band takes the form

$$\hat{S}(t) \pm n^{-1/2}e_{1-\alpha}(\hat{c}_1, \hat{c}_2)\{1 + n[\hat{\sigma}(t)/\hat{S}(t)]^2\}\hat{S}(t). \quad (15)$$

Here $e_{1-\alpha}(\hat{c}_1, \hat{c}_2)$ is the $1 - \alpha$ fractile in the distribution of the supremum of the absolute value of a Brownian bridge over the interval from $\hat{c}_1$ to $\hat{c}_2$; cf. (14). For completely observed survival data the Hall–Wellner band reduces to the well-known Kolmogorov band $\hat{S}(t) \pm n^{-1/2}e_{1-\alpha}(\hat{c}_1, \hat{c}_2)$. For the band (15), one will often let $\tau_1 = 0$, in which case tables of $e_{1-\alpha}(\hat{c}_1, \hat{c}_2) = e_{1-\alpha}(0, \hat{c}_2)$ are given, for example by Koziol & Byar [13] and Hall & Wellner [10] for selected values of α and $\hat{c}_2$. We note that (15) is obtained from (3) by substituting $n^{-1/2}e_{1-\alpha}(\hat{c}_1, \hat{c}_2)\{1 + n[\hat{\sigma}(t)/\hat{S}(t)]^2\}\hat{S}(t)$ for $z_{1-\alpha/2}\hat{\sigma}(t)$. The same substitution in (4) gives the log-minus-log transformed Hall–Wellner band. This transformed band requires $\hat{c}_1 > 0$, so it cannot be extended all the way down to $t = 0$. Owing to the approximation $e_{1-\alpha}(\hat{c}_1, \hat{c}_2) \approx e_{1-\alpha}(0, \hat{c}_2)$, the

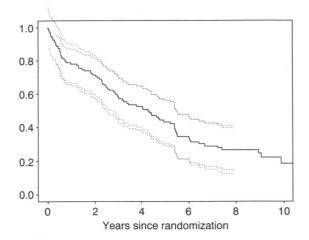

Figure 2 Kaplan–Meier estimate of the survival distribution function for 138 placebo-treated male patients with liver cirrhosis with 95% confidence bands: log-minus-log transformed equal precision band over the interval from 4 months to 8 years (- - - -); Hall–Wellner band over the interval [0, 8] years ($\cdots$)

above-mentioned tables may also be used for the transformed bands when $\hat{c}_1$ is close to zero.

The nontransformed equal precision band tends to achieve too high error rates when the number of observations is low, and the use of transformed bands is recommended, even for samples of a hundred or more. The achieved error rates of the nontransformed Hall–Wellner band are fairly close to the nominal ones even in small samples, and the improvement obtained by using transformed bands is of less importance.

Figure 2 shows the Kaplan–Meier estimate for the liver cirrhosis data with 95% confidence bands. The bands shown are the log-minus-log transformed equal precision band over the interval from 4 months to 8 years and the nontransformed Hall–Wellner band valid from time zero to 8 years. Since $\tau_1 = 1/3$ year and $\tau_2 = 8$ years correspond to $\hat{c}_1 = 0.090$ and $\hat{c}_2 = 0.789$, the fractiles $d_{0.95}(\hat{c}_1, \hat{c}_2) = 2.99$ and $e_{0.95}(0, \hat{c}_2) = 1.36$ were used. It is seen that the equal precision band is narrower than the Hall–Wellner band both for low and high values of t, while the Hall–Wellner band is slightly narrower than the equal precision band for intermediate values.

References

[1]   Andersen, P.K., Borgan, Ø., Gill, R.D. & Keiding, N. (1993). *Statistical Models Based on Counting Processes.* Springer-Verlag, New York.

[2]   Böhmer, P.E. (1912). Theorie der unabhängigen Wahrscheinlichkeiten, *Reports, Memoirs and Proceedings, Seventh International Congress of Actuaries, Amsterdam*, Vol. 2, pp. 327–343.

[3]   Borgan, Ø. & Liestøl, K. (1990). A note on confidence intervals and bands for the survival curve based on transformations, *Scandinavian Journal of Statistics* **17**, 35–41.

[4]   Brookmeyer, R. & Crowley, J.J. (1982). A confidence interval for the median survival time, *Biometrics* **38**, 29–41.

[5]   Cox, D.R. & Oakes, D. (1984). *Analysis of Survival Data*. Chapman & Hall, London.

[6]   Efron, B. (1967). The two sample problem with censored data, in *Proceedings of the Fifth Berkeley Symposium on Mathematical Statistics and Probability*, Vol. 4. Prentice Hall, New York, pp. 831–853.

[7]   Fleming, T.R. & Harrington, D.P. (1991). *Counting Processes and Survival Analysis*. Wiley, New York.

[8]   Gill, R.D. (1983). Large sample behavior of the product-limit estimator on the whole line, *Annals of Statistics* **11**, 49–58.

[9]   Gill, R.D. (1989). Non- and semi-parametric maximum likelihood estimation and the von Mises method (Part 1), *Scandinavian Journal of Statistics* **16**, 97–128.

[10] Hall, W.J. & Wellner, J.A. (1980). Confidence bands for a survival curve from censored data, *Biometrika* **67**, 133–143.

[11] Johansen, S. (1978). The product limit estimator as maximum likelihood estimator, *Scandinavian Journal of Statistics* **5**, 195–199.

[12] Kaplan, E.L. & Meier, P. (1958). Non-parametric estimation from incomplete observations, *Journal of the American Statistical Association* **53**, 457–481, 562–563.

[13] Koziol, J.A. & Byar, D.P. (1975). Percentage points of the asymptotic distributions of one and two sample K-S statistics for truncated or censored data, *Technometrics* **17**, 507–510.

[14] Nair, V.N. (1984). Confidence bands for survival functions with censored data: a comparative study, *Technometrics* **26**, 265–275.

[15] Schlichting, P., Christensen, E., Andersen, P.K., Fauerholdt, L., Juhl, E., Poulsen, H. & Tygstrup, N., for The Copenhagen Study Group for Liver Diseases (1983). Prognostic factors in cirrhosis identified by Cox's regression model, *Hepatology* **3**, 889–895.

[16] Thomas, D.R. & Grunkemeier, G.L. (1975). Confidence interval estimation of survival probabilities for censored data, *Journal of the American Statistical Association* **70**, 865–871.

[17] Turnbull, B.W. (1976). The empirical distribution function with arbitrarily grouped, censored and truncated data, *Journal of the Royal Statistical Society, Series B* **38**, 290–295.

ØRNULF BORGAN

Kappa

In medical research it is frequently of interest to examine the extent to which results of a classification procedure concur in successive applications. For example, two psychiatrists may separately examine each member of a group of patients and categorize each one as psychotic, neurotic, suffering from a personality disorder, or healthy. Given the resulting data, questions may then be posed regarding the diagnoses of the two psychiatrists and their relationship to one another. The psychiatrists would typically be said to exhibit a high degree of agreement if a high percentage of their diagnoses concurred, and poor agreement if they often made different diagnoses. In general, this latter outcome could arise if the categories were ill-defined, the criteria for assessment were different for the two psychiatrists, or their ability to examine these criteria differed sufficiently, possibly as a result of different training or experience. Poor empirical agreement might therefore lead to a review of the category definitions and diagnostic criteria, or possibly retraining with a view to improving agreement and hence consistency of diagnoses and treatment. In another context, one might have data from successive applications of a test for dysplasia or cancer from cervical smears. If the test indicates normal, mild, moderate, or severe dysplasia, or cancer, and the test is applied at two time points in close proximity, ideally the results would be the same. Variation in the method and location of sampling as well as variation in laboratory procedures may, however, lead to different outcomes. In this context, one would say that there is empirical evidence that the test is reliable if the majority of the subjects are classified in the same way for both applications of the test. Unreliable tests would result from the sources of variation mentioned earlier. Again, empirical evidence of an unreliable test may lead to refinements of the testing procedure (*see* **Observer Reliability and Agreement**).

The Kappa Index of Reliability for a Binary Test

For convenience, consider a diagnostic testing procedure generating a binary response variable T indicating the presence ($T = 1$) or absence ($T = 2$) of a particular condition. Suppose this test is applied twice in succession to each subject in a sample of size n. Let T_k denote the outcome for the kth application with the resulting data summarized in the **two-by-two table** (Table 1). where x_{ij} denotes the frequency at which $T_1 = i$ and $T_2 = j$, $x_{i\cdot} = \sum_{j=1}^{2} x_{ij}$, and $x_{\cdot j} = \sum_{i=1}^{2} x_{ij}$, $i = 1, 2, j = 1, 2$. Assuming that test results on different subjects are independent, conditioning on n leads to a **multinomial distribution** for the outcome of a particular table with

$$f(\mathbf{x}; \mathbf{p}) = \begin{pmatrix} n \\ x_{11}\ x_{12}\ x_{21}\ x_{22} \end{pmatrix} \prod_{i=1}^{2} \prod_{j=1}^{2} p_{ij}^{x_{ij}},$$

$\mathbf{x} = (x_{11}, x_{12}, x_{21}, x_{22})'$, $\mathbf{p} = (p_{11}, p_{12}, p_{21}, p_{22})'$, and $p_{22} = 1 - p_{11} - p_{12} - p_{21}$. Let $p_{i\cdot} = \sum_{j=1}^{2} p_{ij}$ and $p_{\cdot j} = \sum_{i=1}^{2} p_{ij}$. Knowledge of $\mathbf{p}$ would correspond to a complete understanding of the reliability of the test. Since knowledge of $\mathbf{p}$ is generally unattainable and estimation of $\mathbf{p}$ does not constitute a sufficient data reduction, indices of reliability/agreement typically focus on estimating one-dimensional functions of $\mathbf{p}$ (*see* **Agreement, Measurement of**).

A natural choice is $p_0 = \sum_{i=1}^{2} p_{ii}$, the probability of raw agreement, which is estimated as $\hat{p}_0 = \sum_{i=1}^{2} x_{ii}/n$. If $p_0 = 1$, then the test is completely reliable since the probability of observing discordant test results is zero. Similarly, if $\hat{p}_0$ is close to unity, then it suggests that the outcomes of the two applications concurred for the vast majority of the subjects. However, several authors have expressed reluctance to base **inferences** regarding reliability on the observed level of raw agreement (see [3] and references cited therein). The purported limitations of $\hat{p}_0$ as a measure of reliability stem from the fact that p_0 reflects both "chance" agreement and agreement over and above that which would be expected by chance. The agreement expected by chance, which we denote by p_e, is computed on the basis of the marginal distribution, defined by $p_1.$ and $p._1$, and under the assumption that the outcomes of the two

tests are independent conditional on the true status. Specifically, $p_e = \sum_{i=1}^{2} p_{i\cdot} p_{\cdot i}$ is estimated by $\hat{p}_e = \sum_{i=1}^{2} x_{1\cdot} x_{\cdot 1}/n^2$. To address concerns regarding the impact of nonnegligible chance agreement, Cohen [3] defined the index kappa which takes the form

$$\kappa = \frac{p_0 - p_e}{1 - p_e},$$

and indicated that it can be interpreted as reflecting "the proportion of agreement *after* chance agreement is removed from consideration". This can be seen by noting that $p_0 - p_e$ is the difference in the proportion of raw agreement and the agreement expected by chance, this being the agreement arising due to factors not driven by chance. If $p_0 - p_e > 0$, then there is agreement arising from nonchance factors; if $p_0 - p_e = 0$, then there is no additional agreement over that which one would expect based on chance; and if $p_0 - p_e < 0$, then there is less agreement than one would expect by chance. Furthermore, $1 - p_e$ is interpreted by Cohen [3] as the proportion "of the units for which the hypothesis of no association would predict disagreement between the judges". Alternatively, this can be thought of as the maximum possible agreement beyond that expected by chance. An estimate of κ, denoted $\hat{\kappa}$, is referred to as the kappa statistic and may be obtained by replacing p_0 and p_e with their corresponding point estimates, giving

$$\hat{\kappa} = \frac{\hat{p}_0 - \hat{p}_e}{1 - \hat{p}_e}. \tag{1}$$

The Kappa Index of Reliability for Multiple Categories

When the classification procedure of interest has multiple nominal categories, assessment of agreement becomes somewhat more involved. Consider a diagnostic test with R possible outcomes and let T_k denote the outcome of the kth application of the test, $k = 1, 2$. Then T_k takes values on $\{1, 2, 3, \ldots, R\}$ and interest lies in assessing the extent to which these outcomes agree for $k = 1$ and $k = 2$. An $R \times R$ **contingency table** may then be constructed (see Table 2), where again x_{ij} denotes the frequency with which the first application of the test led to outcome i and the second led to outcome j, $i = 1, 2, \ldots, R, j = 1, 2, \ldots, R$. A category-specific measure of agreement may be of interest to examine the extent

Table 1

	$T_2 = 1$	$T_2 = 2$	Total
$T_1 = 1$	x_{11}	x_{12}	$x_{1\cdot}$
$T_1 = 2$	x_{21}	x_{22}	$x_{2\cdot}$
Total	$x_{\cdot 1}$	$x_{\cdot 2}$	$x_{\cdot\cdot} = n$

which the two applications tend to lead to consistent conclusions with respect to outcome r, say. In this problem there is an implicit assumption that the particular nature of any disagreements are not of interest. One can then collapse the $R \times R$ table to a 2×2 table constructed by cross-classifying subjects with **binary** indicators such that $T_k = 1$ if outcome r was selected at the kth application, $T_k = 2$ otherwise, $k = 1, 2$. A category-specific kappa statistic can then be constructed in the fashion indicated earlier. This can be repeated for each of the R categories giving R such statistics.

In addition to these category-specific measures, however, an overall summary index of agreement is often of interest. The kappa statistic in (1) is immediately generalized for the $R \times R$ ($R > 2$) table as follows. Let p_{ij} denote the probability of $T_1 = i$ and $T_2 = j$, one of the R^2 multinomial probabilities, $p_{i\cdot} = \sum_{j=1}^{R} p_{ij}$, and $p_{\cdot j} = \sum_{i=1}^{R} p_{ij}, i = 1, 2, \ldots, R, j = 1, 2, \ldots, R$. Then, as before, $\hat{p}_{ij} = x_{ij}/n$, $\hat{p}_{i\cdot} = x_{i\cdot}/n$, $\hat{p}_{\cdot j} = x_{\cdot j}/n$, $\hat{p}_0 = \sum_{i=1}^{R} \hat{p}_{ii}$, $\hat{p}_e = \sum_{i=1}^{R} \hat{p}_{i\cdot}\hat{p}_{\cdot i}$, and the overall kappa statistic takes the same form as in (1). This overall kappa statistic can equivalently be written as a weighted average of category-specific kappa statistics [6].

The kappa statistic has several properties that are widely considered to be attractive for measures of agreement. First, when the level of observed agreement, reflected by $\hat{p}_0$, is equal to the level of agreement expected by chance $(\hat{p}_e)$, $\hat{\kappa} = 0$. Secondly, $\hat{\kappa}$ takes on its maximum value of 1 if and only if there is perfect agreement (i.e. $\hat{p}_0 = 1$ arising from a diagonal table). Thirdly, the kappa statistic is never less than -1. The latter two features require further elaboration, however, as the actual upper and lower limits on $\hat{\kappa}$ are functions of the marginal frequencies. In particular, $\hat{\kappa}$ takes on the value 1 only when

the marginal frequencies are exactly equal and all off-diagonal cells are zero. Values less than 1 occur when the marginal frequencies are the same but there are different category assignments in the table or, more generally, when the marginal frequencies differ (when the marginal frequencies differ there are necessarily nonzero diagonal cells and hence some disagreements). It is natural then to expect the kappa statistic for such a table to be less than unity. Cohen [3] shows that the maximum possible value of $\hat{\kappa}$ takes the form

$$\hat{\kappa}_M = \frac{x_{\cdot\cdot} \sum_{i=1}^{R} \min(x_{i\cdot}, x_{\cdot i}) - \sum_{i=1}^{R} x_{i\cdot}x_{\cdot i}}{x_{\cdot\cdot}^2 - \sum_{i=1}^{R} x_{i\cdot}x_{\cdot i}}, \qquad (2)$$

and argues that this is intuitively reasonable since differences in the marginal frequencies necessarily lead to a reduction in the level of agreement and hence $\hat{\kappa}$. Cohen then suggests that if one is interested in assessing the proportion of the agreement permitted by the margins (correcting for chance), then one computes $\hat{\kappa}/\hat{\kappa}_M$. We return to the topic of marginal frequencies and their influence on the properties of κ later in the article.

If the marginal frequencies for the two tests are uncorrelated (as measured by the product–moment **correlation** of the margins [3]), then the lower bound for $\hat{\kappa}$ is $\hat{\kappa}_L = -(R-1)^{-1}$. When the marginal frequencies are negatively correlated, $\hat{\kappa}_L > -(R-1)^{-1}$. However, when the marginal frequencies are positively correlated, $\hat{\kappa}_L < -(R-1)^{-1}$. It is only as the number of categories reduces to two, the correlation of the marginal frequencies approaches 1, and the **variances** of the marginal frequencies increase, that $\hat{\kappa}_L$ approaches -1 [3].

Having computed a kappa statistic for a given contingency table it is natural to want to characterize the level of agreement in descriptive terms. Landis & Koch [11] provide ranges that suggest, beyond what one would expect by chance, $0.75 < \hat{\kappa}$ typically represents excellent agreement, $0.40 < \hat{\kappa} < 0.75$ fair to good agreement, and $\hat{\kappa} < 0.40$ poor agreement. While there is some appeal to this convenient framework for the interpretation of $\hat{\kappa}$, caution is warranted (*see* **Kappa and Its Dependence on Marginal Rates**).

Frequently, it will be of interest to construct **confidence intervals** for the index kappa. Fleiss et al.

Table 2

	$T_2 = 1$	$T_2 = 2$	$T_2 = 3$	$\cdots$	$T_2 = R$	Total
$T_1 = 1$	x_{11}	x_{12}	x_{13}	$\cdots$	x_{1R}	$x_{1\cdot}$
$T_1 = 2$	x_{21}	x_{22}	x_{23}	$\cdots$	x_{2R}	$x_{2\cdot}$
$T_1 = 3$	x_{31}	x_{32}	x_{33}	$\cdots$	x_{3R}	$x_{3\cdot}$
$\vdots$	$\vdots$	$\vdots$	$\vdots$	$\cdots$	$\vdots$	$\vdots$
$T_1 = R$	x_{R1}	x_{R2}	x_{R3}	$\cdots$	x_{RR}	$x_{R\cdot}$
Total	$x_{\cdot 1}$	$x_{\cdot 2}$	$x_{\cdot 3}$	$\cdots$	$x_{\cdot R}$	$x_{\cdot\cdot} = n$

[8] derive an approximate large sample estimate for the variance of $\hat{\kappa}$, $\widehat{\text{var}}(\hat{\kappa})$, as

$$
\left(\sum_{i=1}^{R} \hat{p}_{ii}[1 - (\hat{p}_{i\cdot} + \hat{p}_{\cdot i})(1 - \hat{\kappa})]^2 \right.
$$
$$
+ (1 - \hat{\kappa})^2 \sum_i \sum_{j \neq i} \hat{p}_{ij}(\hat{p}_{\cdot i} + \hat{p}_{j\cdot})^2
$$
$$
\left. - [\hat{\kappa} - \hat{p}_e(1 - \hat{\kappa})]^2 \right) \Big/ [x_{..}(1 - \hat{p}_e)^2], \quad (3)
$$

and Fleiss [6] recommends carrying out tests (*see* **Hypothesis Testing**) and constructing confidence intervals by assuming approximate **normality** of $(\hat{\kappa} - \kappa)/[\widehat{\text{var}}(\hat{\kappa})]^{1/2}$ and proceeding in the standard fashion. For tests regarding the **null hypothesis** $H_0 : \kappa = 0$, an alternate variance estimate may be derived from (3) by substituting 0 for $\hat{\kappa}$, and $\hat{p}_{i\cdot} \hat{p}_{\cdot j}$ for $\hat{p}_{ij}$, giving

$$
\widehat{\text{var}}_0(\hat{\kappa})
$$
$$
= \left(\sum_{k=1}^{R} \hat{p}_{i\cdot} \hat{p}_{\cdot i}[1 - (\hat{p}_{i\cdot} + \hat{p}_{\cdot i})]^2 + \sum_{i \neq j} \hat{p}_{i\cdot} \hat{p}_{\cdot j} \right.
$$
$$
\left. \times (\hat{p}_{\cdot i} + \hat{p}_{j\cdot})^2 - p_e^2 \right) \Big/ [x_{..}(1 - \hat{p}_e)^2], \quad (4)
$$

with tests carried out as described above.

The Weighted Kappa Index

The discussion thus far has focused on situations in which the test serves as a **nominal** classification procedure (e.g. as in the psychiatric diagnosis example at the beginning of the article). In such settings, since there is no natural ordering to the outcomes, any disagreements are often considered to be equally serious and the methods previously described are directly applicable. In some circumstances with nominal scales, however, certain types of disagreements are more serious then others and it is desirable to take this into account. Furthermore, when the outcome is ordinal (as in the cervical cancer screening example) (*see* **Ordered Categorical Data**), it is often of interest to adopt a measure of agreement that treats disagreements in adjacent categories as less serious than disagreements in more disparate categories. For

the test based on cervical smears designed to classify the condition of the cervix as healthy, mildly, moderately, or severely dysplastic, or cancerous, if on one occasion the test suggested mild dysplasia and on another moderate, this type of disagreement would be considered less serious than if a cervix previously diagnosed as cancerous was subsequently classified as mildly dysplastic. In general, the seriousness reflects clinical implications for treatment and the consequences of wrong decisions.

Weighted versions of the kappa statistic were derived by Cohen [4] to take into account the additional structure arising from ordinal measures or from nominal scales in which certain types of disagreement are of more importance than others. In particular, the objective of adopting a weighted kappa statistic is to allow "different kinds of disagreement" to be differentially weighted in the construction of the overall index. We begin by assigning a weight to each of the R^2 cells; let w_{ij} denote the weight for cell (i, j). These weights may be determined quite arbitrarily but it is natural to restrict $0 \leq w_{ij} \leq 1$, set w_{ii} to unity to give exact agreement maximum weight, and set $0 \leq w_{ij} < 1$ for $i \neq j$, so that all disagreements are given less weight than exact agreement. The selection of the weights plays a key role in the interpretation of the weighted kappa statistic and also impacts the corresponding variance estimates, prompting Cohen [4] to suggest these be specified prior to the collection of the data.

Perhaps the two most common sets of weights are the quadratic weights, with $w_{ij} = 1 - (i - j)^2/(R - 1)^2$, and the so-called Cicchetti weights, with $w_{ij} = 1 - |i - j|/(R - 1)$ [1, 2]. The quadratic weights tend to weight disagreements just off the main diagonal more highly than Cicchetti weights, and the relative weighting of disagreements farther from the main diagonal is also higher with the quadratic weights. Clearly, these two weighting schemes share the minimal requirements cited above. The weighted kappa statistic then takes the form

$$
\hat{\kappa}^{(w)} = \frac{\hat{p}_0^{(w)} - \hat{p}_e^{(w)}}{1 - \hat{p}_e^{(w)}}, \quad (5)
$$

where $\hat{p}_0^{(w)} = \sum_{i=1}^{R} \sum_{j=1}^{R} w_{ij} \hat{p}_{ij}$ and $\hat{p}_e^{(w)} = \sum_{i=1}^{R} \sum_{j=1}^{R} w_{ij} \hat{p}_{i\cdot} \hat{p}_{\cdot j}$. If $\overline{w}_{i\cdot} = \sum_{j=1}^{R} \hat{p}_{\cdot j} w_{ij}$ and $\overline{w}_{\cdot j} = \sum_{i=1}^{R} \hat{p}_{i\cdot} w_{ij}$, then the large-sample variance of $\hat{\kappa}^{(w)}$ is estimated by

$$\widehat{\text{var}}(\hat{\kappa}^{(w)})$$

$$= \left(\sum_{i=1}^{R} \sum_{j=1}^{R} \hat{p}_{ij}[w_{ij} - (\overline{w}_{i.} + \overline{w}_{.j})(1 - \hat{\kappa}^{(w)})]^2 \right. $$

$$\left. - [\hat{\kappa}^{(w)} - \hat{p}_{e}^{(w)}(1 - \hat{\kappa}^{(w)})]^2 \right) \Big/ [x_{..}^2(1 - \hat{p}_{e}^{(w)})^2] \tag{6}$$

and, as before, tests and confidence intervals may be carried out and derived in the standard fashion assuming asymptotic normality of the quantity $(\hat{\kappa}^{(w)} - \kappa^{(w)})/[\widehat{\text{var}}(\hat{\kappa}^{(w)})]^{1/2}$. As in the unweighted case, a variance estimate appropriate for testing H_0 : $\kappa^{(w)} = 0$ may be derived by substituting $\hat{p}_{i.}\hat{p}_{.j}$ for $\hat{p}_{ij}$, and 0 for $\hat{\kappa}^{(w)}$ in (6).

We note in passing that the weighted kappa with quadratic weights has been shown to bear connections to the intraclass correlation coefficient. Suppose that with an ordinal outcome the categories are assigned the integers 1 through R from the "lowest" to "highest" categories, respectively, and assignment to these categories is taken to correspond to a realization of the appropriate integer value. Fleiss & Cohen [7] show that the intraclass correlation coefficient computed by treating these integer responses as coming from a Gaussian **general linear model** for a two-way **analysis of variance**, is asymptotically equivalent to the weighted kappa statistic with quadratic weights.

The Kappa Index for Multiple Observers

Thus far we have restricted consideration to the case of two applications of the classification procedure (e.g. two successive applications of a diagnostic test, two physicians carrying out successive diagnoses, etc.). In many situations, however, there are multiple (> 2) applications and interest lies in measuring agreement on the basis of several applications. Fleiss [5] considered the particular problem in which a group of subjects was examined and classified by a fixed number of observers, but where it was not necessarily the same set of observers carrying out the assessments for each patient. Moreover, Fleiss [5] assumed that it was not possible to identify which observers were involved in examining the patients.

For this problem, we require some new notation. Let M denote the number of subjects, N denote the number of observers per subject, and R denote the number of categories as before. Therefore, NM classifications are to be made. Let n_{ij} denote the number of times the ith subject was assigned to the jth category. A measure of overall raw agreement for the assignments on the ith subject is given by

$$\hat{q}_i = \frac{\sum_{j=1}^{R} n_{ij}(n_{ij} - 1)}{N(N-1)}, \tag{7}$$

which can be interpreted as follows. With N observers per subjects there are $\binom{N}{2}$ possible pairs of assignments. There are $\binom{n_{ij}}{2}$ which agree on category j and hence a total number of $\sum_{j=1}^{R} \binom{n_{ij}}{2}$ pairs of assignments which concur altogether for the ith subject. Thus, (7) simply represents the proportion of all paired assignments on the ith subject for which there was agreement on the category. The overall measure of raw observed agreement over all subjects is then given by $\hat{q}_0 = M^{-1} \sum_{i=1}^{M} \hat{q}_i$, which equals

$$\hat{q}_0 = \frac{\sum_{i=1}^{M} \sum_{j=1}^{R} n_{ij}^2}{MN(N-1)} - \frac{1}{N-1}. \tag{8}$$

As before, however, some agreement would be expected among the observers simply by chance and the kappa statistic in this setting corrects for this. The expected level of agreement is computed by noting that

$$\hat{p}_j = \frac{\sum_{i=1}^{M} n_{ij}}{MN}$$

is the sample proportion of all assignments made to category j, with $\sum_{j=1}^{R} \hat{p}_j = 1$. So if pairs of observers were simply assigning subjects to categories at random and independently one can estimate that they would be expected to agree according to

$$\hat{p}_e = \sum_{j=1}^{R} \hat{p}_j^2, \tag{9}$$

then the kappa statistic is computed by correcting for chance in the usual way as

$$\hat{\kappa} = \frac{\hat{q}_0 - \hat{p}_e}{1 - \hat{p}_e}. \tag{10}$$

The sample variance for (10) is derived by Fleiss et al. [9] to be

$$\widehat{\text{var}}(\hat{\kappa})$$

$$= 2\left[\left(\sum_{j=1}^{R} p_j(1-p_j)\right)^2 - \sum_{j=1}^{R} p_j(1-p_j)\right.$$

$$\left.(1-2p_j)\right] \bigg/ MN(N-1)\left(\sum_{j=1}^{R} p_j(1-p_j)\right)^2 \tag{11}$$

and is typically used for tests or interval estimation in the standard fashion.

When the same set of raters assesses all subjects and individual raters scores are known, it is not possible to use the results of Fleiss [5] without ignoring the rater-specific assignments. For this context, Schouten [13] proposed the use of indices based on weighted sums of pairwise measures of observed and expected levels of agreement. In particular, for a given pair of raters and a given pair of categories, observed and expected measures of agreement may be computed as earlier. Then, for each pair of raters, a measure of overall observed agreement may be obtained by taking a weighted average of such measures over all pairwise combinations of categories. Given a corresponding measure of expected agreement, an overall kappa statistic can be computed in the usual fashion. Schouten [13] then described how to obtain kappa statistics reflecting agreement over all observers, agreement between a particular observer and the remaining observers, and agreement within and between subgroups of observers.

General Remarks

MaClure & Willett [12] provide a comprehensive review and effectively highlight a number of limitations of the kappa statistics. In particular, they stress that for ordinal data derived from categorizing underlying continuous responses, the kappa statistic depends heavily on the often arbitrary category definitions, raising questions about interpretability. They also suggest that the use of weights, while attractive in allowing for varying degrees of disagreement, introduces another component of subjectivity into the computation of kappa statistics. Perhaps the issue of

greatest debate is the so-called prevalence, or base-rate, problem of kappa statistics (*see* **Kappa and Its Dependence on Marginal Rates**). Several other authors have examined critically the properties and interpretation of kappa statistics [10, 14, 15], and the debate of the merits and demerits continues unabated. Despite the apparent limitations, the kappa statistic enjoys widespread use in the medical literature and has been the focus of considerable statistical research.

References

[1]   Cicchetti, D.V. (1972). A new measure of agreement between rank ordered variables, *Proceedings of the American Psychological Association* **7**, 17–18.
[2]   Cicchetti, D.V. & Allison T. (1973). Assessing the reliability of scoring EEG sleep records: an improved method, *Proceedings and Journal of the Electro-physiological Technologists' Association* **20**, 92–102.
[3]   Cohen, J. (1960). A coefficient of agreement for nominal scales, *Educational and Psychological Measurement* **20**, 37–46.
[4]   Cohen, J. (1968). Weighted kappa: nominal scale agreement with provision for scaled disagreement or partial credit, *Psychological Bulletin* **70**, 213–220.
[5]   Fleiss, J.L. (1971). Measuring nominal scale agreement among many raters, *Psychological Bulletin* **76**, 378–382.
[6]   Fleiss, J.L. (1981). *Statistical Methods for Rates and Proportions*, 2nd Ed. Wiley, New York.
[7]   Fleiss, J.L. & Cohen, J. (1973). The equivalence of weighted kappa and the intraclass correlation coefficient as measures of reliability, *Educational and Psychological Measurement* **33**, 613–619.
[8]   Fleiss, J.L., Cohen, J. & Everitt, B.S. (1969). Large sample standard errors of kappa and weighted kappa, *Psychological Bulletin* **72**, 323–327.
[9]   Fleiss, J.L., Nee, J.C.M. & Landis, J.R. (1979). Large sample variance of kappa in the case of different sets of raters, *Psychological Bulletin* **86**, 974–977.
[10]   Kraemer, H.C. & Bloch, D.A. (1988). Kappa coefficients in epidemiology: an appraisal of a reappraisal, *Journal of Clinical Epidemiology* **41**, 959–968.
[11]   Landis, J.R. & Koch, G.G. (1977). The measurement of observer agreement for categorical data, *Biometrics* **33**, 159–174.
[12]   MaClure, M. & Willett, W.C. (1987). Misinterpretation and misuse of the kappa statistic, *American Journal of Epidemiology* **126**, 161–169.
[13]   Schouten, H.J.A. (1982). Measuring pairwise interobserver agreement when all subjects are judged by the same observers, *Statistica Neerlandica* **36**, 45–61.
[14]   Thompson, W.D. & Walter S.D. (1988). A reappraisal of the kappa coefficient, *Journal of Clinical Epidemiology* **41**, 949–958.

[15]   Thompson, W.D. & Walter S.D. (1988). Kappa and the concept of independent errors, *Journal of Clinical Epidemiology* **41**, 969–970.

RICHARD J. COOK

Kappa and Its Dependence on Marginal Rates

The **kappa** statistic was proposed by Cohen [4] as a measure of reliability for **nominal** classification procedures and was constructed specifically to "correct" the proportion of raw agreement for agreement expected purely by random classifications given the marginal rates. Since its introduction there have been many generalizations and extensions developed and it has been applied widely in medical research. There has also been considerable debate about the utility of this index [8, 12, 13], arising in part as a result of a genuine lack of consensus on precisely how to model and measure the reliability of nominal classification procedures. The issues are most easily illustrated in the assessment of the reliability of a simple **binary** test. Let T_k denote the outcome of the kth application of a binary test for which $T_k = 1$ and $T_k = 2$ indicate the presence and absence of disease, respectively, $k = 1, 2$. Upon two applications of this test to a sample of n subjects, cross-classifying the results leads to a **2 × 2 table** (see Table 1), where x_{ij} denotes the frequency with which $T_1 = i$ and $T_2 = j$, $x_{i\cdot} = \sum_{j=1}^{2} x_{ij}$, and $x_{\cdot j} = \sum_{i=1}^{2} x_{ij}$. Conditioning on n leads to a **multinomial distribution** for $\mathbf{x} = (x_{11}, x_{12}, x_{21}, x_{22})'$, where p_{ij} is the probability of $T_1 = i$ and $T_2 = j$, $p_{i\cdot} = \sum_{j=1}^{2} p_{ij}$, and $p_{\cdot j} = \sum_{i=1}^{2} p_{ij}$. The raw agreement is $p_0 = \sum_{i=1}^{2} p_{ii}$ and, given the marginal rates $p_{i\cdot}, i = 1, 2$ and $p_{\cdot j}, j = 1, 2$, and under the assumption of independent classifications, the expected level of agreement is $p_e = \sum_{i=1}^{2} p_{i\cdot} p_{\cdot i}$ The kappa index takes the form $\kappa = (p_0 - p_e)/(1 - p_e)$. The estimate of kappa, subsequently referred to as the kappa statistic and denoted $\hat{\kappa}$, is obtained by replacing p_0 and p_e by the corresponding estimates $\hat{p}_0 = \sum_{i=1}^{2} \hat{p}_{ii}$ and $\hat{p}_e = \sum_{i=1}^{2} \hat{p}_{i\cdot} \hat{p}_{\cdot i}$ respectively, where $\hat{p}_{ii} = x_{ii}/n$, $\hat{p}_{i\cdot} = x_{i\cdot}/n$, and $\hat{p}_{\cdot i} = x_{\cdot i}/n$, $i = 1, 2$.

Table 1

	$T_2 = 1$	$T_2 = 2$	Total
$T_1 = 1$	x_{11}	x_{12}	$x_{1\cdot}$
$T_1 = 2$	x_{21}	x_{22}	$x_{2\cdot}$
Total	$x_{\cdot 1}$	$x_{\cdot 2}$	$x_{\cdot\cdot} = n$

While on the surface the kappa statistic is intuitively appealing as a measure of reliability, paradoxical results can arise from computing the kappa statistic for tables of various configurations. The most often cited paradox with kappa is termed the "base rate" or "prevalence" problem and refers to the fact that for a fixed $\hat{p}_0$, values of $\hat{p}_{1\cdot} \approx \hat{p}_{\cdot 1}$ away from 0.50 in either direction lead to smaller values of $\hat{\kappa}$. Thus, a diagnostic test with fixed **sensitivity** and **specificity** when applied twice to a sample of patients with $\hat{p}_{1\cdot} \approx \hat{p}_{\cdot 1} \approx 0.50$, will generate a kappa statistic larger than would be obtained from a similar application of the test in a very low-risk population (with $\hat{p}_{1\cdot} \approx \hat{p}_{\cdot 1} \approx 0.10$), or in an extremely high-risk population (with $\hat{p}_{1\cdot} \approx \hat{p}_{\cdot 1} \approx 0.90$). Given that the diagnostic instrument is the same in both studies, this result is argued to be counter-intuitive. This paradox also raises concerns about the utility of the ranges for the kappa statistic given by Landis & Koch [9] said to correspond to poor, fair, good, and excellent agreement. Owing to this dependence on the marginal frequencies, a comparison of reliability findings, as measured by $\hat{\kappa}$, is difficult across studies involving populations with different prevalences.

At the population level, some insight can be gained into the reason for this behavior. Let θ denote the **prevalence** of the disease in the population from which the subjects under study were randomly sampled. Let α and β denote the **false positive** and **false negative** error rates for the diagnostic test, respectively. Then, if successive applications of the test may be assumed to be independent, $p_{11} = \theta(1 - \beta)^2 + (1 - \theta)(1 - \alpha)^2$, $p_{12} = \theta(1 - \beta)\beta + (1 - \theta)(1 - \alpha)\alpha$, $p_{21} = \theta(1 - \beta)\beta + (1 - \theta)(1 - \alpha)\alpha$, $p_{22} = \theta\beta^2 + (1 - \theta)\alpha^2$, $p_0 = p_{11} + p_{22} = \theta(1 - 2\beta) + (1 - \theta)(1 - 2\alpha)$, and $p_e = 1 - 2a(1 - a)$, where $a = [\theta(1 - \beta) + (1 - \theta)(1 - \alpha)]^2$. Kraemer [7] derives the relation

$$\kappa = \frac{2\theta(1 - \theta)(1 - \alpha - \beta)^2}{2[(\theta(1 - \beta) + (1 - \theta)\alpha) \times (1 - \theta(1 - \beta) - (1 - \theta)\alpha)]}. \quad (1)$$

For fixed (α, β), plots of κ as a function of θ are concave down taking on the value zero at $\theta = 0$ and $\theta = 1$ [12].

Several solutions to this problem have been proposed ranging from supplementing $\hat{\kappa}$ with additional statistics to facilitate disentangling the nature of the agreement, to entirely new approaches. Feinstein & Cicchetti [6] effectively illustrate the dependence of kappa on the marginal frequencies by considering several sample tables in which the observed raw agreement $\hat{p}_0$ is fixed, but the marginal frequencies vary. In a companion paper, Cicchetti & Feinstein [3] then propose that the kappa statistic should always be reported with two accompanying statistics called the index of average positive agreement, $\hat{q}_{pos} = 2x_{11}/(x_1. + x._1)$, and the index of average negative agreement $\hat{q}_{neg} = 2x_{22}/(x_2. + x._2)$. The motivation is that these statistics may be used to gain insight into the marginal agreement and imbalance in the marginal frequencies and hence allow interpretation of $\hat{\kappa}$ accordingly. Byrt et al. [1] propose using what they refer to as a bias-adjusted kappa, which reduces to an index previously proposed by Scott [11]. Lantz & Nebenzahl [10] suggest that kappa statistics be accompanied with statistics $\hat{\kappa}_{min} = \hat{p}_0^2/[(1 - \hat{p}_0)^2 + 1]$ and $\hat{\kappa}_{max} = \hat{p}_0 - 1/\hat{p}_0 + 1$ for $\hat{p}_0 < 1$, which correspond to the minimum and maximum values of κ for a given level of observed agreement, and $\hat{\kappa}_{nor} = 2\hat{p}_0 - 1$, which is also the so-called prevalence-adjusted, bias-adjusted kappa statistic of Byrt et al. [1].

Much of the work on kappa has been carried out on intuitive, but largely ad hoc, grounds. For example, there is no underlying probability function, and hence **likelihood** function, for which κ is a sole parameter of interest. Rather, it has been proposed as an "index", a function of parameters which may be estimated and, when done so, is thought to have some attractive properties. Thus, it appears that the paradox arises since the kappa statistic is not model-based, and depends in a complicated way on the observed raw agreement and the marginal frequencies. The key factor in the paradoxes is the role of $\hat{p}_e$, which serves as a "correction factor" in the numerator of $\hat{\kappa}$, as well as a rescaling factor in the denominator $1 - \hat{p}_e$. The extent to which the lack of a likelihood function relates to the above prevalence problem is worthy of consideration.

Another difficulty is that it is not generally well understood precisely what is, or should be,

meant by the "reliability" of a **binary** diagnostic test. With a view to exploring this, Cook & Farewell [5] describe a likelihood-based approach for the separate examination of the marginal agreement (relative magnitude of $p_1.$ and $p._1$) and subject-specific agreement (as measured by the **odds ratio**). Likelihood factorizations, conditioning arguments, and exact distributions facilitate detailed examination of well-defined and interpretable aspects of reliability.

In all of the recommended procedures cited above it must be borne in mind that the raw data for the 2×2 table under consideration consist only of four numbers and at most three **degrees of freedom**. Hence, presentation of three or four "summary" statistics does not serve the purpose of data reduction. Nevertheless, there appears to be general agreement that for the purpose of assessing reliability of a diagnostic test with a binary outcome, a single summary statistic is not adequate. The influence of the marginal frequencies on the kappa statistic is also present in the case of multiple nominal categories, but the precise nature of this influence is more difficult to characterize and is not well understood [9]. Chamberlin & Sprott [2] derive a discrete conditional distribution which may be used as a basis for conditional inference (see **Conditionality Principle**) on subject-specific agreement in this context.

References

[1]   Byrt, T., Bishop, J. & Carlin, J.B. (1993). Bias, prevalence and kappa, *Journal of Clinical Epidemiology* **46**, 423–424.

[2]   Chamberlin, S.R. & Sprott, D.A. (1991). On a discrete distribution associated with the statistical assessment of nominal scale agreement, *Discrete Mathematics* **92**, 39–47.

[3]   Cicchetti, D.V. & Feinstein, A.R. (1990). High agreement but low kappa. II. Resolving the paradoxes, *Journal of Clinical Epidemiology* **43**, 551–558.

[4]   Cohen, J. (1960). A coefficient of agreement for nominal scales, *Educational and Psychological Measurement* **20**, 37–46.

[5]   Cook, R.J. & Farewell, V.T. (1995). Conditional inference for subject-specific and marginal agreement: two families of agreement measures, *Canadian Journal of Statistics* **23**, 333–344.

[6]   Feinstein, A.R. & Cicchetti, D.V. (1990). High agreement but low kappa. I. The problems of two paradoxes, *Journal of Clinical Epidemiology* **43**, 543–549.

[7]   Kraemer, H.C. (1979). Ramifications of a population model for κ as a coefficient of reliability, *Psychometrika* **44**, 461–472.

[8]   Kraemer, H.C. & Bloch, A.D. (1988). Kappa coefficients in epidemiology. An appraisal of a reappraisal, *Journal of Clinical Epidemiology* **41**, 959–968.

[9]   Landis, R.J. & Koch, G.G. (1977). The measurement of observer agreement for categorical data, *Biometrics* **33**, 159–174.

[10]   Lantz, C.A. & Nebenzahl, E. (1996). Behaviour and interpretation of the κ statistic: resolution of the two paradoxes, *Journal of Clinical Epidemiology* **49**, 431–434.

[11]   Scott, W.A. (1955). Reliability and content analysis: the case of nominal scale coding, *Public Opinion Quarterly* **19**, 321–325.

[12]   Thompson, W.D. & Walter, S.D. (1988). A reappraisal of the kappa coefficient, *Journal of Clinical Epidemiology* **41**, 949–958.

[13]   Thompson, W.D. & Walter, S.D. (1988). Kappa and the concept of independent errors, *Journal of Clinical Epidemiology* **41**, 969–970.

(*See also* **Agreement, Measurement of; Observer Reliability and Agreement**)

RICHARD J. COOK

Karmarkar's Algorithm *see* Linear Programming

Kendall's Tau *see* Rank Correlation

Kendall, Maurice George

Born: September 6, 1907, in Kettering, UK.
Died: March 29, 1983, in Redhill, UK.

Despite showing only a belated interest in mathematics at school, Maurice Kendall obtained a scholarship to read mathematics at St John's College in Cambridge. He played cricket for his college and was a keen chess player, and gained a first class in both parts of the mathematical tripos.

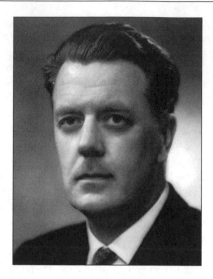

Reproduced by permission of the Royal Statistical Society

After graduating, he entered the administrative class of the Civil Service. Here, at the Ministry of Agriculture and Fisheries, he was responsible for statistical work. A chance meeting with **G. Udny Yule** in 1935 led to Kendall becoming co-author of a revision of Yule's classic textbook [9]. In 1941 Kendall became statistician to the British Chamber of Shipping, and in the following years he published many papers on theoretical statistics. This work was wide-ranging, but major themes were the theory of **rank correlation** coefficients (one of which he discovered in 1938 and now bears his name), **paired comparison** experiments, k statistics, and **time series**. At the same time, Kendall was working on his *Advanced Theory of Statistics*, the first advanced textbook on the subject. This was published as two volumes in 1943 and 1946 [1].

He was appointed professor of statistics at the London School of Economics in 1949, where he founded a research techniques division which carried out large **sample surveys**. In addition to this work and further theoretical research, in this period Kendall published the first important dictionary of statistical terms [4] and worked on the first comprehensive bibliography of statistical literature [5].

In 1961, during his presidency of the **Royal Statistical Society**, he again changed career, becoming scientific director (and ultimately chairman) of a computer consultancy (later called SCICON). During this spell he completed the rewriting of his influential book [1] into three volumes [6].

On retiring in 1972, Kendall embarked on another, testing career as the first director of the World Fertility Survey. This was a huge multinational sample survey project, which fully tested his extraordinary organizational powers. Ill health forced his retirement from this position in 1980.

Kendall was a prolific author, producing 17 books and around 75 papers on theoretical statistics alone. Seventeen of his papers are reprinted in [7], which also contains a bibliography. His other books included [2] and [3].

His interest in language was demonstrated by his literary style – "lucid, balanced, often ironical" [8] – but also by the word play in the spoof story of Lamia Gurdleneck and Sara Nuttal by K.A.C. Manderville in Volume 2 of *The Advanced Theory of Statistics* [6], in which all the names are anagrams of either Maurice (G.) Kendall or Alan Stuart, and his Longfellow pastiche *Hiawatha Designs an Experiment* (reprinted in [1]).

Kendall was much honored. He received the Guy medal in gold from the Royal Statistical Society. In 1974 he was knighted for his services to statistics, and on retiring from the World Fertility Survey he was awarded the United Nations peace medal.

References

[1]   Kendall, M.G. (1943 & 1946). *The Advanced Theory of Statistics*, Vols. 1 & 2. Griffin, London.
[2]   Kendall, M.G. (1948). *Rank Correlation Methods*. Griffin, London.
[3]   Kendall, M.G. (1975). *Multivariate Analysis*. Griffin, London.
[4]   Kendall, M.G. & Buckland, W.R. (1957). *Dictionary of Statistical Terms*. Oliver & Boyd, Edinburgh.
[5]   Kendall, M.G. & Doig, A.G. (1962, 1965, 1968). *Bibliography of Statistical Literature*, Vols. 1–3. Oliver & Boyd, Edinburgh.
[6]   Kendall, M.G. & Stuart, A. (1958, 1961, 1966). *The Advanced Theory of Statistics*, Vols. 1–3. Griffin, London.
[7]   Stuart, A. ed. (1984). *Statistics Theory and Practice. Selected Papers by Maurice Kendall* (1907–1983). Griffin, High Wycombe.
[8]   Stuart, A. (1984). Obituary of Sir Maurice Kendall, *Journal of the Royal Statistical Society, Series A* **147**, 120–122.
[9]   Yule, G.U. & Kendall, M.G. (1937). *An Introduction to the Theory of Statistics*, 11th Ed. Griffin, London.

D. ALTMAN

Kermack–McKendrick Threshold Theorem *see* Epidemic Thresholds

Kernel Estimator *see* Density Estimation

Kernel Regression *see* Nonparametric Regression

Kiefer–Wolfowitz Procedure *see* Stochastic Approximation

Kinship Coefficients *see* Identity Coefficients

Knowledge-Based System *see* Algorithm

Knox's Test *see* Clustering

Kolmogorov Differential Equation *see* Stochastic Processes

Kolmogorov, Andrey Nikolayevich

Born: April 23, 1903, in Tambov, Russia.
Died: October 20, 1987, in Moscow, Russia.

Kolmogorov is widely considered to be one of the greatest mathematicians of the twentieth century. He made important contributions to the theory of functions, topology, **probability theory**, statistics, logic, theory of dynamic systems, information theory, ergodic theory, theory of **algorithms**, mathematical education, and various applications of the above fields

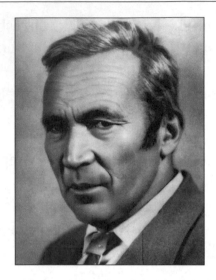

Reproduced by permission of the Royal Statistical Society

of mathematics. His works were mainly concerned with the intermediate areas between several "traditional" branches of mathematics and its applications, and he used fresh and striking ideas illuminating the relations between them. In the field of probability theory and statistics, Kolmogorov's main achievement is perhaps the introduction of the axioms and the clarification, through a rigorous approach, of various basic concepts. He was also famous as the leader of a school of numerous researchers, mainly his students and associates from the former USSR and Eastern block countries, whose work shaped probability theory (and to a lesser extent mathematical statistics) through the 1950s and 1960s.

During his career he held important administrative posts in the Moscow State (Lomonossov) University (MSU) and the USSR Academy of Sciences, including the headship of the Mechanics and Mathematics Department of the MSU, the Laboratory of Statistical Methods of MSU, and the chairmanship of the Mathematics Section of the Academy. Kolmogorov's personality had a great impact on everyone who came into contact with him, and in particular on hundreds of pupils at the specialist mathematical school for gifted children gathered from around the former Soviet Union, which he ran from the 1960s to the early 1980s.

In mathematical statistics, Kolmogorov is acclaimed worldwide for introducing the so-called **Kolmogorov–Smirnov statistic**. Based on this statistic (and its modifications), the Kolmogorov–Smirnov type tests

of **goodness of fit** have been developed, which are among the most widely used in statistical practice. The original references are [5], [8], [12], and [22–24], a detailed account of work done before 1970 can be found in [3], and further developments are commented on in [7].

In Soviet statistics, he is also considered as a founder of the modern approach to the **least squares** method, and his papers [13, 18] are widely quoted. In the West these papers became known much later (see, for example, [20] and [21]). The third direction stemming from Kolmogorov's theoretical work is related to **unbiased** estimators and their relation to **sufficient statistics** [15]. The first application of his approach was connected with industrial quality inspection and discussed in the (almost unobtainable) brochure [14]; it was further developed in [1] (for recent references, see [2]).

Kolmogorov was deeply interested in applied statistics, specifically in regard to the analysis of genetic experiments, turbulence, weather forecasting, analysis of geologic deposits, analysis of artillery fire precision (research conducted before and during the early part of World War II), and analysis of Russian poetry. Many of his ideas were later used in practical recommendations in various fields, including the Soviet nuclear and space programs, although he was never directly involved in any of these projects (unlike most of his contemporaries of a similar stature in the USSR, a fact of which he was rather proud). He was also a keen and original popularizer of statistics, notably through his articles for the *Great Soviet Encyclopedia*. In biostatistics, he was active in commenting on statistical confirmation of **Mendel's law** of genetics (see below) as well as in introducing and developing various mathematical models. For example, in [19] a nonlinear equation was analyzed rigorously in detail, describing the spread of an "advantageous gene". A similar equation was simultaneously proposed by **Fisher** [4], who predicted the long-term behavior of its solution, but did not provide a formal proof; this was done in [19] and subsequent papers. The equations studied in [19] and [4] are now often called Fisher or Kolmogorov–Petrovsky–Piskunov equations (another frequently used name is reaction–diffusion equations); their popularity in combustion theory far surpassed that in the analysis of biologic populations. Another notion connected with Kolmogorov's long-time interest in genetics was that of a **branching process**, introduced for the first time in [17], where the term "branching random processes" was first introduced (for related statistical considerations, see [9], [10], and [16]); again, the popularity of this concept in other applications exceeded that in the original field of theoretical biology.

Kolmogorov's participation in the discussion of the validity of Mendel's laws deserves a detailed account not only as being directly relevant to biostatistics, but also to illustrate the relation between statistics and "real life" at that time. The 1930s and the years following were a period of sharp struggle in Soviet biology. A group led by the infamous T.D. Lysenko started a ferocious campaign against Mendel's theory (and genetics in general) and its use in practice. Capitalizing on the support by Soviet officialdom, the followers of Lysenko denounced genetics as a "bourgeois pseudo-science", useless (or even harmful) for socialism and the future communist society. Their campaigning created an atmosphere of hysteria (matched by the general fear of repression of the period); as a result, many Soviet geneticists lost their jobs and some their lives. Kolmogorov had friendly ties with many of the leading USSR geneticists and was deeply interested in their experiments. In 1939 a collaborator of Lysenko published the results of a series of experiments with plants claiming that they disproved Mendel's 3:1 law. Kolmogorov [11] analyzed her data and, by performing a straightforward **chi-square test**, discovered that the experiments actually confirmed the 3:1 law. Given the circumstances of the time, this was an extraordinarily bold step. The paper [11] provoked an angry reply by Lysenko and his cronies, but luckily it did not cause serious harm to Kolmogorov. [At the same time similar experiments were conducted by another researcher, a follower of Vavilov, the leader of Soviet genetics (by that time dismissed from his positions and replaced by Lysenko; soon after, Vavilov himself was arrested and later died in prison in inhumane conditions). When the results of this series were shown to Kolmogorov, he immediately spotted that the author had "doctored" the data to make them fit exactly to the theoretical curve. I thank Prof. V.M. Tikhomirov, from Moscow State University, for providing me with this episode.] For a detailed account, see, for example, [6] and [25].

This and other episodes served to deter Kolmogorov from further experimentation in the subject. However, he kept a deep interest in biostatistics: in

the 1960s he organized the department of medical statistics in the Laboratory of Statistical Methods and took an active part in its work. His ideas are widely used in medical statistical practice, mostly in Russia, but their detailed account still awaits publication.

References

[1] Belyaev, Yu.K. (1975). *Probability Methods of Sample Control*. Nauka, Moscow (in Russian).

[2] Belyaev, Yu.K. & Lumel'skii, Ya.P. (1992). Unbiased estimators, in *Selected Works of A.N. Kolmogorov*, Vol. 2, A.N. Shiryayev, ed. Kluwer, Dordrecht, pp. 585–587.

[3] Durbin, J. (1973). Distribution theory for tests based on the sample distribution function, in *Regional Conference Series in Applied Mathematics*, Vol. 9, SIAM, Philadelphia.

[4] Fisher, R.A. (1937) The wave of advance of advantageous genes, *Annals of Eugenics* **7**, 355–369.

[5] Glivenko, V. (1933). On the empirical determination of a probability law, *Giornale dell'Istituto Italiano degli Attuari* **4**, 92–99 (in Italian).

[6] Joravsky, D. (1986). *The Lysenko Affair*. University of Chicago Press, Chicago.

[7] Khmaladze, E.V. (1992). Empirical distribution, in *Selected Works of A.N. Kolmogorov*, Vol. 2, A.N. Shiryayev, ed. Kluwer, Dordrecht, pp. 574–582.

[8] Kolmogorov, A.N. (1933). On the empirical determination of a distribution law, *Giornale dell'Istituto Italiano degli Attuari* **4**, 83–91 (in Italian); English translation in *Selected Works of A.N. Kolmogorov*, Vol. 2, A.N. Shiryayev, ed. Kluwer, Dordrecht, 1992, pp. 139–146.

[9] Kolmogorov, A.N. (1935). Deviations from Hardy's formulas under partial isolation, *Doklady Akademii Nauk SSSR* **3**, 129–132 (in Russian); English translation in *Selected Works of A.N. Kolmogorov*, Vol. 2, A.N. Shiryayev, ed. Kluwer, Dordrecht, 1992, pp. 179–181.

[10] Kolmogorov, A.N. (1938). Solution of a biological problem, *Izvestiya NII Matematiki i Mekhaniki Tomskogo Universiteta* **2**(1), 7–12 (in Russian); English translation in *Selected Works of A.N. Kolmogorov*, Vol. 2, A.N. Shiryayev, ed. Kluwer, Dordrecht, 1992, pp. 216–221.

[11] Kolmogorov, A.N. (1940). On a new confirmation of Mendel's laws, *Doklady Akademii Nauk SSSR*. **27**, 38–42 (in Russian); English translation in *Selected Works of A.N. Kolmogorov*, Vol. 2, A.N. Shiryayev, ed. Kluwer, Dordrecht, 1992, pp. 222–227.

[12] Kolmogorov, A.N. (1941). Confidence limits for an unknown distribution function, *Annals of Mathematical Statistics* **12**, 461–463.

[13] Kolmogorov, A.N. (1946). Justification of the method of least squares, *Uspekhi Matematicheskih Nauk* **1**,

57–70 (in Russian); English translation in *Selected Works of A.N. Kolmogorov*, Vol. 2, A.N. Shiryayev, ed. Kluwer, Dordrecht, 1992, pp. 285–302.

[14] Kolmogorov, A.N. (1950). *Statistical Inspection Control When the Admissible Number of Defects is Zero.* Izdatel'stvo Doma Nauchno-Tehnicheskoi Propagandy, Leningrad (in Russian).

[15] Kolmogorov, A.N. (1950). Unbiased estimators, *Izvestiya Akademii Nauk SSSR* **14**, 303–326 (in Russian); English translation in *Selected Works of A.N. Kolmogorov*, Vol. 2, A.N. Shiryayev, ed. Kluwer, Dordrecht, 1992, pp. 369–394.

[16] Kolmogorov, A.N. (1959). Transition of branching processes to diffusion processes and related genetic problems, *Teoriya Veroyatnosteii i E e Primeneniya* **4**, 233–236 (in Russian); English translation in *Selected Works of A.N. Kolmogorov*, Vol. 2, A.N. Shiryayev, ed. Kluwer, Dordrecht, 1992, pp. 466–469.

[17] Kolmogorov, A.N. & Dmitriev, N.A. (1947). Branching random processes, *Doklady Akademii Nauk SSSR* **56**, 7–10 (in Russian); English translation in *Selected Works of A.N. Kolmogorov*, Vol. 2, A.N. Shiryayev, ed. Kluwer, Dordrecht, 1992, pp. 309–314.

[18] Kolmogorov, A.N., Petrov, A.A. & Smirnov, Yu.M. (1947). A formula of Gauss in the method of least squares, *Izvestiya Akademii Nauk SSSR Matematicheskaya* **11**, 561–566 (in Russian); English translation in *Selected Works of A.N. Kolmogorov*, Vol. 2, A.N. Shiryayev, ed. Kluwer, Dordrecht, 1992, 303–308.

[19] Kolmogorov, A.N., Petrovsky, I.G. & Piskunov, N.S. (1937). A study of the diffusion equation with increase in the amount of substance, and its application to a biological problem, *Vestnik Moskovskogo Gosudarstvennogo Universiteta* **1**, 1–26 (in Russian); English translation in *Selected Works of A.N. Kolmogorov*, Vol. 1, V.M. Tikhomirov, ed. Kluwer, Dordrecht, 1991, pp. 242–270.

[20] Linnik, Yu.V. (1961). *Method of Least Squares and Principles of the Theory of Observations.* Oxford.

[21] Scheffé, H. (1959). *Analysis of Variance.* Wiley, New York.

[22] Smirnov, N.V. (1939). An estimate of the discrepancy between empirical distribution curves in two independent samples, *Bulleten' Moskovskogo Gosudarstvennogo Universiteta, Ser. Matematika, Mekhanika* **2**, 3–14 (in Russian).

[23] Smirnov, N.V. (1939). On the deviation of the empirical distribution curve, *Matematicheskii Sbornik* **6**, 3–24 (in Russian).

[24] Smirnov, N.V. (1948). Tables for estimating the goodness of fit of empirical distribution, *Annals of Mathematical Statistics* **19**, 279–281.

[25] Soyfer, V. (1994). *Lysenko and the Tragedy of Soviet Science.* Rutgers University Press, New Brunswick.

YURII SUHOV

Kolmogorov–Smirnov and Cramér–Von Mises Tests in Survival Analysis

The classical one-sample Kolmogorov goodness-of-fit statistic and the two-sample Smirnov statistic are well-known general statistical procedures. They are collectively known as **Kolmogorov–Smirnov (K–S) tests**. Using these techniques in **survival analysis**, modifications have to be made to deal with **censored data**. There are various types of censoring. What is generally known as type I involves observations being known precisely if they are less than a fixed value and only known to exceed the value otherwise. For so-called type II censoring, the smallest r, say, observations out of a possible n are observed. These definitions of censoring are somewhat restricted in terms of survival analysis. Generally, it is assumed that censoring is random for each observation, and special modifications and assumptions are required. For further discussions of censoring see Michael & Schucany [7] for a succinct account, or Andersen et al. [1] for a full account of censoring in the context of survival data.

For type I or type II censoring, adaptations of the Kolmogorov statistic have been made by Barr & Davidson [2], where small-sample percentage points are tabulated; see also Dufour & Maag [3] for modified statistics which can be used with the asymptotic percentage points found by Koziol & Byar [6].

For survival analysis the random censoring case is more commonly met. Fleming et al. [4] proposed one sample and two sample K–S type procedures with randomly censored data. Efficient procedures exist for comparing two populations, such as the **logrank test** for **proportional hazards** and Gehan–Wilcoxon tests (*see* **Nonparametric Methods**), when survival distributions have **proportional odds**. For some alternatives, such as where the difference between two survival curves occurs primarily at a given time, the K–S two-sample statistic should have good power. Examples of this situation occur, for example, in a treatment regime where individuals might obtain short-term benefits but when compared with controls there is no benefit in the longer term. Other examples for which the logrank and Gehan–Wilcoxon tests would have little power include the class of models known as *crossing-hazards*.

Fleming et al. [4] modified the K–S procedures so as to deal with randomly right-censored data. Asymptotic results are obtained for the censoring mechanism being independent of the survival time. The K–S statistics are defined in terms of the difference of two distribution functions, $F_u(t)$ and $F_v(t)$, where $F_u(t)$ is the empirical (sample) distribution function (edf) and, for the one-sample goodness-of-fit statistic, $F_v(t)$ is a hypothesized distribution function and, for the two-sample case, $F_v(t)$ is the edf of the second sample. The classical two-sided K–S statistic is

$$D = \sup_t |F_u(t) - F_v(t)|$$

or, alternatively, with survivor functions $S.(\cdot)$ replacing distribution functions $F.(\cdot)$:

$$D = \sup_t |S_u(t) - S_v(t)|.$$

To obtain statistics which can deal with censored samples, Fleming et al. [4] modify the statistic D and they give computing formulas for the one-sample and two-sample statistics. They also give a simple formula to calculate **P values** based on the asymptotic distribution of the statistic, which, in **simulation** studies, were found to be conservative for the modified two-sample Smirnov statistic with heavily censored data in small samples. Later work of Guilbaud [5] gives exact small sample percentage points for the K–S type statistic.

In **Monte Carlo** simulations, Fleming et al. [4] investigate the power of the modified Smirnov two-sample statistic and compare it with Gehan–Wilcoxon and logrank statistics for various alternatives. For those alternatives purposely designed to have substantial differences between the two survivor functions at a given time and not necessarily at other times, the modified Smirnov statistic had good power. It is suggested that the modified statistics should be used in conjunction with the Gehan–Wilcoxon and logrank statistics and, of course, plots of the survivor functions.

Further results on the **power** of the modified Smirnov statistic are given by Stablein & Koutrouvelis [10] who consider crossing hazards alternatives. For such alternatives the modified Smirnov statistic has very good power, considerably in excess of the logrank statistic.

Schumacher [9] also investigates a Smirnov statistic (called by the author a K–S statistic), which has as its asymptotic distribution the supremum of the Brownian bridge (*see* **Brownian Motion and Diffusion Processes**). In simulation studies the finite sample distributions are found to converge slowly to the asymptotic distribution, and consequently the author is not keen to recommend their use. However, with cheap computing it is a straightforward matter to simulate such statistics, and this is a harsh conclusion.

In the book by Andersen et al. [1] further references are given to more recent work and the authors take an approach which defines statistics having their asymptotic distribution given by distributions derived from the Brownian bridge.

Cramér–von Mises (C–VM) statistics can be defined for the one-sample problem for types I and II censoring as described above. In general form they are defined by

$$\omega^2 = \int [F_u(t) - F_v(t)]^2 \psi(t)\mathrm{d}t,$$

where the same notation is used as above for the K–S statistics and ψ is a weight function. Pettitt & Stephens [8] modify the C–VM statistic to deal with this type of censoring and give computing formulas for the one-sample statistics and tabulate asymptotic distributions when the null hypothesis completely determines the survival function.

Koziol & Green [6] introduce a Cramér–von Mises statistic to test the **goodness of fit** for randomly censored data survival times. They also assume independent censoring where the survival function of the censoring distribution is that of the survival times raised to a positive power, β. They find the asymptotic distribution of the C–VM statistic, which is quite sensitive to the value of β. They discuss how to estimate β from the sample. However, this restiction seems rather harsh for application to survival data found in practice.

Schumacher [9] considers C–VM statistics for the two-sample problem which have their asymptotic distributions given by the standard form, i.e. the integral of the square of the Brownian bridge, and in simulation studies finds that the asymptotic distribution is acceptable for small samples. In a power study, the two-sample C–VM statistic was found to have good power for a crossing survival curve alternative and an "early difference" case. Schumacher [9] also gives references to earlier works and tables of percentage points of various functionals of the Brownian bridge which arise as asymptotic distributions of K–S and C–VM type test statistics.

Values of the various goodness-of-fit and two-sample statistics should be enhanced by plots of data, or vice versa, and Michael & Schucany [7] give details of a number of plots for censored data.

In conclusion, the K–S and C–VM statistics provide useful procedures to detect differences, either in the one- or two-sample cases, which are less likely to be detected using tests based on proportional hazards or proportional odds assumptions.

References

[1]   Andersen, P.K., Borgan, Ø., Gill, R.D. & Keiding, N. (1993). *Statistical Models Based on Counting Processes*. Springer-Verlag, New York.

[2]   Barr, D.R. & Davidson, T. (1973). A Kolmogorov-Smirnov test for censored samples, *Technometrics* **15**, 739–757.

[3]   Dufour, R. & Maag, U.R. (1978). Distribution results for modified Kolmogorov–Smirnov statistics for truncated or censored data, *Technometrics* **20**, 29–32.

[4]   Fleming, T.R.,   O'Fallon, J.R.,   O'Brien, P.C.   & Harrington, D.P. (1980). Modified Kolmogorov–Smirnov test procedures with application to arbitrarily right-censored data, *Biometrics* **36**, 607–625.

[5]   Guilbaud, O. (1988). Exact Kolmogorov-type tests for left-truncated and/or right censored data, *Journal of the American Statistical Association* **83**, 213–221.

[6]   Koziol, J.R. & Byar, D.P. (1975). Percentage points of the asymptotic distribution of one and two sample K–S statistics for truncated or censored data, *Technometrics* **17**, 507–510.

[7]   Michael, J.R. & Schucany, W.R. (1986). Analysis of data from censored samples, in *Goodness-of-Fit Techniques*, R.B. D'Agostino & M.A. Stephens, eds. Marcel Dekker, New York, pp. 461–496.

[8]   Pettitt, A.N.   &   Stephens, M.A.   (1976).   Modified Cramér–von Mises statistics for censored data, *Biometrika* **63**, 291–298.

[9]   Schumacher, M. (1984). Two-sample tests of Cramér–von Mises and Kolmogorov–Smirnov-type for randomly censored data, *International Statistical Review* **52**, 263–281.

[10]   Stablein, D.M. & Koutrouvelis, I.A. (1985). A two-sample test sensitive to crossing hazards in uncensored and singly censored data, *Biometrics* **41**, 643–652.

(*See also* **Hypothesis Testing**)

ANTHONY N. PETTITT

Kolmogorov–Smirnov Test

Consider two independent groups of subjects. To be concrete, suppose an experimental group consists of sons of alcoholic fathers, and each subject consumes a precise amount of alcohol. Suppose some outcome, X, is measured, such as hangover symptoms, and let Y be the outcome for a control group. Let $F(x)$ be the probability that a randomly sampled subject from the experimental group gets a score less than or equal to x. Similarly, let $G(x)$ be the probability that a randomly sampled subject from the control group gets a score less than or equal to x. The Kolmogorov distance between these two distributions is the maximum possible value of $|F(x) - G(x)|$, the maximum being taken over all possible values of x. If the distributions are identical, meaning that $F(x) = G(x)$ for all possible values of x, then the Kolmogorov distance is zero. From a graphical point of view the Kolmogorov distance is the largest vertical distance between the two cumulative distribution functions.

Kolmogorov-type tests are methods for comparing distributions that are based on the Kolmogorov distance function. In some cases one of the distributions might be specified. For example, it might be hypothesized that $F(x)$ is a normal distribution with specified mean and variance, and the goal might be to determine whether this hypothesis is reasonable based on observations that are available. This hypothesis can be tested with what is called a Kolmogorov test. A Kolmogorov–Smirnov test is a Kolmogorov-type test where the goal is to compare two unknown distributions. That is, $F(x)$ and $G(x)$ are not known for any x, but they can be estimated based on randomly sampled subjects from each group, and the goal is to test $H_0 : F(x) = G(x)$, for any x, the hypothesis that the two distributions are identical.

Let $X_1, \ldots, X_m$ be a random sample of observations from the first group, let $Y_1, \ldots, Y_n$ be a random sample from the second, and let $Z_1, \ldots, Z_N$ be the pooled observations, where $N = n + m$. That is, $Z_i = X_i, i = 1, \ldots, m$, and $Z_{n+i} = Y_i, i = 1, \ldots, n$. For any x, let $a_i = 1$ if $X_i \leq x$, otherwise $a_i = 0$. Similarly, let $b_i = 1$ if $Y_i \leq x$, otherwise $b_i = 0$. Let $\hat{F}(x) = \sum a_i/m$ and $\hat{G}(x) = \sum b_i/n$. The Kolmogorov distance between the distributions F and G

is estimated by

$$D = \max |\hat{F}(Z_i) - \hat{G}(Z_i)|,$$

where the maximum is taken over all $i = 1, \ldots, N$. If D is sufficiently large, then reject H_0. When there are no ties, the exact probability of a type I error (*see* **Level of a Test**) can be determined using an algorithm derived by Kim & Jennrich [3]. When there are tied values, results in [4] can be used. Details about these algorithms, together with appropriate software, are summarized in [7].

A common criticism of the Kolmogorov–Smirnov test is that it has low **power** under normality. Table 1 compares its power with several other methods for comparing measures of location. The methods are **Student's t** (T), Welch's adjusted degrees of freedom procedure (W), Yuen's [8] method for trimmed means that reduces to Welch's test when there is no trimming (Y), and a method for comparing one-step M-estimators (*see* **Robustness**) using a **bootstrap method** (OSM). (For details about these tests, see [6].) In Table 1 the first three distributions are normal with variance one, and the difference between the means is δ. The notation CN1 refers to a symmetric heavy-tailed distribution that is a mixture of two normal distributions. It has distribution

$$H(x) = 0.9\Phi(x) + 0.1\Phi\left(\frac{x}{k}\right),$$

with $k = 10$, and where $\Phi(x)$ is the standard normal distribution. That is, with probability 0.9, an observation is sampled from a standard normal distribution, otherwise sampling is from a normal distribution having standard deviation $k = 10$. The difference between the standard normal and CN1 is small as measured by the Kolmogorov distance – it is less than 0.04. Despite this, the variance is equal to 10.9 vs. 1 for the standard normal. The distribution CN2 is the same as CN1, only $k = 20$. Finally, Expo

indicates an **exponential distribution**, and Logn is **lognormal**. The column headed KS (exact) means that the smallest critical value is used such that the probability of a type I error does not exceed $\alpha = 0.05$. The exact probability of a type I error is 0.036. The last column reports power when the critical value is chosen so that the probability of a type I error is as close as possible to 0.05, which in this case is 0.052.

As would be expected, methods for comparing measures of location have more power when sampling from normal distributions, but, with even slight departures from normality (CN1 and CN2), the Kolmogorov–Smirnov test has substantially more power than methods based on means, and it competes well with methods based on robust measures of location.

A criticism of the Kolmogorov–Smirnov test is that when the sample sizes are small, there are situations where the exact probability of a type I error might not be acceptably close to some desired level, because the test statistic, D, has a discrete distribution. Suppose, for example, $\alpha = 0.05$, and consider $n = m = 10$. The exact probability of a type I error, based on the critical value in [1], is 0.035. For $n = m = 11, 12$, and 13 the exact type I error probabilities are 0.036, 0.031, and 0.044, but for $n = m = 14$ it is 0.019, which might be considered too small. However, the next highest significance level is 0.12 which might be considered too high. This problem might be used to argue for comparing some measure of location, but most methods for comparing measures of location can also yield unsatisfactory control over the probability of a type I error, particularly methods based on means (see, for instance [5] and [6]). An exception appears to be a percentile t bootstrap combined with a 20% **trimmed** mean (see [7]).

An advantage of the Kolmogorov–Smirnov test is that it is sensitive to several features of the data which

Table 1 Estimated power, $m = n = 25, \alpha = 0.05$

Distributions	δ	T	W	Y	OSM	KS (exact)	KS ($\alpha = 0.052$)
Normal	0.6	0.529	0.536	0.464	0.531	0.384	0.464
Normal	0.8	0.778	0.780	0.721	0.751	0.608	0.700
Normal	1.0	0.925	0.931	0.890	0.921	0.814	0.872
CN1	1.0	0.326	0.278	0.784	0.788	0.688	0.780
CN2	1.0	0.191	0.162	0.602	0.760	0.698	0.772
Expo	0.6	0.539	0.697	0.623	0.592	0.866	0.867
Logn	0.6	0.232	0.243	0.409	0.363	0.666	0.678

can be revealed using the method described in [2]. This uses the Kolmogorov–Smirnov test statistic to compute a **confidence interval** for the difference between any two **quantiles** such that the simultaneous probability coverage of all such intervals is determined exactly. Note that the 0.2 quantile, for example, of the first group might be larger than the 0.2 quantile of the second, but when the 0.8 quantiles are compared the reverse can be true. That is, the confidence band can indicate a difference between subpopulations of subjects that is completely missed when attention is restricted to a measure of location. Doksum & Sievers [2] suggest plotting the estimated quantiles of the first group vs. the difference between the quantiles. Letting $\hat{x}_q$ and $\hat{y}_q$ be the quantiles of the two groups, plot $\hat{x}_q$ vs. $\delta = \hat{x}_q - \hat{y}_q$. For illustrations and software, see [7].

References

[1]   Conover, W.J. (1980). *Practical Nonparametric Statistics*. Wiley, New York.

[2]   Doksum, K.A. & Sievers, G.L. (1976). Plotting with confidence: graphical comparisons of two populations, *Biometrika* **63**, 421–434.

[3]   Kim, P.J. & Jennrich, R.I. (1973). Tables of the exact sampling distribution of the two-sample Kolmogorov–Smirnov criterion, $D_{mn}, m \leq n$, in *Selected Tables in Mathematical Statistics*, Vol. I, H.L. Harter & D.B. Owen, eds. American Mathematical Society, Providence.

[4]   Schroër, G. & Trenkler, D. (1995). Exact and randomization distributions of Kolmogorov–Smirnov tests for two or three samples, *Computational Statistics and Data Analysis* **20**, 185–202.

[5]   Westfall, P.H. & Young, S.S. (1993). *Resampling-Based Multiple Testing*. Wiley, New York.

[6]   Wilcox, R.R. (1996). *Statistics for the Social Sciences*. Academic Press, San Diego.

[7]   Wilcox, R.R. (1997). *Introduction to Robust Estimation and Hypothesis Testing*. Academic Press, San Diego.

[8]   Yuen, K.K. (1974). The two-sample trimmed t for unequal population variances, *Biometrika* **61**, 165–170.

(*See also* **Nonparametric Methods**)

R. WILCOX

Kosambi Map Function *see* Genetic Map Functions

Kriging *see* Statistical Map

Kruskal–Wallis Test *see* Nonparametric Methods

Kullback–Leibler Information

The Kullback–Leibler [5] information number, $I(P\|Q)$, determined for two probability measures defined on the same measurable space $(\chi, \mathcal{F})$, is a nonnegative number (possibly $+\infty$) which represents "distance" (in a certain sense) between P and Q. This "distance" is not symmetric [in general, $I(P\|Q) \neq I(Q\|P)$], but does have the property that $I(P\|Q) = 0$ if and only if $P = Q$. This quantity is also referred to by a myriad of other names, including information for discrimination, discrimination information, Renyi's information gain, entropy distance, entropy of P relative to Q, cross-entropy, directed divergence, Kullback information.

If P is absolutely continuous with respect to $Q(P \ll Q)$, the **Radon–Nikodým** derivative $P_Q(x)$ is defined almost surely (Q) and serves as a basis for the general definition:

$$I(P\|Q) = \begin{cases} \int_\chi \ln P_Q \, dP = \int_\chi P_Q \ln P_Q \, dQ, \\ \qquad\qquad P \ll Q, \\ +\infty, \qquad P \not\ll Q. \end{cases}$$

Note that, if R is a sigma-finite measure such that $P \ll Q \ll R$, we can also write

$$I(P\|Q) = \int_\chi P_R \ln(P_R/Q_R) \, dR.$$

Thus, for the common situation where P and Q are discrete (and R is the counting measure), the Kullback–Leibler information number reduces to

$$I(P\|Q) = \sum_i p_i \ln\left(\frac{p_i}{q_i}\right),$$

where p_i and q_i are the standard probability mass functions. Note also that, if X is a random vector with probability distribution P, then $I(P\|Q)$ can be interpreted as the expectation of the log of a **likelihood ratio** statistic.

If Q is a uniform measure over a finite set of points and P is a probability measure on the same points, then $I(P\|Q)$ is just the negative of the well-known Shannon entropy [8]. This quantity is very important in statistical information theory, which has its mathematical roots in the concept of entropy in thermodynamics and statistical mechanics.

Given a probability measure Q on a measurable space, the convex set of probability measures defined by

$$S(Q, \rho) = [P : I(P\|Q) < \rho]$$

is often called the I-sphere with center Q and radius ρ. If $\mathcal{E}$ is a convex set of probability measures intersecting $S(Q, \infty)$, a probability measure $R \in \mathcal{E}$ satisfying

$$I(R\|Q) = \inf_{P \in \mathcal{E}} I(P\|Q) \qquad (1)$$

is called the I-projection of Q onto $\mathcal{E}$. Csiszar [1] has shown that the I-projection exists if the convex set $\mathcal{E}$ is closed in variation distance and has also developed an appealing "geometric" approach which characterizes the "tangent hyperplanes" of I-spheres $S(Q, \rho)$.

Problems of the type (1) play a basic role in the information theoretic approach to statistics [4], the theory of large deviations [6], and in statistical physics [3]. Dykstra & Lemke [2] have shown that problems of the form (1) are often equivalent to **multinomial** maximum likelihood problems under various types of constraint regions.

Kullback–Leibler information numbers between distributions in a common family are often quite tractable. Thus, if P and Q are **Poisson distributions** with respective means m_1 and m_2, it is easily shown that $I(P\|Q) = m_1 \ln(m_1/m_2) + m_2 - m_1$.

If P and Q are k-variate normal distributions (*see* **Multivariate Normal Distribution**) with respective mean vectors μ_1 and μ_2 and respective **covariance matrices** Σ_1 and Σ_2, then

$$I(P\|Q) = \tfrac{1}{2} \ln \left(\det \Sigma_2 / \det \Sigma_1 \right)$$
$$+ \tfrac{1}{2} \mathrm{tr} \Sigma_1 \left(\Sigma_2^{-1} - \Sigma_1^{-1} \right)$$
$$+ \tfrac{1}{2} \mathrm{tr} \Sigma_2^{-1} (\mu_1 - \mu_2)(\mu_1 - \mu_2)'.$$

Thus, when $\Sigma_1 = \Sigma_2 = \Sigma$, $I(P\|Q)$ reduces to the natural **Mahalanobis distance** $\tfrac{1}{2}(\mu_1 - \mu_2)' \Sigma^{-1}(\mu_1 - \mu_2)$ between the two mean vectors.

Though Kullback–Leibler information seems very different from the statistical concept of Fisher **information**, there is actually a rather remarkable connection. For example, if we have multinomial distributions whose probabilities $\pi_i(\theta)$, $i = 0, 1, \ldots, k$, depend upon the parameter θ, then

$$\lim_{\Delta\theta \to 0} \frac{I[\Pi(\theta + \Delta\theta)\|\Pi(\theta)]}{(\Delta\theta)^2} = \tfrac{1}{2} I_F(\theta),$$

where I_F denotes the Fisher information and the Kullback–Leibler information number is calculated from the appropriate multinomial distributions [7, Chapter 15].

If P_n denotes an empirical distribution from a random sample and $\mathcal{E}$ denotes a family of possible models, then a natural estimate of a model from the family is the one (in $\mathcal{E}$) closest to P_n. "Closest" here means in the sense of the Kullback–Leibler information number, i.e. the I-projection of P_n onto $\mathcal{E}$.

Moreover, $2n \inf_{P \in \mathcal{E}} I(P\|P_n)$ is often a desirable test statistic (with nice asymptotic properties) for testing whether the actual distribution is contained in $\mathcal{E}$ (*see* **Large-Sample Theory**).

References

[1]   Csiszár, I. (1975). I-divergence geometry of probability distributions and minimization problems, *Annals of Probability* **3**, 146–158.

[2]   Dykstra, R.L. & Lemke, J. (1988). Duality of I-projections and maximum likelihood estimation for log-linear models under cone constraints, *Journal of the American Statistical Association* **83**, 546–554.

[3]   Jaynes, E.T. (1957). Information theory and statistical mechanics, *Physical Review* **106**, 620–630.

[4]   Kullback, S. (1959). *Information Theory and Statistics*. Wiley, New York, 1968; Peter Smith Publisher, Magnolia, 1978.

[5]   Kullback, S. & Leibler, R.A. (1951). On information and sufficiency, *Annals of Mathematical Statistics* **22**, 79–86.

[6]   Sanov, I.N. (1957). On the probability of large deviations of random variables, *Matemateceskii Sbornick N.S.*
42, 11–44.

[7]   Savage, Leonard J. (1972). *The Foundations of Statistics.* Dover, New York.

[8]   Shannon, C.E. (1948). A mathematical theory of
communication, *Bell Systems Technical Journal* **27**,
379–423, 623–656.

RICHARD DYKSTRA

Kurczynski's D^2 *see* Genetic Distance

Kurtosis

Kurtosis is related to the standardized fourth **moment** of a distribution. It is expressed in a number of ways, the most common being

$$\beta_2 = \mu_4/\sigma^4 \quad \text{and} \quad \gamma_2 = \beta_2 - 3,$$

where μ_4 and σ^2 are, respectively, the fourth central moment and the variance of the distribution. Often it is used as a measure to judge the deviation of a distribution from normality. For the **normal distribution**, $\beta_2 = 3$ and $\gamma_2 = 0$. Unimodal distributions with values of β_2 greater than 3 (called *leptokurtic*) usually indicate that the distribution displays a higher "peak" around the mean, and also more probability in the tails of the distribution, than does the normal (see Figure 1). These distributions are also called thick-(or long-)tailed distributions [3, Chapter 9]. Those with β_2 less than 3 (called *platykurtic*) usually are more concentrated about the mean and flatter than the normal. β_2 cannot be less than 1. Those with $\beta_2 = 3$ are called *mesokurtic*.

Sample measures of kurtosis are used in tests of normality. A common test statistic is $b_2 = m_4/m_2^2$, where m_2 and m_4 are the second and fourth moments about the mean (see [3, Chapter 9]). Extensive tables of the **sampling distribution**, as well as approximations, exist for the null distribution of b_2 [3, 4, 7]. Also, it is often used jointly with a measure of **skewness** ($b_1 = m_3/m_2^{3/2}$) to evaluate deviations

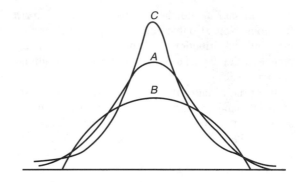

Figure 1   Unimodal   distributions: $A = \beta_2 = 3$; $B = \beta_2 < 3$; $C = \beta_2 > 3$

from normality [2, 3]. D'Agostino & Pearson [2] and D'Agostino et al. [5] developed a **chi-square distribution** approximation that combines b_2 with b_1 for an omnibus test. It is a useful adjunct to normal probability plots [5] (*see* **Normal Scores**).

There have been a number of attempts to generalize kurtosis to the multivariate setting. These have often been in the context of developing **tests of multivariate normality**.

In the case of nonnormality, knowledge of kurtosis is useful in evaluating the **robustness** of standard statistical procedures such as the **Student's t tests** [8] and in developing measures of location [1]. For this latter situation in particular, the tail thickness of a distribution is often very important and some have questioned the usefulness of b_2 for evaluating it. Alternative measures based on sample **quantiles** have been suggested [6, 9].

References

[1]   D'Agostino, R.B. & Lee, A.F. (1977). Robustness of
location estimators under changes of population kurtosis, *Journal of the American Statistical Association* **72**,
393–396.

[2]   D'Agostino, R.B. & Pearson, E.S. (1973). Testing for
departures from normality. I. Fuller empirical results for
the distribution of b_2 and b_1, *Biometrika* **60**, 613–622.

[3]   D'Agostino, R.B. & Stephens, M.A. (1986). *Goodness-
of-Fit Techniques.* Marcel Dekker, New York.

[4]   D'Agostino, R.B. & Tietjen, G.L. (1971). Simulation
probability points for b_2 for small samples, *Biometrika*
58, 669–672.

[5]   D'Agostino, R.B., Belanger, A.J. & D'Agostino, R.B.,
Jr (1990). A suggestion for using powerful and

informative tests of normality, *American Statistician* **44**, 316–321.

[6] Hogg, R.V. (1972). More light on the kurtosis and related statistics, *Journal of the American Statistical Association* **67**, 422–424.

[7] Pearson, E.S. & Hartley, H.O. (1954). *Biometrika Tables for Statisticians*, Vol. 1. Cambridge University Press, Cambridge.

[8] Pearson, E.S. & Please, N.W. (1975). Relation between the shape of a population and the robustness of four simple test statistics, *Biometrika* **62**, 223–241.

[9] Royston, P. (1992). Which measures of skewness and kurtosis are best?, *Statistics in Medicine* **11**, 333–343.

RALPH B. D'AGOSTINO, SR

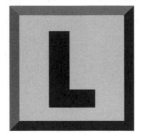

L-Estimator *see* Robustness

L_1 Regression *see* Least Squares

L_p Regression *see* Robust Regression

Laboratory Quality Control

Quality control, or more broadly quality assurance, is an essential part of the conduct of an analytic laboratory. This is especially critical for clinical laboratories since errors in measurement can lead to inappropriate treatment of patients. A full treatment of the many management, planning, record keeping, and audit procedures is beyond the scope of this article (see Garfield [1] for these concerns); we concentrate on a few critical issues in statistical quality control as they impact analytical laboratories.

Estimation of Precision

An important issue in an analytic laboratory involves the attachment of **standard errors** to measured values. Although every effort should be made to avoid bias, it may be difficult to estimate the remaining bias, so standard errors are usually based on the precision of measurements; that is, the standard deviation (sd) of repeat measurements made under identical conditions. This is necessarily only a lower bound on the true error standard deviation.

It will hardly ever be the case that the error standard deviation is constant, independent of the level measured. For large concentrations of the analyte, the standard deviation will often be approximately a multiple of the concentration (more generally, this may be a power function). If small concentrations (near the limit of detection) are not of interest, then a linear equation describing the relationship between the precision and the concentration can be estimated from a series of repeat measurements at several concentrations, by regressing the standard deviation of the repeats on the mean of the repeats. This can often be done during the process of producing a **calibration** curve for the instrument.

If values near the limit of detection are of interest, then a more complex method is called for. Rocke & Lorenzato [10] present a model in which an additive error and a multiplicative error are both present, which allows for realistic behavior at both high and low concentrations. This model can also be estimated during the calibration process.

Control Charts

There are many problems, systematic and sporadic, that can interfere with the accurate determination of values in the analytic laboratory. Reagents may lose potency, temperature or humidity may affect the results, and operators may differ in their technique. There are many methods of statistical quality control that can be used to detect these problems; detailed descriptions may be found in Wadsworth et al. [11] and Montgomery [5]. Two of the most important will be described here. These are Shewhart charts, also known as $\overline{X}$ and R charts, which are used to detect general departure from a state of statistical control, and CUSUM charts, which are used to detect a shift in the mean.

The "state of statistical control" referred to above is, in the context of laboratory errors, one in which measurement errors have zero mean and a standard deviation that does not change with time (although it may differ with the concentration of the analyte), and in which successive measurement errors are not correlated.

Shewhart Charts

Periodically, a small group of repeat measurements is taken on a standard solution. At time t, k replicates are taken, denoted x_{it}, where $1 \leq i \leq k$. The mean $\overline{X}_t$ and the **range** R_t are computed. If the process is in a state of statistical control, and under the additional assumption of normality, each value of the range is an estimate of a multiple of the standard deviation, the value of the multiplier being given in standard tables (see, for example, Wadsworth et al. [11] or Montgomery [5]). After 10 or 20 groups have been accumulated, the mean of the ranges $\overline{R}$, when multiplied by a standardizing constant, is an estimate of the process standard deviation. For example, if $k = 3$, then $\overline{R}/1.693$ is an estimate $\hat{\sigma}$ of the process sd σ.

The group means are then plotted on a chart which has a centerline equal either to the known value for the reference solution or to the average of the group means, and which has two reference lines above and below the centerline at a distance of $\pm 3\hat{\sigma}/\sqrt{k}$ (this whole quantity can be computed as a multiple A_2 of $\overline{R}$). Since the estimate of the process standard deviation is based on the variability of repeats, any factor such as temperature changes, or operator technique, that varies from group to group but not within a group will generate extra variability. If there are no such extra factors (called special causes), and all the variability is caused by the repeat variation (common cause), then the group means will lie outside the two reference lines (called control limits) only very rarely. If, on the other hand,

some extra factor is an important cause of variability, then the group mean will more frequently lie outside the control limits. When this event occurs (a signal, in quality control terminology), the cause of the extra variability should be sought, and eliminated or reduced.

Similarly, the group ranges are plotted on a chart that has a centerline at $\overline{R}$ and control limits at multiples D_3 and D_4 of $\overline{R}$, calculated to be three standard errors above and below the centerline. Any values outside these control limits also indicate a probable departure from a state of statistical control.

Over time, this attention to Shewhart charts, and subsequent investigation of problems, should place the measurement process in a state of statistical control. Continued attention is required to detect later departures from this desirable condition.

CUSUM Charts

Shewhart charts are designed to detect many kinds of departure from a state of statistical control, and are therefore not particularly sensitive to any given one of these. A frequent concern is a shift in the process mean, which would involve, in the laboratory context, the development of a bias in the measurements. Cumulative sum (CUSUM) charts are specifically designed to detect this type of departure, which is often of great concern in the analytic laboratory. More details on this methodology may be found in Wadsworth et al. [11] or in Hawkins & Olwell [3]. Briefly, CUSUM charts achieve their superior detection ability by adding up successive deviations of the group mean $\overline{X}$ from the correct value μ. This allows a small difference to accumulate until a strong signal can be observed; however, it would also allow extremely tiny signals to eventually manifest themselves even if the difference were of no practical importance. The user must therefore specify a critical shift Δ that may be of importance to detect. One then defines the upper CUSUM S_t and the lower CUSUM T_t recursively by

$$S_t = \max(0, S_{t-1} + \overline{X}_t - F),$$

$$T_t = \min(0, T_{t-1} + \overline{X}_t + F),$$

where F is usually taken to be approximately $\Delta/2$. If the mean has shifted by as much as Δ, then the upper (respectively lower) CUSUM will exhibit a trend that will eventually pass any fixed control limits.

Control limits for the upper and lower CUSUMs are derivable from somewhat complicated numerical calculations and must be found in tables in one of the cited references. They are designed so that if the process is in control, the renewal process that would then describe the path of the CUSUM variables would have an expected first passage time (called the *average run length*) that would be sufficiently large not to induce many false alarms. In the form in which we have written the CUSUM, the control limits will be at multiples of the process standard deviation. The originally developed form of the CUSUM chart uses a different, but entirely equivalent, method of determining control limits, called a V-mask. This alternative formulation is described in Wadsworth et al. [11] and Hawkins & Olwell [3].

Proficiency Testing

Proficiency testing is used internally by analytic laboratories to evaluate their own performance and externally to develop new analytic methods or to validate the performance of laboratories. This will usually involve the submission of spiked samples to the analytic process which are blind (the amount present is not known to the analyst) or double-blind (the analyst does not know that the sample is a check sample and not a routine sample). Detailed discussion of these issues may be found Garfield [1] and Youden & Steiner [12].

Intralaboratory Studies

These studies are used by laboratories to check themselves or to improve operations. Blind or double-blind samples can be routinely run and used as the input for control charts or for examination of specific results. Another useful method is Youden's ruggedness testing [12], in which a designed experiment is used deliberately to vary the conditions of the analysis in order to find out what factors influence the variability of the results. An example of this type of study for immunoassays may be found in Jones et al. [4].

Interlaboratory Studies

Interlaboratory studies are an essential component in the development of analytic methods. A proposed method is described to a series of laboratories, each

of which receive a series of samples to analyze. The variability of a measured result then can be partitioned into within-laboratory variance (repeatability or precision) and between-laboratory variance. The total variability, which is the sum of the within- and between-laboratory variances, is called the reproducibility and is a measure of accuracy.

Ideally, the between-laboratory variance would be small, but in practice it is often considerably larger than the within-laboratory variance. This may be due to inadequately described methods, or to the influence of identifiable factors that can be determined with ruggedness testing and controlled in a revised procedure. Poorly performing laboratories may also be identified in an interlaboratory study; Youden & Steiner [12] gives a rank test for this purpose.

Outliers

Outliers can cause a significant disruption in quality control procedures, as well as inaccurate measurement values. Especially, outliers in the initial samples used to determine the control limits for Shewhart charts or to estimate the process standard deviation for CUSUM charts can reduce the effectiveness of these tools. Outliers can also seriously distort the analysis of an interlaboratory study. **Robust** procedures are available for standard Shewhart charts (see Rocke [7] for the technical details and Rocke [9] for practical implementation), CUSUM charts [2], and interlaboratory studies [6, 8]. If outliers are frequent in the check samples used to produce the control charts, it would be essential to discover and eliminate the source of the outliers, since detection of outliers in routine samples would be difficult.

References

[1]   Garfield, F.M. (1991). *Quality Assurance Principles for Analytical Laboratories*, 2nd Ed. Association of Official Analytical Chemists, Washington.

[2]   Hawkins, D.M. (1993). Robustification of cumulative sum charts by winsorization, *Journal of Quality Technology* **25**, 248–261.

[3]   Hawkins, D.M. & Olwell, D.H. (1997). *Cumulative Sum Charts and Charting*. Springer-Verlag, New York.

[4]   Jones, G, Wortberg, M. Kreissig, S.B., Hammock, B.D. & Rocke, D.M. (1995). Sources of experimental variation in calibration curves for enzyme-linked immunosorbent assay, *Analytica Chimica Acta* **313**, 197–207.

[5]   Montgomery, D.C. (1996). *Introduction to Statistical Quality Control*, 3rd Ed. Wiley, New York.

[6]   Rocke, D.M. (1983). Robust statistical analysis of inter-laboratory studies, *Biometrika* **70**, 421–431.

[7]   Rocke, D.M. (1989). Robust control charts, *Technometrics* **31**, 173–184.

[8]   Rocke, D.M. (1991). Robustness and balance in the mixed model, *Biometrics* **47**, 303–309.

[9]   Rocke, D.M. (1992). $\overline{X}_Q$ and R_Q charts: robust control charts, *Statistician* **41**, 97–104.

[10]   Rocke, D.M. & Lorenzato, S, (1995). A two-component model for measurement error in analytical chemistry, *Technometrics* **37**, 176–184.

[11]   Wadsworth, H.M., Stephens, K.S. & Godfrey, A.B. (1986). *Modern Methods of Quality Control and Improvement*. Wiley, New York.

[12]   Youden, W.J. & Steiner, E.H., (1975). *Statistical Manual of the Association of Official Analytical Chemists*. Association of Official Analytical Chemists, Washington.

DAVID M. ROCKE

Lack-of-Fit Sum of Squares *see* Goodness of Fit

Lagged Cumulative Exposure *see* Occupational Health and Medicine

Lagged Dependent Variable

In **longitudinal** studies, several observations are taken from each individual at different time points. Often, an observation depends on previous observations; for example, in a **crossover** clinical trial, observations in one period may depend on the observations in the previous periods. A simple model for this scenario might include a lag-1 dependent variable as an explanatory variable [2]:

$$y_{it} = \gamma y_{i,t-1} + \mathbf{x}_{it}\boldsymbol{\beta} + u_i + e_{it}, \qquad (1)$$

where y_{it} is the observation from subject i in period t, $\mathbf{x}_{it}$ is a vector of **covariates**, u_i is a subject effect,

and e_{it} is an error term. This model can be extended to include multiple lagged variables by replacing $\gamma y_{i,j-1}$ by $\sum_{l=1}^{p} \gamma_l y_{i,t-l}$ in (1). Model (1) is different from a **serially correlated** model with the same covariates. In the latter, $y_{i,t}$ depends on $\mathbf{x}_{it}$ only (not $y_{i,t-1}$), while in the former it depends on all $\mathbf{x}_{i1}, \ldots, \mathbf{x}_{it}$ [4].

Statistical inference based on model (1) includes model fitting, **model checking** and **hypothesis tests**. In biostatistics, the number of subjects is often large, but the number of observations from each subject is small. In this situation we should be careful when using the asymptotic properties of the estimated parameters. For n subjects and times $1, 2, \ldots, T$, and conditional on u_i, the log **likelihood** function of this model can be written as

$$l(\boldsymbol{\beta}, \gamma, \mathbf{u}) = \sum_{i=1}^{n} \sum_{j=1}^{T} \log[p(y_{it}|y_{i,t-1}, \boldsymbol{\beta}, \gamma, u_i)]. \quad (2)$$

When there are no subject effects ($u_i = 0$), this model can be fitted easily using the lagged dependent variables as covariates [3]. When u_i is fixed and $u_i \neq 0$ the **maximum likelihood** estimates (mle) of γ and $\boldsymbol{\beta}$ are not **consistent** for fixed T when the total sample size $n \to \infty$ [2]. To obtain consistent estimates, the **instrumental variable** procedure can be used either for fixed or random u_i. To illustrate how this procedure works we write model (1) as

$$y_{it} - y_{i,t-1} = \gamma(y_{i,t-1} - y_{i,t-2}) + \boldsymbol{\beta}(\mathbf{x}_{it} - \mathbf{x}_{i,t-1})$$
$$+ e_{it} - e_{i,t-1}. \qquad (3)$$

Directly using $(y_{i,t-1} - y_{i,t-2})$ as a covariate may lead to inconsistency, since it and $e_{it} - e_{i,t-1}$ are correlated. However, $(y_{i,t-2} - y_{i,t-3})$ or $y_{i,t-2}$ is independent of $e_{it} - e_{i,t-1}$ and can be used as an instrumental variable. When assuming $u_i \sim \mathrm{N}(0, \sigma_u^2)$ the log likelihood function is more complicated than (2), but the mle can be obtained by the Newton–Raphson method (*see* **Optimization and Nonlinear Equations**). In this case the mle is consistent for fixed T and $n \to \infty$.

Model (1) can be extended to include discrete outcomes. One approach is to discretize y_{ij} by letting $y_{ij}^* = 1$ if $y_{ij} > 0$ and $y_{ij}^* = 0$ otherwise. This approach leads to the autoregressive probit model [1]. A more general approach is to use (1) as the linear predictor in a **generalized linear model**, and a wide range of data such as count data can then be modeled. Again, the model fitting without u_i is easy but the mle for random u_i is very difficult to obtain.

When there are missing data in the repeated measurements we may need to write (1) in another form. For example, when y_{i2} is missing we can write the equation for y_{i3} with y_{i1} as a covariate. This can be done by replacing y_{i2} by its regression model. However, the model becomes nonlinear, and nonlinear regression procedures should be used [4].

There are two special issues in the models with lagged dependent variables. One is the distinction between these models and other models for correlated outcomes. To distinguish these models from the models with random subject effects, we may test for given u_i if y_{ij} depends on the previous outcomes. To distinguish these models from serially correlated models, we may test if y_{ij} depends on previous covariates. Another issue concerns the initial observation y_{i0}. Assuming y_{i0} as fixed leads to a simple model, but it may not be reasonable for models with random u_i. The case when y_{i0} is random is more complicated; see [2] for details.

References

[1]   Hamerle, A. & Ronning, G. (1995). Panel analysis for qualitative variables, in *Handbook of Statistical Modeling for the Social and Behavioral Sciences*, G. Arminger, C.C. Clogg & M.E. Sobel, eds. Plenum, New York.

[2]   Hsiao, C. (1986). *Analysis of Panel Data*. Cambridge University Press, Cambridge, Chapter 4.

[3]   Jones, B. & Kenward, M.G. (1989). *Design and Analysis of Cross-over Trials*. Chapman & Hall, London.

[4]   Rosner, B. & Munoz, A. (1992). Conditional linear models for longitudinal data, in *Statistical Models for Longitudinal Studies of Health*, J.H. Dwyer, M. Feinleib, P. Lippert & H. Hoffmeister, eds. Oxford University Press, New York.

B. JONES & J. WANG

Lagrangian Poisson Distribution *see* Contagious Distributions

Laguerre Polynomials *see* Polynomial Approximation

Lambda Criterion, Wilks'

In 1932, Wilks [35] proposed the **likelihood ratio test** criterion, known usually as Wilks' Λ criterion, for testing the equality of the mean vectors of k p-variate normal distributions with common but unknown **covariance matrix** (*see* **Multivariate Normal Distribution**). Later, Wilks [36] and Bartlett [2] extended its use for testing regression coefficients; see Anderson [1] (*see* **Multiple Linear Regression**).

The problem in its canonical form can be expressed as follows. Let $(\mathbf{X}) : p \times r, \mathbf{Y} : p \times m$, and $\mathbf{Z} : p \times n$ be random matrices such that the columns of $\mathbf{X}, \mathbf{Y}$, and $\mathbf{Z}$ are independently distributed as p-variate normal distributions with the same covariance matrix $\boldsymbol{\Sigma}$. The problem is to test $H_0 : \boldsymbol{\Theta} \equiv E(\mathbf{X}) = \mathbf{0}$ against $H_1 : \boldsymbol{\Theta} \neq \mathbf{0}$, given that $E(\mathbf{Z}) = \mathbf{0}$, $\boldsymbol{\Sigma}$ being unknown. The likelihood-ratio test, evaluated by Wilks [34], rejects H_0 if and only if

$$V_{p,r,n} \equiv \frac{\det(\mathbf{ZZ'})}{\det(\mathbf{XX'} + \mathbf{ZZ'})}$$

is too small; here "det" denotes the determinant. The Λ criterion is the $\frac{1}{2}(r + m + n)$th power of $V_{p,r,n}$. In the context of the original problem or the **multivariate analysis of variance** (MANOVA) problem, the matrices $\mathbf{XX'}$ and $\mathbf{ZZ'}$ denote the sums of products and cross products matrices due to the hypothesis H_0 and due to error, respectively. It is tacitly assumed that $n \geq p$.

Wilks [35] derived the null distribution of $V_{p,r,n}$ explicitly for $p = 1, 2, 3$ with $r = 3$, and for $p = 4$ with $r = 4$; see also Consul [5] and Mathai [17].

The null distribution of $V_{p,r,n}$ can be expressed as the distribution of $U_1, U_2, \ldots, U_p$, where the U_is are independently distributed, with the distribution of U_i being the **beta distribution** $B(\frac{1}{2}(n + 1 - i), r/2)$; moreover, the distribution of $V_{p,r,n}$ is the same as that of $V_{r,p,n+r-p}$; see [1]. For $p = 1, 2$ and $r = 1, 2$ the distributions of $V_{p,r,n}$ take simple *F* **distribution** forms as follows [1]:

$$\frac{1 - V_{1,r,n}}{V_{1,r,n}} \frac{n}{r} \sim F_{r,n},$$

$$\frac{1 - V_{p,1,n}}{V_{p,1,n}} \frac{n + 1 - p}{p} \sim F_{p,n+1-p},$$

$$\frac{1 - (V_{2,r,n})^{1/2}}{(V_{2,r,n})^{1/2}} \frac{n - 1}{r} \sim F_{2r,2(n-1)},$$

$$\frac{1 - (V_{p,2,n})^{1/2}}{(V_{p,2,n})^{1/2}} \frac{n+1-p}{p} \sim F_{2p,2(n+1-p)}.$$

Wald & Brookner [37] presented a method for obtaining the null distribution of $V_{p,r,n}$ for even values of p and r; see also Schatzoff [29] and Anderson [1]. For other results on the null distribution, see Pillai & Gupta [24] and the books by Seber [32] and Muirhead [20].

Tables for significance points of $V_{p,r,n}$ are obtained by Schatzoff [29], Pillai & Gupta [24], Lee [16] and Davis [9, 10]; see also Anderson [1], Muirhead [20], and Pearson & Hartley [22].

Bartlett [3] has shown that the null distribution of $-[n - \frac{1}{2}(p - r + 1)] \log V_{p,r,n}$ tends to the **chi-square distribution** with pr **degrees of freedom** as $n \to \infty$; see [1]. Mudholkar & Trivedi [19] have suggested a normal approximation to the distribution of $- \log V_{p,r,n}$ for large p or r; see [1]. This approximation is better than the chi-square approximation when n is small. Rao [27] has suggested an F approximation as follows:

$$\frac{1 - V^{1/s}}{V^{1/s}} \frac{ks - q}{pr} \sim F_{pr,ks-q},$$

where $s = [(p^2 r^2 - 4)/(p^2 + r^2 - 5)]^{1/2}$, $q = (pr/2) - 1$, and $k = r - (p - r + 1)/2$. For small r, this approximation is more accurate than the chi-square approximation.

An asymptotic expansion of the null distribution of $V_{p,r,n}$ (in powers of $1/n$) in terms of chi-square distributions has been given in Rao [26], Anderson [1], and Muirhead [20].

Constantine [4] has obtained the moments of the nonnull distribution of $V_{p,r,n}$. For asymptotic expansion of the nonnull distribution in terms of noncentral chi-square distributions, see Muirhead [20], Suguira [33], Suguira & Fujikoshi [34], Fujikoshi [12], and Pillai [23].

Schwarz [31] has shown that the likelihood ratio test is **Bayes** and admissible; see also Anderson [1]. The **power** function of this test depends on the parameters only through the characteristic roots (**eigenvalues**) $v_1, \ldots, v_p$ of $\Theta\Theta'\Sigma^{-1}$. DasGupta et al. [8] have shown that the power of the likelihood ratio test monotonically increases as each v_i increases; see also a review paper by DasGupta [6]. The power of this test has been studied by DasGupta & Perlman [7].

The power functions of the likelihood ratio test, the **Lawley–Hotelling trace** test, and **Pillai's trace test** for the MANOVA problem have been compared by Rothenburg [28] on the basis of asymptotic expansions. It is shown that if the coefficient of variation of the v_is is large enough, then the power of the Lawley–Hotelling trace test is greater than that of the likelihood ratio test, which in turn is greater than that of Pillai's test; in the opposite situation, the ordering of power is reversed. For comparisons of the power function of the likelihood ratio test with the power functions of other standard tests for the MANOVA, see Itô [13], Lee [15], Mikhail [18], Olson [21], Pillai & Jayachandran [25], and Schatzoff [30]. Olson's study [21] indicates that the likelihood ratio test is quite robust under departure from covariance homogeneity. For a review of results on **robustness**, see Itô [14] (*see* **Robustness of Multivariate Techniques**).

References

[1]   Anderson, T.W. (1984). *An Introduction to Multivariate Statistical Analysis*, 2nd Ed. Wiley, New York.

[2]   Bartlett, M.S. (1934). The vector representation of a sample, *Proceedings of the Cambridge Philosophical Society* **30**, 327–340.

[3]   Bartlett, M.S. (1938). Further aspects of the theory of multiple regression, *Proceedings of the Cambridge Philosophical Society* **34**, 33–40.

[4]   Constantine, A.G. (1963). Some noncentral distributional problems in multivariate analysis, *Annals of Mathematical Statistics* **34**, 1270–1285.

[5]   Consul, P.C. (1966). On the exact distributions of the likelihood ratio criterion for testing linear hypothesis about regression coefficients, *Annals of Mathematical Statistics* **37**, 1319–1330.

[6]   DasGupta, S. (1980). Monotonicity and unbiasedness property of ANOVA and MANOVA tests, in *Handbook of Statistics*, Vol. 1, P.R. Krishnaiah, ed. North-Holland, New York, pp. 179–198.

[7]   DasGupta, S. & Perlman, M.D. (1973). On the power of Wilks' U-test for MANOVA, *Journal of Multivariate Analysis* **3**, 220–225.

[8]   DasGupta, S., Anderson, T.W. & Mudholkar, G.S. (1964). Monotonicity of the power functions of some tests of multivariate linear hypothesis, *Annals of Mathematical Statistics* **35**, 200–205.

[9]   Davis, A.W. (1971). Percentile approximations for a class of likelihood ratio criteria, *Biometrika* **58**, 349–356.

[10]   Davis, A.W. (1979). On the differential equation for Meijer's $G_{p,p}^{p,0}$ function and further tables of Wilks's likelihood ratio criterion, *Biometrika* **66**, 519–531.

[11] Davis, A.W. (1980). On the effects of moderate multivariate abnormality on Wilks's likelihood ratio criterion, *Biometrika* **67**, 419–427.

[12] Fujikoshi, Y. (1973). Asymptotic formulas for the distributions of three statistics for multivariate linear hypothesis, *Annals of the Institute of Statistical Mathematics* **25**, 423–437.

[13] Itô, K. (1962). A comparison of the powers of two multivariate analysis of variance tests, *Biometrika* **49**, 455–482.

[14] Itô, P.K. (1980). Robustness of ANOVA and MANOVA test producers, in *Handbook of Statistics*, Vol. 1, P.R. Krishnaiah, ed. North-Holland, New York, pp. 199–236.

[15] Lee, Y.S. (1971). Asymptotic formulae for the distribution of a multivariate test statistic: power comparisons of certain multivariate tests, *Biometrika* **58**, 647–651.

[16] Lee, Y.S. (1972). Some results on the distribution of Wilks' likelihood ratio criterion, *Biometrika* **59**, 649–664.

[17] Mathai, A.M. (1971). On the distribution of the likelihood ratio criterion for testing linear hypothesis on regression coefficients, *Annals of the Institute of Statistical Mathematics* **23**, 181–197.

[18] Mikhail, N.N. (1965). A comparison of tests of the Wilks–Lawley hypothesis in multivariate analysis, *Biometrika* **52**, 149–156.

[19] Mudholkar, G.S. & Trivedi, M.C. (1981). A normal approximation for the multivariate likelihood ratio statistics, in *Statistical Distributions in Scientific Work*, Vol. 5, C. Tallie et al., eds. Reidel, Dordrecht pp. 219–230.

[20] Muirhead, R.J. (1982). *Aspects of Multivariate Statistical Theory*. Wiley, New York.

[21] Olson, C.L. (1974). Comparative robustness of six tests in multivariate analysis of variance, *Journal of the American Statistical Association* **69**, 874–908.

[22] Pearson, E.S. & Hartley, H.O. (1972). *Biometrika Tables for Statisticians*, Vol. II. Cambridge University Press, Cambridge.

[23] Pillai, K.C.S. (1977). Distributions of characteristic roots in multivariate analysis, part II: non-null distributions, *Canadian Journal of Statistics* **5**, 1–62.

[24] Pillai, K.C.S. & Gupta, A.K. (1969). On the exact distribution of Wilks's criterion, *Biometrika* **56**, 109–118.

[25] Pillai, K.C.S. & Jayachandran, K. (1967). Power comparisons of tests of two multivariate hypotheses based on four criteria, *Biometrika* **54**, 195–210.

[26] Rao, C.R. (1948). Tests of significance in multivariate analysis, *Biometrika* **35**, 58–79.

[27] Rao, C.R. (1956). An asymptotic expansion of the distribution of Wilks' criterion, *Bulletin of the International Statistical Institute* **33**, 177–180.

[28] Rothenburg, T.J. (1977). Edgeworth expansions for multivariate test statistics, *IP-255*, Center for Research in Management Science, University of California, Berkeley.

[29] Schatzoff, M. (1966). Exact distribution of Wilks's likelihood ratio criterion, *Biometrika* **53**, 347–358.

[30] Schatzoff, M. (1966). Sensitivity comparisons among tests of the general linear hypotheses, *Journal of the American Statistical Association* **61**, 415–435.

[31] Schwarz, R. (1967). Admissible tests in multivariate analysis of variance, *Annals of Mathematical Statistics* **38**, 698–710.

[32] Seber, G.A.F. (1984). *Multivariate Observations*. Wiley, New York.

[33] Sugiura, N. (1973). Further asymptotic formulas for the non-null distributions of three statistics for multivariate linear hypothesis, *Annals of the Institute of Statistical Mathematics* **25**, 153–163.

[34] Sugiura, N. & Fujikoshi, Y. (1969). Asymptotic expansions of the non-null distributions of the likelihood ratio criteria for multivariate linear hypothesis and independence, *Annals of Mathematical Statistics* **40**, 942–952.

[35] Wilks, S.S. (1932). Certain generalizations in the analysis of variance, *Biometrika* **24**, 471–494.

[36] Wilks, S.S. (1935). On the independence of *k* sets of normally distributed statistical variables, *Econometrica* **3**, 309–326.

[37] Wald, A. & Brookner, R.J. (1941). On the distribution of Wilks' statistic for testing the independence of several groups of variables, *Annals of Mathematical Statistics* **12**, 137–152.

(*See also* **Multivariate Analysis, Overview**)

SOMESH DASGUPTA

Lambda Measure of Association *see* Goodman–Kruskal Measures of Association

Laplace, Pierre-Simon

Born: March 23, 1749, in Beaumont-en-Auge, France.
Died: March 5, 1827, in Paris, France.

"Laplace was among the most influential scientists in all history" [1]. The son of a well-to-do tradesman, he entered the University of Caen in 1766 to study theology, but left prematurely to study mathematics in Paris under d'Alembert. He secured an appointment at the Ecole Militaire (where he examined Napoleon), and was elected to the Académie des Sciences in 1773. His career continued to flourish after the Revolution, and for a short time he was Napoleon's Minister of the Interior. He became Chancellor of the Senate in 1803 and a Marquis in 1806.

During the first 20 years of his academic life, he worked prolifically in several areas of mathematical science, notably celestial mechanics, differential equations, and probability and statistics. These remained the central themes throughout his career. As his research findings proliferated and matured, Laplace incorporated them into two major treatises, *Mécanique céleste* (1799–1825) and *Théorie analytique des probabilités* (1812). The second edition of the latter, in 1814, was accompanied by a new introduction, *Essai philosophique sur les probabilités*.

Laplace's early work on probability adopted a **Bayesian** approach. Laplace had discovered **Bayes' theorem**, possibly unaware in 1774 of Bayes' posthumous publication of 1763. He applied this to combinatorial and demographic problems, and used the **beta** prior distribution for **binary data**. Other techniques and results introduced by Laplace included **generating functions** for discrete distributions, **characteristic functions**, the Laplace transform (at least in embryo), a form of the **central limit theorem**, and various aspects of **regression** and **least squares**. Commentators on his career usually refer to his somewhat cavalier attitude towards results obtained by other workers. According to [1], "not a single [contemporary] testimonial bespeaking congeniality survives". Nevertheless, as Gratton-Guiness [2] remarks,

Laplace's contributions to probability and statistics were fundamental . . . He . . . changed the emphasis of probability from its preoccupation with moral sciences and jurisprudence to include also applications in scientific contexts, wither it had hitherto infrequently strayed. His most important early successors were Quetelet and Poisson; after them, both probability and statistics moved to adulthood in the family of sciences, and the heritage from Laplace began to be recognized.

The major memoir [1], written in collaboration with others, contains extensive bibliographic information. The relation between Laplace's work and that of his near-contemporaries, especially **Gauss**, is described in [3].

References

[1]   Fox, R., Gillispie, C.C. & Gratton-Guinness, J. (1981). Laplace, Pierre-Simon, Marquis de, in *Dictionary of Scientific Biography*, Vol. 15, C.C. Gillispie, ed. Scribner, New York, pp. 273–403.

[2]   Grattan-Guiness, I. (1983). Laplace, Pierre Simon, in *Encyclopedia of Statistical Sciences*, Vol. 4, S. Kotz & N.L. Johnson, eds. Wiley, New York, pp. 469–473.

[3]   Stigler, S.M. (1986). *The History of Statistics: the Measurement of Uncertainty before 1900*. Belknap Press, Cambridge, Mass.

P. ARMITAGE

Large-Sample Theory

Large-sample theory (LST) plays a fundamental role in biostatistics in the prescription of fruitful methodology that can be well adapted in practical applications, often under conditions weaker than in standard (finite sample) parametrics. The basic clause of *large samples* is usually satisfied in real biostatistical applications, especially in investigations involving large-scale data collection. The advent of modern computers has strengthened the case for LST. The research literature on LST has gone through a phenomenal growth during the past three decades wherein delicate concepts from **probability** theory and **stochastic processes** have been blended towards a unified resolution, though at the cost of mathematical abstractions and sophistications often beyond the normal range of comprehension in biostatistics. Moreover, in biostatistics, various experimental or observational factors generally impose certain constraints on underlying statistical models, so that the classical parametric theory may not be universally adoptable, and increasingly **nonparametrics** and **semiparametrics** are being used; the LST has an even more dominant role in this setup. Yet there is a hierarchy in the methodological developments within the domain of LST with respect to their validity in moderate sample sizes, and many modern developments are geared toward a better resolution for moderate to large sample sizes. The interesting point in this context is the interplay between *validity robustness* and *efficiency robustness*; modern LST addresses this aspect quite well.

The basic concepts in probability theory underlying the evolution of LST in biostatistics are the following:

1. *stochastic, almost sure*, and other *modes of* **convergence**;
2. *probability inequalities*, and **laws of large numbers**; and
3. *weak convergence* or *convergence in distribution (law)*.

In the classical sense these concepts were mostly developed for sample *statistics* that are generally expressible as the sum or average of independent random elements. Yet, in applications one often encounters more general forms of statistics violating this postulation, and even sometimes sample functions that are *stochastic processes* in a general sense. The *empirical distribution* (*see* **Goodness of Fit**) and *survival* functions (*see* **Survival Distributions and Their Characteristics**) are classical examples of this type. In this context the emergence of *martingales, reverse martingales* and related *dependent sequences* has greatly reshaped the adaptability of LST in diverse setups, and our discussion remains somewhat incomplete without their introduction and role (*see* **Counting Process Methods in Survival Analysis**). The intricate role of LST in **transformations** on variables or statistics also deserves a closer look.

The main theme of LST relates to the *asymptotic distribution theory* for various statistics that arise in statistical analysis in biostatistics, where *point* and *confidence set* **estimation**, and **hypothesis testing** occupy a focal point. In this context, *linear*, **generalized linear, categorical data** models, and some semiparametric and nonparametric models deserve detailed discussion. LST in survival analysis is also a vital component of this development. For a comprehensive view, we also briefly present some *invariance principles* that play a fundamental role in these developments.

Stochastic Convergence

Let T_n be a statistic based on a sample of size N from a population with distribution function F, and let θ be a parameter which can generally be defined as a function of F. Then T_n is said to converge in probability (or stochastically) to θ if, for every positive η and ε, there exists a positive integer $n_0 = n_0(\eta, \varepsilon)$, such that

$$\Pr\{|T_n - \theta| > \eta\} < \varepsilon, \quad \text{for all } n \geq n_0. \quad (1)$$

If we view T_n as an estimator of θ, then the above definition coincides with the notion of (*weak*) **consistency** in estimation theory. Similarly, T_n converges almost surely (or strongly) to θ if

$$\Pr\{|T_n - \theta| > \eta, \text{ for some } N \geq n\} < \varepsilon,$$
$$\text{for all } n \geq n_0. \quad (2)$$

Again, in estimation theory this corresponds to the notion of *strong consistency*. In the same vein, T_n is said to converge in the rth mean, for some $r > 0$, if

$$\mathrm{E}\{|T_n - \theta|^r\} \to 0, \quad \text{as } n \to \infty. \quad (3)$$

Note that both almost sure convergence and convergence in the rth mean imply convergence in probability, but the converse may not be true generally. These definitions extend readily for the case of vectors T_n and θ where we need to use the Euclidean or other norms, and also to more general cases by using suitable norms. As an example consider the case of T_n being the sample distribution function defined as $F_n(\cdot)$, and consider the *sup-norm* $||F_n - F|| = \sup\{|F_n(x) - F(x)| : x \in \mathbf{R}\}$. With respect to this metric, the definitions all extend to this case of functional statistics and parameters.

Probability Inequalities

The *Chebyshev inequality*. For a nonnegative random variable U with $\mu = \mathrm{E}U$, $\Pr\{U \geq \mu t\} \leq t^{-1}$, for all $t > 0$, provides the genesis of all probability inequalities. Letting $U = (T_n - \theta)^2$ and denoting by $\sigma_n^2 = \mathrm{E}\{(T_n - \theta)^2\}$, we have the derived Chebyshev inequality:

$$\Pr\{|T_n - \theta| \geq \varepsilon\} \leq \varepsilon^{-2}\sigma_n^2, \quad \text{for every } \varepsilon > 0, \quad (4)$$

so that a sufficient condition for the stochastic convergence of T_n is that $\sigma_n \to 0$ as $n \to \infty$. Although this characterization does not require T_n to have independent summands, in fact it is the second (and generally rth) mean convergence property. For almost sure convergence and related results some sharper inequalities are useful. Among these, special mention may be made of (i) the *Bernstein inequality*, (ii) the *Kolmogorov–Hájek–Rényi inequality*, and

(iii) the *Hoeffding inequality*, all of which were initially formulated for independent summands, but later were generalized to some dependent cases as well. Other useful inequalities in probability theory include the c_r inequality ($r > 0$), the *Holder inequality*, the *Cauchy–Schwarz inequality*, and the *Jensen inequality*. For details we refer the reader to Sen & Singer [21] and Ferguson [7], where other pertinent references are all cited.

Laws of Large Numbers (LLN)

For independent and identically distributed (iid) random variables, the *Khintchine Strong LLN* asserts the almost sure convergence of the sample mean to the population mean whenever the latter exists. The *Borel SLLN* refers to the particular case of Bernoulli variables (*see* **Binary Data**). However, without the iid clause, extra regularity conditions are needed for such LLNs to hold. The *Kolmogorov SLLN*, in the case of independent but not necessarily identically distributed summands, is based on the convergence of the series $\sum_{n \geq 1} n^{-2} \sigma_n^2$, where σ_n^2 stands for the variance of X_n, for $n \geq 1$. These LLNs have also been extended to some dependent sequences. The *Markov LLN* relates to stochastic convergence for the possibly nonidentically distributed case, and does not require the second moment condition, but a condition slightly more stringent than the first.

Martingales and Reversed Martingales

Let $\{T_n; n \geq 1\}$ be a sequence of random variables with finite expectations. If $E\{T_n | T_j, j \leq n - 1\} = T_{n-1}$ almost everywhere for every $n \geq 1$ (where T_0 can be taken as a constant), then $\{T_n; n \geq 1\}$ is termed a martingale. If in the above (conditional) expectation, for all n, the $=$ is replaced by a $\geq$ (or $\leq$), then we have a submartingale (or supermartingale) sequence. A sequence $\{T_n\}$ forms a reversed martingale if for every n, $E\{T_n | T_{n+1}, T_{n+2}, \ldots\} = T_{n+1}$, almost everywhere, and a similar definition holds for reversed sub (or super) martingales. The sample mean, U-**statistics** and many other symmetric estimators can be characterized as reversed martingales. Similarly, sample sums, **likelihood ratio test statistics**, and other forms of **rank** statistics can be characterized as martingales. Score statistics, arising

in parametric models [16] as well as in various nonparametric and semiparametric applications [10], are abundant in biostatistics (*see* **Likelihood**). In most of these cases, either a reversed martingale or a forward martingale characterization holds. The empirical distribution function F_n is also a reversed martingale (process). Such dependent sequences show up frequently in survival analysis and other areas in biostatistics. Most of the probability inequalities and LLNs have been extended to such dependent sequences, and hence they enjoy similar convergence properties. We refer to some of these later in the article.

Weak Convergence and CLT

Consider a sequence $\{T_n; n \geq n_0\}$ of random variables or statistics with distribution functions $\{G_n; n \geq n_0\}$. Then T_n is said to converge weakly (or in distribution/law) to a possibly degenerate random variable T with distribution function G, if $\|G_n - G\| \to 0$ as $n \to \infty$, i.e. G_n converges to G at all points of continuity of G. Of particular interest is the classical **central limit theorem** (CLT) which relates to the case of a normal G. In the case of iid random variables $\{X_i, i \geq 1\}$ with finite mean μ and variance σ^2, $T_n = n^{-1/2} \sum_{i=1}^n (X_i - \mu)/\sigma$ converges in law to T, where T has the standard normal distribution function. The *Liapounoff* theorem established this weak convergence result in the nonidentically distributed case under a moment condition of order higher than 2, while the classical *Lindeberg–Feller* CLT pertains to the same result under a less stringent *uniform integrability* condition: for all $\varepsilon > 0$.

$$s_n^{-2} \sum_{i=1}^n E[(X_i - EX_i)^2 I(|X_i - EX_i| > \varepsilon s_n)] \to 0,$$
$$\text{as } n \to \infty \qquad (5)$$

where $s_n^2 = \sum_{i=1}^n \text{var}(X_i)$. These CLTs have been extended to more general *triangular* schemes as well as to some multivariate situations. In this context, it may not be necessary to assume that the limiting distribution is of full rank, i.e. degenerate limit laws are also allowed. Moreover, the CLTs hold for various dependent summands, including the martingales and reverse martingales, under some extra mild regularity conditions [5]. In general, in biostatistics, often a statistic T_n does not have independent summands, and may not even be strictly a martingale or reversed martingale, so a CLT may not be applied on it. However, in this context the well-known *Slutsky* theorem, presented below, provides an easily verifiable approach.

Let $\{X_n\}$ and $\{Y_n\}$ be sequences of random variables not necessarily independent, such that $X_n \overset{\mathcal{D}}{\longrightarrow} X$ and $Y_n \overset{\mathcal{P}}{\longrightarrow} c$, a constant. Then the following results hold:

$$X_n + Y_n \overset{\mathcal{D}}{\longrightarrow} X + c,$$

$$X_n Y_n \overset{\mathcal{D}}{\longrightarrow} cX,$$

and

$$X_n / Y_n \overset{\mathcal{D}}{\longrightarrow} X/c, \quad \text{if } c \neq 0. \tag{6}$$

In a variety of situations, we have the following *projection* result:

$$T_n = T_n^0 + R_n; \quad T_n^0 = \sum_{i=1}^{n} \mathrm{E}[T_n|X_i]$$
$$- (n-1)\mathrm{E}[T_n], \tag{7}$$

and the remainder term, R_n, having the nice property that $\mathrm{E}(R_n^2) = \mathrm{E}(T_n - \theta)^2 - \mathrm{E}(T_n^0 - \theta)^2$, stochastically converges to 0 at a rate faster than the standard error of T_n^0, whenever the projection technique yields an asymptotic quadratic mean equivalence. In such a case, the CLT holds for $\{T_n^0\}$ (which has independent summands), while the Slutsky theorem leads to the asymptotic normality of the standardized form of T_n. Hoeffding [8] used this projection result for U-statistics, where T_n^0 is a sample average of iid random variables, and he also indicated how the nonidentically distributed clause can be accommodated in the same vein. During the past 50 years a vast amount of research work has been accomplished in this direction. We refer to Jurečková & Sen [10] for deeper results on *asymptotic representations* of possibly nonlinear statistics in terms of T_n^0 and a remainder term, wherein the algebraic complications underlying the projection technique's asymptotic quadratic mean equivalence has further been replaced by a less stringent weaker expansion. As a simple illustration, consider the case of the sample variance $S_n^2 = n^{-1}\sum_{i=1}^{n}(X_i - \overline{X}_n)^2$, where $\overline{X}_n = n^{-1}\sum_{i=1}^{n} X_i$ is the sample mean. Here $T_n^0 = n^{-1}\sum_{i=1}^{n}(X_i - \mu)^2$ and $R_n = O_p(n^{-1})$. Thus, the CLT applies to $\sqrt{n}(S_n^2 - \sigma^2)$, though it is itself not an average of iid random variables.

Some weak convergence results allied to the above CLTs deserve mention. First, the asymptotic version of the *Cochran* theorem. Let $\sqrt{n}(\mathbf{T}_n - \boldsymbol{\theta}) \overset{\mathcal{D}}{\longrightarrow} \mathcal{N}_p(\mathbf{0}, \boldsymbol{\Gamma})$, and let $\mathbf{A}_n$ be a possibly stochastic matrix, converging (in probability) to $\mathbf{A}$, a generalized inverse of $\boldsymbol{\Gamma}$, with $\mathrm{Tr}(\mathbf{A}) = q(\leq p)$. Then $n(\mathbf{T}_n - \boldsymbol{\theta})'\mathbf{A}_n(\mathbf{T}_n - \boldsymbol{\theta})$ has an asymptotically **chi-square distribution** with q **degrees of freedom**. This theorem has many uses in biostatistics, and we will discuss some of them later in the article. As an illustration, we consider the case of the **Hotelling T^2 statistic** (in the multivariate one-sample model):

$$T_n^2 = n(\overline{\mathbf{X}}_n - \boldsymbol{\mu})'\mathbf{S}_n^{-1}(\overline{\mathbf{X}}_n - \boldsymbol{\mu}), \tag{8}$$

where $\boldsymbol{\mu}$ and $\boldsymbol{\Sigma}$ are the population mean vector and **covariance matrix**, and $\overline{\mathbf{X}}_n$ and $\mathbf{S}_n$ are their sample counterparts. Whenever the underlying distribution function has finite second-order moments, $\mathbf{S}_n \overset{\mathcal{P}}{\longrightarrow} \boldsymbol{\Sigma}$ and the multivariate CLT applies for $\sqrt{n}(\overline{\mathbf{X}}_n - \boldsymbol{\mu})$. Therefore, by the above version of the Cochran theorem, we claim that as n increases, T_n^2 has closely the central chi-square distribution function with p degrees of freedom. This result is useful in testing suitable null hypotheses on $\boldsymbol{\mu}$ as well as for obtaining *confidence sets* for $\boldsymbol{\mu}$, without specifically making the multinormality assumption. In the general context of linear models (without normality of the errors), the conventional least squares procedures lead to various estimates and test statistics where the Slutsky theorem and the above version of the Cochran theorem provide access to related asymptotic distribution theory. We refer to Sen & Singer [21] for most of these details.

Secondly, under the same setup, consider a real valued function $Z_n = g(\mathbf{T}_n)$ and define $\nu = g(\boldsymbol{\theta})$. Then under differentiability of $g(\cdot)$ at $\boldsymbol{\theta}$, we have

$$\sqrt{n}(Z_n - \nu) \overset{\mathcal{D}}{\longrightarrow} \mathcal{N}(0, \gamma^{*2}), \tag{9}$$

where $\gamma^{*2} = (\dot{g})'\boldsymbol{\Gamma}(\dot{g})$, and $\dot{g}$ is the gradient (vector) of $g(\cdot)$ at $\boldsymbol{\theta}$, which is assumed to be nonnull (as otherwise we would have a degenerate normal law). This basic CLT result has numerous applications in biostatistics. As a simple illustration, we consider the case of the sample *coefficient of variation*, $V_n = $

$S_n/\overline{X}_n$, where it is assumed that the population mean, μ, is nonnull (usually taken to be positive). Thus, V_n is a function of $(\overline{X}_n, S_n^2)$, and the above result directly yields the asymptotic normality of $\sqrt{n}(V_n - \xi)$, where $\xi = \sigma/\mu$. Sample correlation and regression coefficients are also notable examples of this type of statistics.

Thirdly, it should be clearly kept in mind that such *weak convergence results may not imply moment convergence*, i.e. the convergence of the mean, variance, and other moments of the statistics T_n or $g(T_n)$ to their asymptotic counterparts as specified by their asymptotic distributions. A simple example to this effect is the parameter θ, the reciprocal of the binomial (probability) parameter π, where T_n is the sample proportion, and $g(T_n) = T_n^{-1}$ is the natural plug-in estimator of θ. This model arises in the context of the well known **Capture-mark-release-recapture** (CMRR) procedure for estimating the size of a finite population; see, for example, Sen & Singer [21]. Since T_n can assume the value 0 with a positive probability $(1 - \pi)^n$, no matter how large n is, $g(T_n)$ does not have any finite positive order moment. However, the asymptotic normality result pertains to $g(T_n)$ as long as $\pi > 0$. As a historical note it may be mentioned that during the 1940s and 1950s considerable attempts were made to obtain the exact **skewness** and **kurtosis** coefficients of sampling distributions of various statistics (or estimators) in showing that they are asymptotically null, so that their asymptotic distribution would be normal. While the *Fréchet–Shohat* theorem (based on moment convergence of all order) justifies such an approach, obviously, the convergence of the first four moments may not suffice. Moreover, this limits the scope to a more restricted class of statistics which have finite moments all of finite order. In (bio-)statistical applications, for example, for setting a (large-sample) confidence interval for a parameter or testing a null hypothesis on the same, all we need is the asymptotic distribution and estimates of the parameter(s) that appear in these laws. Thus, weak convergence results are generally enough, and moment convergence is usually not needed. Finally, in such applications we may like to have some deeper weak convergence results which can match with more complexities and also may accelerate the goodness of fit of the asymptotics for moderate to large samples. These are presented separately in the following three sections.

Weak Convergence: Conditional Distributions

In the context of *resampling plans*, such as **jackknifing** and **bootstrapping**, one encounters a somewhat different asymptotic situation which requires additional care. We illustrate this with the simple bootstrap methodology. Let $X_1, \dots, X_n$ be n iid random variables drawn from a distribution function F, and let $T_n = T(X_1, \dots, X_n)$ be a suitable statistic whose population counterpart is denoted by θ. In a variety of cases it may be possible to establish that under suitable regularity assumptions, the distribution function $G_n(\cdot)$ of $\sqrt{n}[T_n - \theta]$ converges to a limiting distribution function $G(\cdot)$ as n becomes large; however this distribution function G may not be normal, or even if it is so, it may have a scale parameter γ which is an involved functional of F. Therefore, we may like to estimate G_n in a nonparametric manner. From $(X_1, \dots, X_n)$, we draw with replacement a sample of n observations, and denote these by $X_1^*, \dots, X_n^*$, respectively. Let $T_n^* = T(X_1^*, \dots, X_n^*)$ be the bootstrap version of T_n, and let us denote by $Z_n^* = \sqrt{n}[T_n^* - T_n]$. Note that under the conditional law $\Pr\{X_i^* = X_k | X_1, \dots, X_n\} = n^{-1}$, for all $i, k = 1, \dots, n$, the exact (conditional) distribution of Z_n^* can be obtained by enumeration, though such a task becomes prohibitively laborious as n increases (check the growth of the number n^n). Moreover, this conditional (bootstrap law) is intended as an estimator of the unconditional law G_n. This naturally imposes some restraints on the type of G_n for which a passage from the conditional to the unconditional distribution is well lighted. For example, if G_n is not attracted by a normal limit, then this postulation may not be true. This objective often precludes small sample size cases, even when G_n has a normal limit. As such, when n is large, M (a large number of) repetitions of the bootstrapping yields conditionally independent and identically distributed copies of Z_n^*, and this set is used to estimate G_n as well as a measure of its scale parameter. A very similar case arises in multivariate nonparametrics where conventional rank statistics are not usually genuinely distribution-free even under suitable null hypotheses (of invariance), and hence, their permutation distribution (*see* **Randomization Tests**) (corresponding to the case of simple random **sampling without replacement** (SRSWOR)) is used to generate the (conditional) null distribution of such rank statistics. In such applications, too, the passage from the conditional to unconditional distributions is generally fortified for large samples when the asymptotic (multi-)normality can be incorporated in a suitable manner; we refer to Puri & Sen [15] for a detailed account of such permutational LST. In jackknifing, a similar SRSWOR scheme arises, and it rests on the permutational probability measure generated by the $n!$ equally likely permutations of the observations. In such a case, the classical weak convergence results may not directly hold, though under additional mild regularity assumptions, the passage from the conditional limit law to an unconditional one can be fortified. Usually the (multi-)normality of the conditional distribution and its asymptotic homoscedasticity suffice for the purpose. But that may exclude some important applications in practice. For example, if the limit distribution is (scale) mixed-normal, this convergence of conditional limit laws to their unconditional forms may not generally hold. A word of caution: contrary to the belief and heuristic practice of using such resampling schemes for moderate to small sample sizes as well, there is no sound methodological justification for such usages. In many cases, they may be misleading.

Weak Invariance Principles

Let $X_1, \ldots, X_n$ be n iid random variables with finite mean μ and variance σ^2. Set $S_k = \sum_{i \le k}(X_i - \mu), k \ge 1$, and let $S_0 = 0$. Then the CLT asserts that for large n, $S_n/\{\sqrt{n}\sigma\}$ has closely a standard normal distribution. Let us construct a stochastic process $W_n = \{W_n(t), t \in (0, 1)\}$, by letting $W_n(k/n) = \{S_k/\{\sigma\sqrt{n}\}, k = 0, 1, \ldots, n\}$ and completing the definition by linear interpolation on $(0, 1)$. This way we map the *partial sum process* $\{S_k; k \le n\}$ into a stochastic process W_n with continuous sample paths on the unit interval $(0, 1)$. Now let $W = \{W(t), t \in (0, 1)\}$ be a *Gaussian process* on the unit interval $(0, 1)$, such that $EW(t) = 0$ and $E[W(s)W(t)] = \min(s, t), s, t \in (0, 1)$. Then W is termed a *standard* **Brownian motion process** on (0,1). As a generalization of the CLT, we have the following:

$$W_n \xrightarrow{\mathcal{D}} W, \quad \text{as } n \to \infty. \tag{10}$$

The implications of this weak convergence result are (i) the finite dimensional distributions of W_n converge to those of W, and (ii) like W, W_n is *tight*

or relatively compact. The first result follows by using a multivariate version of the CLT, while (ii) can be established by using some maximal inequalities, and both accomplished under no extra regularity conditions. This result extends directly to martingales/reversed martingales and to the nonidentically distributed case as well.

A second weak invariance principle having a profound impact on LST in biostatistics is the following. Let $F_n(x) = n^{-1} \sum_{i=1}^{n} I(X_i \le x), x \in \mathbf{R}$, be the sample distribution function, and define a stochastic process $W_n^0 = \{W_n^0(t), t \in (0, 1)\}$ by letting $W_n^0(t) = \sqrt{n}[F_n(x) - F(x)]$, at $t = F(x)$, for $t \in (0, 1)$. Also, let $W^0 = \{W^0(t), t \in (0, 1)\}$ be a Gaussian function on $(0, 1)$, such that $EW^0(t) = 0$ and $E[W^0(s)W^0(t)] = \min(s, t) - st, s, t \in (0, 1)$. W^0 is termed a *standard Brownian bridge* or a *tied-down* Brownian motion. Note that at $t = 0$ or 1, $W_n^0(t)$ is equal to 0 with probability 1, and hence the term *tied-down* has been affixed. Here also, we have for all continuous F,

$$W_n^0 \xrightarrow{\mathcal{D}} W^0, \quad \text{as } n \to \infty, \tag{11}$$

and the implications of this weak convergence result are the same as in (10). Extensions to higher dimensional distribution functions and more general functionals of the sample distribution functions have been considered at great depth. We refer to Jurečková & Sen [10], for some details. Some applications of these invariance principles will be discussed later in the article.

Variance Stabilizing Transformations

In a general setup, whenever $\sqrt{n}(T_n - \theta) \xrightarrow{\mathcal{D}} \mathcal{N}(0, \sigma^2)$, the asymptotic variance σ^2 may depend on the unknown parameter θ; therefore, we write $\sigma^2 = h(\theta)$ and assume that the form of $h(\cdot)$ is known. To use the above result for drawing a confidence interval for θ or to test a suitable null hypothesis on θ, it may be more desirable to consider a transformation: $T_n \to g(T_n)$, such that $\sqrt{n}(g(T_n) - g(\theta)) \xrightarrow{\mathcal{D}} \mathcal{N}(0, c^2)$, where $g(\cdot)$ is a manageable function and c does not depend on θ. While in general such a transformation may not exist, but for the single parameter case there are some well-known cases where it has worked out well; these are therefore termed variance stabilizing transformations (*see* **Delta Method**). It follows from (9) that a sufficient condition for this to be achieved is that

$$g'(\theta) = c\{h(\theta)\}^{-1/2} \quad \text{or} \quad g(\theta) = c \int \{h(y)\}^{-1/2} dy. \tag{12}$$

For **binomial**, **Poisson**, normal variance and **correlation** coefficient parameters, (12) work out well, and furthermore, in all these cases, some small corrections have been incorporated, mostly on empirical grounds, to provide a faster rate of convergence of the asymptotic normality result: the statistical motivation, however, stems primarily from LST. We refer to Sen & Singer [21, Chapter 3] for details. There are, however, some impasses in the multiparameter case where the dependence pattern of the coordinate estimators may violate the applicability of the variance stabilizing transformation for their covariance terms. A classical example is the **multinomial** distribution where for each cell probability one may use the arc-sin transformation to stabilize its asymptotic variance but then their covariances would still be dependent on the unknown cell probabilities.

Order Statistics and Empirical Distribution

Order statistics and empirical distribution functions are interrelated (one-to-one) in the classical univariate setup, and together they play a fundamental role in LST, particularly in *robust* as well as *nonparametric* inference problems. In biostatistics, in the active area of **survival analysis**, their role is overwhelming. The order statistics are neither independent nor identically distributed, even when the unordered collection relates to iid random variables. Hence LST pertaining to sums of independent random variables may not be directly applicable here. But with a reformulation in terms of indicator functions, most of these standard LST's can be adopted for order statistics, for sample quantiles, as well as extreme values. For example, for LLNs for sample quantiles, the Borel SLLN applies with little modification, while for the CLT, under the positivity and continuity of the density function at the population quantile, this approach via Bernoulli variables works out better, not only for a single quantile in a univariate setup but also for multiple quantiles in a general multivariate setup. More conveniently with adaptations from weak invariance principles for the empirical distributional processes,

the related LST for order statistics and empirical distributions has emerged in a very elegant form. Interestingly enough, reversed martingales also play a very prominent role in this context. We refer to Sen & Singer [10, Chapter] for some details. In **robust** estimation, covering both parametric and nonparametric models, we often use *L-estimators*, which are linear combinations of functions of order statistics, and *M-estimators*, which are solutions of implicit equations involving suitable *score functions* and the empirical distribution function. Likewise, *R-estimators* of location and regression parameters are based on suitable *rank-order* statistics which can be expressed as functionals of the empirical distributions. In this way we can conceive of a statistic $T_n = T(F_n)$ as a general functional of the empirical distribution function, F_n, and use LST pertaining to invariance principles for such processes, as outlined in (11). Naturally, the nature of $T(\cdot)$ will dictate the LST approach, and suitable differentiability properties of such functionals provide the necessary tools. A detailed treatment of this area of LST is beyond the scope of this article, but we refer the reader to Jurečková & Sen [10, Chapters 3 and 7], where an up-to-date and unified account has been provided. Hoeffding's [8] *U-statistics*, von Mises [23] statistical functionals and their (multi-sample) generalizations occupy a prominent place in nonparametrics, and they are abundant in biostatistics applications. Fortunately, they are statistical functionals and there are various martingale–reversed martingale representations for such statistics, discussed in detail in Sen [19], which pave the way for adoption of standard LST tools for the study of asymptotics for such statistics.

LST for MLE and BAN Estimators

In biostatistics, in actual applications, often, for easier interpretations and simpler statistical analysis, suitable parametric statistical models are postulated, and this approach naturally tilts the flavor to using optimal parametric statistical estimators (and tests) for the model parameters. *Maximum likelihood estimators* (MLE) are known to have various optimality properties, at least asymptotically, and in this depiction LST plays a basic role. In the case of the so-called **exponential family** *of densities*, granted *sufficiency* and *continuous differentiability* of the *likelihood function* (of the sample observations), the LST is generally based on the standard tools described earlier.

However, for a density not belonging to such a class (namely the **Cauchy**, *Laplace*), the treatment of LST becomes more complex and involves additional regularity assumptions. Basically the approach is to explore a *quadratic approximation* for the likelihood ratio statistic in a suitable neighborhood of the true parameter point, and this in turn provides an asymptotic representation for the MLE in terms of the *likelihood score statistics* which yield the desired asymptotic normality, consistency, as well as asymptotic efficiency properties of the MLE $\hat{\theta}_n$ (in the regular case). Basically, if we denote the score statistics $(\partial/\partial\theta) \ln L_n(X_1, \ldots, X_n)$ by $U_n(\theta)$, and the *Fisher* **information** *per observation* by $I(\theta) = n^{-1}\mathrm{E}\{U_n^2(\theta)\}$, then under appropriate regularity conditions we have a first-order asymptotic representation:

$$\hat{\theta}_n - \theta = \{nI(\theta)\}^{-1}U_n(\theta) + o_p(n^{-1/2}), \quad (13)$$

where $U_n(\theta)$ involves independent summands with zero mean and variance $I(\theta)$, and hence the CLT applies there. This leads to the following:

$$\sqrt{n}[\hat{\theta}_n - \theta] \xrightarrow{\mathcal{D}} \mathcal{N}(0, I^{-1}(\theta)), \quad (14)$$

where by the classical Fréchet–**Cramér–Rao information** inequality, $[nI(\theta)]^{-1}$ is the lower bound to the mean square error of an unbiased estimator of θ; this yields the asymptotic efficiency (and asymptotic unbiasedness) of the MLE. A similar situation holds in the multiparameter case. The regularity conditions, clasically known as the *Cramér conditions*, have gone through some evolution during the past 50 years. Although least stringent regularity conditions may be formulated as in LeCam [12], from a biostatistical applications point of view, a somewhat intermediate set of conditions hinging on the following compactness condition of the second derivative of the log density function provides a much simpler and more easily verifiable scenario. As $\delta(>0)$ approaches 0,

$$\mathrm{E}\{\sup(|(\partial^2/\partial\theta^2)\ln f(X, \theta+h) - (\partial^2/\partial\theta^2)$$
$$\ln f(X, \theta)|) : |h| < \delta\} \to 0; \quad (15)$$

Cramér's conditions involve the third derivative instead of this compactness of the second derivative.

For the exponential family of densities, the above condition follows from the continuity of the parametric functions, and in many other cases it can be verified by standard manipulations; we refer to Sen & Singer [21, Chapter 5] for details.

It is quite pertinent here to make some comments about LST for the MLE. First, in a nonregular case, the MLE may not be asymptotically normal, and may even lose its asymptotic efficiency property. Secondly, the MLE may not be the only estimator that is asymptotically efficient in the above sense. There are alternate estimators which may often share the asymptotic normality and efficiency properties along with the MLE; such estimators are termed best asymptotically normal **(BAN) estimators**. In the context of *categorical data models*, such BAN estimators based on the *minimum chi-square* and *modified minimum chi-square* criteria have been extensively studied in the literature (see for example, Agresti [1] and Sen & Singer [21] where detailed references are also cited); often, they are computationally less cumbersome than the MLE. Thirdly, the MLE are generally not robust to plausible model departures, and in that respect, alternative estimators, particularly *adaptive* estimators, may combine the BAN property with robustness to a greater extent. Finally, with the increase in the number of parameters, the performance characteristics of the MLE may deteriorate, and they may even become inconsistent or inefficient; the classical Neyman–Scott problem with a large number of nuisance parameters is a glaring example. Hence, modifications are often made to enhance the efficiency of the MLE. Among various such modifications, we refer to (*partial*) PMLE based on suitable partial likelihood functions [4], and quasi- and profile MLE based on **quasi-** and **profile likelihood** functions, which in a semiparametric context will be treated briefly later in the article.

LST and WLSE

Linear models (*see* **General Linear Model**) and *linear statistical inference* are household words in biostatistics. With the primary objective of interacting with researchers in biomedical and environmental sciences, in biostatistics it is customary to pose simple linear models that can be easily interpreted to collaborative scientists and can thereby be adapted to conventional linear statistical inference tools. Yet, in many cases the basic assumptions underlying such conventional procedures may not be tenable, and hence suitable modifications are often necessary to cope with the valid and efficient use of statistical inference tools. In biostatistics often we have nonnegative response variables where suitable transformations are used to induce linearity of the model to a greater extent, albeit at the cost of having nonnormal distributions (or vice versa). Therefore in linear statistical inference the basic assumption of normality of the errors may not be always tenable, and without this, the MLE based on the normality assumption may lose its appeal of validity and efficiency. The classical least squares estimators (LSE) and (large-sample) tests based on them occupy a focal point in this situation, and for such linear statistics, standard LST applies well. Weighted (WLSE) and generalized (GLSE) least squares estimators are the hybrids of the LSE that suit such nonstandard applications to a greater extent. The *heteroscedastic* linear model, $\mathbf{Y} = \mathbf{X}\boldsymbol{\beta} + \mathbf{e}$, $E(\mathbf{e}) = \mathbf{0}$, $V(\mathbf{e}) = \text{diag}(\sigma_1^2, \ldots, \sigma_n^2)$, provides a typical application of the WLSE when the σ_j^2 are not equal but known up to an unknown scalar constant (*see* **Scedasticity**). Thus, if we take $\sigma_j^2 = c_j\sigma^2$, $j \geq 1$, where the c_j are known constants, not all equal, while σ^2 is unknown, and if we denote the ith row of $\mathbf{X}$ by $\mathbf{x}_i'$, $i = 1, \ldots, n$, then we can consider the weighted sum of squares due to residuals:

$$\sum_{i=1}^{n} c_i^{-1}\{Y_i - \mathbf{x}_i'\boldsymbol{\beta}\}^2 \qquad (16)$$

and minimize this with respect to $\boldsymbol{\beta}$. This leads to the WLSE of $\boldsymbol{\beta}$. This procedure extends readily to the multivariate case where the $\mathbf{Y}_i$ are p vectors for some $p \geq 1$, provided the covariance matrices of the associated error vectors satisfy a similar heteroscedastic condition. In that setup it is generally referred to as the (generalized) GLSE, and if such a matrix is diagonal, it is termed the WLSE. The GLSE or WLSE are linear estimators, and hence the LLNs, CLTs, and other standard asymptotics apply here under some extra mild conditions on the c_i. However, in biostatistical applications, such as in **loglinear models** for categorical data, the exact variance–covariances of the transformed response statistics are not known, and are estimated from the sample itself. That brings the relevance of LST into a broader perspective. Estimated variance–covariances are used in the above minimization problem, often requiring an iterative procedure to update these estimates along with the estimates of the main parameters of interest. The two-step (Aitken) estimator belongs to this class. For details of related LST we refer to Sen & Singer [21, Chapter 7]. Other related procedures for linear (as well as location) models include the so called **trimmed** *LSE* (TLSE) and *regression quantiles* (*see* **Quantile Regression**); these are discussed in detail in Jurečková & Sen [10], and the related LST runs parallel to the case of WLSE. From a robustness prospect, however, such TSLE or regression quantiles are more appealing than the classical LSE.

LST of Statistical Tests

For testing a simple null hypothesis H_0 against a simple alternative H_1, the **Neyman–Pearson** *Fundamental Lemma* characterizes the *likelihood ratio test* (LRT) as most powerful, and this extends to *uniformly* **most powerful** (UMP) tests for *one-sided* alternatives. However, in a general multiparameter case with possibly **nuisance parameters**, one has typically composite null and composite alternative hypotheses. Here an exact (similar) test may not always exist, and even if one exists, it may be difficult to characterize one that will be uniformly best. For this reason, characterizations of optimality of statistical tests have often been made in an asymptotic framework, and there are competing tests sharing such properties in some way or other. Among such classes of tests, the following (parametric) deserve special mention: (i) likelihood ratio test, (ii) Rao's score test, and (iii) Wald's test; we refer to Rao [16] for a nice comparative account. The LRT is based on two sets of MLE, computed under H_0 and H_1, respectively, providing the ratio of the two maximized likelihood functions. LST pertaining to such LRTs, covering their null as well as alternative hypothesis distributions, is interlinked with the LST for the MLE, and hence they involve parallel regularity assumptions. Rao's score test, on the other hand, is based on the likelihood score statistics and their modifications, so that their asymptotics can be studied directly by using the standard LST tools. Computationally, Rao's score test is usually less cumbersome than the LRT. Wald's test is directly based on the MLE and the parametric constraints imposed by the hypotheses, and hence the general asymptotics for the MLE provide the access for parallel results for this type of tests. For local alternatives all the three types of tests share common asymptotic properties (*see* **Locally Most Powerful Tests**), although for nonlocal alternatives the LRT may have some advantages in a special way of interpretation [9]. Here also, on robustness considerations, such likelihood-based tests may not be very suitable. Moreover, for *restricted alternatives*, such as one-sided multiparameter hypotheses, such tests may have quite complicated forms and may even lose their asymptotic optimality properties to a greater extent (*see* **Isotonic Inference**). Roy's [17] **union–intersection principle** has added a lot of flexibility to this testing scenario, and their asymptotics have been studied under similar regularity assumptions. From robustness and nonparametric considerations, alternative tests based on *L*-, *M*- and *R*-estimators and suitable *U*-statistics have been extensively studied in the literature; we refer to Jurečková & Sen [10, Chapter 10] for a good account of these. In these developments, naturally, the asymptotics for such estimators play a basic role. In passing, we should also comment on **sequential** and *multistage* tests which have been considered in the literature. In this context, the classical Wald [25] *sequential probability ratio test* (SPRT) and its generalizations are all aimed at capturing some optimality properties in an interpretable manner. In the general multiparameter (composite hypothesis testing) case, again such optimality properties in an exact sense are hard to establish, and there is a good deal of asymptotics in the interpretation and derivation of such plausible optimality properties. The domain is by no means restricted to classical parametric setups, and nonparametric as well as robust procedures have been developed along the same vein. These procedures exploit the weak convergence and invariance principles introduced earlier and inherit the robustness aspects of the estimators or test statistics on which they are based. For details, we refer to Sen [19]. Group sequential procedures and related repeated significance testing (RST) procedures in **clinical trials** and biomedical studies have received considerable attention during the past two decades (*see* **Data and Safety Monitoring**). In this domain, too, the development of the methodology inherits a lot of asymptotics, and LST plays a vital role. In these developments, exact computations of boundary crossing probabilities, even for binomial or normal distributions, may become prohibitively laborious, if not impossible, and weak convergence of the encountered stochastic processes to suitable Gaussian functions (e.g. Brownian motion or Brownian bridge) provides the adaptability of standard results for Gaussian processes, and a general account of these developments is given in Sen [19, Chapters 9 and 10]. There are some other variations of such schemes, and we shall refer to some of them later in the article.

Semiparametric and Generalized Linear Models

Linear models are abundant in biostatistics, and yet in many applications the *normality* of the error components, their *homoscedasticity*, or even the basic *linearity of the model* may not be tenable. The classical MLE in the normal case agree with the *least squares estimators* (LSE), and for such linear estimators, standard LST can be adopted without many problems [21, Chapter 7]. Nevertheless, the optimality of the LSE may no longer be true when there are model departures. Therefore alternate models have been introduced to deemphasize the three basic assumptions underlying the normal theory MLE or the LSE, and in that way alternative classes of estimators have evolved.

Box–Cox Type Transformations

In biomedical applications the response variables are mostly nonnegative with (highly) positively skewed distributions. Although in such a case asymptotic normality of the LSE can be justified methodologically, in applications it may require an enormously large sample size. For this reason, logarithm, square-root, or cube-root transformations (*see* **Power Transformations**) are used to induce more symmetry in these response distributions so that moderate sample asymptotics can be justified to a greater extent. On the other hand, if the original model is closely linear, such nonlinear transformations can affect the regression relation considerably. Thus, one may require some **nonlinear regression** *models* to validate such transformations in practice. Either way, the LSE may not retain their normal-theory optimality, even asymptotically, although consistency and asymptotic normality would be retained under fairly general conditions [21, Chapter 7].

Generalized Linear Models

In **biological assays** and many survival analysis models, a response variable may be *quantal* (i.e. all or nothing) in nature (*see* **Quantal Response Models**). For such dichotomous (or even polychotomous) response variables, standard LSE may not work out well. *Logit* (**logistic regression**), *probit* and other models in bioassay are the precursors of **generalized linear models** (GLM). A more unified approach to such GLMs is outlined in McCullagh & Nelder [14]; their treatment addresses mostly the finite sample (or exact) methodology, and the findings are quite relevant to a general exponential family of densities. Nevertheless, in biostatistical applications such exact GLMs may not be tenable in all cases, and often (weighted) WLSE methodology is incorporated to falicitate suitable large-sample solutions (see [21, Chapter 7]). Such GLMs yield suitable *estimating equations* (EEs) (*see* **Estimating Functions**) which provide the estimators (mostly) as implicit solutions; this way the situation is similar to the case of the MLE. However, to cope with variations from most ideal situations, such EEs are replaced by suitable **generalized estimating equations** (GEE), and in their asymptotic treatment one needs additional regularity assumptions and manipulations too; see [21, Chapter 7]. Viewed from a practical perspective in a biostatistics context, such as in bioassays, dosimetric and mechanistic models in *toxicological* studies, the doses may be subject to *measurement errors* (*see* **Errors in Variables**) or latent effects, so that even if a simple GLM were pertinent to the basic dose–response pattern, such perturbations may cause great damage to their adoption without reservation. In this manner, one ignores the GLM methodology and has to take recourse in alternative LST where robustness and nonparametrics may dominate the scenario.

Nonparametric Linear Models

While assuming the linearity or additivity of the basic model, no specific distributional assumption is made on the response variables. An extensive literature relates to *L*-, *M*- and *R*- procedures in a variety of linear models, and an up-to-date treatment of the related asymptotics is contained in Jurečková & Sen [10]. Such procedures are generally more robust, consistent, and have asymptotic normality properties. Within this bigger class, one can also have suitable

adaptive estimators which are asymptotically efficient and robust as well.

Semiparametric Models

The **Cox model** [3] or **proportional hazards model** (PHM) is a very simple illustration of a semiparametric model. In a simple two-sample model, if F and G are the respective distribution functions, and we denote the corresponding survival functions by $\overline{F}(x) = 1 - F(x)$ and $\overline{G}(x) = 1 - G(x), x \in \mathbf{R}$, then in a Lehmann [13] model (*see* **Lehmann Alternatives**), we set $\overline{G}(x) = [\overline{F}(x)]^c$, for some $c > 0$. The null hypothesis of the homogeneity of F and G then reduces to $c = 1$. If the distribution functions are absolutely continuous with densities f and g, respectively, then we define equivalently the **hazard** *functions* $h_F(x)$ and $h_G(x)$ as $f(x)/\overline{F}(x)$ and $g(x)/\overline{G}(x)$, respectively. Then the Lehmann model can be put equivalently as $h_G(x) = ch_F(x)$, for all x, i.e. the two hazard functions are proportional. Motivated by this simple observation, Cox [3] considered a general situation where conditionally on a set of concomitant variates, say, $\mathbf{z}$, the hazard function for the primary variate, denoted by $h(y|\mathbf{z})$, is assumed to satisfy the following model:

$$h(y|z) = h_0(y)\exp\{\boldsymbol{\beta}'\mathbf{z}\}, \qquad (17)$$

where the nonnegative $h_0(y)$, the baseline hazard rate, is independent of the concomitant variates and is of arbitrary form (i.e. nonparametric in nature), and the regression on the concomitant variates is of a specified parametric form. This also leads to the following:

$$\ln h(y|\mathbf{z}) = \ln h_0(y) + \boldsymbol{\beta}'\mathbf{z}; \qquad (18)$$

in the literature this is known as the *hazard regression*. In either setup, note that $h_0(y)$ is a functional while β is a finite dimensional (regression) parameter. For this reason, this is referred to as a semiparametric model. Typically, in a general setup one may have a functional parameter space, and in that way the MLE or other conventional estimators may lose their efficacy, and often, consistency properties too. It may be possible in some cases to reparameterize in such a way that the parameters of interest constitute a finite-dimensional vector, while the nuisance parameter space may be very large. In this setup, often a conditional approach leads to a **partial**

likelihood function whereby the finite-dimensional parameters of interest can be estimated consistently by the (partial) PMLE and with reasonable efficacy. Martingale methods play a basic role in the related asymptotics, and in this context, *counting processes* have evolved to be of prime interest in the study of general asymptotics; we refer to Andersen et al. [2] for a nice account of related asymptotics.

Nonparametric Regression and Smoothing Techniques

The past 20 years have witnessed a phenomenal growth of research literature in this domain, and these developments are of considerable use in biostatistics. Both the *kernel* and *nearest neighbor* methods are popular in this context (*see* **Density Estimation**). In terms of model flexibility, such models are the most desirable ones. However, in terms of precision of derived estimators, such a model may have the opposite flavor. Compared to the usual $\sqrt{n}$-consistency of the classical estimators in the parametric or semiparametric models, here one has n^{λ}-consistency for some positive $\lambda < 1/2$. Moreover, the asymptotic bias and asymptotic standard error may be of comparable order of magnitude, and hence *adaptive bandwidth* selection procedures are often prescribed to achieve asymptotic optimality within this class. Generally, much larger sample size is required for the adaptibility of asymptotics in the nonparametric regression case than in other models; we refer to Thompson & Tapia [22] for a treatise of **nonparametric regression** and function estimation problems.

LST for Time-Sequential Schemes

This is one of the most important areas of current research activities in biostatistics, and LST has a fundamental role in this field. In clinical trials or medical investigations, generally one obtains data sets accumulating over time, so that statistical conclusions are drawn at the termination of the study. On the contrary, most of these studies relate to comparisons of different treatments or subgroups, and involve human beings. Thus, for ethical reasons, it is often advised that if there is any real difference in the response patterns for the various subgroups, then the trial should be able to detect it as early as possible, and the better treatment be made available to the

entire set of subjects for their better prospects. On the other hand, lacking any real difference, the trial, if conducted up to the end of the planned duration, may contain valuable information for other scientific studies as well. This motivates the need for *interim analysis* in such clinical trials, and these may be made either on a periodic (namely fixed calendar-month/year interval) basis or on a monitoring basis resulting in the so called time-sequential procedures. The main points of difference between the classical sequential and time-sequential procedures are the following:

1. The number of subjects to be included in the study is prefixed in a time-sequential scheme, but is itself a random variable in a sequential one. Thus the formulation of an average sample number (ASN) is quite different in the two schemes.
2. The observations in a sequential scheme are typically iid, whereas in a time-sequential one they typically represent the ordered failure points along with other concomitant variables, and hence the iid clause generally is not tenable.
3. The emphasis on type I and type II errors in a sequential test is somewhat different from that in a time-sequential one.
4. **Censoring** (of various types) is a typical phenomenon in a time-sequential scheme, and to a greater extent the statistical modeling and analysis depend on such deviations.
5. Typically, in view of point 4, nonparametrics and semiparametrics play a more dominant role in time-sequential schemes than in the classical sequential schemes, where the probability (or likelihood) ratio statistics have a more visible parametric flavor.

Nonparametric and semiparametric procedures for time-sequential schemes have been studied extensively in the literature during the past two decades. The basic foundation was laid down by the development of martingale methodology for various rank statistics [19], as well as for counting processes related to such stochastic events [2]. In this context the classical LST may not be directly applicable; nevertheless, they are quite pertinent and justifiable through the modifications based on adoption of martingale theory. We conclude this discussion with a brief introduction to LST pertinent to the

Kaplan–Meier [11] *product-limit* (PL) estimator of the survival function under random censoring. In random censoring schemes the set of censoring variables $T_1, \ldots, T_n$ are iid according to a distribution function G, and T_i and X_i are stochastically independent for every i; note that the X_i are iid with a survival function $\overline{F}$. The observable random elements are $Z_i = \min(X_i, T_i)$ and $I_i = I(Z_i = X_i)$, $i = 1, \ldots, n$. Define $N_n(t) = \sum_{i \le n} I(Z_i > t)$, t real, and set $\alpha_i(t) = I(Z_i \le t, I_i = 1)$, $i \ge 1$, t real, and let $\tau_n = \max\{Z_i : i \le n\}$. Then the PL-estimator of $\overline{F}$ is given by

$$\overline{P}_n(t) = \prod_{i=1}^{n} \left\{ \frac{N_n(Z_i)}{N_n(Z_i) + 1} \right\}^{\alpha_i(t)} I(t \le \tau_n)$$

$$= \prod_{\{i : Z_i \le t\}} \left\{ \frac{n\overline{H}_n(Z_i)}{n\overline{H}_n(Z_i) + 1} \right\}^{I_i}, \qquad (19)$$

where $\overline{H}_n(t) = n^{-1} N_n(t)$, t real. Thus, this estimator (a stochastic process) can be viewed as a functional of the counting process $\{N_n(t), t \text{ real}\}$, and hence LST relating to such counting processes can be imported here to study the asymptotic properties of the PL-estimator. Alternatively, suitable martingale characterizations of the PL-estimator can also be incorporated in the study of related LST. We refer to Andersen et al. [2] for details, albeit at a much higher level of mathematical sophistication. Generally test statistics or estimators in time-sequential schemes are functionals of the PL-estimator (in the censored case) or the original empirical survival function (in the uncensored case), having some sort of time-sequential flavor, and hence suitable stochastic processes relating to such functionals can be incorporated to formulate the *stopping* and *decision rules*. For example, in survival analysis, the *mean residual life* (MRL) is an important tool to measure the effectiveness of treatment protocols (*see* **Life Table**). Corresponding to the population measure

$$\mu(x) = \{\overline{F}(x)\}^{-1} \int_x^\infty \overline{F}(y) \mathrm{d}y, \qquad (20)$$

the sample measure is defined by $\hat{\mu}_n = \{\overline{P}_n(x)\}^{-1} \int_x^\infty \overline{P}_n(y) \mathrm{d}y$, and one may like to study the weak or strong consistency and asymptotic normality of $\hat{\mu}_n(x)$ for a given x, and more generally for a range of values of x. Weak convergence of such stochastic processes naturally provides the key to subsequent developments, and a systematic account of this type of LST in the context of clinical trials is given in Sen [20].

References

[1] Agresti, A. (1990). *Categorical Data Analysis*. Wiley, New York.

[2] Andersen, P.K., Borgan, O., Gill, R.D. & Keiding, N. (1993). *Statistical Models Based on Counting Processes*. Springer-Verlag, New York.

[3] Cox, D.R. (1972). Regression models and life tables (with discussion), *Journal of the Royal Statistical Society, Series B* **34**, 187–220.

[4] Cox, D.R. (1975). Partial likelihood, *Biometrika* **62**, 269–276.

[5] Dvoretzky, A. (1971). Asymptotic normality for sums of dependent random variables, *Proceedings of the Sixth Berkeley Symposium on Mathematical Statistics and Probability*, Vol. 2. University of California Press, Berkeley, pp. 513–535.

[6] Efron, B. & Tibshirani, R.J. (1993). *An Introduction to the Bootstrap*. Chapman & Hall, London.

[7] Ferguson, T. (1996). *Large Sample Theory*. Chapman & Hall, London.

[8] Hoeffding, W. (1948). A class of statistics with asymptotically normal distribution, *Annals of Mathematical Statistics* **19**, 293–325.

[9] Hoeffding, W. (1965). Asymptotically optimal tests for multinomial distributions (with discussion), *Annals of Mathematical Statistics* **36**, 369–408.

[10] Jurečková, J. & Sen, P.K. (1996). *Robust Statistical Procedures*. Wiley, New York.

[11] Kaplan, E.L. & Meier, P. (1958). Nonparametric estimation from incomplete observations, *Journal of the American Statistical Association* **53**, 457–481, 562–563.

[12] LeCam, L. (1986). *Asymptotic Methods in Statistical Decision Theory*. Springer-Verlag, New York.

[13] Lehmann, E.L. (1953). The power of rank tests, *Annals of Mathematical Statistics* **24**, 23–43.

[14] McCullagh, P. & Nelder, J.A. (1989). *Generalized Linear Models*, 2nd Ed. Chapman & Hall, London.

[15] Puri, M.L. & Sen, P.K. (1971). *Nonparametric Methods in Multivariate Analysis*. Wiley, New York.

[16] Rao, C.R. (1948). Large sample tests of statistical hypotheses concerning several parameters with applications to problems of estimation, *Proceedings of the Cambridge Philosophical Society* **44**, 50–57.

[17] Roy, S.N. (1953). On a heuristic method of test construction and its use in multivariate analysis, *Annals of Mathematical Statistics* **24**, 220–238.

[18] Sen, P.K. (1968). Estimates of the regression coefficient based on Kendall's tau, *Journal of the American Statistical Association* **63**, 1379–1389.

[19] Sen, P.K. (1981). *Sequential Nonparametrics*. Wiley, New York.

[20]   Sen, P.K. (1985). *Theory and Applications of Sequential Nonparametrics*, CBMS/NSF Ser. 49. SIAM, Philadelphia.

[21]   Sen, P.K. & Singer, J.M. (1993). *Large Sample Methods in Statistics*. Chapman & Hall, London.

[22]   Thompson, J.R. & Tapia, R.A. (1990). *Nonparametric Function Estimation, Modeling and Simulation*. SIAM, Philadelphia.

[23]   von Mises, R. (1947). On the asymptotic distribution of differentiable statistical functions, *Annals of Mathematical Statistics* **18**, 309–348.

[24]   Wald, A. (1943). Tests of statistical hypotheses concerning several parameters when the number of observations is large, *Transactions of the American Mathematical Society* **54**, 426–482.

[25]   Wald, A. (1947). *Sequential Analysis*. Wiley, New York.

(*See also* **Limit Theorems**)

PRANAB K. SEN

Lasso *see* Variable Selection

Last Value Carried Forward *see* Clinical Trials of Antibacterial Agents

Last Value Imputation *see* Missing Data in Clinical Trials

Latent Class Analysis

Latent class analysis is a discrete variable analog of **factor analysis**. Latent class analysis was originally developed [11, 16] to investigate the classification of subjects according to an underlying categorical trait, such as an attitude or psychological state, that is not directly observable. Membership in a particular class of the underlying variable is estimated from a subject's responses to a set of categorical items. Overviews of latent class modeling are given by Lazarsfeld & Henry [17], Andersen [3], Henry [13], McCutcheon [19], and Clogg [6].

Examples

The following example is a simplified version of the items considered by Rimer [20] in a study of methods for promoting smoking cessation. Subjects were asked to agree or disagree with a series of items, a subset of which are:

1. Smoking cigarettes relieves your tension.
2. Smoking helps you concentrate and do better work.
3. You are more relaxed and more pleasant when smoking.
4. You like the image of yourself as a smoker.

In principle, responses to these items reveal an underlying attitude towards smoking, perhaps reflecting a subject's "resistance" to quitting smoking. The trait of "resistance" could be dichotomized into the categories: not resistant or resistant. The observed items, 1–4 above, are called the manifest variables, while the underlying trait is the latent variable. In the example, both the manifest variables and the latent variable are dichotomous, but latent class models can be applied more generally, with manifest and latent variables that are ordinal or polytomous categorical variables (*see* **Ordered Categorical Data; Polytomous Data**).

A fundamental assumption in latent class modeling is "local independence", which states that given the latent class membership, the manifest variables are conditionally independent. A numerical example serves to illustrate this assumption. Consider a population that can be cross-classified according to the manifest variables, A and B, in the proportions displayed in Table 1. Suppose that the population can be divided into equal proportions by a binary latent variable, and that within levels of the latent variable the population can be cross-classified according to the manifest variables A and B as displayed in Table 2. The values in the cells of the table represent

Table 1   Cross-classification of two manifest variables

		A		Total
		Agree	Disagree	Total
B	Agree	0.4	0.2	0.6
	Disagree	0.2	0.2	0.4
	Total	0.6	0.4	1

Table 2 Illustration of local independence of manifest variables (*A* and *B*) given the latent variable, *Z*

Z = 1

		B		
		Agree	Disagree	Total
A	Agree	0.64	0.16	0.80
	Disagree	0.16	0.04	0.20
	Total	0.80	0.20	1

Z = 0

		B		
		Agree	Disagree	Total
A	Agree	0.16	0.24	0.40
	Disagree	0.24	0.36	0.60
	Total	0.40	0.60	1

the conditional probabilities associated with *A* and *B*, given the level of *Z*. Despite the marginal association between variables *A* and *B* displayed in Table 1, the variables *A* and *B* are conditionally independent, given the level of the latent variable.

In practice, displays such as Table 2 cannot be constructed because the latent variable is unobservable directly. In many cases, however, the existence of a latent variable can be derived from theoretical models of attitudes, behavior, or psychology. Latent class analysis can be used to investigate the degree to which inferences about the unobservable latent trait can be derived from the manifest or observed variables. The next section provides a mathematical formulation of latent class analysis.

Mathematical Model

Suppose that each of *n* subjects is observed on *K* categorical manifest variables, $\mathbf{Y} = (Y_1, \ldots, Y_K)$, with each variable taking on one of *C* categories. The cells of the *K*-way cross-classification table are indexed by $\mathbf{y} = (y_1, \ldots, y_k)$, with $n_\mathbf{y}$ denoting the observed number of subjects and $\pi_\mathbf{y}$ denoting the probability associated with response profile $\mathbf{y}$. The cell frequencies are assumed to have a **multinomial distribution** with $\mathrm{E}(n_\mathbf{y}) = n\pi_\mathbf{y}$ and $\Sigma_\mathbf{y} \pi_\mathbf{y} = 1$. The latent variable, *Z*, is assumed to take on one of *T* classes, with θ_z denoting the proportion of the population in class $z, z = 1, \ldots, T, \sum_{z=1}^{T} \theta_z = 1$. In the segment of the population in latent class $Z = z$, the proportion of the population classified into the cell indexed by $\mathbf{y}$ is denoted $\pi_{\mathbf{y}|t} = \Pr(\mathbf{Y} = \mathbf{y}|T = t)$. The assumption of local independence states that given the latent class membership, the manifest variables are conditionally independent:

$$\Pr[\mathbf{Y} = \mathbf{y}|Z = z] = \prod_{i=1}^{K} \Pr[Y_i = y_i|Z = z]. \quad (1)$$

Estimates of the conditional response probabilities, $\Pr[Y_i = y_i|Z = z], i = 1, \ldots, K$, and the latent class proportions, $\theta_z, z = 1, \ldots, T$, are derived from the observed counts, $n_\mathbf{y}$, through the equations $\mathrm{E}(n_\mathbf{y}) = n\pi_\mathbf{y}$ and

$$\pi_\mathbf{y} = \sum_{z=1}^{T} \prod_{i=1}^{K} \Pr[Y_i = y_i|Z = z]\theta_z. \quad (2)$$

The latent class model can also be viewed as a **loglinear model** [10, 12] for the expected counts in a $(K + 1)$-way cross-classification of the *K* manifest variables $(Y_1, Y_2, \ldots, Y_K)$ and the latent variable, *Z*. Denoting the expected counts by $m_{y,z}$, and with the usual constraints on the parameters of the loglinear model [1], the loglinear model

$$\ln m_{y,z} = \mu + \lambda_z^Z + \lambda_{y_1}^{Y_1} + \cdots + \lambda_{y_K}^{Y_K} + \lambda_{y_1,z}^{Y_1 Z}$$
$$+ \cdots + \lambda_{y_K,z}^{Y_K Z} \quad (3)$$

expresses conditional independence of the manifest variables, $\mathbf{Y}$, given the latent class. Although the cell frequencies in the $(K + 1)$-way classification are not observed, estimates in the loglinear model (3), are derived from the observed frequencies in the *K*-way cross-classification of the manifest variables, n_y.

Maximum likelihood is the most widely used method for estimating the parameters of the latent class model. Goodman [10] proposed an iterative algorithm for obtaining maximum likelihood estimates; the algorithm is an example of a general procedure now known as the **EM algorithm** [8]. Once the maximum likelihood estimates, $\hat{m}_{y,z}$, have been computed, the goodness-of-fit of the latent class model can be tested. The most commonly used statistics for testing goodness-of-fit are the generalized **likelihood ratio test** statistic,

$$G^2 = 2 \sum_\mathbf{y} n_y \ln(n_y/\hat{m}_y),$$

and the Pearson X^2 statistic,

$$X^2 = \sum_y \frac{(n_y - \hat{m}_y)^2}{\hat{m}_y},$$

where $\hat{m}_y = \Sigma_z \hat{m}_{y,z}$ (see **Chi-Square Tests**). Under the null hypothesis that the latent class model fits, the statistics are asymptotically distributed as a χ^2 random variable, with degrees of freedom equal to the number of cells in the table cross-classifying the manifest variables, minus the number of parameters being estimated in (3). With K manifest variables, each representing C categories, and with one latent trait having T classes, the degrees of freedom for testing the goodness-of-fit of the model equals $C^K - T[1 + K(C-1)]$. A comparison of these statistics is given in [14].

Despite the similarity in form to standard loglinear model analysis, fitting a latent class model involves the additional issue of the **identifiability** of parameters. For example, with K binary manifest variables ($C = 2$) and T latent classes, for $T > 2^K/(1 + K)$, the number of parameters in the model exceeds the number of "observations", the number of cells in the cross-classification of the manifest variables. Having more observations than parameters is a necessary condition for all parameters to be identifiable, but it is not sufficient. The identifiability of parameters is discussed in [10] and [18].

Extensions and Other Applications

Clogg & Goodman [7] extended the single population latent class analysis to simultaneous modeling of latent classes across several populations. Latent class methods specific to ordinal manifest variables were considered by Clogg [5]. In addition to its original applications in the study of attitudes, latent class modeling has been applied to the study of inter-rater reliability [2, 23] (see **Observer Reliability and Agreement**), survey response errors [4], incomplete data [9, 24], chronic disease epidemiology [15], medical diagnosis [21], and repeated measurements (see **Longitudinal Data Analysis, Overview**) [22].

References

[1]   Agresti, A. (1990). *Categorical Data Analysis*. Wiley, New York.

[2]   Agresti, A. & Lang, J. (1993). Quasi-symmetric latent class models, with application to rater agreement, *Biometrics* **49**, 131–139.

[3]   Andersen, E.B. (1982). Latent structure analysis: a survey, *Scandinavian Journal of Statistics* **9**, 1–12.

[4]   Bye, B. & Schechter, E. (1986). A latent Markov model approach to the estimation of response errors in multiwave panel data, *Journal of the American Statistical Association* **81**, 375–380.

[5]   Clogg, C. (1979). Some latent structure models for the analysis of Likert-type data, *Social Science Research* **8**, 297–301.

[6]   Clogg, C. (1992). The impact of sociological methodology on statistical methodology (with discussion), *Statistical Science* **7**, 183–196.

[7]   Clogg, C. & Goodman, L. (1984). Latent structure analysis of a set of multidimensional contingency tables, *Journal of the American Statistical Association* **79**, 762–771.

[8]   Dempster, A., Laird, N. & Rubin, D. (1977). Maximum likelihood from incomplete data via the EM algorithm (with discussion), *Journal of the Royal Statistical Society, Series B* **39**, 1–38.

[9]   Espeland, M. & Handelman, S. (1989). Using latent class models to characterize and assess relative error in discrete measurements, *Biometrics* **45**, 587–599.

[10]   Goodman, L. (1974). Exploratory latent structure analysis using both identifiable and unidentifiable models, *Biometrika* **61**, 215–231.

[11]   Green, B.F. (1952). Latent structure analysis and its relation to factor analysis, *Journal of the American Statistical Association* **47**, 71–76.

[12]   Hagenaars, J. (1993). *Log-Linear Models with Latent Variables*. Sage, Newbury Park.

[13]   Henry, N. (1983). Latent structure analysis in *Encyclopedia of Statistical Sciences*, Vol. 4, S. Kotz and N.L. Johnson, eds. Wiley, New York, pp. 497–504.

[14]   Holt, J. & Macready, G. (1988). Comparison of maximum likelihood and Pearson chi-square statistics for assessing latent class models, in *American Statistical Association 1988 Proceedings of the Section on Social Statistics*. American Statistical Association, Alexandria, pp. 167–171.

[15]   Kaldor, J. & Clayton, D. (1985). Latent class analysis in chronic disease epidemiology, *Statistics in Medicine* **4**, 327–335.

[16]   Lazarsfeld, P.F. (1950). The logical and mathematical foundations of latent structure analysis, in *Measurement and Prediction*, S.A. Stouffer et al., eds. Princeton University Press, Princeton.

[17]   Lazarsfeld, P.F. & Henry, N.W. (1968). *Latent Structure Analysis*. Houghton-Mifflin, Boston.

[18]   Lindsay, B., Clogg, C. & Grego, J. (1991). Semiparametric estimation in the Rasch model and related exponential response models, including a simple latent class model for item analysis, *Journal of the American Statistical Association* **86**, 96–107.

[19]   McCutcheon, A. (1987). *Latent Class Analysis*. Sage, Newbury Park.

[20]   Rimer, B. (1993). Enhancing Cancer Control in a Community Health Center, *R01 CA59734-03*. National Cancer Institute.

[21]   Rindskopf, D. & Rindskopf, W. (1986). The value of latent class analysis in medical diagnosis, *Statistics in Medicine* **5**, 21–27.

[22]   Skene, A. & White, S. (1992). A latent class model for repeated measurements experiments, *Statistics in Medicine* **11**, 2111–2122.

[23]   Uebersax, J. & Grove, W. (1993). A latent trait finite mixture model for the analysis of rating agreement, *Biometrics* **49**, 823–835.

[24]   Winship, C. & Mare, R. (1989). Loglinear models with missing data: a latent class approach, *Sociological Methodology* **7**, 331–367.

(*See also* **Contingency Table; Rasch Models**)

MARK R. CONAWAY

Latent Failure Times Model *see* Competing Risks

Latent Period

Latency or *latent period* is defined as the time interval between the initiation time, say t_0, of a disease process and the time, say t_1, of the first occurrence of a specifically defined manifestation of the disease. For infectious diseases (*see* **Communicable Diseases**), t_0 is the time of infection by the infectious agent and the manifestation may either be a specific serologic marker, or a laboratory abnormality, or a symptom [31]. If the manifestation is the occurrence of a symptom, then the latent period is the same as the **incubation period**, which is the term usually used by statisticians for infectious diseases (e.g. Alcabes [1]). In the case of cancer epidemiology, t_0 is the time of initial exposure to a carcinogen (cancer initiation) and t_1 the time of the first clinical occurrence of the disease [3, 14]. For example, the initial exposure may be the time of exposure to **radiation** or the time of exposure to a chemical carcinogen, and the

first clinical occurrence may be detected by a biological marker for cancer or by clinical evidence of a tumor [15]. For A-bomb survivors such as those from Hiroshima or Nagasaki, Japan, t_0 is thus the actual time of explosion of the bomb whereas t_1 is the time the disease first appears.

Other Definitions

For infectious diseases, Bailey [5] and Anderson & May [2] have used "the time to first become infectious" as the specified manifestation so that they define the latent period of the disease as the time interval from the point of infection to the beginning of the state of infectiousness of the infected host. This latter definition is not necessarily synchronous with the incubation period except in cases (e.g. yellow fever) in which both the average intervals from the point of infection to the infectiousness of the host and from the point of infection to the onset of a symptom are very short. For many infectious diseases caused by parasites, a distinction can usually be made between infection according to some laboratory criteria and symptoms of illness [2]. For infectious diseases caused by viruses and bacteria, however, such a distinction may be difficult; furthermore, for some viral diseases such as smallpox and yellow fever, an infected individual may be immune to the disease so that illness may never occur in some individuals [2, 30].

For exposure to a carcinogen, distinctions have been made between the biologic latent period and the epidemiologic latent period. For exposure to radiation, such as in A-bomb survivors, the biologic latent period is defined in [39] as the interval during which an elevation of the risk of the disease occurs between the exposed and nonexposed individuals (see Example 3 in the next section for illustration), whereas the epidemiologic latent period is defined in [39] as the interval between the first exposure and the time of death from the cause of interest. For exposure to a chemical carcinogen, the beginning of the biologic latent period is the time that a DNA adduct of the carcinogen first appears because carcinogenesis starts with the interaction between the DNA adduct of the carcinogen and the genome of the host [18, 37]. The endpoint of the biologic latent period is the time of first occurrence of a cancer tumor cell; see [36]. For the epidemiologic latent period, the initial time is the time of first exposure to the carcinogen, whereas the endpoint is the time of first appearance of a detectable cancer tumor. It is shown in [18] that it is not the exposed dose but the dose of the DNA adduct of the agents that gives a linear **dose–response** curve for small doses; furthermore, detectable cancer tumors arise by clonal expansion from cancer tumor cells [45]. Thus, in most cases there are significant differences between the biologic latent period and the epidemiologic latent period.

Some Examples

The latent period of a disease may be very short and fairly constant. In some chronic infectious diseases, and in cancer, the latent period may be very long and varies greatly among individuals, in which case one should treat it as a **random variable** and work with the probability distribution of this variable.

Example 1. Yellow Fever

Yellow fever is an infectious disease caused by a yellow fever virus which is the prototype of the flavivirus genus (family Flaviviridae). It is an acute, mosquito-borne viral infection that occurs in epidemic and endemic form in tropical America and Africa. Clinical symptoms of this disease include fever, headache, malaise, and lassitude which persist for 2 to 4 days and occur in 10%–20% of the infected individuals. For this disease, the incubation period is very short (3 to 6 days) and can be considered as fairly constant [30].

Example 2. Malaria

Malaria is an infectious disease caused by parasites called Plasmodia. This disease occurs mainly in tropical areas and is transmitted to humans by the bite of malaria-infected female Anopheles mosquitoes. The four major *Plasmodium* species are *P. falciparum* (Africa, Asia, Oceania, Central America, and South America), *P. vivax* (Asia, Oceania, Central America, and South America), *P. ovale* (Africa and Oceania), and *P. malariae* (Africa and South America). The incubation periods for these four *Plasmodium* species are 8–27 days (average 12 days), 8–27 days (average 14 days), 9–17 days (average 15 days), and 16–28 days, respectively [33]. For this disease the

human host becomes infectious with the accumulation of gametocytes in the blood. Hence the interval from infection to infectiousness is the time from initial infection to the first appearance of gametocytes in the blood. (This is the definition of latent period used by Anderson & May [2].) For the above four species, this period is given by 9–10 days, 9–10 days, 10–14 days, and 15–16 days, respectively [2].

Example 3. Leukemia in A-Bomb Survivors

Land & Norman [24] have studied the biologic latent periods of radiogenic cancers occurring among Japanese A-bomb survivors in Hiroshima and Nagasaki, Japan. The leukemias (acute leukemia and chronic granulocytic leukemia) are particularly interesting since the cumulative distributions of those who have been exposed to an A-bomb with kerma doses of 100 rads or more lie on the far left of those who have not been exposed to an A-bomb or those who have been exposed to an A-bomb but with the kerma doses of 0–9 rads. The magnitude of the elevation of the cumulative probability of leukemia over the biologic latent period depends on the age of the survivor at the time of exposure, with the age group 10–19 years at exposure having the largest elevation followed by the age groups 20–34 and 35–49 years at exposure. The biologic latent periods for leukemia are intervals from five years since exposure (time of explosion of the bomb) to an endpoint, say t_1, which is less than 29 years since exposure and which depends on the age of the survivor at the time of exposure. For the age groups 10–19 and 20–34 years at exposure, t_1 is 29 years since exposure, but for age groups 0–9 and 35–49 years at exposure, t_1 is approximately 25 years since exposure.

Example 4. Incubation Period of AIDS

The infectious chronic disease **AIDS** is caused by a retrovirus called HIV (human immunodeficiency virus). This is an endemic fatal infectious disease without cure at the present time. (For a summary of basic facts about AIDS, see [34].) Following infection by HIV, it usually takes several months to develop HIV antibodies in the blood. (For the time interval from infection to the development of antibodies, the estimate by Horsburgh et al. [20] is 3.5

months.) According to the 1993 surveillance definition of AIDS used by the US **Centers for Disease Control** and Prevention (CDC), the incubation period is the time interval between infection by HIV and the first time that the total CD4 T-cell counts falls below $200/\text{mm}^3$ or the first time that the absolute percentage of CD4 T-cells falls below 14% or the first time that one of the 25 symptoms listed in [12] appears. This period is usually several years and depends on age [35], treatment with antiviral drugs [29], the presence of mutations of the gene CCR5 [16] (long or short AIDS survivors), and possibly other **covariates**. For untreated subjects aged 20–50 years at infection, the average incubation period is about 10 years. Note, however, that the AIDS definition used by CDC has been broadened three times, first in June 1985, next in July 1987, and then in December 1992. Hence, the incubation times measured before 1993 tend to be longer than the incubation times based on the 1993 AIDS definition.

The Latent Period of Infectious Diseases

For some infectious diseases such as yellow fever and malaria, the incubation period is relatively short and can be regarded as approximately constant. However, for some chronic infectious diseases such as AIDS, the incubation period is long and variable. In this latter case it makes more sense to treat the incubation period as a random variable, rather than as a fixed constant "latency", and to describe the process in terms of the probability distribution of incubation times. For example, the probability distribution of the incubation period of AIDS has been studied extensively, as summarized in Brookmeyer & Gail [9], Becker & Motika [6], and Tan et al. [38]. This probability distribution has been estimated by both parametric and **nonparametric methods**. However, all the estimates in the literature are based on the 1987 definition of AIDS: estimates of the HIV incubation period based on data and the 1993 AIDS definition have yet to be published.

The Latent Period of Cancer

Some researchers have used the concept of latency and average latent period to describe the interval between exposure to the A-bomb and the subsequent cancer onset in Hiroshima and Nagasaki, Japan [24, 7]. For example, leukemias tend to arise about five years following exposure to nuclear radiation [7]. However, Brookmeyer [8] pointed out that such estimates might be misleading because of censoring (*see* **Censored Data**) and competing causes (*see* **Competing Risks**) of death.

Many investigators prefer to consider the distribution of time to cancer onset, especially investigators who study cancer onset in animals exposed to low doses of a carcinogen [15]. In such cases the latent period is usually very long, and the expected time-to-tumor may exceed vastly the normal life span of the animal. In such circumstances, information on the mean latent period is not sufficient to determine the probability of developing a tumor before dying of some other causes. Moreover, different distributions may have the same **mean** time to tumor in the high dose range but give vastly different risk estimates when extrapolated to low doses [17, 43]. Thus, some scientists have avoided the use of mean latency for risk assessment based on low dose extrapolation (*see* **Extrapolation, Low-Dose**) [15]; rather, they describe carcinogens as altering the probability distribution of time to detectable cancer. This probability distribution depends on the mechanism of carcinogenesis and is influenced by many factors. In particular, the incidence of cancer is altered by changing the dose of the carcinogen to which the individual is exposed.

Armitage & Doll [4] developed the first stochastic model of carcinogenesis for the time-to-tumor distribution. This model is referred to as the multistage model (*see* **Multistage Carcinogenesis Models**) as described in reviews by Whittemore & Keller [42] and Kalbfleish et al. [21]. The Armitage–Doll multistage model (*see* **Dose–Response Models in Risk Analysis**) assumes that a tumor develops from a normal stem cell by k ($k \geq 2$) consecutive and irreversible genetic changes. These assumptions and the assumptions of low transition rates imply a **Weibull** model for the cancer **incidence rate**, $\lambda(t)$, and the following dose–response relationship between cancer incidence rate and the dose, d, of carcinogen:

$$\lambda(t) \propto \eta(d) \times t^{k-1}, \tag{1}$$

where $\eta(d)$ is a function of the dose d and is independent of time t.

The Armitage–Doll multistage model has been widely used by statisticians to assess how exposure to carcinogens alters the cancer incidence rates and the distributions of time-to-tumor. Breslow & Day [7] and others [13, 10] applied this model to study the effects of cigarette smoking on lung cancer risk, of asbestos exposure on risk of lung cancer and mesothelioma, and of radiation exposure on risks of leukemia, breast cancer, and bone cancer. While it is widely accepted that cancer results from a multistage process, recent results from molecular biology and molecular genetics have raised questions about some details of the assumptions in the Armitage–Doll multistage model (see [36] and [19]).

For risk assessment of carcinogens by low dose extrapolation, it has been documented that the same observable data can be fitted equally well by different models that yield very different estimates of risk at low doses [41]. Such extrapolation should be based on biologically plausible models, preferably models suggested by data. Thorslund et al. [40] and Moolgavkar et al. [32] proposed the MVK two-stage model (see [36]) for risk assessment. In this model, the first stage is a **Poisson process** describing how normal stem cells are changed into initiated cells by mutation (initiation); in the second stage the model incorporates stochastic birth and death (*see* **Stochastic Processes**) for proliferation of initiated cells (promotion), that change into malignant tumor cells by another mutation. Dose–response curves based on the MVK two-stage model have been developed by Chen & Moini [11], and by Krewski & Murdoch [23]. They have used these dose–response curves to assess how a carcinogen alters cancer incidence through its effects on initiating mutations or on the rate of proliferation of initiated cells. If the carcinogen is a pure initiator, then the dose–response curve for cancer incidence can be factorized as a product of a function of dose and a function of time and age; in these cases, the pattern of dose–response curves of the MVK model is quite similar to that of the Armitage–Doll multistage model. However, if the carcinogen is a promoter or a complete carcinogen, then the dose–response curves of the MVK model cannot be factorized, and they differ qualitatively from the Armitage–Doll model.

The MVK two-stage model, and extensions of it, together with many other biologically supported models have been analyzed in Tan [36] and in Yakovlev & Tsodikov [44]. Some extensions and modifications have recently been developed by Little and his colleagues [25]–[28]. (Little [25, 26] has called the

multievent model in Tan [36] the generalized MVK model.) By merging initiation and promotion, alternate modeling approaches have been proposed by Klebanov et al. [22] for radiation carcinogenesis.

References

[1]   Alcabes, P. (1993). The incubation period of human immunodeficiency virus, *Epidemiologic Reviews* **15**, 303–318.

[2]   Anderson, R.M. & May, R.M. (1992). *Infectious Diseases of Humans: Dynamics and Control*. Oxford University Press, Oxford.

[3]   Armitage, P. & Doll, R. (1961). Stochastic models for carcinogenesis, in *Proceedings of the Fourth Berkeley Symposium on Mathematical Statistics and Probability: Biology and Problems of Health*. University of California Press, Berkeley, pp. 19–38.

[4]   Armitage, P. & Doll, R. (1954). The age distribution of cancer and a multi-stage theory of carcinogenesis, *British Journal of Cancer* **8**, 1–12.

[5]   Bailey, N.T.J. (1975). *The Mathematical Theory of Infectious Diseases and Its Applications*. Griffin, London.

[6]   Becker, N.G. & Motika, M. (1993). Smoothed nonparametric back-projection of AIDS incidence data with adjustment for therapy, *Mathematical Biosciences* **118**, 1–23.

[7]   Breslow, N.E. & Day, N.E. (1987). *Statistical Methods in Cancer Research*, Vol. II: *The Design and Analysis of Cohort Studies*. International Agency for Research on Cancer, Lyon.

[8]   Brookmeyer, R. (1988). Time and latency considerations in the quantitative assessment of risk, in *Epidemiology and Health Risk Assessment*, L. Gordis, ed. Oxford University Press, Oxford, pp. 178–188.

[9]   Brookmeyer, R. & Gail, M.H. (1994). *AIDS Epidemiology: A Quantitative Approach*. Oxford University Press, Oxford.

[10] Brown, C.C. & Chu, K.C. (1983). Implications of multistage theory of carcinogenesis applied to occupational arsenic exposure, *Journal of the National Cancer Institute* **70**, 455–463.

[11] Chen, C.W. & Moini, A. (1990). Cancer dose–response models incorporating clonal expansion, in *Scientific Issues in Quantitative Cancer Risk Assessment*, S.H. Moolgavkar, ed. Birkhauser, Boston, pp. 153–175.

[12] CDC (1992). Revised classification system for HIV infection and expanded surveillance case definition for AIDS among adolescents and adults, *Morbidity and Mortality Weekly Report* **41** (RR-17), 1–19.

[13] Day, N.E. & Brown, C.C. (1980). Multistage models and primary prevention of cancer, *Journal of the National Cancer Institute* **64**, 977–989.

[14] Druckrey, H. (1967). Quantitative aspects of carcinogenesis, in *Potential Carcinogenic Hazards from Drugs,*

R. Truhaut, ed. UICC Monograph Series, Vol. 7, Springer-Verlag, New York, pp. 60–78.

[15] Guess, H.A. & Hoel, D.G. (1977). The effect of dose on cancer latency period, *Journal of Environmental Pathology and Toxicology* **1**, 279–286.

[16] Hill, C.M. & Littman, D.R. (1996). Natural resistance to HIV, *Nature* **382**, 668–669.

[17] Hoel, D.G., Gaylor, D.W., Kirschstein, R.L. & Saffiotti, U. (1975). Estimation of risks of irreversible delayed toxicity, *Journal of Toxicology and Environmental Health* **1**, 133–151.

[18] Hoel, D.G., Kaplan, N.L. & Anderson, N.W. (1983). Implication of nonlinear kinetics on risk estimation in carcinogenesis, *Science* **210**, 1032–1037.

[19] Hopkin, K. (1996). Tumor evolution: survival of the fittest cells, *Journal of NIH Research* **8**, 37–41.

[20] Horsburgh, C.R. Jr, Qu, C.Y. & Jason, I.M. (1989). Duration of human immunodeficiency virus infection before detection of antibody, *Lancet* **2**, 637–640.

[21] Kalbfleisch, J.D., Krewski, D.R. & Van Ryzin, J. (1983). Dose-response models for time-to-response toxicity data, *Canadian Journal of Statistics* **11**, 25–50.

[22] Klebanov, L.B. Rachev, S.T. & Yakovlev, A.Y. (1993). A stochastic model of radiation carcinogenesis: latent time distributions and their properties, *Mathematical Biosciences* **113**, 51–75.

[23] Krewski, D.R. & Murdoch, D.J. (1990). Cancer modeling with intermittent exposure, in *Scientific Issues in Quantitative Cancer Risk Assessment*, S.H. Moolgavkar ed. Birkhauser, Boston, pp. 196–214.

[24] Land, C.E. & Norman, J.E. (1978). Latent periods of radiogenic cancers occurring among Japanese A-bomb survivors, in *Late Biological Effects of Ionizing Radiation*, Vol. 1. International Atomic Energy Agency, Vienna.

[25] Little, M.P. (1995). Are two mutations sufficient to cause cancer? Some generalizations of the two-mutation model of carcinogenesis of Moolgavkar, Venzon and Knudson, and of the multistage model of Armitage and Doll, *Biometrics* **51**, 1278–1291.

[26] Little, M.P. (1996). Generalizations of the two-mutation and classical multi-stage models of carcinogenesis fitted to the Japanese atomic bomb survivor data, *Journal of Radiology Protection* **16**, 7–24.

[27] Little, M.P., Muirhead, C.R., Boice, J.D. & Kleinerman, R.A. (1995). Using multistage models to describe radiation-induced leukaemia, *Journal of Radiology Protection* **15**, 315–334.

[28] Little, M.P., Muirhead, C.R. & Stiller, C.A. (1996). Modeling lymphocytic leukaemia incidence in England and Wales using generalizations of the two-mutation model of carcinogenesis of Moolgavkar, Venzon and Knudson, *Statistics in Medicine* **15**, 1003–1022.

[29] Longini, I.R. Jr, Clark, W.S. & Karon, J. (1993). The effect of routine use of therapy in showing the clinical course of human immunodeficiency virus (HIV) infection in population-based cohort, *American Journal of Epidemiology* **137**, 1229–1240.

[30] Monath, T.P. (1994). Yellow fever, in *Infectious Disease: A Treatise of Infectious Diseases*, 5th Ed. P.D. Hoeprich, M.C. Jordan & A.R. Ronald, eds. Lippincott, Philadelphia pp. 826–828.

[31] Mosley, J.W. (1994). Epidemiology, in *Infectious Disease: A Treatise of Infectious Diseases*, 5th Ed. P.D. Hoeprich, M.C. Jordan & A.R. Ronald, eds. Lippincott, Philadelphia pp. 20–31.

[32] Moolgavkar, S.H. Cross, F.T. & Luebeck, E.G. (1990). A two-mutation model for radon-induced lung tumors in rats, *Radiation Research* **121**, 28–37.

[33] Redd, S.C. & Campbell, C.C. (1994). Malaria, in *Infectious Disease: A Treatise of Infectious Diseases*, 5th Ed. P.D. Hoeprich, M.C. Jordan & A.R. Ronald, eds. Lippincott, Philadelphia, pp. 1335–1344.

[34] Rhame, F.S. (1994). Acquired immunodeficiency syndrome, in *Infectious Disease: A Treatise of Infectious Diseases*, 5th Ed. P.D. Hoeprich, M.C. Jordan & A.R. Ronald, eds. Lippincott, Philadelphia, pp. 628–652.

[35] Rosenberg, P.S. (1995). Scope of the AIDS epidemic in the United States, *Science* **270**, 1372–1375.

[36] Tan, W.Y. (1991). *Stochastic Models of Carcinogenesis*. Marcel Dekker, New York.

[37] Tan, W.Y. & Singh, K.P. (1987). Assessing the effects of metabolism of environmental agents on cancer tumor development by a two-stage model of carcinogenesis, *Environmental Health Perspective* **74**, 203–210.

[38] Tan, W.Y. Tang, S.C. & Lee, S.R. (1996). Characterization of the HIV incubations and some comparative studies, *Statistics in Medicine* **15**, 197–220.

[39] Thomas, D.C. & McNeill, K.G. (1982). Risk estimates for the health effects of alpha radiation, in *Appendix M, Research Report*. Atomic Energy Control Board, Ottawa.

[40] Thorslund, T.W., Brown, C.C. & Charnley, C. (1987). Biologically motivated cancer risk models, *Risk Analysis* **7**, 109–119.

[41] Van Ryzin, J. (1980). Quantitative risk assessment, *Occupational Medicine* **22**, 321–326.

[42] Whittemore, A.S. & Keller, J.B. (1978). Quantitative theories of carcinogenesis, *SIAM Review* **20**, 1–30.

[43] Whittemore, A. & Altshuler, B. (1976). Lung cancer incidence in cigarette smokers: further analysis of Doll and Hill's data for British physicians, *Biometrics* **32**, 805–816.

[44] Yakovlev, A.Y. & Tsodikov, A.D. (1996). *Stochastic Models of Tumor Latency and Their Biostatistical Applications*. World Scientific, Singapore.

[45] Yang, G.L. & Chen, C.W. (1991). A stochastic two-stage carcinogenesis model: a new approach to computing the probability of observing tumor in animal bioassays, *Mathematical Biosciences* **104**, 247–258.

WAI-YUAN TAN & CHAO W. CHEN

Latent Predictor *see* Measurement Error in Epidemiologic Studies

Latent Variable *see* Path Analysis

Latin Square Designs

A Latin square design is a **balanced incomplete block design** for comparing t treatments in which heterogeneity is eliminated in two ways. It is an **incomplete block design** insofar as not every combination of row, column, and treatment is assigned to an experimental unit. It is a *balanced* design insofar as the number of treatments is equal in each row and in each column.

Example 1

Suppose a toxicologist wants to compare a series of t treatments. Suppose the experiments are to be carried out in r different laboratories $L_1, \ldots, L_r$ on c different animal species $S_1, \ldots, S_c$. The experimenter wants to take into account the heterogeneity coming from both these factors. The simplest experimental design would be a **randomized complete blocks design** in which every treatment is assigned to every combination of both heterogeneity factors. In this whole experiment we would have rct experimental units corresponding to rc blocks and t treatments. This number of experimental units can become enormous, even for moderate r, c, and t. If $r = c = t$, this design can be replaced by a Latin Square Design (LSD) in which each treatment, traditionally denoted with Latin letters, occurs exactly once in each row and once in each column, so that the number of experimental units is only t^2.

In other settings a complete block design is physically impossible, as in Examples 2 and 3, and Latin square designs are a natural alternative.

Example 2

In a field experiment where the experimental field exhibits a gradient in two orthogonal directions, each spot can only be assigned to a single treatment.

Example 3

In a **clinical trial** the **blocking** factors may be the individual subject and successive time periods. If the objective of the trial is to compare treatments, then only one treatment can be given to a given subject at a given time. This design is called a **crossover** trial (see [5]).

Construction of the Design

If we want to use an LSD, we have first to choose a Latin square. A Latin square of order t is an arrangement of t letters or numbers (representing the treatments) in a square of t columns and t rows (representing the two heterogeneity factors), such that each letter appears once and only once in each column and each row (whence the balance of the design). Latin squares of any order exist, as can be seen from Figure 1.

The enumeration of all the Latin squares of any order t becomes tedious as t increases. However, permuting rows, columns or treatments of a Latin square gives another Latin square. Particular Latin squares are those for which the first column and the first row are ordered (A, B, C, ...); these are called *standard* Latin squares. By permuting rows and columns of a standard Latin square we can obtain $t!(t-1)!$ different Latin squares.

Thus, sampling a Latin square consists in:

1. sampling a standard Latin square with equiprobability among all the standard Latin squares;
2. randomly permuting the t rows, the $t-1$ first columns and the t treatments.

For more details of this procedure and tables of standard Latin squares, see [2]; for tables of random permutations, see [1].

The **randomization** procedure of a Latin square is equivalent to the observation of the t^3 random variables δ_{ijk}, where $\delta_{ijk} = 1$ if the treatment k

$$
\begin{array}{cccccc}
1 & 2 & 3 & \ldots & t-1 & t \\
2 & 3 & 4 & \ldots & t & 1 \\
3 & 4 & 5 & \ldots & 1 & 2 \\
\ldots & & & & & \ldots \\
t & 1 & 2 & \ldots & & t-1
\end{array}
$$

Figure 1 Example of Latin square of order t

is affected in row i and column j, and 0 otherwise. These random variables have the following properties:

$$\sum_i \delta_{ijk} = \sum_j \delta_{ijk} = \sum_k \delta_{ijk} = 1. \qquad (1)$$

$$E(\delta_{ijk}) = \frac{1}{t}, \quad \text{for all } i, j, k. \qquad (2)$$

$$E(\delta_{ijk}\delta_{i'j'k'})$$

$$= \begin{cases} 1/t, & \text{if } i = i' \text{ and } j = j' \\ & \text{and } k = k', \\ 0, & \text{if either } i \neq i' \text{ or } j \neq j' \\ & \text{or } k \neq k', \\ 1/t(t-1), & \text{if either } i = i' \text{ or } j = j' \\ & \text{or } k = k', \\ 1/t(t-1)^2(t-2), & \text{if } i \neq i' \text{ and } j \neq j' \\ & \text{and } k \neq k'. \end{cases}$$

$$(3)$$

Estimation and Analysis of Variance

Let Y_{ijk} be the response that would be observed if the kth treatment were assigned on the ith row and the jth column. Under unit-treatment additivity (in the terminology of Hinkelmann & Kempthorne [3]), i.e. under the hypothesis that there are no **interactions** between the treatments on one side and rows or columns on the other side, we can write:

$$Y_{ijk} = \mu + \alpha_i^{C} + \alpha_j^{R} + \alpha_k^{T} + \alpha_{ij}^{RC} + \varepsilon_{ijk}, \qquad (4)$$

where superscripts C, R, and T indicate columns, rows, and treatments respectively. The technical errors ε_{ijk} are assumed independent with zero **mean** and equal **variance** σ_ε^2, and are independent of the randomization procedure. We can also write the usual side conditions which imply no loss of generality:

$$\alpha_{\cdot}^{C} = \alpha_{\cdot}^{R} = \alpha_{\cdot}^{T} = \alpha_{i\cdot}^{RC} = \alpha_{\cdot j}^{RC} = 0, \quad \text{for all } i, j. \qquad (5)$$

We note that within an LSD not all Y_{ijk} are actually measured but only those for which the **random variable** δ_{ijk} is equal to 1.

The observed means can thus be written:

$$Y_{i\cdot\cdot} = \frac{1}{t}\sum_j\sum_k \delta_{ijk}Y_{ijk},$$

$$Y_{\cdot j\cdot} = \frac{1}{t}\sum_i\sum_k \delta_{ijk}Y_{ijk},$$

$$Y_{\cdot\cdot k} = \frac{1}{t}\sum_i\sum_j \delta_{ijk}Y_{ijk},$$

$$Y_{\cdots} = \frac{1}{t^2}\sum_{ijk} \delta_{ijk}Y_{ijk}. \qquad (6)$$

If we substitute Y_{ijk} in (6) by its expression from (4), then, after applying the side conditions (5) and the relations (1), we obtain:

$$Y_{i\cdot\cdot} = \mu + \alpha_i^{R} + \frac{1}{t}\sum_j\sum_k \delta_{ijk}\varepsilon_{ijk},$$

$$Y_{\cdot j\cdot} = \mu + \alpha_j^{C} + \frac{1}{t}\sum_i\sum_k \delta_{ijk}\varepsilon_{ijk},$$

$$Y_{\cdot\cdot k} = \mu + \alpha_k^{T} + \frac{1}{t}\sum_i\sum_j \delta_{ijk}\varepsilon_{ijk},$$

$$Y_{\cdots} = \mu + \frac{1}{t^2}\sum_i\sum_j\sum_k \delta_{ijk}\varepsilon_{ijk}. \qquad (7)$$

The total sum of squares $SS_{\text{tot}} = \sum_{ijk}\delta_{ijk}(\varepsilon_{ijk})^2$ can be decomposed as follows:

$$SS_{\text{tot}} = t\sum_i (Y_{i\cdot\cdot} - Y_{\cdots})^2 + t\sum_j (Y_{\cdot j\cdot} - Y_{\cdots})^2$$

$$+ t\sum_k (Y_{\cdot\cdot k} - Y_{\cdots})^2 + SS_e. \qquad (8)$$

The **expectations** of these sums of squares depend on the **moments** of the δ_{ijk} given in (2) and (3). Somewhat tedious computations yield the **analysis of variance** table given in Table 1 where:

$$\sigma_R^2 = \frac{1}{t-1}\sum_i (\alpha_i^{R})^2,$$

$$\sigma_C^2 = \frac{1}{t-1}\sum_j (\alpha_j^{C})^2,$$

$$\sigma_T^2 = \frac{1}{t-1}\sum_k (\alpha_k^{T})^2, \qquad (9)$$

and

$$\sigma_{RC}^2 = \frac{1}{(t-1)^2}\sum_i\sum_j (\alpha_{ij}^{RC})^2.$$

To test the hypothesis (*see* **Hypothesis Testing**) of equality of the treatment effects (i.e. $\sigma_T^2 = 0$), we are

Table 1 Analysis of variance of an LSD

Source	df	SS	E(MS)
Rows	$t-1$	$t\sum_i(Y_{i..}-Y_{...})^2$	$\mathrm{E}(MS_\mathrm{T})=\sigma_\varepsilon^2+t\sigma_\mathrm{R}^2$
Columns	$t-1$	$t\sum_j(Y_{.j.}-Y_{...})^2$	$\mathrm{E}(MS_\mathrm{C})=\sigma_\varepsilon^2+t\sigma_\mathrm{C}^2$
Treatments	$t-1$	$t\sum_k(Y_{..k}-Y_{...})^2$	$\mathrm{E}(MS_\mathrm{T})=\sigma_\varepsilon^2+\sigma_\mathrm{RC}^2+t\sigma_\mathrm{T}^2$
Error	t^2-3t+2	by subtraction $=SS_\mathrm{e}$	$\mathrm{E}(MS_\mathrm{e})=\sigma_\varepsilon^2+\sigma_\mathrm{RC}^2$
Total	t^2-1	$\sum_{ijk}\delta_{ijk}(Y_{ijk}-Y_{...})^2$	

led by Table 1 to consider the ratio

$$F=\frac{MS_\mathrm{T}}{MS_\mathrm{e}}. \tag{10}$$

This statistic can be referred to $F(t-1, t^2-3t+2)$ under normal theory (*see* **F Distribution**). Nevertheless, Welch [6] investigates its distribution under the randomization process for LSD described above and Hinkelmann & Kempthorne [3], reviewing this work, "assume that normal theory gives satisfactory approximations to corresponding randomization tests".

Another immediate consequence of Table 1 is that there do not exist any legitimate tests for row and column effects unless we suppose absence of interaction between them ($\sigma_\mathrm{RC}^2=0$).

Other Topics

Departure from Additivity

The effects of row × treatment, column × treatment, row × column × treatment can severely affect the results obtained above, as discussed in detail by Scheffé [4]. Nevertheless, Wilk & Kempthorne [7] show that the usual F test is still appropriate, even in the presence of interactions, if the t rows have been sampled from a population of R rows, the t columns have been sampled from a population of C columns, the t treatments have been sampled from a population of T treatments with $R >> t, C >> t$, and $T >> t$ (*see* **Random Effects**).

Limitations of the LSD and Some Extensions

It can be argued that the LSD is limited from a practical point of view. Some extensions have been proposed for the following problems (see [3]):

1. the numbers of rows, columns and treatments have to be the same (**Youden squares** and Latin rectangles are some alternatives);
2. for small values of t the number of **degrees of freedom** for error is insufficient (this can be mended by replicating the LSDs);
3. the number of heterogeneity factors is restricted to two (**Graeco–Latin squares** deal with three or more heterogeneity factors).

References

[1]   Cochran, W.G. & Cox, G.M. (1957). *Experimental Designs*, 2nd Ed. Wiley, New York.

[2]   Fisher, R.A. & Yates, F. (1963). *Statistical Tables for Biological, Agricultural and Medical Research*. Oliver & Boyd, Edinburgh.

[3]   Hinkelmann, K. & Kempthorne, O. (1994). *Design and Analysis of Experiments*, Vol. 1. Wiley, New York.

[4]   Scheffé, H. (1959). *The Analysis of Variance*. Wiley, New York.

[5]   Senn, S. (1994). The AB/BA crossover: past, present and future?, *Statistical Methods in Medical Research* **3**, 303–324.

[6]   Welch, B.L. (1937). On the z-test in randomized blocks and Latin squares, *Biometrika* **29**, 21–52.

[7]   Wilk, M.B. & Kempthorne, O. (1957). Non-additivities in a Latin square design, *Journal of the American Statistical Society* **52**, 218–236.

PASCAL WILD & MICHEL GRZEBYK

Lattice Designs

The term *lattice design* encompasses two different types of equireplicate designs. The first type, *square lattice designs* and their extensions, are resolvable (0, 1) incomplete block designs. The second type, *lattice squares* and their extensions, are nested *row-column designs* (*see* **Youden Squares and Row-Column Designs**) for which each block is a complete replicate.

An **incomplete block design** for t treatment each replicated r times with all blocks of size $k < t$ is *resolvable* if the b blocks can be grouped into $r = bk/t$ sets of $s = t/k$ blocks, such that each set is a complete replicate. A $(0, 1)$-*design* has each pairwise treatment concurrence equal to 0 or 1. A square lattice design, introduced by **F. Yates** in 1936, has $t = k^2$ and $s = k$. It can be constructed by writing the numbers 1 to t in a $k \times k$ array. The *simple square lattice design* has $r = 2$. The k blocks of the first replicate are the rows of the array. The second replicate uses the columns. The *triple square lattice design* has $r = 3$. The third replicate is found by superimposing a **Latin square** of order k on the array, and using the Latin square symbols to define the blocks.

If $k \neq 6$, then the Greek letters of a **Graeco-Latin square** can be used to get a fourth replicate (*quadruple square lattice design*). If $k \neq 3, 6, 10$, then at least five replicates can be obtained using *mutually* **orthogonal** *Latin squares* (MOLS). If k is a prime power, a complete set of $k - 1$ MOLS exist, and up to $k + 1$ replicates are possible. If, in this case, $k + 1$ replicates are used, then the variance-balanced design, called a *balanced square lattice*, is a symmetric **balanced incomplete block design** BIBD $[k^2, k(k + 1), k]$.

For example, using the three MOLS of order 4:

$$
\begin{array}{|cccc|}
\hline
1 & 2 & 3 & 4 \\
2 & 1 & 4 & 3 \\
3 & 4 & 1 & 2 \\
4 & 3 & 2 & 1 \\
\hline
\end{array}
\quad
\begin{array}{|cccc|}
\hline
1 & 2 & 3 & 4 \\
3 & 4 & 1 & 2 \\
4 & 3 & 2 & 1 \\
2 & 1 & 4 & 3 \\
\hline
\end{array}
\quad
\begin{array}{|cccc|}
\hline
1 & 2 & 3 & 4 \\
4 & 3 & 2 & 1 \\
2 & 1 & 4 & 3 \\
3 & 4 & 1 & 2 \\
\hline
\end{array}
$$

on the array

$$
\begin{array}{|cccc|}
\hline
1 & 2 & 3 & 4 \\
5 & 6 & 7 & 8 \\
9 & 10 & 11 & 12 \\
13 & 14 & 15 & 16 \\
\hline
\end{array}
$$

gives the balanced square lattice design (parentheses denote blocks, each replicate is a row):

(1 2 3 4),   (5 6 7 8),   (9 10 11 12),   (13 14 15 16);
(1 5 9 13),   (2 6 10 14),   (3 7 11 15),   (4 8 12 16);
(1 6 11 16),   (2 5 12 15),   (3 8 9 14),   (4 7 10 13);
(1 7 12 14),   (2 8 11 13),   (3 5 10 16),   (4 6 9 15);
(1 8 10 15),   (2 7 9 16),   (3 6 12 13),   (4 5 11 14).

For $r < 5$, the first r replicates (say) can be used.

The need for t to be a perfect square (and not 36 if more than three replicates are required) can be a severe restriction. In some experiments, such as variety trials which often use a large number of varieties and few replicates (two or three), it may be possible to add a few extra treatments, or even remove some, to get $t = k^2$. Various extensions have been proposed to allow some other values of t. *Cubic lattices* have $t = k^3$ and $s = k^2$ in a similar way using a cubic array and orthogonal Latin cubes; and m-dimensional lattices with $t = k^m$ for $m > 3$ are possible if k is prime. A *rectangular lattice* with $t = k(k + 1)$ and $s = k + 1$ can be constructed in a similar way to the square lattices using the numbers 1 to t in a $(k + 1) \times (k + 1)$ array with the leading diagonal omitted. For $r > 2$ the Latin squares used must have each symbol occurring on the main diagonal. The idea for constructing the rectangular lattice can be used for any $s > k + 1$ by, if possible, omitting further (wrap-around) diagonals. The α-*designs* are an extension to resolvable designs with any s – see John [3, Section 4.8] and John & Williams [4, Sections 4.4 and 4.5]. Optimal two-replicate resolvable designs are discussed by John & Williams [4, Section 4.7].

Although specific formulas can be given, as in John [3, Section 3.4], John & Williams [4, Sections 4.2 and 4.3], the usual *intrablock* analysis for the model with fixed treatment and block effects – see John [3, Sections 1.3–1.5] and John & Williams [4, Sections 1.4–1.6] – is easily carried out on a computer. If s is not small, then it may be worth using the *interblock* information also. Various methods are available for combining the information, but a good choice nowadays would be to use a computer package (*see* **Software, Biostatistical**) such as GENSTAT or SAS which performs REML (**restricted maximum likelihood**) estimation – see John & Williams [4, Sections 7.5 and 7.6].

Lattice squares, introduced by F. Yates in 1940, are nested row-column designs for $t = k^2$ in $r > 1$ complete blocks (or groups) of k rows and k columns. If k is a prime power, then a variance-balanced design, the *balanced lattice square*, is possible. This needs $r = (k + 1)/2$ for k odd, and $r = k + 1$ for k even. The balanced lattice square can be constructed from the balanced square lattice design. If k is odd, then each replicate of a balanced square lattice forms either the rows or the columns of one block. If k is even, then each replicate of a balanced square lattice forms the rows of one block, and the columns of another. For example, the balanced lattice square with $t = 3$ is

$$
\begin{array}{ccc}
1 & 2 & 3 \\
4 & 5 & 6 \\
7 & 8 & 9
\end{array}
\qquad
\begin{array}{ccc}
1 & 6 & 8 \\
9 & 2 & 4 \\
5 & 7 & 3
\end{array}
$$

and one with $t = 4$ is

$$
\begin{array}{cccc}
1 & 2 & 3 & 4 \\
5 & 6 & 7 & 8 \\
9 & 10 & 11 & 12 \\
13 & 14 & 15 & 16
\end{array}
\qquad
\begin{array}{cccc}
1 & 5 & 9 & 13 \\
6 & 2 & 14 & 10 \\
11 & 15 & 3 & 7 \\
16 & 12 & 8 & 4
\end{array}
$$

$$
\begin{array}{cccc}
1 & 6 & 11 & 16 \\
12 & 15 & 2 & 5 \\
14 & 9 & 8 & 3 \\
7 & 4 & 13 & 10
\end{array}
\qquad
\begin{array}{cccc}
1 & 7 & 12 & 14 \\
8 & 2 & 13 & 11 \\
10 & 16 & 3 & 5 \\
15 & 9 & 6 & 4
\end{array}
$$

$$
\begin{array}{cccc}
1 & 8 & 10 & 15 \\
2 & 7 & 9 & 16 \\
3 & 6 & 12 & 13 \\
4 & 5 & 11 & 14
\end{array}
$$

If k is odd, then a balanced lattice square with $r = k + 1$ repeats the original design with the rows and columns interchanged.

Lattice squares which are not variance-balanced are obtained if other numbers of replicates are used. Care is then needed in the choice of the r replicates to ensure that the combined row and column treatment concurrences are as equal as possible – see Cochran & Cox [1, Section 12.12] and John & Williams [4, Section 6.2]. Designs may be possible for some $r > 1$ if k is not a prime power, depending on the maximum number of MOLS of order k. Balanced lattice squares for $k = 3, 4, 5, 7, 8, 9, 11, 13$ are given by Cochran & Cox [1, Chapter 12].

As before, the restriction on the possible values of t may be severe. Extensions to *lattice rectangles* are possible. John & Williams [4] discuss other resolvable nested row–column designs: α-designs (Section 6.3), two-replicate designs (Section 6.6), and designs generated using **algorithms** (Section 6.4). If the design is not balanced, then the usual intrablock analysis can again be easily carried out on a computer. There is no interblock information when each block is a complete replicate, but there may sometimes be useful interrow or intercolumn information, which again is best combined using REML estimation.

The lattice square designs and square lattices can be used for replicated blocked **factorial experiments** if the product of the levels is k^2 – see Cochran & Cox [1, Sections 10.12 and 12.11]. For the balanced designs, main effects and **interactions** are equally partially **confounded**. If $t_1 = t_2 = k$, then the first replicate of the square lattice design confounds one main effect, and the second replicate confounds the other.

Some further details on lattice designs are given by Cornelius [2].

References

[1] Cochran, W.G. & Cox, G.M. (1957). *Experimental Designs*, 2nd Ed. Wiley, New York.

[2] Cornelius, P.L. (1983). Lattice designs, in *Encyclopedia of Statistical Sciences*, Vol. 4, S. Kotz & N.L. Johnson, eds. Wiley, New York, pp. 510–518.

[3] John, J.A. (1987). *Cyclic Designs*. Chapman & Hall, London.

[4] John, J.A. & Williams, E.R. (1995). *Cyclic and Computer Generated Designs*, 2nd Ed. of [3]. Chapman & Hall, London.

(*See also* **Experimental Design in Biostatistics**)

R.J. MARTIN

Law of Independence *see* Mendel's Laws

Law of Large Numbers

The first theorem recognizable as a precise form of a limiting-frequency statement (or "law of large numbers" in the terminology introduced by Poisson) is the famous *"weak law of large numbers for Bernoulli trials"* of James Bernoulli (1654–1705) [2] (*see* **Bernoulli Family**). In our current notation and terminology his theorem, published posthumously in *Ars Conjectandi* (1713), now reads as follows. Let $X_1, \ldots, X_n$ be the outcomes of n independent 0–1 trials (Bernoulli trials) with success probability p. With $S_n = \sum_{i=1}^{n} X_i$ the number of successes (the number of ones) and $\overline{X}_n = S_n/n$, we have for each $\varepsilon > 0$

$$\lim_{n \to \infty} \Pr\left(|\overline{X}_n - p| > \varepsilon\right) = 0.$$

In words: the ratio of the number of successes and the number of trials or the proportion of successes **converges in probability** to the success probability p. A universally applied notation is $\overline{X}_n \xrightarrow{\text{Pr}} p$ (i.e. $\overline{X}_n$ converges to p in probability).

Remark 1.   The result provides some empirical confirmation for the axioms of probability theory [7, Chapter 1] (*see* **Foundations of Probability**). See also [3, pp. 20–21] for an introductory discussion.

Remark 2.   The proof is a simple application of the Chebyshev inequality:

$$\Pr\left(|\overline{X}_n - p| > \varepsilon\right) \le \frac{1}{\varepsilon^2} \mathrm{E}\left(\overline{X}_n - p\right)^2$$
$$= \frac{p(1-p)}{n\varepsilon^2} \to 0, \quad n \to \infty.$$

For $X_1, \ldots, X_n$ a sequence of independent random variables with common distribution function F, let $S_n = \sum_{i=1}^{n} X_i, \overline{X}_n = S_n/n$ and $\mu = \mathrm{E}(X_1)$. Then the following generalization of Bernoulli's theorem has been obtained.

Theorem 1.   Khinchin's law of large numbers

$$\mathrm{E}|X_1| < \infty \text{ implies } \overline{X}_n \xrightarrow{\text{Pr}} \mu.$$

In words: the sample mean $\overline{X}_n$ is a "weakly consistent" estimator of the population mean μ.

A refined version of this result is the following characterization due to Kolmogorov (see [2] for further details).

Theorem 2.   In order that there exist constants μ_n such that for each $\varepsilon > 0$

$$\lim_{n \to \infty} \Pr\left(|\overline{X}_n - \mu_n| > \varepsilon\right) = 0,$$

it is necessary and sufficient that

$$n\Pr\left(|X_1| > n\right) \to 0, \quad n \to \infty.$$

In this case, $\mu_n = \int_{-n}^{n} x \mathrm{d}F(x)$.

Strong Law of Large Numbers

Almost sure (a.s.) convergence is a mode of convergence that describes the behavior of a statistic (e.g. the sample mean, $\overline{X}_n$) outside an unspecified set of probability zero. Almost sure convergence is stronger than convergence in probability (see Remark 4 below). Synonyms for almost sure convergence are convergence with probability one and convergence almost everywhere.

The Kolmogorov strong law of large numbers, the a.s. version of Khinchin's law, reads as follows.

Theorem 3.   For $X_1, \ldots, X_n$ a sequence of independent random variables with common distribution function F:

$$\mathrm{E}|X_1| < \infty \text{ if and only if } \Pr\left(\lim_{n \to \infty} \overline{X}_n = \mu\right) = 1$$

with $\mu = \mathrm{E}(X_1)$.

Remark 3.   The standard way to write this result is $\mathrm{E}|X_1| < \infty$ if and only if $\overline{X}_n \to \mu$ a.s.

In words: the sample mean $\overline{X}_n$ is a "strongly **consistent**" estimator of the population mean μ.

Remark 4.   This simple characterization of strong convergence makes it clear why probabilists like the a.s. convergence mode. For statisticians the difference between the weak and the strong law of large numbers is subtle and cannot be adequately explained without measure theory. See [3, p. 233] for an intuitive discussion and some amusing quotations. From an applied point of view, most statisticians seem to be satisfied with convergence in probability.

Applications

Application 1

For $X_1, \ldots, X_n$ a sequence of independent random variables with common distribution function F let $\mathbb{F}_n$ denote the empirical distribution function, i.e.

$$\mathbb{F}_n(x) = \frac{\#\{i : X_i \leq x\}}{n} = \frac{1}{n} \sum_{i=1}^{n} I\{X_i \leq x\}, \quad x \in \mathbb{R}$$

(*see* **Goodness of Fit**). For fixed x, $\mathbb{F}_n(x) \to F(x)$ a.s. by the strong law of large numbers. This property strengthens to almost sure convergence uniform in x.

Theorem 4.   Glivenko–Cantelli theorem.

$$\sup_{x \in \mathbb{R}} |\mathbb{F}_n(x) - F(x)| \to 0 \text{ a.s.}$$

In words: uniformly in x we can rediscover F from the data. Taking n large enough, this can be done to any desired degree of precision.

Application 2

We now discuss the statistical relevance of the consistency results given in the previous sections. Many problems in statistics are of the following type: for a given (unknown) parameter θ ($\mathbb{R}$-valued, $\mathbb{R}^d$-valued, or a function), find a consistent estimator T_n and obtain the limit distribution of $n^\gamma(T_n - \theta)$. Typical values for γ are $\gamma = 1/2$ for the classical **central limit theorem** (normality) and $\gamma = 1$ for a limit distribution that corresponds to a weighted sum of centered **chi-square distributed** random variables. Typically, $\text{var}[n^\gamma(T_n - \theta)] \to \sigma^2$, with σ^2 a **nuisance parameter** that needs to be estimated in a consistent way in order to construct, for example, approximate **confidence intervals** for θ.

To make this point clear, consider the following simple example. Given a sequence of independent identically distributed random variables $X_1, \ldots, X_n$ let $\theta = \mu$ and $T_n \equiv \overline{X}_n$. If $0 < \sigma^2 = \text{var}(X_1) < \infty$, then the limit distribution of $n^{1/2}(\overline{X}_n - \mu)$ is a zero mean **normal distribution** with variance σ^2. The sample variance

$$S_n^2 = \frac{1}{n-1} \sum_{i=1}^{n} (X_i - \overline{X}_n)^2$$

$$= \frac{n}{n-1} \left\{ \frac{1}{n} \sum_{i=1}^{n} X_i^2 - \overline{X}_n^2 \right\}$$

is a (strongly) consistent estimator for σ^2. To see this note that

$$\overline{X}_n \to \mu \text{ a.s. implies } \overline{X}_n^2 \to \mu^2,$$

and that the strong law of large number gives

$$\frac{1}{n} \sum_{i=1}^{n} X_i^2 \to EX_1^2 = \sigma^2 + \mu^2.$$

Hence we have $S_n^2 \to \sigma^2$ a.s.

We therefore obtain, using Slutsky's theorem (for which weak consistency is sufficient) that the limit distribution of $n^{1/2}(\overline{X}_n - \mu)/S_n$ is standard normal. Hence, an approximate $100(1 - \alpha)\%$ confidence interval for μ is of the form $\overline{x}_n \pm z_{1-(\alpha/2)}(s_n/n^{1/2})$ with $\overline{x}_n$ and s_n^2 the actual values of $\overline{X}_n$ and S_n^2 and $z_{1-(\alpha/2)}$ the $[1 - (\alpha/2)]$-percentile of the standard normal distribution.

Extensions

Extension 1

Let $X_1, X_2, \ldots$ be a sequence of random variables with a common distribution function F and replace the independence assumption by the **stationarity** assumption: for every n the joint distribution of $X_1, \ldots, X_n$ is the same as the joint distribution of $X_{1+k}, \ldots, X_{n+k}$ for all positive integers k.

On the basis of general results from ergodic theory one can show that, given the stationary process, $X_1, X_2, \ldots, \overline{X}_n$ still obeys laws of large numbers. Note that ergodic theory applies to a large number of problems in probability theory and analysis. See [8] for further reading.

Extension 2

Given a sequence of independent zero-mean random variables $\Delta_1, \Delta_2, \ldots$, define $X_n = \sum_{i=1}^{n} \Delta_i$. With $\mathcal{F}_n = \sigma(X_1, \ldots, X_n)$, the σ-algebra generated by $X_1, \ldots, X_n$, we then have that

$$E(X_{n+1}|\mathcal{F}_n) = X_n.$$

This simple property delineates a very useful class of **stochastic processes**: martingales. The study of laws of large numbers for martingales is an intrinsic part of modern probability theory and the results are extremely important for a variety of applications in, for example, survival analysis [5] (*see* **Counting**

Process Methods in Survival Analysis). Further discussion is beyond the scope of this article; we refer to [1, Section 35] for an excellent introductory discussion and a number of interesting examples. A specialized reference is [6].

Finally, note that thorough discussions on the law of large numbers can be found in [4], [9], and [10].

References

[1]   Billingsley, P. (1979). *Probability and Measure*. Wiley, New York.

[2]   Bingham, N.H. (1989). *Theory of Probability and Its Applications* **34**, 129–139.

[3]   Chung, K.L. (1975). *Elementary Probability Theory with Stochastic Processes*. Springer-Verlag, New York.

[4]   Doob, J.L. (1953). *Stochastic Processes*. Wiley, New York.

[5]   Fleming, T.R. & Harrington, D.P. (1991). *Counting Processes and Survival Analysis*. Wiley, New York.

[6]   Hall, P. & Heyde, C.C. (1980). *Martingale Limit Theory and its Applications*. Academic Press, New York.

[7]   Kolmogorov, A.N. (1950). *Foundations of the Theory of Probability*. Chelsea, New York.

[8]   Krengel, U. (1985). *Ergodic Theorems*. Walter de Gruyter, Berlin.

[9]   Révész, P. (1968). *The Laws of Large Numbers*. Academic Press, New York.

[10]   Stout, W.F. (1974). *Almost Sure Convergence*. Academic Press, New York.

(*See also* **Limit Theorems**)

PAUL JANSSEN

Law of Segregation *see* Mendel's Laws

Law of the Iterated Logarithm *see* Limit Theorems

Lawley–Hotelling Trace

To test the equality of mean vectors of k p-variate normal distributions (*see* **Multivariate Normal Distribution**) with common but unknown covariance matrix, Hotelling [14] proposed a test, known as the Hotelling's generalized trace (or T_0^2) test, which could be considered as a generalization of **Hotelling's T^2 test** proposed for $k = 2$. This test statistic was also considered by Lawley [21], Bartlett [4], and Hsu [16]; it is often known as the Lawley–Hotelling trace. The test can be expressed as follows in its canonical form.

Consider random matrices $\mathbf{U} : p \times r$, $\mathbf{V} : p \times m$, and $\mathbf{W} : p \times n$, such that the columns of $\mathbf{U}$, $\mathbf{V}$ and $\mathbf{W}$ are independently distributed as p-variate normal distributions with a common covariance matrix $\boldsymbol{\Sigma}$. The problem is to test $\mathrm{H}_0 : \boldsymbol{\Theta} \equiv \mathrm{E}(\mathbf{U}) = \mathbf{0}$ against $\mathrm{H}_1 : \boldsymbol{\Theta} \neq \mathbf{0}$, given that $\mathrm{E}(\mathbf{W}) = \mathbf{0}$, $\boldsymbol{\Sigma}$ being unknown. The Lawley–Hotelling's trace test rejects H_0 if and only if

$$T_0^2 \equiv \mathrm{trace}[(\mathbf{U}\mathbf{U}')(\mathbf{W}\mathbf{W}')^{-1}]n$$

is too large; it is assumed that $n \geq p$. The **multivariate analysis of variance** (MANOVA) problem can be reduced to the above canonical form; in that case, $\mathbf{U}\mathbf{U}'$ and $\mathbf{W}\mathbf{W}'$ denote the sums of products and cross products matrices due to the hypothesis H_0 and due to error, respectively. This trace test can be deduced from Roy's **union–intersection principle**; see Mudholkar et al. [25].

The Lawley–Hotelling trace criterion can be considered for testing independence between two sets of variates jointly distributed as a normal distribution, as well as for testing equality of covariance matrices of two p-variate normal distributions; for this correspondence, see the article on **Pillai's trace test** and the review papers by Pillai [30, 31].

Hotelling [15] derived an explicit form of the null distribution of T_0^2 for $p = 2$; see Hsu [16] and Anderson [1]. Constantine [5] expressed the density of T_0^2 as an infinite series in generalized Laguerre polynomials, and also as an infinite series in zonal polynomials; for details, see Muirhead [27]. Pillai [29] suggested to approximate the null distribution of T_0^2 as follows:

$$F_{\nu_1, \nu_2} = \frac{\nu_2}{\nu_1} \times \frac{T_0^2}{ns},$$

where $s = \min(p, r)$, $\nu_1 = s(t + s + 1)$, $\nu_2 = s(n - p - 1)$, $t = |r - p| - 1$, and $F_{a,b}$ denotes the **F distribution** with a and b df; for details on this approximation, see Pillai [29].

Tables of the significance points of T_0^2 have been given by Grubbs [13] for $p = 2$, and by Davis [7–9] for $p = 3(1)10$; see Anderson [1]. Approximate significance points of T_0^2 have been suggested by Pillai [29]; see also Pillai & Samson [33] and Hughes & Saw [17].

The asymptotic (as $n \to \infty$) null distribution of T_0^2 is the **chi-square distribution** with rp **degrees of freedom**. For asymptotic expansion and approximation of the null (nonnull) distribution of T_0^2 in terms of chi-square (noncentral chi-square) distributions, see Itô [18, 19], Fujikoshi [10, 11], Siotani [37], Davis [8], Pillai [30, 31], Khatri & Pillai [20], Pillai & Young [35], and Muirhead [26, 27], in particular.

The power function of the Lawley–Hotelling trace test depends on the parameters through the characteristic roots $v_1, \ldots, v_p$ of $\Theta\Theta'\Sigma^{-1}$ in the above set-up (*see* **Eigenvalue**). Ghosh [12] has shown that this test is admissible; for a different proof, see Anderson [1]. DasGupta et al. [6] have shown that the **power** of this test increases monotonically as each of the v_i's increases. For monotonicity of the power function of the trace test for testing independence between two sets of variates, see Anderson & DasGupta [3], and for testing equality of covariance matrices, see Anderson & DasGupta [2]. Simultaneous confidence regions for Θ based on the Lawley–Hotelling's trace criterion are given in [1].

The power of the Lawley–Hotelling test has been compared with the powers of the other standard tests for the MANOVA problem by a number of authors; see Mikhail [24], Schatzoff [36], Pillai & Jayachandran [32], Fujikoshi [11], and Lee [22]. If the characteristic roots v_i are substantially unequal such that the coefficient of variation of the roots is large enough, then the Lawley–Hotelling test is more powerful than the **likelihood ratio test**, which, in turn is more powerful then Pillai's trace test; the reverse is true if the v_i's are close. Lee [22] has noted that the power of the Lawley–Hotelling test is nearly constant on the region trace $[\Theta\Theta'\Sigma^{-1}]$ = constant. For **robustness** of the Lawley–Hotelling test, see Mardia [23], Olson [28], Pillai & Sudjana [34], the review papers by Pillai [30, 31], and the article on **robustness of multivariate techniques**.

References

[1]   Anderson, T.W. (1984). *An Introduction to Multivariate Statistical Analysis*, 2nd Ed. Wiley, New York.

[2]   Anderson, T.W. & DasGupta S. (1964). A monotonicity property of the power functions of some tests of the equality of two covariance matrices, *Annals of Mathematical Statistics* **35**, 1059–1063.

[3]   Anderson, T.W. & DasGupta, S. (1964). Monotonicity of power functions of some tests of independence between two sets of variates, *Annals of Mathematical Statistics* **35**, 206–208.

[4]   Bartlett, M.S. (1934). A note on tests of significance in multivariate analysis, *Proceedings of the Cambridge Philosophical Society* **34**, 33–40.

[5]   Constantine, A.G. (1966). The distribution of Hotelling's generalized T_0^2. *Annals of Mathematical Statistics* **37**, 215–225.

[6]   DasGupta, S., Anderson, T.W. & Mudholkar, G.S. (1964). Monotonicity of the power functions of some tests of multivariate linear hypothesis, *Annals of Mathematical Statistics* **36**, 1174–1184.

[7]   Davis, A.W. (1970). Exact distribution of Hotelling's generalized T_0^2, *Biometrika* **57**, 187–191.

[8]   Davis, A.W. (1970). Further applications of a differential equation for Hotelling's generalized T_0^2, *Annals of the Institute of Statistical Mathematics* **22**, 77–87.

[9]   Davis, A.W. (1980). Further tabulation of Hotelling's generalized T_0^2, *Communications in Statistics – Simulation and Computation* **9**, 321–336.

[10] Fujikoshi, Y. (1970). Asymptotic expansions of the distributions of test statistics in multivariate analysis, *Journal of Science Hiroshima University, Series A-1* **32**, 293–299.

[11] Fujikoshi, Y. (1973). Asymptotic formulas for the distributions of three statistics for multivariate linear hypothesis, *Annals of the Institute of Statistical Mathematics* **25**, 423–437.

[12] Ghosh, M.N. (1964). On the admissibility of some tests of MANOVA, *Annals of Mathematical Statistics* **35**, 789–794.

[13] Grubbs, G.E. (1954). Tables of 1% and 5% probability levels of Hotelling's generalized T^2 statistic, *Technical note no. 926*, Ballistic Research Laboratory, Aberdeen, Proving Ground, Maryland.

[14] Hotelling, H. (1947). Multivariate quality control, illustrated by the air-testing of sample bombsights, in *Techniques of Statistical Analysis*, C. Eisenhart, M.W. Hastay & W.A. Wallis, eds. McGraw-Hill, New York, pp. 111–184.

[15] Hotelling, H. (1951). A generalized T test and measure of multivariate dispersion, in *Proceedings of the Second Berkeley Symposium on Mathematical Statistics and Probability*, J. Neyman, ed. University of California Press, Berkeley, pp. 23–41.

[16] Hsu, P.L. (1940). On generalized analysis of variance (I), *Biometrika* **31**, 221–237.

[17] Hughes, D.T. & Saw, J.G. (1972). Approximating the percentage points of Hotelling's generalized T_0^2 statistic, *Biometrika* **59**, 224–226.

[18]   Itô, K. (1956). Asymptotic formulae for the distribution of Hotelling's generalized T_0^2 statistic, *Annals of Mathematical Statistics* **27**, 1091–1105.

[19]   Itô, K. (1960). Asymptotic formulae for the distribution of Hotelling's generalized T_0^2 statistic, II, *Annals of Mathematical Statistics* **31**, 1148–1153.

[20]   Khatri, C.G. & Pillai, K.C.S. (1966). On the moments of trace of a matrix and approximations to its noncentral distribution, *Annals of Mathematical Statistics* **37**, 1312–1318.

[21]   Lawley, D.N. (1938). A generalization of Fisher's Z-test, *Biometrika* **30**, 180–187.

[22]   Lee, Y.S. (1971). Asymptotic formulae for the distributions of a multivariate test statistic: power comparison of some multivariate tests, *Biometrika* **58**, 647–651.

[23]   Mardia, K.V. (1971). The effect of non-normality on some multivariate tests and robustness to non-normality in the linear model, *Biometrika* **58**, 105–127.

[24]   Mikhail, N.N. (1965). A comparison of tests of the Wilks–Lawley hypothesis in multivariate analysis, *Biometrika* **52**, 149–156.

[25]   Mudholkar, G.S., Davidson, M.L. & Subbiah, P. (1974). A note on the union–intersection character of some MANOVA procedures, *Journal of Multivariate Analysis* **4**, 486–493.

[26]   Muirhead, R.J. (1970). Asymptotic distributions of some multivariate tests, *Annals of Mathematical Statistics* **41**, 1002–1010.

[27]   Muirhead, R.J. (1982). *Aspects of Multivariate Statistical Theory*. Wiley, New York.

[28]   Olson, C.L. (1974). Comparative robustness of six tests in multivariate analysis of variance, *Journal of the American Statistical Association* **69**, 894–908.

[29]   Pillai, K.C.S. (1955). Some new test criteria in multivariate analysis, *Annals of Mathematical Statistics* **26**, 117–121.

[30]   Pillai, K.C.S. (1976). Distributions of characteristic roots in multivariate analysis, part I: null distributions, *Canadian Journal of Statistics* **4**, 157–184.

[31]   Pillai, K.C.S. (1977). Distributions of characteristic roots in multivariate analysis, part II: non-null distributions, *Canadian Journal of Statistics* **5**, 1–62.

[32]   Pillai, K.C.S. & Jayachandran, K. (1967). Power comparisons of tests of two multivariate hypotheses based on four criteria, *Biometrika* **54**, 195–210.

[33]   Pillai, K.C.S. & Samson, P. (1959). On Hotelling's generalization of T^2, *Biometrika* **46**, 160–168.

[34]   Pillai, K.C.S. & Sudjana (1975). Exact robustness studies of tests of two multivariate hypotheses based on four criteria and their distribution problems under violations, *Annals of Statistics* **3**, 617–638.

[35]   Pillai, K.C.S. & Young, D.L. (1966). On the exact distribution of Hotelling's generalized T_0^2, *Journal of Multivariate Analysis* **1**, 90–107.

[36]   Schatzoff, M. (1966). Sensitivity comparisons among tests of the general linear hypotheses, *Journal of the American Statistical Association* **61**, 415–435.

[37]   Siotani, M. (1971). An asymptotic expansion of the non-null distributions of Hotelling's generalized T_0^2 statistic, *Annals of Mathematical Statistics* **42**, 560–571.

(*See also* **Lambda Criterion, Wilks'; Multivariate Analysis, Overview**)

SOMESH DASGUPTA

LD$_{50}$ *see* Median Effective Dose

Lead Time Bias *see* Screening Benefit, Evaluation of

League Tables *see* Quality of Care

Least Significant Difference Procedure *see* Multiple Comparisons

Least Squares

Because of the controversy between Legendre and **Gauss** about the priority in the discovery of least squares, it is useful to distinguish between the principle of least squares and the theory of least squares.

Let $\mathbf{y}$, $\boldsymbol{\xi}(\boldsymbol{\theta})$, and $\mathbf{e}$, be $n \times 1$ vectors of observations, of known parametric functions of $\boldsymbol{\theta}$, and of random observational or experimental errors, respectively, where $\boldsymbol{\theta}$ is a $k \times 1$ vector of unknown parameters, $k < n$. The model is

$$\mathbf{y} = \boldsymbol{\xi}(\boldsymbol{\theta}) + \sigma \mathbf{e}, \qquad (1)$$

where σ is a scalar parameter specifying the measurement scale. The problem is to estimate $\boldsymbol{\theta}$. If the observations were free from errors, $\mathbf{e} \equiv \mathbf{0}$, and if the model were exactly correct, the resulting n equations $\mathbf{y} = \boldsymbol{\xi}(\boldsymbol{\theta})$ in the k parameters $\boldsymbol{\theta}$ would have to be consistent in the mathematical sense that there exists a value of $\boldsymbol{\theta}$ satisfying all n equations. However, in general this is not the case, and the equations are inconsistent – there is no value of θ satisfying (1). The observations are assumed to have been taken with equal care, so that all observations should contribute equally to the estimation of θ. The problem is therefore to combine the observations to extract all of their information about θ. This problem used to be referred to as the combination of observations. There is no value of θ that in general minimizes the errors **e** uniformly. They therefore have to be minimized in some global sense. Laplace suggested minimizing the sum of absolute deviations $\sum |e_i|$, sometimes called L_1 regression (*see* **Robust Regression**). The principle of least squares minimizes the sum of squared deviations $Q = \sum e_i^2 = \sum [y_i - \xi_i(\theta)]^2$. The resulting least squares estimate, $\hat{\theta}$, is a solution of the least square equations $\partial Q / \partial \theta_j = \sum (y_i - \xi_i) \partial \xi_i / \partial \theta_j = 0$.

In the special but widespread case where $\xi(\theta)$ is a linear function of θ, $\xi = \mathbf{X}\theta$, $\mathbf{X}$ being an $n \times k$ matrix of rank k of known constants x_{ij}, (1) becomes

$$\mathbf{y} = \mathbf{X}\theta + \sigma\mathbf{e}, \qquad (2)$$

the Gauss linear model, discussed in text books as linear regression. The corresponding least squares equation and least squares estimate are

$$(\mathbf{X}'\mathbf{X})\hat{\theta} = \mathbf{X}'\mathbf{y}, \qquad \hat{\theta} = (\mathbf{X}'\mathbf{X})^{-1}\mathbf{X}'\mathbf{y}. \qquad (3)$$

Legendre has priority in the principle of least squares, having published in 1805 [4], whereas Gauss's first publication on least squares was in 1809 [2]. Legendre derived the models $\mathbf{y} = \xi + \sigma\mathbf{e}$ and the special case (2), and the corresponding least squares equations including (3). But Gauss [2, 3] went on to develop the theory of least squares, producing the treatment of linear regression as given in textbooks today. In fact, according to Fisher [1, p.88], Gauss's method only lacked for completeness the refinement of the use of **Student's** t **distribution**, appropriate for samples of rather small numbers of observations.

Standard Normal Errors

This is Gauss's first, or parametric inferential, approach [2]. Gauss assumed the errors **e** to be n independent random variables having density function $\prod f(e_i) = \prod f(y_i - \xi_i)$. He then used a typically Bayesian argument assuming independent uniform prior distributions for θ_i to obtain a posterior

density function for θ. The estimate $\hat{\theta}$ was chosen to be the mode of this posterior density function. Since the posterior distribution of θ is proportional to $\prod f(e_i)$, which is proportional to the likelihood function of θ, the resulting equations of estimation are

$$\sum_{i=1}^{n} [\partial f(y_i - \xi_i) / \partial \xi_i] (\partial \xi_i / \partial \theta_j), \quad j = 1, \ldots, n, \quad (4)$$

which are equivalent to the equations of maximum likelihood, and $\hat{\theta}$ is the **maximum likelihood** estimate. To proceed further requires specifying f. To do this Gauss assumed that for the single-parameter model in which $\xi_i \equiv \theta$, $i = 1, \ldots, n$, the appropriate estimate of the scalar θ is $\bar{y}$. This was the procedure commonly used in the physical sciences, such as astronomy. Substituting $\xi_i \equiv \theta$ into (4), and requiring the solution $\hat{\theta}$ to be $\bar{y}$, implies that $f(e_i)$ is the normal $N(0, 1)$ density. Then $\prod f(e_i) \propto \exp(-Q^2/2)$, where $Q = \sum (y_i - \xi_i)^2$. Maximizing f is equivalent to minimizing Q, which is the method of least squares. Gauss then specialized to the linear model (2), produced (3), and went on to develop the theory of normal linear regression as presented in textbooks today. He also generalized (1) to $\sigma = \text{diag}(\sigma_i)$, where the observations have different scale parameters σ_i. This results in weighted least squares in which $Q = \sum [y_i - \xi_i(\theta)]^2 / \sigma_i^2$ is to be minimized. This approach to least squares can be considered as a generalization of the use of the arithmetic **mean**. It is based upon the normal error distribution, in which case its use is equivalent to the use of the more general method of maximum likelihood.

Unspecified Distribution

This is Gauss's second, or nonparametric decision-theoretic, approach [3] based on the following assumptions.

1. The model. The model is (2) where the errors have zero means, unit variances, and are uncorrelated.
2. Linear estimates. The measuring instrument is sufficiently precise that the squares and higher powers of the errors **e** can be ignored, thus restricting attention to linear error-consistent estimates

$$\tilde{\theta} = \mathbf{C}\mathbf{y}, \quad \text{where } \mathbf{C}\mathbf{X} = \mathbf{I}, \qquad (5)$$

and $\mathbf{C}$ is a $k \times n$ matrix. The error-consistency requirement, $\mathbf{CX} = \mathbf{I}$, is to ensure that when the observations are free from errors, $\mathbf{e} \equiv \mathbf{0}$, the estimate should be the true value, $\tilde{\theta} \equiv \theta$.

3. Squared error loss. Estimation is a game with a potential loss (see **Loss Function**) and no hope for gain. The loss is taken to be proportional to the squared error $(\tilde{\theta} - \theta)^2$.

The requirement is that the estimate (5) should minimize the expected loss, the well-known **mean square error** (EMS) criterion, $\mathrm{E}(\tilde{\theta} - \theta)^2$. Gauss's Theorem proves that among all estimates (5), the least squares estimate $\hat{\theta}$ minimizes the EMS.

Gauss then went on to examine various decompositions of sums of squares, and essentially develop the **analysis of variance**. He also showed that if $Q_m = (\mathbf{y} - \mathbf{X}\hat{\theta})'(\mathbf{y} - \mathbf{X}\hat{\theta})$ is the residual or minimum sum of squares, then $\mathrm{E}(Q_m) = (n - k)\sigma^2$. He thus recommended $s = [Q_m/(n - k)]^{1/2}$ as the appropriate estimate of σ. Notice that while s^2 is an unbiased estimate of σ^2, s is a biased estimate of σ. Thus Gauss did not seem to be preoccupied with unbiased estimates.

Discussion

This last point is particularly relevant as textbooks almost always treat (5) as a requirement of **unbiasedness**, implying that the purpose of least squares is to seek **minimum variance unbiased estimates**. The resulting formalized theorem is usually referred to as the Gauss–Markov Theorem.

Textbooks also usually ignore the justification of the linearity requirement (assumption 2), and assume it is simply reasonable to restrict attention to linear estimates. This, together with unbiasedness and variance, lead to best linear unbiased estimates (BLUEs) and uniformly minimum variance (UMV) estimates. Justification for such estimates thus appears to be based more on their mathematical convenience than on their scientific relevance.

The domain of the application of least squares to parametric models is (1) where $\mathbf{e}$ is a vector of independent N(0,1) errors. In this case least squares is identical to maximum likelihood. When $\mathbf{e}$ is not normal, least squares is no longer relevant, but maximum likelihood usually is applicable to the estimation of components θ_i if due attention is paid to the shape of the likelihood functions of θ_i.

The domain of application of the nonparametric approach, where the model is not specified, is to areas where it is appropriate to assume $\mathbf{e}$ is small, so that it makes sense to restrict attention to linear estimates and to a squared error loss function. For example, Gauss originally applied least squares to the calculation of a planetary orbit, and the prediction of where the planet will be seen. He also used it in map-making, or geodesy, where the above assumptions are fulfilled. These assumptions may not be generally appropriate in many applications in biology and the life sciences, and hence in biostatistics. There the principal source of error is usually the variability of the experimental material, which may be large and asymmetric.

These considerations make it seem unlikely that least squares, as a method of estimation per se, has a widespread application in biostatistics. However, *weighted* least squares has computational applications in iterative procedures required to find the maximum likelihood estimate (see **Optimization and Nonlinear Equations**). In particular it is useful in obtaining an initial value θ_0 to start the iterations using the Newton–Raphson or Fisher's scoring methods. For example, consider the binomial **logistic regression** $\mathbf{y} \sim \mathrm{bin}(\mathbf{s}, \mathbf{p})$, where $\zeta = \log[\mathbf{p}/(1 - \mathbf{p})] = \mathbf{X}\theta$. If $\hat{\zeta} = \log[\hat{\mathbf{p}}/(1 - \hat{\mathbf{p}})] = \log[\mathbf{y}/(\mathbf{s} - \mathbf{y})]$, an initial value $\theta^{(0)}$ is the weighted least squares estimate of θ in the regression of $\hat{\zeta}$ on $\mathbf{X}$. This is obtained by minimizing with respect to θ the weighted sum of squares

$$Q = \sum_{i=1}^{n} \left(\hat{\zeta} - \sum_{j=1}^{k} x_{ij}\theta_j \right)^2 n_i \hat{p}_i(1 - \hat{p}_i)$$
$$= (\hat{\zeta} - \mathbf{X}\theta)' D (\hat{\zeta} - \mathbf{X}\theta),$$

where D is the diagonal matrix of elements $n_i \hat{p}_i(1 - \hat{p}_i)$, the reciprocals of the estimated variances of the $\hat{\zeta}_i$. The successive correction terms in the Newton–Raphson iterations can be obtained in a similar way (see **Optimization and Nonlinear Equations**).

For further details on Gauss and least squares, see Sprott [5].

References

[1]   Fisher, R.A. (1973). *Statistical Methods and Scientific Inference.* Hafner, New York.

[2] Gauss, C.F. (1809). *Theoria Motus Corporum Coeles-tium*. Werke 7. (English translation: C.H. Davis. Dover, New York, 1963.)

[3] Gauss, C.F. (1821, 1823, 1826). *Theoria Combinationis Erroribus Minimis Obnoxiae*, Parts 1, 2, and Supplement. Werke 4, pp. 1–108.

[4] Legendre, A.M. (1805). Nouvelles méthodes pour la determination des orbits des cométes. (Appendix: Sur la méthode des moindres carrés.)

[5] Sprott. D.A. (1978). Gauss's contributions to statistics, *Historia Mathematica* **5**, 183–203.

(*See also* **Estimation**)

D.A. SPROTT

Leave-One-Out *see* Cross-Validation

Lee–Coulson Distribution *see* Bacterial Growth, Division, and Mutation

Left Truncation *see* Truncated Survival Times

Legendre Polynomials *see* Polynomial Approximation

Lehmann Alternatives

To study the effect of a drug one often needs to make a **nonparametric** comparison of the cumulative distribution function, G, of **scores** from treated subjects, with the distribution, F, of scores from the untreated control group. In such comparisons, Lehmann [5] pointed out that under any alternative hypothesis the test is not distribution-free. To overcome this difficulty, Lehmann suggested a functional relationship $G = f(F)$, where f is a specified function between G and F. The importance of this formulation is that the distribution of the **rank** vector under the alternative hypothesis will depend only on f and hence every rank statistic will have a nonparametric distribution-free property. As an illustration, Lehmann derived the power of various rank tests for simple alternatives $G = F^2$ and $G = F^3$.

One of the major applications of the Lehmann alternatives has been in the formulation of the alternative hypothesis for testing the effect of a drug when some subjects in the treatment group are not affected by the treatment. This so-called "nonresponse" phenomenon occurs, for example, in the development of a new drug. In such studies, one may exhibit greater variability as well as mean response in the treatment group. This increased variability can be considered to be due to the presence of subjects in the treatment group who are unaffected by the treatment. Thus, if p is the proportion of subjects in the treatment group who respond to the treatment, then Salsburg [9] suggests testing the null hypothesis of no treatment effect,

$$H_0: G(x) = F(x), \tag{1}$$

against a Lehmann-type alternative of the form

$$H_1: G(x) = (1 - p)F(x) + p[F(x)]^\gamma, \tag{2}$$

where $\gamma > 1$ is a known constant. Salsburg's argument is based on maintaining the same range of observations in the treatment and control groups. In this form of the Lehmann alternative the response of each subject in the treatment group who is affected by treatment is assumed to have the same distribution as the maximum of γ responses in the control group. Salsburg suggests using a rank test, where the two samples are ranked together and the score for a given subject is

$$s(i) = \left(\frac{i}{N + 1}\right)^k, \quad k > 1, \tag{3}$$

where i is the combined rank of that subject and N is the total number of subjects in the combined set. Conover & Salsburg [1] show that when $\gamma = 5$ and $k = \gamma - 1 = 4$, then a rank test based on (3) provides a test with maximum **asymptotic relative efficiency**. The recommended value of $\gamma = 5$ is based on some empirical results. Razzaghi & Nanthakumar [8] formulated the problem of testing for treatment effect in terms of the parameter p as

$$H_0: p = 0$$

against

$$H_1: p > 0$$

and derived a **locally most powerful test**. Such a test is based on the statistic

$$S_{n,m} = \sum_{i=1}^{n} F_m^{\gamma-1}(y_i), \qquad (4)$$

where m is the number of subjects in the control group and F_m is the empirical distribution of the control observations defined at any point x as the proportion of the control observations not exceeding x, and $y_1, \ldots, y_n$ are the observations from the treatment group. The test of H_0 against H_1 will reject the hypothesis of no treatment effect when

$$S_{n,m} > \frac{n}{\gamma} + \frac{\gamma-1}{\gamma} \left(\frac{n}{2\gamma-1} \right)^{1/2} Z_\alpha,$$

where Z_α is the $100(1-\alpha)$th fractile (or **quantile**) of the **standard normal distribution**. The power of the test based on (4) increases as the proportion of the responders, p, rises. A value of $\gamma = 5$ is again recommended on the basis of an analysis of the **power** of the test.

Conover & Salsburg [1] also present an argument for using the other form of the Lehmann alternative and expressed the distribution of the treatment in the presence of nonresponders as the hypothesis

$$H_2: (1-p)F(x) + p\{1 - [1 - F(x)]^{1/\gamma}\}, \quad \gamma > 1, \qquad (5)$$

which implies that the distribution of each control score is assumed to have the same distribution as the minimum of γ responses from the treatment group. Razzaghi & Nanthakumar [7] proposed a locally

optimal test for the alternative (5). The test is based on the score statistic (*see* **Likelihood**)

$$T_n = \sum_{i=1}^{n} [1 - F(y_i)]^{-(\gamma-1)/\gamma}. \qquad (6)$$

It is shown that when $\gamma = 2$, the asymptotic distribution of T_n under the null hypothesis is normal, while for $\alpha > 2$ this distribution is in the domain of attraction of a stable distribution. More specifically, a locally most powerful test of H_0 against H_2 with $\gamma = 2$ rejects the null hypothesis, H_0, when

$$T_n > 2n \left[1 - (n \ln n)^{-1/2} \right] + (n \ln n)^{1/2} Z_\alpha, \qquad (7)$$

and the test for $\gamma > 2$ rejects H_0 when

$$\{T_n - n\gamma(1 - a_n^{-(\gamma-1)^{-1}})\}/a_n \qquad (8)$$

exceeds the $(1-\alpha)$th fractile of a stable distribution with indices $\gamma/(\gamma-1)$ and -1. In (8), a_n is given by

$$a_n = \{[8\gamma n / \ln n]^{(\gamma-1)/\gamma}$$
$$- [16n / \ln n]^{1/2}\}/(\gamma-2)^{2(\gamma-1)/\gamma}. \qquad (9)$$

Example

To illustrate the methodologies described here, we use a data set from an experiment on **pain** scores. The data first appeared in Conover & Salsburg [1]. Values for patients from a study of acute painful diabetic neuropathy were recorded at baseline and after four weeks of treatment on an analog scale. The changes from baseline were described as the natural logarithm of the ratio of baseline to final scores. Table 1 is reproduced from Conover & Salsburg for

Table 1   Pain scores ln(baseline/final)

Treated patients, Y_i						
−1.535	−0.547	−0.201	−0.201	−0.154	−0.095	−0.049
0.000	0.000	0.000	0.105	0.111	0.201	0.251
0.310	0.406	0.511	0.531	0.575	0.575	0.773
0.981	1.299	1.299	1.322	1.386	1.792	2.398

Controls, X_i						
−1.490	−0.021	−0.128	−0.087	−0.054	0.000	0.000
0.000	0.000	0.000	0.028	0.039	0.049	0.061
0.080	0.105	0.134	0.193	0.216	0.223	0.273
0.288	0.330	0.357	0.487	0.541	0.793	1.042
1.099	1.609					

Reproduced from [1] by permission of the publisher.

completeness. For these data using $\gamma = 5$, the value of $s(i)$ is 0.261 for the treated patients and 0.133 for the control subjects, leading to a P value of 0.031. The value of $S_{n,m}$ is 2.10, leading to a P value of 0.0179. Computation of T_n for these data gives

$$T_n = \begin{cases} 100.13, & \gamma = 2, \\ 210.31, & \gamma = 3, \\ 421.28, & \gamma = 5, \end{cases}$$

and in all cases the test indicates a highly significant treatment effect. The fractiles of a stable distribution may be obtained from Cross [3].

There is a vast body of literature on the theoretical development and applications of Lehmann alternatives. Wijsman [10] provides a comprehensive and thorough list of early references. Halperin & Ware [4], Cox [2], and Peto [6] discuss the use of Lehmann alternatives in the analysis of data from **clinical trials**. The intent here has been to demonstrate more recent applications in biostatistical problems.

References

[1]   Conover, W.J. & Salsburg, D.S. (1988). Locally most powerful tests for detecting treatment effects when only a subset of patients can be expected to "respond to treatment", *Biometrics* **44**, 189–196.
[2]   Cox, D.R. (1972). Regression models and life-tables, *Journal of the Royal Statistical Society, Series B* **39**, 79–85.
[3]   Cross, M.J. (1973). Tables of finite-mean nonsymmetric stable distributions as computed from their convergent and asymptotic series, *Journal of Statistical Computation and Simulation* **3**, 1–27.
[4]   Halperin, M. & Ware, J. (1974). Early decisions in a censored Wilcoxon two-sample test for accumulating survival data, *Journal of the American Statistical Association* **69**, 414–422.
[5]   Lehmann, E.L. (1953). The power of rank tests, *Annals of Mathematical Statistics* **24**, 23–43.
[6]   Peto, R. (1972). Rank tests of maximal power against Lehmann-type alternatives, *Biometrika* **59**, 467–471.
[7]   Razzaghi, M. & Nanthakumar, A. (1992). On using Lehmann alternatives with nonresponders, *Mathematical Biosciences* **109**, 69–83.
[8]   Razzaghi, M. & Nanthakumar, A. (1994). A locally most powerful test for detecting a treatment effect in the presence of nonresponders, *Biometrical Journal* **3**, 373–384.
[9]   Salsburg, D.S. (1986). Alternative hypotheses for the effects of drugs in small-scale clinical studies, *Biometrics* **42**, 671–674.
[10]   Wijsman, R.A. (1985). Lehmann alternatives, in *Encyclopedia of Statistical Sciences*, Vol. 5, S. Kotz & N.L. Johnson, eds. Wiley, New York.

(*See also* **Cure Models; Proportional Hazards, Overview**)

MEHDI RAZZAGHI

Lehmann–Scheffé Theorem *see* Sufficient Statistic

Length Bias

The length-biased distribution is a **probability** distribution resulting from a biased sampling scheme in which the probability of observing a positive-valued **random variable** is proportional to the value of the variable.

Length Bias in Renewal Theory

The presence of length bias is a natural phenomenon in **renewal** theory. Consider a sequence of random variables

$$X_1, \quad X_1 + X_2, \quad X_1 + X_2 + X_3, \ldots,$$

where the Xs are positive-valued, nondegenerate, independent and identically distributed (iid) random variables. Suppose the process starts from time 0 and is observed at the time τ_0, where τ_0 is a positive constant. Let α be the index so that

$$\sum_{i=1}^{\alpha-1} X_i < \tau_0 \le \sum_{i=1}^{\alpha} X_i.$$

Let Y, T, and R respectively denote the length of the interval containing τ_0, the backward recurrence time, and the forward recurrence time, or equivalently,

$$Y = X_\alpha, \qquad T = \tau_0 - \left\{ \sum_{i=1}^{\alpha-1} X_i \right\},$$

$$R = \left\{ \sum_{i=1}^{\alpha} X_i \right\} - \tau_0.$$

Let f, S, and μ represent the density function, survivorship function, and mean of X_1, respectively. When τ_0 is sufficiently large so that an *equilibrium condition* is reached [3], the joint density of (T, R) can then be derived as

$$p_{T,R}(t, r) = f(t + r)I(t \geq 0, r \geq 0)/\mu. \quad (1)$$

The marginal density functions of Y, T, and R can be derived, based on (1), as

$$p_Y(y) = yf(y)I(y \geq 0)/\mu, \quad (2)$$

$$p_T(t) = S(t)I(t \geq 0)/\mu, \quad (3)$$

$$p_R(r) = S(r)I(r \geq 0)/\mu. \quad (4)$$

The distribution of (2) is generally referred to as the *length-biased distribution*.

Although the length-biased distribution in renewal theory is usually derived under the iid assumption on the Xs, as a general result the independence assumption can be removed and the density formulas (1)–(4) still remain valid [6].

Statistical Methods

Length-biased sampling is recognized in many research fields including epidemiology, ecology, and reliability. A number of methods for length-biased data have been developed in the statistical literature. Cox [4] proposed estimating the survivorship function by a weighted empirical distribution function (*see* **Goodness of Fit**), with weight inversely proportional to y_i:

$$\hat{S}_n(y) = n^{-1}\hat{\mu} \sum_{i=1}^{n} \left[y_i^{-1}I(y_i > y) \right],$$

where $\hat{\mu} = \{n^{-1}\sum_j y_j^{-1}\}^{-1}$ serves as an appropriate estimate of μ, since $n^{-1}\sum_j y_j^{-1}$ estimates μ^{-1}. The estimator $\hat{S}_n$ can be proven to be the **nonparametric maximum likelihood estimator** of S, a special case under Vardi's **selection bias** models [12, 13]. Following the same weighting procedure, a kernel estimator of the density function f (*see* **Density Estimation**)

was proposed in [7] as

$$\hat{f}_n(y) = n^{-1}\hat{\mu} \sum_{i=1}^{n} \left[y_i^{-1}K_h(y - y_i) \right],$$

where $K_h(x) = h^{-1}K(h^{-1}x)$, $h > 0$, with K a kernel function. Alternatively, one could first estimate the length-biased density, (2), by an ordinary kernel estimator and then use the relationship of (2) and f to obtain an estimator of f [2]. Under the proportional hazards model [5], a risk set sampling technique was developed in [17] for estimating regression parameters. For $y_j \geq y_i$, let $\Delta_j(y_i)$ be a binary variable which equals 1 with probability y_i/y_j, and 0 with probability $1 - (y_i/y_j)$. The indicators $\Delta_j(y_i)$ are used to identify bias-adjusted **risk sets** and to construct **pseudo-likelihood** equations. Regression parameter estimates are then derived by solving the score equations (*see* **Likelihood**).

Length Bias in Prevalent Cohorts

Length-biased sampling could arise in many epidemiologic studies when survival data are collected from a disease population (*see* **Prevalent Case**). As an illustration, suppose a random sample of women with breast cancer (b.c.) are recruited for observation of survival. Assume (i) the rate of occurrence of b.c. remains constant over time, and (ii) the density function of the time from b.c. to death, f, is independent of the calendar time when b.c. occurred. Conditions (i) and (ii) together are referred to as the *equilibrium condition*. Denote by τ_i the calendar time when woman i with b.c. is recruited, t_i the time from the initial diagnosis of b.c. to τ_i, and y_i the time from the initial diagnosis of b.c. to death. Under the equilibrium condition, the joint density of (t_i, y_i) is an equivalent of (1), namely

$$p_{T,Y}(t, y) = f(y)I(y \geq t \geq 0)/\mu, \quad (5)$$

and the distribution of y_i is length-biased with density (2). Suppose a sample of iid $(t_1, y_1), \ldots, (t_n, y_n)$ is observed. By the factorization theorem, the observed failure times $\{y_i\}$ serve as **sufficient statistics** for parameters of f. In this case, the variables $\{t_i\}$ do not contain additional information for f.

The preceding length-biased sample can be described more generally as disease prevalent data. Suppose there are two chronologically ordered and nonrecurrent events, termed the initiating and terminating events. Replacing the events of b.c. and death by the initiating and terminating events, the sample $\{y_i\}$ is length-biased when study individuals are recruited from those who have experienced the initiating event but have not experienced the terminating event [16]. Samples of this type could also be collected in a **screening** program for chronic diseases. It was indicated by Zelen & Feinleib [20] that the screen does not detect people at random, but detects people with longer preclinical **sojourn times**.

Although statistical methods can be formulated on the basis of length-biased observations as discussed earlier, the analysis could be further complicated by the presence of right **censoring**. We next make connection between length-biased sampling and left **truncation** in this context.

Length Bias and Left Truncation

Using formula (5), the density function of y_i given t_i can be derived as $f(y)I(y > t)/S(t)$, a truncated density function. The observed t_i in left truncation models [8, 10, 11, 15, 16, 19] is usually termed the *truncation time* and has density function $S(t)I(t > 0)/\mu$. Given the observations $(t_1, y_1), \ldots, (t_n, y_n)$, the full density can be expressed as the product of the marginal density of the t_i,

$$\prod_{i=1}^{n} \left[S(t_i)/\mu \right],$$

and the conditional density of y_i given the t_i,

$$\prod_{i=1}^{n} \left[f(y_i)/S(t_i) \right]. \tag{6}$$

In length-biased models the truncation times in general do not serve as **ancillary statistics** for parameters of f, and thus the conditional likelihood (6) is used subject to loss of information.

Suppose now the observation of the terminating event is subject to right-censoring. Assume the following independent censoring condition: conditional on the observed t_i, the time from τ_i to the terminating event, r_i, is independent of the time from τ_i to censoring, d_i. This independent censoring condition does not, however, imply independence between the length-biased time, $y_i(= t_i + r_i)$, and the censoring time, $c_i(= t_i + d_i)$ [14, 16]. Let $w_i = \min\{y_i, c_i\}$

be the time from the initiating event to the end of observation, and $\delta_i = I(w_i = y_i)$ the censoring indicator. Conditional on t_i, under the independent censoring condition the density of (w_i, δ_i) is proportional to $f(w_i)^{\delta_i} S(w_i)^{1-\delta_i}/S(t_i)$. Given a sample of iid observations $(t_1, w_1, \delta_1), \ldots, (t_n, w_n, \delta_n)$, statistical approaches based on the conditional likelihood,

$$\prod_{i=1}^{n} \left[f(w_i)^{\delta_i} S(w_i)^{1-\delta_i}/S(t_i) \right],$$

are considered as methods for left-truncated and right-censored data. These approaches replace the usual risk sets $R(w) = \{w_i : w_i \geq w\}$ by $R^*(w) = \{w_i : t_i \leq w \leq w_i\}$ and result in an interesting contrast with the familiar techniques used in survival analysis [11, 15, 16, 19]. These methods can be alternately derived using **counting process** techniques with left-filtering [1, 8, 10]. The connection between renewal processes and left truncation can also be made by various approaches [9, 18]. While the methods provide "simple solutions" for analyzing censored length-biased data, these conditional approaches, similar to the left-truncation case, are used subject to loss of **efficiency** because marginal information from the truncation times is not used in the construction of the methods. Furthermore, the applicability of these methods requires that the truncation time, t_i, be observable, and such a requirement might not be met in some applications.

Length Bias and Cross-Sectional Sampling

In the example of prevalent cohorts, the initiating and terminating events are required to be nonrecurrent. Nevertheless, the problem of length bias could also be encountered in studies that adopt **cross-sectional** sampling techniques to collect failure times from univariate or bivariate recurrent event processes (*see* **Repeated Events**). In these studies the outcome variable of interest is the length between two successive events. The crucial condition assumed, for the validity of length-biased distribution, is the equilibrium condition for the recurrent events. With cross-sectional samplings, the intervals which contain the sampling times are observed and form the length-biased sample. Examples include cross-sectional samples of (i) fibre length [4], where the recurrent events are of the same type and the location of an event is specified as the left end of a fibre, and (ii) length of stay in a hospital, in which the bivariate recurrent events are admission to and discharge from a hospital.

References

[1]   Andersen, P.K., Borgan, O., Gill, R.D. & Keiding, N. (1992). *Statistical Models Based on Counting Processes*. Springer-Verlag, New York.

[2]   Bhattacharyya, B.B., Franklin, L.A. & Richardson, G.D. (1988). A comparison of nonparametric unweighted and length-biased density estimation of fibres, *Communications in Statistics – Theory and Methods*, **17**, 3629–3644.

[3]   Cox, D.R. (1962). *Renewal Theory*. Methuen, London.

[4]   Cox, D.R. (1969). Some sampling problems in technology, in *New Development in Survey Sampling*, N.L. Johnson & H. Smith, Jr, eds. Wiley–Interscience, New York, pp. 506–527.

[5]   Cox, D.R. (1972). Regression models and life tables (with discussion), *Journal of the Royal Statistical Society, Series B* **34**, 187–220.

[6]   Cox, D.R. & Isham, V. (1980). *Point Processes*. Chapman & Hall, London.

[7]   Jones, M.C. (1991). Kernel density estimation for length biased data, *Biometrika* **78**, 511–519.

[8]   Keiding, N. (1992). Independent delayed entry, in *Survival Analysis: State of the Art*, J.P. Klein & P.K. Goel, eds. Kluwer, Dordrecht, pp. 309–326.

[9]   Keiding, N. & Gill, R.D. (1988). Random truncation models and Markov processes. *Technical Report*. Centre for Mathematics and Computer Science, Amsterdam, The Netherlands.

[10]   Keiding, N. & Gill, R.D. (1990). Random truncation models and Markov processes, *Annals of Statistics* **18**, 582–602.

[11]   Lai, T.-L. & Ying, Z. (1991). Rank regression methods for left-truncated and right-censored data, *Annals of Statistics* **19**, 417–442.

[12]   Vardi, Y. (1982). Nonparametric estimation in the presence of length bias, *Annals of Statistics* **10**, 616–620.

[13]   Vardi, Y. (1985). Empirical distributions in selection bias models, *Annals of Statistics* **13**, 178–203.

[14]   Vardi, Y. (1989). Multiplicative censoring, renewal processes, deconvolution and decreasing density: nonparametric estimation, *Biometrika* **76**, 751–761.

[15]   Wang, M.-C., Jewell, N.P. & Tsai W.-Y. (1986). Asymptotic properties of the product-limit estimate under random truncation, *Annals of Statistics* **14**, 1597–1605.

[16]   Wang, M.-C. (1991). Nonparametric estimation from cross-sectional survival data, *Journal of the American Statistical Association* **86** 130–143.

[17]   Wang, M.-C. (1996). Hazards regression analysis for length-biased data, *Biometrika* **83**, 343–354.

[18]   Winter, B.B. & Foldes, A. (1988). A product-limit estimator for use with length-biased data, *Canadian Journal of Statistics* **16**, 337–355.

[19]   Woodroofe, M. (1985). Asymptotic properties of the product-limit estimate under random truncation, *Annals of Statistics* **13**, 163–177.

[20]   Zelen, M. & Feinleib, M. (1969). On the theory of screening for chronic diseases, *Biometrika* **56**, 601–614.

(*See also* **Weighted Distributions**)

MEI-CHENG WANG

Leptokurtic *see* Kurtosis

Leukemia Clusters

Interest in the possibility that cases of cancer and leukemia tend to occur in clusters has a long history [6]. Early reports were of cancer in particular families or houses; more recently interest has centred on spatial and space–time **clustering**. Most recent interest concerns leukemia in children and has been stimulated by suspicions of an environmental etiology.

The possible explanation of clusters most considered is that environmental **radiation** might be responsible for leukemia in children, and public concern is so great that it has had a major impact on the development of civil nuclear power programs. Natural though such apprehensions may be, they are out of all proportion to the strength of the epidemiologic evidence. Radiation is certainly a known leukemogen, but most environmental doses are too low to account for significant risk. Recently, other leukemogenic mechanisms have been receiving more attention, notably the possibility of an infectious etiology. Although there is some evidence of geographical clustering, this is not strong and, despite intensive investigation, no actual leukemia cluster has led to the identification of a specific cause.

The Nature of Leukemia

Acute leukemia is a malignant disease characterized by rapid proliferation of leucocytes from a single malignant clonal cell; chronic forms develop slowly over a long period of time but are capable of becoming acute. The tumor is relatively rare in adults, but commonest in children, accounting for around a third of all cases of malignant disease under the age of 15. The most distinctive of the numerous forms is acute lymphocytic leukemia (ALL). In practice, many epidemiologic investigations distinguish only between ALL and acute nonlymphocytic leukemia (ANLL).

Types of cancer generally, and leukemia in particular, show very different relative frequencies in children and adults. Thus ALL accounts for around 80% of all leukemia in children, with a peak at around 3 years of age [15]. Most of the remaining cases are of ANLL, chronic leukemia being rare in childhood. Among adults, however, the commonest form is chronic lymphocytic leukemia, ALL being less common than either the chronic or acute myelocytic forms [25].

Reported **incidence rates** of leukemia show some variation internationally; these may be partly due to genetic factors, but are probably also a consequence of differences in reporting and diagnostic procedures [25]. In addition, the disease tends to be masked by acute infections, which may explain some of the international differences and the more marked historical trends [24]. Intranational rates show less variation for children [14] than for adults [7].

The Etiology of Leukemia

The etiology of leukemia is only partly understood. The importance of genetic factors is clear from its association with certain conditions having a clear genetic etiology, notably Down's syndrome (trisomy 21), in which the risk of childhood leukemia is increased about 15-fold [35].

Of the various exogenous factors that have been proposed as having etiological significance for leukemia, ionizing radiation is by far the most important. That it causes leukemia in high doses (of the order of 100 mSv or more) has been established beyond doubt by various epidemiologic studies [29, 34], which, however, predominantly involved adults. There is also significant evidence that the much lower doses exposing the fetus in obstetric X-ray investigations (typically 2–20 mSv) are leukemogenic [4, 13]. The epidemiologic evidence therefore justifies

the interest in environmental radiation, especially the possibility of a risk near nuclear installations [33] or following nuclear accidents. In most cases, however, the excess radiation levels in such environments are small compared with the natural background radiation and are unlikely to explain observed excesses of leukemia [11].

A viral component of the etiology has also been suspected for a long time. The first strong epidemiologic evidence relates to a cohort of children born in March 1958 in the UK [17], for which there was a ninefold increase in the risk of leukemia and lymphoma among children whose mothers contracted influenza during pregnancy. Chance may have at least partly exaggerated the finding, and it is noteworthy also that the relevant exposure was to a particularly virulent epidemic of the Asian strain; in any event, subsequent corroboration was only partial [30]. More recently, Greaves [21] has postulated that children exposed to below average levels of infection postnatally may fail to develop a fully effective immune system, making them more vulnerable to tumor initiation. Such a mechanism might explain the known association between childhood leukemia and high socieconomic status [14] and also the population-mixing phenomena demonstrated by Kinlen [23] and discussed below.

Other known or possible causes of leukemia include chemotherapeutic agents [12]; exposure to chemical carcinogens, which is normally occupational and may be parental [28]; and exposure to electromagnetic fields [10]. With the exception of the last of these, for which the evidence is least convincing, a genuine causal relationship would be unlikely to result in demonstrable **geographic patterns**.

The Nature of Clustering

Clustering may be defined as the tendency of observations to be situated closer to one another than would be expected. The reference space within which a cluster appears may be discrete or continuous, the former being exemplified by clustering within families. The problem of analyzing excesses within family or other groups raises few special problems, however. Greater interest, both theoretically and practically, attaches to clustering in a continuum, which is normally taken to be geographical space, time, or their product, the latter giving rise to space–time clustering.

Clustering in time only would presumably be indicative of a widely dispersed short-term hazard; few instances of such hazards have been proposed for leukemia. Seasonal variation (*see* **Seasonal Time Series**) could also induce this form of clustering, though the term would not normally be taken to include such an effect and specific, period-related methods of analysis would be more appropriate than general tests. Rather little evidence of seasonality in leukemia incidence has been advanced [16].

Clustering in space could be ascribed to a number of possible mechanisms, mostly involving geographical variation of risk. Local variation of genetic factors could in principle produce spatial clustering, but there is little or no evidence of this in the case of leukemia. Spatial variation is more likely to be due to local variation in risk due to some environmental factor.

Space–time clustering – i.e. an **interaction** between the space and time distributions – could be indicative of some infective mechanism in the etiology of the disease. The evidence for this is briefly summarized below. Space–time interaction tests have the apparent attraction that they can be executed without knowledge of the marginal distributions in time and space, the latter being particularly hard to estimate accurately. However, they are vulnerable to space–time interactions in the denominators, i.e. to changes in population distribution over the study period (*see* **Denominator Difficulties**). Little work has been done on how sensitive they are to such changes and how much this may affect published findings.

Assessment of clusters is inevitably bound up with the methods used to detect them (*see* **Geographical Analysis**). Here we emphasize only the importance of distinguishing between situations where there is or is not a hypothesis identified a priori; the distinction crucially affects the choice of method as well as the interpretation of the results.

Evidence of Leukemia Clustering

Most of the study of leukemia clustering has concentrated on childhood leukemia, and this is reflected in the following brief review.

Nuclear Installations

The specific environmental issue that has received greatest attention is that of possible risk in proximity to nuclear installations. Early concern following the accident at Three Mile Island in the US gained new impetus in the UK, particularly after a television program in 1983 identified an abnormally large number of cases in Seascale, a village near the nuclear reprocessing plant at Sellafield in Cumbria.

Although Sellafield is one of the largest nuclear reprocessing plants in the world and has released significant quantities of radiation into the environment, detailed radiologic analyses considering available estimates of risk coefficients and parallel exposures from nuclear fallout make it very unlikely that radiation alone could account for the observed **relative risks** [11, 33]. The hypothesis that paternal preconception irradiation might be the crucial pathway [19] is inconsistent with current dosimetric estimates of genetic risk and with other epidemiologic studies [26].

Nevertheless, public concern remains high and a number of clusters in the vicinity of other nuclear installations have been reported more or less anecdotally; significantly, perhaps, these include excesses at other reprocessing plants at Dounreay in Scotland [8] and La Hague in France [32]. Public concern has extended to nuclear power generating stations although they normally have very much lower emissions. This concern has prompted a number of studies of nuclear installations in the UK [5], the US [22], and Canada [27]. These studies have not generally uncovered further significant excesses.

The excess in Seascale is particularly difficult to interpret in view of the mode of its discovery and initial reporting. Its statistical significance is in some measure diluted by the observation that Seascale is one of almost 10 000 similar areal units in the UK. The fact remains, however, that the Sellafield plant is unique in terms of its history and activity and any prior hypothesis would presumably have put high odds on this being the most likely location of any excess. It is disturbing too that, since the initial finding, further cases have occurred: between 1984 and 1992 there were a further three cases of ALL and non-Hodgkin lymphoma, bringing the total since 1963 to eight, compared with around 0.65 expected [9]. A useful collection of abstracts and papers on childhood cancers near nuclear installations was published in 1993 and dedicated to the late **Martin J. Gardner** [3].

Viral Etiologies

The difficulty of explaining the Seascale cluster in terms of radiation has prompted a search for other possibilities. Foremost of these is the possibility that the risk of childhood leukemia is increased by exposure to an infective agent consequent on increased levels of "population mixing". In a remarkable series of papers, Kinlen and colleagues studied other populations in which a similar mixing effect could be expected [23]. These include new towns, the vicinities of major construction sites, and communities receiving wartime evacuees; they showed consistently raised risks of childhood leukemia. An explanation might be that children in the indigenous population are vulnerable to an infectious agent or agents not previously encountered or, in line with Greaves' argument [21], that they have a generally higher susceptibility to leukemogenesis resulting from a reduced exposure to infections in the postnatal period. The geographic data do not permit the identification of a specific organism and are consequently unlikely to throw more light on these possible mechanisms.

Generalized Clustering of Childhood Leukemia

The evidence discussed above is noteworthy, and perhaps more convincing, because it stands out from the relative uniformity of childhood leukemia incidence. Attempts to demonstrate widespread and generalized clustering have not, generally speaking, produced striking results. An atlas of leukemia incidence covering around a third of the population of England and Wales in the years 1984–88 [7] demonstrates moderate variation between counties; this is probably largely due to the contribution for adults, which was not separated out. Tests of spatial clustering at a more local level, however, were broadly negative.

As far as childhood leukemia is concerned, the largest register of data in the world is the (UK) National Registry of Childhood Tumours maintained by the Childhood Cancer Research Group in Oxford (*see* **Disease Registers**). Geographically referenced cases occurring in Britain in the years 1966-1983 were made available to a group of researchers, who tried out their different methodologies; the results were reported in a monograph [14]. The evidence of generalized spatial clustering was rather slight, was related to ALL under the age of 5 and appeared

to be strongest in rural areas [1]; the latter association may be a reflection of the socioeconomic effect already noted. An analysis of space–time clustering by Gilman et al. [20] reported some statistically significant results, but these were hard to interpret because of the problems of multiple testing (*see* **Multiple Comparisons**) and of sensitivity to population changes referred to above; the latter problem is especially severe in the analysis of large data sets, where statistically significant results may correspond to very small real effects. The overview by Gardner [18] concluded: "Overall, there are apparently no dramatic findings in the results of the analyses carried out for this volume."

This negative view of the importance of generalized clustering is consistent with many other papers and reviews [25, 31], though the review by Alexander [2] concludes that the data as a whole are "consistent with their interpretation as an imperfect reflection of some underlying population infective process". It is only to be expected that some significant findings will be reported. They should certainly not be discounted, but need critical appraisal, particularly where there may be doubts about the methodology.

Discussion

We conclude from this review that the evidence for any significant general tendency of leukemia to exhibit clustering is equivocal at best. It would be as unsatisfactory to conclude that there is no such effect as to conclude that the evidence is strong enough to provide real pointers toward the etiology. Although there is some evidence of geographic and of space–time clustering, the effects are at most weak and the scope for methodologic and data error is considerable. Methodologic limitations work both ways: it is possible that some stronger effects are being masked by inefficient methods and inadequate data. In particular, it is likely that place of birth is at least as important as place of residence in the etiology of childhood leukemia; unfortunately, it is in practice harder to obtain extensive data on place of birth and most published results relate to residence at diagnosis or death.

There is no particular reason why geography should hold the clue to the etiology of leukemia. Even if environmentally varying factors were known to be very important, the mobility of the population will inevitably dilute the impact on individuals. In practice, so little is known about the etiology of the disease that we cannot assume prima facie that environment should be significant. None of this is likely to allay the anxieties of people who believe that their own form of the disease is directly related to their own circumstances. If only to put their anxieties into perspective and offer the best possible reassurance, it is necessary to maintain research effort on the possibility that there is a much stronger environmental component in the etiology of the disease than appears likely at present.

References

[1] Alexander, F.E. (1991). Investigations of localized spatial clustering, and extra-Poisson variation, in *The Geographical Epidemiology of Childhood Leukaemia and non-Hodgkin Lymphomas in Great Britain, 1966-83. Studies on Medical and Population Subjects, No. 53*, G. Draper, ed. HMSO, London, pp. 69-76.

[2] Alexander, F.E. (1993). Viruses, clusters and clustering of childhood leukaemia: a new perspective?, *European Journal of Cancer, Series A* **29**, 1424-1443.

[3] Beral, V., Roman, E. & Bobrow, M., eds (1993). *Childhood Cancer and Nuclear Installations*. British Medical Journal Publishing Group, London.

[4] Bithell, J.F. & Stewart, A.M. (1975). Pre-natal irradiation and childhood malignancy: a review of British data from the Oxford survey, *British Journal of Cancer* **31**, 271-287.

[5] Bithell, J.F., Dutton, S.J., Draper, G.J. & Neary, N.M. (1994). The distribution of childhood leukaemias and non-Hodgkin lymphomas near nuclear installations in England and Wales, *British Medical Journal* **309**, 501-505.

[6] Boyle, P., Walker, A.M. & Alexander, F.E. (1996). Historical aspects of leukaemia clusters, in *Methods for Investigating Localized Clustering of Disease*, F.E. Alexander & P. Boyle, eds. IARC, Lyon, pp. 1-20.

[7] Cartwright, R.A., Alexander, F.E., McKinney, P.A. & Ricketts, T.J. (1990). *Leukaemia and Lymphoma: An Atlas of Distribution within Areas of England and Wales 1984-1988*. Leukaemia Research Fund, London.

[8] Committee on Medical Aspects of Radiation in the Environment (COMARE) (1988). *Second Report. Investigation of the Possible Increased Incidence of Leukaemia in Young People near the Dounreay Nuclear Establishment, Caithness, Scotland*. HMSO, London.

[9] Committee on Medical Aspects of Radiation in the Environment (COMARE) (1996). *Fourth Report. The Incidence of Cancer and Leukaemia in Young People in the Vicinity of the Sellafield Site, West Cumbria*. HMSO, London.

[10] Committee on the Possible Effects of Electromagnetic Fields on Biologic Systems (1966). *Possible Health Effects of Exposure to Residential Electric and Magnetic Fields*. National Academy Press, Washington.

[11] Darby, S.C. & Doll, R. (1987). Fallout, radiation doses near Dounreay, and childhood leukaemia, *British Medical Journal* **294**, 603-607.

[12] Doll, R. (1989). The epidemiology of childhood leukaemia, *Journal of the Royal Statistical Society, Series A* **152**, 341-351.

[13] Doll, R. & Wakeford, R. (1997). Risk of childhood cancer from fetal irradiation, *British Journal of Radiology* **70**, 130-139.

[14] Draper, G., ed. (1991). *The Geographical Epidemiology of Childhood Leukaemia and non-Hodgkin Lymphomas in Great Britain, 1966-83. Studies on Medical and Population Subjects, No. 53*. HMSO, London.

[15] Draper, G.J., Birch, J.M., Bithell, J.F., Kinnier Wilson, L.M., Leck, I., Marsden, H.B., Morris Jones, P.H., Stiller, C.A. & Swindell, R. (1982). *Childhood Cancer in Britain: Incidence, Survival and Mortality. Studies on Medical and Population Subjects, No. 37*. HMSO, London.

[16] Ederer, F., Myers, M.H. & Mantel, N.A. (1964). A statistical problem in space and time: do leukemia cases come in clusters?, *Biometrics* **20**, 626-638.

[17] Fedrick, J. & Alberman, E.D. (1972). Reported influenza in pregnancy and subsequent cancer in the child, *British Medical Journal* **ii**, 485-488.

[18] Gardner, M.J. (1991). Overview of the geographical approach to investigating childhood leukaemia, in *The Geographical Epidemiology of Childhood Leukaemia and non-Hodgkin Lymphomas in Great Britain, 1966-83. Studies on Medical and Population Subjects, No. 53*, G.Draper, ed. HMSO, London, pp. 127-131.

[19] Gardner, M.J., Snee, M.P., Hall, A.J., Powell, C.A., Downes, S. & Terrell, J.D. (1990). Results of case-control study of leukaemia and lymphoma among young people near Sellafield nuclear plant in West Cumbria, *British Medical Journal* **300**, 423-429.

[20] Gilman, E.A. & Knox, E.G. (1991). Temporal-spatial distribution of childhood leukaemias and non-Hodgkin lymphomas in Great Britain, in *The Geographical Epidemiology of Childhood Leukaemia and non-Hodgkin Lymphomas in Great Britain, 1966-83. Studies on Medical and Population Subjects, No. 53*, G. Draper, ed. HMSO, London, pp. 77-99.

[21] Greaves, M.F. (1997). Aetiology of acute leukaemia, *Lancet* **349**, 344-349.

[22] Jablon, S, Hrubec, Z. & Boice, J.D. (1991). Cancer in populations living near nuclear facilities - a survey of mortality nationwide and incidence in 2 states, *Journal of the American Medical Association* **265**, 1403-1408.

[23] Kinlen, L.J. (1995). Epidemiological evidence for an infective basis in childhood leukaemia, *British Journal of Cancer* **71**, 1-5.

[24] Kneale, G.W. (1971). Excess sensitivity of pre-leukaemics to pneumonia, *British Journal of Preventive and Social Medicine* **25**, 152-159.

[25] Linet, M.S. (1985). *The Leukemias: Epidemiologic Aspects*. Oxford University Press, New York.

[26] Little, M.P., Charles, M.W. & Wakeford, R. (1995). A review of the risks of leukemia in relation to parental pre-conception exposure to radiation, *Health Physics* **68**, 299–310.

[27] McLaughlin, J.R., King, W.D., Anderson, T.W., Clarke, E.A. & Ashmore, J.P. (1993). Paternal radiation exposure and leukaemia in offspring: the Ontario case–control study, *British Medical Journal* **307**, 959–966.

[28] O'Leary, L.M., Hicks, A.M., Peters, J.M. & London, S. (1991). Parental occupational exposures and risk of childhood cancer: a review, *American Journal of Industrial Medicine* **20**, 17–35.

[29] Preston, D.L., Kusumi, S., Tomonaga, M., Izumi, S., Ron, E., Kuramoto, A., Kamada, N., Dohy, H., Matsui, T., Nonaka, H., Thompson, D.E., Soda, M. & Mabuchi, K. (1994). Cancer incidence in atomic bomb survivors. Part III: Leukemia, lymphoma and multiple myeloma, 1950–1987, *Radiation Research* **137**, S68–S97.

[30] Shore, R.E., Pasternack, B.S. & McCrea Curnen, M.G. (1976). Relating influenza epidemics to childhood leukemia in tumor registries without a defined population base: a critique with suggestions for improved methods, *American Journal of Epidemiology* **103**, 527–535.

[31] Smith, P.G. (1982). Spatial and temporal clustering, in *Cancer Epidemiology and Prevention*, D. Schottenfeld & J.F. Fraumeni, eds. W.B. Saunders, Philadelphia.

[32] Viel, J.-F., Pobel, D. & Carré, D. (1995). Incidence of leukemia in young people around the La Hague nuclear waste reprocessing plant: a sensitivity analysis, *Statistics in Medicine* **14**, 2459–2472.

[33] Wakeford, R. & Binks, K. (1989). Childhood leukaemia and nuclear installations, *Journal of the Royal Statistical Society, Series A* **152**, 61–86.

[34] Weiss, H.A., Darby, S.C., Fearn, T. & Doll, R. (1995). Leukemia mortality after X-ray treatment for ankylosing spondylitis, *Radiation Research* **142**, 1–11.

[35] Zipursky, A., Poon, A. & Doyle, J. (1992). Leukemia in Down syndrome: a review, *Pediatric Hematology and Oncology* **9**, 139–149.

JOHN F. BITHELL

Level of a Test

The level of a statistical test, often called the level of significance, is the probability of rejecting the **null hypothesis** of "no effect" when in fact it is true. In classical **hypothesis testing** a null hypothesis, denoted by H_0, is assumed to be true, and the observed data are evaluated by a statistical test procedure to decide if the data provide sufficient evidence to reject this hypothesis. The possible outcomes of this test procedure are summarized in Table 1.

The level of the test is the probability of making a type I error. The decision to accept or reject H_0 is based on a comparison of the prespecified level of the test (generally 0.05 or 0.01) with the test procedure's **P value**, i.e. the calculated probability of finding a difference at least as great as the one actually observed, assuming that H_0 is true. If the *P* value is less than the level of the test, then the experimental data are considered to be inconsistent with the null hypothesis, H_0 is rejected, and the result is declared to be "statistically significant" at that particular level. If the *P* value is greater than the level of the test, then H_0 is accepted. A statistically significant departure from the null hypothesis may or may not be of practical importance in a given study.

Although the level of a test is traditionally taken as 0.05 or 0.01, this choice may vary, depending upon the probability of type I and type II errors that the experimenter is willing to accept. The level of a test is also one of several factors (together with sample size, the magnitude of the difference to be detected and the underlying variability) that determine the **power** of a test procedure for detecting departures from the null hypothesis (power is defined as one minus the probability of a type II error). Thus, for example, if 0.01 rather than 0.05 is selected as the level of the test, the probability of a type I error is reduced, but so is the power for detecting departures from H_0.

Other statistical terms that are often used to refer to the level of a test include the size of the test, the alpha error, and the **false positive rate**.

Table 1

		State of Nature	
		H_0 true	H_0 false
Decision	Accept H_0	Correct	Type II error
	Reject H_0	Type I error	Correct

J.K. HASEMAN

Leverage *see* Diagnostics

Lexis Diagram

A Lexis diagram is a (time, age) coordinate system, representing individual lives by line segments of unit slope, joining (time, age) of birth and death [13] (see Table 1 and Figure 1). The Lexis diagram is an important descriptive tool in epidemiology and **demography**. However, it also has several applications in **survival analysis** and analytical epidemiology as a tool for several classes of statistical models, as surveyed by Keiding [8]. These uses of the Lexis diagram are less common and it is the aim of this article to indicate some recent developments.

Lexis [13] in his Figure 1, reproduced here as Figure 2, originally considered a diagram of (calendar time at birth, age) in which life lines will be vertical rather than having unit slope. In his Figure 2,

Table 1 Five lives illustrated in Figure 1

Born	Died	Age at death
1918	1966	48
1926	1944	18
1934	1992	58
1944	1978	34
1954	1968	14

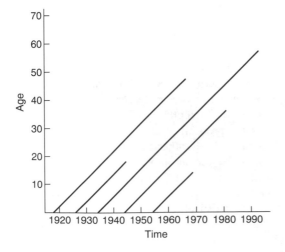

Figure 1 A Lexis diagram representing the five lives of Table 1

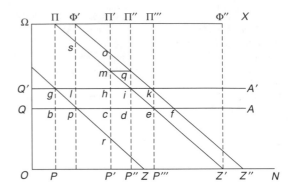

Figure 2 Lexis's diagram [13, Figure 1]

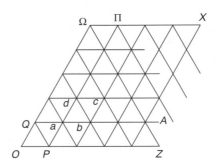

Figure 3 Lexis's equilateral diagram [13, Figure 2]

reproduced here as Figure 3, he also mentioned an equilateral diagram in which the time units in the calendar time, age, and cohort (i.e. time of birth) directions are of the same length. Lexis further discussed a three-dimensional extension allowing for an intermediate (irreversible) life event, in Lexis's case exemplified by marriage. This corresponds to the three-state model basic to the modern statistical description of **incidence** and **prevalence** (cf. [9]).

Despite its long history, the Lexis diagram is still being rediscovered among statisticians, cf. Goldman [6] for the standard Lexis diagram and Weinkam & Sterling [18] for the equilateral Lexis diagram.

Applications of the Lexis Diagram in Survival Analysis and Analytical Epidemiology

Clinical Trials with Staggered Entry

In many **clinical trials** patients arrive sequentially in calendar time but the substantive interest is on survival time since entry. As explained in the articles

Interim Analysis of Censored Data and **Staggered Entry**, the resulting interplay between the two time scales (calendar time and duration) has generated considerable complications in the development of a satisfactory statistical theory, particularly if comparisons between treatments are intended along the way at certain fixed time points (interim analysis) or sequentially (*see* **Data and Safety Monitoring**).

As mentioned by Keiding et al. [11] (*see* **Delayed Entry**), it is sometimes feasible to exploit the remaining life times of individuals (counted with delayed entry) from an interim analysis to supplement new individuals in a confirmatory analysis. This idea is explained in the Lexis diagram of Figure 4.

Disease Incidence Studies

Lexis diagram representations of classical (often historically) prospective studies (*see* **Cohort Study; Cohort Study, Historical**) of (calendar time, age)-specific disease incidence are common, and we return to some of the statistical issues below. More intricate sampling plans may also take advantage of this representation, such as the **retrospective** incidence study of a **cross-sectional** sample of prevalent diabetics by Keiding et al. [12], where each incident and surviving

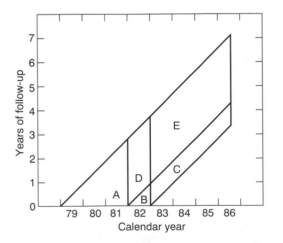

Figure 4 Lexis diagram of the DBCG-77 clinical trials on adjuvant treatment of breast cancer. The traditional independent data set for verifying an unexpected finding in A would be based on B and C. However, much more information is obtained by including also D and E, and in fact B and D already would have yielded the independent confirmation not achieved by B and C. Reproduced from Keiding et al. [11] by permission of John Wiley & Sons Ltd

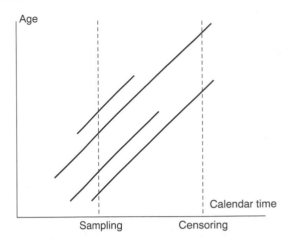

Figure 5 Lexis diagram of a prevalent cohort study. Four patients are sampled and their disease onset is known. During the follow-up period two of them die; the other two are still alive at the end of follow-up, where they are censored

case needed to be weighted (in a **Horvitz–Thompson** fashion) by its inverse survival probability from disease onset to the sampling date.

Prevalent Cohort Studies

A prevalent cohort study is based on a cross-sectional sample of diseased patients, with or without retrospective information on disease onset. Patients are followed until death or a fixed later calendar time, whichever comes first, (see Figure 5, and also [7] for additional examples and the link to the Arjas–Haara theory of innovative and noninnovative marks in the marked **point process** that accounts for the partial observation). The articles **Biased Sampling of Cohorts in Epidemiology** and **Delayed Entry** provide surveys of design and analysis problems for such studies.

Statistical Inference in the Lexis Diagram

Piecewise Constant Intensity Models

Many disease incidence and mortality studies (perhaps particularly in cancer) have taken piecewise constant intensity models (*see* **Grouped Survival Times**) as method of choice (see Clayton & Schifflers [4, 5] for a definitive survey). As is also well known in sociology, there is an inherent unidentifiability of the linear component in a model allowing for dependence on both **age, period and cohort** (*see* **Identifiability**), although Nakamura [15] showed that a **Bayesian** framework allowed roughness penalties in the three directions to decide the matter.

Point Processes, Continuous Time

Brillinger [3] initiated an exact use of point processes as a basis for statistical models for incidence and mortality in the Lexis diagram, generalized to morbidity (incidence) and prevalence by Keiding [9, 10] (see also [17]). Without parametric assumptions, statistical analysis requires smoothing formally studied by McKeague & Utikal [14] and embedded in an **empirical Bayes** interpretation of **penalized likelihood** by Berzuini et al. [2], Berzuini & Clayton [1] and Ogata et al. [16], who reanalyzed the retrospective diabetes incidence study by Keiding et al. [12] quoted above.

References

[1]   Berzuini, C. & Clayton, D. (1994). Bayesian analysis of survival on multiple time scales, *Statistics in Medicine* **13**, 823–838.

[2]   Berzuini, C., Clayton, D. & Bernardinelli, L. (1993). Bayesian inference on the Lexis diagram, *Bulletin of the International Statistics Institute* **55**, 149–165; with discussion **55**, 42–43.

[3]   Brillinger, D.R. (1986). The natural variability of vital rates and associated statistics (with discussion), *Biometrics* **42**, 693–734.

[4]   Clayton, D. & Schifflers, E. (1987). Models for temporal variation in cancer rates. I: age-period and age-cohort models, *Statistics in Medicine* **6**, 449–467.

[5]   Clayton, D. & Schifflers, E. (1987). Models for temporal variation in cancer rates. II: age–period–cohort models, *Statistics in Medicine* **6**, 469–481.

[6]   Goldman, A.I. (1992). Eventcharts: Visualizing survival and other timed-events data, *American Statistician* **46**, 13–18.

[7]   Keiding, N. (1989). Discussion of E. Arjas: Survival models and martingale dynamics, *Scandinavian Journal of Statistics* **16**, 209–213.

[8]   Keiding, N. (1990). Statistical inference in the Lexis diagram, *Philosophical Transaction of the Royal Society of London, Series A* **332**, 487–509.

[9]   Keiding, N. (1991). Age-specific incidence and prevalence: a statistical perspective (with discussion), *Journal of the Royal Statistical Society, Series A* **154**, 371–412.

[10]   Keiding, N. (1992). Independent delayed entry (with discussion), *Survival Analysis: State of the Art*, J.P. Klein & P.K. Goel, eds. Kluwer, Dordrecht, pp. 309–326.

[11]   Keiding, N., Bayer, T. & Watt-Boolsen, S. (1987). Confirmatory analysis of survival data using left truncation of the life times of primary survivors, *Statistics in Medicine* **6**, 939–944.

[12]   Keiding, N., Holst, C. & Green, A. (1989). Retrospective estimation of diabetes incidence from information in a prevalent population and historical mortality, *American Journal of Epidemiology* **130**, 588–600.

[13]   Lexis, W. (1875). *Einleitung in die Theorie der Bevölkerungsstatistik.* Trübner, Strassburg.

[14]   McKeague, I.W. & Utikal, K.J. (1990). Inference for a nonlinear counting process regression model, *Annals of Statistics* **18**, 1172–1187.

[15]   Nakamura, T. (1986). Bayesian cohort models for general cohort table analyses, *Annals of the Institute of Statistical Mathematics* **38**, 353–370.

[16]   Ogata, Y., Katsura, K., Keiding, N., Holst, C. & Green, A. (1996). Age–period–cohort analysis of incidence from incompletely detected retrospective data, *Research Report 96/2*. Department of Biostatistics, University of Copenhagen.

[17]   Wang, M.-C., Brookmeyer, R. & Jewell, N.P. (1993). Statistical models for prevalent cohort data, *Biometrics* **49**, 1–11.

[18]   Weinkam, J.J. & Sterling, T.D. (1991). A graphical approach to the interpretation of age-period-cohort data, *Epidemiology* **2**, 133–137.

NIELS KEIDING

Life Expectancy

Life expectancy is both the most summary and the most significant measure derived from a **life table**. Life expectancy at age **x** is the average number of years a person aged **x** will live if subject to the mortality rates contained in the life table.

In life table notation, life expectancy at age **x**, $\mathring{e}_x$, is given by

$$\mathring{e}_x = T_x / l_x,$$

where T_x is the total years lived in the life table population after exact age **x**, and $l_x =$ the number of survivors in the life table population at exact age **x**. The method for calculating these quantities can be found in standard textbooks [3].

Like the life table itself, life expectancy is determined by the force of mortality or mortality hazard function, $\mu(x)$, over the entire age range (*see* **Hazard**

Rate). In continuous notation

$$\mathring{e}(x) = \int_x^\infty l(x)dx/l(x),$$

and since

$$l(x) = \exp\left[-\int_0^x \mu(u)d(u)\right],$$

it can be seen that life expectancy at age **x** reflects both the **cumulative hazard** from birth to age **x** (through l_x), and the cumulative hazard from **x** to the oldest age (through T_x, itself an integral of l_x).

In **actuarial** analysis it is normal to distinguish between the complete (exact) expectation of life and the curtate or whole year expectation, but in **demography** and epidemiology the complete expectation is universally employed.

In most populations $\mathring{e}(x)$ tends to rise between birth and age 1, and to decline linearly thereafter, although in very low mortality countries the decline is virtually linear throughout the age range.

The most common life expectancy encountered is $\mathring{e}(0)$, the expectation of life at birth. Because $\mathring{e}(0)$ incorporates the entire mortality experience of the cohort or life table population, it may be considered as an age standardized (*see* **Standardization Methods**) measure of mortality, where the standard age distribution is derived from the age pattern of mortality itself.

Life expectancy at birth has increased substantially with modernization, rising from a preindustrial level of perhaps 40 years to current levels of over 80 in countries like Japan. Because of its cumulative impact throughout the age range, improved survival in infancy has made the greatest contribution to this increase.

In recent years there have been unexpected gains in expectation of life at older ages in some very low mortality countries, leading to predictions that expectation of life could rise to 100 years, with significant effects on social security and pension systems. However, 85 seems a more likely upper limit [2].

Traditionally, life table theory has not had a strong statistical component: the focus has primarily been on the average expectation of life, rather than on its distribution. However, Chiang [1] has addressed the **sampling** theory of the life table, and more recently the homogeneity/heterogeneity of life expectancy has received renewed attention, particularly in the context of expectation of life at advanced ages.

Life expectancy is also used as a powerful tool in association with multistate or multilevel life tables. Expectations of working life, of a healthy life, or of a life free of disability are examples of this. Unlike death, individuals may move in and out of these states, requiring modifications to the logic of the life table to incorporate nonabsorbing states.

References

[1] Chiang, C.L. (1984). *The Life Table and Its Applications*. Krieger, Malabar.
[2] Olshansky, S.J. & Carnes, B.A. (1994). Demographic perspectives on human senescence, *Population and Development Review* **20**, 57–80.
[3] Shryock, H.S. & Siegel, J.S. (1973). *The Methods and Materials of Demography*. US Department of Commerce, Bureau of the Census, Washington.

L. SMITH

Life Table

A life table is a tabular representation of central features of the distribution of a positive **random variable**, say T, with an absolutely continuous distribution. It may represent the lifetime of an individual, the failure time of a physical component, the remission time of an illness, or some other duration variable. In general, T is the time of occurrence of some event that ends individual survival in a given status. Let its cumulative distribution function (cdf) be $F(t) = \Pr(T \le t)$ and let the corresponding survival function be $S(t) = 1 - F(t)$, where $F(0) = 0$. If $F(\cdot)$ has the probability density function (pdf) $f(\cdot)$, then the risk of event occurrence is measured by the **hazard** $\mu(t) = f(t)/S(t)$, for t where $S(t) > 0$. Because of its sensitivity to changes over time and to risk differentials between population subgroups, $\mu(t)$ is a centerpiece of interest in empirical investigations.

In applications to human mortality, which is where life tables originated, the time variable normally is a person's attained age and is denoted x. The function $\mu(x)$ is then called the *force of mortality* or *death intensity* (*see* **Hazard Rate**). The life-table function $l_x = 100\,000\,S(x)$ is called the *decrement function* and is tabulated for integer x in *complete life tables*; in *abridged life tables* it is tabulated for sparser values of x, most often for five-year intervals of age. The *radix* l_0 is selected to minimize the need for decimals in the l_x table; a value different from $100\,000$ is sometimes chosen. Other life-table functions are the expected number of deaths $d_x = l_x - l_{x+1}$ at age x (i.e. between age x and age $x + 1$), the single-year death probability $q_x = \Pr(T \le x + 1 | T > x) = d_x/l_x$, and the corresponding survival probability $p_x = 1 - q_x$. Simple integration gives

$$q_x = 1 - \exp\left[-\int_x^{x+1} \mu(s)\mathrm{d}s\right]. \qquad (1)$$

Life-table construction consists in the estimation and tabulation of functions of this nature from empirical data. If ungrouped individual-level data are available, then the **Kaplan–Meier estimator** can be used to estimate l_x for all relevant x and estimators of the other life-table functions can then be computed subsequently. Alternatively, a segment of the **Nelson–Aalen estimator** can be used to estimate $\int_x^{x+1} \mu(s)\mathrm{d}s$; (1) can then be used to estimate q_x for each x, and the rest of the computations follow suit. From any given schedule of death probabilities $q_0, q_1, q_2, \ldots$, the l_x table is easily computed sequentially by the relation $l_{x+1} = l_x(1 - q_x)$ for $x = 0, 1, 2, \ldots$. Much of the effort in life-table construction therefore is concentrated on providing such a schedule $\{q_x\}$.

More conventional methods of life-table construction use **grouped survival times**. Suppose for simplicity that the range of the lifetime T is subdivided into intervals of unit length and that the number of failures observed during interval x is D_x. Let the corresponding total person-time recorded under risk of failure in the same interval be R_x. Then, if $\mu(t)$ is constant over interval x (the assumption of *piecewise constancy*), then the *death rate* $\hat{\mu}_x = D_x/R_x$ is the **maximum likelihood** estimator of this constant. Relation (1) can again be used to provide an estimator

$$\hat{q}_x = 1 - \exp(-\hat{\mu}_x), \qquad (2)$$

and the crucial first step in the life-table computation has been achieved. Instead of (2), $\hat{\mu}_x/\left(1 + \frac{1}{2}\hat{\mu}_x\right)$ is often used to estimate q_x. This solution is of older vintage and may be regarded as an approximation to (2).

Two kinds of problems may arise: (i) the exact value of R_x may not be known, and (ii) the constancy assumption for the hazard may be violated.

When the exact risk time R_x is not known, some approximation is often used. An Anglo-Saxon tradition is to use the mid-year population in the age interval. Alternatively, suppose that the number N_x of survivors to exact age x and the number W_x of withdrawals (losses to follow-up) in the age interval are known. What has become known as the **actuarial method** then consists in approximating R_x by $N_x - \frac{1}{2}(D_x + W_x)$. If there are no withdrawals and N_x is known, then D_x/N_x is the maximum likelihood estimator of q_x, and this provides a suitable starting point for the life-table computations.

For the case where only grouped data are available and the piecewise-constancy assumption for the intensity function is implausible, various methods have been developed to improve on (2). For an overview, see Keyfitz [12]. Even if single-year age groups are used, mortality drops too fast in the first year of life to merit an assumption of constancy over this interval. Demographers often use $\hat{\mu}_0/[1 + (1 - a_0)\hat{\mu}_0]$ to estimate q_0, where a_0 is some small figure, say between 0.1 and 0.15 [2]. If it is possible to partition the first year of life into subintervals in each of which mortality *can* be taken as constant, then it is statistically more efficient essentially to build up a life table for this year. This leads to an estimate like $\hat{q}_0 = 1 - \exp(-\sum_i \hat{\mu}_i)$, where the sum is taken over the first-year intervals. See Dublin et al. [5, p. 24] for an example.

The force of mortality is sometimes represented by a function $h(x; \theta)$, where θ is a vector of parameters. Actuaries most often use the classical Gompertz–Makeham function $h(x; a, b, c) = a + bc^x$ for the force of mortality in their life tables (*see* **Parametric Models in Survival Analysis**). When individual-level data are available, it would be statistically most efficient to estimate the parameters by the maximum likelihood method, but most often they are estimated by fitting $h(\cdot; \theta)$ to a schedule of death rates $\{\hat{\mu}_x\}$, perhaps by **least squares**, minimum chi-square (*see* **BAN Estimates**), or some **method of moments**. This approach is called *analytic graduation*; for its statistical theory, see [11]. One of many alternatives to modeling the force of mortality is to let [10]

$$q_x/p_x = A^{(x+B)^C} + D\exp[-E(\ln x - \ln F)^2] + GH^x.$$

So far we have tacitly assumed that the data come from a group of independent individuals who have all been observed in parallel and whose lifetimes have the same cdf. **Staggered** (delayed) **entries** into the study population and voluntary exits (withdrawals) from it are permitted provided they contain no information about the risk in question, be it death, recurrence of a disease, or something else. Nevertheless, the basic idea is that of a connected cohort of individuals that is followed from some significant starting point (like birth or the onset of some disease) and which is diminished over time due to *decrements (attrition)* caused by the risk's operation. In demography, this corresponds to following a **birth cohort** through life or a marriage cohort while their marriages last, and the ensuing tables are called *cohort life tables.*

Because such tables can only be terminated at the end of a cohort's life, it is more common to compute age-specific attrition rates $\hat{\mu}_x$ from data collected for the members of a population during a limited period and to use the mechanics of life-table construction to produce a *period life table* for the population from such rates. If mortality patterns are tied to cohorts, then individuals who live at widely differing ages in the period of observation cannot be expected to have the same risk structure, and the period table is said to reflect the patterns of a *synthetic* (fictitious) cohort exposed to the risk of the period at the various ages.

Multiple-Decrement Tables

When two or more mutually exclusive risks operate on the study population (*see* **Competing Risks**), one may correspondingly compute a *multiple-decrement table* to reflect this. For instance, a period of sickness can end in death or, alternatively, in recovery. Suppose that an integer random variable K represents the *cause of decrement* and define $F_k(t) = \Pr(T \leq t, K = k)$, $f_k(t) = dF_k(t)/dt$, and $\mu_k(t) = f_k(t)/S(t)$, assuming that all $F_k(\cdot)$ are absolutely continuous. Then $\mu_k(\cdot)$ is the cause-specific hazard (intensity) for risk cause k and $\mu(t) = \sum_k \mu_k(t)$ is the total risk of decrement at time t. For the multiple-decrement table, we define the decrement probability

$$q_x^{(k)} = \Pr(T \leq x + 1, K = k | T > x)$$

$$= \int_0^1 \exp\left[-\int_0^t \mu(x+s)ds\right] \mu_k(x+t)dt. \quad (3)$$

For given risk intensities, $q_x^{(k)}$ can be computed by numerical integration in (3). The expected number

of decrements at age x as a result of cause k is $d_x^{(k)} = l_x q_x^{(k)}$. When estimates are available for the cause-specific risk intensities, one or two columns can therefore be added to the life table for each cause to include estimates of $d_x^{(k)}$ and possibly $q_x^{(k)}$.

Several further life-table functions can be defined by formal reduction or elimination of one or more of the intensity functions in formulas like those above. In this manner, a *single-decrement life table* can be computed for each cause k, depicting what the normal life table would look like *if* cause k were the only one that operated in the study population and *if* it did so with the risk function estimated from the data. The purpose is to see the effect of the risk cause in question without interference from other causes. Some demographers call this abstraction the risk's *pure* effect. No assumption is made that in practice the total attrition risk can actually be reduced to the level of the one which is in focus or that this cause operates independently of other causes. For instance, a single-decrement life table of recovery from an illness reflects the pure timing effect of the duration structure of the intensity of recovery even though the elimination of mortality is unattainable.

A single-decrement life table is at an extreme end of a class of tables produced by deleting one (or more) of the cause intensities in formulas like those above. To obtain a *cause-deleted life table*, where only cause k has been eliminated, one may introduce $\mu_{-k}(t) = \mu(t) - \mu_k(t)$,

$$q_x^{(-k)} = \int_0^1 \exp\left[-\int_0^t \mu_{-k}(x+s)ds\right] \mu_{-k}(x+t)dt$$

$$= 1 - \exp\left[\int_x^{x+1} \mu_{-k}(s)ds\right], \quad (4)$$

and so on, and a "normal" life table may be computed with $\mu(t)$ replaced by $\mu_{-k}(t)$ everywhere. A corresponding cause-deleted multiple-decrement life table may be based on reduced cause-specific decrement probabilities like

$$\int_0^1 \exp\left[-\int_0^t \mu_{-k}(x+s)ds\right] \mu_j(x+t)dt,$$

for $j \neq k$.

Such a table would show what a normal table would look like *if* it were possible to eliminate cause k without changing the risk of any other cause. Again no assumption needs to be made about the feasibility of such elimination in real life nor about cause independence. The computations are based on a pure abstraction. The interpretation for real-life applications must be based on substantive considerations and is a different matter.

Life Expectancy

An individual's **life expectancy** (at birth) is the expected value

$$\mathring{e}_0 = \mathrm{E}(T) = \int_0^\infty [1 - F(x)]\mathrm{d}x = \int_0^\infty l_x/l_0\mathrm{d}x$$

of his or her lifetime T, computed for the probability distribution $F(\cdot)$ operating at the time of birth. When the individual has survived to (exact) age x, his or her remaining lifetime, $U = T - x$, is positive and has the survival function $S_x(u) = S(x + u)/S(x) = l_{x+u}/l_x$, and the *residual life expectancy* is

$$\mathring{e}_x = \mathrm{E}(T - x | T > x) = \int_0^\infty S_x(u)\mathrm{d}u = \int_0^\infty \frac{l_{x+u}}{l_x}\mathrm{d}u.$$

If $L_x = \int_0^1 l_{x+t}\mathrm{d}t$, we get $L_x \cong \frac{1}{2}(l_x + l_{x+1})$ by the trapezoidal rule of numerical integration, and

$$\mathring{e}_x = \sum_{t=0}^\infty L_{x+t} \cong \sum_{t=0}^\infty \frac{l_{x+t}}{l_x} - \frac{1}{2}, \qquad (5)$$

which is normally used to compute values for $\mathring{e}_x$.

Equivalent names for the life expectancies are *mean survival time* for $\mathring{e}_0$ and *mean residual survival time at age x* for $\mathring{e}_x$. The *median length of life* is the median in the distribution of T; it used to be called the *probable length of life* (*see* **Median Survival Time**). Correspondingly, the *median residual length of life* at age x used to be called the *probable residual length of life*. If we denote the latter by ξ_x, then it is defined by the relation $l_{x+\xi_x} = \frac{1}{2}l_x$.

The above functions can be computed for cohort life tables and for period life tables. Figure 1 shows plots of the function $\mathring{e}_x$ according to the mortality experience for Swedish women in 1891–1900 and 1990–1994. The life expectancy at birth has increased from 53.6 years in the older table to 80.8 some one hundred years later. Note that in the older table $\mathring{e}_x$ increases with x up to age 2 and remains above $\mathring{e}_0$ up through age 11. When mortality is high at very young ages, surviving the first part of life *increases* your expected remaining lifetime. As a consequence of mortality improvements for very young children,

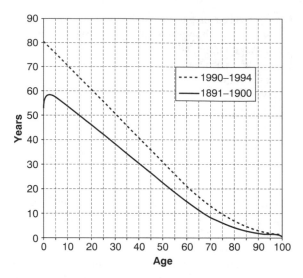

Figure 1   Residual life expectancy for Swedish women, 1891–1900 and 1990–1994

these features have disappeared in the younger table. Note that the expected *total* lifetime, $x + \mathring{e}_x$, always increases with x throughout the human lifespan. (One can show that the derivative of this function is always positive.) The longer you have lived already, the longer you can expect the total length of your life to be.

In a multiple-decrement situation, formula (5) can be used to compute a residual life expectancy $\mathring{e}_x^{(-k)}$ from the decrement series of the cause-deleted life table for risk k. The difference $\mathring{e}_x^{(-k)} - \mathring{e}_x$ is the gain one would get in residual life expectancy at age x if it were possible to eliminate risk cause k without changing the risk intensity of any other cause of decrement. Dublin et al. [5, p. 96] note that according to the cause-specific mortality of the US in 1939–1941 the gain would be 9.01 years for white men and 8.80 years for white women at age 0 if one could eliminate the risk of death due to cardiovascular–renal diseases at all ages (and change no other cause-specific mortality risks). The gains from eliminating the risk of death in cancer alone were much less (1.39 years for men and 2.05 years for women).

History and Literature

The first step toward the development of the life table was taken when **Graunt** [9] published his famous

Bills of Mortality. There were subsequent contributions by **Halley**, Huygens, Leibniz, Euler, and others. Deparcieux [4] clarified the definition of the life expectancy and identified the need for separate tables for men and women. Wargentin [17] was the first to publish real age-specific death rates, and the first to do so for a whole country. Price [14] included most of the columns now associated with the life table, and the tables by Duvillard [7] contained them all. The basic notions of cause-eliminated life tables go back to Bernoulli [1]. Cournot [3] developed the essentials of their mathematics. See Dupâquier [6] and Seal [15] for historical overviews. Smith & Keyfitz [16] have collected extracts from many original texts.

Life-table techniques are described in most introductory textbooks on the methods of actuarial statistics, biostatistics, demography, or epidemiology. See for example, Chiang [2], Elandt-Johnson & Johnson [8], or Manton & Stallard [13].

References

[1]   Bernoulli, D. (1766). Essai d'une nouvelle analyse de la mortalité causée par la petite vérole, et des avantages de l'inoculation pour la prévenir. *Histoire de l'Académie Royale des Sciences, Mémoires, Année 1760*, pp. 1–45.

[2]   Chiang, C.L. (1984). *The Life Table and its Applications*. Krieger, Malabar.

[3]   Cournot, A. (1843). *Exposition de la théorie des chances et des probabilités*. Hachette, Paris.

[4]   Deparcieux, A. (1746). *Essai sur les probabilités de la durée de la vie humaine*. Guérin Frères, Paris.

[5]   Dublin, L.I., Lotka, A.J. & Spiegelman, M. (1947). *Length of Life*. Ronald Press, New York.

[6]   Dupâquier, J. (1996). *L'invention de la table de mortalité*. Presses Universitaires de France, Paris.

[7]   Duvillard, E. (1806). *Analyse des tableaux de l'influence de la petite vérole, et de celle qu'un préservatif tel que la vaccine peut avoir sur la population et la longévité*. Paris.

[8]   Elandt-Johnson, R.C. & Johnson, N.L. (1980). *Survival Models and Data Analysis*. Wiley, New York.

[9]   Graunt, J. (1662). *Natural and Political Observations Made Upon the Bills of Mortality*. London.

[10]   Heligman, L. & Pollard, J. (1980). The age pattern of mortality, *Journal of the Institute of Actuaries* **107**, 49–75.

[11]   Hoem, J.M. (1972). Analytic graduation, in *Proceedings of the Sixth Berkeley Symposium on Mathematical Statistics and Probability 1970*, Vol. 1, L.M. Le Cam, J. Neyman & E.L. Scott, eds. University of California Press, Berkeley, pp. 569–600.

[12]   Keyfitz, N. (1982). Keyfitz method of life-table construction, in *Encyclopedia of Statistical Sciences*, Vol. 4, S. Kotz & N.L. Johnson, eds. Wiley, New York, pp. 371–372.

[13]   Manton, K.G. & Stallard, E. (1984). *Recent Trends in Mortality Analysis*. Academic Press, New York.

[14]   Price, R. (1783). *Observations of Reversionary Payments: On Schemes for Providing Annuities for Widows, and for Persons in Old Age; and on the National Debt*. Cadell & Davies, London.

[15]   Seal, H. (1977). Studies in the history of probability and statistics, XXV: multiple decrements or competing risks, *Biometrika* **64**, 429–439.

[16]   Smith, D. & Keyfitz, N. (1977). *Mathematical Demography: Selected Papers*. Springer-Verlag, Heidelberg.

[17]   Wargentin, P. (1766). *Mortaliteten i Sverige, i anledning af Tabell-Verket*. Kongl. Vetenskaps-Academiens Handlingar, Stockholm.

(*See also* **Demography; Vital Statistics, Overview**)

Jan M. Hoem

Likelihood

In general use the word *likelihood* is a synonym for **probability** but in statistics it has a more specific meaning; it is the probability (or probability density) of the observed data given the probability model which gave rise to the data. Likelihood is used to compare different possible candidate values for the *parameters* of the model, and for this purpose it needs to be defined only up to a constant of proportionality: any constant multiple of the likelihood serves equally well. When comparing two candidate values for a parameter, the one with the greater likelihood is said to be *more likely*, and parameter values for which the probability of the observed data is greatest are known as *most likely* values, or **maximum likelihood** estimates. The concept of likelihood is central to both the *frequency* and the **Bayesian** theory of **inference**. In addition there have been many attempts to found a theory of inference on likelihood alone.

A Simple Example

Let 10 subjects be followed for five years, and a record made of whether they die (fail) or survive. A simple probability model is that the outcome for each subject is independently random with probability π for failure and $1 - \pi$ for survival. The probability π is the *parameter* of the model. When four subjects fail, and six survive, the probability of the observed data is found from the **binomial distribution** to be

$$L(\pi) = 210\pi^4(1 - \pi)^6.$$

Suppose we wish to compare $\pi = 0.1$ with $\pi = 0.5$ as possible values for the true value which gave rise to the data. The two likelihoods are $L(0.1) = 0.0112$ and $L(0.5) = 0.2051$, so $\pi = 0.5$ is more likely than $\pi = 0.1$. The most likely value is $\pi = 0.4$, which has likelihood 0.2508. Since the likelihood can be scaled by any constant without altering such comparisons it is often convenient to scale it to take the value 1 when π takes its most likely value. The scaled likelihood for π is then the **likelihood ratio** $L(\pi)/L(\hat{\pi})$, where $\hat{\pi}$ is the most likely value for π.

Part (a) of Figure 1 shows the likelihood ratio for a range of possible values for π. Values of π corresponding to a high likelihood ratio are said to be *supported* by the data; those with a low likelihood ratio are not supported. The distinction between supported and not supported depends on where the cut-point is placed on the likelihood ratio scale. A convenient summary of the information about π in the data is

provided by the most likely value of π and a range of values which are supported at a given cut-point. The choice of cut-point can be regarded as a matter of convention; for example, we might all agree that parameter values with likelihood ratios above 0.15 are supported, while those with values below are not supported. Another approach is to choose the cut-point in terms of how well the supported range works when evaluated for repeated samples from the probability model assumed to have given rise to the data. This is called the *frequency* approach to statistics.

For any particular value of π the cut-point 0.1465 produces a supported range which includes the value of π in approximately 95% of repeated samples, provided the likelihood curve has roughly a *normal* bell shape. For this cut-point, then, the range of supported values corresponds to a 95% **confidence interval**. The supported range may also be thought of as a Bayesian *plausibility* interval based on a uniform *prior* belief about the true value of π. With a cut-point 0.1465 the area under the curve in part (a) of Figure 1, between the two verticals, is approximately 95% of the total area, so the *posterior* probability that π lies between the two limits is approximately 0.95. For all but very small studies the likelihood will have a normal bell shape (this is called the **central limit theorem**), and the three approaches (given likelihood

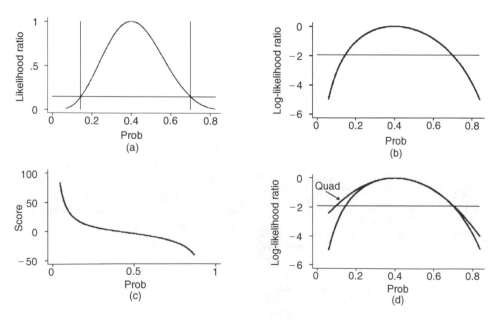

Figure 1   (a) Likelihood, (b) log likelihood, (c) score, and (d) quadratic approximation

ratio, given confidence level, and given posterior probability) will lead to almost the same range of values for the parameter.

Likelihood ratios are most easily studied as differences in log likelihoods. In this example the log likelihood is

$$l(\pi) = 4\log(\pi) + 6\log(1 - \pi),$$

and the log of the likelihood ratio is $l(\pi) - l(\hat{\pi})$. This log-likelihood function is shown in part (b) of Figure 1; the cut point for the supported range is now $\log(0.1465) = -1.921$ and the shape of the log-likelihood ratio curve is quadratic rather than a bell. The shape can be further explored by examining the gradient at each value of the parameter, given by

$$l'(\pi) = 4/\pi - 6/(1 - \pi).$$

This is called the *score* function and it is usually written as $u(\pi)$. The graph of the score function is shown in part (c) of Figure 1; note that the score is zero when π takes its most likely value of 0.4.

Some General Definitions

Let the data consist of observations $x_1, x_2, \ldots, x_N$, with probability model $f(x; \theta)$, which depends on a parameter θ. When there are only a limited number of possible values for x the function $f(x; \theta)$ specifies the probability of each outcome, and when there are infinitely many outcomes $f(x; \theta)$ specifies the probability density. The log likelihood for θ is

$$l(\theta) = \sum_{i=1}^{N} \log f(x_i; \theta),$$

and the score function is

$$u(\theta) = l'(\theta) = \sum_{i=1}^{N} \frac{f'(x_i; \theta)}{f(x_i; \theta)}.$$

The most likely value of θ is $\hat{\theta}$, satisfying $u(\hat{\theta}) = 0$.

In the neighborhood of $\theta = \hat{\theta}$ the score function is approximately linear [see part (c) of Figure 1], and using Taylor's expansion

$$u(\theta) \approx u(\hat{\theta}) + (\theta - \hat{\theta})u'(\hat{\theta}).$$

The quantity $u'(\hat{\theta}) = l''(\hat{\theta})$ is negative, and its numerical value, namely $-l''(\hat{\theta})$, is called the observed

information and is referred to as $j(\hat{\theta})$, or j for short. Since $u(\hat{\theta}) = 0$ the linear approximation can be written as

$$u(\theta) \approx -j(\theta - \hat{\theta}).$$

In part (c) of Figure 1 j is the numerical value of the gradient of the score function at $\pi = 0.4$. The steeper this gradient the more precise $\hat{\theta}$ is as an estimate of θ.

When considering the frequency properties of $\hat{\theta}$ as an estimate of θ it is best to write the function $l(\theta)$ as $l(\theta; x)$, stressing that it is a function of both the parameter values and the data. In a strictly likelihood approach the data are fixed and θ varies, which is why we write the function as $l(\theta)$. In the frequency approach it is x (the data) which varies and θ which is fixed, so that $l(\theta; x)$ is a **random variable**. The value of θ should be thought of as fixed at its true value, i.e. the value which gave rise to the data. The score $u(\theta; x)$ is now also a random variable, and is particularly important in frequency theory because its mean is zero and its variance can be calculated from the log likelihood. In fact

$$\mathrm{var}(u) = -\mathrm{E}[l''(\theta; x)].$$

The quantity $-\mathrm{E}\{l''(\theta; x)\}$ is called the *expected* or *Fisher information* and referred to as $i(\theta)$. When evaluated at $\theta = \hat{\theta}$ the expected information usually reduces to the same thing as the observed information, i.e. $i(\hat{\theta}) = j(\hat{\theta})$. Using the approximation $u(\theta) \approx -j(\theta - \hat{\theta})$, it follows that

$$\hat{\theta} - \theta \approx j^{-1}u(\theta),$$

and

$$\mathrm{var}(\hat{\theta}) \approx j^{-1}\,\mathrm{var}(u)\,j^{-1}.$$

Since $\mathrm{var}(u) \approx j$, the right-hand side of this equation becomes $j^{-1}jj^{-1} = j^{-1}$, so the variance of $\hat{\theta}$ in repeated samples is approximately j^{-1}, the inverse of the observed information.

The expression $\mathrm{var}(\hat{\theta}) \approx j^{-1}\,\mathrm{var}(u)\,j^{-1}$ is called the *information sandwich*. There are situations when it is unwise to assume that $\mathrm{var}(u) = j$, and better to replace $\mathrm{var}(u)$ by an empirically based estimate, using the individual values $u(\hat{\theta}; x_i)$. In this case the sandwich does not reduce to j^{-1} but provides instead a more robust estimate of the variance of $\hat{\theta}$.

When combining data from several sources, about the same parameter, the total log likelihood is obtained by adding the log likelihoods from the different sources. Since the score is the first derivative of the log likelihood, the total score is also found by adding the scores from the different sources, and since the information is the second derivative of the log likelihood it too is found by adding over sources. This additive property of the log likelihood and its derivatives makes the combining of data from different sources straightforward.

Approximate Log Likelihoods

The function $l(\theta)$ can be expanded around $\theta = \hat{\theta}$ using Taylor's expansion:

$$l(\theta) \approx l(\hat{\theta}) + (\theta - \hat{\theta})l'(\hat{\theta}) + \tfrac{1}{2}(\theta - \hat{\theta})^2 l''(\hat{\theta}).$$

Since $l'(\hat{\theta}) = 0$ and $j = -l''(\hat{\theta})$, it follows that

$$l(\theta) - l(\hat{\theta}) \approx -\tfrac{1}{2}j(\theta - \hat{\theta})^2.$$

This may also be written as

$$l(\theta) - l(\hat{\theta}) \approx -\frac{1}{2}\left(\frac{\theta - \hat{\theta}}{S}\right)^2,$$

where $S^2 = j^{-1}$ is the variance of $\hat{\theta}$. The fact that the log likelihood is approximately quadratic shows that the frequency distribution of $\hat{\theta}$ is approximately normal. A 95% confidence interval for θ is therefore given by $\hat{\theta} \pm 1.960S$. Alternatively, solving

$$-\frac{1}{2}\left(\frac{\theta - \hat{\theta}}{S}\right)^2 = \log(0.1465) = -1.921$$

for θ leads to the same expression.

Two or More Parameters

Extending the results from one parameter to two or more parameters is largely a question of notation. For simplicity we concentrate on two parameters $\boldsymbol{\theta} = (\theta_1, \theta_2)$. The log likelihood $l(\theta)$ is now a function of both parameters, and there are two score functions $\mathbf{u} = (u_1, u_2)$, where u_1 is the derivative of $l(\theta_1, \theta_2)$ with respect to θ_1, and u_2 is the derivative of $l(\theta_1, \theta_2)$ with respect to θ_2. Similarly, there are two most likely values $\hat{\boldsymbol{\theta}} = (\hat{\theta}_1, \hat{\theta}_2)$ which together maximize

the value of $l(\theta)$. The observed information becomes

$$j_{11}(\hat{\boldsymbol{\theta}}) = \frac{-\partial^2 l(\boldsymbol{\theta})}{\partial \theta_1^2},$$

$$j_{22}(\hat{\boldsymbol{\theta}}) = \frac{-\partial^2 l(\boldsymbol{\theta})}{\partial \theta_2^2},$$

$$j_{12}(\hat{\boldsymbol{\theta}}) = j_{21}(\hat{\boldsymbol{\theta}}) = \frac{-\partial^2 l(\boldsymbol{\theta})}{\partial \theta_1 \partial \theta_2},$$

where all the derivatives are evaluated at $\boldsymbol{\theta} = \hat{\boldsymbol{\theta}}$. These quantities are often written as a 2×2 information matrix $\mathbf{j}(\hat{\boldsymbol{\theta}})$ with elements $j_{rs}(\hat{\boldsymbol{\theta}})$, where $r = 1, 2$ and $s = 1, 2$. Similarly, the expected information becomes a 2×2 matrix $\mathbf{i}(\boldsymbol{\theta})$ with elements

$$i_{rs}(\boldsymbol{\theta}) = -\mathrm{E}[\partial^2 l(\boldsymbol{\theta})/\partial \theta_r \partial \theta_s].$$

All the results for one parameter extend in a fairly straightforward way to two or more parameters. In particular, the distribution of $\mathbf{u} = (u_1, u_2)$ has zero mean $(0, 0)$, and covariance matrix equal to $\mathbf{i}(\boldsymbol{\theta})$, the expected information matrix. When evaluated at $\boldsymbol{\theta} = \hat{\boldsymbol{\theta}}$ this becomes equal to $\mathbf{j}(\hat{\boldsymbol{\theta}})$, the observed information matrix. The linear approximation to the score functions becomes

$$u_1 \approx -j_{11}(\theta_1 - \hat{\theta}_1) - j_{12}(\theta_2 - \hat{\theta}_2),$$

$$u_2 \approx -j_{12}(\theta_1 - \hat{\theta}_1) - j_{22}(\theta_2 - \hat{\theta}_2),$$

which may be written in matrix terms as

$$\mathbf{u} \approx -\mathbf{j}(\boldsymbol{\theta} - \hat{\boldsymbol{\theta}}), \qquad \hat{\boldsymbol{\theta}} - \boldsymbol{\theta} = \mathbf{j}^{-1}\mathbf{u}.$$

The mean of the distribution of $\hat{\boldsymbol{\theta}}$ is approximately $(0, 0)$ and the covariance matrix is approximately

$$\mathbf{j}^{-1}\,\mathrm{var}(\mathbf{u})\mathbf{j}^{-1},$$

which reduces to $\mathbf{j}^{-1}$ when $\mathrm{var}(\mathbf{u})$ is replaced by $\mathbf{j}$.

Finally, the quadratic approximation to the log likelihood in the neighborhood of $(\hat{\theta}_1, \hat{\theta}_2)$ is

$$l(\theta_1, \theta_2) - l(\hat{\theta}_1, \hat{\theta}_2) \approx -\tfrac{1}{2}j_{11}(\theta_1 - \hat{\theta}_1)^2$$
$$-\tfrac{1}{2}j_{22}(\theta_2 - \hat{\theta}_2)^2 - j_{12}(\theta_1 - \hat{\theta}_1)(\theta_2 - \hat{\theta}_2),$$

which shows that the joint distribution of $(\hat{\theta}_1, \hat{\theta}_2)$ is approximately bivariate normal with mean $(0, 0)$ and covariance matrix $\mathbf{j}^{-1}$.

Nuisance Parameters

A supported *region* for (θ_1, θ_2) can be found by solving $l(\theta_1, \theta_2) = -1.921$, but in most practical applications one of the two parameters (say θ_1) is of interest and the other is a *nuisance*; so one wants a supported range for θ_1. It is straightforward to find a supported range for θ_1 for a given value θ_2^0 for θ_2, by solving $l(\theta_1, \theta_2^0) = -1.921$ for θ_1, but the answer will in general depend on θ_2^0. Only rarely will the supported range be independent of the value chosen for θ_2^0.

There are two possible ways of obtaining a supported range for θ_1 which is not dependent on choosing a particular value of θ_2. The first way is to find some aspect of the data which, when held fixed, leads to a *conditional* log likelihood which depends only on θ_1. Provided the aspects of the data which are held fixed are uninformative about θ_1, no information is lost by using the conditional log likelihood.

The second way is to replace the nuisance parameter θ_2 by its most likely value given θ_1, that is by $\hat{\theta}_2(\theta_1)$. The resulting log likelihood, $l_p(\theta_1) = l(\theta_1, \hat{\theta}_2(\theta_1))$, is called the *profile* log likelihood for θ_1, and can be used to find a confidence interval for θ_1 by solving $l_p(\theta_1) = -1.921$, as before. The idea of profile log likelihood extends to more than one nuisance parameter, but should not be used when there are many nuisance parameters to be eliminated, but not very much data. This is because each $\hat{\theta}_2(\theta_1)$ is too poorly estimated for the resulting profile log likelihood to be useful. A well-known example where this happens is a matched case–control study where there is a nuisance parameter for each new matched set. In this situation it is necessary to use a conditional log likelihood, and indeed this is generally the best thing to do provided one is available. Unfortunately there are many situations where it is not possible to find a conditional likelihood which depends only on the parameter of interest.

A quadratic approximation to the **profile likelihood** for θ_1 is found by starting from the quadratic approximation to $l(\theta_1, \theta_2)$, in the neighborhood of $(\hat{\theta}_1, \hat{\theta}_2)$, and then obtaining the profile likelihood for θ_1. This gives a quadratic approximation to $l_p(\theta_1)$, the profile likelihood for θ_1, of the form

$$l_p(\theta_1) \approx -\frac{1}{2} \left(\frac{\theta_1 - \hat{\theta}_1}{S} \right)^2,$$

where S is given by

$$S^2 = \frac{j_{22}}{j_{11} j_{22} - j_{12}^2}.$$

This is the first diagonal element in the inverse of j, the observed information matrix, so the quadratic approximation to the profile likelihood for θ_1 coincides with the normal approximation to $\hat{\theta}_1$.

Hypothesis Testing

From a strictly likelihood point of view, support for a specific *null* value of a parameter, say θ^0, is measured by the likelihood ratio for this value in the same way as for any other value of θ. The likelihood ratio is a measure of how different θ^0 is from $\hat{\theta}$. Cut-points on the likelihood ratio scale are a matter of convention; some useful ones are shown in Table 1.

From a frequency point of view we measure how far θ^0 is from $\hat{\theta}$ in terms of how often the value of some statistic in repeated samples exceeds the value observed. To do this requires a statistic whose distribution when $\theta = \theta^0$ is known, and a natural one to choose is the score $u(\theta^0; x)$. When the true value of θ is θ^0, the score has mean zero and variance $i(\theta^0)$, so the distribution of

$$z = \frac{u(\theta^0) - 0}{[i(\theta^0)]^{1/2}}$$

is approximately N(0, 1), a normal distribution with unit variance, and the probability of observing a value greater than $|z|$ is obtained by looking z^2 up in a χ^2 distribution with one degree of freedom (df). This probability is called the **P value**, and the test is called a *score test*.

Another candidate for the choice of statistic is $\hat{\theta}$, the most likely value of θ. When the true value of θ is θ^0, this statistic has an approximately normal distribution with mean θ^0 and variance j^{-1}. The probability of observing a value greater than $|z|$,

Table 1

Likelihood ratio	Evidence against the null value
>0.25	None
0.15–0.25	Slight
0.05–0.15	Strong
<0.05	Very strong

where z is now

$$z = \frac{\hat{\theta} - \theta_0}{j^{-1/2}},$$

is obtained by looking z^2 up in a χ^2 distribution with one df. The test is now called a *Wald test*.

The last and generally the best statistic which is used is the log-likelihood ratio itself. Provided the log-likelihood curve is reasonably close to a quadratic shape, the distribution of

$$d = 2[l(\hat{\theta}) - l(\theta^0)]$$

is approximately χ^2 with one df. The probability of observing a value of d which is greater than the one actually observed is found by looking up d in tables of the **chi-square distribution** on 1 df. The test is now called the (log) **likelihood ratio test**.

All three tests extend to null hypotheses in which several parameters take their null values; for example the distribution of

$$2[l(\hat{\theta}_1, \hat{\theta}_2) - l(\theta_1^0, \theta_2^0)]$$

is approximately χ^2 on two df.

Further Reading

The concept of likelihood was introduced to statistics by Fisher in 1925, but the first book to discuss statistical inference from an exclusively likelihood point of view is Edwards [4]. More recent accounts which stress the central role of likelihood in statistical inference are given by Lindsey [5] at an elementary level, Azzalini [1] at an intermediate level, and Barndorff-Nielson & Cox [2] at an advanced level. An elementary account of the use of likelihood in the context of epidemiology is given by Clayton & Hills [3].

References

[1] Azzalini, A. (1996). *Statistical Inference Based on the Likelihood*. Chapman & Hall, London.
[2] Barndorff-Nielson, O.E. & Cox, D.R. (1994). *Inference and Asymptotics*. Chapman & Hall, London.
[3] Clayton, D.G. & Hills, M. (1993). *Statistical Models in Epidemiology*. Oxford University Press, Oxford.
[4] Edwards, A.W.F. (1972). *Likelihood*. Cambridge University Press, London.
[5] Lindsey, J.K. (1995). *Introductory Statistics: The Modeling Approach*. Oxford University Press, Oxford.

(*See also* **Foundations of Probability; Hypothesis Testing**)

MICHAEL HILLS

Likelihood Principle *see* Foundations of Probability

Likelihood Ratio

Let x_{obs} be a vector of observed data. To analyze the data, one often assumes that x_{obs} has been randomly drawn from a population whose distribution is described by a joint density function $f(x; \theta)$ depending on an unknown parameter vector θ. The distribution may be discrete or continuous or may have both discrete and continuous components, such as occurs with some censored data. The **likelihood** of the parameter vector θ based on the data vector x_{obs} is defined to be $L(\theta) = f(x_{obs}; \theta)$. Given two possible values of the parameter vector, the one with the greater likelihood is regarded as being more likely to be the true parameter value. That is to say, the value θ_1 is more likely than the value θ_2 if the *likelihood ratio* $L(\theta_1)/L(\theta_2)$ is greater than 1. In fact, the likelihood ratio can be used as a quantitative measure of the strength of support that the data provide for θ_1 in comparison with θ_2.

For example, consider an urn containing 10 balls, θ of which are red and $10 - \theta$ are green. Suppose we draw two balls at random without replacement from the urn and both balls are red. The probability of such an outcome is $f(2; \theta) = (\theta/10)[(\theta - 1)/9] = \theta(\theta - 1)/90$. To compare the possibility that $\theta = 6$ with the possibility that $\theta = 5$, we can calculate the likelihood ratio $L(6)/L(5) = f(2; 6)/f(2; 5) = 1.5$ and state that $\theta = 6$ is 1.5 times as likely as $\theta = 5$.

The likelihood ratio $L(\theta_0)/L(\theta_1)$ is a sensible test statistic for testing the simple null hypothesis $H_0: \theta = \theta_0$ vs. the simple alternative hypothesis $H_1: \theta = \theta_1$ (*see* **Hypothesis Testing**). If the ratio is small, then the likelihood of θ_0 is small in comparison with the likelihood of θ_1, and so it makes sense that we should reject H_0. Moreover, Neyman & Pearson [2] showed that this test is the most powerful one among all tests having the same level (*see* **Neyman–Pearson Lemma**). For testing a general null hypothesis $H_0: \theta \in \Theta_0$ vs. a general alternative hypothesis $H_1: \theta \in \Theta_1$, Neyman & Pearson [1] proposed the test statistic $\lambda = L(\hat{\theta}_0)/L(\hat{\theta})$, where $L(\hat{\theta}_0)$ is the maximum value of the likelihood as θ varies over Θ_0 and $L(\hat{\theta})$ is the maximum value of the likelihood as θ varies over Θ_0 and Θ_1 (*see* **Likelihood Ratio Tests**). The null hypothesis is rejected if λ is small. Some authors call λ a *likelihood ratio* but it is also called a *likelihood ratio criterion* or *generalized likelihood ratio* or *maximum likelihood ratio* or *likelihood ratio test statistic*. The quantity $-2\log\lambda$ is also sometimes called a *likelihood ratio test statistic*.

Other Interpretations of the Likelihood Ratio

Although the concept of likelihood is distinct from the concept of probability, it is possible to give the likelihood ratio $L(\theta_1)/L(\theta_2)$ a direct probability interpretation if we take a **Bayesian** viewpoint. Suppose that, on the basis of past experience, it can be assumed that the true parameter is either θ_1 or θ_2 and that both are equally probable. Then our **prior distribution** is given by $\Pr(\theta_1) = \Pr(\theta_2) = 0.5$. The likelihood ratio coincides with the ratio $\Pr(\theta_1|\mathbf{x}_{\text{obs}})/\Pr(\theta_2|\mathbf{x}_{\text{obs}})$ of the posterior probabilities of the two parameters.

If the likelihood ratio is viewed as a random function, in the manner indicated below, then it is a minimal sufficient statistic (*see* **Sufficient Statistic**). Choose a fixed parameter vector θ_0 and, for each fixed value of $\mathbf{x}$, regard the likelihood ratio $R(\mathbf{x})(\theta) = L(\theta; \mathbf{x})/L(\theta_0; \mathbf{x}) = f(\mathbf{x}; \theta)/f(\mathbf{x}; \theta_0)$ as a real-valued function of θ. Let $\mathbf{X}$ be a random vector with density $f(\mathbf{x}; \theta)$. It is a consequence of the factorization theorem for sufficient statistics that $R(\mathbf{X})$ is a minimal sufficient statistic.

References

[1]   Neyman, J. & Pearson, E.S. (1928). On the use and interpretation of certain test criteria for purposes of statistical inference, *Biometrika* **20A**, 175–240, 263–295.

[2]   Neyman, J. & Pearson, E.S. (1933). On the problem of the most efficient tests of statistical hypotheses, *Philosophical Transactions of the Royal Society, Series A* **231**, 289–337.

D. BIRKES

Likelihood Ratio Tests

Suppose $\mathbf{x}_{\text{obs}}$ is a vector of data that have been collected in order to test a hypothesis. The likelihood ratio test is a hypothesis testing procedure that can be performed in a wide variety of situations. To apply the procedure, we must be able to regard the observed data $\mathbf{x}_{\text{obs}}$ as having been drawn at random from a population whose distribution is described by a joint density function $f(\mathbf{x}; \theta)$ depending on an unknown parameter vector θ, and we must formulate the hypothesis as a statement about θ. The distribution of the population may be discrete or continuous or may have both discrete and continuous components, such as occurs with some censored data.

The function $L(\theta) = f(\mathbf{x}_{\text{obs}}; \theta)$ is called the **likelihood** function. Let Θ denote the set of possible parameter vectors and let Θ_0 be a subset of Θ. For testing the null hypothesis $H_0: \theta \in \Theta_0$ vs. the alternative hypothesis $H_a: \theta \notin \Theta_0$, Neyman & Pearson [12] introduced the *likelihood ratio test* (abbreviated as *LR test*; also called the *generalized likelihood ratio test* or *maximum likelihood ratio test*). Let $L(\hat{\theta})$ be the maximum value of the likelihood as θ varies over Θ, let $L(\hat{\theta}_0)$ be the maximum as θ varies over Θ_0, and let

$$\lambda = \frac{L(\hat{\theta}_0)}{L(\hat{\theta})}.$$

The maximizing value $\hat{\theta}$ of the parameter vector is called the maximum likelihood estimator (MLE) of θ (*see* **Maximum Likelihood**), and $\hat{\theta}_0$ is the MLE under the null hypothesis. We can expect the MLE $\hat{\theta}$ to be close to the true parameter vector. If the null hypothesis were true, i.e. if the true parameter vector were in Θ_0, then we would expect both $\hat{\theta}$ and $\hat{\theta}_0$ to be close to the true parameter vector, and hence we would expect λ to be close to 1. The likelihood ratio test rejects the null hypothesis if λ is significantly smaller than 1, i.e. if the maximum likelihood under the null hypothesis is significantly smaller than the maximum likelihood under the alternative hypothesis.

In special situations the **P value** of a likelihood ratio test can be calculated exactly, but in general it must be approximated. If $f(\mathbf{x};\boldsymbol{\theta})$ satisfies certain regularity conditions (discussed below), then an approximate P value can be obtained as the proportion of a **chi-square distribution** that is larger than $-2\log\lambda$, where the number of **degrees of freedom** is the number of independent conditions that the null hypothesis imposes on the parameter vector $\boldsymbol{\theta}$. This proportion can be calculated by using the chi-square cumulative distribution function that is available in some computer packages, or bounds can be put on it by using a chi-square table.

Example 1

The diastolic blood pressures of 15 patients with moderate essential hypertension were measured immediately before and two hours after taking the drug captopril [5, p. 72]. A common way to analyze such data is to calculate the differences ("after" minus "before") and regard them as a random sample from a normally distributed population with unknown mean, δ, and unknown standard deviation, σ. The null hypothesis that the drug has no effect on blood pressure can be formulated as H_0: $\delta = 0$. The likelihood function is

$$L(\delta, \sigma) = \frac{1}{(2\pi)^{n/2}\sigma^n} \exp\left[-\frac{1}{2\sigma^2}\sum_{i=1}^{n}(x_i - \delta)^2\right],$$

where n is the sample size and the x_is are the differences. For the observed blood pressure data this becomes

$$L(\delta, \sigma) = \frac{1}{(2\pi)^{15/2}\sigma^{15}}$$
$$\times \exp\left[-\frac{1}{2\sigma^2}(15\delta^2 + 278\delta + 2327)\right].$$

The likelihood attains its maximum value, $L(\hat{\delta}, \hat{\sigma})$, at $\hat{\delta} = -9.27$ and $\hat{\sigma} = 8.32$. Under the null hypothesis, the likelihood attains a maximum value, $L(0, \hat{\sigma}_0)$, at $\hat{\sigma}_0 = 12.46$. Then $-2\log\lambda = 2[\log L(-9.27, 8.32) - \log L(0, 12.46)] = 12.10$. Since the null hypothesis imposes only one condition on the parameters, the number of degrees of freedom is 1. From a chi-square table we see that the approximate P value is less than 0.001, and we conclude that the drug has an effect.

Example 1 is simple enough that there are explicit formulas for the MLEs: $\hat{\delta} = \bar{x}$, where $\bar{x}$ is the sample mean; $\hat{\sigma} = [(n-1)/n]^{1/2}s$, where s is the sample standard deviation; and $\hat{\sigma}_0 = (\sum x_i^2/n)^{1/2}$. Therefore there are explicit formulas for $L(\hat{\delta}, \hat{\sigma})$ and $L(0, \hat{\sigma}_0)$ and hence for λ, namely $\lambda = (\hat{\sigma}/\hat{\sigma}_0)^n$. In general, however, $L(\hat{\boldsymbol{\theta}})$ and $L(\hat{\boldsymbol{\theta}}_0)$ must be calculated by numerical optimization methods (*see* **Optimization and Nonlinear Equations**).

In Example 1 the LR test is equivalent to the usual t test. In fact, if $x_1, \ldots, x_n$ is a random sample from a normally distributed population with unknown mean μ and unknown standard deviation σ, then the LR test statistic, $-2\log\lambda$, for testing H_0: $\mu = \mu_0$, is an increasing function of the **Student's t statistic** $|t| = |\bar{x} - \mu_0|/(s/\sqrt{n})$. Therefore, in this situation it is possible to obtain the exact P value of the LR test. (But of course it is exact only if the population is exactly normally distributed.) From a t table it is seen that the exact P value also is less than 0.001.

Example 2

For the data in Example 1, the assumption that the blood pressure differences come from a normally distributed population can be justified by arguing that the data contain no outliers and that the t test is robust against nonnormality. But if one felt uncomfortable about assuming normality, a different test of the null hypothesis of no drug effect could be performed by regarding the differences as a random sample from a continuous population with an unknown proportion π of positive values. Here we are assuming nothing about the population other than that it is continuous. The null hypothesis can be formulated as H_0: $\pi = 0.5$. Let x denote the number of patients whose blood pressure differences were positive. The likelihood function is

$$L(\pi) = \frac{n!}{x!(n-x)!}\pi^x(1-\pi)^{n-x}.$$

This is another simple example in which the MLE has an explicit formula: $\hat{\pi} = x/n$. For the blood pressure data, $-2\log\lambda = 2[\log L(2/15) - \log L(0.5)] = 9.01$. The number of degrees of freedom is 1. From a chi-square table we see that the approximate P value is between 0.01 and 0.001, and we again conclude that the drug has an effect.

Another test based on the same assumptions (i.e. that the differences are a random sample from a continuous population) is the **sign test**. For the blood pressure data, the sign test has a P value of about 0.005. For large sample sizes n, the two tests are almost equivalent. An exact test is also available in this example, using the fact that, under our assumptions, the exact distribution of x is **binomial**. The P value of the exact test is 0.007, and so the P values from the three tests are in approximate agreement.

Example 3

One half of a group of 42 leukemia patients were treated with the drug 6-mercaptopurine and the other half were given a placebo [4]. Their remission times, in weeks, were recorded during a period of one year. At the end of the year some patients still had had no remission, and so these observations were censored. Let us assume that the patients were selected and treated independently of one another. A reasonable model for such data is that they are two independent **censored** random samples from two **Weibull** distributions. The likelihood function is

$$L(\kappa_1, \rho_1, \kappa_2, \rho_2) = L_1(\kappa_1, \rho_1)L_2(\kappa_2, \rho_2),$$

where

$$L_i(\kappa_i, \rho_i) = \kappa_i^{d_i} \rho_i^{d_i \kappa_i}$$
$$\times \exp\left[(\kappa_i - 1) \sum_{\text{unc}} \log x_{ij} - \rho_i^{\kappa_i} \sum_{\text{all}} x_{ij}^{\kappa_i}\right],$$

in which x_{ij} is the jth observation in the ith subgroup ($i = 1, 2, j = 1, \ldots, 21$), d_i is the number of uncensored observations in the ith subgroup, "unc" indicates summation over the uncensored observations, and "all" indicates summation over all the observations, including the censored ones. The null hypothesis of no treatment effect can be expressed as $H_0: \kappa_1 = \kappa_2$ and $\rho_1 = \rho_2$.

No explicit expression for λ is available in this example. However, there is an explicit expression for the MLE $\hat{\rho}_i$ as a function of κ_i, namely $\hat{\rho}_i = (d_i/\sum_{\text{all}} x_{ij}^{\kappa_i})^{1/\kappa_i}$. Substitute this into $L_i(\kappa_i, \hat{\rho}_i)$ to obtain the **profile likelihood** $L_{Pi}(\kappa_i)$. A numerical procedure must be used to maximize the profile likelihood, yielding the MLE $\hat{\kappa}_i$, from which we obtain $L(\hat{\kappa}_1, \hat{\rho}_1, \hat{\kappa}_2, \hat{\rho}_2) = L_{P1}(\hat{\kappa}_1)L_{P2}(\hat{\kappa}_2)$. Similarly, combining the two subgroups into a single sample under the assumption that H_0 is true, we can obtain $L_{P0}(\hat{\kappa}_0)$ and then $-2\log\lambda = 2[\log L_{P1}(\hat{\kappa}_1) +$

$\log L_{P2}(\hat{\kappa}_2) - \log L_{P0}(\hat{\kappa}_0)] = 66.17$. The number of degrees of freedom is 2. From a chi-square table we see that the approximate P value is less than 0.001, and we conclude that the treatment has an effect.

Likelihood ratio tests are commonly used in a number of different statistical areas. In **multiple linear regression** and **analysis of variance** for models with independent and identically normally distributed errors, the usual F **tests** are equivalent to LR tests. In **multivariate analysis**, tests using the Wilks lambda criterion (*see* **Discriminant Analysis, Linear**) are equivalent to LR tests. In the analysis of **generalized linear models**, the reduction in deviance between a model and an extended model is equal to the LR test statistic $-2\log\lambda$ for testing whether the two models are significantly different. To test hypotheses about **contingency tables**, one typically uses either the Pearson **chi-square test** or the LR test.

Likelihood ratio tests have been proposed in many other areas too. For any parametric statistical model that satisfies certain, fairly general, regularity conditions, the null distribution of $-2\log\lambda$ is well approximated by a chi-square distribution, and so it is straightforward, at least in theory, to apply the LR test to test the parameters of the model. In practice, calculation of the likelihood ratio often requires numerical optimization, which can involve substantial computation; but computation is becoming less of a concern as computer capabilities increase. The regularity conditions mentioned above assume that the support $\{\mathbf{x} : f(\mathbf{x}; \theta) > 0\}$ does not depend on θ, and that $f(\mathbf{x}; \theta)$ is differentiable with respect to θ, and other more technical requirements concerning first-order and higher-order derivatives. Under such conditions the null distribution of the LR test statistic can be approximated by a chi-square distribution with d degrees of freedom, where d is the difference in the dimensions of Θ and Θ_0. By the dimension of Θ is meant the number of "freely varying" components in the vector θ. More precisely, the dimension of Θ is k if it contains a solid k-dimensional cube and does not contain a solid $(k+1)$-dimensional cube. The degrees of freedom d can also be described as the number of independent conditions that the null hypothesis imposes on the parameter vector θ.

The chi-square approximation for the null distribution of the LR test statistic is based on asymptotic theory (*see* **Large-Sample Theory**) and so it may not work well if the sample size is small. For example, for small **categorical data** sets the chi-square approximation is usually poor [1] and produces inaccurate P values. The approximation may also be inadequate if the number of parameters is large, such as when testing the **goodness of fit** of a **generalized linear model** against a saturated model [6], or if the null parameters are on the boundary of the parameter set, such as when testing whether a **variance component** is zero [10, p. 501].

In situations where the chi-square distribution poorly approximates the null distribution of the likelihood ratio test statistic it is sometimes possible to obtain a better approximation, or even the exact distribution. For example, for the Wilks lambda criterion, its null distribution is better approximated by using an F distribution rather than a chi-square distribution [14], and there are numerical procedures for calculating its exact critical values to any desired precision. General higher-order asymptotic methods, such as Bartlett adjustment [11] (*see* **Bartlett's Test**) or modified profile likelihood [9, 13], can be used to adjust a likelihood ratio so that its null distribution can be well approximated.

Likelihood ratio tests have been shown to have certain asymptotic optimality properties in many situations [2, 3], although they typically lack certain other desirable asymptotic properties such as **Pitman efficiency** [7] (*see* **Asymptotic Relative Efficiency (ARE)**) and asymptotic **robustness** [8]. In some simple situations the LR test, using the exact distribution of λ, is optimal for small as well as large sample sizes. In the case when the null and alternative hypotheses are both simple, i.e. when testing $H_0: \theta = \theta_0$ vs. $H_a: \theta = \theta_1$, the **Neyman–Pearson lemma** states that the LR test is the **most powerful test** for any given **level**. In a one-parameter **exponential family** the LR test of a one-sided hypothesis is a uniformly most powerful test. In general, the LR test is not necessarily optimal, but it has wide applicability and has given reasonable results in a large number of cases in which its performance has been studied.

References

[1]   Agresti, A. (1990). *Categorical Data Analysis*. Wiley, New York.

[2]   Bahadur, R.R. (1965). An optimal property of the likelihood ratio statistic, *Proceedings of the Fifth Berkeley Symposium on Mathematical Statistics and Probability*, Vol. 1, University of California Press, Berkeley, pp. 13–26.

[3]   Cox, D.R. & Hinkley, D.V. (1974). *Theoretical Statistics*. Chapman & Hall, London.

[4]   Cox, D.R. & Oakes, D. (1984). *Analysis of Survival Data*. Chapman & Hall, New York.

[5]   Cox, D.R. & Snell, E.J. (1981). *Applied Statistics: Principles and Examples*. Chapman & Hall, New York.

[6]   Firth, D. (1991). Generalized linear models, in *Statistical Theory and Modelling*, D.V. Hinkley, N. Reid & E.J. Snell, eds. Chapman & Hall, New York, pp. 55–82.

[7]   Kallenberg, W.C.M. (1983). Intermediate efficiency, theory and examples, *Annals of Statistics* **11**, 170–182.

[8]   Kent, J.T. (1982). Robust properties of likelihood ratio tests, *Biometrika* **69**, 19–27.

[9]   Lindsey, J.K. (1996). *Parametric Statistical Inference*. Oxford University Press, Oxford.

[10] Littell, R.C., Milliken, G.A., Stroup, W.W. & Wolfinger, R.D. (1996). *SAS System for Mixed Models*. SAS Institute Inc., Cary.

[11] McCullagh, P. & Nelder, J.A. (1989). *Generalized Linear Models*, 2nd Ed. Chapman & Hall, New York.

[12] Neyman, J. & Pearson, E.S. (1928). On the use and interpretation of certain test criteria for purposes of statistical inference, *Biometrika* **20A**, 175–240, 263–295.

[13] Pierce, D.A. & Peters, D. (1992). Practical use of higher order asymptotics for multiparameter exponential families (with discussion), *Journal of the Royal Statistical Society, Series B* **54**, 710–737.

[14] Rao, C.R. (1973). *Linear Statistical Inference and Its Applications*, 2nd Ed. Wiley, New York.

(*See also* **Likelihood Ratio**)

D. BIRKES

Likelihood Ratio with Diagnostic Tests

The use of **sensitivity** and **specificity** to quantify the performance of a diagnostic test in relation to the true presence or absence of a specific disease is now well established in the medical literature. The emphasis on the formal evaluation of the information yielded by a diagnostic test and its incorporation into the diagnostic process has been an important theme in what is now called **clinical epidemiology** [4]. A renewed methodologic interest in the evaluation of diagnostic tests has led to alternative approaches being proposed, both to quantify test performance and to compare more easily the relative merits of competing tests [2]. One of these newer techniques is the use of **likelihood ratios** [1]. The objective of this article is to define the likelihood ratio in the context of a diagnostic test, to explain its use in the diagnostic process, and to contrast it with other techniques (*see* **Diagnostic Tests, Evaluation of**).

The Diagnostic Process

The term "diagnostic test" is used here to denote any item of diagnostic information derived from patient history, physical examination, biochemical or histologic examination of tissue, blood, or urine, or some sort of imaging. For example, a clinician might use the presence or absence of heart murmur to help diagnose a defective heart valve or a test that detects the presence of a normally intracellular enzyme in the blood of a suspected heart attack victim. In these situations the clinician would modify his/her degree of belief that the patient has the disease of interest on the basis of the test result. This might lead in turn to the immediate application of therapy, a decision to conduct further diagnostic testing which is usually more costly and/or more invasive (e.g. a coronary angiogram or ultrasound) but more definitive, or possibly to cease further workup on the grounds that the disease is unlikely to be present.

The result of the diagnostic test may be inherently dichotomous (e.g. the presence or absence of a physical sign), ordinal (e.g. the grade of murmur), or purely quantitative, as in the case of many laboratory tests. Despite this quantification, test results are often dichotomized into so-called positive and negative results based on some predetermined cutpoint. The choice of cutpoint may be fairly arbitrary (e.g. the 95th percentile for "normal" patients) or selected to yield the best discrimination between truly diseased and not diseased subgroups. Optimally chosen cutpoints would, in addition, take into account the

"costs" associated with the consequences of subsequent clinical decisions and the true disease status.

Clearly, the dichotomization of a test result discards some of the diagnostic information but it allows the clinician to incorporate more easily the test information into the diagnostic process. Dichotomization allows the performance of the test to be quantified and the straightforward computation of post-test probability of disease by **Bayes' theorem** [3].

Sensitivity, Specificity, and Predictive Value

In the context of a dichotomous diagnostic test, sensitivity and specificity define the test's inherent ability to be positive when disease is truly present and negative when it is absent. In other words

$$\text{sensitivity} = \Pr(\text{positive test} \mid \text{disease present})$$
$$= 1 - \beta,$$
$$\text{specificity} = \Pr(\text{negative test} \mid \text{disease not present})$$
$$= 1 - \alpha.$$

The complementary probabilities are analogous to the type I (α) and type II (β) errors in the context of **hypothesis testing**, hence the notation.

Suppose we have a population of patients in which a proportion, p, truly have a particular disease and the remainder, $1 - p$, do not. In other words, the background **prevalence** of disease is p. If the diagnostic test was conducted on each member of the population, then the distribution of the test results that would occur is displayed in Table 1. The expression within each cell of the table represents the proportion of the population with a particular combination of test result and true disease status. Note that the tacit assumption here is that the sensitivity and specificity are known for the test *in this population*.

Table 1 Test results in patients with and without disease

Diagnostic test result	Disease status		Predictive value (post-test probability)
	Present	Absent	
Positive	$p(1-\beta)$	$(1-p)\alpha$	$\dfrac{p(1-\beta)}{p(1-\beta)+(1-p)\alpha}$
Negative	$p\beta$	$(1-p)(1-\alpha)$	$\dfrac{p\beta}{p\beta+(1-p)(1-\alpha)}$

Faced with a diagnostic challenge for an individual patient in this population, the physician would start from the prior expectation, p, that the disease is present. This would then be modified in the light of the test result for the patient, increasing the probability of disease if the test was positive and reducing it if it was negative. Exactly how much the *prior probability* is modified in the light of the test result depends on the test's sensitivity and specificity. In the population as a whole, the proportion $p(1 - \beta) + (1 - p)\alpha$ would test positive; of this total, $p(1 - \beta)$ would actually have the disease (true positives) and $(1 - p)\alpha$ would not (false positives). Thus, given a positive test, a proportion $p(1 - \beta)/[p(1 - \beta) + (1 - p)\alpha]$ would truly have the disease. Similarly, a proportion $p\beta/[p\beta + (1 - p)(1 - \alpha)]$ would have the disease in those who tested negative. These quantities are referred to either as post-test probabilities or **predictive values** and by inspection can be seen to result from a direct application of Bayes' theorem.

Post-Test Odds

Odds are an alternative way of expressing the likelihood of an event. Saying that an event has odds of one to three of occurring (i.e. an odds of 1/3) is equivalent to saying the probability is one quarter. Probabilities are thus converted to odds by the relationship

$$\text{odds} = \text{probability}/(1 - \text{probability}),$$

and odds back to probability by

$$\text{probability} = \text{odds}/(1 + \text{odds}).$$

If, in the diagnostic situation above, we express the post-test chance of disease in terms of odds, then we produce the following expressions:

post-test odds(positive test)

$$= \frac{p(1 - \beta)/[p(1 - \beta) + (1 - p)\alpha]}{(1 - p)\alpha/[p(1 - \beta) + (1 - p)\alpha]}$$

$$= \frac{p}{1 - p} \times \frac{1 - \beta}{\alpha}$$

$$= \text{pre-test odds} \times \frac{\text{sensitivity}}{1 - \text{specificity}}.$$

The quantity sensitivity/(1 − specificity) is called the *likelihood ratio* (LR) for a positive test result. A

similar calculation for the odds of disease given a negative test result leads to

post-test odds(negative test)

$$= \frac{p}{1 - p} \times \frac{\beta}{1 - \alpha}$$

$$= \text{pre-test odds} \times \frac{1 - \text{sensitivity}}{\text{specificity}}$$

and the quantity $(1 - \text{sensitivity})/\text{specificity}$ is called the *likelihood ratio* for a negative test result.

A Numerical Example

The present-day horseshoe crab *(Limulus Polyphemus)* remains virtually unchanged from its primeval ancestors. Its primitive defenses include a blood-clotting mechanism designed to isolate and encapsulate certain types of bacteria infecting its blood stream. A purified extract of horseshoe crab blood forms the basis of the limulus lysate test for detecting the presence of gram-negative infections in humans. This test can yield a result in about one hour compared with two or three days for the definitive blood culture. In a recent study of febrile patients, the limulus test was found to have sensitivity 79% and specificity 96% in a population with a 4% prevalence of septicemia [6]. Thus, using the post-test probability expressions above, we have

Pr(septicemia | positive test)

$$= (0.04 \times 0.79)/[0.4 \times 0.79$$

$$+ (1 - 0.04)(1 - 0.96)] = 0.4514,$$

Pr(septicemia | negative test)

$$= 0.04 \times (1 - 0.79)/[0.04 \times (1 - 0.79)$$

$$+ (1 - 0.04) \times 0.96)] = 0.0090.$$

In other words, a positive test would increase the probability of septicemia from 4% to 45%, whereas a negative test would reduce it to less than 1%. From the quoted sensitivity and specificity:

$$\text{LR(positive test)} = \frac{\text{sensitivity}}{1 - \text{specificity}} = \frac{0.79}{1 - 0.96}$$

$$= 19.75,$$

$$\text{LR(negative test)} = \frac{1 - \text{sensitivity}}{\text{specificity}} = \frac{1 - 0.79}{0.96}$$

$$= 0.2188.$$

A pre-test probability of 0.04 corresponds to an odds of $0.04/(1 - 0.04) = 0.0417$. The post-test odds are then:

$$\text{post-test odds (positive test)} = 0.0417 \times 19.75$$

$$= 0.8236,$$

$$\text{post-test odds (negative test)} = 0.0417 \times 0.2188$$

$$= 0.0091.$$

Conversion from odds back to probability yields the same probabilities as above. Note that a positive test causes the odds to be multiplied by almost 20, whereas a negative test requires the odds to be reduced by a factor of about five.

Generalization of the LR

The initial objective of the diagnostic workup is to determine the probability that the patient has the disease in the light of the test result. While sensitivity and specificity are simple statistics that describe test performance, their combined influence on post-test probability is not obvious. By contrast, LR has a direct multiplicative effect on pre-test odds, making the impact of the additional diagnostic evidence provided by the test more apparent. The calculation of post-test odds can be done approximately using a little mental arithmetic. Alternatively, simple nomograms are available which convert pre-test to post-test probability via the appropriate LR [4].

The most important advantage of LR is that it can be generalized to handle ordinal (*see* **Ordered Categorical Data**) or purely quantitative tests [1]. While the computation of post-test probability via Bayes' theorem can incorporate a quantitative test result, the terms sensitivity and specificity can only be directly applied if the quantitative test is first dichotomized at some cutpoint into positive and negative categories. Other than for simplicity, there seems little justification for collapsing a quantitative test into this dichotomy. A patient whose test result was only just over the cutpoint for positivity would be assigned the same post-test probability as a patient whose test result was extremely elevated. At some stage the physician must make the decision whether the patient has, or does not have, the disease. However, this ultimate dichotomization should be based on actual post-test probability, not on the intermediate test result. This issue would be especially important if the current test was only one step in a more extensive sequential diagnostic workup.

For a continuous test result, X, the definition of LR is

$$\text{LR}(X) = \frac{\Pr(X| \text{ patient diseased})}{\Pr(X| \text{ patient not diseased})}.$$

These probabilities, and thus the LR, can be estimated empirically for an inherently ordinal test (e.g. the traditional $+$, $++$, $+++$ grading of heart murmur) or, for a purely quantitative test, by dividing the test result into subranges. In either case, the post-test odds are computed as the product of pre-test odds and LR, but now the LR is computed for the patient's own test result, as opposed to an average LR for all test results above or below a cutpoint.

Empirical LR Estimates

Table 2 shows LR computed for various ranges of creatine kinase (CK) for patients with and without myocardial infarction (MI) from a study by Smith [5]. Now, by using the LR for the range of the test result obtained, one can compute a more specific post-test probability. Obviously, the more extreme CK value of ≥ 280 would lead to a higher post-test probability of MI compared with a relatively mildly elevated CK at say 150.

Table 2 Creatine kinase (CK) in patients with and without myocardial infarction (MI)

CK range	Proportion of MI patients (A)	Proportion of non-MI patients (B)	LR (A/B)
≥ 280	97/230 0.4217	1/130 0.0077	54.8
200–279	37/230 0.1609	2/130 0.0154	10.5
120–199	51/230 0.2217	5/130 0.0385	5.8
40–119	43/230 0.1870	34/130 0.2613	0.71
<40	2/230 0.0087	88/130 0.6769	0.013

Purely Continuous LR

Although going some way to creating a LR for each level of the test result, in the example above we have had to combine patients within a range of CKs to provide enough data points to estimate the LR. Conceptually, the purely continuous test result situation is depicted in Figure 1. The individual test results for patients with and without the disease form two continuous *distributions* where the *heights* of the curves at any point are the relative frequencies of that test result for the populations of patients with and without the disease. By definition, the LR at any value of the test result, X, is the ratio of the relative frequency (i.e. probability density) of X in the diseased to nondiseased distributions. If the data for the test results from representative samples of diseased and nondiseased patients can be adequately described by some appropriate mathematical model, then the LR can in turn be described mathematically at each X. For example, if both samples of test results were **normally distributed** with different **means** and **variances** so that

$$X \sim N(\mu_1, \sigma_1^2) \text{ for diseased patients,}$$

$$X \sim N(\mu_2, \sigma_2^2) \text{ for nondiseased patients,}$$

then the LR would be

$$LR(X) = \frac{\left(2\pi\sigma_1^2\right)^{-1/2} \exp\left[-\frac{(X-\mu_1)^2}{2\sigma_1^2}\right]}{\left(2\pi\sigma_2^2\right)^{-1/2} \exp\left[-\frac{(X-\mu_2)^2}{2\sigma_2^2}\right]},$$

which simplifies a little to

$$LR(X) = \frac{\sigma_2}{\sigma_1} \exp\left[-0.5(z_1^2 - z_2^2)\right],$$

where the z_1 and z_2 are the standardized deviates (*see* **Standard Normal Deviate**) of the test result X with respect to the diseased and nondiseased distributions, respectively.

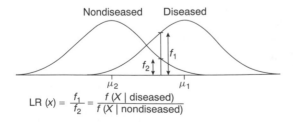

$$LR(x) = \frac{f_1}{f_2} = \frac{f(X \mid \text{diseased})}{f(X \mid \text{nondiseased})}$$

Figure 1   Likelihood ratio for a quantitative test

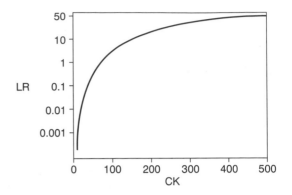

Figure 2   Continuous likelihood ratio curve

The CK data from Smith are almost perfectly **lognormally distributed** with $\log_e$ CK having mean $= 5.45$ and SD $= 0.737$ for MI patients and mean $= 3.19$, SD $= 1.030$ for noninfarct patients. Substitution of these parameter estimates into the expression above leads to the continuous curve (Figure 2), which provides a value for LR corresponding to each individual value of the CK test.

Summary

In its simplest form, LR is a useful measure of the diagnostic information conveyed by a diagnostic test. Compared with sensitivity and specificity, it offers a more interpretable measure of the impact of the test result on the probability of disease and also a simplification in the calculation, especially if one is prepared to think in terms of odds rather than probability. More importantly, it allows a natural extension to accommodate truly quantitative test results. The LR can reflect the diagnostic information at any level of test result. This leads to a post-test probability for the actual test result observed in the patient as opposed to a less specific post-probability computed from a test result which has been first dichotomized into positive and negative categories. Full utilization of the diagnostic information would require knowledge of the LR at each value of X and this may be quite feasible in many clinical situations.

References

[1]   Albert, A. (1982). On the use and computation of likelihood ratios in clinical chemistry, *Clinical Chemistry* **28**, 1113–1119.

[2]   Begg, C.C. (1991). Advances in statistical methodology for diagnostic medicine in the 1980s, *Statistics in Medicine* **10**, 1887–1895.

[3]   Brown, B.W., Jr (1977). *Statistics – A Biomedical Introduction*. Wiley, New York, pp. 25–30.

[4]   Sackett, D.L., Haynes, R.B. & Tugwell, P. (1985). *Clinical Epidemiology: A Basic Science for Clinical Medicine*. Little, Brown & Company, Boston.

[5]   Smith, A.F. (1967). Diagnostic value of serum creatine-kinase in a coronary care unit, *Lancet* **2**, 178–182.

[6]   van Deventer, S.J., Büller, H.R., ten Cate, J.W., Sturk, A. & Pauw, W. (1988). Endotoxaemia: an early predictor of septicaemia in febrile patients, *Lancet* **1**, 605–609.

ROBIN S. ROBERTS

Likert Scale

A Likert scale, or summated rating scale, is computed by summing responses over several items hypothesized to measure the same latent variable or construct [1]. Likert scales are often used to measure opinions, beliefs, or attitudes regarding a particular underlying construct. Items that comprise Likert scales are often measured on Likert response formats, which represent degrees of endorsement of those items [2]. For example, consider the following item measured on a five-point Likert response format:

Item:	Diet is an important part of a healthy lifestyle				
Response options:	Strongly agree	Agree	Neither	Dis- agree	Strongly disagree
	1	2	3	4	5

Items measured on Likert response formats are generally presented as declarative statements. For respondents to discriminate among response options, it is recommended that the items be presented as strong declarative statements.

Likert response formats may have three, four, five or more response options. An example of a six-point Likert response format which could have been used for the sample item above is: Strongly agree, Moderately Agree, Mildly agree, Mildly Disagree, Moderately disagree, and Strongly disagree. The five-point Likert response format is widely used. The number of response options for a given item depend upon the item being measured and subjects' abilities to discriminate between response options. Investigators should try to provide respondents with response options that are approximately equally spaced across the continuum of endorsement.

Many applications involve the measurement of a single underlying construct using multiple items, since in many cases single items are not adequate to measure the construct with sufficient precision. A Likert scale is constructed by summing or averaging responses over the set of all items to produce an overall score. In constructing the Likert scale, usually each item is equally weighted. If an investigation involves k such items, each measured on the same r-point Likert response format (responses coded as $1, 2, \ldots, r$, with higher scores reflecting more endorsement of each item), then the theoretic range of the Likert scale is k to kr.

Assumptions underlying the construction of multiple-item Likert scales are that each item is linearly related to the overall scale score, and that each item comprising the scale has approximately the same distribution (e.g. similar means and standard deviations). As an aside, when investigators present a set of items related to a single construct to respondents, some of the items should be reverse coded so as to reduce the likelihood that respondents consistently select the same response (e.g. strongly agree) for each item.

There are a number of techniques used to evaluate the **reliability** and validity (*see* **Validation Study**) of multiple-item Likert scales. These include, for example, the internal consistency reliability of the Likert scale, which is generally assessed using the **Cronbach's alpha** coefficient, and construct validity, which is assessed through **factor analysis**.

References

[1]   DeVellis, R.F. (1991). *Scale Development: Theory and Applications*, Sage, Newbury Park.

[2]   Stewart, A.L. & Ware, J.E., Jr (1992). *Measuring Functioning and Well-Being: the Medical Outcomes Study Approach*. Duke University Press, Durham.

(*See also* **Principal Components Analysis; Psychometrics, Overview**)

KIMBERLY A. DUKES

Limit Theorems

The earliest results in mathematical probability (dating from 1654) involved computations for finite sample spaces having equally likely outcomes, and thus could be regarded merely a branch of elementary combinatorics. The subject took a major step forward, however, both in the depth of its results and the sophistication of its methods after the discovery of its first limit theorems: James Bernoulli's **law of large numbers** (c. 1685, published posthumously in his *Ars conjectandi* of 1713) and Abraham De Moivre's **central limit theorem** [5] for sequences of dichotomous **binary** trials. These results extracted order from chaos by demonstrating that random phenomenon in the small (a limited number of observations) can exhibit regularities and deterministic behavior in the large.

Such results were often motivated by, and provided a theoretical basis for, the process of statistical **estimation**; in modern terminology, the law of large numbers amounts to nothing other than a statement that the sample mean is a **consistent** estimator of the population mean. If, for example, S_n denotes the number of successes in n dichotomous trials having probability of success p, then Bernoulli proved that $\lim_{n\to\infty} S_n/n = p$; using Stirling's approximation (including correction terms) to estimate the individual terms in the **binomial distribution** and then summing, De Moivre dramatically refined Bernoulli's result to discover the remarkable fact that

$$\lim_{n\to\infty} \Pr\left[a \le \frac{S_n - np}{[np(1-p)]^{1/2}} \le b \right]$$
$$= \frac{1}{(2\pi)^{1/2}} \int_a^b \exp\left(-\frac{1}{2}x^2 \right) dx.$$

During the nineteenth and twentieth centuries, this result was extended far beyond the simple coin-tossing setup considered by De Moivre, important contributions being made by the French school of **Laplace** and **Poisson**, the Russian school of Chebyshev, Markov, Liapunov, Bemstein, Khinchin, and **Kolmogorov**, and the varied contributions of von Mises, Cantelli, Lindeberg, Lévy, and Feller in the period between the two world wars. Fueling these advances were the use of increasingly sophisticated methods such as the introduction of **characteristic functions** (by Laplace) and the **method of moments** (by Markov). The introduction

of measure theory by Lebesgue and its use in the axiomatization of mathematical probability by Kolmogorov (*see* **Probability Theory**) led in turn to a sharp distinction between different forms of limit theorem, corresponding to different concepts of convergence: most commonly, **convergence in distribution**, probability, almost sure, and in L^p.

It is useful to regard a sequence of random variables as a single function $X(n, \omega)$, n being an integer and ω an element of a sample space. If one first fixes n, the result is a **random variable** $X_n(\cdot)$ (a function on the sample space), and one can then investigate the behavior of the distribution of X_n as $n \to \infty$; limiting behavior in this case corresponds to convergence in distribution. If, on the other hand, one first fixes ω, the result is a sequence $\omega(\cdot)$ (a function on the set of integers), and one can investigate the behavior of this *sample path* for typical values of ω; this corresponds to the case of almost sure convergence provided that the sequence converges except on a set of ω having probability 0.

The two behaviors can be very different. If, for example, the sequence represents an aperiodic finite **Markov chain**, then the distribution of X_n converges to the stationary distribution of the chain, but the sample paths $\omega(\cdot)$ cycle endlessly among the finite states of the chain; thus, in one sense, the chain exhibits ordered behavior over time, but in another it remains chaotic. (This phenomenon was first pointed out by Paul Ehrenfest, who introduced his celebrated urn model to illustrate that the Zermelo *recurrence paradox* does not contradict Boltzmann's demonstration that in statistical mechanics the entropy of a system, properly understood, is an increasing function of time. One can, in fact, prove some limit theorems in probability by first showing that an associated entropy function for a sequence of random variables increases with time.)

Thus, the law of large numbers has two versions, weak and strong, corresponding to convergence in probability and almost sure convergence. Just as the central limit theorem can be regarded as a refinement of the weak law of large numbers, the *law of the iterated logarithm* may be regarded as a refinement of the strong law of large numbers (almost sure convergence of the sequence of sample means to the population mean). This result (due in increasing generality to Khinchin, Kolmogorov, and Hartmann–Wintner), one of the three pearls of the classical limit theorems, states that the sample path behavior for a sum of independent and identically distributed random variables, properly normalized, is at once both simple and unexpected: if $X_1, X_2, X_3, \ldots$ are independent and identically distributed random variables, such that $E[X_k] = 0$, $\text{var}[X_k] = 1$ and $S_n = X_1 + \cdots + X_n$, then

$$\Pr\left[\lim_{n \to \infty} \sup \frac{S_n}{(2n \log \log n)^{1/2}} = 1\right] = 1.$$

(It is simple to deduce from this that the set of limit points for the normalized sequence is almost surely the closed interval $[-1, 1]$.) Other such "zero–one" laws include the celebrated Borel–Cantelli lemmas used to prove the strong law.

This classical theory was subsequently extended to the study of sums and triangular arrays of sequences of random variables not having two **moments**, and using forms of normalization other than the mean and standard deviation. The stable and infinitely divisible distributions then arise as possible limiting distributions; the entire edifice is summarized in spare and elegant fashion in the classic and beautiful book of Gnedenko & Kolmogorov [8]. Lamperti [9] provides an attractive and accessible account of many of the key features of this classical theory.

Other generalizations of the classical theorems include the Birkhoff *ergodic theorem* and the *martingale convergence theorem*. The ergodic theorem (a direct descendant of Ehrenfest's attempts to explain and justify Boltzmann's theories) extended convergence of sample means from the domain of independence to that of stationary sequences (sequences invariant under shift); the martingale convergence theorem extracts a key property of centered sums (that one's expected future gain in a sequence of fair games is the same as one's present fortune) to derive other limiting forms of behavior. In the hands of Doob [6] and his successors, the martingale concept and its use became a fundamental and pervasive aspect of modern probability theory.

Two important modern advances in limit theorems after this classical period were the concepts of invariance principles and functional limit theorems. *Invariance principles* establish that if one sequence in a class of possible sequences converges to a limit, then all sequences in that class must converge to the same limit. Thus, one proof of the central limit theorem demonstrates that if the normalized sum of a sequence of independent and identically distributed random variables having a second moment (such as Bernoulli

trials) converges to the standard normal distribution, then all sequences in this class must also converge to this limit (see [4]). *Functional central limit theorems* generalize the central limit theorem by considering functionals of sample paths (such as the maximum) and determining their limiting distribution by computing the distribution of that functional applied to the limiting distribution of sample paths: **Brownian motion**. The abstraction of these two theories led to the creation of the subject of *weak convergence* (see [2]).

There is a simple hierarchy that applies to the most common modes of convergence for a sequence of random variables: convergence almost surely $\Rightarrow$ convergence in probability $\Rightarrow$ convergence in distribution. These implications admit of limited reversal: if a sequence of random variables converges in probability, then every subsequence contains a further subsequence converging almost surely; if a sequence of random variables converges in distribution, then one can find a sequence of random variables having the same one-dimensional distributions that converges almost surely (*Skorokhod's theorem*).

This last result is related to a distinctively modern element in the proof of limit theorems: the use of *coupling methods* to construct versions of the random elements in question that live on the same probability space. Due originally to the gifted French probabilist Doeblin (who died tragically at the beginning of the Second World War), the method only gained currency decades later. Its use provides perhaps the most elegant derivation of the limiting behavior for countable Markov chains (see, for example, [3]).

The increasing use of the **bootstrap** [7], **Markov chain Monte Carlo**, simulated annealing, and other **computer-intensive methods** only recently possible, points to an emerging post-modern period of limit theorems in mathematical probability, the outlines of which are only just beginning to be clear. For a number of interesting applications of modern limit theorems to the biological sciences, see Waterman [10]. Such applications include methods as diverse as the Aldous [1] Poisson clumping heuristic, the Erdös–Renyi law of large numbers, and the theory of large deviations.

References

[1]   Aldous, D. (1989). *Poisson Approximations via the Poisson Clumping Heuristic*. Springer-Verlag, New York.

[2]   Billingsley, P. (1968). *Convergence of Probability Measures*. Wiley, New York.

[3]   Billingsley, P. (1995). *Probability and Measure*. Wiley, New York.

[4]   Breiman, L. (1968). *Probability*. Addison-Wesley, Reading.

[5]   De Moivre, A. (1738). *The Doctrine of Chances*, 3rd Ed., 1756. Reprinted Chelsea, New York, 1967.

[6]   Doob, J.L. (1953). *Stochastic Processes*. Wiley, New York.

[7]   Efron, B. & Tibshirani, R. (1993). *An Introduction to the Bootstrap*. Chapman & Hall, New York.

[8]   Gnedenko, B.V. & Kolmogorov, A.N. (1949). *Limit Distributions for Sums of Independent Random Variables*, 2nd English Ed.; translated, annotated, and revised by K.L. Chung. Addison-Wesley, Reading, 1968.

[9]   Lamperti, J. (1996). *Probability*, 2nd Ed. Wiley, New York.

[10] Waterman, M.S. (1995). *Introduction to Computational Biology: Maps, Sequences, and Genomes*. Chapman & Hall, New York.

(*See also* **Large-Sample Theory**)

S.L. ZABELL

Limits of Agreement *see* Observer Reliability and Agreement

Linder, Forrest E.

Born: November 21, 1906, in Waltham, Massachusetts.

Died: August 18, 1988, in Washington, DC.

Forrest E. Linder devoted a lifetime of service to the worldwide development of vital and health statistics (*see* **Vital Statistics, Overview**). Although born in Massachusetts, he grew up in Iowa where, at Iowa State University, he received a doctorate in mathematics and statistics. Following a brief assignment with a foundation in Massachusetts, he moved to Washington, DC, in 1935, where he served until 1944 as a statistician with the US Bureau of the Census. In 1939 he spent a year in Montevideo assisting the Uruguayan government in establishing a vital statistics system. This was the beginning of Linder's interest in international vital statistics. He subsequently established an international vital statistics program at the Bureau of the Census, which provided training in civil registration and vital statistics to foreign national officials as well as an on-site consulting program for Latin American countries.

During World War II he served as Assistant Chief of the Medical Statistics Division of the US Navy, where he was responsible for establishing a morbidity reporting system, including the necessary data-processing support to provide current estimates of morbidity and mortality for the personnel of a greatly expanded wartime navy. After the war, Linder joined the United Nations where he became the first Chief of the Demographic and Social Statistics Branch of the UN Statistical Office. There, his contributions to the improvement of the **demographic** statistics of developing countries included projects he conceived and inspired, such as the world **censuses** of population and housing of 1950 and 1960 and a series of regional seminars on vital and health statistics. He was instrumental in designing and producing the first *United Nations Demographic Yearbook, Principles for a Vital Statistics System*, and the *Handbook of Vital Statistics Methods*.

In 1957, Linder returned to the federal civil service in Washington, DC, to become the director of the newly established National Health Survey, a program of the US Public Health Service. When the National Office of Vital Statistics was merged with the National Health Survey in 1960 to form the **National Center for Health Statistics (NCHS)**, Linder was named as its first director, a post he held until his retirement in 1967.

Upon leaving the Public Health Service, he joined the faculty at the University of North Carolina where he was both professor of biostatistics and the first director of the International Program of Laboratories for Population Statistics, popularly known as POPLAB [3]. While at POPLAB, he began to lay the groundwork for an international organization that would address the professional interests and needs of national officials responsible for civil registration. Recognizing that these officials were a diverse group, often working in isolation and without an international focus for information exchange and guidance, he founded the International Institute for Vital Registration in 1974, an organization to encourage and promote the improvement of civil registration throughout the world with special attention to lesser developed countries. When he retired from the university he served as President and Executive Director of the Institute until his death in 1988.

During a career that spanned half a century, Forrest Linder had an impressive list of important technical publications; these covered a wide range of topics in demography and health, such as fertility measurement, morbidity and mortality analysis, and survey methodology applied to public health (*see* **Surveys, Health and Morbidity; Sample Surveys**) [1, 2, 4–7]. He served on international and national advisory committees, such as the World Fertility Survey Steering Committee, US Agency for International Development Research Advisory Committee, **World Health Organization** Expert Committees on Health Statistics, and the US National Committee on Vital and Health Statistics; and he received the Distinguished Service Award from the US Department of Health, Education and Welfare and the Bronfman Prize from the **American Public Health Association**.

In each of his professional endeavors Forrest Linder exhibited a strong pioneering spirit at the highest technical level. Throughout his career he continued his abiding interest in the improvement of national and international vital and health statistics and he had an unfailing belief in the importance of his undertakings. His work has had a positive influence not only on civil registration and vital statistics programs throughout the world, but also on the many statisticians, demographers and others with whom he came in contact.

References

[1]   Linder, F.E. (1965). National health interview surveys, in *Trends in the Study of Morbidity and Mortality*, Public Health Papers, No. 27. World Health Organization, Geneva.

[2]   Linder, F.E. (1967). Sources of data on health in the United States, in *Preventive Medicine*, D. Clark & B. MacMahon, eds. Little, Brown & Company, Boston, pp. 55–56.

[3]   Linder, F.E. (1971). *The Concept and the Program of the Laboratories for Population Statistics*, International Program of Laboratories for Population Statistics, Scientific Series No. 1. University of North Carolina, Chapel Hill.

[4]   Linder, F.E. (1971). Fertility and family planning in relation to public health, *Milbank Memorial Fund Quarterly*, Vol. XLIX, No. 4, Part 2, New York.

[5]   Linder, F.E. (1974). The dual-record system of collecting demographic data, *United Nations Publication ST/ECLA/Conf. 47/L.3*. United Nations, New York.

[6]   Linder, F.E. & Grove, R. (1965). Techniques of Vital Statistics, Reprint of Chapters I–IV, *Vital Statistics Rates in the United States, 1900–1940*. National Center for Health Statistics, Washington.

[7]   Linder, F.E. & Lingner, J.W. (1975). *Systems of Demographic Measurement: General Evaluation – The Measurement Problem*, International Program of Laboratories for Population Statistics, Scientific Series No. 22. University of North Carolina, Chapel Hill.

ROBERT A. ISRAEL

Lindley's Paradox

A sharp **null hypothesis** may be strongly rejected by a standard sampling theory test of significance (*see* **Hypothesis Testing**) and yet be awarded high odds by a **Bayesian** analysis based on a small **prior probability** for the null hypothesis and a diffuse distribution of one's remaining probability over the **alternative hypothesis**. This disagreement between sampling theory and Bayesian methods was first studied by Jeffreys [2], and it was first called a paradox by Lindley [3].

The paradox can be exhibited in the simple case where we are testing $\theta = 0$ using a single observation Y from a **normal distribution** with variance one and mean θ. If we observe a large value y for Y ($y = 3$, for example), then standard sampling theory allows us to reject confidently the null hypothesis. But the Bayesian approach advocated by Jeffreys can give quite a different result. Jeffreys advised that we assign a nonzero prior probability π_0 to the null hypothesis and distribute the rest of our probability over the real line according to a fairly flat probability density, $\pi_1(\theta)$. If the range of possible values for θ is very wide, then the set of values within a few units of y will be very unlikely under $\pi_1(\theta)$, and consequently the overall **likelihood** of the alternative hypothesis,

$$L_1 = \int_{-\infty}^{\infty} \frac{1}{(2\pi)^{1/2}} \exp\left[-\frac{1}{2}(y - \theta)^2\right] \pi_1(\theta)\mathrm{d}\theta,$$

will be very small. It may even be so much smaller than the likelihood of the null hypothesis,

$$L_0 = \frac{1}{(2\pi)^{1/2}} \exp(-y^2/2),$$

that the odds in favor of the null hypothesis,

$$\frac{\Pr(\theta = 0 | Y = y)}{\Pr(\theta \neq 0 | Y = y)} = \frac{\pi_0}{1 - \pi_0} \frac{L_0}{L_1}, \qquad (1)$$

are substantial.

We can think of (1) as a way of balancing arguments for and against the null hypothesis. *Against* the null hypothesis is its small initial probability (small π_0) and the unlikeliness of the observation under the null hypothesis (small L_0). *For* the null hypothesis is the unlikeliness of alternative values of θ near y [small $\pi_1(\theta)$, leading to small L_1]. There is no strong constraint between the arguments for and against. No matter how small π_0 and L_0 are, a sufficiently diffuse $\pi_1(\theta)$ can make L_1 small enough to counterbalance them.

If we are confident of the specified prior distribution – if, for example, we are working with a series of problems involving θs that are zero about π_0 of the time and distributed roughly according to $\pi_1(\theta)$ the rest of the time – then the Bayesian analysis is unassailable, and hence we must reject the standard sampling theory. An observation three standard deviations from the null hypothesis is not adequate to reject the null hypothesis if that observation is even more unlikely under the alternative hypothesis. This has led many authors to suggest that we make tests increasingly stringent as measurements become more precise relative to the range of possible values for what is being measured. We should, for example, lower the significance level (*see* **Level of a Test**) as the sample size grows. More sophisticated suggestions are made by Berger & Delampady [1].

However, if diffuseness of $\pi_1(\theta)$ reflects merely a wide uncertainty about θ rather than a positive prior confidence that values of θ near y are likely to occur, then the conflict seems to constitute a criticism of the Bayesian analysis. If we have no idea how θ arises, then our mere ignorance cannot justify a skepticism about values close to y so strong as to outweigh real evidence against the value of zero. This has motivated non-Bayesian approaches discussed by Shafer [4].

References

[1]   Berger, J. & Delampady, M. (1987). Testing precise hypotheses (with discussion), *Statistical Science* **2**, 317–352.

[2]   Jeffreys, H. (1939). *Theory of Probability*. Oxford University Press, Oxford.

[3]   Lindley, D.V. (1957). A statistical paradox, *Biometrika* **44**, 187–192.

[4]   Shafer, G. (1982). Lindley's paradox (with discussion), *Journal of the American Statistical Association* **77**, 325–351.

GLENN SHAFER

Linear Discriminant Function *see* Discriminant Analysis, Linear

Linear Filter *see* ARMA and ARIMA Models

Linear Modeling *see* General Linear Model

Linear Predictor *see* Generalized Linear Model

Linear Programming

Linear programming (LP) is a decision model (*see* **Decision Theory**) that was developed early in the history of **operations research** and has wide applicability. It is a technique for finding optimal solutions, i.e. solutions to a decision problem that optimize some objective (maximize profit, minimize cost, etc.) subject to a set of constraints. In health care, LP has been applied both to management decision making and to decisions regarding clinical care. A few examples of LP are: (i) to improve breast cancer diagnosis on the basis of cell characteristics from a fine needle biopsy and to model the likelihood of recurrence in surgically treated patients [10]; (ii) to optimize scheduling nurses to meet coverage needs at the lowest cost [7]; (iii) to develop a model of costs and revenues based on patient diagnostic groups for strategic planning at a major university medical center [1]; (iv) to identify underutilized resources and inefficient production of services at the Department of Veterans Affairs medical centers [14]; (v) to develop a severity index for emergency medicine patients with cardiac problems [11]; (vi) to determine a treatment plan for radiation therapy that optimizes tumor exposure while reducing the exposure of healthy tissue [12]; and (vii) to compare alternative methods to develop a state rate-setting formula for nursing homes [2]. Greenberg [3–6] provides a tutorial with an overview of LP methodology and applications, while Hillier & Lieberman [8] is an excellent basic reference.

Although LP is the decision model most widely used by corporations, health care applications have been limited in the past by inaccessible software, unavailable data and low demand. Charge based fee-for-service clinical practice and cost-plus reimbursement for hospitals coupled with less competition in the past produced a low perceived need to optimize. The growth of managed care with its emphasis on global budgets and capitation for the care of populations is changing this situation; consequently, LP is likely to become more important in health care management and in **health services research** (*see* **Health Services Organization in the US**).

Model

An LP model has three main components: (i) a set of *decision variables* which represent quantities over which management has control; (ii) an *objective function*, defined on the decision variables, representing the quantity that the decision maker wishes to optimize; and (iii) a set of *constraints* representing the limitations imposed on the decision choices. The word *linear* refers to the form of the functions of the decision variables appearing in the objective function and in the constraints. The form of these functions is a summation of terms, each term being a single decision variable multiplied by a coefficient. Thus, linear programming, strictly defined, does not permit forms that have variables raised to powers or multiplied by other variables. There are techniques for nonlinear programming, but they involve different algorithms. The term *programming* refers to the iterative nature of solution techniques, not to computer programming.

Solving an LP problem involves finding a set of values to assign to the decision variables that will maximize (or minimize) the objective function

without violating any of the constraints. Constraints may reflect limitations on resources, policy requirements, proportional relationships that must be maintained, or other requirements of the situation. There are three types of functional constraints: requirements – "greater than or equal to", limitations – "less than or equal to", and strict equality. Sign constraints are requirements that a variable be nonnegative.

There are three stages in LP analysis: formulation, solution, and interpretation. Formulation involves expressing the decision problem as an LP model in *standard form*. In standard form the constraints have the variables on the left-hand side of the operator and a constant on the right-side (known as RHS or right-hand-side quantities). Next, the "optimal solution" is found and its general properties are determined, including sensitivity to parameter variations (*see* **Sensitivity Analysis**) and shadow prices for all constraints. Then, interpretation involves translating the numbers produced by the solution technique into their meaning in the context of the decision to be made.

Solution Techniques

Once an LP model has been formulated, a solution is sought. Some LP models do not have solutions. Actually, with any LP model exactly one of the following will be the case: (i) it will have at least one optimal solution; (ii) it will be infeasible; or (iii) it will be unbounded. An *infeasible model* is one in which there is no solution that satisfies all of the constraints. An *unbounded model* is one in which the objective function can move infinitely far in the desired direction. In the latter case, it is likely that the model was formulated incorrectly, or does not represent a real-life situation. There are three widely known *techniques for solving* LP problems: the Graphical Solution Technique, the **Simplex** Method, and the Interior Point Method (also known as "Karmarkar's Algorithm").

Graphical Solution Technique

This technique is generally used only for problems that contain two variables; its value is more as a teaching tool than as a practical problem-solving technique. Coordinate axes represent the decision variables and constraints are plotted, often resulting in an enclosed area; assuming that a feasible solution does exist, the set of all feasible solutions in this enclosed area is called the *feasible region* (Figure 1). Each corner of this enclosed area is known as a *corner-point feasible* (CPF) solution; the importance of CPF solutions is that the optimal value of the objective function will come from this set. The objective function is then set to an arbitrary constant, yielding an equation which is plotted as a line (called a contour line or isoquant). Another arbitrary constant is then used to generate a parallel line with the same slope and in the direction of improving the objective function. The last CPF solution to intersect an isoquant line as it leaves the feasible region in the direction of optimization is the optimal solution. The optimal solution(s) will become apparent from this analysis. If there is an optimal solution, then there will be at least one corner point optimal solution; if two corner points are optimal, then all of the points in between them are also optimal.

If constraints do not stop the contour lines from moving infinitely far in the desired direction, then the problem is *unbounded*. An unbounded problem has failed to include or appropriately value at least one relevant constraint.

If there is no simultaneous optimal solution to all of the constraints in the problem as formulated, then the model may be infeasible, also known as *inconsistent*, or misspecified. Infeasible LP problems result from the constraint equations, not the objective function, and they should be reviewed if the model is infeasible. In practice, constructing large LP models may involve constraint inputs from many different individuals or teams, so initial infeasibility of a model is not uncommon.

As mentioned above, this technique is applied to two variable problems. LP models with only one decision variable are not of practical significance. With three decision variables, the feasible region would typically be a three-dimensional figure with flat surfaces, and the objective function would be represented by contour planes finding the best corners of this figure. With more than three variables, visual representation becomes impracticable.

Example

A simplified problem that could be solved by the graphical technique is the decision for assigning the mix of appointment slots for two types of patients in a fee-for-service Nurse Practitioner clinic to produce the optimal amount of revenue. Assume that the revenue from a hypertensive patient visit (H) is \$10 and for a patient with diabetes (D) \$18, that Nurse Practitioners (NP) see the former on average for six minutes and the latter for 15 minutes while Nursing Assistants (NA) are with both types of patients for 18 minutes, and that total available Nurse Practitioner hours equals 7000 while those for Nursing Assistants equals 14 000. The objective function is then $10H + 18D$, the first constraint is $0.1H + 0.25D \leq 7000$, and the second constraint is $0.3H + 0.3D \leq 14\,000$. The optimal solution is to schedule 31 111 hypertension patients and 15 555 diabetes patients.

The Simplex Method

George Dantzig developed the Simplex Method in the 1940s and it has proven to be both robust and versatile. This method produces successive outputs, known as tableaus, as part of its iterative search for an optimal solution. To establish an initial tableau, remove inequalities and satisfy the nonnegativity constraints of the model, additional variables are introduced: *slack* variables for constraint equations ("≤") and *surplus* variables for requirements ("≥"). In the optimal solution to the LP, slack or surplus variables will be zero for active constraints and positive for inactive constraints.

The standard equation constraint form of the LP in matrix notation is then

$$\text{optimize } Z = c\mathbf{x}$$

$$\text{subject to } A\mathbf{x} + \mathbf{s} = \mathbf{b}$$

$$\mathbf{x}, \mathbf{s} \geq 0.$$

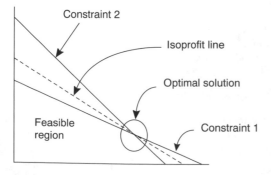

Figure 1 Graphical method for solving linear programming problems

Continuing with the graphical analogy, the Simplex Method first identifies a corner point; if there is none, then the problem is said to be *inconsistent*, or infeasible. Once a corner point is identified, then the **algorithm** moves from corner point to adjacent corner point of the feasible region, with each successive iteration produced by the Gaussian elimination equaling or improving the value of the objective function. The algorithm terminates when an optimal CPF solution is identified; the resulting basic feasible solution consists of the nonnegative variables in the set.

Example

In an article on hospital financial planning [1] linear programming is used at a leading academic medical center to evaluate the resource and revenue implications of changes in patient acuity level and primary insurer. The goal in this formulation is to maximize net revenue after variable expenses:

$$\max \sum_j (r_j - vc_j)^* x_j,$$

where r_j = total revenue from patient type j, vc_j = total variable cost from patient type j, and x_j = number of patients of type j. Here, the decision variables can be optimized for a given situation or varied to explore the financial impact under differing scenarios, for example, in contract negotiations, in considering major capital renovations, or in considering a shift in patient mix based on marketing emphases or regulations. Examples of constraints in this model include the number of beds in each clinical service, ancillary services, requirements that the institution meet at least minimum levels of demand for admission by populations it has traditionally served, and limits on patient demand by various groups – based on the output from a separate forecasting study.

For an LP (the *primal*) there also exists an alternate formulation of the problem, called the *dual*, in which the number of decision variables in the primal equals the number of constraints in the dual and the number of constraints in the primal equals the number of decision variables in the dual. Optimization of the primal also results in optimization of the dual; however, if the primal is a maximization model, then the dual will be a minimization model and vice versa. When the optimal solution contains fewer positive variables than constraints, it is said to be *degenerate*.

One result of degeneracy is that there is restricted ability to do postoptimality analyses.

Most problems of practical significance are too large to be solved manually, so specialized software has been written to perform this function. The time to solve an LP is essentially determined by the number of constraints in the problem rather than the number of decision variables; therefore, using the relationship between the primal and dual specifications, solving the formulation with the smaller number of constraints will be faster. Although computing speed and power continue to increase, this is a useful observation since the sizes of the problems to be solved are also increasing.

Beyond computational efficiency there is economic information contained in the correspondence between the primal and dual. Much of the value of an LP solution comes from post-optimality, or sensitivity, analysis. The typical computer output for an optimized LP model will contain values for the objective function, for basic structural variables (those having nonzero values), shadow prices for the constraints and change vectors for Right-Hand-Side and objective ranging or sensitivity analyses. These *change vectors* report how much the basic variables change when the Right-Hand-Side constraints are increased or decreased; *shadow prices* show how much the value of the objective function will change as the values of the RHS change. Taken together, these results answer the questions of how much of which resources should be purchased, if any, and at what price.

The range of values over which these sensitivity analyses are valid is restricted: information on the lower and upper bounds of these ranges for each variable will be included in the printout under sensitivity analysis. If the quantities being considered in the sensitivity analyses lie outside these ranges, then the model must be rerun with different inputs since the original optimal solution would no longer be valid. Finally, sensitivity results are only correct when the values reported lie within the upper and lower bounds, and only when one variable is changed at a time. If the analyst is interested in simultaneous changes to more than one variable, again the model must be rerun with these changes in the input.

Interior Point Method

An alternative to the Simplex Method was reported by Narendra Karmarkar in 1984. Karmarkar's approach and similar barrier algorithms are based on progressing along successive points interior to the feasible region toward an optimal solution. Since the algorithm does not move from corner to corner as the Simplex does, it is potentially much faster for very large problems and may be the only option for extremely large problems. Research continues on interior point algorithms for LP; however, they are currently inferior to the Simplex Method in supporting sensitivity analysis [8, 9].

Software

Few problems of practical significance can be solved manually; fortunately, developments in hardware and software have moved the ability to solve large linear programming problems to the desktop. Depending on the operating system, size of the problem, price, data input source(s), and other features desired, many options exist to support a knowledgeable user; however, online support for a novice is infrequently provided [15].

Perhaps the most immediately useful of the LP software to a broad audience are the **spreadsheet** packages that include optimization routines or have transparent "add-ins" for this function. These functions, coupled with stored models and report writer capability, allow users easy import of data into widely used applications packages to produce outputs clearly on the basis of an array of scenarios or assumptions. Some commercial packages, e.g. SAS OR [13] (*see* **Software, Biostatistical**) employ enhancements that allow the user greater flexibility of features than the Simplex Method alone would permit.

Quantitative management courses, such as those typically taught in masters programs in business or health administration, increasingly rely on spreadsheet applications to teach these methods – increasing the likelihood that the techniques may be applied more often than in the past.

Internet

Typical LP resources on the **internet** include web sites for professional associations, university courses on LP, computer routines that permit LP problems to be solved over the internet, and other areas of specialization. Although the internet is dynamic, a useful overview of resources and potential uses is provided by Sodhi [16].

Summary

Until recent advances in data availability, hardware, software, and trained users, the tradeoff between the time and cost of modeling, obtaining the data, and the likely payoff for what might be one-time efforts, discouraged widespread use of LP in health care. As the expectations for efficient, quality health care increase and integrated financing and delivery systems look for ways to address simultaneously demands for lower cost and higher quality, the opportunities for the application of LP should increase.

References

[1] Brandeau, M.L. & Hopkins, D.S.P. (1984). A patient mix model for hospital financial planning, *Inquiry* **21**, 32–44.

[2] Diehr, G. & Tamura, H. (1989). Linear programming models for cost reimbursement, *Health Services Research* **24**, 329–347.

[3] Greenberg, H.J. (1993). How to analyze the results of linear programs – part 1: preliminaries, *Interfaces* **23**, 56–67.

[4] Greenberg, H.J. (1993). How to analyze the results of linear programs – part 2: price interpretation, *Interfaces* **23**, 97–114.

[5] Greenberg, H.J. (1993). How to analyze the results of linear programs – part 3: infeasibility diagnosis, *Interfaces* **23**, 120–139.

[6] Greenberg, H.J. (1993). How to analyze the results of linear programs – part 4: forcing substructures, *Interfaces* **24**, 121–130.

[7] Harmeier, P.E. (1991) Linear programming for optimization of nurse scheduling, *Computers in Nursing* **9**, 149–151.

[8] Hillier, F.S. & Lieberman, G.J. (1995). *Introduction to Operations Research*, 6th Ed. McGraw-Hill, New York.

[9] Hooker, J.N. (1986). Karmarkar's linear programming algorithm, *Interfaces* **13**, 75–90.

[10] Mangasarian, O.L., Street, W.N. & Wolberg, W.H. (1995). Breast cancer diagnosis via linear programming, *Operations Research* **43**, 570–577.

[11] Nagurney, F. (1992). A regression-like approach to developing a severity index for EMS patients, *Computers in Biology and Medicine* **22**, 123–133.

[12] Rosen, I.I., Lane, R.G., Morrill, S.M. & Belli, J.A. (1991). Treatment plan optimization using linear programming, *Medical Physics* **18**, 141–152.

[13] SAS Institute Inc. (1989). *SAS/OR® User's Guide, Version 6*, 1st Ed. SAS Institute Inc., Cary.

[14] Sexton, T.R., Leiken, A.M., Nolan, A.H., Liss, S., Hogan, A. & Silkman, R.H. (1989). Evaluating managerial efficiency of Veterans Administration medical centers

using data envelopment analysis, *Medical Care* **27**, 1175–1188.

[15]   Sharda, R. (1995). Linear programming solver software for personal computers: 1995 report, *OR/MS Today* **22**, 49–57.

[16]   Sodhi, M.S. (1995). An OR/MS guide to the internet, *Interfaces* **25**, 14–29.

ALAN LYLES

Linear Rank Statistic *see* Ranks

Linear Rank Tests in Survival Analysis

Linear rank tests for survival data are generalized **nonparametric methods** for testing the null hypothesis of equal **survival distributions** among groups.

A number of approaches to generalizing rank tests to censored data have appeared in the literature – approaches which are often quite different from one another. The earliest statistic to reach widespread use was that of Gehan [13], who generalized the **Wilcoxon–Mann–Whitney** scores for the two-group problem. Mantel [24] used arguments based on the construction of the **Mantel–Haenszel** test for stratified $2 \times K$ contingency tables to propose a test that later became known as the **logrank test**. Efron [8] then proposed a statistic based on combining the values of the estimated survival distributions of two groups across time. In 1970 Breslow [5] provided a generalization of the Kruskal–Wallis statistic that reduced to the Gehan–Wilcoxon statistic in two samples. The work of Peto & Peto [25] made important progress in studying the properties of these and other tests. In 1972, the **proportional hazards** model of Cox [6] (*see* **Cox Regression Model**) provided a setting in which the logrank test could be derived as a **partial likelihood** score test from a regression model. Prentice [26] showed in 1978 that many of these tests were asymptotically equivalent to tests that were natural generalizations of the classical linear rank tests for uncensored data described in Hájek & Šidák [17]. In his seminal doctoral thesis and later published work, Aalen [1, 2] showed that the theory

of **counting processes** and martingales could be used to recast two-sample tests with right-censored data in the multiplicative intensity model and to study their asymptotic theory. Gill [14] extended this work to a complete study of the operating characteristics of two-sample tests with censored data, and Andersen et al. [3] illustrated the use of this methodology for tests used to compare more than two groups. Remarkably, all these approaches point to essentially the same tests.

Censored data rank tests are most well-developed for right-censored failure time data. Data are right-censored if, for each subject in a study, the underlying data consist of the time, T, to some event and a censoring time, U, while the observable data are $X = \min(T, U)$ and $\delta = I(T \leq U)$, where $I(A)$ is the usual indicator random variable of the event A. The variable T is commonly called a failure time or a survival time. The underlying survival function, $\Pr(T > t)$, is usually denoted by $S(t)$, the cumulative hazard, $-\log S(t)$, by $\Lambda(t)$ for continuous T, and the hazard function for absolutely continuous T by $\lambda(t)$ (*see* **Survival Distributions and Their Characteristics**). If S has discontinuities or is otherwise not differentiable, the cumulative hazard function is given more generally by $\Lambda(t) = -\int_0^t [S(u-)]^{-1} dS(u)$. We let $\pi(t) = \Pr(X \geq t)$, the probability that a subject is at risk at time t.

Linear rank tests are most commonly used when making comparisons among K groups, $K \geq 2$, or when comparing a single group with a known or hypothesized population. For the K-group problem, the observable data consist of the pairs (X_{ij}, δ_{ij}), $1 \leq j \leq n_i, i = 1, \ldots, K$; that is, there are n_i observations in the ith of K groups, with underlying survival distribution $S_i(t)$ and probability $\pi_i(t)$ of being at risk. The validity of all the tests discussed below depends centrally on the assumption that the observed failure rate among cases at risk of failure is the same rate that would be observed if censoring were not present. This is satisfied if T_{ij} and U_{ij} are independent random variables for all pairs i, j, and we assume this condition throughout.

We use the counting process setting here. That methodology is not only the most recent and the most successful in studying the asymptotic theory of these tests, but it also provides a surprisingly useful framework for a less formal exploration of their properties. The theory for these tests is best understood for the two-sample problem, and, since the two-group comparison problem is the most prevalent testing problem with censored data, we discuss that case in greater detail.

Gill [15] provides an accessible and intuitive introduction to the martingale approach to survival analysis in the context of the proportional hazards model.

The Counting Process Approach

Counting process methods are now widely used for survival data, and these methods have a particularly simple form when used to study rank tests. Generally, a **stochastic process** $N = [N(t) : t \geq 0]$ is a counting process if $N(0) = 0$ and it has increasing, right-continuous step functions for paths, with jumps of size 1 at each discontinuity. The process

$$N_{ij} = [N_{ij}(t) = I(X_{ij} \leq t, \delta_{ij} = 1); t \geq 0]$$

has simple right-continuous step functions for paths, beginning at 0 at $t = 0$ and taking a single jump to 1 at time t if and only if $T_{ij} = t$ and $T_{ij} \leq U_{ij}$. The information in the pair (X_{ij}, δ_{ij}) is equivalent to that in the complete path of N_{ij} as well as in the path of the process $N_{ij}^{U}(t) = I(X_{ij} \leq t, \delta_{ij} = 0)$. Formally, the information up to time t in the pair N_{ij}, N_{ij}^{U} is represented as the σ-algebra $\mathcal{F}_t^{ij}$ generated by the set of variables $[N_{ij}(u), N_{ij}^{U}(u); 0 \leq u \leq t]$. The **information** in all K groups up to time t is the product σ-algebra $\mathcal{F}_t = \otimes_{ij} \mathcal{F}_t^{ij}$. Since that information increases with time, the collection of σ-algebras $\mathcal{F} = (\mathcal{F}_t; t \geq 0)$ forms a filtration, i.e. an increasing sequence (in t) of σ-algebras.

The counting process approach uses the stochastic calculus of martingales in its representation of test statistics and the martingale **central limit theorems** [29] for the asymptotic theory (*see* **Large-Sample Theory**). A process $M = [M(t); t \leq 0]$ is a martingale with respect to a filtration $(\mathcal{G}_t; t \geq 0)$ if

1. $M(t)$ is adapted to $\mathcal{G}_t$ for each t
2. $E|M(t)| < \infty$ for all $t < \infty$, and
3. $E[M(t + s)|\mathcal{G}_t] = M(t)$ a.s. for all $s \geq 0, t \geq 0$.

Condition 3 implies that $E[M(t) - M(u)|\mathcal{G}_u] = 0$ for all $u \leq t$, and this is sometimes written informally as $E[dM(t)|\mathcal{G}_{t-}] = 0$. A process M is called a submartingale if the equation for the conditional

expectation in condition 3 above is replaced by the inequality $E[M(t + s)|\mathcal{G}_t] \geq M(t)$. Because the martingale property depends on the underlying filtration, we sometimes say that M is a $\mathcal{G}_t$-martingale. The martingale definition implies that a linear combination of processes which are martingales with respect to a common filtration $\mathcal{G}$ will itself be a $\mathcal{G}_t$-martingale.

It is possible to show that, when T_{ij} and U_{ij} are independent for all pairs i, j, the process

$$M_{ij}(t) = N_{ij}(t) - \int_0^t Y_{ij}(u) d\Lambda_i(u) \qquad (1)$$

is a martingale with respect to the filtration $\mathcal{F}$ defined above, where $Y_{ij}(u) = I(X_{ij} \geq u)$ is the process denoting whether or not subject i, j has failed or been censored before time t (cf. Theorems 1.3.1 and 1.3.2 in Fleming & Harrington [10]). The integral on the right-hand side of (1) is called the compensator for the process N_{ij}. For simplicity of notation we usually write (1), and others like it, as

$$M_{ij} = N_{ij} - \int Y_{ij} d\Lambda_i.$$

It is not surprising that M_{ij} is an $\mathcal{F}_t$-martingale. Conditional on the history of the failure and censoring processes before time t, the conditional probability of a jump in N_{ij} at t is approximately $Y_{ij}(t) d\Lambda_i(t)$, so that $E(dN_{ij} - Y_{ij} d\Lambda_i|\mathcal{F}_{t-}) = 0$. This result is an example of the more general Doob–Meyer decomposition for submartingales (cf. [9]), which states that for any submartingale Z (subject to boundedness conditions) there exists a predictable process A, called the compensator for Z, such that $Z - A$ is a martingale.

Nearly all commonly used linear rank statistics for survival data can, under H_0, be represented, or at least approximately so, as $\sum_{ij} \int H_{ij} dM_{ij}$, or as sums of stochastic integrals of "predictable" processes with respect to the fundamental martingale processes. This construction allows the use of the stochastic calculus for martingales outlined below. More detail may be found in Fleming & Harrington [10] and Andersen et al. [4]. To keep the technical material to a minimum, we have not given the most general versions of these results.

There are several definitions of a predictable process; the following is one of the more accessible.

Definition.   A stochastic process $H = [H(t); t \geq 0]$ defined on a probability space $(\Omega, \mathcal{A}, P)$ is predictable with respect to a filtration $\mathcal{F} = (\mathcal{F}_t; t \geq 0)$ on that space if H is measurable with respect to the smallest σ-algebra on $[0, \infty) \times \Omega$ generated by the adapted left-continuous processes.

This definition implies that any left-continuous $\mathcal{F}_t$-adapted process will be $\mathcal{F}_t$-predictable; operationally, that is how predictability is checked.

Slightly more general versions of the following theorems appear in Fleming & Harrington [10, cf. Theorem 2.4.1].

Theorem 1. Suppose H is a bounded, $\mathcal{F}_t$-predictable process and M an $\mathcal{F}_t$-martingale with $M(0+) - M(0) = 0$. Then the process

$$\int H \, \mathrm{d}M = \left[\int_0^t H(u) \mathrm{d}M(u); t \geq 0 \right]$$

is an $\mathcal{F}_t$-martingale.

Theorem 2. Suppose M_1 and M_2 are square integrable $\mathcal{F}_t$-martingales (i.e. $\sup_{t \geq 0} \mathrm{E}M_i^2(t) < \infty$, $i = 1, 2$). Then there exists a unique $\mathcal{F}_t$-predictable process $\langle M_1, M_2 \rangle$ such that $M_1 M_2 - \langle M_1, M_2 \rangle$ is an $\mathcal{F}_t$-martingale.

The process $\langle M_1, M_2 \rangle$ is called the predictable covariation process for the martingales M_1 and M_2. When M_1 and M_2 are the same process M, $\langle M, M \rangle$ is called the predictable quadratic variation process, and is often denoted by $\langle M \rangle$. Since martingales have constant expected value, $\mathrm{E}M_1(t)M_2(t) = \mathrm{E}\langle M_1, M_2 \rangle(t)$ whenever $M_1(0)M_2(0) - \langle M_1, M_2 \rangle(0) = 0$. This formula is particularly valuable for computing second **moments** when the quadratic variation process takes a simple form, as it does for the counting process martingales arising in survival analysis.

It is possible to show that

$$\left\langle \int H_1 \mathrm{d}M_1, \int H_2 \mathrm{d}M_2 \right\rangle = \int H_1 H_2 \mathrm{d}\langle M_1, M_2 \rangle$$

(cf. Fleming & Harrington [10, Theorem 2.4.2]).

The following summarizes results on quadratic variation processes for counting process martingales.

Definition. A k-dimensional counting process $(N_1, N_2, \ldots, N_k)$ is called a multivariate counting process

if each component N_j is a counting process and no two component processes jump at the same time.

Theorem 3. Let $(N_1, N_2, \cdots, N_k)$ be a multivariate counting process, and let A_j be the compensator of N_j. Then $\langle M_j, M_j \rangle = \int (1 - \Delta A_j) \mathrm{d}A_j$ and $\langle M_i, M_j \rangle = -\int \Delta A_i \mathrm{d}A_j$ for $i \neq j$.

When a survival distribution is continuous, $\Delta A = 0$, and these formulas are particularly simple. In that case $\langle M_i, M_j \rangle = 0$ and the martingales M_i and M_j are called orthogonal. The more general formula is useful, however, in estimating second moments when there are **ties** in observed failure times, even when the underlying model is continuous, as will be seen below.

Common Linear Rank Tests

Despite its demanding technical foundation, the martingale approach to rank tests is a useful setting for formulating tests. This is most easily seen for two-sample tests. Suppose two groups have survival functions S_1 and S_2 and cumulative hazard functions Λ_1 and Λ_2. Let $\overline{N}_i = \sum_j N_{ij}$, $\overline{Y}_i = \sum_j Y_{ij}$, and $\overline{M}_i = \overline{N}_i - \int \overline{Y}_i \mathrm{d}\Lambda_i$, $i = 1, 2$. The observed number of failures at time t in group 1 is $\mathrm{d}N_1(t)$; with independent censoring and under H$_0$: $\Lambda_1 = \Lambda_2$, the conditionally expected number of failures in group 1 at t, given that a failure has been observed at t, is

$$\overline{Y}_1(t)\{\mathrm{d}[\overline{N}_1(t) + \overline{N}_2(t)]\}/[\overline{Y}_1(t) + \overline{Y}_2(t)].$$

A simple test of H$_0$ can be constructed by comparing

$$\int_0^\infty \mathrm{d}\overline{N}_1 - \overline{Y}_1 \frac{\mathrm{d}(\overline{N}_1 + \overline{N}_2)}{\overline{Y}_1 + \overline{Y}_2} \qquad (2)$$

with 0. This statistic is the numerator of the logrank statistic. Simple algebra shows that under H$_0$ the above expression is equal to

$$\int_0^\infty \frac{\overline{Y}_1 \overline{Y}_2}{\overline{Y}_1 + \overline{Y}_2} \left(\frac{\mathrm{d}\overline{N}_1}{\overline{Y}_1} - \frac{\mathrm{d}\overline{N}_2}{\overline{Y}_2} \right) = \int_0^\infty \frac{\overline{Y}_1 \overline{Y}_2}{\overline{Y}_1 + \overline{Y}_2}$$
$$\times \left[\left(\frac{\mathrm{d}\overline{N}_1}{\overline{Y}_1} - \mathrm{d}\Lambda_1 \right) - \left(\frac{\mathrm{d}\overline{N}_2}{\overline{Y}_2} - \mathrm{d}\Lambda_2 \right) \right]$$
$$= \int_0^\infty \frac{\overline{Y}_2}{\overline{Y}_1 + \overline{Y}_2} \mathrm{d}\overline{M}_1 - \int_0^\infty \frac{\overline{Y}_1}{\overline{Y}_1 + \overline{Y}_2} \mathrm{d}\overline{M}_2$$

$$= \sum_{j=1}^{n_1} \int_0^\infty \frac{\overline{Y}_2}{\overline{Y}_1 + \overline{Y}_2} dM_{1j}$$

$$- \sum_{j=1}^{n_2} \int_0^\infty \frac{\overline{Y}_1}{\overline{Y}_1 + \overline{Y}_2} dM_{2j}. \tag{3}$$

Gill [14] used an expression similar to (3) as a foundation for a generalized class of statistics that includes many previously discussed in the literature.

Definition. Suppose one has two samples of right-censored observations (X_{ij}, δ_{ij}), $1 \le j \le n_i$, $i = 1, 2$, giving rise to the counting and at risk processes $\overline{N}_i, \overline{Y}_i, i = 1, 2$, and let $(\mathcal{F}_t; t \ge 0)$ be the filtration generated by $[N_{ij}(u), Y_{ij}(u); 0 \le u \le t, 1 \le j \le n_i, i = 1, 2]$. Let K be a bounded nonnegative $\mathcal{F}_t$-predictable process satisfying $K(t) = 0$ whenever $\overline{Y}_1(t)\overline{Y}_2(t) = 0$. Then

$$G_K = \int_0^\infty K \left(\frac{d\overline{N}_1}{\overline{Y}_1} - \frac{d\overline{N}_2}{\overline{Y}_2} \right)$$

is called a statistic of the class $\mathcal{K}^+$. When

$$K = \left(\frac{n_1 + n_2}{n_1 n_2} \right)^{1/2} W \left(\frac{\overline{Y}_1 \overline{Y}_2}{\overline{Y}_1 + \overline{Y}_2} \right)$$

$$= \left(\frac{n_1 n_2}{n_1 + n_2} \right)^{1/2} W \frac{\overline{Y}_1}{n_1} \frac{\overline{Y}_2}{n_2} \frac{n_1 + n_2}{\overline{Y}_1 + \overline{Y}_2},$$

the statistic is called a weighted logrank statistic. The fraction $\overline{Y}_1 \overline{Y}_2 / (\overline{Y}_1 + \overline{Y}_2)$ appears in the usual logrank statistic; as will be seen later, the terms involving sample sizes ensure **convergence** under null and alternative hypotheses. The function W reweights the observed minus expected increments in (2). Although weighted logrank statistics are a subset of the statistics of class $\mathcal{K}^+$, they are the most common in applications, and we give those somewhat more attention here. Since the function W is the important part of the weight function in these statistics, we denote weighted logrank statistics by G_W.

The upper limit of integration in the integral representation for statistics of class $\mathcal{K}^+$ occasionally causes confusion. Because the weight function in the two-sample statistic takes value 0 as soon as at least one of the **risk sets** is empty, the integral as written denotes a statistic computed for the portion of the time axis over which there are cases at risk in both groups. Contributions to the statistic stop when all

cases in either one of the groups have failed or have been censored; that is the most natural way for the practitioner to think of these nonparametric statistics. In the asymptotic theory for some of these statistics, the integral may be computed only over a prespecified time interval for which the probability of a subject being at risk at the right end point is bounded away from zero. That is not necessary for most of the statistics discussed here. Finally, the upper limit of integration may be thought of as a variable t when the statistic is considered a process with changing values as time increases. This last perspective is used in the martingale calculus.

If W is a predictable process, a weighted logrank statistic can, under H_0, be represented as sums of stochastic integrals of predictable processes with respect to martingales, so that G_W is itself a martingale. This representation and its quadratic variation process can be used to derive formulas for the first two moments of these test statistics. The following summarizes Theorems 3.3.1 and 3.3.2 in Fleming & Harrington [10]; except for some regularity conditions and tedious algebra, it follows directly from Theorems 1 and 2.

Theorem 4. Let G_K be a statistic of the class $\mathcal{K}$. When $\Lambda_1 = \Lambda_2 = \Lambda$, $EG_K = 0$ and

$$EG_K^2 = E \sum_{i=1}^2 \int_0^\infty \frac{K^2}{\overline{Y}_i} (1 - \Delta\Lambda) d\Lambda.$$

The variance estimator

$$\hat{\sigma}^2 = \int_0^\infty \sum_{i=1}^2 \frac{K^2}{\overline{Y}_i} \left(1 - \frac{\Delta\overline{N}_1 + \Delta\overline{N}_2 - 1}{\overline{Y}_1 + \overline{Y}_2 - 1} \right)$$

$$\times \frac{d(\overline{N}_1 + \overline{N}_2)}{\overline{Y}_1 + \overline{Y}_2} \tag{4}$$

is an **unbiased** estimate of EG_K^2.

When Λ is continuous, $\Delta\Lambda = 0$ in the expression for EG_K^2, and the second term in the sum comprising the integrand in $\hat{\sigma}^2$ would seem unnecessary. That term is present only when two or more observed failure times are equal, however, and seems to improve the small-sample behavior of the estimator in tied data.

When $W = 1$, the statistic is the logrank statistic originally proposed by Mantel [24]. The same statistic arises as a partial likelihood score statistic in a proportional hazards regression model with a single binary covariate, although that approach leads to the variance estimate which assumes $\Delta \Lambda$ is identically 0. When $W(t)$ is a function of the proportion of cases at risk at time t, $[\overline{Y}_1(t) + \overline{Y}_2(t)]/(n_1 + n_2)$, the statistic is a member of the family proposed by Tarone & Ware [32]. If W is exactly the proportion of cases at risk, then G_W is the Gehan [13] generalization of the Wilcoxon statistic. If $W = \hat{S}^-$, the left-continuous version of the **Kaplan–Meier** [19] estimator computed with the two groups combined, then the statistic is asymptotically equivalent to the Wilcoxon generalization proposed by Prentice [26] and to a similar statistic proposed by Peto & Peto [25]. When $W = (\hat{S}^-)^\rho$, $\rho > 0$, the resulting family of statistics is that proposed by Harrington & Fleming [18]. In this family, the logrank statistic corresponds to $\rho = 0$ and the Prentice–Wilcoxon to $\rho = 1$. Gray & Tsiatis [16] have shown that this family may be extended to allow $\rho < 0$. The statistic proposed by Efron [8] is equivalent to one with weight

$$W = (\overline{Y}_1 + \overline{Y}_2)\hat{S}_1^- \hat{S}_2^- I(\overline{Y}_1 \overline{Y}_2 > 0)/(\overline{Y}_1 \overline{Y}_2).$$

Since both $\overline{Y}_1$ and $\overline{Y}_2$ are $\mathcal{F}_t$-adapted and left-continuous, the use of the left-continuous version of the Kaplan–Meier estimator in these statistics ensures predictability of the integrand K.

The counting process representation of these statistics provides insight into the term "linear rank tests". In uncensored data, where $X_{ij} = T_{ij}$ for all pairs i, j, a classical linear rank statistic as discussed in Hájek & Šidák [17] has the form $\sum_{i,j} a(R_{ij})$, where R_{ij} is the rank of T_{ij} in the combined sample and a is function assigning scores to the ranks. When the weight function W in a weighted logrank statistic depends only on the order of the possibly censored observations in the combined sample, as in all the statistics discussed above, then the Stieltjes integral representation of the statistic consists of a linear combination of scores assigned to observed failures according to the ordering of the observations X_{ij}.

The counting process representation also sheds light into the operating characteristics of these two-sample tests. The weighted logrank statistics can be written as

$$c \int_0^\infty W \left[d\overline{N}_1 - \overline{Y}_1 \frac{d(\overline{N}_1 + \overline{N}_2)}{\overline{Y}_1 + \overline{Y}_2} \right],$$

where c is a constant depending only on sample size. When W is constant, the observed minus expected failures are weighted equally, so that deviations from 0 in these terms in the right tail of the observations, where the risk sets are small, have as much influence on the value of the statistic as early deviations at times with large risk sets. If S_1 and S_2 are absolutely continuous and $\lambda_1 - \lambda_2$ changes sign at some time t, i.e. the underlying distributions have crossing hazard functions, then the logrank statistic may have a value that is not significantly different from zero, regardless of sample size (cf. Fleming et al. [11] for an example from a clinical study and Prentice & Marek [27] for an extended discussion). If W decreases when the observations increase, as in the Harrington–Fleming family when $\rho > 0$, then earlier differences in the observed minus expected failures will be emphasized. Gill [14] shows that statistics of the class $\mathcal{K}^+$ are consistent as long as $\Lambda_1(t) \geq \Lambda_2(t)$ for all t or vice versa, with strict inequality on at least one interval containing nonzero mass for the two distributions. Formal results about asymptotic operating characteristics under alternative hypotheses are summarized later.

The K-sample, $K > 2$, statistics are natural generalizations of the two-sample tests. Let $\overline{N}_i$, $\overline{Y}_i$, $i = 1, \ldots, K$, be defined as with two groups, and let $\overline{N} = \sum_i \overline{N}_i$ and $\overline{Y} = \sum_i \overline{Y}_i$. Under H_0: $\Lambda_1 = \Lambda_2 = \cdots = \Lambda_K$, the K-dimensional statistic with the ith component given by

$$G_{W,i} = \int_0^\infty W \left(d\overline{N}_i - \overline{Y}_i \frac{d\overline{N}}{\overline{Y}} \right)$$

is, for each group, a weighted sum of observed minus conditionally expected number of failures. It is not difficult to show that $\sum_i G_{W,i} = 0$, so that there are only $K - 1$ linearly independent components in the statistic. More detailed information about the covariance of the components of the statistic comes from the equivalent (under H_0) martingale representation

$$G_{W,i} = \sum_{l=1}^{K} \int_0^\infty W \left(r_{il} - \frac{\overline{Y}_i}{\overline{Y}} \right) d\overline{M}_l,$$

where $r_{il} = 1$ when $i = l$ and 0 otherwise. If we assume that the underlying cumulative hazard functions are continuous and that there are no ties in the observed data, the components of the statistic can be written as a sum of integrals with respect to orthogonal martingales. The simpler formulas for quadratic variation and covariation can be used to show that, under the hypothesis that all groups have a common cumulative hazard Λ,

$$\langle G_{W,i} \rangle = \sum_{l=1}^{K} \int_0^\infty W^2 \left(r_{il} - \frac{\overline{Y}_i}{\overline{Y}} \right)^2 \overline{Y}_l d\Lambda$$

and

$$\langle G_{W,i}, G_{W,k} \rangle = \sum_{l=1}^{K} \int_0^\infty W^2 \left(r_{il} - \frac{\overline{Y}_i}{\overline{Y}} \right)$$

$$\times \left(r_{kl} - \frac{\overline{Y}_k}{\overline{Y}} \right) \overline{Y}_l d\Lambda$$

$$= \int_0^\infty W^2 \frac{\overline{Y}_i}{\overline{Y}} \left(r_{ik} - \frac{\overline{Y}_i}{\overline{Y}} \right) \overline{Y} d\Lambda.$$

The last expression leads to a natural estimator $\hat{\Sigma}$ of the **covariance matrix** of the statistic, with elements $\hat{\sigma}_{ik}$ given by

$$\hat{\sigma}_{ik} = \int_0^\infty W^2 \frac{\overline{Y}_i}{\overline{Y}} \left(r_{ik} - \frac{\overline{Y}_k}{\overline{Y}} \right) d\overline{N}. \qquad (5)$$

As with the two-sample statistic, it is possible to show that $E(\hat{\sigma}_{ik}) = \text{cov}(G_{W,i}, G_{W,k})$.

The basic martingale may also be used to construct a statistic for comparing a single sample with a known or hypothesized population distribution with failure rate $d\Lambda_0$. The natural analog of the weighted logrank statistic is

$$c \int_0^\infty W(d\overline{N}_1 - \overline{Y}_1 d\Lambda_0 du).$$

These statistics are discussed in detail in Andersen et al. [4] and Woolson [33].

Asymptotic Distribution Theory

Large-sample normality for the K-sample statistics under both null and alternative distributions has been established by a number of authors. The original derivations of these tests by Gehan, Mantel, and others contained strong plausibility arguments for asymptotic distributions, and Schoenfeld [31] may have been one of the first to establish formally the asymptotic **efficiency** of the logrank test under proportional hazards alternatives. Using the original martingale formulation of Aalen and the martingale

central limit theorem of Rebolledo [29], Gill provided a thorough study of the large-sample operating characteristics of the two-sample tests under both null and alternative hypotheses (*see* **Power**). Andersen et al. [3] used the same methodology to study the large-sample behavior of tests for more than two samples. The theorems below summarize the major results in this area. The first results provide asymptotic distributions under the null hypothesis, first for the two-sample case, and then for the general K-sample statistics.

The most general theorems about the convergence of these statistics require more regularity conditions than might at first be expected. Beyond the usual conditions needed for central limit theorems, the asymptotic normality in these statistics can be disturbed if the weight function W becomes too large or if the cumulative hazard approaches infinity too quickly. The following theorem for the two-sample case covers nearly all the statistics used in practice and, because of the form of the weight function, does not require many conditions. This theorem appears as Theorem 7.2.1 in Fleming & Harrington [10], and relies for its proof on the more general result of Corollary 4.3.1 in Gill [14].

Theorem 5. In the two-sample testing problem with right-censored data (as described above), let $\hat{S}(t)$ denote the Kaplan–Meier estimator computed from the combined samples. Let $\hat{\pi}(t)$ denote the pooled sample estimator of the probability that a subject is alive and uncensored at time t, i.e. $\hat{\pi}(t) = [\overline{Y}_1(t) + \overline{Y}_2(t)]/(n_1 + n_2)$. Let f be a nonnegative bounded continuous function of bounded variation on $[0, 1]$. Suppose the weighted logrank statistic G_W has weight function of the form

$$\left(\frac{n_1 n_2}{n_1 + n_2} \right)^{1/2} W(t) \frac{\overline{Y}_1(t)}{n_1} \frac{\overline{Y}_2(t)}{n_2} \frac{n_1 + n_2}{\overline{Y}_1 + \overline{Y}_2},$$

where $W(t) = f[\hat{S}(t-)]$ or $W(t) = f[\hat{\pi}(t)]$. Suppose that $\lim_n n_i/n = a_i$ exists and lies in $(0, 1)$, and let $\hat{\sigma}$ be as in (4). Then under H_0: $\Lambda_1 = \Lambda_2$, $G_W/\hat{\sigma}$ converges in distribution, as $n \to \infty$, to a normally distributed random variable with mean 0 and variance 1.

Theorem 6 follows from Theorem V.2.1 and Example V.2.10 in Andersen et al. [4]. Because of the linear dependence of the terms in the K-dimensional statistic, the last component is usually dropped when computing the quadratic form for a Wald test (*see* **Likelihood**).

Theorem 6. In the K-sample testing problem with right-censored data (as described above), let $\hat{S}(t)$ denote the Kaplan–Meier estimator computed from the combined samples. Let $\hat{\pi}(t)$ denote the pooled sample estimator of the probability that a subject is at risk at time t, i.e.

$$\hat{\pi}(t) = [\overline{Y}_1(t) + \cdots + \overline{Y}_K(t)]/(n_1 + \cdots + n_K).$$

Let f be a nonnegative bounded continuous function of bounded variation on $[0, 1]$. Suppose the weight function W in the K-sample weighted logrank statistic is of the form $W(t) = f[\hat{S}(t-)]$ or $W(t) = f[\hat{\pi}(t)]$, and let the ith component of the standardized statistic be given by

$$G_{W,i} = \left[\frac{n}{n_i(n - n_i)} \right]^{1/2} \int_0^\infty W \left(d\overline{N}_i - \overline{Y}_i \frac{d\overline{N}}{\overline{Y}} \right),$$

where $n = \sum_i n_i$. Let the column vector $\mathbf{G}$ be given by $\mathbf{G}' = (G_{W,1}, \ldots, G_{W,K-1})$, and let the estimated covariance matrix for this $(K - 1)$ dimensional vector be denoted by $\hat{\mathbf{\Sigma}}_{K-1}$ with elements given in (5). Suppose that $\lim_n n_i/n$ exists and lies in $(0, 1)$ for each i. Then, under H_0: $\Lambda_1 = \cdots = \Lambda_k$, and as $n \to \infty$, the quadratic form $\mathbf{G}' \hat{\mathbf{\Sigma}}_{K-1}^{-1} \mathbf{G}$ converges in distribution to a χ^2 random variable with $K - 1$ **degrees of freedom** (*see* **Chi-Square Distribution**).

When all K components of the statistic are used in the quadratic form, a generalized inverse of the complete, singular covariance matrix may be used (*see* **Matrix Algebra**).

Asymptotic distributions under alternative hypotheses provide information about the power of the statistics. Gill [14] has shown that all two-sample tests of class $\mathcal{K}^+$ have asymptotic power 1, i.e. are consistent, under ordered hazards alternatives. Consequently, asymptotic power comparisons must be made under sequences of alternatives approaching the null hypothesis. Results with the counting process formulation are again simplest in the two-sample case. If a test statistic is asymptotically normal under a sequence of alternative hypotheses converging to the null hypothesis as the sample size increases, then the ratio of the square of the asymptotic mean to the asymptotic variance is called the (asymptotic)

efficacy. The efficacy will be the noncentrality parameter in the χ^2 distribution for the square of the statistic, and the ratio of efficacies for two statistics, computed under the same sequence of alternatives, has the same value as the asymptotic ratio of the sample sizes needed for the two tests to have equal power. To avoid technical details, we will argue only heuristically here. Generally, much more care must be taken when establishing limiting distributions under sequences of alternative distributions. Gill [14] contains detailed results for the two-sample problem; the results for the K-sample problem may be found in Andersen et al. [3, 4]. The asymptotic theory of testing, especially for rank-based methods, may be found in Randles & Wolfe [28] and Hájek & Šidák [17].

For simplicity, we assume that the underlying survival distributions are absolutely continuous. We let $n = n_1 + n_2$ index the underlying survival and hazard functions in the sequence of alternative distributions. When the two hazard functions λ_1^n and λ_2^n are not equal, a two-sample statistic of the class $\mathcal{K}^+$ can be written

$$
\begin{aligned}
G_K &= \int_0^\infty K \left(\frac{d\overline{N}_1}{\overline{Y}_1} - \frac{d\overline{N}_2}{\overline{Y}_2} \right) = \int_0^\infty K \left(\frac{d\overline{N}_1}{\overline{Y}_1} - \lambda_1^n \right) \\
&\quad - \int_0^\infty K \left(\frac{d\overline{N}_2}{\overline{Y}_2} - \lambda_2^n \right) + \int_0^\infty K(\lambda_1^n - \lambda_2^n) \\
&= \int_0^\infty \frac{K}{\overline{Y}_1} d\overline{M}_1 - \int_0^\infty \frac{K}{\overline{Y}_2} d\overline{M}_2 \\
&\quad + \int_0^\infty K \left(\frac{\lambda_1^n}{\lambda_0} - \frac{\lambda_2^n}{\lambda_0} \right) \lambda_0,
\end{aligned}
\tag{6}
$$

where λ_0 is the hypothetical common hazard function under the null hypothesis. For the weighted logrank statistics,

$$K = \left(\frac{n_1 n_2}{n_1 + n_2} \right)^{1/2} W \frac{\overline{Y}_1}{n_1} \frac{\overline{Y}_2}{n_2} \frac{n_1 + n_2}{\overline{Y}_1 + \overline{Y}_2},$$

where W is usually a function converging to some deterministic function w. The martingale central limit theorem implies that the first two terms in (6) converge to a mean zero Gaussian (**normal**) random variable, and the **strong law of large numbers** implies that the last two terms in the equation for K above converge collectively to $\pi_1 \pi_2/(a_1 \pi_1 + a_2 \pi_2)$. Loosely speaking, the convergence of the statistic to a Gaussian variable under a sequence of alternatives will depend on the convergence of

$$\int_0^\infty \frac{\pi_1\pi_2}{a_1\pi_1 + a_2\pi_2} w \left(\frac{n_1 n_2}{n_1 + n_2}\right)^{1/2} \left(\frac{\lambda_1^n}{\lambda_0} - \frac{\lambda_2^n}{\lambda_0}\right) \lambda_0.$$

The last three terms in the integrand above may be written as

$$\left(\frac{n_1 n_2}{n_1 + n_2}\right)^{1/2} \left[\left(\frac{\lambda_1^n}{\lambda_0} - 1\right) - \left(\frac{\lambda_2^n}{\lambda_0} - 1\right)\right] \lambda_0.$$

Convergence under the sequence of alternative distributions will thus depend on convergence of

$$[n_1 n_2/(n_1 + n_2)]^{1/2}[(\lambda_i^n/\lambda_0) - 1]$$

to a function $g_i, i = 1, 2$. This implies when $i = 1$, for instance, that the ratio of functions λ_1^n/λ_0 must converge to 1 at rate $n_1^{1/2}$, and that λ_1^n/λ_2^n must also converge to 1 at the same rate. If $g = g_1 - g_2$, then the asymptotic mean of the statistic under this sequence of alternatives will be

$$\mu = \int_0^\infty \frac{\pi_1\pi_2}{a_1\pi_1 + a_2\pi_2} wg\lambda_0.$$

The asymptotic variance of the statistic will be determined by the first two integrals in (6), and turns out to equal the asymptotic variance under the null hypothesis,

$$\sigma^2 = \int_0^\infty \frac{\pi_1\pi_2}{a_1\pi_1 + a_2\pi_2} w^2\lambda_0.$$

The asymptotically best weighted logrank test statistic is the member of that class that maximizes this efficacy with respect to the asymptotic weight function w. Gill [14] uses a Lagrange multiplier argument to show that, in fact, the asymptotic efficacy is maximized over all of $\mathcal{K}^+$ when a statistic is a weighted logrank statistic with weight function W converging to an asymptotic weight function w proportional to g. This result can be used to calculate the best test from $\mathcal{K}^+$ against particular types of alternatives.

Suppose that $\lambda_i^n = \lambda_{\theta_i^n}$. Then,

$$\left(\frac{n_1 n_2}{n_1 + n_2}\right)^{1/2} \left(\frac{\lambda_1^n}{\lambda_0} - 1\right)$$

$$= \frac{\lambda_{\theta_i^n} - \lambda_{\theta_0}}{\theta_i^n - \theta_0} \times \left(\frac{n_1 n_2}{n_1 + n_2}\right)^{1/2} \frac{\theta_i^n - \theta_0}{\lambda_{\theta_0}}. \qquad (7)$$

If $\theta_i^n \to \theta_0$ such that

$$\lim_{n\to\infty} \left(\frac{n_1 n_2}{n_1 + n_2}\right)^{1/2} (\theta_i^n - \theta_0) = c_i^*,$$

then both sides in (7) will approach $c_i^* \partial/\partial\theta \log \lambda_\theta$, where the derivative with respect to θ is evaluated at θ_0. Consequently, the function g appearing in the asymptotic mean and efficacy under a sequence of alternatives will be proportional to

$$\frac{\partial}{\partial\theta}\bigg|_{\theta=\theta_0} \log \lambda_\theta.$$

This result confirms that, for instance, when $\lambda_{\theta_i^n}(t) = \lambda_0(t) \exp(\theta_i^n)$, $i = 1, 2$ (i.e. proportional hazards alternatives), the most efficient statistic of class $\mathcal{K}^+$ has a constant weight function W (i.e. is the logrank statistic).

Computing asymptotic relative efficiencies against optimal tests for parametric models is more difficult, but uses the same approach. Gill [14] shows that, when the hazard function in the two-sample problem is known up to a single parameter $\theta_i^n, i = 1, 2$, satisfying

$$\theta_i^n - \theta_0 = (-1)^{i+1} c \left[\frac{n_{i'}}{n_i(n_1 + n_2)}\right]^{1/2}, \quad i \ne i',$$

then the asymptotic efficacy of the **likelihood ratio test** of equality of the two hazard functions is given by

$$\int_0^\infty \left(\frac{\partial}{\partial\theta} \log \lambda_\theta\big|_{\theta=\theta_0}\right)^2 (a_2\pi_1 + a_1\pi_2)\lambda_{\theta_0}).$$

Gill also shows that the ratio of the asymptotic efficacies comparing an optimal test of class $\mathcal{K}^+$ to the likelihood ratio test is bounded above by 1, as expected, but that the ratio may equal 1 when $\pi_1 = \pi_2$. Under random censoring, $\pi_i(t) = \Pr(T_{ij} \ge t)\Pr(U_{ij} \ge t)$. Since in the limit $\Pr(T_{1j} \ge t) = \Pr(T_{2j} \ge t)$, fully efficient tests of the class $\mathcal{K}^+$ can be found when asymptotic censoring distributions are equal.

The study of asymptotic operating characteristics of general K-sample tests uses similar tools; the interested reader can find a detailed treatment in Andersen et al. [4].

The counting process and martingale framework provides methods for a rigorous study of the operating characteristics of linear rank tests for censored data, but a variety of other approaches have been used in special cases. As mentioned in the introduction, Gehan [13] originally generalized the two-sample Wilcoxon test by extending the notion of the scores used in the Mann–Whitney version of the Wilcoxon statistic. Gehan then used a permutation argument to compute a distribution under the null hypothesis, conditional on the observed pattern of censorship (*see* **Randomization Tests**), and argued that the permutation distribution would approach normality in large samples. Since the Gehan–Wilcoxon statistic corresponds to a weighted logrank statistic with weight function $W(t) = [\overline{Y}_1(t) + \overline{Y}_2(t)]/(n_1 + n_2)$, which asymptotically depends on both the underlying survival and censoring distributions in the groups, Gill's results show that this version of the Wilcoxon statistic has operating characteristics that depend on the censoring distribution. Leurgans [22, 23] also provides extensive applied and theoretical discussions of the asymptotic operating characteristics of rank statistics for censored data.

Mantel's [24] original derivation of the two-sample logrank statistic treated the observations as a series of 2×2 **contingency tables**, with one table at each observed failure time. The marginal classifications of the tables denoted the number of subjects at risk in each group just prior to the observed failure time, and the numbers of subjects failing or not failing at the observed time. Mantel argued that, conditional on the risk sets in the two groups at the observed failure times, the set of observed minus conditionally expected number of failures in group 1 were independent, and that standard central limit theorems could be used to justify asymptotic normality. Mantel's arguments were heuristic, but the differences between observed and conditionally expected failures in the tables are exactly the increments in the integral representation, (2). The martingale representation shows that these increments are uncorrelated and consequently asymptotically independent. Mantel also argued that, since the Mantel–Haenszel statistic on which the logrank test is based is efficient at detecting a constant **odds ratio** different from 1 in stratified 2×2 tables, the logrank should have good power against proportional hazards alternatives.

Prentice [26] generalized the theory of linear rank tests, as described in Hájek & Šidák [17], to censored observations by suggesting a modification to the efficient score. This approach outlined a general context for linear rank tests for censored data, and showed that many of the statistics finding widespread use could be thought of as special cases of this general approach. Prentice was the first to show that Gehan's generalization of the Wilcoxon statistic was not the only natural way to create a Wilcoxon-type statistic for censored data. The Wilcoxon statistic in uncensored data arises from the optimal scoring function for shift alternatives in the **logistic distribution** [17], and Prentice's generalized scoring function for censored data led to a statistic that was approximately the weighted logrank statistic with weight function $\hat{S}(t-)$. Cuzick [7] later showed that many of the asymptotic results on linear rank tests for uncensored data could be extended to test statistics using the Prentice scoring function.

Because of space constraints, many important contributions to this field have necessarily been omitted. First, in the interest of simplicity, we have suppressed much of the generality that results from the use of martingale theory. The more complete treatments in [4], [14], and elsewhere discuss the use of local martingales, which relax some of the implicit boundedness conditions in the martingale definition. Local martingales allow more general weight functions in $\mathcal{K}^+$ statistics and also are used, sometimes in subtle ways, in the proofs of many of the results stated here. The asymptotic theory for these tests has been described only briefly (with mathematical details kept to a minimum) and small-sample properties not at all. It is possible to derive a permutation distribution for tests such as the logrank under the null hypothesis and the assumption of equal censoring in both groups, but most small-sample studies have relied on **simulation** (cf. Lee et al. [21] and Latta [20]). Alternative variance estimators to those given here are discussed in Andersen et al. [4]. Stratified tests are available for situations when differences among groups within strata are constant but baseline failure rates across strata differ (cf. [4]) (*see* **Stratification**). Gastwirth [12] and others have discussed the problem of how to combine linear rank tests for censored data when it is difficult to specify clearly the form of an alternative hypothesis. Robins & Rotnitzky [30] have proposed tests that relax the independent censoring assumption so prominently used here. Many authors have studied nonparametric estimates of survival distributions with left- or interval-censored data, and these estimates often lead to test statistics. Several nonlinear rank tests based on the sample path behavior of statistics from $\mathcal{K}^+$ have been proposed; some generalize the classical **Kolmogorov–Smirnov test**. There is an extensive literature on **sequential** methods that can be used with censored data linear rank tests in clinical trials and other prospective studies (*see* **Interim Analysis of Censored Data**). Finally, many more linear rank tests have been proposed than just those discussed in this article.

References

[1]   Aalen, O.O. (1975). Statistical Inference for a Family of Counting Processes, *Ph.D. Dissertation*. University of California, Berkeley.

[2]   Aalen, O.O. (1978). Nonparametric inference for a family of counting processes, *Annals of Statistics* **6**, 701–726.

[3]   Andersen, P.K., Borgan, Ø., Gill, R.D. & Keiding, N. (1982). Linear nonparametric tests for comparison of counting processes with application to censored survival data (with discussion), *International Statistical Review* **50**, 219–258.

[4]   Andersen, P.K., Borgan, Ø., Gill, R.D. & Keiding, N. (1992). *Statistical Models Based on Counting Processes*. Springer-Verlag, New York.

[5]   Breslow, N.E. (1970). A generalized Kruskal-Wallis test for comparing K samples subject to unequal patterns of censorship, *Biometrika* **57**, 579–594.

[6]   Cox, D.R. (1972). Regression models and life-tables (with discussion), *Journal of the Royal Statistical Society, Series B* **34**, 187–220.

[7]   Cuzick, J. (1985). Asymptotic properties of censored linear rank tests, *Annals of Statistics* **13**, 133–141.

[8]   Efron, B. (1967). The two-sample problem with censored data, *Proceedings of the Fifth Berkeley Symposium on Mathematics, Statistics & Probability*, Vol. 4, Prentice Hall, New York, pp. 831–853.

[9]   Elliot, R.J. (1982). *Stochastic Calculus and Applications*. Springer-Verlag, New York.

[10]   Fleming, T.R. & Harrington, D.P. (1991). *Counting Processes and Survival Analysis*. Wiley, New York.

[11]   Fleming, T.R., O'Fallon, J.R., O'Brien, P.C. & Harrington, D.P. (1980). Modified Kolmogorov-Smirnov test procedures with application to arbitrarily right censored data, *Biometrics* **36**, 607–626.

[12]   Gastwirth, J.L. (1985). The use of maximum efficiency robust tests in combining contingency tables and survival analysis, *Journal of the American Statistical Association* **80**, 380–384.

[13]   Gehan, E.A. (1965). A generalized Wilcoxon test for comparing arbitrary singly-censored samples, *Biometrika* **52**, 203–223.

[14]   Gill, R.D. (1980). *Censoring and Stochastic Integrals*. Mathematical Centre Tracts 124, Mathematisch Centrum, Amsterdam.

[15]   Gill, R.D. (1984). Understanding Cox's regression model: A martingale approach, *Journal of the American Statistical Association* **79**, 441–447.

[16]   Gray, R.J. & Tsiatis, A.A. (1989). A linear rank test for use when the main interest is in differences in cure rates, *Biometrics* **45**, 899–904.

[17]   Hájek, J. & Šidák, Z. (1967). *Theory of Rank Tests*. Academic Press, New York.

[18]   Harrington, D.P. & Fleming, T.R. (1982). A class of rank test procedures for censored survival data, *Biometrika* **69**, 133–143.

[19]   Kaplan, E.L. & Meier, P. (1958). Nonparametric estimator from incomplete observations, *Journal of the American Statistical Association* **53**, 457–481.

[20]   Latta, R.B. (1981). A Monte Carlo study of some two-sample rank tests with censored data, *Journal of the American Statistical Association* **76**, 713–719.

[21]   Lee, E.T., Desu, M.M. & Gehan, E.A. (1973). A Monte Carlo study of the power of some two-sample tests, *Biometrika* **62**, 425–432.

[22]   Leurgans, S. (1983). Three classes of censored data rank tests: Strengths and weaknesses under censoring, *Biometrika* **70**, 651–658.

[23]   Leurgans, S. (1984). Asymptotic behavior of two-sample rank tests in the presence of random censoring, *Annals of Statistics* **12**, 572–589.

[24]   Mantel, N. (1966). Evaluation of survival data and two new rank order statistics arising in its consideration, *Cancer Chemotherapy Reports* **50**, 163–170.

[25]   Peto, R. & Peto, J. (1972). Asymptotically efficient rank invariant test procedures (with discussion), *Journal of the Royal Statistical Society, Series A* **135**, 185–206.

[26]   Prentice, R.L. (1978). Linear rank tests with right censored data, *Biometrika* **65**, 167–179.

[27]   Prentice, R.L. & Marek, P. (1979). A qualitative discrepancy between censored data rank tests, *Biometrics* **35**, 861–867.

[28]   Randles, R.H. & Wolfe, D.A. (1979). *Introduction to the Theory of Nonparametric Statistics*. Wiley, New York.

[29]   Rebolledo, R. (1980). Central limit theorems for local martingales, *Zeitschrift für Wahrlichtkeitstheorie und Verwandte Gebeite* **51**, 269–286.

[30]   Robins, J. & Rotnitzky, A. (1992). Recovery of information and adjustment for dependent censoring, in *AIDS Epidemiology: Methodologic Issues*, N. Jewell, K. Dietz & V. Farewell, eds. Birkhauser, New York, pp. 297–331.

[31]   Schoenfeld, D.A. (1981). The asymptotic properties of nonparametric tests for comparing survival distributions, *Biometrika* **68**, 316–319.

[32]   Tarone, R.E. & Ware, J. (1977). On distribution free tests for equality of survival distributions, *Biometrika* **64**, 156–160.

[33]   Woolson, R.F. (1981). Rank tests and a one-sample logrank test for comparing observed survival data to a standard population, *Biometrics* **37**, 687–696.

(*See also* **Survival Analysis, Overview**)

DAVID HARRINGTON

Linear Regression, Simple

Historically, the term "regression" was introduced by **Galton** [3, p. 246] to describe the tendency for the offspring of seeds "to be always more mediocre [i.e. more average] than their parent seeds . . . . The experiments showed further that the mean filial regression towards mediocrity was directly proportional to the parental deviation from it". Pearson & Lee [4] subsequently collected data on the heights of 1078 father–son pairs in order to study Galton's "law of universal regression" which they summarized as "Each peculiarity in a man is shared by his kinsmen, but on the average in a less degree" (*see* **Regression to the Mean**).

Modern applications rarely involve the element of "regression" as Galton meant it; however, the word is now too established to change. Consequently, regression now describes any relationship between a **response** (dependent) variable, Y, and a **covariate** or **explanatory** (independent, predictor) variable, X. Strictly speaking, only the response, Y, is assumed to vary randomly; however, in many applications the observed values of X are not known or fixed. We assume that any inherent variation in the measurement of X can be ignored. If this is not the case, we strongly advise resorting to methods that are appropriate when there is measurement error in an explanatory variable (*see* **Errors in Variables**). Simple linear regression involves finding the best-fitting curve that relates $E(Y|X)$, the mean value of Y given X, and X, using an equation with a suitable functional form, such as $E(Y|X) = \beta_0 + \beta_1 X$. This regression equation is called linear because $E(Y|X)$ is a linear (straight-line) function with respect to the unknown model parameters, β_0 and β_1. It is not essential that $E(Y|X)$ also depend linearly on X, although this is frequently the case in applications. For example, the model $E(Y|X) = \beta_0 + \beta_1 X^2$ describes a linear regression model that is a straight-line function of β_0 and β_1,

but is quadratic in X (*see* **Polynomial Regression**). Whatever the model form, the goals of regression modeling are

1.   to determine whether Y and X are associated in some systematic way; and/or
2.   to estimate or **predict** the value of Y, or its mean, corresponding to a known value of X.

The unknown parameters, β_0 and β_1, are estimated from data – ordered pairs $(X_1, Y_1), \ldots, (X_n, Y_n)$ – using the method of **least squares**, which was discovered independently by **Gauss** and Legendre; see Plackett [5].

Estimating β_0 and β_1

Before fitting a linear regression model to data, it is wise to examine a scatterplot of Y vs. X in order to ensure that the proposed relationship is a sensible one (*see* **Graphical Displays**). Such a scatterplot is shown in Figure 1 for measurements of systolic blood pressure and age obtained from 21 males between the ages of 25 and 80. For these data, the notion that average systolic blood pressure increases systematically, in a roughly linear manner, with age seems plausible.

All linear regression models consist of a systematic component – the model equation, $E(Y|X) = \beta_0 + \beta_1 X$ – and a residual (random, error) component, ε; the sum, $\beta_0 + \beta_1 X + \varepsilon$, constitutes the regression model for Y. The **residual**, $\varepsilon = Y - \beta_0 - \beta_1 X$, represents the amount by which an observed value of Y deviates from the predicted mean, $\beta_0 + \beta_1 X$.

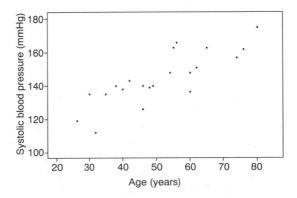

Figure 1   A scatterplot of systolic blood pressure (Y) vs. age (X) for a sample of 21 males between 25 and 80 years old

Not all (X_j, Y_j) pairs for a given set of data will lie on the predicted line (curve). The method of least squares identifies the unique values of β_0 and β_1 that minimize the average of the squared residuals. Specifically, $\hat{\beta}_1 = S_{xy}/S_{xx}$ and $\hat{\beta}_0 = \bar{y} - \hat{\beta}_1 \bar{x}$, where $\bar{x} = \sum_{i=1}^{n} x_i/n$, $\bar{y} = \sum_{i=1}^{n} y_i/n$, $S_{xy} = \sum_{i=1}^{n}(x_i - \bar{x})(y_i - \bar{y})$, and $S_{xx} = \sum_{i=1}^{n}(x_i - \bar{x})^2$. The equation of the estimated regression of Y on X is

$$\hat{Y} = \hat{\beta}_0 + \hat{\beta}_1 X = \bar{y} + \hat{\beta}_1(X - \bar{x}).$$

Least squares estimates can be derived based only on the assumptions that the residuals, $\varepsilon_1, \ldots, \varepsilon_n$, are uncorrelated and have a mean value of zero and constant variance, σ^2. We use the estimated residuals $\hat{\varepsilon}_i = Y_i - \hat{Y}_i = Y_i - \hat{\beta}_0 - \hat{\beta}_1 X_i$, $i = 1, \ldots, n$, to estimate σ^2. The formula

$$\hat{\sigma}^2 = \frac{1}{n-2} \sum_{i=1}^{n} \hat{\varepsilon}_i^2,$$

which involves $\sum_{i=1}^{n} \hat{\varepsilon}_i^2$, the estimated residual sum of squares, emphasizes that two parameters, β_0 and β_1, are estimated; hence the divisor $n - 2$. Adopting the additional assumption that the residuals are **normally distributed** gives rise to various statistical procedures that we will discuss subsequently. First, however, we examine linear regression as an explanation for the observed variability in the response, Y.

Partitioning the Variability in Y

To account for the variability in Y, we can always resort to the simplest explanation, namely that Y varies about a fixed mean, μ. The corresponding linear regression model is $Y_i = \beta_0 + \varepsilon_i$, where $\beta_0 = \mu$. In this case, the residuals, i.e. $\varepsilon_i = Y_i - \beta_0 = Y_i - \mu$, are usually large, and result in a substantial estimate of σ^2. For the data concerning blood pressure and age, these estimated residuals are shown in Figure 2(a). In the absence of additional information, this is the only explanation we can devise for the variability in Y.

However, when Y appears to depend systematically on X, we can use the known values of X that were measured concurrently with Y to estimate $E(Y|X)$. Using $\hat{Y} = E(Y|X)$, we can partition the observed variability in Y into two components – the change in $E(Y|X)$ accounted for by the change in X, and the residual variability of Y values that have the same value of X, and hence the same value

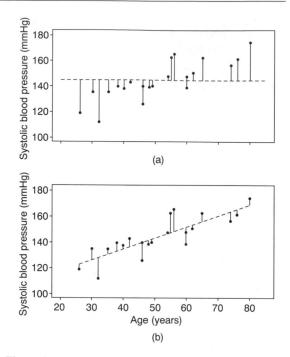

Figure 2   Estimated residuals (solid lines) for systolic blood pressure measurements (Y) in a sample of 21 males between 25 and 80 years old. (a) Based on the simple model, $Y = \mu + \varepsilon$; the dashed line indicates $\hat{\mu} = 144.7$. (b) Based on the linear regression model, $Y = \beta_0 + \beta_1 X + \varepsilon$, relating Y and age (X); the dashed line indicates the least squares estimated regression equation $\hat{Y} = 100.6 + 0.86X$

of $E(Y|X)$. These two components of variability correspond to the systematic component, $\beta_0 + \beta_1 X$, and the residual component, ε, respectively, in the linear regression model $Y = \beta_0 + \beta_1 X + \varepsilon$. By estimating $E(Y|X) = \beta_0 + \beta_1 X$, we can reduce the estimated residuals and hence the estimate of σ^2, the residual variation. Clearly, the estimated residual sum of squares in Figure 2(b) will be much less than the corresponding value based on the estimated residuals in Figure 2(a). Equivalently, knowing a subject's age provides important information about what his blood pressure is likely to be.

This partition of the variability in Y is usually summarized in an **analysis of variance** (ANOVA) table, such as the one corresponding to the example shown in Table 1. This partitioning is represented by the equation

$$\sum_{i=1}^{n}(Y_i - \bar{Y})^2 = \sum_{i=1}^{n}(\hat{Y}_i - \bar{Y})^2 + \sum_{i=1}^{n}(Y_i - \hat{Y}_i)^2,$$

Table 1 An ANOVA table summarizing the partition of observed variability in blood pressure measurements into the systematic (model) component represented by the estimated regression model, $\hat{Y} = \hat{\beta}_0 + \hat{\beta}_1 X$, and the residual component. The value of R^2 for these data is 0.69

Source	SS	df	MS
Model	3453.5	1	3453.5
Residual	1545.8	19	81.36
Total	4999.3	20	

which is alternatively described by the relationship

total sum of squares = model sum of squares
+ residual sum of squares.

The ratio of the model sum of squares to the total sum of squares is called R^2, and represents the proportion of the observed variability in Y that is accounted for by modeling the mean response for Y as the function, $\beta_0 + \beta_1 X$, of X.

Interpreting the Regression Estimates

If two values of the explanatory variable differ by one unit, the corresponding values of the model equation differ by β_1. Therefore, $\hat{\beta}_1$ represents the estimated change in the mean response associated with a unit increase in the explanatory variable. Of course, this estimate and its interpretation are only valid within the range of X values used in fitting the linear regression model.

The value β_0 represents the mean response when $X = 0$. Frequently, this mean response may be of no interest, or may not belong to the range of X values used in fitting the model to data. A more useful parameter in many situations is $\gamma = \beta_0 + \beta_1 \bar{x}$, which represents the mean response when $X = \bar{x}$, the observed average of the explanatory variable. The estimated value is $\hat{\gamma} = \hat{\beta}_0 + \hat{\beta}_1 \bar{x} = \bar{y}$, the sample mean of Y.

The estimates of β_0 and β_1 for the example are 100.6 and 0.86, respectively. From these data we conclude that 0.86 mmHg is the estimated increase in mean blood pressure associated with each additional year of age for men 25–80 years old. At an age of $\bar{x} = 51.1$ years, the estimated mean blood pressure is $\hat{\gamma} = \bar{y} = 145$ mmHg.

Statistical Inference in Linear Regression

Under the additional assumption that the residuals, $\varepsilon_1, \ldots, \varepsilon_n$, are normally distributed, the estimators of β_0 and β_1 have normal sampling distributions. Estimated **standard errors** (est. se) for $\hat{\beta}_0$ and $\hat{\beta}_1$ are routinely produced by most computing packages (*see* **Software, Biostatistical**). The ratio of each estimate to its corresponding estimated standard error follows a **Student's t distribution** with $n - 2$ **degrees of freedom** (df). From these results, **hypothesis tests** and/or **confidence intervals** for β_0 and β_1 can be evaluated. Likewise, the **sampling distribution** of $\hat{\gamma} = \bar{Y}$ is normal, and the corresponding estimated standard error is $s/\sqrt{n}$, where $s^2 = \hat{\sigma}^2$.

A test of the null hypothesis, $H_0 : \beta_1 = 0$, is routinely used to assess the significance of the regression; that is, to determine whether the data constitute statistical evidence of an association between Y and X. This test can be based either on the ratio $\hat{\beta}_1/$est. se$(\hat{\beta}_1)$, which has a Student's t distribution with $n - 2$ df, or on $[\hat{\beta}_1/$est. se$(\hat{\beta}_1)]^2$, which has an **F distribution** with 1 and $n - 2$ df. The latter test statistic is equal to the ratio of the model mean square to the residual mean square in the corresponding ANOVA table for the regression analysis, and usually appears in an additional column labelled F ratio.

For the blood pressure vs. age example, the estimated standard errors for $\hat{\beta}_0, \hat{\beta}_1$ are 7.05 and 0.13, respectively. The 95% confidence interval for β_1 is (0.58, 1.14), and for γ the interval is (136, 153).

Model Diagnostics

A fitted regression model and associated statistical inferences are based on various assumptions concerning the functional form of the model for $E(Y|X)$ and distributional properties of the residuals. Violations of these assumptions may invalidate conclusions based on the regression analysis. Therefore, it is essential to check these assumptions, using various types of **diagnostic** plots.

The estimated residuals, $\hat{\varepsilon}_i = Y_i - \hat{\beta}_0 - \hat{\beta}_1 X_i$, $i = 1, \ldots, n$, play an essential role in model diagnostics. Many computer packages offer the option of using these ordinary residuals or the corresponding standardized or studentized residuals, which have a common variance. Use of either of the latter two is preferable, since the $\hat{\varepsilon}_i$s do not all have the same variance.

The following diagnostic plots furnish graphical evidence that one or more of the model assumptions may be contradicted by the data:

1. Residuals vs. the fitted values, $\hat{Y}_i$. An unsuitable functional form is usually revealed by the systematic appearance of this plot, as is nonconstant variance.
2. Residuals vs. the explanatory variable, X_i. Systematic patterns in this plot can indicate violations of the mean 0, constant variance assumptions, or inappropriate model form.
3. Normal probability plot of the residuals. This plot checks the normal distribution assumption from which all the statistical inference procedures arise (*see* **Normal Scores**).
4. Residuals vs. the temporal/spatial order of data collection. Unexpected regularity in this plot suggests that the Y_is may be correlated. To prepare this diagnostic check, it is essential to record the temporal/spatial ordering when data are first collected.
5. Index plots (plot against the case number, i.e. the observation label) of the leverages and Cook's distance (*see* **Diagnostics**). The former are a measure of the amount of influence exerted on $\hat{Y}_i$ by the corresponding observed response, Y_i. Cook's distance is a summary measure of the influence that each case exerts on the estimated regression coefficients. These two diagnostic plots can reveal outliers (values of Y that are anomalous with respect to the rest of the data) or influential points (values of (X_j, Y_j) that strongly influence the estimated values of $\hat{\beta}_0$, $\hat{\beta}_1$ and s^2).

Deviations from the expected (null) pattern in any of these plots may indicate problems that require further investigation or remedial action. For additional details concerning model diagnostics, see Belsley et al. [1] or Cook & Weisberg [2]. Further details concerning examination of the adequacy of a fitted regression model are found in the article on **Goodness of Fit**.

References

[1] Belsley, D.A., Kuh, E. & Welsch, R.E. (1980). *Regression Diagnostics: Identifying Influential Data and Sources of Collinearity*. Wiley, New York.

[2] Cook, R.D. & Weisberg, S. (1982). *Residuals and Influence in Regression*. Chapman & Hall, London.

[3] Galton, F. (1885). Regression towards mediocrity in hereditary stature, *Journal of the Anthropological Institute* **15**, 246–263.

[4] Pearson, K. & Lee, A. (1903). On the laws of inheritance in man. I. Inheritance of physical characters, *Biometrika* **2**, 357–462.

[5] Plackett, R.L. (1972). Studies in the history of probability and statistics, XXIX: the discovery of the method of least squares, *Biometrika* **59**, 239–251.

(*See also* **Multiple Linear Regression**)

DAVID E. MATTHEWS

Linear-by-Linear Association *see* Categorical Data Analysis

Linearization Methods of Variance Estimation

The **variance** of a linear function of variables is a linear function of variables. An approximation by a linear function of a nonlinear function enables one to derive an approximate variance of a complex nonlinear function. The most common approach consists of taking linear terms of Taylor series expansion of the nonlinear function of the observations around their expected values. The approach has been widely used for approximating large-sample variances (*see* **Large-Sample Theory**), and is referred to as Taylor Series Linearization or the **Delta method**. Another linearization approach was suggested by Quenouille [6] and made well known by Tukey [10] as **jackknife**. A good review of the jackknife and other methods appears in [7].

Tepping [9] suggested the use of Taylor series linearization for estimating variances in complex **sample surveys**. Applications to **mean** and **linear regression** coefficients for complex surveys were presented by Kish & Frankel [4] and Folsom [3]. Some **simulation** results were presented by Shah et al. [8]. Woodruff [11] presented a general application of the linearization method to explicit functions of observed data. Binder [1] extended the results to parameters defined as implicit functions or estimating equations. Binder also proved the asymptotic **normality** of the estimates. Binder [2] presented an application of Taylor series linearization to the estimation of parameters for Cox's **proportional hazard** model for the survival data collected from a complex sample survey. We present here a brief summary of the results by Woodruff [11] and Binder [1].

The Taylor series linearization method is illustrated here for statistics that can be defined explicitly as functions of linear statistics estimated from a survey sample. Means, totals, proportions, general ratios of the form $\sum wx / \sum wy$, and linear regression coefficients all fall into this category of functions. A linearized variable, Z_i, is defined on the basis of the Taylor series expansion of the function, and then substituted into the variance formula appropriate under the specified design for any linear statistic estimated from the sample.

The technique will be illustrated for a statistic which is a function of two linear statistics, although it extends to any number of linear statistics and to statistics that are vectors. Let $\hat{\theta}$ be an estimate of the population parameter θ, with $\hat{\theta} = F(X, Y)$ where X and Y are two linear sample statistics. Let $\mu_x = \mathrm{E}(X)$ and $\mu_y = \mathrm{E}(Y)$, where the **expectation** operator E denotes averaging over repeated sampling from the **target population**. θ can be expanded in a Taylor series about μ_x and μ_y, so that

$$\hat{\theta} = F(\mu_x, \mu_y) + \partial F_x(\mu_x, \mu_y)(X - \mu_x)$$
$$+ \partial F_y(\mu_x, \mu_y)(Y - \mu_y)$$
$$+ \text{ higher order terms},$$

where the $\partial F_x(\mu_x, \mu_y)$ and $\partial F_y(\mu_x, \mu_y)$ functions are first-order partial derivatives of F with respect to X and Y evaluated at their respective expectations, μ_x and μ_x. If the higher order terms are negligible, then

$$\mathrm{var}[\hat{\theta}] \doteq \mathrm{E}[\hat{\theta} - F(\mu_x, \mu_y)]^2$$
$$= \{(\partial F_x)^2 \mathrm{E}(X - \mu_x)^2 + (\partial F_y)^2 \mathrm{E}(Y - \mu_y)^2$$
$$+ 2(\partial F_x)(\partial F_y)$$
$$\times \mathrm{E}[(X - \mu_x)(Y - \mu_y)](Y - \mu_y)]\}$$
$$\times \{(\partial F_x)^2 \mathrm{var}(X) + (\partial F_y)^2 \mathrm{var}(Y)$$
$$+ 2(\partial F_x)(\partial F_y)\mathrm{cov}(X, Y)\},$$

where $\partial F_x = \partial F_x(\mu_x, \mu_y)$ and $\partial F_y = \partial F_y(\mu_x, \mu_y)$.

An equivalent computational procedure for producing the Taylor series variance estimate suggested by Woodruff [11] recognizes that the variable portion of the linearization in his Eq. (3.2) is

$$Z = (\partial F_x)X + (\partial F_y)Y,$$

and therefore

$$\mathrm{var}[\hat{\theta}] \doteq \mathrm{var}[(\partial F_x)X + (\partial F_y)Y]$$
$$= \mathrm{var}(Z).$$

Noting that X and Y are linear statistics formed from the corresponding response variates x_i and y_i, measured on the ith sample unit, the variance approximation can be produced by substituting the linearized variable

$$Z_i = (\partial F_x)X_i + (\partial F_y)Y_i$$

for x_i or y_i in the variance formula appropriate for computing $\mathrm{var}(X)$ or $\mathrm{var}(Y)$ under the specified sample design. To obtain a sample estimate for the Taylor series variance approximation, one replaces the population-evaluated derivative functions in Z_i with the corresponding sample analog, i.e.

$$Z_i = [\partial F_x(X, Y)]x_i + [\partial F_y(X, Y)]y_i.$$

Binder [1, 2] proposed and justified using an implicit differentiation method for estimating the variance for a vector of survey statistics. Binder's results are particularly useful when the parameters are implicitly defined, but the results also cover the explicit case.

Logistic regression coefficients and survival models (*see* **Survival Analysis, Overview**) fall into this category of parameters that are implicitly defined.

Let $\theta = (\theta_1, \ldots, \theta_p)'$ be the finite population parameter vector which is defined by

$$W(\theta) = \sum_{k=1}^{N} U(Z_k; \theta) - v(\theta) = 0,$$

where $Z_k = (z_{1k}, \ldots, z_{qk})$ are the data values for the kth unit, and $W(\theta)$ is a vector with the ith element:

$$W_i(\theta) = \sum_{k=1}^{N} V_i(Z_k; \theta) - v_i(\theta) = 0.$$

Let $U(\theta) = \sum_{k=1}^{N} U(Z_k; \theta)$ be estimated from the sample by $\hat{U}(\theta)$. $\hat{U}(\theta)$ is the estimator of the total based on the functions of data values $U(Z_1; \theta), \ldots,$ $U(Z_n; \theta)$, for example $\hat{U}(\theta) = \sum_{i \in S} w_i U(Z_i; \theta)$. Then,

$\hat{W}(\theta) = \hat{U}(\theta) - v(\theta)$. Assuming that a unique solution exists, $\hat{\theta}$, the estimate of θ, is defined as the solution to

$$\hat{W}(\hat{\theta}) = 0.$$

To approximate the variance of $\hat{\theta}$, Binder expands $\hat{W}(\hat{\theta})$ in a Taylor series about the point $\hat{\theta} = \theta$, where θ is the true unknown parameter. Defining $\hat{J}(\theta) = \partial \hat{W}(\theta)/\partial \theta$ as the $p \times p$ matrix whose ij element is the partial derivative $\partial \hat{W}_i(\theta)/\partial \theta_j$, and expanding $\hat{W}(\hat{\theta})$ about $\hat{\theta} = \theta$, gives

$$0 = \hat{W}(\hat{\theta}) \approx \hat{W}(\theta) + \hat{J}(\theta)(\hat{\theta} - \theta),$$

or, if $\hat{J}^{-1}(\theta)$ exists,

$$\hat{\theta} - \theta \doteq \hat{J}^{-1}(\theta)\hat{W}(\theta).$$

This leads to the approximation of the variance matrix of $\hat{\theta}$:

$$V(\hat{\theta}) \doteq [\hat{J}^{-1}(\theta)][V(\hat{W}(\theta))][\hat{J}^{-1}(\theta)]',$$

where $V(\hat{W}(\theta))$ is the **covariance matrix** of $\hat{W}(\theta)$. Finally, θ is replaced by its estimator $\hat{\theta}$, in both $\hat{J}^{-1}(\theta)$ and $V(\hat{W}(\theta))$ to obtain the estimator of the covariance matrix of $\hat{\theta}$:

$$\hat{V}(\hat{\theta}) = [\hat{J}^{-1}(\hat{\theta})][\hat{V}(\hat{W}(\hat{\theta}))][\hat{J}^{-1}(\hat{\theta})]'.$$

Binder [1] gives regularity conditions that are needed to ensure the asymptotic normality of the parameters $W_i(\hat{\theta})$ and the consistency of $\hat{V}(\hat{\theta})$. These conditions include:

1. the existence of a parameter space that contains a neighborhood of the parameter θ;
2. the existence of a sequence of sample designs and populations which admits asymptotically normal estimators for certain population totals and consistent estimators for the variance of the estimate of the totals: in particular, $\hat{W}(\theta)$ is approximately normally distributed for fixed θ;
3. some continuity and limiting conditions on $W(\theta)$ and its partial derivatives, and a continuity condition on the variance of the estimated total.

Furthermore, Binder [1, Corollary 2] shows that the asymptotic distribution of $\sqrt{n}(\hat{\theta} - \theta)$ is the same as the asymptotic distribution of a **random variable** that is **multivariate normal** with mean zero and variance–covariance matrix $n[\hat{J}^{-1}(\hat{\theta})][\hat{V}\hat{W}(\hat{\theta})][\hat{J}^{-1}(\hat{\theta})]'$.

The question is often raised as to how good the linearization method is compared with other alternatives. There are basically three major competing methods: balanced repeated replication (BRR), jackknife, and **bootstrap** methods.

The drawbacks of the linearization methods are:

1. Linearization methods require computation of derivatives, and hence are more difficult to program than BRR or jackknife. Linearization methods are also limited to smooth functions of observations.
2. The impact of weight adjustments, such as **poststratification** or **nonresponse**, on variance estimation is difficult to account for, and is often ignored in most implementations.

The advantages for the linearization method are:

1. They require substantially less computational resources than jackknife and BRR and are most suitable for large datasets.
2. They are applicable to a large number of situations, and can be applied to **multistage** designs with or without replacements. BRR and jackknife are somewhat limited in this respect.

Kreswki & Rao [5], and Rao & Wu [7] have compared the three methods. Linearization methods are less **biased** and more stable than BRR or jackknife methods. Asymptotically, all of the methods provide **consistent estimators** of the variances, and hence the differences between them get smaller as the sample size increases. Overall there are no compelling reasons to choose one method over the others, and the decision to select a method should be based on convenience and available software. Currently, three software packages have implemented variance estimation using the linearization method. These are: SUDAAN, by Research Triangle Institute; PCCARP, by Iowa State University; and STATA, by Stata Corporation (*see* **Software, Biostatistical**).

References

[1]   Binder, D.A. (1983). On the variances of asymptotically normal estimators from complex surveys, *International Statistical Review* **51**, 279–292.

[2]   Binder, D.A. (1992). Fitting Cox's proportional hazards models from survey data, *Biometrika* **79**, 139–147.

[3] Folsom, R.E. (1974). *National Assessment Approach to Sampling Error Estimation, Sampling Error Monograph*, Prepared for National Assessment of Educational Progress, Denver.

[4] Kish, L. & Frankel, M.R. (1974). Inference from complex surveys, *Journal of Royal Statistical Society, Series B* **36**, 1–37.

[5] Krewski, D. & Rao, J.N.K. (1981). Inference from stratified samples: properties of the linearization, jackknife and balanced repeated replication methods, *Annals of Statistics* **9**, 25–45.

[6] Quenouille, M.H. (1956). Note on bias in estimation, *Biometrika* **43**, 353–360.

[7] Rao, J.N.K. & Wu, C.F.J. (1985). Inference from stratified samples: second order analysis of three methods for nonlinear statistics, *Journal of the American Statistical Association* **80**, 620–630.

[8] Shah, B.V., Holt, M.M. & Folsom, R.E. (1977). Inference about regression models from survey data, *Bulletin of the International Statistical Institute* **47**, 43–57.

[9] Tepping, B.J. (1968). The estimation of variance in complex surveys, in *American Statistical Association 1968 Proceedings of the Section on Social Statistics*. American Statistical Association, Alexandria, pp. 11–18.

[10] Tukey, J.W. (1958). Bias and confidence in not quite large samples, *Annals of Mathematical Statistics* **29**, 614.

[11] Woodruff, R.S. (1971). A simple method for approximating the variance of a complicated estimate, *Journal of the American Statistical Association* **66**, 411–414.

BABUBHAI V. SHAH

Lineweaver–Burk Plot *see* Michaelis–Menten Equation

Link Function *see* Generalized Linear Model

Linkage Analysis, Model-Based

In the field of **human genetics**, the main goal has been to identify the **genes** that are responsible for various phenotypes (*see* **Genotype**) – typically diseases. The primary method for doing so has been through looking at phenotypically silent marker loci that are randomly distributed in the genome (*see* **Polymorphism**), and trying to determine which such loci have alleles that tend to cosegregate in families with the trait of interest. In linkage analysis one tries to estimate the frequency with which the marker and disease gene segregate together in families. When we talk of model-based linkage analysis, it is assumed that one can fully describe the mode of action of the disease gene, i.e. its allele frequency (*see* **Gene Frequency Estimation**) and the **penetrances** for each disease locus genotype (*see* **Gene**). When one does not know these quantities accurately, one often applies model-free linkage analysis methods (*see* **Linkage Analysis, Model-Free**), which effectively correspond to special cases of model-based linkage analysis. Similarly, it can be shown that other methods for detecting correlations between a marker locus and disease gene on a population level through **linkage disequilibrium** analysis can also be considered as special cases of model-based linkage analysis. For this reason, it is important to understand the principles of model-based linkage analysis, because their principles are behind all statistical gene mapping techniques (*see* **Genetic Map Functions**).

Biological Basis of Linkage

The human genetic material is composed of large linear units of deoxyribonucleic acid (DNA) called chromosomes, each of which contains a long linear sequence of genes. These genes are **DNA sequences** that tell the cell how to construct a specific protein, and thus these genes provide the blueprint from which a person is assembled. There are 22 pairs of chromosomes in each human cell, plus a pair of sex chromosomes (X and Y) which determine the sex of an individual (XX individuals are female, and XY individuals are male). Each person receives one copy of each chromosome from his mother and one copy from his father, and thus each person has 50% of his DNA inherited from each parent. Since 50% of one's genes come from each parent, there is a **correlation** between related individuals at the phenotypic level, and thus the common observation that certain diseases "run in families". The male sperm cell and the female egg cell each contain one copy of each chromosome (haploid state) from the father and mother, respectively, instead of two copies of each chromosome as in a normal somatic cell (diploid state). When the sperm and egg combine to form a new child, this infant again has two copies of each chromosome. The important step in determining the genetic makeup of the new child is to look at how the single copy of each chromosome is selected for each gamete. The process by which these haploid gametes are generated is called meiosis. If we label the two copies of chromosome N that a given parent has as N_a and N_b (where this individual received chromosome N_a from his father and chromosome N_b from his mother), then **Mendel's laws** dictate that which copy of each chromosome is transmitted to any given gamete is determined at random, and that each chromosome is inherited independently of every other. Thus, the probability that a gamete receives chromosome 1_b equals the probability that it receives 1_a, and the same holds for chromosomes 2,3, and so on. In this simplified model of inheritance, if an allele located somewhere on chromosome 1_a was received by a given gamete, then the probability of another allele on chromosome 1_a also being inherited would be 1, while the probability of an allele located on chromosome 2_a being inherited would be 0.5. If life were this simple, then we could easily test whether or not two genes were on the same chromosome (syntenic) by checking whether any gamete ever received the a allele at one gene and the b allele at the other. Under the **null hypothesis** that two genes are on different chromosomes, 50% of gametes would receive the a allele at one gene and the b allele at the other, and it would thus be very easy to test for synteny.

In human meiosis, however, it is not as simple as this. There is an additional source of variation in the genetic material. During meiosis the two copies of each chromosome line up next to each other and undergo a random process called recombination in which the two copies of each chromosome can exchange their genetic material with each other (as illustrated in Figure 1). In fact, there may be many such crossover events per chromosome in each meiotic event, and thus there is a great deal of variation between even the most tightly related people. When an odd number of crossover events occur between two genes, the alleles from different ancestral chromosome are received (i.e. allele a

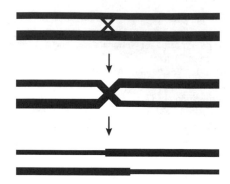

Figure 1 Pictorial representation of recombination. The (thick and thin) lines represent homologous chromosomes during meiosis; the black X in the top of the figure represents a recombination event, one outcome of which is indicated in the figure

at one locus and allele b at the other) – in this situation we say that a recombination of the genetic material has occurred between these two loci – the combination of alleles a at one locus and b at the other is a new combination that was not present on either parental chromosome. If an even number of crossovers occurs between two genes, then the same combination of alleles as in the parents is present in the gamete – this is termed a nonrecombination. If two loci are on different chromosome, they recombine with probability 50% (since, as was indicated earlier, given allele a was inherited at a given point on chromosome 1, the probability of an allele on chromosome 2 being present in the gamete in its b form is 50%). Similarly, if two loci are very far apart on the same chromosome (and we assume an absence of chromatid interference) they also recombine with probability 50%, but when two loci are very close together on the same chromosome, the probability of a recombination between them tends toward 0 as the distance between them decreases. Thus it becomes possible to devise a means of testing for linkage between two loci by looking at whether they recombine with probability 50% or less.

There are a large number of loci spread randomly throughout the human genome called marker loci that have no known function, but that are very variable from person to person, and whose positions in the genome are well known. It is straightforward to determine the genotype of any individual at these polymorphic DNA sequence variations, and thus we can look for genes with unknown position in the genome by testing whether the gene of interest recombines with a marker locus with probability less than 50%. Since there are marker loci spread throughout the genome, at least one of them should be linked to any new gene we wish to isolate. The goal of linkage analysis is to identify marker loci that recombine with our trait locus with low probability, such that we may significantly narrow down the portion of the total genome where this gene can be found by subsequent labor-intensive molecular analysis. The closer we can get to the gene through the simple process of linkage analysis, the easier it will be to identify, though typically it is impossible to get within less than 2 cM – approximately 2 000 000 base pairs – through linkage analysis with a disease having a known mode of inheritance, while for complex traits with an unknown mode of inheritance, it may be difficult to get within less than 10 cM (10 000 000 base pairs), further complicating the subsequent molecular analyses required. The next Sections introduce the mathematical techniques employed in the testing and estimation of linkage in humans, starting from the simplest situations and continuing through to the general case.

Lod Score Analysis

The most commonly employed statistic in human genetic linkage analysis is based on the principle of **maximum likelihood**. In this, we compute the probability of the observed data under different assumptions about the unknown parameter – here the recombination fraction (typically denoted as θ). The null hypothesis is that $\theta = 0.5$, and the alternative is that $\theta < 0.5$, so the test statistic is based on the maximum of the **likelihood ratio** $\Lambda(\theta) = L(\theta)/L(\theta = \frac{1}{2})$. For purely historical reasons, the lod score function commonly used is $Z(\theta) = \log_{10}[\Lambda(\theta)]$; however, the quantity $2 \ln \Lambda$ is much more theoretically pleasing since, asymptotically, $\max_\theta[2 \ln \Lambda(\theta)](= \Lambda_{\max})$ is distributed as a mixture of a 50% point mass at 0 and 50% $\chi^2_{(1)}$ – the 50% point mass at zero because of the one-sided alternative, $\theta < 0.5$ (if $\hat{\theta} = 0.5$, $\Lambda_{\max} = 0$) and other arguments (cf. [15], [20], and [7]). The conventional critical value used in linkage analysis for calling a test significant is $Z \geq 3$, which corresponds to a *P* **value** of 0.0001 if we assume the distribution given above. The reason for insisting on such a small *P* value is due to the multiple testing

employed (*see* **Multiple Comparisons**) if one were to conduct a full genome scan with many markers, and the low prior probability of linkage to a randomly selected marker locus (see [6], [11], [16], and [21] for more details).

Counting Recombinants and Nonrecombinants – Phase-Known Pedigrees

In some situations it is possible to directly observe whether a recombination occurred or not between two loci in a given meiosis. This is commonly the case in animal crosses, where you can breed animals to the point where you know which of their offspring are the results of recombinant meioses and which are nonrecombinant. Let us assume that our data are in the form of genotypes, so we can write the pedigree **likelihood** as

$$L(\theta) = \Pr(\text{genotypes}_{\text{parents}})$$
$$\times \Pr(\text{genotypes}_{\text{offspring}}|\text{genotypes}_{\text{parents}}),$$

and the lod score can then be written as

$$\log_{10} \frac{L(\theta)}{L\left(\theta = \frac{1}{2}\right)} \log_{10} =$$

$$\frac{\Pr(\text{genotypes}_{\text{parents}})}{\times \Pr(\text{genotypes}_{\text{offspring}}|\text{genotypes}_{\text{parents}}; \theta)}{\Pr(\text{genotypes}_{\text{parents}})}$$
$$\times \Pr\left(\text{genotypes}_{\text{offspring}}|\text{genotypes}_{\text{parents}}; \theta = \frac{1}{2}\right)$$

Note that in the ratio we can factor out $\Pr(\text{genotypes}_{\text{parents}})$, since this factor is independent of the recombination fraction, as the genotypes are known and identical in numerator and denominator. Therefore, assuming we can count the number, k, of recombinants out of n meioses (leaving $n - k$ nonrecombinants), the likelihood is simply $L(\theta) = \theta^k(1 - \theta)^{n-k}$. The maximum likelihood estimate of the recombination fraction in this case is trivial to compute as $\hat{\theta} = k/n$ if $k < n/2$; $\hat{\theta} = 0.5$ if $k \geq n/2$ (since values of $\theta > 0.5$ are inadmissible). While this estimate of θ is biased (because of the inadmissibility of estimates of $\theta > 0.5$), it can be shown to be asymptotically unbiased (cf. [16]). It is possible to count recombinants and nonrecombinants in situations when the phase is known. When we say the

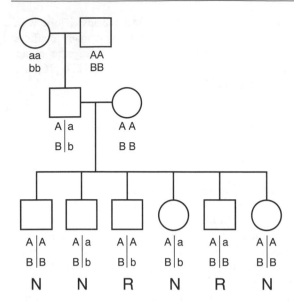

Figure 2 Sample phase-known pedigree with two codominant loci indicated – the first locus has two alleles (A and a) and the second locus has alleles B and b. Nonrecombinant meioses are indicated by "N" and recombinant meioses by "R"

phase is known we mean that it is possible to tell which alleles were inherited from each grandparent. Consider the pedigree shown in Figure 2; in that pedigree it is apparent that allele A at the first locus and allele B at the second locus in the father were inherited together from the grandfather; and similarly alleles a and b were inherited together from the grandmother. If the two loci are syntenic, it would mean they are on the same chromosome in the father. In this case, among the children all A B or a b haplotypes are nonrecombinants (parental types), while all children who received haplotypes A b or a B are recombinants (or nonparental types). In this example, there are four nonrecombinant children and two recombinants, so our lod score is computed as

$$Z(\theta) = \log_{10} \frac{\theta^2(1-\theta)^4}{(0.5)^2(0.5)^4} = \log_{10} 2^6 \theta^2 (1-\theta)^4.$$

In this pedigree, the maximum likelihood estimate of θ is $2/6 = 1/3$, so the maximum lod score is $Z(1/3) = 0.1475$. Note that the information coming from alleles inherited from the mother by the offspring was not included in this computation. This is because there is no linkage information coming from the mother as she is homozygous (*see*

Heterozygosity) at both loci, and thus she transmits alleles A and B to all children with probability 1, independently of the recombination fraction. In fact, a parent has to be heterozygous at both loci to be informative for linkage. If the mother were Aa at the first locus and BB at the second, then every child would receive a B allele with probability 1, and at the other locus A is inherited with probability 0.5, independently of the recombination fraction (since the inheritance of the B allele is ubiquitous).

Lod Scores in Phase-Unknown Pedigrees

Often there is some ambiguity about the parental phase – for example, if the grandparents were unavailable for genotyping. Consider the same pedigree without the grandparents having been typed (as shown in Figure 3). In this situation, there are two possible phases for the father – either he could have phase A B/a b or he could have phase A b/a B. A priori these two phases are equally likely (assuming an absence of linkage disequilibrium), so we either have four recombinants and two nonrecombinants or we have four nonrecombinants and two recombinants. Early human geneticists would throw these pedigrees

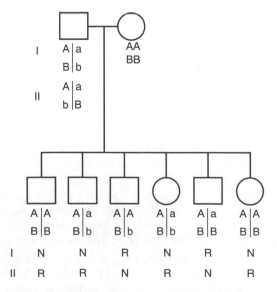

Figure 3 Sample phase-unknown pedigree with two possible phases for the father – indicated as I and II – under each of his offspring is an indication of whether the individual had a recombination or not between these two loci under each possible phase for the father

away because it was thought that they contained no useful information about linkage. However, there is information in these families. The likelihood is computed as

$$L(\theta) = \Pr(\text{parents})\Pr(\text{off}|\text{parents}; \theta)$$

$$= \sum_{\text{phases}} \Pr(\text{phase}_{\text{father}})$$

$$\times \Pr(\text{genotypes}_{\text{off}}|\text{phase}_{\text{father}}; \theta),$$

since the only ambiguity in the parental genotypes is in the paternal phase. In this example, each phase has probability 0.5, so

$$L(\theta) = \tfrac{1}{2}\theta^4(1-\theta)^2 + \tfrac{1}{2}\theta^2(1-\theta)^4$$

$$= \tfrac{1}{2}\theta^2(1-\theta)^2[\theta^2 + (1-\theta)^2].$$

Note that the maximum likelihood estimate (MLE) of θ is not trivial to compute by hand, although it can be estimated using numerical maximization techniques; using the ILINK program of the LINKAGE package [13] (*see* **Software for Genetic Epidemiology**), the MLE is found to be 0.5. Even though there are not 50% of meioses in this case showing evidence of recombination, as analyzed in detail by Nordheim et al. [15], there are an enormous number of potential phase-unknown pedigrees that all yield an estimate of $\theta = 0.5$. That is not to say that phase-unknown pedigrees do not provide information about linkage in general. Consider a phase-unknown pedigree with N children all of whom received the identical alleles at both loci – this would either represent N recombinants or N nonrecombinants. The likelihood would then be equal to $L(\theta) = \tfrac{1}{2}\theta^N + \tfrac{1}{2}(1-\theta)^N$, which can be shown to be maximized when $\theta = 0$, giving a lod score of

$$Z_{\text{PU}}(\theta = 0) = \log_{10} \frac{\tfrac{1}{2}(0)^N + \tfrac{1}{2}(1)^N}{\tfrac{1}{2}\left(\tfrac{1}{2}\right)^N + \tfrac{1}{2}\left(\tfrac{1}{2}\right)^N}$$

$$= \log_{10} \frac{\tfrac{1}{2}}{\left(\tfrac{1}{2}\right)^N} = (N-1)\log_{10}(2),$$

where the subscript PU stands for phase-unknown. If the pedigree were phase-known with six nonrecombinants, then the likelihood would be $L(\theta) = (1 - \theta)^N$, which is also maximized when $\theta = 0$, but giving a lod score of $Z_{\text{PK}}(\theta = 0) = \log_{10}(1)^N/\left(\tfrac{1}{2}\right)^N =$

$N\log_{10}(2)$, where the subscript PK indicates phase-known. So, in each pedigree there is a cost of one meiosis when the phase is unknown if there is no recombination – when there is recombination in the pedigree the cost is even higher, as was illustrated by the previous example. It may seem like a small cost initially, but if you consider that the average sibship size is between two and three, the cost can be huge in a large set of pedigrees. The lod score in each phase-unknown pedigree is $Z_{\text{PU}}(\theta = 0) = [(N-1)/N]Z_{\text{PK}}(\theta = 0)$ when all sibs are nonrecombinant. Note that this is an upper bound on the phase-unknown lod score as a function of the phase-known lod score. In general, $Z_{\text{PU}}(\hat{\theta}) \leq [(N-1)/N]Z_{\text{PK}}(\tilde{\theta})$, where θ is estimated separately in the phase-known and phase-unknown cases, and there is linkage. In the US, most sibships are of size two or three, so that the lod scores in each pedigree are at least 1.5–2 times higher for phase-known pedigrees than for phase-unknown pedigrees, when there is linkage between the two loci. Since lod scores can be added across pedigrees at the same recombination fraction values (since all pedigrees are independent, and independent likelihoods can be multiplied), the sum over a large set of pedigrees will also be 1.5–2 times larger or more if there is linkage and the phase can be established unequivocally.

Genotypes Unknown

We are often confronted with the complication that not all individuals' genotypes are known. Remember that, when we know the genotypes of the parents, the pedigree likelihood for a phase-known nuclear pedigree is

$$L(\theta; \text{data}) = \Pr(g_{\text{pa}})\Pr(g_{\text{ma}}) \prod_{\text{offspring}}$$

$$\times \Pr(g_{\text{offs}}|g_{\text{ma}}, g_{\text{pa}}; \theta),$$

where g_{ma} is the genotype of the mother, etc.; and in the case of unknown phase it is just

$$L(\text{data})$$

$$= \sum_{\text{phase}} \Pr(g_{\text{ma}}, \text{Phase}_{\text{ma}})\Pr(g_{\text{pa}}, \text{Phase}_{\text{pa}})$$

$$\times \prod_{\text{offspring}} P(g_{\text{offs}}|g_{\text{pa}}, g_{\text{ma}}, \text{Phase}_{\text{pa}}, \text{Phase}_{\text{ma}}; \theta).$$

If we were interested in the actual probability of the data, then we would have to use the allele frequencies at each marker locus in order to compute $\Pr(g_{pa})$ from the allele frequencies for the two loci. For example, if g_{ma} were AA at one locus and BB at the other, then $\Pr(g_{ma})$ would be $\Pr(A)\Pr(A)\Pr(B)\Pr(B)$ if we assume **Hardy–Weinberg equilibrium** and absence of linkage disequilibrium. Note that, in the phase-known situation, the lod score is

$$Z(\theta) = \log_{10} \frac{\Pr(g_{ma})\Pr(g_{pa}) \times \displaystyle\prod_{\text{offspring}} \Pr(g_{\text{offs}}|g_{ma}, g_{pa}; \theta)}{\Pr(g_{ma})\Pr(g_{pa}) \times \displaystyle\prod_{\text{offspring}} \Pr\left(g_{\text{offs}}|g_{ma}, g_{pa}; \theta = \tfrac{1}{2}\right)},$$

and we do not need to worry about the exact values of the probability of the parental genotypes, since they can be factored out of this ratio and have no effect on the lod score – this makes sense because the parental genotypes tell us nothing in and of themselves about the recombination fraction. Similarly, in the phase-unknown case, we also know the genotypes of the parents, so we can factor the independent genotype and phase probabilities as $\Pr(g_{ma}, \text{Phase}_{ma}) = \Pr(g_{ma})\Pr(\text{Phase}_{ma})$, assuming absence of linkage disequilibrium, and so

$$
\begin{aligned}
Z(\theta) = \log_{10} & \left(\Pr(g_{ma})\Pr(g_{pa}) \sum_{\text{phase}_{ma}} \Pr(\text{Phase}_{ma}) \right. \\
& \times \sum_{\text{phase}_{pa}} \Pr(\text{Phase}_{pa}) \prod_{\text{offspring}} \Pr(g_{\text{offs}}|g_{ma}, g_{pa}, \\
& \text{Phase}_{ma}, \text{Phase}_{pa}; \theta) \Big/ \Pr(g_{ma})\Pr(g_{pa}) \\
& \times \sum_{\text{phase}_{ma}} \Pr(\text{Phase}_{ma}) \sum_{\text{phase}_{pa}} \Pr(\text{Phase}_{pa}) \\
& \times \prod_{\text{offspring}} \Pr\left(g_{\text{offs}}|g_{ma}, g_{pa}, \text{Phase}_{ma}, \right. \\
& \left. \left. \text{Phase}_{pa}; \theta = \tfrac{1}{2}\right) \right).
\end{aligned}
$$

Again, the parental genotype probabilities factor out of this equation, but the phase probabilities do not.

In fact, it is possible to consider the phase as an integral part of the parental genotype, and in that case we see that we are effectively taking the sum over all possible parental genotypes (with phase), and weighting them by their probabilities. This argument can be easily extended to cover situations in which we known nothing about the genotype of the parents. In that case, the likelihood can be written as

$$
\begin{aligned}
L(\theta; \text{data}) = \sum_{G_{ma}} \sum_{G_{pa}} & \Pr(G_{ma})\Pr(G_{pa}) \\
& \times \prod_{\text{offspring}} \Pr(g_{\text{offs}}|G_{ma}, G_{pa}; \theta),
\end{aligned}
$$

where G_i is the genotype with the phase of individual i; note that for the offspring we do not know the phase. If we wished to express this formula in terms of each offspring's genotype with phase, then it would be

$$
\begin{aligned}
L(\theta; \text{data}) = \sum_{G_{ma}} \Pr(G_{ma}) & \sum_{G_{pa}} \Pr(G_{pa}) \\
& \times \prod_{\text{offspring}} \sum_{G_{\text{offs}}} \Pr(G_{\text{offs}}|G_{ma}, G_{pa}; \theta).
\end{aligned}
$$

In this way we can also include offspring whose genotype is unknown, or who have some ambiguity in their genotypes. Only the parental genotypes are functions of the allele frequencies, while the genotypes of their children are dependent solely on the parental genotypes and the recombination fraction in each case.

Genotype Unknown – Phenotype Known

It is important to note that thus far we have been dealing only with genotypes, and we have assumed that we can either identify the genotype or else we know nothing. In reality we are usually somewhere in the middle; the most important way linkage analysis is used is to identify genes which affect the expression of some trait, typically by increasing the probability of becoming affected with some disease. In this situation, there are additional parameters needed to perform the linkage analysis – we need to quantify the probability of the phenotype conditional on each of the possible genotypes at the locus in question. For example, if we have a dominant disease with full penetrance, then this means that we have a disease-predisposing locus with, typically, two alleles, D and +, where Pr(disease|DD) = Pr(disease|D+) = 1; Pr(disease|++) = 0. Note that this also uniquely determines the penetrances for the phenotype "unaffected" as well, because Pr(disease|DD) + Pr (unaffected|DD) = 1. In this case Pr(unaffected|DD) = Pr(unaffected|D+) = 0, and Pr(unaffected|++) = 1. For a fully penetrant recessive disease, Pr (disease|DD) = 1, and Pr(disease|D+) = Pr(disease| ++) = 0. These are the two most classical situations in which the genotypes are not uniquely determined by the phenotypes. These penetrances can be factored into the likelihood in a straightforward manner as

$$L(\theta; \text{data}) = \Pr(\text{Ph}_{\text{ma}})\Pr(\text{Ph}_{\text{pa}})$$
$$\times \prod_{\text{offspring}} \Pr(\text{Ph}_{\text{offs}}|\text{Ph}_{\text{ma}}, \text{Ph}_{\text{pa}}; \theta),$$

where Ph_i is the observed phenotype for individual i at all loci. If we allow for the penetrances as described above, we know that $\Pr(\text{Ph}) = \sum_G \Pr(G)\Pr(\text{Ph}|G)$. For parents, $\Pr(G)$ can be computed from the allele frequencies at each locus, and $\Pr(\text{Ph}|G)$ is the penetrance that must be specified for each locus. The sum is taken over all possible genotypes at all loci. If the individual is an offspring in the pedigree, then $\Pr(G)$ is replaced by $\Pr(G|G_{\text{ma}}, G_{\text{pa}}; \theta)$, and the penetrance remains unchanged, since this is considered to depend only on the individual's genotype. In this way we can take into account any possible relationships between genotype and phenotype. Note that many genotypes will not be possible, as they are incompatible with Mendelian laws – for example, you cannot have parents who are AA and AA having a child who has genotype aa. For this reason, many terms will have zero probability. Complicated computer programs have been written to perform these calculations for any set of penetrances and general pedigree structures. For further details about the technical aspects of likelihood calculations in linkage analysis the reader is referred to [1] and [16]. The important thing here is to see why it is necessary to specify all the parameters, and how they affect the analysis.

Fully Penetrant Recessive Traits

The simplest mode of inheritance to consider for a disease is one with full penetrance and no phenocopies. Let us start by considering a simple

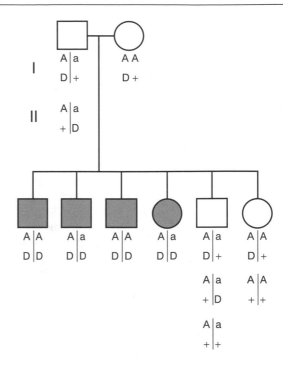

Figure 4 Sample pedigree with a fully penetrant autosomal recessive disease segregating. Solid shapes indicate affected individuals with this trait, and open figures are unaffected

recessive trait, which means that Pr(affected|DD) = 1 and Pr(affected|D + or ++) = 0. Look at the pedigree in Figure 4. In this pedigree, the possible genotypes (with phase) for each individual are indicated – the probabilities of all other genotypes can be shown to be 0. Because the trait is fully penetrant recessive, all affected individuals must have genotype DD, and all unaffected individuals are either D + or ++. Because the parents have affected children, they must each have at least one D allele, and because they are unaffected, they cannot have two – therefore, they are D|+. The only ambiguous cases are the two unaffected children, who could be either ++ or D+, since both of these are compatible with the parental genotypes and the phenotype unaffected. Because the mother is not heterozygous at both loci, we cannot tell whether recombination occurred between the trait and marker loci (since all children must receive the A allele from her with probability 1, irrespective of what disease allele they received). Because there is no ambiguity in the genotype of the affected individuals, it is clear that they provide most of the information about linkage.

The ambiguity of the other sibs' disease locus genotypes adds noise to the analysis. Because disease alleles are typically rare, and recessive diseases are quite often lethal, it is rare for parents to be affected themselves, and thus the majority of pedigrees which one will ascertain (*see* **Ascertainment**) are either nuclear pedigrees, as in Figure 4, or inbred (*see* **Inbreeding**) pedigrees, where the disease alleles in the affected kids are identical by descent from some common ancestor.

In the case of inbred pedigrees, most affected children would be homozygous at a marker locus tightly linked to the recessive trait locus [19] (this is also the fundamental cause of linkage disequilibrium if one thinks of populations as large extended inbred pedigrees). Smith [19] proposed that an efficient strategy for detecting linkage with rare recessive traits in inbred pedigrees would be to look for marker loci at which affected individuals are more frequently homozygous than expected – a technique that has come to be known as homozygosity mapping. It is critical to point out that homozygosity mapping is not a different statistical technique to analyze data – in fact, one normally applies standard model-based linkage analysis to the pedigree in question. It is merely an efficient technique for minimizing the amount of genotyping one needs to detect linkage, by only typing one affected child from a consanguineous marriage segregating a recessive disease in the initial genome screen – later, of course, one should go back and genotype the parents and other family members to make sure that the individual has received the marker alleles identical by descent (IBD) from one common ancestor.

Fully Penetrant Dominant Disease

The second classical model for trait inheritance is fully penetrant dominant, in which $\Pr(\text{affected}|DD \text{ or } D+) = 1$ and $\Pr(\text{affected}|++) = 0$. The majority of affected individuals in such a disease are going to have genotype $D+$, because the disease allele is typically very rare, and all affected children have at least one affected parent. As a result of this, pedigrees segregating fully penetrant dominant diseases are typically large and extend over multiple generations, with smaller sibships than in recessive disease pedigrees. This is because, in recessive diseases, when we ascertain pedigrees to have more than one affected child, we are biased toward large sibships,

whereas for dominant diseases there are typically affected individuals in many generations. For this reason, dominant traits are often transmitted in phase-known meioses, whereas most meioses in recessive pedigrees are phase-unknown (typically only the bottom generation has affected individuals).

Complex Disease

A complex disease is one for which either the mode of inheritance is unknown, there are multiple genes involved, diagnosis is uncertain, or environmental factors are the entire cause of the disease, and no genes are involved at all [12]. Typically, the penetrances are not 0 and 1, but somewhere in the middle, even for single gene disorders. It may be that a disease has a late age of onset, which is variable from individual to individual, or it may be that certain environmental factors are necessary in combination with the genes to produce a phenotype, etc. (*see* **Penetrance**).

When such complexities are present, it becomes difficult to do a good model-based linkage analysis, because the linkage analysis is based on specified parameters, as indicated above. When these parameters are incorrectly specified, the recombination fraction is usually overestimated, and the lod scores may be smaller than if the model was correct. That is not to say the power is always highest when analysis is done under the correct model – power to detect linkage often tends to be higher when the genetic effect of a locus on the trait is overestimated, especially if the mode of inheritance is actually very weak – hence the high power of **"model-free" linkage methods**, which are in many cases mathematically equivalent to lod score analyses under models with very strong genetic effects, as shown later in this article. However, when the mode of inheritance is incorrectly specified, it is impossible to get accurate estimates of the location of a disease gene from the recombination fraction estimates, and the test statistic itself is the only means of determining the location of the disease gene. For this and other reasons it is very difficult to fine-map a disease gene for a complex trait in an equivalently sized dataset, and the accuracy will be orders of magnitude less with complex traits. As an extension of this argument, it will also probably be very difficult to find linkage disequilibrium with complex trait predisposing genes, as those genes are often very common, thus leading to extreme allelic and nonallelic heterogeneity in the population-as-pedigree.

Testing for Linkage – Positive and Negative

Originally, the lod score method was proposed as a sequential procedure in which one would continue to add more and more families until the lod score at some predetermined recombination fraction either exceeded 3, in which case linkage was accepted, or fell below −2, in which case linkage was said to be excluded [14]. However, the common practice changed such that people now maximize the lod score over the recombination fraction to prove linkage with greater **power**, while to exclude linkage they simply look at all values of θ for which the lod score remains below −2 (all points to the left of the upward pointing arrow in Figure 5). The example shown in Figure 5 would allow for the conclusion that there is linkage with MLE of a recombination fraction equal to $\hat{\theta}$, as indicated in the Figure, and yet linkage is also excluded at small recombination fractions in the same pedigree. Since it is known, for linkage analysis under an incorrect mode of inheritance assumption, that the recombination fraction MLEs are biased in an upward direction [17], such decision rules for "exclusion" mapping are not very useful when the mode of inheritance is not well characterized and correctly modeled.

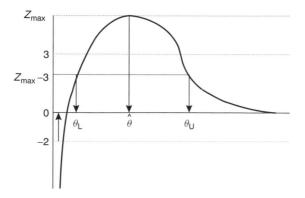

Figure 5 Sample graph of two-point lod scores as a function of the recombination fraction, with: indicators of the maximum lod score, Z_{max}; the maximum likelihood estimate of the recombination fraction, $\hat{\theta}$; the upper and lower limits of its 3-unit support interval, (θ_U and θ_L); and the exclusion region (to the right of the upwardly pointing arrow)

In modern human genetic linkage studies a large number of markers are tested in a fixed set of pedigrees. In this context, the spirit of lod score analysis has changed dramatically since the days of Morton [14]. We are no longer testing one specific marker, but an entire genome-wide set of markers, typically spaced at intervals from 5–10 cM, in which case there would be about 600 such markers in a full genomic scan. In analyzing this situation, there is a multiple testing problem to be taken into account. If there is a single gene disorder, it has been argued that the gene must be somewhere, and thus as more markers are shown to be unlinked, the prior probability that one of the remaining markers is linked is increased, and this would theoretically compensate for the large number of tests. However, this argument does not hold if we are using linkage analysis to prove there is a gene. For certain complex diseases we have no proof of a genetic component at all, despite the best efforts of **segregation analysis**. If there is no gene, the prior probabilities of linkage are not increased after many markers are all found to be unlinked to the trait.

The current theoretical arguments about critical values are based on the null hypothesis distribution of the lod score maximized over all markers in the genome. If there is no linkage, different analyses have predicted the probability of a lod score of 3 arising by chance for some marker to be between 0.005 and 1, depending on the pedigree structure, marker informativeness, and other assumptions (e.g. [9] and [22]). For example, for a fixed critical value, with more informative markers, there is a lower rate of **false** (and true) **positives** over the whole genome. There is thus a small but nontrivial chance of getting at least one false positive in a genome screen with a large number of markers. In practice, one might consider how their best lod scores compare with the lod scores at other markers throughout the genome – obviously the highest lod scores are the most promising, and the lower ones are less so (cf. [22]). There are no hard and fast rules, because molecular technology has progressed to the point where one can feasibly obtain genotypes for as many markers as one wants. Ideally, one should consider the lod scores for all markers in a completed genome scan jointly before interpreting borderline results, in contrast to the old days (i.e. 3–4 years ago) of linkage analysis where typing small numbers of markers was a huge chore. For complex diseases, a lod score of

3 is not so convincing today, unless it is with a **candidate gene**, or it is interpreted in the context of a full genome scan.

Estimation of the Recombination Fraction

When the mode of inheritance is known, it is possible to compute the exact likelihood for the data, and the maximum likelihood estimates of the recombination fraction, while typically biased, are consistent. To demonstrate the **bias** in a very simple example, let us consider a phase-known pedigree with four informative meioses, and let us assume that the recombination fraction is 0.50. Then we compute the expectation of the MLE. The possible outcomes are given in Table 1. Because $E(\hat{\theta}) = \sum_{\text{Data}} \hat{\theta} \Pr(\text{data})$, where the sum is taken over all possible outcomes, in this case, while $\theta = 0.5$, $E(\hat{\theta}) = 0.40625$, which shows a considerable downward bias. However, asymptotically, as the number of informative meioses approaches infinity, the **expectation** of the estimate approaches its true value, and therefore the MLE of θ is **consistent**.

That the MLE of the recombination is consistent is valuable to researchers in human genetics, as it gives a means not only to detect linkage through use of the lod score as a test statistic, but also to estimate the distance between the marker locus and the disease-predisposing gene. Normally, because these estimates are not very accurate in small samples, we construct support intervals around the MLE, and say that the true recombination lies somewhere in that interval with reasonable certainty. The k-lod-unit support interval for the MLE of the recombination fraction consists of all values of θ for which $Z(\theta) \geq Z(\hat{\theta}) - k$. Historically, researchers used $k = 1$ to construct a support interval which asymptotically was approximately equivalent to a 95% confidence interval. However, an inconsistency arises when the maximum lod score is greater than 1 and less than 3, because in that case a 1-unit support interval would exclude the null hypothesis $\theta = 0.5$, even though the null hypothesis has not been rejected. Two possible solutions to this problem are in common practice. The original recommendation was to think of linkage analysis as a two-step procedure, i.e. first one tests the null hypothesis of no linkage, and if this null hypothesis is rejected, then and only then do you consider the estimates of the recombination fraction and its 1-unit support interval [3]. Another argument suggests that, since testing and estimation are based on the same statistic, it is impossible to separate the two logically, and for this reason, a 3-lod-unit support interval should be constructed (because the test is typically performed with the critical value of $Z > 3$) [21]. Fundamentally, either argument works, and it all depends on what the end-user wants to believe – the latter procedure will allow support intervals to be constructed even without significant test results, while the former does not; however, the latter procedure gives much wider support intervals, and thus does not narrow down the region in which the investigators would have to look for the gene as much as a 1-unit support interval would. The counter argument is that 1 in 20 times (approximately) the gene would be outside the 1-unit support interval, while only 1 in 10 000 times would the gene fall outside the 3-unit support interval. The choice of support criteria is dependent largely on the desires of the investigator and whether one thinks a 5% chance of missing the gene is a gamble worth taking.

The caveat of all this discussion about estimating recombination fractions is that it is dependent on the accuracy of the parametric model for the disease *and* the marker locus. It presumes that the allele frequencies are all accurately estimated and that the

Table 1 Sample demonstration of the bias in estimates of the recombination fraction in small samples

Pedigree	Outcome			
Recombinants	Nonrecombinants	Pr(data)	$\hat{\theta}$	Pr(data)*$\hat{\theta}$
0	4	(0.5)	0	0
1	3	4(0.5)	0.25	0.0625
2	2	6(0.5)	0.50	0.1875
3	1	4(0.5)	0.50	0.1250
4	0	(0.5)	0.50	0.03125
Total		1		0.40625

penetrances are correct as well. For complex diseases, this is never the case, especially at the trait locus. In many cases, it is impossible to do this correctly when we are restricted to the confines of a single-locus parametric model of disease with no environmental cofactors. There have been attempts made to extend linkage analysis methods to multiple gene traits, and to mixed environmental/genetic models, but they are computationally intensive, and do not tend to increase the power of the test statistic greatly. The only gain from these complications, for most cases studied thus far, is an increase in the accuracy of the recombination fraction estimates. However, in practice, if one is using a single gene model which is known with certainty to be incorrect, one will find that the recombination fraction is always overestimated, and loses all of its meaning; in those situations, the value of the test statistic itself is all we have to use in fine-mapping the trait locus.

Relationships Between "Model-Free" and "Model-Based" Methods

In linkage analysis, **nonparametric methods** have been employed to "increase robustness" [9] and to make the calculations fast and simple [2]. Initially it was impossible to do likelihood-based analysis on complex pedigrees, as for general pedigrees the likelihoods could not be computed in the absence of recent technological and theoretical innovations, while most sib-pair and relative pair analyses could be performed on the back of an envelope. However, as soon as there were additional affected relatives beyond the initial affected relative pair, the analyses become problematic, as there are higher-order correlations among the marker genotypes of multiple affected individuals within a single pedigree. In special situations the multiple relative pairs may be asymptotically pairwise-independent [2], but it is still an approximation to looking at the entire set of affected individuals jointly, as in likelihood-based pedigree analysis.

Recent theoretical studies have demonstrated that one can often use model-based likelihood methods to compute statistics with equivalent properties to the pairs-based statistics, in which the entire set of affected individuals in a pedigree are analyzed jointly, e.g. [8]. Below, the simplest cases are examined in detail for sib-pair analysis and extended-pedigree identity-by-descent (IBD) analyses (*see* **Linkage Analysis, Model-Free**).

Sib-Pair Analysis

It has recently been demonstrated [7, 8] that there is an algebraic equivalence between the sib-pair mean test [2] and parametric linkage analysis under a recessive model. More accurately, it has the same statistical properties as a likelihood-based linkage analysis between the marker locus of interest and a "pseudo-marker", which has genotype 1–2 in the mother, 3–4 in the father, and 2–3 in each affected child. If one sets $\theta = 1/2$ between these two loci, then from each parent the children share one allele at the marker locus IBD with probability $p = \theta^2 + (1 - \theta)^2 = 0.5$, which is the null hypothesis of the sib-pair mean test statistic. When θ is allowed to take on all values between 0 and 0.5, there is a 1:1 mapping of the interval $[\theta : 0, 0.5] \to [p : 0.5, 1]$, and the lod score between the marker locus and this "pseudo-marker" is a simple transformation of the sib-pair mean test statistic, $R = (x - y)^2/(x + y)$, where $Z_{\max} = R/2\ln(10)$, x is the number of alleles shared IBD over all sib-pairs, and y is the number of alleles not shared IBD across all sib-pairs). In light of this equivalence when one is analyzing only sibling pairs, the analogy can be extended to multiplex sibships [10, 18] by computing the lod scores between a marker locus and such a "pseudo-marker" where all affected siblings in a sibship have genotype 2/3. The statistic $R = 2\ln[L(\hat{\theta})/L(\theta = 0.5)]$ has a well-defined distribution which converges rapidly, in as few as 20 sibpairs, to a 50–50 mixture of $\chi^2_{(1)}$ and a point mass at $R = 0$. The traditional mean test, no matter what weighting function is assumed for multiplex sibships [2], has a skewed distribution when larger sibships are analyzed. Analysis of the power of this likelihood-based extension has been shown to be consistently robust and powerful over a wide variety of modes of inheritance [4].

Other Affected Relative Pairs

In other "model-free" methods based on extended pedigrees, it is customary to select a set of pairs of relatives and see if they share more alleles IBD than would be expected if there were no linkage. Traditionally, this has been most frequently done by breaking multiplex pedigrees into all possible pairs of affected relatives, and pretending they are independent of each other, when really there is a complicated set of interdependencies which only go away asymptotically (i.e. in unrealistically large datasets). Ultimately, one is interested in testing whether or not a given marker locus segregates independently of the trait in the entire pedigree. Following the aforementioned logic, in pedigrees without consanguinities, any pair of individuals who are not sibs can share at most one allele IBD. If we have a simple pedigree with only two affected individuals, an artificial "pseudo-marker" locus can be created in which they share the one marker allele IBD that is the most they could possibly share, i.e. they each are assigned a pseudo-marker genotype 1/2, where all founder individuals who are not ancestors of all affected individuals are given genotype 1/1. Performing a likelihood-based analysis of this locus (setting the allele frequency of the 2 allele to be very small) against a marker would represent a test equivalent to an IBD test on this relative pair because the recombination fraction again is a 1:1 transformation of the probability that the two relatives share an allele IBD. The model of the trait "pseudo-marker" genotypes is essentially a rare dominant mode of inheritance in the likelihood calculations. In this way it is possible to develop statistics with properties analogous to various nonparametric IBD methods within the unified context of likelihood-based lod score analysis, giving us a common currency and a feel for the underlying symmetries between conceptually different methods of linkage analysis.

Linkage Disequilibrium

Ultimately, linkage disequilibrium analysis is very similar to the extended pedigree analysis described above. In linkage disequilibrium analyses, the population under study is thought of as one giant pedigree, in which the disease predisposing allele is assumed to have entered a population once, or very few times (*see* **Linkage Disequilibrium**). Then, many generations later, at tightly linked marker loci, the allele which was on the founder chromosome would still be present with a higher frequency among affected individuals. In essence, the null hypothesis is that the marker locus genotypes are independent of the disease, i.e. the disease and marker alleles have segregated independently in this population. Under the alternative hypothesis, however, the assumption is that the affected individuals would share more alleles IBD from this common ancestor than any two randomly selected individuals from the population.

Again, an analogy can be made to likelihood-based linkage analysis in the population, following the paradigm from the previous section, assuming each individual had received 2 alleles IBD (i.e. we typically have to look at genotypes in **case–control** disequilibrium studies). However, in a population, we assume that the individuals under study are so distantly related that we can approximate the linkage analysis by simply comparing the genotype frequencies in affecteds and unaffecteds. If there are known to be closer relationships between certain sets of individuals in the population, it would behoove the analyst to take these correlations into account where relationships can be identified, to avoid erroneous assumptions that all genotypes within case and control samples are really iid.

Algebraic Equivalence ≠ Identical Assumptions

It is, of course, erroneous to say that IBD analysis in sib-pairs "assumes" the mode of inheritance to be recessive – rather, it is more appropriate to say that the sib-pair mean test statistic is algebraically equivalent to lod score analysis under a recessive model (with additional assumptions). The subtle difference between these two statements is critical to appreciate, for the null hypothesis properties of likelihood-based lod score analyses do not depend in any way on the true mode of inheritance, and are valid irrespective of the true state of nature. This same statement holds for nonparametric tests as well: under the null hypothesis, the marker is assumed to segregate randomly and independently of the trait, and thus the true mode of inheritance is irrelevant to the validity of any of these tests.

Conclusion

Likelihood-based parametric linkage analysis is the **gold standard** for detecting disease genes through reverse genetics in pedigree data. There are a number of other procedures (*see* **Linkage Analysis, Model-Free**) which provide simple and rapid approximations to this type of analysis, but ultimately it remains the standard which the nonparametric methods attempt to emulate. Bearing in mind the **Neyman–Pearson lemma**, which states that if there is a best test of a given hypothesis it will be in the form of a likelihood ratio, and also the manner in which full likelihood analysis can use all of the data and not just a small subset thereof, it remains the method of choice. It has been very successful in mapping hundreds of disease-predisposing genes, and while there are no easy answers to the questions of the future – involving common complex diseases – it seems likely that it will be the best unified framework at our disposal to build upon in answering these more complicated but very important problems.

References

[1]   Bailey, N.T.J. (1961). *Introduction to the Mathematical Theory of Genetic Linkage*. Clarendon Press, Oxford.

[2]   Blackwelder, W.C. & Elston, R.C. (1985). A comparison of sib-pair linkage tests for disease susceptibility loci, *Genetic Epidemiology* **2**, 85–97.

[3]   Conneally, P.M., Edwards, J.H., Kidd, K.K., Lalovel, J.M., Morton, N.E., Ott, J. & White, R. (1985). Report on the committee on methods of linkage analysis and reporting, *Cytogenetics and Cell Genetics* **40**, 356–359.

[4]   Davis, S. & Weeks, D.E. (1996). Comparison of non-parametric statistics for detecting linkage in affected-sir-pair data, *American Journal of Human Genetics* **59**, A216.

[5]   Doerge, R.W. (1995). Testing for linkage: phase known/unknown, *Journal of Heredity* **86**, 61–62.

[6]   Ginsburg, E.Kh., Axenovich, T.I. & Goodman, D.W. (1996). On estimation of linkage test power, *Genetic Epidemiology* **13**, 355–366.

[7]   Hyer, R.N., Julier, C. Buckley, J.D. Trucco, M., Rotter, J., Spielman, R., Barnett, A., Bain, S., Boitard, C., Deschamps, I., Todd, J.A., Bell, J.I. & Lathrop, G.M. (1991). High-resolution linkage mapping for susceptibility genes in human polygenic disease: insulin-dependent diabetes mellitus and chromosome 11q, *American Journal of Human Genetics* **48**, 243–257.

[8]   Knapp, M., Seuchter, S.A. Baur, M.P. (1994). Linkage analysis in nuclear families: relationship between affected sib-pair tests and lod score analysis, *Human Heredity* **44**, 44–51.

[9]   Kruglyak, L. & Lander, E.S. (1995). Complete multipoint sib-pair analysis of qualitative and quantitative traits, *American Journal of Human Genetics* **57**, 439–454.

[10]   Kuokkanen, S., Sundvall, M., Terwilliger, J.D., Tienari, P.J. Wikström, J., Holmdahl, R., Pettersson, U. & Peltonen, L. (1996). A putative vulnerability locus to multiple sclerosis maps to 5p14-p12 in a region syntenic to the murine locus EAE2, *Nature Genetics* **13**, 447–480.

[11]   Lander, E. & Kruglyak, L. (1995). Genetic dissection of complex traits: guidelines for interpreting and reporting linkage results, *Nature Genetics* **11**, 241–247.

[12]   Lathrop, G.M., Terwilliger, J.D. & Weeks, D.E. (1996). Multifactorial inheritance and genetic analysis of multifactorial disease, in *Emory & Rimoin's Principles and Practice of Medical Genetics*, 3rd Ed., D.L. Rimoin, J.M. Connor & R.E. Pyeritz, eds. Churchill Livingstone, New York, pp. 333–346.

[13]   Lathrop, G.M., Lalouel, J.M. Julier, C. & Ott, J. (1984). Strategies for multilocus linkage analysis in humans, *Proceedings of the National Academy of Sciences* **81**, 3443–3446.

[14]   Morton, N.E. (1955). Sequential tests for the detection of linkage, *American Journal of Human Genetics* **7**, 277–318.

[15]   Nordheim, E.V. (1984). On the performance of a likelihood ratio test for genetic linkage, *Biometrics* **40**, 785–790.

[16]   Ott, J. (1984). *Analysis of Human Genetic Linkage*, 1st Ed. Johns Hopkins University Press, Baltimore.

[17]   Risch, N. & Giuffra, L. (1992). Model misspecification and multipoint linkage analysis, *Human Heredity* **42**, 77–92.

[18]   Satsangi, J., Parkes, M., Louis, E., Hashimoto, L., Kato, N., Welsh, K., Terwilliger, J.D., Lathrop, G.M., Bell, J.I. & Jewell, D.P. (1996). Two-stage genome-wide search in inflammatory bowel disease provides evidence for susceptibility loci on chromosomes 3,7, and 12, *Nature Genetics* **14**, 199–202.

[19]   Smith, C.A.B. (1953). The detection of linkage in human genetics, *Journal of the Royal Statistical Society, Series B* **15**, 153–184.

[20]   Tai, J.J. & Chen, C.L. (1989). Asymptotic distribution of the lod score for familial data, *Proceedings of the National Science Council of the Republic of China, Series B* **13**, 38–41.

[21]   Terwilliger, J.D. & Ott, J. (1994). *Handbook of Human Genetic Linkage*. Johns Hopkins University Press, Baltimore.

[22]   Terwilliger, J.D., Shannon, W.D. Lathrop, G.M. Nolan, J.P. Goldin, L.R. Chase, G.A. & Weeks, D.E. (1997). True and false positive peaks in genome-wide scans: applications of length-biased sampling to linkage mapping *American Journal of Human Genetics* **61**, 430–438.

J.D. TERWILLIGER

Linkage Analysis, Model-Free

Model-free linkage methods, in contrast to **model-based linkage methods**, do not depend on prior specification of a model of inheritance for the disease or trait of interest. In other words, the frequencies and **penetrances** of disease **genotypes** need not be known in advance, and functions of these quantities may in fact be estimated in conjunction with linkage parameters. It is important to recognize, however, that many of the methods do rely on assumptions about the underlying genetic model and some methods are in fact parametric and semiparametric in nature. In this Section, two general types of model-free linkage methods will be distinguished – those designed for qualitative traits and those designed for quantitative traits – although both theory and applications of these two groups of methods overlap. Model-free linkage methods typically evaluate marker locus identity-by-descent (IBD) relationships among family members, often pairs of siblings, and thus are often referred to as relative-pair, or sib-pair, methods.

Identity by Descent

A pair of related individuals shares an allele IBD if that allele has a common ancestral source, i.e. the same chromosome of the same ancestor. In the context of linkage analysis, the common ancestor is taken to be a recent ancestor – one within the sampled pedigree. For example, if the pair are siblings, the common ancestors are their parents, and the sibs may have inherited the same paternal allele and/or maternal allele. Let f_i, $i = 0, 1, 2$, be the prior (unconditional) probability that a relative pair shares i alleles IBD at a single marker locus, and $\hat{f}_i$ the estimate of f_i conditional on available marker data (*see* **Genetic Markers**). Now, let π be the proportion of alleles a relative pair shares IBD at a single locus, and $\hat{\pi} = \frac{1}{2}\hat{f}_1 + \hat{f}_2$ the estimate of π conditional on available marker data. Table 1 gives the prior (unconditional) distribution of π for different types of relative pairs.

Computation of the $\hat{f}_i$ for a single marker locus, using available pedigree marker data, was first proposed by Haseman & Elston [24] for nuclear families,

and later by Amos et al. [3] for extended pedigrees. Let I_m represent the available family marker data. Then

$$\hat{f}_i = \frac{\Pr(\pi = i/2, I_m)}{\Pr(I_m)}$$

is a general form for estimating $\hat{f}_i$. The denominator is the probability, or likelihood, of the pedigree marker data, and may be computed using an **Elston–Stewart** ("peeling") **algorithm**; the numerator can be written as a sum of the terms of the denominator consistent with sharing i alleles IBD, each term representing a phase-known pedigree genotype. More detailed algorithms for computing $\hat{f}_i$ for different types of relative pairs were given by Amos et al. [3]. Whittemore & Halpern [52] also presented a peeling algorithm for computing the probabilities of IBD relationships among the genes of pedigree members, and then showed how to use these probabilities to calculate the probability of any combination of genotypes or phenotypes for the pedigree members.

Estimation of multipoint IBD probabilities has also been explored. Let d represent the **genetic distance** from an arbitrary origin on a marker map with known intermarker distances. To compute the $\hat{f}_{di}$, the estimated allele-sharing distribution at location d, Kruglyak & Lander [29] employed a hidden **Markov chain** model that assumes that the π at consecutive loci behave in a first-order Markov manner; i.e. $\Pr(\pi_k|\pi_1, \pi_2, \ldots, \pi_{k-1}) = \Pr(\pi_k|\pi_{k-1})$, for loci ordered 1 through k on a chromosome. Inheritance at each location d is represented by an inheritance vector $V(d)$, in which each component corresponds to a particular meiosis in the pedigree and the component takes a value of 0 or 1 according to whether the paternal or maternal allele is transmitted. Computation of the probability distribution for $V(d)$ conditional on the marker data can be accomplished by considering pairs of loci successively. Additional computational speed is achieved by taking advantage of the fact that phase differences in the founders are equivalent and have equal probabilities [31]. An even faster algorithm uses a divide-and-conquer method and allows for meiosis-specific recombination fractions at virtually no additional cost [27]. These algorithms are all modifications of the Lander–Green algorithm [30, 32]. Sobel & Lange [46] developed a **Markov chain Monte Carlo** algorithm to approximate multipoint IBD-sharing estimates in larger pedigrees.

Table 1 Prior distribution of π for relative pairs

Type of relative pair	π			$E(\pi)$
	0	$\frac{1}{2}$	1	
Sibling	$\frac{1}{4}$	$\frac{1}{2}$	$\frac{1}{4}$	$\frac{1}{2}$
Second degree	$\frac{1}{2}$	$\frac{1}{2}$	0	$\frac{1}{4}$
Third degree	$\frac{3}{4}$	$\frac{1}{4}$	0	$\frac{1}{8}$

Table 2 Regression parameters in the expressions for $\hat{\pi}_d$ and $\hat{f}_{1d}^a$

ρ_0	$(1 - \psi_1)(1 - \psi_2)/\psi_m$
ρ_1	$-\psi_2(1 - \psi_2)(1 - 2\psi_1)/[\psi_m(1 - \psi_m)]$
ρ_2	$-\psi_1(1 - \psi_1)(1 - 2\psi_2)/[\psi_m(1 - \psi_m)]$
ω_0	$2\psi_1(1 - \psi_1)\psi_2(1 - \psi_2)/\psi_m^2$
ω_1	$2(1 - 2\psi_1)(1 - 2\psi_2)\psi_1(1 - \psi_1)\psi_2(1 - \psi_2)/[\psi_m^2(1 - \psi_m^2)]$
ω_2	$(1 - 2\psi_1)^2\psi_2^2(1 - \psi_2)^2/[\psi_m^2(1 - \psi_m^2)]$
ω_3	$(1 - 2\psi_2)^2\psi_1^2(1 - \psi_1)^2/[\psi_m^2(1 - \psi_m^2)]$
ω_4	$(1 - 2\psi_1)^2(1 - 2\psi_2)^2\psi_1(1 - \psi_1)\psi_2(1 - \psi_2)/[\psi_m^2(1 - \psi_m^2)(1 - 2\psi_m)^2(1 - 2\psi_m + 2\psi_m^2)]$

[a]From Olson [34], reproduced by permission of the publisher; $\psi_j = \theta_j^2 + (1 - \theta_j)^2$, $j = 1, 2, \ldots, m$.

Given multipoint IBD-sharing estimates at marker locus locations, **regression** models can also be used to obtain IBD-sharing estimates at points between two markers. Let f_{ij} be the prior (unconditional) joint probability that a sib-pair shares i alleles IBD at one marker locus and j alleles IBD at a second, usually linked, marker locus, and let $\hat{f}_{ij}$ be estimates, conditional on the available marker data, that account for the recombination fraction, assumed to be known, between the two markers. Let $\hat{f}_{i.} = \sum_j \hat{f}_{ij}$, $\hat{f}_{.j} = \sum_i \hat{f}_{ij}$, $\hat{\pi}_1 = \hat{f}_{1.}/2 + \hat{f}_{2.}$, $\hat{\pi}_2 = \hat{f}_{.1}/2 + \hat{f}_{.2}$, and $\widehat{\pi_1\pi_2} = \hat{f}_{11}/4 + (\hat{f}_{12} + \hat{f}_{21})/2 + \hat{f}_{22}$. Given these multipoint estimates of IBD-sharing at two adjacent loci and assuming no crossover interference (*see* **Genetic Map Functions**), IBD-sharing at a point d between the two loci can be obtained using the regression equations

$$\hat{\pi}_d = \rho_0 + \rho_1\hat{\pi}_1 + \rho_2\hat{\pi}_2$$

and

$$\hat{f}_{1d} = \omega_0 + \omega_1(\hat{\pi}_1 + \hat{\pi}_2 - 2\widehat{\pi_1\pi_2})$$
$$+ \omega_2\hat{f}_{1.} + \omega_3\hat{f}_{.1} + \omega_4\hat{f}_{11},$$

where expressions for the regression parameters in terms of the recombination fractions between the two loci (θ_m), between the first marker and $d(\theta_1)$, and between the second marker and $d(\theta_2)$ are given in Table 2 [34].

Linkage Between Marker and Qualitative Trait

Model-free linkage methods designed for qualitative traits often consider samples of affected sib-pairs or

sibships with at least two affected members. If a trait and marker are linked, affected sib-pairs should share more alleles IBD than expected by chance. Under the **null hypothesis** of no linkage, sib-pairs are expected to share exactly 0, 1, or 2 alleles IBD at a single marker locus with respective probabilities $\frac{1}{4}$, $\frac{1}{2}$, and $\frac{1}{4}$. Early test statistics generally assumed that the marker IBD state can be determined with certainty, so that a sample of n pairs can be partitioned into n_0, n_1, and n_2 pairs corresponding to sharing 0, 1, or 2 alleles IBD. Day & Simons [14] and Suarez et al. [48], assuming such a fully informative marker locus, proposed a one-sided (*see* **Alternative Hypothesis**) **nonparametric** test statistic (T_2) that compares the observed proportion of sib-pairs that share exactly two marker alleles IBD to its null value of $\frac{1}{4}$:

$$T_2 = \frac{n_2/n - 1/4}{[3/(16n)]^{1/2}}.$$

Green & Woodrow [22] proposed a one-sided nonparametric test statistic (T_m) that compares the observed mean proportion of marker alleles shared IBD to its null value of $\frac{1}{2}$:

$$T_m = \frac{n_2 + n_1/2 - 1/2}{[1/(8n)]^{1/2}}.$$

Extensions for use with larger sibships were proposed by Green & Woodrow [22] and deVries et al. [15]. These more general test statistics can substitute $\bar{\hat{\pi}} = \sum_{j=1}^n \hat{\pi}_j/n$ for $n_2 + n_1/2$ and an empirical variance estimate for the denominator when IBD sharing cannot be determined with certainty.

A **goodness-of-fit** statistic that compares the observed IBD distribution to that expected by chance was proposed by Weitkamp et al. [50]. Blackwelder

& Elston [5] compared the **power** of this test statistic, T_2, and T_m and found that T_m has greater power for most one-locus genetic models; T_2 has more power for some recessive models. Schaid & Nick [44] studied the asymptotically most powerful linear combination of the $\hat{f}_i$ and determined that T_m has power close to optimal for a broad range of single-locus models. Knapp et al. [28] determined that, provided $\delta_1^2 = \delta_0 \delta_2$, where $\delta_s = \mathrm{Pr}$ (affected|trait genotype with s susceptibility alleles), T_m is uniformly most powerful in θ, the recombination fraction between trait and marker loci.

Suarez et al. [48] characterized the distribution of sib-pair IBD sharing in terms of the population trait prevalence K, additive genetic variance σ_a^2, dominance genetic variance σ_d^2, and θ, the recombination fraction between trait and marker loci. Suarez et al. [44] determined the boundaries of this parameter space under a one-locus model. Risch [38–41] developed a parametric strategy for detecting linkage to complex diseases using affected sib-pairs and extended the methodology to multilocus trait models and to other types of relative pairs. Let z_{ri} be parameters defined as the probability that an affected relative pair of type r shares i marker alleles IBD. Then the lod score [the log base 10 of the ratio of the likelihoods under the alternative and the null hypothesis of no linkage (*see* **Likelihood Ratio**)] for the pedigree marker data I_m given **ascertainment** of an affected relative pair of type r (arp_r) can be written

$$Z(I_m | \mathrm{arp}_r) = \log_{10} \sum_{i=0,1,2} \frac{\hat{f}_i z_{ri}}{f_{ri}}. \quad (1)$$

Under the null hypothesis $\theta = \frac{1}{2}$, $z_{ri} = f_{ri}$, for $i = 0, 1, 2$, and $Z(I_m | \mathrm{arp}_r) = 0$. The lod score (1) is maximized over the z_{ri} at regular (e.g. 1 cM) intervals in a chromosomal region containing the typed markers. Alternatively, Hauser et al. [25] maximized the lod score over both the z_{ri} and the recombination fraction between one of two flanking markers and a disease locus assumed to lie between them.

Now define K_r to be the probability that a relative of type r of an affected individual is also affected, and let $\lambda_r = K_r/K$ be the **relative risk** of disease to a relative of type r. Let the subscripts s, o, and m denote sibling, parent/offspring, and monozygotic twins (*see* **Heterozygosity**), respectively. Under the assumption that a single locus confers susceptibility to disease, the z_{ri} are related to the relative risks and the recombination fraction as shown in Table 3 [39]. For affected sib-pairs, when $\theta = 0$, $z_{s0} = 1/(4\lambda_s)$, $z_{s1} = \lambda_o/(2\lambda_s)$, and $z_{s2} = \lambda_m/(4\lambda_s)$. Constraints on the z_{si} consistent with a one-locus genetic model are: $z_{s0} \geq 0$, $z_{s2} + z_{s0} \geq z_{s1}$, and $z_{s1} \geq 2z_{s0}$. Holmans [26] determined the asymptotic distribution of the maximum lod score under these constraints to be a mixture of χ_1^2 and χ_2^2 random variables; a lod score of 2.3 corresponds to a significance level of 10^{-3}. For various types of relative pairs, Lander & Kruglyak [33] proposed that pointwise significance levels (*see* **Hypothesis Testing**) and lod scores corresponding to a genome-wide significance of 0.05 be considered "significant" evidence in favor of linkage, assuming a single disease locus and an infinitely dense marker map. Davis et al. [13] developed **simulation**-based nonparametric statistics that condition on the marker

Table 3   Parameters of z_{ri} for relative pairs[a]

Type of relative pair	z_{r0}	z_{r1}	z_{r2}
Full sibling	$\frac{1}{4} - \frac{1}{4\lambda_s}(2\psi - 1)[(\lambda_s - 1)$ $+ 2(1-\psi)(\lambda_s - \lambda_o)]$	$\frac{1}{2} - \frac{1}{2\lambda_s}(2\psi - 1)^2(\lambda_s - \lambda_o)$	$\frac{1}{4} + \frac{1}{4\lambda_s}(2\psi - 1)[(\lambda_s - 1)$ $+ 2\psi(\lambda_s - \lambda_o)]$
Grandparental	$\frac{1}{2} - \frac{1}{2\lambda_g}(1 - 2\theta)(\lambda_g - 1)$	$\frac{1}{2} + \frac{1}{2\lambda_g}(1 - 2\theta)(\lambda_g - 1)$	–
Avuncular	$\frac{1}{2} - \frac{1}{2\lambda_a}(1 - \theta)(1 - 2\theta)^2(\lambda_a - 1)$	$\frac{1}{2} + \frac{1}{2\lambda_a}(1 - \theta)(1 - 2\theta)^2(\lambda_a - 1)$	–
Half-sibling	$\frac{1}{2} - \frac{1}{2\lambda_h}(2\psi - 1)(\lambda_h - 1)$	$\frac{1}{2} + \frac{1}{2\lambda_h}(2\psi - 1)(\lambda_h - 1)$	–
First cousin	$\frac{3}{4} - \frac{1}{2\lambda_c}[(1 - \theta)^4 + \theta^2(1 - \theta)^2$ $+ \frac{\theta^2}{2} - \frac{1}{4}](\lambda_c - 1)$	$\frac{1}{4} + \frac{1}{2\lambda_c}[(1 - \theta)^4 + \theta^2(1 - \theta)^2$ $+ \frac{\theta^2}{2} - \frac{1}{4}](\lambda_c - 1)$	–

[a]From Risch [39], reproduced by permission of the publisher; $\psi = \theta^2 + (1 - \theta)^2$; s = full sibling, g = grandparental, a = avuncular, h = half-sibling, c = first cousin, o = parent/offspring.

genotypes of the unaffected family members. For samples of affected sib-pairs, a test statistic with more power than the lod score for some recessive models is

$$T_{z2} = \left(\hat{z}_{s2} - \tfrac{1}{4} \right) \Big/ \mathrm{var}(\hat{z}_{s2}),$$

where $\mathrm{var}(\hat{z}_2)$ is obtained from the observed **information matrix** [35].

Affected sib-pair methods are particularly useful in detecting linkage to complex diseases, which are expected to be oligogenic. The single-locus lod score provides a valid test of linkage even if other loci contribute to a disease. Multilocus models are also of interest. A general two-locus lod score with eight free parameters may be written as

$$Z(I_\mathrm{m}|\mathrm{arp_s}) = \log_{10} \sum_{i=0,1,2} \sum_{j=0,1,2} \frac{z_{ij} \hat{f}_{i1} \hat{f}_{j2}}{f_{i1} f_{j2}},$$

where the subscripts 1 and 2 refer to the two loci, and z_{ij} are parameters representing the probability that an affected sib-pair shares i alleles IBD and the first locus and j at the second locus. The two disease loci are assumed to be unlinked. If the two loci interact in a multiplicative fashion, then $z_{ij} = z_i z_j$ by definition, and four free parameters are required. Let λ_{ki} be the relative risk to a relative that shares i alleles IBD with an affected individual at disease locus k, and let K_k and λ_{ks} be the contributions to the overall prevalence and sibling relative risk due to locus k. If the two loci interact in an additive fashion, then

$$\frac{z_{ij}}{f_{1i} f_{2j}} - 1 = \frac{1}{\lambda_\mathrm{s}} \left(\frac{K_1}{K} \right)^2 (\lambda_{1i} - \lambda_{1\mathrm{s}})$$
$$+ \frac{1}{\lambda_\mathrm{s}} \left(\frac{K_2}{K} \right)^2 (\lambda_{2j} - \lambda_{2\mathrm{s}}),$$

an additive property [39]; this formulation also requires four free parameters.

The lod score (1) may also be written as

$$Z(I_\mathrm{m}|\mathrm{arp_s}) = \log_{10} \left[1 + \beta \left(\hat{\pi} - \tfrac{1}{2} \right) + \gamma \left(\hat{f}_1 - \tfrac{1}{2} \right) \right],$$

where $\beta = (\sigma_\mathrm{a}^2 + \sigma_\mathrm{d}^2)/(KK_\mathrm{s}) = 4(z_2 - z_0)$ and $\gamma = -\sigma_\mathrm{d}^2/(2KK_\mathrm{s}) = 2(z_1 - z_0 - z_2)$. The general two-locus model may similarly be parameterized in terms of **variance components** $\sigma_{\mathrm{a}_j}^2, \sigma_{\mathrm{d}_j}^2, \sigma_{\mathrm{a}_1\mathrm{a}_2}^2, \sigma_{\mathrm{d}_1\mathrm{d}_2}^2$, and $\sigma_{\mathrm{a}_j\mathrm{d}_{3-j}}^2$ – the contribution to the total genetic variance due to the **interaction** between the additive

(a) or dominance (d) component of the jth locus, $j = 1, 2$ [11, 16, 23, 35]. One such model [35] is

$$Z(I_\mathrm{m}|\mathrm{arp_s}) = \log_{10} \Big\{ 1 + (KK_\mathrm{s})^{-1} \Big[B_1 \left(\hat{\pi}_1 - \tfrac{1}{2} \right)$$
$$+ C_1 \left(\hat{f}_{11} - \tfrac{1}{2} \right) + B_2 \left(\hat{\pi}_2 - \tfrac{1}{2} \right)$$
$$+ C_2 \left(\hat{f}_{12} - \tfrac{1}{2} \right) + D \left(\hat{\pi}_1 \hat{\pi}_2 - \tfrac{1}{4} \right)$$
$$+ F_1 \left(\hat{\pi}_1 \hat{f}_{12} - \tfrac{1}{4} \right) + F_2 \left(\hat{\pi}_2 \hat{f}_{11} - \tfrac{1}{4} \right)$$
$$+ G \left(\hat{f}_{11} \hat{f}_{12} - \tfrac{1}{4} \right) \Big] \Big\},$$

where

$$B_j = \sigma_{\mathrm{a}_j}^2 + \sigma_{\mathrm{d}_j}^2, \quad j = 1, 2,$$
$$C_j = -\sigma_{\mathrm{d}_j}^2/2, \quad j = 1, 2,$$
$$D = \sigma_{\mathrm{a}_1\mathrm{a}_2}^2 + \sigma_{\mathrm{a}_1\mathrm{d}_2}^2 + \sigma_{\mathrm{a}_2\mathrm{d}_1}^2 + \sigma_{\mathrm{d}_1\mathrm{d}_2}^2,$$
$$F_j = -\sigma_{\mathrm{a}_j\mathrm{d}_{3-j}}^2 + \sigma_{\mathrm{d}_1\mathrm{d}_2}^2/2, \quad j = 1, 2,$$

and

$$G = \sigma_{\mathrm{d}_1\mathrm{d}_2}^2/4.$$

When K and K_s are known, the variance components may be estimated directly; otherwise, the model can be fitted by reparameterizing so that $B_1^* = B_1/(KK_\mathrm{s})$, and similarly for the remaining parameters. **Additive** and **multiplicative models** can also be fitted using variance components parameterizations [35].

For linkage analysis using small pedigrees, Kruglyak et al. [31] proposed calculating a scoring function $S(v, \Psi)$ (*see* **Scores**) that depends on an inheritance vector v and the observed disease phenotypes Ψ in the pedigree. When the inheritance vector is unknown, one computes its conditional expectation

$$\overline{S}(\Psi) = \sum_v S(v, \Psi) P(v),$$

where $P(v)$ is estimated using available marker data. The authors further discuss a model-free scoring function that considers IBD-sharing among sets of affected family members; this scoring function was first proposed by Whittemore & Halpern [51]. Let a denote the number of affected individuals in a pedigree, let h be a collection of alleles obtained by choosing one allele from each of these individuals, and let $b_i(h)$ denote the number of times that the ith founder allele appears in h. The scoring function is defined as

$$S_{\text{all}}(v) = 2^{-a} \sum_{h} \left[\prod_{i} b_i(h)! \right],$$

where the sum is over the 2^a possible ways to choose h. Kruglyak et al. then standardize the score to obtain $Z(v) = [S(v) - \mu]/\sigma$, where μ and σ are the mean and standard deviation of S under the **uniform distribution** of inheritance vectors. A global score is obtaining by taking a weighted average of standardized scores; weights depend on pedigree size.

The affected-pedigree-member (APM) method of Weeks & Lange [49] can also be used to analyze extended pedigrees, and uses identity-by-state sharing to incorporate information from multiple markers; this method is less powerful than methods based on IBD sharing [21]. Curtis & Sham [12] proposed comparing observed and expected numbers of alleles shared IBD between all affected relative pairs in a pedigree. Guo [23] proposed plotting $\hat{\pi}$ over each chromosomal interval and examining further regions for which $\hat{\pi}$ is substantially larger than $\frac{1}{2}$.

Elston [17] and Elston et al. [18] developed and studied two-stage global search designs for linkage analysis to complex diseases using pairs of affected relatives. In the first of the two stages, a genome scan is performed on n affected pairs using m equally spaced marker loci. For each marker with a pointwise **P value** less than α^*, k additional markers in the region are typed and a more stringent significance level α applied. Given the relative risk λ_r for a particular trait locus, the desired power of the study, and the ratio of the cost of recruiting one person into the study to the cost of performing one marker assay, n, m, k, and α may be chosen to minimize the total cost of the study. Typically, an optimal two-stage procedure halves the cost of a study, compared to a procedure involving only the first stage and the criterion α.

Linkage analysis may also be done using discordant pairs, i.e. pairs in which one member is affected and the other unaffected. Such pairs provide good power for linkage if the disease is rare and dominant, or if the disease is common. The lod score takes the same form as (1), except that the z_{ri} are now the probabilities that a discordant pair of type r share i alleles IBD. For discordant sib-pairs, genetic constraints are obtained by reversing the roles of z_{s0} and z_{s2} in the inequalities given above for affected sib-pairs.

Linkage Between Marker and Quantitative Trait

The problem of detecting linkage between a marker locus and a locus underlying a quantitative trait using sib-pair data was first considered by Penrose [37], who proposed comparing the covariance of the sib-pair trait and marker differences with that expected when the trait and marker are not linked. Haseman & Elston [24] and Blackwelder [4] expanded this idea and included available marker information from the parents.

Assume that a single locus with alleles T and t underlies a quantitative trait. For an observation X from the trait distribution, the genetic model may be written

$$X = \mu + g + e,$$

where μ is an overall mean, g is a major gene effect such that $g = a, d$, or $-a$ for trait genotypes TT, Tt, or tt, respectively, and e is a residual effect with an unspecified distribution. Putting $p = \Pr(T)$ and $q = 1 - p$,

$$\sigma_a^2 = 2pq[a - d(p - q)]^2,$$
$$\sigma_d^2 = 4p^2q^2d^2,$$

and $\sigma_g^2 = \sigma_a^2 + \sigma_d^2$. Also, let $\sigma_\varepsilon^2 = E(e_1 - e_2)^2$, for a pair of sibs indexed 1 and 2, and let $\psi = \theta^2 + (1 - \theta)^2$, where θ is the recombination fraction between trait and marker loci.

The squared difference $Y = (X_1 - X_2)^2$ between the measurements of a quantitative trait for a randomly sampled pair of siblings is a linear function of the **Bayesian** estimate of the proportion of marker alleles shared IBD between the members of the pair ($\hat{\pi}$) and the estimated probability that the pair share exactly one marker allele IBD ($\hat{f}_1$), i.e.

$$E(Y|I_m) = \alpha_s + \beta_s\hat{\pi} + \gamma_s\hat{f}_1,$$

where

$$\alpha_s = \sigma_\varepsilon^2 + 2\sigma_g^2\psi + 2\sigma_d^2\psi(1 - \psi),$$
$$\beta_s = 2\sigma_g^2(1 - 2\psi),$$

and

$$\gamma_s = \sigma_d^2(1 - 2\psi)^2.$$

If $\theta = \frac{1}{2}$ or $\sigma_g^2 = 0$, then $\beta = 0$; otherwise, $\beta < 0$. After fitting the regression model using **least squares**, an asymptotically normal one-sided test of linkage may be constructed.

Similar regression relationships have been developed for other types of relative pairs, specifically half-sib, grandparental, avuncular, and cousin pairs [2]; all take the form

$$E(Y|I_m) = \alpha_r + \beta_r \hat{\pi},$$

where α_r and β_r are functions of $\sigma_a^2, \sigma_d^2, \sigma_\varepsilon^2$, and θ that are specific to relative pair type r (Table 4). Olson & Wijsman [36] used **generalized estimating equations** to combine information from different types of relative pairs in a set of pedigree data. Assume that p types of relative pairs are of interest and that the data set consists of N pedigrees, each with n_i relative pairs. Under a working independence model, α_r and β_r are estimated separately for each type of relative pair; the robust **covariance matrix** of these estimates is given by

$$var(\alpha, \beta) = \left(\sum_{i=1}^{N} \mathbf{D}_i' \mathbf{D}_i\right)^{-1} \left(\sum_{i=1}^{N} \mathbf{D}_i' \hat{\mathbf{S}}_i \hat{\mathbf{S}}_i' \mathbf{D}_i\right)$$

$$\times \left(\sum_{i=1}^{N} \mathbf{D}_i' \mathbf{D}_i\right)^{-1},$$

where $\mathbf{D}_i$ is an $n_i \times 2p$ matrix containing the $\hat{\pi}_r$ and $\hat{f}_1$ (analogous to the design matrix in a linear regression model), and $\mathbf{S}_i$ is a vector of length n_i with elements $y - \alpha_r - \beta_r \hat{\pi}_r$. A one-sided, asymptotically normal, test of linkage takes the form

$$T = N^{1/2} \mathbf{c}^T \hat{\beta} / [\mathbf{c}^T \, var(\hat{\beta}) \mathbf{c}]^{1/2},$$

where $\mathbf{c}$ is a p-dimensional vector of weights, chosen a priori, with elements $var(\pi_r) n_r$, n_r is the total number of pairs of type r, and $\hat{\beta}$ is a vector of the regression estimates $\hat{\beta}_r$. In a multipoint setting, or when a candidate locus is being tested, the model

with common slope

$$E(Y|I_m) = \alpha_r + \beta \hat{\pi}$$

may be fitted; $\mathbf{D}_i$ becomes an $n_i \times p + 1$ matrix and no a priori weights are required to test linkage. Because $\beta_s = \beta_h$ for all values of the recombination fraction, sib-pairs and half-sib-pairs may be combined in a similar manner for a genome scan using single markers. Schaid et al. [45] combine these two types of pairs into a single test of linkage, using an empirically derived adjustment to the **degrees of freedom** of the t-statistic (*see* **Student's t Distribution**) to allow for correlated pairs.

Regression models have been developed for sampling schemes other than random sampling. Assume that probands are sampled from the upper tail of the trait distribution. Let $X_1 > c$ be the proband trait value, and X_2 the trait value for the proband's sibling. **Consistent estimates** of regression coefficients may be obtained by fitting

$$X_2 = A + B_1 X_1 + B_2 \left(\hat{\pi} - \tfrac{1}{2}\right)$$

$$+ B_3 \left(\left|\hat{\pi} - \tfrac{1}{2}\right| - \tfrac{1}{4}\right),$$

[7]. $B_2 = 0$ if $\theta = \tfrac{1}{2}$; otherwise, $B_2 > 0$. ($B_2 < 0$ if probands are sampled from the lower tail of the trait distribution.) Conditioning on the ascertainment process, rather than the proband's trait value, gives

$$E(X_2|I_m, X_1 > c) = A^* + B_2^* \left(\hat{\pi} - \tfrac{1}{2}\right)$$

$$+ B_3^* \left(\left|\hat{\pi} - \tfrac{1}{2}\right| - \tfrac{1}{4}\right).$$

Use of this sampling scheme greatly increases the power to detect linkage [6, 7], particularly for a rare allele with a large effect.

This "selected sampling" scheme provides excellent power provided that one samples probands from

Table 4 Coefficients of the regression of squared pair differences on the proportion of alleles shared IBD for relative pairs[a]

Type of relative pair	α_r	β_r
Half-sibling	$\sigma_\varepsilon^2 + 2\sigma_g^2 - 2\theta(1-\theta)\sigma_a^2$	$-2(1-2\theta)^2 \sigma_a^2$
Grandparental	$\sigma_\varepsilon^2 + 2\sigma_g^2 - \theta\sigma_a^2$	$-2(1-2\theta)\sigma_a^2$
Avuncular	$\sigma_\varepsilon^2 + 2\sigma_g^2 - (\tfrac{5}{2}\theta - 4\theta^2 + 2\theta^3)\sigma_a^2$	$-2(1-2\theta)^2(1-\theta)\sigma_a^2$
First cousin	$\sigma_\varepsilon^2 + 2\sigma_g^2 - (\tfrac{4}{3}\theta - \tfrac{5}{3}\theta^2 + 2\theta^3 - \tfrac{2}{3}\theta^4)\sigma_a^2$	$-2(1-2\theta)^2(1 - \tfrac{4}{3}\theta + 2\theta^2)\sigma_a^2$

[a]From Amos & Elston [2], reproduced by permission of the publisher.

the tail of the distribution with the rarer allele. A second design, which is uniformly powerful in all genetic situations, is sampling of extreme discordant sib-pairs – pairs such that one sib has a trait value from the upper tail and the other from the lower tail. For example, given a large sample of probands with an extreme value in one direction (usually that indicating disease), one might genotype only those pairs for which the sibling has a trait value in the opposite tail. Such extreme discordant pairs provide good power for detecting linkage for additive, dominant, and recessive models [42, 43]. As there may be little trait variation within each tail, it is useful to ignore this variation and model

$$z_i \equiv \Pr(\pi = i/2|\text{edsp}), \quad i = 0, 1, 2,$$

where edsp denotes "extreme discordant sib-pair". The lod score is the same as in the case of sampling sib-pairs discordant for a dichotomous trait, which may be considered a special case of edsp for which the two tails share the same cutpoint, with different constraints on the z_i.

Other approaches to quantitative trait linkage have been proposed. To assess evidence for genetic linkage from pedigrees, Amos [3] modeled the covariance matrix of pedigree trait values in terms of variance components, IBD sharing and the recombination fraction. Let a general model for trait values X be

$$X_i = \mu + g_i + G_i + \boldsymbol{\beta}^\mathrm{T}\mathbf{w}_i + e_i,$$

where μ, g_i, and e_i are the overall mean, major genotype effect, and environmental error, as before, G_i is a random effect of polygenes (*see* **Polygenic Inheritance**), $\mathbf{w}_i$ a vector of fixed covariates, and $\boldsymbol{\beta}$ a set of regression parameters. Without loss of generality, take $\mathrm{E}(g_i) = \mathrm{E}(e_i) = \mathrm{E}(G_i) = 0$. Then

$$\mathrm{E}(X_i) = \mu + \boldsymbol{\beta}^\mathrm{T}\mathbf{w}_i,$$

$$\mathrm{var}(X_i) = \sigma_\mathrm{a}^2 + \sigma_\mathrm{d}^2 + \sigma_\mathrm{G}^2 + \sigma_\mathrm{e}^2,$$

and

$$\mathrm{cov}(X_i, X_j|\pi_{ij}) = f(\theta, \pi_{ij})\sigma_\mathrm{a}^2 + g(\theta, f_{2ij})\sigma_\mathrm{d}^2 + \phi_{ij}\sigma_\mathrm{G}^2 \quad \text{for } i \neq j,$$

where ϕ_{ij} is the coefficient of relationship between family members i and j (*see* **Inbreeding**), $f(\theta, \pi_{ij})$ is given for various relative pairs in Table 5, and $g(\theta, f_{2ij})$ equals 0 for all but sib-pairs, in which case

Table 5 Expressions for $f(\theta, \pi_{ij})^\mathrm{a}$

Relative pair	$f(\theta, \pi_{ij})$
Sibling	$\frac{1}{2} + (1 - 2\theta)^2(\pi_{ij} - \frac{1}{2})$
Half-sibling	$\frac{1}{4} + (1 - 2\theta)^2(\pi_{ij} - \frac{1}{4})$
Avuncular	$\frac{1}{4} + (1 - 2\theta)^2(1 - \theta)(\pi_{ij} - \frac{1}{4})$
Grandparental	$\frac{1}{4} + (1 - 2\theta)(\pi_{ij} - \frac{1}{4})$
First cousin	$\frac{1}{8} + (1 - 2\theta)^2(1 - \frac{4}{3}\theta + \frac{2}{3}\theta^2)(\pi_{ij} - \frac{1}{8})$

[a]From Amos [1], reproduced by permission of the publisher.

$$\mathrm{cov}(X_i, X_j|\pi_{ij}) = 2\theta(1 - \theta)\sigma_\mathrm{g}^2$$
$$+ 2(\theta - 1)\theta(1 - 2\theta + 2\theta^2)\sigma_\mathrm{d}^2$$
$$+ [(1 - 2\theta)^2\sigma_\mathrm{g}^2 - (1 - 2\theta)^4\sigma_\mathrm{d}^2]\pi_{ij}$$
$$+ (1 - 2\theta)^4\sigma_\mathrm{d}^2 f_{2ij}.$$

Parameters may be estimated using **maximum likelihood** methods, if **multivariate normality** of errors is assumed, or by estimating-equation approaches.

Another approach, the weighted pairwise correlation (WPC) statistic, was proposed by Commenges [8]. This score test may be applied to sets of large pedigrees with several types of relative pairs. Consider a set of F pedigrees, each with n_f members. For an individual pedigree, a general form for the score statistic is

$$S_\mathrm{L} = \sum_{i<j} W_{ij}U_iU_j,$$

where $W_{ij} = \hat{\pi}_{ij} - \overline{\hat{\pi}}_{rij}$ are centered IBD-sharing estimates for the pair of relatives i and j, and U_i is the residual $x_i - \mathrm{E}(X_i|\text{covariates})$, based on some parametric model for the mean of X. If more **robustness** is desired, the U_i may be replaced by their centered **ranks**, to give

$$S_\mathrm{R} = \sum_{i<j} W_{ij}(R_i - \overline{R})(R_j - \overline{R}),$$

where R_i is the rank of the ith residual, and $\overline{R}$ is the mean of the ranks. For a set of F pedigrees, linkage may be tested using

$$S = \frac{\sum_{f=1}^{F}[S_{\mathrm{Rf}} - \mathrm{E}(S_{\mathrm{Rf}})]}{\left(\sum_{f=1}^{F}\mathrm{var}\,S_{\mathrm{Rf}}\right)^{1/2}},$$

where

$$E(S_{Rf}) = -\frac{n_f + 1}{12} \sum_{i<j} W_{ijf},$$

$$var(S_{Rf}) = A \sum_{i<j} W_{ijf}^2 + B \sum_{i<j} \sum_{r<s; r,s \neq i,j}$$
$$\times W_{ijf} W_{rsf} - 2C \sum_{i,j \neq i} \sum_{r \neq i,j} W_{irf} W_{jrf},$$

$A = (n_f+1)(n_f-2)(5n_f^2+n_f-8)/720$, $B = (n_f+1)(10n_f+16)/720$, and $C = (n_f+1)(5n_f^2-3n_f-16)/720$. This test is called the weighted pairwise rank correlation (WPRC) test. Simulations show that the WPRC can be more powerful than the Haseman–Elston test for single large pedigrees, or in the presence of genotype-by-environment interaction (*see* **Gene–Environment Interaction**) or family-specific residual variance [10]. For larger samples of small pedigrees, the Haseman–Elston test is generally the more powerful, particularly for highly heritable dominant traits. The WPC or WPRC can be applied to dichotomous traits as well as to quantitative traits and can substitute identity-by-state sharing for IBD sharing estimates. Commenges & Abel [9] proposed a **transformation** that yields uncorrelated **residuals** and a more robust test statistic.

Goldgar [19] proposed a multipoint IBD method that assumes that the quantitative trait is due to additive genetic effects and a normally distributed random environmental component. The method is parameterized using the proportion of the total trait variance due to additive genetic effects (h^2) and the proportion (P) of the genetic variance due to loci in the chromosomal interval defined by the marker loci. For each sib-pair, the proportion of the chromosomal region shared IBD, conditional on the marker data, is estimated. A covariance matrix of the sibship trait values is then constructed as a function of the IBD-sharing estimates, h^2, and P. The likelihood for the trait values, conditional on IBD-sharing, is assumed to be multivariate normal; numerical maximum-likelihood techniques are used to estimate P and to test the null hypothesis $P = 0$. Limited simulation suggests that this multipoint method is more powerful than the single-marker Haseman–Elston method. The method also has power comparable to model-based linkage analysis when parental data are unknown, the effect of the major locus is small and there is additional

genetic variation, or the parameters of the model-based analysis are misspecified [20].

Software

Estimates of multipoint IBD-sharing may be obtained using MAPMAKER/SIBS (nuclear families) and GENEHUNTER (small pedigrees). These programs also apply a variety of parametric and nonparametric tests of linkage for both quantitative and qualitative data. For single markers, the SAGE program SIBPAL performs nonparametric tests of linkage for affected sib-pairs, and applies the Haseman–Elston regression method for sib and half-sib pairs. The SAGE program RELPAL estimates single-marker allele-sharing probabilities for large pedigrees and applies the Olson–Wijsman test of linkage. The SAGE program DESPAIR provides optimal two-stage designs for genome searches using affected relative pairs. Other software, including APM, ASPEX, ERPA, ESPA, GAS, MFLINK, MIM, NOPAR, and SIMIBD, that perform various aspects of model-free linkage analysis, are available from their respective authors (*see* **Software for Genetic Epidemiology**).

References

[1]   Amos, C.I. (1994). Robust variance-components approach for assessing genetic linkage in pedigrees, *American Journal of Human Genetics* **54**, 535–543.

[2]   Amos, C.I. & Elston, R.C. (1989). Robust methods for the detection of genetic linkage for quantitative data from pedigrees, *Genetic Epidemiology* **6**, 349–360.

[3]   Amos, C.I., Dawson, D.V. & Elston, R.C. (1990). The probabilistic determination of identity-by-descent sharing for pairs of relatives from pedigrees, *American Journal of Human Genetics* **47**, 842–853.

[4]   Blackwelder, W.C. (1977). Statistical Methods for Detecting Genetic Linkage from Sibship Data, *Institute of Statistics Mimeo Series No. 1114*. Department of Biostatistics, University of North Carolina, Chapel Hill.

[5]   Blackwelder, W.C. & Elston R.C. (1985). A comparison of sib-pair linkage tests from disease susceptibility loci, *Genetic Epidemiology* **2**, 85–97.

[6]   Cardon, L.R. & Fulker, D.W. (1994). The power of interval mapping of quantitative trait loci using selected sib pairs, *American Journal of Human Genetics* **55**, 825–833.

[7]   Carey, G. & Williamson, J.A. (1991). Linkage analysis of quantitative traits: increased power by using selected samples, *American Journal of Human Genetics* **49**, 786–796.

[8] Commenges, D. (1994). Robust genetic linkage analysis based on a score test of homogeneity: the weighted pairwise correlation statistic, *Genetic Epidemiology* **11**, 189–200.

[9] Commenges, D. & Abel, L. (1996). Improving the robustness of the weighted pairwise correlation test for linkage analysis, *Genetic Epidemiology* **13**, 559–574.

[10] Commenges, D., Olson, J. & Wijsman, E. (1994). The weighted pairwise correlation statistic for linkage analysis: simulation study and application to Alzheimer's disease, *Genetic Epidemiology* **11**, 201–212.

[11] Cordell, H.J., Todd, J.A., Bennett, S.T., Kawaguchi, Y. & Farrall, M. (1995). Two-locus maximum lod score analysis of a multifactorial trait: joint consideration of IDDM2 and IDDM4 in type 1 diabetes, *American Journal of Human Genetics* **57**,920–934.

[12] Curtis, D. & Sham, P.C. (1994). Using risk calculation to implement an extended relative pair analysis, *Annals of Human Genetics* **58**,151–162.

[13] Davis, S., Schroeder, M., Goldin, L.R. & Weeks, D.E. (1996). Nonparametric simulation-based statistics for detecting linkage in general pedigrees, *American Journal of Human Genetics* **58**, 867–880.

[14] Day, N.E. & Simons, M.J. (1976). Disease susceptibility genes – their identification by multiple case family studies, *Tissue Antigens* **8**, 109–119.

[15] deVries, R.R.P., Fat, R.F.M., Lai, A., Nijenhuis, L.E. & van Rood, J.J. (1976). HLA-linked genetic control of host response to *Mycobacterium leprae, Lancet* **ii**, 1328–1330.

[16] Dupuis, J., Brown, P.O. & Siegmund, D. (1995). Statistical methods for linkage analysis of complex traits from high-resolution maps of identity by descent, *Genetics* **140**, 843–856.

[17] Elston, R.C. (1992). Designs for the global search of the human genome by linkage analysis, in *Proceedings of the Sixteenth International Biometric Conference*, Hamilton, New Zealand, December 7–11, pp. 39–51.

[18] Elston, R.C., Guo, X. & Williams, L.V. (1996). Two-stage global search designs for linkage analysis using pairs of affected relatives, *Genetic Epidemiology* **13**, 535–558.

[19] Goldgar, D.E. (1990). Multipoint analysis of human quantitative genetic variation, *American Journal of Human Genetics* **47**, 957–967.

[20] Goldgar, D.E. & Oniki, R.S. (1992). Comparison of a multipoint identity-by-descent method with parametric multipoint linkage analysis for mapping quantitative traits, *American Journal of Human Genetics* **50**, 598–606.

[21] Goldin, L.R. & Weeks, D.E. (1993). Two-locus models of disease: comparison of likelihood and nonparametric linkage methods, *American Journal of Human Genetics* **53**, 908–915.

[22] Green, J.R. & Woodrow, J.C. (1977). Sibling method for detecting HLA-linked genes in a disease, *Tissue Antigens* **9**, 31–35.

[23] Guo, S.-W. (1995). Detection of genome similarity as an exploratory tool for mapping complex traits, *Genetic Epidemiology* **12**, 877–882.

[24] Haseman, J.K. & Elston, R.C. (1972). The investigation of linkage between a quantitative trait and a marker locus, *Behavior Genetics* **2**, 3–19.

[25] Hauser, E.R., Boehnke, M., Guo, S.-W. & Risch, N. (1996). Affected-sib-pair interval mapping and exclusion for complex genetic traits: sampling considerations, *Genetic Epidemiology* **13**, 117–137.

[26] Holmans, P. (1993). Asymptotic properties of affected-sib-pair linkage analysis, *American Journal of Human Genetics* **52**, 362–374.

[27] Idury, R.M. & Elston, R.C. (1997). A faster and more general hidden Markov model algorithm for multipoint likelihood calculations, *Human Heredity* **47**, 197–202.

[28] Knapp, M., Seuchter, S.A. & Baur, M.P. (1994). Linkage analysis in nuclear families. 1: Optimality criteria for affected sib-pair tests, *Human Heredity* **44**, 37–43.

[29] Kruglyak, L. & Lander, E.S. (1995). Complete multipoint sib-pair analysis of qualitative and quantitative trait data, *American Journal of Human Genetics* **57**, 439–454.

[30] Kruglyak, L., Daly, M.J. & Lander, E.S. (1995). Rapid multipoint linkage analysis of recessive traits in nuclear families, including homozygosity mapping, *American Journal of Human Genetics* **56**, 519–527.

[31] Kruglyak, L., Daly, M.J., Reeve-Daly, M.P. & Lander, E.S. (1996). Parametric and nonparametric linkage analysis: a unified multipoint approach, *American Journal of Human Genetics* **58**, 1347–1363.

[32] Lander, E.S. & Green, P. (1987). Construction of multilocus genetic maps in humans, *Proceedings of the National Academy of Sciences* **84**, 2363–2367.

[33] Lander, E. & Kruglyak, L. (1995). Genetic dissection of complex traits: guidelines for interpreting and reporting linkage results, *Nature Genetics* **11**, 241–247.

[34] Olson, J.M. (1995). Robust multipoint linkage analysis: an extension of the Haseman-Elston method, *Genetic Epidemiology* **12**, 177–193.

[35] Olson, J.M. (1997). Likelihood-based models for linkage analysis using affected sib pairs, *Human Heredity* **47**, 110–120.

[36] Olson, J.M. & Wijsman, E.M. (1993). Linkage between quantitative trait and marker loci: methods using all relative pairs, *Genetic Epidemiology* **10**, 87–102.

[37] Penrose, L.S. (1938). Genetic linkage in graded human characters, *Annals of Eugenics* **6**, 133–138.

[38] Risch, N. (1990). Linkage strategies for genetically complex traits. I. Multilocus models, *American Journal of Human Genetics* **46**, 222–228.

[39] Risch, N. (1990). Linkage strategies for genetically complex traits. II. The power of affected relative pairs, *American Journal of Human Genetics* **46**, 229–241.

[40] Risch, N. (1990). Linkage strategies for genetically complex traits. III. The effect of marker polymorphism on analysis of affected relative pairs, *American Journal of Human Genetics* **46**, 242–253.

[41] Risch, N. (1992). Corrections to "Linkage strategies for genetically complex traits. III. The effect of marker polymorphism on analysis of affected relative pairs", *American Journal of Human Genetics* **51**, 673–675.

[42] Risch, N. & Zhang, H. (1995). Extreme discordant sib pairs for mapping quantitative trait loci in humans, *Science* **268**, 1584–1589.

[43] Risch, N. & Zhang, H. (1996). Mapping quantitative trait loci with extreme discordant sib pairs: sampling considerations, *American Journal of Human Genetics* **58**, 836–843.

[44] Schaid, D.J. & Nick, T.G. (1990). Sib-pair linkage tests for disease susceptibility loci: Common tests vs. the asymptotically most powerful test, *Genetic Epidemiology* **7**, 359–370.

[45] Schaid, D.J., Elston, R.C., Wilson, A.F. & Tran, L. (1994). In *SAGE Statistical Analysis for Genetic Epidemiology, Release 2.2*. Computer program available from the Department of Epidemiology and Biostatistics, Case Western Reserve University, Cleveland, Ohio, USA.

[46] Sobel, E. & Lange, K. (1996). Descent graphs in pedigree analysis: applications to haplotyping, location scores, and marker-sharing statistics, *American Journal of Human Genetics* **58**, 1323–1337.

[47] Suarez, B.K., Reich, T. & Trost, J. (1976). Limits of the general two-allele single locus model with incomplete penetrance, *Annals of Human Genetics* **40**, 231–243.

[48] Suarez, B.K., Rice, J. & Reich, T. (1978). The generalized sib paid IBD distribution: its use in the detection of linkage, *Annals of Human Genetics* **42**, 87–94.

[49] Weeks, D.E. & Lange, K. (1988). The affected-pedigree-member method of linkage analysis, *American Journal of Human Genetics* **42**, 315–326.

[50] Weitkamp, L.R., Stancer, H.C., Persad, E., Flood, C. & Guttormsen, S. (1981). Depressive disorders and HLA: a gene on chromosome 6 that can affect behavior, *New England Journal of Medicine* **305**, 1301–1306.

[51] Whittemore, A.S. & Halpern, J. (1994). A class of tests for linkage using affected pedigree members, *Biometrics* **50**, 118–127.

[52] Whittemore, A.S. & Halpern, J. (1994). Probability of gene identity by descent: computation and applications, *Biometrics* **50**, 109–117.

(*See also* **Identity Coefficients**)

JANE M. OLSON

Linkage Disequilibrium

Linkage disequilibrium, more appropriately termed allelic association or allelic disequilibrium, refers to the nonrandom association between the alleles at two or more genetic loci in a natural breeding population (see **Gene**). The concept of linkage disequilibrium was postulated by population geneticists in theoretical studies of the consequences of random mating on the distribution of alleles and allelic combinations (**genotypes**) at multiple loci. Further theoretical studies have shown that in most instances this nonrandom association declines rapidly with evolutionary time, and as a function of the recombination frequency between the loci. However, with natural selection, allelic associations may persist in a population for long evolutionary time periods. With the availability of high-resolution genetic maps in the human and many other species, empirical studies of linkage disequilibrium in different genomic segments have been initiated. These studies have not only shed light on the distribution of alleles and allelic combinations in the genome, but also on the **population genetic** mechanisms that are likely to lead to the observed distribution of linkage disequilibrium across loci. In particular, these studies suggest that in certain circumstances, linkage disequilibrium can be used to infer the location of a disease-causing gene by studying **disease–marker associations**.

Hardy–Weinberg Law

The rediscovery of Mendelism (*see* **Mendel's Laws**) coincided with the identification of hundreds of phenotypes, in diverse species, whose inheritance could be explained by a dominant or recessive allele. In crosses, the familiar 3:1 segregation ratio (*see* **Segregation Analysis, Classical**) was consistently observed for these phenotypes, leading to the suggestion that the population frequency of dominant to recessive genotypes should also be in the 3:1 ratio. This suggestion was, however, easily refuted by observations in natural populations. This dilemma was resolved by Hardy and Weinberg who showed by theoretical analysis that the frequency of genotypes in populations, under the simplifying assumptions of random mating in a population of infinite size and the absence of mutation, migration and selection, was solely determined by the frequencies of the constituent alleles [6] (*see* **Hardy–Weinberg Equilibrium**). Thus, if the allele frequencies of the dominant, D, and recessive, d, alleles at an autosomal locus were p and q, respectively, then the frequencies of the genotypes DD, Dd, and dd are p^2, $2pq$, and q^2, respectively. The same results apply to females at an X-linked locus, with males having alleles in proportion to their population frequencies. In the presence of dominance, the dominant and recessive phenotypes have population frequencies of $p^2 + 2pq = 1 - q^2$ and q^2, respectively. Under these assumptions, Hardy and Weinberg also showed that, irrespective of the initial genotype frequency distributions, one generation of random mating generates the above genotype frequencies and that these allele and genotype frequencies do not change further over time, i.e. the frequencies are at an equilibrium state.

Shortly after, in the 1910s, with the discovery of genetic linkage, theoretical studies were initiated to investigate the consequences of random mating when two linked loci were considered, and under the same simplifying assumptions used by Hardy [6]. Jennings [9] and Robbins [17] showed that with two linked genes, the population, once again, approached an equilibrium state in which the alleles at the two loci associated at random; Geiringer [5] solved the problem with three linked factors. If two loci, one with alleles D and d with frequencies p and q, respectively, and a second with alleles E and e with frequencies r and s, respectively, arc linkcd with rccombination frequency θ ($0 \leq \theta \leq 1/2$), then, at equilibrium, the frequency of homozygotes such as DDEE is $p^2 r^2$, the frequency of single **heterozygotes** such as DdEE is $2pqr^2$, and the frequency of the double heterozygote DdEe is $4pqrs$. In random mating populations, the equilibrium population frequency of any genotype, at one or more loci, is determined solely by the constituent allele frequencies at individual loci.

Linkage Disequilibrium

Jennings [9], Robbins [17], and Geiringer [5] also determined the rate of approach to equilibrium when more than one locus is involved and gave the genotypic distributions after any finite number of generations. These authors showed that, under random mating, the frequency of any multilocus genotype, g generations from an initial condition, is determined by the products of frequencies of the four haplotypes (allele combinations) DE, De, dE, and de, and that the haplotype frequencies change over time. After g generations, the haplotype frequencies are:

$$DE : h_1 = pr + \varepsilon,$$
$$De : h_2 = ps - \varepsilon,$$
$$dE : h_3 = qr - \varepsilon,$$
$$de : h_4 = qs + \varepsilon.$$

In each generation there is a specific departure of the haplotype frequencies from the equilibrium values; this excess or deficiency is denoted as ε and termed the coefficient of allelic association or linkage disequilibrium. Note that the numerical value of ε is bounded, since each haplotype frequency is nonnegative, less than unity, and the four haplotype frequencies add to 1, as follows:

$$-\min(pr, qs) \leq \varepsilon \leq \min(ps, qr).$$

With genetic recombination between the D and E locus, the coefficient of allelic association declines every generation so that in successive generations they are related as:

$$\varepsilon' = (1 - \theta)\varepsilon.$$

Thus, in g generations, the total decline is,

$$\varepsilon_g = (1 - \theta)^g \varepsilon_0,$$

where ε_0 is the coefficient of allelic association at generation zero (initial condition). Note that in any generation, $\varepsilon = h_1 h_4 - h_2 h_3$.

The above equations suggest that linkage disequilibrium occurs only as a nonequilibrium phenomenon since it always declines to zero. However, the rate of decline is determined by the recombination value with a half-life of $-\ln 2/\ln(1 - \theta)$; the inverse relationship with the recombination value suggests that, for very close linkage, disequilibrium may persist for long evolutionary time periods.

Causes of Linkage Disequilibrium

An extensive body of population genetics literature shows how various forms of natural selection acting on individual genes can lead to permanent, equilibrium association of the alleles at two loci, even in the absence of linkage [14]. Additionally, when two loci are linked, natural selection at one locus can lead to the apparent selection at a linked locus ("hitchhiking") and permanent linkage disequilibrium. However, and as stated earlier, in the absence of natural selection no permanent associations are expected at two linked loci. Thus, the term linkage disequilibrium is a misnomer since linkage is neither necessary nor sufficient for permanent associations to occur; the descriptive term allelic (nonrandom) association is more appropriate. Other circumstances under which allelic associations can occur, although not permanently, are population admixture and population subdivision (*see* **Admixture in Human Populations**). In the latter case, a population with hidden subpopulations, each of which differs in allele frequencies and/or allelic associations, but treated as a single population, can also create allelic disequilibrium. Further details on these and other theoretical models are provided in [13]–[15].

In many large, random mating populations allelic associations are nevertheless observed. In humans, such observations, restricted to very closely linked **blood group** genes, such as those within the Rhesus (C, D, and E loci) and MNS (M and S loci), or within the **HLA system** of genes, have been known for a long time [1]. More recently, with the availability of multiple DNA **polymorphisms** in a small genomic region, these studies have gained in popularity. In fact, polymorphic alleles at multiple sites all within 20–30 kilobases of DNA demonstrate allelic associations [3]. These observations are best explained by the nonequilibrium state of the human population and the expectation of a slow decay of linkage disequilibrium when the maximal recombination rate within a region is less than 0.0005 per generation [3]. These observations have found multiple uses such as for associating specific mutations with a molecular haplotype in a genomic region [11] and for mapping the location of a mutation to a small genetic interval [12].

Parameterization and Estimation

Allelic associations, parameterized as the coefficient of linkage disequilibrium ε, are most easily and efficiently estimated from haplotype data. However, for most diploid organisms it is not possible to derive haplotypes from diploid two-locus genotypes unless family data (i.e. parents, offspring, and other relatives are sampled and studied) are also available (*see* **Haplotype Analysis**). Then, haplotype frequencies are estimated from the relative frequencies of haplotypes in a sample of independent families and by counting only independent haplotypes within each family. Tests of allelic associations (H$_0$: $\varepsilon = 0$) are based on the significance of a chi-squared statistic with 1 df comparing the observed and expected (under equilibrium) haplotype frequencies. In a sample of n haplotypes studied, if allelic associations are present, the expected value of this **chi-square** statistic is $\chi^2 = n\rho^2$, where,

$$\rho = \frac{\varepsilon}{(pqrs)^{1/2}}.$$

Thus, the **correlation** in the chi-square **contingency table** of observations is another measure of linkage disequilibrium, one that is a natural measure based on the test of association. In many investigations, this latter measure has been used since ρ appears to be less dependent on the allele frequencies than ε. A measure that is not dependent on allele frequencies and finding more popular use in these studies is Yule's measure of association [12]:

$$A = \frac{h_1 h_4 - h_2 h_3}{h_1 h_4 + h_2 h_3}.$$

The above results are for loci with two alleles per locus, whereas many polymorphic markers have multiple alleles. Then, coefficients for allelic association have to be defined for each allele pair at two loci, allele triples for three loci, and so on. A discussion of these multiple disequilibria and tests of hypotheses on them is discussed in [18].

When family data are unavailable, linkage disequilibrium parameters can be efficiently estimated from population samples using iterative methods such as the **EM algorithm**. In the genetic context, this was first proposed by Hill [8] for two loci; additional methods and calculations of sample size for predefined statistical **power** was studied by Brown [2]. In addition, Brown [2] considers the appropriate parameterization of disequilibria for multiple loci taken together (i.e. the nonrandom association of alleles at multiple loci) once the pairwise disequilibria have been considered. Tests of significance (*see* **Hypothesis Testing**) are performed by appropriate modifications of the chi-square test alluded to above. Of greater importance, particularly with DNA polymorphism data, is the existence of multiple alleles at each locus studied. In this circumstance there are several possible tests of disequilibrium, such as an omnibus test or conditional tests on specific collection of alleles. Weir & Cockerham [18] have provided a theoretical and statistical account of this situation.

It is clear that accurate estimates of allelic associations require very large sample sizes when the allele frequencies, at one of the two loci studied, are close to 0 or 1. This occurs whenever **disease–marker associations** are evaluated. In these circumstances a conditional sampling strategy, in which marker genotypes are evaluated within classes of affected and unaffected individuals, is very efficient. Chakravarti et al. [4] have provided a **maximum likelihood** method for estimation of linkage disequilibrium statistics from conditional marker genotype data. These methods are useful for mapping disease genes with respect to a map of DNA markers (*see* **Genetic Map Functions**) [10, 12].

Current Applications

Studies of allelic associations across the genome and in various natural populations are now beginning, with the availability of high-resolution genetic maps in a number of species. So far, the primary purpose of these studies has been to probe the population structure of natural populations. Since in large randomly mating populations no allelic associations are expected, the finding of widespread associations will suggest that these populations are either not in equilibrium or that they have been recently established from a small number of founders. The fitting of specific population genetic models can then elucidate whether the nonequilibrium nature of these populations is due to genetic drift, natural selection, subdivision, or migration. In the human, these types of studies all suggest that modern humans have descended from a limited pool of founders ($\sim$10 000) approximately 200 000 years or so before the present.

In the human, the greatest application of studies of allelic association is to find the location of a disease gene with respect to a map of DNA markers, once the gene has been genetically localized to a DNA segment under 1000 kilobases. This was first demonstrated with the molecular cloning of the gene for cystic fibrosis [12]. A theoretical basis for disease–marker associations owing to common descent of a specific mutation from an ancestor, such as for cystic fibrosis, has been given by Hastbacka et al. [7] and Puffenberger et al. [16]. The prospects for such disease mapping, as an aid to the molecular cloning of the mutant gene, has also been discussed by Jorde [10].

References

[1]   Bodmer, W.F. & Cavalli-Sforza, L.L. (1976). *Genetics, Evolution, and Man*. W.H. Freeman, San Francisco.

[2]   Brown, A.H.D. (1975). Sample sizes required to detect linkage disequilibrium between two or three loci, *Theoretical Population Biology* **8**, 184–201.

[3]   Chakravarti, A., Buetow, K.H., Antonarakis, S.E., Waber, P.G., Boehm, C.D. & Kazazian, H.H. (1984). Nonuniform recombination within the human β-globin gene cluster, *American Journal of Human Genetics* **36**, 1239–1258.

[4]   Chakravarti, A., Li, C.C. & Buetow, K.H. (1984). Estimation of the marker gene frequency and linkage disequilibrium from conditional marker data, *American Journal of Human Genetics* **36**, 177–186.

[5]   Geiringer, H. (1945). Further remarks on linkage in Mendelian heredity, *Annals of Mathematical Statistics* **16**, 390–393.

[6]   Hardy, G.H. (1908). Mendelian proportions in a mixed population, *Science* **28**, 49–50.

[7]   Hastbacka, J., de la Chapelle, A., Kaitial, I., Sistonen, P., Weaver, A. & Lander, E.S. (1992). Linkage disequilibrium mapping in isolated founder populations: diastrophic dysplasia in Finland, *Nature Genetics* **2**, 204–211.

[8]   Hill, W.G. (1974). Estimation of linkage disequilibrium in randomly mating populations, *Heredity* **33**, 229–239.

[9]   Jennings, H.S. (1917). The numerical results of diverse systems of breeding with respect to two pairs of characters, linked or independent, with special relation to the effects of linkage, *Genetics* **12**, 97–154.

[10]   Jorde, L.B. (1995). Linkage disequilibrium as a gene-mapping tool, *American Journal of Human Genetics* **56**, 11–14.

[11]   Kazazian, H.H., Stuart, O.H., Markham, A.F., Chapman, C.R., Youssoufian, H. & Waber, P.G. (1984). Quantification of the close association between DNA haplotypes and specific β-thalassaemia mutations in mediterraneans, *Nature* **310**, 152–154.

[12]   Kerem, B., Rommens, J.M., Buchanan, J.A., Markiewicz, D., Cox, T.K., Chakravarti, A., Buchwald, M. & Tsui, L.C. (1989). Identification of the cystic fibrosis gene: Genetic analysis, *Science* **245**, 1073–1808.

[13]   Kimura, M. & Crow, J.F. (1970). *An Introduction to Population Genetics Theory*. Harper & Row, New York.

[14]   Kimura, M. & Ohta, T. (1971). *Theoretical Aspects of Population Genetics*, Princeton University Press, Princeton.

[15]   Li, C.C. (1976). *First Course in Population Genetics*. The Boxwood Press, Pacific Grove.

[16]   Puffenberger, E.G., Kauffman, E.R., Bolk, S., Matise, T.C., Washington, S.S., Angrist, M., Weissenbach, J., Garver, K.L., Mascari, M., Ladda, R., Slaugenhaupt, S.A. & Chakravarti, A. (1994). Identity-by-descent and association mapping of a recessive gene for Hirschsprung disease on human chromosome 13q22, *Human Molecular Genetics* **3**, 1217–1225.

[17] Robbins, R.B. (1918). Some applications of mathematics to breeding problems. III, *Genetics* **3**, 375–389.

[18] Weir, B.S. & Cockerham, C.C. (1978). Testing hypotheses about linkage disequilibrium with multiple alleles, *Genetics* **88**, 633–642.

ARAVINDA CHAKRAVARTI

Linked Plots *see* Multivariate Graphics

LISREL

The acronym LISREL was coined by Jöreskog [5–7]: it is derived from LInear Structural RELations. Researchers use the term LISREL to refer either to **structural equations models** or to Jöreskog & Sörbom's [8] popular **software** program to estimate such statistical models. The LISREL *model* consists of two primary parts: a latent variable model and a measurement model. The former allows linear relationships between latent (unobserved) variables. This is much like a simultaneous equation model used in econometrics, except that it has latent rather than observed variables. It formulates the relation between the latent variables free of the confounding effects of measurement errors. The measurement model provides the linkages between the latent and observed variables. This model enables a researcher to use multiple indicators of the latent variables and to assess the "quality" of the measures. Many popular linear models (e.g. simultaneous equations, **confirmatory factor analysis, multiple regression, analysis of variance, analysis of covariance,** etc.) are special cases of Jöreskog's LISREL model.

In the original LISREL model, linear relations were assumed between continuous latent and continuous observed variables. Extensions of the LISREL model (see, for example, [8] and [11]) maintain the assumption of continuous latent variables but allow noncontinuous observed variables; for example, **censored**, ordinal (*see* **Ordered Categorical Data**), or dichotomous variables (*see* **Binary Data**). The relation between the latent variables and the noncontinuous observed variables is nonlinear. Other

extensions allow equations that are nonlinear in the latent variables [3, 9, 10]. The article **Structural Equation Models** gives a more complete description of the LISREL model.

The second use of the term LISREL refers to a computer software program. One of the primary reasons for the rise in popularity of structural equation models was the availability of Jöreskog & Sörbom's [8] LISREL software package. For many years, LISREL was the only widely available program capable of estimating and testing these models. It is partly for this reason that both the structural equation model and the software were referred to by the same LISREL term. Since about the mid-1980s, other structural equation software programs have become more common (e.g. [1], [2], [4], and [12]). In addition, Jöreskog & Sörbom have continuously updated the LISREL program. The greater availability of software has contributed both to the further spread of these models as well as to the trend to refer to the statistical models as "structural equation models". The latter term helps to distinguish the model from the software needed to analyze the model.

References

[1] Arbuckle, J.L. (1997). *AMOS User's Guide, Version 3.6.* Small Waters Company, Chicago.

[2] Bentler, P.M. (1992). *EQS Structural Equations Program Manual.* BMDP Statistical Software, Los Angeles.

[3] Bollen, K.A. (1995). Structural equation models that are nonlinear in latent variables: a least-squares estimator, in *Sociological Methodology 1995*, P.M. Marsden, ed. American Sociological Association, Washington, pp. 223–251.

[4] Hartmann, W.M. (1990). *The CALIS Procedure: Extended User's Guide.* SAS Institute, Cary.

[5] Jöreskog, K.G. (1973). A general method for estimating a linear structural equation system, in *Structural Equation Models in the Social Sciences*, A.S. Goldberger & O.D. Duncan, eds. Academic Press, New York, pp. 85–112.

[6] Jöreskog, K.G. (1977). Structural equation models in the social sciences: specification estimation, and testing, in *Applications of Statistics*, P.R. Krishnaiah, ed. North-Holland, Amsterdam, pp. 265–287.

[7] Jöreskog, K.G. & Sörbom, D. (1981). LISREL V: *Analysis of Linear Structural Relationships by the Method of Maximum Likelihood.* National Educational Resources, Chicago.

[8] Jöreskog, K.G. & Sörbom, D. (1993). *LISREL 8.* Scientific Software, Mooresville.

[9]   Jöreskog, K.G. & Yang, F. (1996). Nonlinear structural equation models: the Kenny–Judd model with interaction effects, in *Advanced Structural Equation Modeling*, G. Marcoulides & R. Schumacker, eds. Lawrence Erlbaum, Mahwah, pp. 57–88.

[10] Kenny, D.A. & Judd, C.M. (1984). Estimating the nonlinear and interactive effects of latent variables, *Psychological Bulletin* **96**, 201–210.

[11] Muthén, B. (1984). A general structural equation model with dichotomous, ordered categorical, and continuous latent variable indicators, *Psychometrika* **49**, 115–132.

[12] Muthén, B. (1988). *LISCOMP: Analysis of Linear Structural Equations with a Comprehensive Measurement Model*, 2nd Ed. Scientific Software, Mooresville.

KENNETH A. BOLLEN

List-Assisted Method *see* Random Digit Dialing Sampling for Case–Control Studies

Listwise Deletion for Missing Data *see* Missing Data Estimation, "Hot Deck" and "Cold Deck"

Litter Effect *see* Preclinical Treatment Evaluation

Little's Equation in Queuing Theory *see* Incidence–Prevalence Relationships

Lo(w)ess *see* Graphical Displays

Locally Most Powerful Tests

The classical **Neyman–Pearson Lemma** gives a **most powerful (MP) test** for the problem of testing a simple null hypothesis $\theta = \theta_0$ against a simple alternative hypothesis $\theta = \theta_1$. The Neyman–Pearson tests turn out to be uniformly most powerful (UMP) in some situations, but this is not true in general. For example, when $H_0: \theta \in \Theta_0 \subset \Theta$ and $H_1: \theta \in \Theta_1 \subset \Theta$ are one-sided, then the existence of a UMP test for every level α is essentially equivalent to the requirement that the joint density function has a monotone **likelihood ratio** property [11].

When a UMP test does not exist, one may restrict the class of tests to, say, the class of **unbiased** and/or invariant tests, and then look for a UMP test in this smaller class. Alternatively, one may look for tests that have maximum power against alternatives in a subset of Θ_1. The case when the subset of alternatives is "close" to the null parameter values has received a good deal of attention, presumably because tests that have good power for "local alternatives", which are the hardest to detect, may also retain good power for "nonlocal" alternatives.

Locally Most Powerful Tests

We focus attention to the case when θ is a real parameter, and use the Neyman & Pearson [8, 9] framework. Consider the problem of testing $H_0: \theta \leq \theta_0$ against $H_1: \theta > \theta_0$. Let ϕ_0 be a test function with **power** function $\beta_{\phi_0}(\theta) = E_\theta \phi_0(X)$. Then ϕ_0 is a locally most powerful (LMP) test of size α if there exists a $\Delta > 0$ such that for any other test ϕ with $\alpha = \sup_{\theta \leq \theta_0} \beta_{\phi_0}(\theta) \geq \sup_{\theta \leq \theta_0} \beta_\phi(\theta)$, $\beta_{\phi_0}(\theta_0) \geq \beta_\phi(\theta)$ for every $\theta \in (\theta_0, \theta_0 + \Delta]$. Thus, an LMP test maximizes

$$\left. \frac{\mathrm{d}}{\mathrm{d}\theta} \beta(\theta) \right|_{\theta=\theta_0} = \left. \beta'(\theta) \right|_{\theta=\theta_0}$$

subject to the size constraint. Under some smoothness conditions one can show that any test of the form $\phi_0(\mathbf{x}) = 1$ if $\partial \log f(\mathbf{x};\theta)/\partial\theta|_{\theta=\theta_0} > k, = 0$ if $\partial \log f(\mathbf{x};\theta)/\partial\theta|_{\theta=\theta_0} < k$ will maximize $\beta'(\theta)|_{\theta=\theta_0}$. Here $f(\mathbf{x};\theta)$ is the joint probability density function (pdf) of a **random sample** $X_1, X_2, \ldots, X_n$ with common pdf $f(\mathbf{x};\theta)$.

Consider for example, the problem of testing $H_0: \theta \leq 0$ against $H_1: \theta > 0$, where θ is the **median** of a **Cauchy** density function $f(x;\theta) = \pi^{-1}[1 + (x-\theta)^2]^{-1}$, $-\infty < x < \infty$. Let $x_1, x_2, \ldots, x_n$ be n observations. It is easy to see that MP size α tests of $\theta = 0$ against $\theta = \theta_1, \theta_1 > 0$, depend on θ_1 and hence a UMP test for testing H_0 against H_1 does not exist. An LMP test of H_0 against H_1 is of form

$$\phi_0(\mathbf{x}) = \begin{cases} 1, & \text{if } \sum_{i=1}^n 2x_i/(1+x_i^2) > k, \\ 0, & \text{elsewhere,} \end{cases}$$

where one chooses k so that the size of ϕ_0 is α (*see* **Critical Region**).

This LMP test, although good at detecting small departures from H_0: $\theta \le 0$, is quite unsatisfactory in detecting values of θ much larger than 0. In fact, $\beta_{\phi_0}(\theta) \to 0$ as $\theta \to \infty$ if $\alpha < 1/2$.

Locally Most Powerful Unbiased Tests

The definition of an LMP test can be extended to the case of two-sided alternatives. In general, there do not exist LMP tests for two-sided alternatives. The LMP test ϕ_0 above is trivially unbiased in some interval $[\theta_0, \theta_0 + \Delta)$. It follows that $\beta'_{\phi_0}(\theta_0) \ge 0$, suggesting that for testing $\theta = \theta_0$ against $\theta \ne \theta_0$ we seek a test ϕ_0 with power function

$$\beta_{\phi_0}(\theta_0) = \alpha, \quad \beta'_{\phi_0}(\theta_0) = 0 \quad \text{and}$$

$$\beta''_{\phi_0}(\theta_0) \text{ maximum.}$$

Such a test is called LMP unbiased of size α for testing H_0: $\theta = \theta_0$ against H_1: $\theta \ne \theta_0$.

An LMP unbiased test is of the form

$$\phi_0(\mathbf{x}) = \begin{cases} 1, & \text{if } \left.\dfrac{\partial^2}{\partial\theta^2} f(\mathbf{x};\theta)\right|_{\theta=\theta_0} \\[2mm] & > k_1 f(\mathbf{x};\theta_0) + k_2 \left.\dfrac{\partial}{\partial\theta} f(\mathbf{x};\theta)\right|_{\theta=\theta_0}, \\[3mm] \gamma(\mathbf{x}), & \text{if } \left.\dfrac{\partial^2}{\partial\theta^2} f(\mathbf{x};\theta)\right|_{\theta=\theta_0} \\[2mm] & = k_1 f(\mathbf{x};\theta_0) + k_2 \left.\dfrac{\partial}{\partial\theta} f(\mathbf{x};\theta)\right|_{\theta=\theta_0}, \\[3mm] 0, & \text{if } \left.\dfrac{\partial^2}{\partial\theta^2} f(\mathbf{x};\theta)\right|_{\theta=\theta_0} \\[2mm] & < k_1 f(\mathbf{x};\theta_0) + k_2 \left.\dfrac{\partial}{\partial\theta} f(\mathbf{x};\theta)\right|_{\theta=\theta_0}, \end{cases}$$

where k_1, k_2, and $\gamma(\cdot)$ are chosen to satisfy $\beta_{\phi_0}(\theta_0) = \alpha$ and $\beta'_{\phi_0}(\theta_0) = 0$.

For the Cauchy density function in the first section, the critical region of the LMP test is the set of points

$\mathbf{x}$ such that

$$2\sum_{i=1}^n \frac{x_i^2 - 1}{(1+x_i^2)^2} + \left[\sum_{i=1}^n \frac{2x_i}{1+x_i^2}\right]^2 > k_1,$$

where k_1 is chosen to satisfy $\beta_{\phi_0}(\theta_0) = \alpha$. This test is not a two-sided version of the LMP test given in the first section.

Locally Most Powerful Invariant Tests

Similar considerations apply when attention is restricted to the class of tests that are invariant under a group of transformations on the sample space. Then it is sufficient to consider test statistics that are functions of the maximal invariant and local optimality criteria may be applied to its density.

Consider, for example, the **nonparametric** two-sample problem. Let $X_1, X_2, \ldots, X_m$ and $Y_1, Y_2, \ldots, Y_n$ be random samples from respective (continuous) distribution functions F and G. Suppose we wish to test H_0: $F(x) \ge G(x)$ for all x against H_1: $F(x) \le G(x)$ for all x $[F(x) \ne G(x)$ for some $x]$. Restricting attention to the **sufficient statistics** $X_{(1)} < X_{(2)} < \cdots < X_{(m)}$ and $Y_{(1)} < Y_{(2)} < \cdots < Y_{(n)}$, the problem is invariant under continuous monotone transformations and a maximal invariant is the set of ranks $(R_1, R_2, \ldots, R_m, S_1, S_2, \ldots, S_n)$, where $R_i = $ **rank** of X_i in the combined sample and $S_j = $ rank of Y_j in the combined sample. Invariance considerations lead us to focus attention on tests that depend only on $R_1, R_2, \ldots, R_m$. Again, a UMP rank test of H_0 does not exist, but one can obtain LMP rank tests.

Suppose, for example, that we fix g, the probability density function corresponding to G and consider the location problem of testing H_0: $f(x) = g(x)$ against H_1: $f(x) = g(x - \theta)$ for values of $\theta > 0$. Then the methods of the first section lead to the LMP test: reject H_0: $\theta = 0$ against H_1: $\theta > 0$ for large values of the linear rank statistic $\sum_{i=1}^m a(R_i)$, where

$$a(i) = E\left[-\frac{g'(G^{-1}(U_{(i)}))}{g(G^{-1}(U_{(i)}))}\right], \quad i = 1, 2, \ldots, m,$$

and $U_{(1)} < U_{(2)} < \cdots < U_{(N)}$ are the **order statistics** for a random sample of size $N = m + n$ from a **uniform** $(0, 1)$ distribution. The special case when g is normal $(0, 1)$ leads to the well-known Fisher–Yates test (*see* **Normal Scores**), while when g is logistic, the resulting test is the **Wilcoxon–Mann–Whitney test**.

LMP rank tests are especially useful when the data are **censored**. Rank tests with type II censored data have been discussed by Johnson [4] and Mehrotra et al. [6], and by Prentice [12] and Peto & Peto [10] for arbitrarily censored data.

Ferguson [1, Sections 5.5 and 5.7] is an easily accessible source for LMP tests. Both Lehmann [5] and Schmetterer [14, Section III.6], give a more measure-theoretic treatment. Hájek & Šidák [2, Section III.4] give a fairly general treatment of LMP rank tests for various hypotheses of invariance. At a somewhat lower level, one can refer to Randles & Wolfe [13, Section 9.1]. For the multiparameter case, see Isaacson [3], Schmetterer [14], Neyman [7], and Neyman & Pearson [9].

References

[1]   Ferguson, T. (1967). *Mathematical Statistics*. Academic Press, New York.

[2]   Hájek, J. & Šidák, Z. (1967). *Theory of Rank Tests*. Academic Press, New York.

[3]   Isaacson, S.L. (1951). On the theory of unbiased tests of simple statistical hypotheses specifying the values of two or more parameters, *Annals of Mathematical Statistics* **22**, 217–234.

[4]   Johnson, R. (1974). *Reliability and Biometry*. SIAM, Philadelphia.

[5]   Lehmann, E. (1986). *Testing of Statistical Hypotheses*. Wiley, New York.

[6]   Mehrotra, K., Johnson, R. & Bhattacharya, G. (1977). Locally most powerful tests for multiple-censored data, *Communications in Statistics – Theory and Methods* **6**, 459–470.

[7]   Neyman, J. (1935). Sur la vérification des hypothèses statistiques composées, *Bulletin de la Société Mathematique de France, Paris* **63**, 246–266.

[8]   Neyman, J. & Pearson, E. (1936). Contributions to the theory of testing statistical hypotheses, *Statistical Research Memoirs* **1**, 1–37.

[9]   Neyman, J. & Pearson, E. (1938). Contributions to the theory of testing statistical hypotheses, *Statistical Research Memoirs* **2**, 25–57.

[10] Peto, R. & Peto, J. (1972). Asymptotically efficient rank invariant test procedures, *Journal of the Royal Statistical Society, Series A* **135**, 185–198.

[11] Pfanzagl, J. (1963). Überall trennscharfe tests und monotone Dichtequotienten, *Zeitschrift für Wahrscheinlichkeitstheorie und Verwandte Gebiete* **1**, 109–115.

[12] Prentice, R.L. (1978). Linear rank tests with right censored data, *Biometrika* **65**, 167–179.

[13] Randles, R. & Wolfe, D. (1979). *Introduction to the Theory of Nonparametric Statistics*. Wiley, New York.

[14] Schmetterer, L. (1974). *Introduction to Mathematical Statistics*. Springer-Verlag, New York.

(*See also* **Large-Sample Theory; Linear Rank Tests in Survival Analysis**)

EDSEL A. PEÑA & VIJAY K. ROHATGI

Location Model for Discrimination *see* Discriminant Analysis, Linear

Location Score *see* Multipoint Linkage Analysis

Location–Scale Family

A set of random variables $X_1, \ldots, X_n$ is said to have a location–scale family distribution with parameter (μ, σ) if their joint cumulative distribution function (cdf) can be expressed as

$$F(x_1, \ldots, x_n | \mu, \sigma) = F\left(\frac{x_1 - \mu}{\sigma}, \ldots, \frac{x_n - \mu}{\sigma}\right),$$
$$\mu \text{ real}, \sigma > 0,$$

for some cdf $F(\cdot)$. Equivalently $(X_1, \ldots, X_n)$ has a location–scale family with parameter (μ, σ) if the joint cdf of $(T_1, \ldots, T_n)$ is $F(t_1, \ldots, t_n)$, where $T_i = (X_i - \mu)/\sigma$, $F(t_1, \ldots, t_n)$ is any n-dimensional cdf, and different $F(\cdot)$s correspond to different location–scale families. The parameter μ is the location parameter and σ is the scale parameter. The parameter (μ, σ) is defined as the location-scale parameter of a random variable X if and only if the distribution of $(x - \mu)/\sigma$ under (μ, σ) is free from μ and σ.

From any location–scale family of distributions, two important subfamilies are obtained; namely, a location family with the parameter μ when σ is fixed (and without loss of generality $\sigma = 1$), and a scale family with the parameter σ when μ is fixed (and without loss of generality $\mu = 0$).

Corresponding to any location–scale family $F(x_1, \ldots, x_n | \mu, \sigma)$, the member of the family with $\mu = 0$ and $\sigma = 1$ has a cdf $F(x_1, \ldots, x_n)$ and is referred to as the "standard" or "generator" of the family, generated through a group of location and scale transformations. If $F(x_1, \ldots, x_n)$ has a probability density function (pdf) $f(x_1, \ldots, x_n)$ with respect to a Lebesgue measure, then the continuous location–scale family has a pdf

$$\frac{1}{\sigma^n} f\left(\frac{x_1 - \mu}{\sigma}, \ldots, \frac{x_n - \mu}{\sigma}\right).$$

Some important examples of location–scale family distributions are **uniform** $(\mu - \sigma, \mu + \sigma)$, **normal** (μ, σ) (here σ is the standard deviation), and **Cauchy** (μ, σ).

Parameter Estimation

Least Squares Estimation

Order statistics play an important role in the estimation of μ and σ. We assume that $X_1, \ldots, X_n$ are independent, identically distributed (iid) with a location scale pdf $(1/\sigma)h[(x - \mu)/\sigma]$, where $h(\cdot)$ is known. From the property of the location–scale family, it follows that $X_i = \mu + \sigma Z_i$, $i = 1, \ldots, n$, where $Z_1, \ldots, Z_n$ are iid with pdf $h(z)$. If $Y_1, \ldots, Y_n$ are the order statistics based on $X_1, \ldots, X_n$, and $Z_{(1)}, \ldots, Z_{(n)}$ are the order statistics based on $Z_1, \ldots, Z_n$, then $Y_i = \mu + \sigma Z_{(i)}$, $i = 1, \ldots, n$. Since $h(\cdot)$ is a known pdf, $E(Z_{(i)}) = \alpha_i$, and $\text{cov}(Z_{(i)}, Z_{(j)}) = w_{ij}$, $i, j = 1, \ldots, n$, are known [assuming the first two moments of $h(\cdot)$ exist]. Then, we get

$$E(\mathbf{Y}) = \mu \mathbf{1} + \sigma \boldsymbol{\alpha} = \mathbf{A}\boldsymbol{\theta},$$

where $\mathbf{Y} = (Y_1, \ldots, Y_n)^T$, $\boldsymbol{\alpha} = (\alpha_1, \ldots, \alpha_n)^T$, and $\mathbf{1}$ is a vector with unit elements, $\mathbf{A} = (\mathbf{1}, \boldsymbol{\alpha})$, $\boldsymbol{\theta} = (\mu, \sigma)^T$ and $\text{var}(\mathbf{Y}) = \sigma^2 \mathbf{w}$, where $\mathbf{w}$ is the matrix of the elements w_{ij}. Then weighted **least squares** estimates of μ and σ are given by

$$\hat{\mu} = -\boldsymbol{\alpha}^T \boldsymbol{\Gamma} \mathbf{Y}, \quad \hat{\sigma} = \mathbf{1}^T \boldsymbol{\Gamma} \mathbf{Y},$$

where $\boldsymbol{\Gamma} = \boldsymbol{\Omega}(\mathbf{1}\boldsymbol{\alpha}^T - \boldsymbol{\alpha}\mathbf{1}^T)\boldsymbol{\Omega}/\Delta$, $\boldsymbol{\Omega} = \mathbf{w}^{-1}$ and $\Delta = |\mathbf{A}^T \boldsymbol{\Omega} \mathbf{A}|$. The variance–**covariance matrix** of these

estimates is given by

$$\frac{\sigma^2}{\Delta}\begin{pmatrix} \boldsymbol{\alpha}^T \boldsymbol{\Omega} \boldsymbol{\alpha} & -\mathbf{1}^T \boldsymbol{\Omega} \boldsymbol{\alpha} \\ -\mathbf{1}^T \boldsymbol{\Omega} \boldsymbol{\alpha} & \mathbf{1}^T \boldsymbol{\Omega} \mathbf{1} \end{pmatrix}.$$

For details, see Lloyd [6].

Minimum Risk Equivariant Estimation

Since a location–scale family is a group family (see [4, pp. 19–21]), invariance consideration plays an important role in inference. For a location family of distributions $f(x_1 - \mu, \ldots, x_n - \mu)$ and a group of location transformations, a maximal invariant statistic is given by $(x_1 - x_n, \ldots, x_{n-1} - x_n)$. This is an **ancillary statistic** since its distribution does not depend on μ.

Under a squared error **loss**, the minimum risk equivariant (MRE) estimate (if it exists) of μ is given by (see, for example, [4, p. 160])

$$\frac{\int \mu f(x_1 - \mu, \ldots, x_n - \mu)\, d\mu}{\int f(x_1 - \mu, \ldots, x_n - \mu)\, d\mu}, \tag{1}$$

and is known as the Pitman estimate of μ. If $X_1, \ldots, X_n$ are iid $N(\mu, \sigma)$ with σ known, then the above estimate reduces to $\bar{x}$. In this case, it is also the uniformly **minimum variance unbiased estimate** (UMVUE) of μ.

Similarly, for a scale family of distributions $(1/\sigma^n)f(x_1/\sigma, \ldots, x_n/\sigma)$ and a group of scale transformations, a maximal invariant statistic is given by $(x_1/x_n, \ldots, x_{n-1}/x_n, x_n/|x_n|)$ (see [4, p. 174]) which is an ancillary statistic. Under the loss function $(a/\sigma^r - 1)^2$, the MRE estimate (if it exists) of σ^r is given by (see, [4, p. 177])

$$\frac{\int_0^\infty \sigma^{n+r-1} f(\sigma x_1, \ldots, \sigma x_n)\, d\sigma}{\int_0^\infty \sigma^{n+2r-1} f(\sigma x_1, \ldots, \sigma x_n)\, d\sigma}. \tag{2}$$

For $X_1, \ldots, X_n$ iid $N(0, \sigma)$ and $r = 2$, the above estimate reduces to $\sum x_i^2/(n + 2)$.

For a location–scale family of distributions $(1/\sigma^n)f[(x_1 - \mu)/\sigma, \ldots, (x_n - \mu)/\sigma]$ and a group of location–scale transformations, a maximal invariant statistic is given by (see [4, p. 179])

$$\left(\frac{x_1 - x_n}{x_{n-1} - x_n}, \dots, \frac{x_{n-2} - x_n}{x_{n-1} - x_n}, \frac{x_{n-1} - x_n}{|x_{n-1} - x_n|} \right).$$

Estimation of $\beta\mu + \gamma\sigma$ for known β and γ is important. (The case $\beta = 1$, $\gamma = 0$, corresponds to the estimation of μ, whereas $\beta = 0$, $\gamma = 1$, corresponds to the estimation of σ, and $\beta = 1$ and given γ corresponds to the estimation of a certain percentile.)

Under an invariant loss function $L(\mu, \sigma, a) = w[(a - \beta\mu - \gamma\sigma)/\sigma]$, the MRE estimator (if it exists) of $\beta\mu + \gamma\sigma$ has been discussed in detail in Datta & Ghosh [2]. For the loss function $w(x) = x^2$, and for $X_1, \dots, X_n$ iid $N(\mu, \sigma)$, the MRE estimator of $\beta\mu + \gamma\sigma$ is given by $\beta\overline{X} + \gamma kS$, where

$$k = \frac{(n-1)^{1/2}\Gamma(n/2)}{\sqrt{2}\Gamma[(n+1)/2]},$$

$$S^2 = \frac{1}{n-1}\sum(X_i - \overline{X})^2$$

(see [3, p. 182]). The UMVUE of μ and σ^2 for the $N(\mu, \sigma)$ problem are $\overline{X}$ and S^2, respectively.

It follows from Berger [1, p. 410] that the MRE estimates for μ in (1), for σ^r in (2), and for $\beta\mu + \gamma\sigma$ are generalized Bayes estimates with respect to the right invariant Haar density for the respective group of location, scale, and location–scale transformations (*see* **Decision Theory**).

Hypothesis Tests

To test for location and scale parameters, the most widely used assumption is that $X_1, \dots, X_n$ are iid $N(\mu, \sigma)$. In this setup, to test $H_0 : \mu = \mu_0$ vs. $H_1 : \mu \neq \mu_0$, for example, the rejection region for known σ is

$$\left| \frac{n^{1/2}(\overline{X} - \mu_0)}{\sigma} \right| \geq z_{\alpha/2},$$

where $z_{\alpha/2}$ is the $100(1 - \alpha/2)$th percentile point of a **standard normal** distribution. For unknown σ, the corresponding rejection region is obtained by replacing σ and $z_{\alpha/2}$ in the preceding rejection region by S and $t_{\alpha/2}$, the $100(1 - \alpha/2)$th percentile point of **Student's t distribution**, with $n - 1$ degrees of freedom, respectively. The above tests can be shown to be uniformly most powerful unbiased (UMPU)

tests and can be derived as **likelihood ratio tests**. To test for σ^2, $H_0 : \sigma^2 = \sigma_0^2$ vs. $H_1 : \sigma^2 \neq \sigma_0^2$, the widely used test which rejects if

$$\frac{(n-1)S^2}{\sigma_0^2} \leq \chi^2_{1-\alpha/2} \quad \text{or} \quad \frac{(n-1)S^2}{\sigma_0^2} \geq \chi^2_{\alpha/2}$$

is an approximate (for large n) UMPU size α test, where $\chi^2_{\alpha/2}$ is the $100(1 - \alpha/2)$th percentile of the χ^2_{n-1} distribution (**chi-square distribution** with $n - 1$ **degrees of freedom**). For details on these tests and other distribution-free tests for the location and scale parameters, the reader is referred to Lehmann [5].

References

[1]   Berger, J.O. (1985). *Statistical Decision Theory and Bayesian Analysis*, Springer-Verlag, New York.

[2]   Datta, G.S. & Ghosh, M. (1988). Minimum risk equivariant estimators of percentiles in location–scale families of distributions, *Calcutta Statistical Association Bulletin* **37**, 201–207.

[3]   Ferguson, T.S. (1967). *Mathematical Statistics: A Decision Theoretic Approach*. Academic Press, New York.

[4]   Lehmann, E.L. (1983). *Theory of Point Estimation*. Wiley, New York.

[5]   Lehmann, E.L. (1986). *Testing Statistical Hypotheses*. Wiley, New York.

[6]   Lloyd, E.H. (1952). Least squares estimation of location and scale parameters using order statistics, *Biometrika* **39**, 88–95.

GAURI SANKAR DATTA

Locus *see* Gene

Lod Score *see* Linkage Analysis, Model-Based

Log Link Function *see* Generalized Linear Model

Log-Logistic Distribution *see* Parametric Models in Survival Analysis

Logarithmic Scoring Rule *see* Multivariate Classification Rules: Calibration and Discrimination

Logarithmic Series Distribution *see* Negative Binomial Distribution

Logarithmic Series Distribution, Multivariate *see* Multivariate Distributions, Overview

Logarithmic Transformation *see* Power Transformations

Logistic Distribution

The logistic **random variable** X with mean μ and variance σ^2 has a cumulative distribution function

$$F(x, \mu, \sigma) = \{1 + \exp[-\pi(x - \mu)/(\sigma\sqrt{3})]\}^{-1},$$

$$-\infty < x < \infty,$$

$$-\infty < \mu < \infty, \quad \sigma > 0, \qquad (1)$$

and density function f, which is simply related to its distribution function by

$$f(x, \mu, \sigma) = \frac{\pi}{\sigma\sqrt{3}} F(x, \mu, \sigma)[1 - F(x, \mu, \sigma)]. \quad (2)$$

We denote this distribution by $\mathcal{L}(\mu, \sigma^2)$. These functions may also be expressed as

$$F(x, \mu, \sigma) = \frac{1}{2}\left\{1 + \tan h\left[\frac{\pi}{2}(x - \mu)/(\sigma\sqrt{3})\right]\right\} \qquad (3)$$

and

$$f(x, \mu, \sigma) = \frac{\pi}{4\sigma\sqrt{3}}\operatorname{sech}^2\left[\frac{\pi}{2}(x - \mu)/(\sigma\sqrt{3})\right], \quad (4)$$

with the latter expression providing the logistic with the sech-square(d) distribution label. The density f is bell-shaped and symmetrical, with heavier tails than a normal density with the same mean and variance.

To describe some of the basic properties of the logistic distribution, it is simpler to use the "canonical form", $\mathcal{L}(0, \pi^2/3)$, which corresponds to the random variable Z, with mean $\mu = 0$ and variance $\sigma^2 = \pi^2/3$, and has cumulative distribution and density functions

$$G(z) = \frac{1}{1 + e^{-z}}, \qquad (5)$$

$$g(z) = G(z)[1 - G(z)], \qquad (6)$$

and a monotonic *hazard* function

$$\lambda(z) = \frac{g(z)}{1 - G(z)} = G(z). \qquad (7)$$

Eq. (6), and therefore (2), characterizes the logistic distribution and is equivalent to the linearity of the **transformation**

$$\log\left[\frac{G(z)}{1 - G(z)}\right] = z. \qquad (8)$$

This transformation, which is labeled *logit* by Berkson [7], is perhaps the single best known and most popular application of the logistic distribution, especially in the context of modeling **quantal response** data, and performing **logistic regression**.

The distribution function of the standardized random variable $Z/(\pi/\sqrt{3})$, is very close to the **standard normal** distribution, and even closer to the distribution function of a normal random variable with zero mean and standard deviation 15/16 [31]. However, this distribution function is even better approximated by that of a standardized **Student's t distribution** with nine **degrees of freedom** [37]. Moreover, unlike the normal distribution, the sum of independent logistic random variables is not a logistic random variable. Goel [22] and George & Mudholkar [19] give closed-form expressions for the distribution function, and the latter authors also propose a simple Student's t approximation.

Characteristic Function

The **characteristic function** of Z may be expressed in the forms

$$\phi_Z(t) = \Gamma(1 - it)\Gamma(1 + it) = \prod_{j=1}^{\infty}\left(1 - \frac{t^2}{j^2}\right)^{-1} \qquad (9)$$

and

$$\phi_Z(t) = \sum_{k=1}^{\infty} (-1)^{k-1} \frac{2(2^{2k}-1)}{(2k)!} B_{2k}(\pi it)^{2k}, \quad (10)$$

where the B_{2k}s are Bernoulli numbers [53]. The characteristic function (9), or direct integration, may be used to obtain the absolute **moments**

$$E|Z|^k = 2\Gamma(k+1)\left[1 - \frac{1}{2^{k+1}}\zeta(k)\right], \quad (11)$$

where $\zeta(k) = \sum_{j=1}^{\infty} j^{-k}$, is the zeta function.

From (9), we get the following equalities in distribution [17]:

$$Z \overset{\mathcal{D}}{=} \sum_{j=1}^{\infty} W_j$$

$$\overset{\mathcal{D}}{=} \sum_{j=1}^{\infty} (E_{1j} - E_{2j}) \overset{\mathcal{D}}{=} Y_1 - Y_2, \quad (12)$$

where the W_js are independent Laplace or double exponential random variables, and the E_{ij}s are independent **exponential** random variables with respective densities $f_{W_j}(w) = (j/2)\exp(-j|w|)$, $-\infty < \omega < \infty$, $f_{E_{ij}}(x) = j\exp(-jx)$, $i = 1, 2$; $j = 1, 2, \ldots$ and Y_1, Y_2 are iid **extreme value** random variables with density $h(y) = e^{-y}\exp(-e^{-y})$, $-\infty < y < \infty$. The logistic distribution is also obtained from a mixture of the extreme value distribution and the exponential distribution [12]. From (12) we may conclude immediately that the logistic distribution is infinitely divisible.

Order Statistics

Let $Z_{1:n} \le Z_{2:n} \le \cdots \le Z_{n:n}$ be **order statistics** of a random sample from $\mathcal{L}(0, \pi^2/3)$. Then it can be shown that the characteristic function of $Z_{r:n}$ may be expressed as

$$\phi_{r:n}(t) = \prod_{j=1}^{r-1}\left(1 + \frac{it}{j}\right) \prod_{k=1}^{n-r}\left(1 - \frac{it}{k}\right)\phi_Z(t) \quad (13)$$

(see [10], [28], [45], and [46]). Consequently,

$$Z_{r:n} + \sum_{k=1}^{n-r} E_{1k} - \sum_{j=1}^{r-1} E_{2j} \overset{\mathcal{D}}{=} Z_1, \quad (14)$$

where the E_{ij}s are independent exponential random variables with densities $f_{E_{ij}}$ given above, $i = 1, 2$, $j = 1, \ldots, n-1$. Gupta & Shah [28] provide percentage points for the rth order statistics, $Z_{r:n}$, for $1 \le n \le 25$. Shah [51] and Gupta & Balakrishnan [26] provide an extensive list of recurrence relations for the moments of order statistics of the logistic distribution. Gupta & Shah [28] and Malik [36] give closed-form expressions for the **range**, $R_n = Z_{n:n} - Z_{1:n}$, and the rth quasi-range, $Z_{n-r:n} - Z_{r+1:n}$. By expressing the distribution of the range in terms of an associated Legendre function, George & Rousseau [21] obtain the recurrence relation

$$nP(R_{n+2} \le x) = (2n+1)\left(\frac{1+e^{-x}}{1-e^{-x}}\right)$$
$$\times \Pr(R_{n+1} \le x) - (n+1)$$
$$\times \Pr(R_n \le x). \quad (15)$$

George & Rousseau [20] show that the characteristic function of the midrange $(Z_{n:n} + Z_{1:n})/2$ may be expressed as

$$\varphi_n(t) = \begin{cases} \displaystyle\prod_{j=1}^{p-1}\left(1 + \frac{t^2}{4j^2}\right)[\phi_Z(t/2)]^2, \\ \qquad \text{if } n = 2p, \\[2mm] \displaystyle\prod_{j=1}^{p}\left[1 + \frac{t^2}{(2j-1)^2}\right]\phi_Z(t), \\ \qquad \text{if } n = 2p+1, \end{cases} \quad (16)$$

and obtain a closed-form expression for its distribution. For a sample of size three, they establish the rather interesting relationship

$$\frac{Z_{1:3} + Z_{3:3}}{2} \overset{\mathcal{D}}{=} Z_{2:3}. \quad (17)$$

Gumbel [23], relating the logistic to extreme value distributions, shows that, for a large family of symmetric distributions satisfying a general set of conditions that are formalized by de Haan [11], the limiting distribution of the midrange is logistic [16]. This result is extended by Gumbel to the "mth midrange", i.e. $(Z_{m:n} + Z_{n-m+1:n})/2$. In this case, the asymptotic distribution is a generalized logistic. Gumbel & Keeney [25] show that the logistic is the asymptotic distribution of a family of extremal quotients.

Generalized Logistic

It is easy to see that if U is **uniformly distributed** on the unit interval $(0,1)$, then the logit transform of U, $\log\left[U/(1-U)\right]$, has the logistic distribution function G. In fact, one of the many generalizations of the logistic distribution is obtained by simply replacing the uniform random variable U (which is equal in distribution to a **beta** $(1,1)$ random variable), with a beta (α, β) random variable, [18, 47]. When $\alpha = \beta$, the symmetric generalized logistic is obtained. Like the logistic distribution, the generalized logistic is used for modeling binary response data [47] and the log of survival times [34]. In the context of application to quantal assay data, Stukel [52] proposes another generalization of the logistic distribution by introducing different shape parameters at the tails of the distribution (*see* **Quantal Response Models**).

Parametric Estimation

The simplicity of the logistic distribution, as expressed by (1)-(6), belies the complexity of the process of estimating its parameters. No closed forms exist for the MLE (**maximum likelihood** estimator), BLUE (best linear **unbiased** estimators), or UMVUE (uniform **minimum variance unbiased estimators**) of the mean μ and variance σ^2. For example, given a random sample $X_1, \ldots, X_n$ from an $\mathcal{L}(\mu, \sigma^2)$ population, the estimating equations for the MLE of μ and σ^2, which must be solved iteratively, may be expressed by

$$\frac{1}{n}\sum_{i=1}^{n}\frac{1}{1+\exp[\pi(X_i-\mu)/(\sigma\sqrt{3})]}=\frac{1}{2} \quad (18)$$

and

$$\frac{1}{n}\sum_{i=1}^{n}\left(\frac{X_i-\mu}{\sigma}\right)\left(\frac{1-\exp[\pi(X_i-\mu)/(\sigma\sqrt{3})]}{1+\exp[\pi(X_i-\mu)/(\sigma\sqrt{3})]}\right)$$
$$=\frac{\sqrt{3}}{\pi}. \quad (19)$$

From Gupta & Gnanadesikan [27] (in which explicit approximate expressions for the BLUE estimates of μ and σ are given based on selected order statistics $X_{n_1:n} \leq X_{n_2:n} \leq \cdots \leq X_{n_k:n}$), Gupta et al. [29] and Harter & Moore [30] (in which linear estimates are calculated from censored data), a vast literature has

evolved on the use of **censored** logistic random variables to estimate μ and σ. Using the large sample variance–**covariance matrix** of the MLEs, Antle et al. [1] construct **confidence intervals** for μ and σ. Bain [4], Eastman [13], Schafer & Sheffield [49], and Bain et al. [5] discuss applications in life-testing using complete and censored data. Other accounts involving the use of linear functions of order statistics for estimating the logistic parameters are given by several authors in Balakrishnan [6, Chapter 4].

Multivariate Distributions

A model for a **bivariate distribution** with logistic marginals first proposed by Gumbel [24] is extended by Malik & Abraham [37] to an m-dimensional multivariate distribution function

$$F_{\mathbf{Z}} = (\mathbf{z}) = F_{Z_1,\ldots,Z_m}(z_1,\ldots,z_m)$$
$$= \left(1+\sum_{i=1}^{m}\exp(-z_i)\right)^{-1}, \quad (20)$$

with density function

$$f_{\mathbf{Z}}(\mathbf{z}) = m!\,\frac{\exp\left(-\sum_{i=1}^{m}z_i\right)}{\left[1+\sum_{i=1}^{m}\exp(-z_i)\right]^{m+1}}, \quad (21)$$

where $\mathbf{Z} = (Z_1,\ldots,Z_m)$ and $\mathbf{z} = (z_1,\ldots,z_m)$. This distribution, which is sometimes referred to as the Gumbel–Malik–Abraham model, suffers from the restriction that the **correlation** between any pair Z_i, Z_j, is 1/2.

The joint **moment generating function** of $\mathbf{Z}$ is given by

$$M_{\mathbf{Z}}(t_1,\ldots,t_m) = \Gamma\left(1+\sum_{j=1}^{m}t_j\right)\prod_{j=1}^{m}\Gamma(1-t_j). \quad (22)$$

From this generating function, Arnold [3] observes that, analogous to the univariate logistic distribution, the joint distribution of $(Z_1,\ldots,Z_m)$ is the same distribution as $(Y_1 - Y_0,\ldots,Y_m - Y_0)$, where $Y_0, Y_1,\ldots,Y_m$ are independent, identically distributed (iid) extreme value random variables with density given by $h(y) = e^{-y}\exp(-e^{-y})$, $-\infty < y < \infty$.

The Gumbel–Malik–Abraham model is one example of a multivariate logistic distribution that can be constructed by using a multivariate analog of a property of the univariate logistic distribution. Others are described by Arnold [3]. These include a representation in terms of a multivariate survival function:

$$\Pr(\mathbf{Z} \geq \mathbf{z})$$
$$= \left[1 + \sum_{j=1}^{m} \exp(z_i) + \sum_{j_1 \neq j_2} c_{j_1 j_2} \exp(z_{j_1} + z_{j_2})\right.$$
$$\left. + \cdots + c_{1 \ldots m} \exp(z_1 + z_2 + \cdots + z_m)\right]^{-1}, (23)$$

where $\mathbf{Z} \geq \mathbf{z}$ denotes the event $Z_1 \geq z_1, Z_2 \geq z_2, \cdots, Z_m \geq z_m$ and the cs are chosen to satisfy conditions that make (23) a true survival function [2] (*see* **Survival Distributions and Their Characteristics**). This expression can be obtained from a multivariate analog of the following result: if $Z_1, Z_2, \ldots,$ are iid $\mathcal{L}(0, \pi^2/3)$ variables and N is a **geometric** random variable with $\Pr(N = n) = pq^{n-1}, q = 1 - p$, then

$$Z_{1:N} - \log p \overset{\mathcal{D}}{=} Z_{N:N} + \log p \overset{\mathcal{D}}{=} Z_1. \quad (24)$$

Eq. (23) clearly generalizes the Gumbel–Malik–Abraham representation. As an example, the bivariate logistic distribution function obtained from (23) is given by

$$F_{Z_1, Z_2}(z_1, z_2)$$
$$= [1 + \exp(-z_1) + \exp(-z_2) + \theta \exp(-z_1 - z_2)]^{-1},$$
$$(25)$$

where $0 \leq \theta \leq 2$.

Another representation given by Arnold [3] uses the concept of **frailty** from survival analysis to obtain

$$\Pr(\mathbf{Z} \geq \mathbf{z}) = \Lambda_F \left\{\sum_{j=1}^{m} \Lambda_F^{-1}[1 + \exp(z_j)]^{-1}\right\}, (26)$$

where Λ_F denotes the Laplace transform of a given distribution function F. Using distribution functions instead of survival functions leads to a different, but related, family of multivariate logistic distribution

functions

$$\Pr(\mathbf{Z} \leq \mathbf{z}) = \Lambda_F \left\{\sum_{j=1}^{m} \Lambda_F^{-1}[1 + \exp(-z_j)]^{-1}\right\}. \quad (27)$$

Examples of multivariate logistic distributions from these models are:

$$\Pr(\mathbf{Z} \geq \mathbf{z}) = \left\{\sum_{j=1}^{m}[1 + \exp(z_j)]^{(1/\alpha)} - m + 1\right\}^{-\alpha} \quad (28)$$

and

$$\Pr(\mathbf{Z} \leq \mathbf{z}) = \left\{\sum_{j=1}^{m}[1 + \exp(-z_j)]^{(1/\alpha)} - m + 1\right\}^{-\alpha}, \quad (29)$$

corresponding to a choice of **gamma** $(\alpha, 1)$ for F and

$$\Pr(\mathbf{Z} \leq \mathbf{z})$$
$$= \exp\left[-\left(\sum_{j=1}^{m}\{\log[1 + \exp(-z_j)]\}^{(1/\alpha)}\right)^{\alpha}\right], (30)$$

corresponding to choosing $\Lambda_F(t) = \exp(-t^\alpha), \alpha \leq 1$.

The Farlie–Gumbel–Morgenstern model of a multivariate logistic [3, 32, 33] is yet another representation. This model may be described by

$$\Pr(\mathbf{Z} \leq \mathbf{z}) = \prod_{j=1}^{m} G(z_j) \left\{1 + \alpha \prod_{j=1}^{m}[1 - G(z_j)]\right\}, \quad (31)$$

where $|\alpha| < 1$ and $G(z) = (1 + e^{-z})^{-1}$. This model suffers from a restriction in correlation: $\rho(Z_i, Z_j) = 3\alpha/\pi^2$ for every pair Z_i, Z_j. The correlation structure limits the use of the model. The bivariate version of this model is due to Gumbel [24].

Historical Notes and Applications

The logistic function is one of the oldest models for analyzing **demographic** and organismic growth data. Verhulst [55], Pearl [42, 43], Pearl & Reed [44], Yule [56], and, more recently, Oliver [40, 41] and Leach [35] discuss applications to **population growth**. Other biological applications of the logistic function include the modeling of the growth of yeast cells [39, 44, 50] and the use of the logistic function in analysis of survival data [46].

Reed & Berkson [48], are usually credited with the logistic label, and Berkson [7–9] has championed the use of the logistic distribution function for modeling **dose–response** curves in **bioassay** (see also Finney [14, 15]). Berkson's minimum logit chi-square estimates are easier to compute than maximum likelihood estimates. However, with the availability of sophisticated software, this is no longer a significant advantage. From the limited use of the logistic distribution for quantal bioassay has emerged logistic regression analysis, which is currently a very popular **generalized linear model** procedure for analyzing **binary data**. In the context of applications of logistic regression to health and social sciences, Tsokos & DiCroce [54] give an extensive bibliography.

References

[1] Antle, C., Klimko, L. & Harkness, W. (1970). Confidence intervals for the parameters of the logistic distribution, *Biometrika* **57**, 397–402.

[2] Arnold, B.C. (1990). A flexible family of multivariate Pareto distributions, *Journal of Statistical Planning and Inference* **24**, 249–258.

[3] Arnold, B.C. (1992). Multivariate logistic distributions, in *Handbook of the Logistic Distribution*, N. Balakrishnan, ed. Marcel Dekker, New York, Chapter 11.

[4] Bain, L.J. (1978). *Statistical Analysis of Reliability and Life-Testing Models – Theory and Practice*. Marcel Dekker, New York.

[5] Bain, L.J., Balakrishnan, N., Eastman, J.A., Engelhart, M. & Antle, C.A. (1992). Reliability estimation based on MLEs for complete and censored samples, in *Handbook of the Logistic Distribution*, N. Balakrishnan, ed. Marcel Dekker, New York, Chapter 5.

[6] Balakrishnan, N. (1992). Maximum likelihood estimation based on complete and Type II censored samples, *Handbook of the Logistic Distribution*, N. Balakrishnan, ed. Marcel Dekker, New York, Chapter 3.

[7] Berkson, J. (1994). Application of the logistic function to bioassay, *Journal of the American Statistical Association* **37**, 357–365.

[8] Berkson, J. (1951). Why I prefer logits to probits, *Biometrics* **7**, 327–339.

[9] Berkson, J. (1953). A statistically precise and relatively simple method of estimating the bioassay and quantal response, based on the logistic function, *Journal of the American Statistical Association* **48**, 565–599.

[10] Birnbaum, A. & Dudman, J. (1963). Logistic order statistics, *Annals of Mathematical Statistics* **34**, 658–663.

[11] de Haan, L. (1975). *On Regular Variation and Its Application to Weak Convergence of Sample Extremes*, 3rd Ed. Mathematical Center Tracts, Vol. 32, Amsterdam.

[12] Dubey, S.D. (1969). A new derivation of the logistic distribution, *Naval Research Logistics Quarterly* **16**, 37–40.

[13] Eastman, J.A. (1972). Statistical Issues of Various Time-to-Fail Distributions, *Doctoral Thesis*. University of Missouri-Rolla, Missouri.

[14] Finney, D.J. (1947). The principles of biological assay, *Journal of the Royal Statistical Society, Series B* **9**, 46–91.

[15] Finney, D.J. (1952), *Statistical Methods in Biological Assay*. Hafner, New York

[16] Galambos, J. (1987). *The Asymptotic Theory of Extreme Order Statistics*, 2nd Ed. Krieger, Melbourne, Florida.

[17] George, E.O. & Devidas, M. (1992). Some related distributions, in *Handbook of the Logistic Distribution*, N. Balakrishnan, ed. Marcel Dekker, New York, Chapter 10.

[18] George, E.O. & Ojo, M.O. (1980). On a generalization of the logistic distribution, *Annals of the Institute of Statistical Mathematics* **32**, 161–169.

[19] George, E.O. & Mudholkar, G.S. (1983). On the convolution of logistic random variables, *Metrika* **30**, 1–13.

[20] George, E.O. & Rousseau, C.C. (1987). On the logistic midrange, *Annals of the Institute of Statistical Mathematics* **39**, 627–635.

[21] George, E.O. & Rousseau, C.C. (1992). Asymptotics of the logistic range, *Sankhyā, Series B* **54**, 165–169.

[22] Goel, P.K. (1975). On the distribution of standardized mean samples from the logistic population, *Sankhyā, Series B* **37**, 165–172.

[23] Gumbel, E.J. (1944). Ranges and midranges, *Annals of Mathematical Statistics* **15**, 414–422.

[24] Gumbel, E.J. (1961). Bivariate logistic distributions, *Journal of the American Statistical Association* **56**, 335–349.

[25] Gumbel, E.J. & Keeney, R.D. (1950). The extremal quotient, *Annals of Mathematical Statistics* **21**, 523–538.

[26] Gupta, S.S. & Balakrishnan, N. (1992). Logistic order statistics and their properties, in *Handbook of the Logistic Distribution*, N. Balakrishnan, ed. Marcel Dekker, New York, Chapter 2.

[27] Gupta, S.S. & Gnanadesikan, M. (1966). Estimation of the parameters of the logistic distribution, *Biometrika* **53**, 565–570.

[28] Gupta, S.S. & Shah, B.K. (1965). Exact moments and percentage points of the order statistics and the distribution of the range from the logistic distribution, *Annals of Mathematical Statistics* **36**, 907–920.

[29] Gupta, S.S., Qureishi, A.S. & Shah, B.K. (1967). Best linear unbiased estimators of the parameters of the logistic distribution using order statistics, *Technometrics* **9**, 43–56.

[30] Harter, H.L. & Moore, A.H. (1967). Maximum likelihood estimation, from censored samples, of the parameters of a logistic distribution, *Journal of the American Statistical Association* **62**, 675–684.

[31] Johnson, N.L. & Kotz, S. (1970). *Distribution in Statistics, Continuous Univariate Distributions*, Vol. 2. Wiley, New York.

[32] Johnson, N.L. & Kotz, S. (1975). On some generalized Farlie-Gumbel-Morgenstern distributions, *Communications in Statistics – Theory and Methods* **4**, 415–427.

[33] Johnson, N.L. & Kotz, S. (1977). On some generalized Farlie-Gumbel-Morgenstern distributions, II: Regression, correlations and further generalizations, *Communications in Statistics – Theory and Methods* **6**, 485–496.

[34] Kalbfleisch, J.D. & Prentice, R.L. (1980). *The Statistical Analysis of Failure Time Data*. Wiley, New York.

[35] Leach, D. (1981). Re-evaluation of the logistic curve for human populations, *Journal of the Royal Statistical Society, Series A* **144**, 94–103.

[36] Malik, H.J. (1980). Exact formula for the cumulative distribution function of the quasi-range from the logistic distribution, *Communications in Statistics – Theory and Methods* **9**, 1527–1534.

[37] Malik, H.J. & Abraham, B. (1973). Multivariate logistic distribution, *Annals of Statistics* **1**, 588–590.

[38] Mudholkar, G.S. & George, E.O. (1978). A remark on the shape of the logistic distribution, *Biometrika* **65**, 667–668.

[39] Oliver, F.R. (1964). Methods of estimating the logistic growth function, *Applied Statistics* **13**, 57–66.

[40] Oliver, F.R. (1966). Aspects of maximum likelihood estimation of the logistic growth function, *Journal of the American Statistical Association* **61**, 697–705.

[41] Oliver, F.R. (1982). Notes on the logistic curve for human populations, *Journal of the Royal Statistical Society, Series A* **145**, 359–363.

[42] Pearl, R. (1925). *The Biology of Population Growth*, Knopf, New York.

[43] Pearl, R. (1940). *Medical Biometry and Statistics*, Sanders, Philadelphia.

[44] Pearl, R. & Reed, L.J. (1920). On the rate of growth of the population of the United States since 1790 and its mathematical representation, *Proceedings of the National Academy of Sciences* **6**, 275–288.

[45] Plackett, R.L. (1958). Linear estimation from censored data, *Annals of Mathematical Statistics* **29**, 131–142.

[46] Plackett, R.L. (1959). The analysis of life test data, *Technometrics* **1**, 9–19.

[47] Prentice, R.L. (1976). A generalization of the probit and logit methods for dose-response curves, *Biometrics* **32**, 761–768.

[48] Reed, L.J. & Berkson, J. (1929). The application of the logistic function to experimental data, *Journal of Physical Chemistry* **33**, 760–779.

[49] Schafer, R.E. & Sheffield, T.S. (1973). Inferences on the parameters of the logistic distribution, *Biometrika* **29**, 449–455.

[50] Schultz, H. (1930). The standard error of a forecast from a curve, *Journal of the American Statistical Association* **25**, 139–185.

[51] Shah, B.K. (1970). Note on the moments of a logistic order statistics, *Annals of Mathematical Statistics* **41**, 2151–2152.

[52] Stukel, T. (1988). Generalized logistic models, *Journal of the American Statistical Association* **83**, 426–431.

[53] Tarter, M.E. & Clark, V.A. (1965). Properties of the median and other order statistics of the logistic variates, *Annals of Mathematical Statistics* **36**, 1779–1786.

[54] Tsokos, C.P. & DiCroce, P.S. (1992). Applications in health and social sciences, in *Handbook of the Logistic Distribution*, N. Balakrishnan, ed. Marcel Dekker, New York, Chapter 17.

[55] Verhulst, P.J. (1845). Recherches mathematiques sur la loi d'accroissement de la population. *Académie de Bruxelles* **18**, 1–38.

[56] Yule, G.U. (1925). The growth of population and factor which controls it, *Journal of the Royal Statistical Society, Series A* **88**, 1–58.

E. OLUSEGUN GEORGE

Logistic Regression

The goal of a logistic regression analysis is to find the best fitting and most parsimonious, yet biologically reasonable, model to describe the relationship between an outcome (dependent or response variable) and a set of independent (predictor or explanatory) variables. What distinguishes the logistic regression model from the **linear regression** model is that the outcome variable in logistic regression is categorical and most usually *binary* or *dichotomous* (*see* **Binary Data**).

In any regression problem the key quantity is the mean value of the outcome variable, given the value of the independent variable. This quantity is called the *conditional mean* and will be expressed as $E(Y|x)$, where Y denotes the outcome variable and x denotes a value of the independent variable. In linear regression we assume that this mean may be expressed as an equation linear in x (or some transformation of x or Y), such as

$$E(Y|x) = \beta_0 + \beta_1 x.$$

This expression implies that it is possible for $E(Y|x)$ to take on any value as x ranges between $-\infty$ and $+\infty$.

Many distribution functions have been proposed for use in the analysis of a dichotomous outcome variable. Cox & Snell [2] discuss some of these.

There are two primary reasons for choosing the logistic distribution. These are: (i) from a mathematical point of view it is an extremely flexible and easily used function, and (ii) it lends itself to a biologically meaningful interpretation.

To simplify notation, let $\pi(x) = E(Y|x)$ represent the conditional mean of Y given x. The logistic regression model can be expressed as

$$\pi(x) = \frac{\exp(\beta_0 + \beta_1 x)}{1 + \exp(\beta_0 + \beta_1 x)}. \quad (1)$$

The *logit transformation*, defined in terms of $\pi(x)$, is as follows:

$$g(x) = \ln\left[\frac{\pi(x)}{1 - \pi(x)}\right] = \beta_0 + \beta_1 x. \quad (2)$$

The importance of this transformation is that $g(x)$ has many of the desirable properties of a linear regression model. The logit, $g(x)$, is linear in its parameters, may be continuous, and may range from $-\infty$ to $+\infty$ depending on the range of x.

The second important difference between the linear and logistic regression models concerns the conditional distribution of the outcome variable. In the linear regression model we assume that an observation of the outcome variable may be expressed as $y = E(Y|x) + \varepsilon$. The quantity ε is called the *error* and expresses an observation's deviation from the conditional mean. The most common assumption is that ε follows a normal distribution with mean zero and some variance that is constant across levels of the independent variable. It follows that the conditional distribution of the outcome variable given x is normal with mean $E(Y|x)$, and a variance that is constant. This is not the case with a dichotomous outcome variable. In this situation we may express the value of the outcome variable given x as $y = \pi(x) + \varepsilon$. Here the quantity ε may assume one of two possible values. If $y = 1$, then $\varepsilon = 1 - \pi(x)$ with probability $\pi(x)$, and if $y = 0$, then $\varepsilon = -\pi(x)$ with probability $1 - \pi(x)$. Thus, ε has a distribution with mean zero and variance equal to $\pi(x)[1 - \pi(x)]$. That is, the conditional distribution of the outcome variable follows a binomial distribution with probability given by the conditional mean, $\pi(x)$.

Fitting the Logistic Regression Model

Suppose we have a sample of n independent observations of the pair $(x_i, y_i), i = 1, 2, \ldots, n$,

where y_i denotes the value of a dichotomous outcome variable and x_i is the value of the independent variable for the ith subject. Furthermore, assume that the outcome variable has been coded as 0 or 1 representing the absence or presence of the characteristic, respectively. To fit the logistic regression model (1) to a set of data requires that we estimate the values of β_0 and β_1, the unknown parameters.

In linear regression the method used most often to estimate unknown parameters is **least squares**. In that method we choose those values of β_0 and β_1 that minimize the sum of squared deviations of the observed values of Y from the predicted values based upon the model. Under the usual assumptions for linear regression the least squares method yields estimators with a number of desirable statistical properties. Unfortunately, when the least squares method is applied to a model with a dichotomous outcome the estimators no longer have these same properties.

The general method of estimation that leads to the least squares function under the linear regression model (when the error terms are normally distributed) is **maximum likelihood**. This is the method used to estimate the logistic regression parameters. In a very general sense the maximum likelihood method yields values for the unknown parameters that maximize the probability of obtaining the observed set of data. To apply this method we must first construct a function called the *likelihood function* (*see* **Likelihood**). This function expresses the probability of the observed data as a function of the unknown parameters. The *maximum likelihood estimators* of these parameters are chosen to be those values that maximize this function. Thus, the resulting estimators are those that agree most closely with the observed data.

If Y is coded as 0 or 1, then the expression for $\pi(x)$ given in (1) provides (for an arbitrary value of $\beta' = (\beta_0, \beta_1)$, the vector of parameters) the conditional probability that Y is equal to 1 given x. This will be denoted $\Pr(Y = 1|x)$. It follows that the quantity $1 - \pi(x)$ gives the conditional probability that Y is equal to zero given x, $\Pr(Y = 0|x)$. Thus, for those pairs (x_i, y_i), where $y_i = 1$, the contribution to the likelihood function is $\pi(x_i)$, and for those pairs where $y_i = 0$, the contribution to the likelihood function is $1 - \pi(x_i)$, where the quantity $\pi(x_i)$ denotes the value of $\pi(x)$ computed at x_i. A convenient way to express the contribution to the likelihood function for the pair

(x_i, y_i) is through the term

$$\xi(x_i) = \pi(x_i)^{y_i}[1 - \pi(x_i)]^{1-y_i}. \qquad (3)$$

Since the observations are assumed to be independent, the likelihood function is obtained as the product of the terms given in (3) as follows:

$$l(\beta) = \prod_{i=1}^{n} \xi(x_i). \qquad (4)$$

The principle of maximum likelihood states that we use as our estimate of β the value that maximizes the expression in (4). However, it is easier mathematically to work with the log of (4). This expression, the *log likelihood*, is defined as

$$L(\beta) = \ln[l(\beta)]$$
$$= \sum\{y_i \ln[\pi(x_i)] + (1 - y_i) \ln[1 - \pi(x_i)]\}. (5)$$

To find the value of β that maximizes $L(\beta)$ we differentiate $L(\beta)$ with respect to β_0 and β_1 and set the resulting expressions equal to zero. These equations are as follows:

$$\sum_{i=1}^{n} [y_i - \pi(x_i)] = 0 \qquad (6)$$

and

$$\sum_{i=1}^{n} x_i[y_i - \pi(x_i)] = 0, \qquad (7)$$

and are called the *likelihood equations*.

In linear regression, the likelihood equations, obtained by differentiating the sum of squared deviations function with respect to β, are linear in the unknown parameters, and thus are easily solved. For logistic regression the expressions in (6) and (7) are nonlinear in β_0 and β_1, and thus require special methods for their solution. These methods are iterative in nature and have been programmed into available logistic regression software. McCullagh & Nelder [6] discuss the iterative methods used by most programs. In particular, they show that the solution to (6) and (7) may be obtained using a generalized weighted least squares procedure.

The value of β given by the solution to (6) and (7) is called the maximum likelihood estimate, denoted as $\hat{\beta}$. Similarly, $\hat{\pi}(x_i)$ is the maximum likelihood estimate of $\pi(x_i)$. This quantity provides an estimate of the conditional probability that Y is equal to 1,

given that x is equal to x_i. As such, it represents the fitted or predicted value for the logistic regression model. An interesting consequence of (6) is that

$$\sum_{i=1}^{n} y_i = \sum_{i=1}^{n} \hat{\pi}(x_i).$$

That is, the sum of the observed values of y is equal to the sum of the predicted (expected) values.

After estimating the coefficients, it is standard practice to assess the significance of the variables in the model. This usually involves testing a statistical hypothesis to determine whether the independent variables in the model are "significantly" related to the outcome variable. One approach to testing for the significance of the coefficient of a variable in any model relates to the following question. *Does the model that includes the variable in question tell us more about the outcome (or response) variable than does a model that does not include that variable?* This question is answered by comparing the observed values of the response variable with those predicted by each of two models; the first with and the second without the variable in question. The mathematical function used to compare the observed and predicted values depends on the particular problem. If the predicted values with the variable in the model are better, or more accurate in some sense, than when the variable is not in the model, then we feel that the variable in question is "significant". It is important to note that we are not considering the question of whether the predicted values are an accurate representation of the observed values in an absolute sense (this would be called *goodness of fit*). Instead, our question is posed in a relative sense.

For the purposes of assessing the significance of an independent variable we compute the value of the following statistic:

$$G = -2 \ln \left(\frac{\text{likelihood without the variable}}{\text{likelihood with the variable}} \right). \qquad (8)$$

Under the hypothesis that β_1 is equal to zero, the statistic G will follow a chi-square distribution with one degree of freedom. The calculation of the log likelihood and this generalized **likelihood ratio test** are standard features of any good logistic regression package. This makes it possible to check for the significance of the addition of new terms to the model as a matter of routine. In the simple case of a single independent variable, we can first fit a model containing only the constant term. We can then fit a model containing the independent variable along with the constant. This gives rise to a new log likelihood. The likelihood ratio test is obtained by multiplying the difference between the log likelihoods of the two models by -2.

Another test that is often carried out is the Wald test, which is obtained by comparing the maximum likelihood estimate of the slope parameter, $\hat{\beta}_1$, with an estimate of its standard error (*see* **Likelihood**). The resulting ratio

$$W = \frac{\hat{\beta}_1}{\widehat{\text{se}}(\hat{\beta}_1)},$$

under the hypothesis that $\beta_1 = 0$, follows a standard normal distribution. Standard errors of the estimated parameters are routinely printed out by computer software. Hauck & Donner [3] examined the performance of the Wald test and found that it behaved in an aberrant manner, often failing to reject when the coefficient was significant. They recommended that the likelihood ratio test be used. Jennings [5] has also looked at the adequacy of inferences in logistic regression based on Wald statistics. His conclusions are similar to those of Hauck & Donner.

Both the likelihood ratio test, G, and the Wald test, W, require the computation of the maximum likelihood estimate for β_1. For a single variable this is not a difficult or costly computational task. However, for large data sets with many variables, the iterative computation needed to obtain the maximum likelihood estimates can be considerable.

The logistic regression model may be used with matched study designs. Fitting **conditional logistic regression** models requires modifications, which are not discussed here. The reader interested in the conditional logistic regression model may find details in [4, Chapter 7].

The Multiple Logistic Regression Model

Consider a collection of p independent variables which will be denoted by the vector $\mathbf{x}' = (x_1, x_2, \ldots, x_p)$. Assume for the moment that each of these variables is at least interval scaled. Let the conditional probability that the outcome is present be denoted by $\Pr(Y = 1|\mathbf{x}) = \pi(\mathbf{x})$. Then the logit of the

multiple logistic regression model is given by

$$g(\mathbf{x}) = \beta_0 + \beta_1 x_1 + \beta_2 x_2 + \cdots + \beta_p x_p, \quad (9)$$

in which case

$$\pi(x) = \frac{\exp[g(\mathbf{x})]}{1 + \exp[g(\mathbf{x})]}. \quad (10)$$

If some of the independent variables are discrete, nominal scaled variables (*see* **Nominal Data**) such as race, sex, treatment group, and so forth, then it is inappropriate to include them in the model as if they were interval scaled. In this situation a collection of *design variables* (or **dummy variables**) should be used. Most logistic regression software will generate the design variables, and some programs have a choice of several different methods.

In general, if a nominal scaled variable has k possible values, then $k - 1$ design variables will be needed. Suppose, for example, that the jth independent variable, x_j has k_j levels. The $k_j - 1$ design variables will be denoted as D_{ju} and the coefficients for these design variables will be denoted as $\beta_{ju}, u = 1, 2, \ldots, k_j - 1$. Thus, the logit for a model with p variables and the jth variable being discrete is

$$g(\mathbf{x}) = \beta_0 + \beta_1 x_1 + \cdots + \sum_{u=1}^{k_j-1} \beta_{ju} D_{ju} + \beta_p x_p.$$

Fitting the Multiple Logistic Regression Model

Assume that we have a sample of n independent observations of the pair $(\mathbf{x}_i, y_i), i = 1, 2, \ldots, n$. As in the univariate case, fitting the model requires that we obtain estimates of the vector $\boldsymbol{\beta}' = (\beta_0, \beta_1, \ldots, \beta_p)$. The method of estimation used in the multivariate case is the same as in the univariate situation, i.e. maximum likelihood. The likelihood function is nearly identical to that given in (4), with the only change being that $\pi(\mathbf{x})$ is now defined as in (10). There are $p + 1$ likelihood equations which are obtained by differentiating the log likelihood function with respect to the $p + 1$ coefficients. The likelihood equations that result may be expressed as follows:

$$\sum_{i=1}^{n} [y_i - \pi(\mathbf{x}_i)] = 0$$

Table 1   Code sheet for the variables in the low birth weight data set

Variable	Abbreviation
Identification code	ID
Low birth weight (0 = birth weight $\geq$2500 g, 1 = birth weight <2500 g)	LOW
Age of the mother in years	AGE
Weight in pounds at the last menstrual period	LWT
Race (1 = white, 2 = black, 3 = other)	RACE
Smoking status during pregnancy (1 = yes, 0 = no)	SMOKE
History of premature labor (0 = none, 1 = one, etc.)	PTL
History of hypertension (1 = yes, 0 = no)	HT
Presence of uterine irritability (1 = yes, 0 = no)	UI
Number of physician visits during the first trimester (0 = none, 1 = one, 2 = two, etc.)	FTV
Birth weight (g)	BWT

and

$$\sum_{i=1}^{n} x_{ij}[y_i - \pi(\mathbf{x}_i)] = 0,$$

for $j = 1, 2, \ldots, p$.

As in the univariate model, the solution of the likelihood equations requires special purpose software which may be found in many packaged programs. Let $\hat{\beta}$ denote the solution to these equations. Thus, the fitted values for the multiple logistic regression model are $\hat{\pi}(\mathbf{x}_i)$, the value of the expression in (13) computed using $\hat{\beta}$ and $\mathbf{x}_i$.

Before proceeding further we present an example that illustrates the formulation of a multiple logistic regression model and the estimation of its coefficients.

Example

To provide an example of fitting a multiple logistic regression model, consider the data for the low birth weight study described in Appendix 1 of Hosmer & Lemeshow [4]. The code sheet for the data set is given in Table 1.

The goal of this study was to identify risk factors associated with giving birth to a low birth weight baby (weighing less than 2500 g). In this study data were collected on 189 women; $n_1 = 59$ of them delivered low birth weight babies and $n_0 = 130$ delivered normal birth weight babies. In this example the variable race has been recoded using the two design variables shown in Table 2. FTV was recoded to 0 = some, 1 = none, and PTL was recoded to

Table 2   Coding of design variables for RACE

RACE	RACE 1	RACE 2
White	0	0
Black	1	0
Other	0	1

0 = none, 1 = one or more. The two newly coded variables are called FTV01 and PTL01.

The results of fitting the logistic regression model to these data are given in Table 3.

In Table 3 the estimated coefficients for the two design variables for race are indicated in the lines denoted by "RACE 1" and "RACE 2". The estimated logit is given by

$$\hat{g}(\mathbf{x}) = 0.545 - 0.035 \times \text{AGE} - 0.015 \times \text{LWT}$$
$$+ 0.815 \times \text{SMOKE} + 1.824 \times \text{HT} + 0.702$$
$$\times \text{UI} + 1.202 \times \text{RACE 1} + 0.773 \times \text{RACE 2}$$
$$+ 0.121 \times \text{FTV01} + 1.237 \times \text{PTL01}.$$

The fitted values are obtained using the estimated logit, $\hat{g}(\mathbf{x})$, as in (10).

Testing for the Significance of the Model

Once we have fit a particular multiple (multivariate) logistic regression model, we begin the process of assessment of the model. The first step in this process is usually to assess the significance of the variables

Table 3 Estimated coefficients for a multiple logistic regression model using all variables from the low birth weight data set

Logit estimates

Number of obs. =   189
$\chi^2(9) = 37.94$
Prob $> \chi^2 = 0.0000$

Log likelihood $= -98.36$

Variable	Coeff.	Std. error	z	Pr $> |z|$	[95% conf. interval]	
AGE	−0.035	0.039	−0.920	0.357	−0.111	0.040
LWT	−0.015	0.007	−2.114	0.035	−0.029	−0.001
SMOKE	0.815	0.420	1.939	0.053	−0.009	1.639
HT	1.824	0.705	2.586	0.010	0.441	3.206
UI	0.702	0.465	1.511	0.131	−0.208	1.613
RACE 1	1.202	0.534	2.253	0.024	0.156	2.248
RACE 2	0.773	0.460	1.681	0.093	−0.128	1.674
FTV01	0.121	0.376	0.323	0.746	−0.615	0.858
PTL01	1.237	0.466	2.654	0.008	0.323	2.148
cons	0.545	1.266	0.430	0.667	−1.937	3.027

in the model. The likelihood ratio test for overall significance of the p coefficients for the independent variables in the model is performed based on the statistic G given in (8). The only difference is that the fitted values, $\hat{\pi}$, under the model are based on the vector containing $p + 1$ parameters, $\hat{\beta}$. Under the null hypothesis that the p "slope" coefficients for the covariates in the model are equal to zero, the distribution of G is **chi-square** with p **degrees of freedom**.

As an example, consider the fitted model whose estimated coefficients are given in Table 3. For that model the value of the log likelihood is $L = -98.36$. A second model, fit with the constant term only, yields $L = -117.336$. Hence $G = -2[(-117.34) - (-98.36)] = 37.94$ and the **P value** for the test is Pr$[\chi^2(9) > 37.94] < 0.0001$ (see Table 3). Rejection of the **null hypothesis** (that all of the coefficients are simultaneously equal to zero) has an interpretation analogous to that in multiple linear regression; we may conclude that at least one, and perhaps all p coefficients are different from zero.

Before concluding that any or all of the coefficients are nonzero, we may wish to look at the univariate Wald test statistics, $W_j = \hat{\beta}_j / \hat{se}(\hat{\beta}_j)$. These are given in the fourth column (labeled z) in Table 3. Under the hypothesis that an individual coefficient is zero, these statistics will follow the **standard normal** distribution. Thus, the value of these statistics may give us an indication of which of the variables in the model may or may not be significant. If we

use a critical value of 2, which leads to an approximate level of significance (two-tailed) of 0.05, then we would conclude that the variables LWT, SMOKE, HT, PTL01 and possibly RACE are significant, while AGE, UI, and FTV01 are not significant.

Considering that the overall goal is to obtain the best fitting model while minimizing the number of parameters, the next logical step is to fit a reduced model, containing only those variables thought to be significant, and compare it with the full model containing all the variables. The results of fitting the reduced model are given in Table 4.

The difference between the two models is the exclusion of the variables AGE, UI, and FTV01 from the full model. The likelihood ratio test comparing these two models is obtained using the definition of G given in (8). It has a distribution that is chi-square with three degrees of freedom under the hypothesis that the coefficients for the variables excluded are equal to zero. The value of the test statistic comparing the models in Tables 3 and 4 is $G = -2[(-100.24) - (-98.36)] = 3.76$ which, with three degrees of freedom, has a P value of $P[\chi^2(3) > 3.76] = 0.2886$. Since the P value is large, exceeding 0.05, we conclude that the reduced model is as good as the full model. Thus there is no advantage to including AGE, UI, and FTV01 in the model. However, we must not base our models entirely on tests of statistical significance. Numerous other considerations should influence our decision to include or exclude variables from a model.

Table 4 Estimated coefficients for a multiple logistic regression model using the variables LWT, SMOKE, HT, PTL01 and RACE from the low birth weight data set

Logit estimates					Number of obs. = 189	
					$\chi^2(6) =$ 34.19	
					Prob $> \chi^2 = 0.0000$	

Log likelihood = 100.24

Variable	Coeff.	Std. error	z	$Pr > |z|$	[95% conf. interval]	
LWT	−0.017	0.007	−2.407	0.016	−0.030	−0.003
SMOKE	0.876	0.401	2.186	0.029	0.091	1.661
HT	1.767	0.708	2.495	0.013	0.379	3.156
RACE 1	1.264	0.529	2.387	0.017	0.226	2.301
RACE 2	0.864	0.435	1.986	0.047	0.011	1.717
PTL01	1.231	0.446	2.759	0.006	0.357	2.106
cons	0.095	0.957	0.099	0.921	−1.781	1.970

Interpretation of the Coefficients of the Logistic Regression Model

After fitting a model the emphasis shifts from the computation and assessment of significance of estimated coefficients to interpretation of their values. The interpretation of any fitted model requires that we can draw practical inferences from the estimated coefficients in the model. The question addressed is: *What do the estimated coefficients in the model tell us about the research questions that motivated the study?* For most models this involves the estimated coefficients for the independent variables in the model. The estimated coefficients for the independent variables represent the slope or rate of change of a function of the dependent variable per unit of change in the independent variable. Thus, interpretation involves two issues: (i) determining the functional relationship between the dependent variable and the independent variable, and (ii) appropriately defining the unit of change for the independent variable.

For a linear regression model we recall that the slope coefficient, β_1, is equal to the difference between the value of the dependent variable at $x + 1$ and the value of the dependent variable at x, for any value of x. In the logistic regression model $\beta_1 = g(x + 1) - g(x)$. That is, the slope coefficient represents the change in the logit for a change of one unit in the independent variable x. Proper interpretation of the coefficient in a logistic regression model depends on being able to place meaning on the difference between two logits. Consider the interpretation of the coefficients for a univariate logistic regression model for each of the possible measurement scales of the independent variable.

Dichotomous Independent Variable

Assume that x is coded as either 0 or 1. Under this model there are two values of $\pi(x)$ and equivalently two values of $1 - \pi(x)$. These values may be conveniently displayed in a **2 × 2 table**, as shown in Table 5.

The **odds** of the outcome being present among individuals with $x = 1$ is defined as $\pi(1)/[1 - \pi(1)]$. Similarly, the odds of the outcome being present among individuals with $x = 0$ is defined as $\pi(0)/[1 - \pi(0)]$. The **odds ratio**, denoted by ψ, is defined as the ratio of the odds for $x = 1$ to the odds for $x = 0$, and is given by

$$\psi = \frac{\pi(1)/[1 - \pi(1)]}{\pi(0)/[1 - \pi(0)]}. \tag{11}$$

The log of the odds ratio, termed log odds ratio, or *log odds*, is

$$\ln(\psi) = \ln \left\{ \frac{\pi(1)/[1 - \pi(1)]}{\pi(0)/[1 - \pi(0)]} \right\} = g(1) - g(0),$$

which is the *logit difference*, where the log of the odds is called the logit and, in this example, these are

$$g(1) = \ln\{\pi(1)/[1 - \pi(1)]\}$$

and

$$g(0) = \ln\{\pi(0)/[1 - \pi(0)]\}.$$

Using the expressions for the logistic regression model shown in Table 5 the odds ratio is

Table 5   Values of the logistic regression model when the independent variable is dichotomous

			Independent variable X	
			$x = 1$	$x = 0$
Outcome variable	Y	$y = 1$	$\pi(1) = \dfrac{\exp(\beta_0 + \beta_1)}{1 + \exp(\beta_0 + \beta_1)}$	$\pi(0) = \dfrac{\exp\beta_0}{1 + \exp\beta_0}$
		$y = 0$	$1 - \pi(1) = \dfrac{1}{1 + \exp(\beta_0 + \beta_1)}$	$1 - \pi(0) = \dfrac{1}{1 + \exp\beta_0}$
		Total	1.0	1.0

$$\psi = \frac{\left(\dfrac{\exp(\beta_0 + \beta_1)}{1 + \exp(\beta_0 + \beta_1)}\right)\left(\dfrac{1}{1 + \exp(\beta_0)}\right)}{\left(\dfrac{\exp(\beta_0)}{1 + \exp(\beta_0)}\right)\left(\dfrac{1}{1 + \exp(\beta_0 + \beta_1)}\right)}$$

$$= \frac{\exp(\beta_0 + \beta_1)}{\exp(\beta_0)} = \exp(\beta_1).$$

Hence, for logistic regression with a dichotomous independent variable

$$\psi = \exp(\beta_1), \qquad (12)$$

and the logit difference, or log odds, is

$$\ln(\psi) = \ln[\exp(\beta_1)] = \beta_1.$$

This fact concerning the interpretability of the coefficients is the fundamental reason why logistic regression has proven such a powerful analytic tool for epidemiologic research. A confidence interval (CI) estimate for the odds ratio is obtained by first calculating the endpoints of a **confidence interval** for the coefficient β_1, and then exponentiating these values. In general, the endpoints are given by

$$\exp\left[\hat{\beta}_1 \pm z_{1-\alpha/2} \times \widehat{se}(\hat{\beta}_1)\right].$$

Because of the importance of the odds ratio as a measure of association, point and interval estimates are often found in additional columns in tables presenting the results of a logistic regression analysis.

In the previous discussion we noted that the estimate of the odds ratio was $\hat{\psi} = \exp(\hat{\beta}_1)$. This is correct when the independent variable has been coded as 0 or 1. This type of coding is called "reference cell" coding. Other coding could be used. For example, the variable may be coded as -1 or $+1$. This type

of coding is termed "deviation from means" coding. Evaluation of the logit difference shows that the odds ratio is calculated as $\hat{\psi} = \exp(2\hat{\beta}_1)$ and if an investigator were simply to exponentiate the coefficient from the computer output of a logistic regression analysis, the wrong estimate of the odds ratio would be obtained. Close attention should be paid to the method used to code design variables.

The method of coding also influences the calculation of the endpoints of the confidence interval. With deviation from means coding, the estimated standard error needed for confidence interval estimation is $\widehat{se}(2\hat{\beta}_1)$, which is $2 \times \widehat{se}(\hat{\beta}_1)$. Thus the endpoints of the confidence interval are

$$\exp\left[2\hat{\beta}_1 + z_{1-\alpha/2} \times 2 \times \widehat{se}(\hat{\beta}_1)\right].$$

In summary, for a dichotomous variable the parameter of interest is the odds ratio. An estimate of this parameter may be obtained from the estimated logistic regression coefficient, regardless of how the variable is coded or scaled. This relationship between the logistic regression coefficient and the odds ratio provides the foundation for our interpretation of all logistic regression results.

Polytomous Independent Variable

Suppose that instead of two categories the independent variable has $k > 2$ distinct values (*see* **Polytomous Data**). For example, we may have variables that denote the county of residence within a state, the clinic used for primary health care within a city, or race. Each of these variables has a fixed number of discrete outcomes and the scale of measurement is nominal.

Table 6 Cross-classification of hypothetical data on RACE and CHD status for 100 subjects

CHD status	White	Black	Hispanic	Other	Total
Present	5	20	15	10	50
Absent	20	10	10	10	50
Total	25	30	25	20	100
Odds ratio ($\hat{\psi}$)	1.0	8.0	6.0	4.0	
95% CI		(2.3, 27.6)	(1.7, 21.3)	(1.1, 14.9)	
$\ln(\hat{\psi})$	0.0	2.08	1.79	1.39	

Suppose that in a study of coronary heart disease (CHD) the variable RACE is coded at four levels, and that the cross-classification of RACE by CHD status yields the data presented in Table 6. These data are hypothetical and have been formulated for ease of computation. The extension to a situation where the variable has more than four levels is not conceptually different, so all the examples in this section use $k = 4$.

At the bottom of Table 6 the odds ratio is given for each race, using white as the reference group. For example, for hispanic the estimated odds ratio is $(15 \times 20)/(5 \times 10) = 6.0$. The log of the odds ratios are given in the last row of Table 6. This display is typical of what is found in the literature when there is a perceived referent group to which the other groups are to be compared. These same estimates of the odds ratio may be obtained from a logistic regression program with an appropriate choice of design variables. The method for specifying the design variables involves setting all of them equal to zero for the reference group, and then setting a single design variable equal to one for each of the other groups. This is illustrated in Table 7.

Table 7 Specification of the design variables for RACE using white as the reference group

RACE (code)	D_1	D_2	D_3
White (1)	0	0	0
Black (2)	1	0	0
Hispanic (3)	0	1	0
Other (4)	0	0	1

Use of any logistic regression program with design variables coded as shown in Table 7 yields the estimated logistic regression coefficients given in Table 8.

A comparison of the estimated coefficients in Table 8 with the log odds in Table 6 shows that $\ln[\hat{\psi}(\text{black, white})] = \hat{\beta}_{11} = 2.079$, $\ln[\hat{\psi}(\text{hispanic, white})] = \hat{\beta}_{12} = 1.792$, and $\ln[\hat{\psi}(\text{other, white})] = \hat{\beta}_{13} = 1.386$.

In the univariate case the estimates of the standard errors found in the logistic regression output are identical to the estimates obtained using the cell

Table 8 Results of fitting the logistic regression model to the data in Table 6 using the design variables in Table 7

Variable	Coeff.	Std. error	z	$P > \|z\|$	[95% conf. interval]	
RACE 1	2.079	0.632	3.288	0.001	0.840	3.319
RACE 2	1.792	0.645	2.776	0.006	0.527	3.057
RACE 3	1.386	0.671	2.067	0.039	0.072	2.701
cons	−1.386	0.500	−2.773	0.006	−2.367	−0.406

Variable	Odds ratio				[95% conf. interval]	
RACE 1	8				2.32	27.63
RACE 2	6				1.69	21.26
RACE 3	4				1.07	14.90

frequencies from the contingency table. For example, the estimated standard error of the estimated coefficient for design variable (1), $\hat{\beta}_{11}$, is $0.6325 = (1/5 + 1/20 + 1/20 + 1/10)^{1/2}$. A derivation of this result appears in Bishop et al. [1].

Confidence limits for odds ratios may be obtained as follows:

$$\hat{\beta}_{ij} \pm z_{1-\alpha/2} \times \widehat{se}(\hat{\beta}_{ij}).$$

The corresponding limits for the odds ratio are obtained by exponentiating these limits as follows:

$$\exp[\hat{\beta}_{ij} \pm z_{1-\alpha/2} \times \widehat{se}(\hat{\beta}_{ij})].$$

Continuous Independent Variable

When a logistic regression model contains a continuous independent variable, interpretation of the estimated coefficient depends on how it is entered into the model and the particular units of the variable. For purposes of developing the method to interpret the coefficient for a continuous variable, we assume that the logit is linear in the variable.

Under the assumption that the logit is linear in the continuous covariate, x, the equation for the logit is $g(x) = \beta_0 + \beta_1 x$. It follows that the slope coefficient, β_1, gives the change in the log odds for an increase of "1" unit in x, i.e. $\beta_1 = g(x + 1) - g(x)$ for any value of x. Most often the value of "1" will not be biologically very interesting. For example, an increase of 1 year in age or of 1 mmHg in systolic blood pressure may be too small to be considered important. A change of 10 years or 10 mmHg might be considered more useful. However, if the range of x is from zero to one, as might be the case for some created index, then a change of 1 is too large and a change of 0.01 may be more realistic. Hence, to provide a useful interpretation for continuous scaled covariates we need to develop a method for point and interval estimation for an arbitrary change of c units in the covariate.

The log odds for a change of c units in x is obtained from the logit difference $g(x + c) - g(x) = c\beta_1$ and the associated odds ratio is obtained by exponentiating this logit difference, $\psi(c) = \psi(x + c, x) = \exp(c\beta_1)$. An estimate may be obtained by replacing β_1 with its maximum likelihood estimate, $\hat{\beta}_1$. An estimate of the standard error needed for confidence interval estimation is obtained by multiplying the estimated standard error of $\hat{\beta}_1$ by c. Hence the endpoints

of the $100(1 - \alpha)\%$ CI estimate of $\psi(c)$ are

$$\exp[c\hat{\beta}_1 \pm z_{1-\alpha/2}c\widehat{se}(\hat{\beta}_1)].$$

Since both the point estimate and endpoints of the confidence interval depend on the choice of c, the particular value of c should be clearly specified in all tables and calculations.

Multivariate Case

Often logistic regression analysis is used to *adjust statistically* the estimated effects of each variable in the model for differences in the distributions of and associations among the other independent variables. Applying this concept to a multiple logistic regression model, we may surmise that each estimated coefficient provides an estimate of the log odds adjusting for all other variables included in the model. The term confounder is used by epidemiologists to describe a covariate that is associated with both the outcome variable of interest and a primary independent variable or risk factor. When both associations are present the relationship between the risk factor and the outcome variable is said to be *confounded* (*see* **Confounding**). The procedure for adjusting for confounding is appropriate when there is no interaction.

If the association between the covariate and an outcome variable is the same within each level of the risk factor, then there is no interaction between the covariate and the risk factor. When interaction is present, the association between the risk factor and the outcome variable differs, or depends in some way on the level of the covariate. That is, the covariate modifies the effect of the risk factor (*see* **Effect Modification**). Epidemiologists use the term effect modifier to describe a variable that interacts with a risk factor.

The simplest and most commonly used model for including interaction is one in which the logit is also linear in the confounder for the second group, but with a different slope. Alternative models can be formulated which would allow for other than a linear relationship between the logit and the variables in the model within each group. In any model, interaction is incorporated by the inclusion of appropriate higher order terms.

An important step in the process of modeling a set of data is to determine whether or not there is evidence of interaction in the data. Tables 9 and 10

Table 9 Estimated logistic regression coefficients, log likelihood, and the likelihood ratio test statistic (G) for an example showing evidence of confounding but no interaction

Model	Constant	SEX	AGE	SEX × AGE	Log likelihood	G
1	−1.046	1.535			−61.86	
2	−7.142	0.979	0.167		−49.59	24.54
3	−6.103	0.481	0.139	0.059	−49.33	0.52

Table 10 Estimated logistic regression coefficients, log likelihood, and the likelihood ratio test statistic (G) for an example showing evidence of confounding and interaction

Model	Constant	SEX	AGE	SEX × AGE	Log likelihood	G
1	−0.847	2.505			−52.52	
2	−6.194	1.734	0.147		−46.79	11.46
3	−3.105	0.047	0.629	0.206	−44.76	4.06

present the results of fitting a series of logistic regression models to two different sets of hypothetical data. The variables in each of the data sets are the same: SEX, AGE, and CHD. In addition to the estimated coefficients, the log likelihood for each model and minus twice the change (deviance) is given. Recall that minus twice the change in the log likelihood may be used to test for the significance of coefficients for variables added to the model. An interaction is added to the model by creating a variable that is equal to the product of the value of the sex and the value of age.

Examining the results in Table 9 we see that the estimated coefficient for the variable SEX changed from 1.535 in model 1 to 0.979 when AGE was added in model 2. Hence, there is clear evidence of a confounding effect owing to age. When the interaction term "SEX × AGE" is added in model 3 we see that the change in the deviance is only 0.52 which, when compared with the chi-square distribution with one degree of freedom, yields a P value of 0.47, which clearly is not significant. Note that the coefficient for sex changed from 0.979 to 0.481. This is not surprising since the inclusion of an interaction term, especially when it involves a continuous variable, will usually produce fairly marked changes in the estimated coefficients of dichotomous variables involved in the interaction. Thus, when an interaction term is present in the model we cannot assess confounding via the change in a coefficient. For these data we would prefer to use model 2 which suggests that age is a confounder but not an effect modifier.

The results in Table 10 show evidence of both confounding and interaction due to age. Comparing model 1 with model 2 we see that the coefficient

for sex changes from 2.505 to 1.734. When the age by sex interaction is added to the model we see that the deviance is 4.06, which yields a P value of 0.04. Since the deviance is significant, we prefer model 3 over model 2, and should regard age as both a confounder and an effect modifier. The net result is that any estimate of the odds ratio for sex should be made with respect to a specific age.

Hence, we see that determining if a covariate, X, is an effect modifier and/or a confounder involves several issues. Determining effect modification status involves the parametric structure of the logit, while determination of confounder status involves two things. First, the covariate must be associated with the outcome variable. This implies that the logit must have a nonzero slope in the covariate. Secondly, the covariate must be associated with the risk factor. In our example this might be characterized by having a difference in the mean age for males and females. However, the association may be more complex than a simple difference in means. The essence is that we have incomparability in our risk factor groups. This incomparability must be accounted for in the model if we are to obtain a correct, unconfounded estimate of effect for the risk factor.

In practice, the confounder status of a covariate is ascertained by comparing the estimated coefficient for the risk factor variable from models containing and not containing the covariate. Any "biologically important" change in the estimated coefficient for the risk factor would dictate that the covariate is a confounder and should be included in the model, regardless of the statistical significance of the estimated coefficient for the covariate. On the other hand, a covariate is an effect modifier only when the interaction term added to the model is both biologically meaningful and statistically significant. When a covariate is an effect modifier, its status as a confounder is of secondary importance since the estimate of the effect of the risk factor depends on the specific value of the covariate.

The concepts of adjustment, confounding, interaction, and effect modification may be extended to cover the situations involving any number of variables on any measurement scale(s). The principles for identification and inclusion of confounder and interaction variables into the model are the same regardless of the number of variables and their measurement scales.

Much of this article has been abstracted from [4]. Readers wanting more detail on any topic should consult this reference.

References

[1]   Bishop, Y.M.M., Fienberg, S.E. & Holland, P. (1975). *Discrete Multivariate Analysis: Theory and Practice*. MIT Press, Boston.

[2]   Cox, D.R. & Snell, E.J. (1989). *The Analysis of Binary Data*, 2nd Ed. Chapman & Hall, London.

[3]   Hauck, W.W. & Donner, A. (1977). Wald's Test as applied to hypotheses in logit analysis, *Journal of the American Statistical Association* **72**, 851–853.

[4]   Hosmer, D. & Lemeshow, S. (1989). *Applied Logistic Regression*. Wiley, New York.

[5]   Jennings, D.E. (1986). Judging inference adequacy in logistic regression, *Journal of the American Statistical Association* **81**, 471–476.

[6]   McCullagh, P. & Nelder, J.A. (1983). *Generalized Linear Models*. Chapman & Hall, London.

(*See also* **Categorical Data Analysis; Loglinear Models; Proportional-Odds Model; Quantal Response Models**)

STANLEY LEMESHOW & DAVID W. HOSMER, JR

Logistic Regression, Conditional

An important extension of the **logistic regression** model is the analysis of data from stratified samples (*see* **Stratification**). Examples of this application include studies where data are collected from several different sites such as schools, hospitals, or clinics as well as analyses where **covariates** are controlled for by defining *post hoc* stratification variables. The most frequently encountered stratified study design employing the logistic regression model is the matched **case–control study** used in epidemiology (*see* **Matched Analysis**). A discussion of the rationale for these matched studies may be found in epidemiology texts such as Breslow & Day [1], Kleinbaum et al. [5], Schlesselman [8], Kelsey et al. [4], and Rothman [7].

The basic idea is to expand the logistic model by inclusion of stratification variables. Assume the sampled data may be represented as a triple $(y_{kj}, \mathbf{x}_{kj}, \mathbf{z}_k)$, where $j = 1, 2, \ldots, n_k$ represents the particular subject observed within stratum $k = 1, 2, \ldots, K$, $y_{kj} = 0$ or 1 is the observed value of the binary outcome variable for subject j in stratum k, $\mathbf{x}'_{kj} = (x_{kj1}, x_{kj2}, \ldots, x_{kjp})$ is a vector of p nonconstant covariates, and $\mathbf{z}'_k = (z_{k1}, z_{k2}, \ldots, z_{kq})$ is a vector of q covariates defining stratum characteristics. The quantity n_k denotes the number of observations in stratum k. The vector $\mathbf{z}$ may simply contain one variable to indicate the stratum, $z_k = k$, or a set of values of q covariates may be used to define strata. For example, if one defined strata by gender and race coded at three levels, then $\mathbf{z}'_k = (z_{k1}, z_{k2})$ with $z_{k1} = 0$ or 1, $z_{k2} = 1, 2,$ or 3, and $k = 1, 2, \ldots, 6$.

A number of different stratified logistic regression models are possible. The simplest logistic regression model has a logit function with one design variable for the stratum specific effect and constant slope across strata for the covariates, namely

$$g(\mathbf{x}_{kj}, z_k) = \beta_0 + \alpha_k + \boldsymbol{\beta}' \mathbf{x}_{kj}. \tag{1}$$

The logit function is discussed in detail in the article on **Logistic Regression**. It is defined in terms of the model conditional probability as $g(\mathbf{x}_{kj}, z_k) = \ln\{\pi(\mathbf{x}_{kj}, z_k)/[1 - \pi(\mathbf{x}_{kj}, z_k)]\}$ and $\pi(\mathbf{x}_{kj}, z_k) = \Pr(Y_{kj} = 1 | \mathbf{x}_{kj}, z_k)$. In the parameterization in (1) one may think of the values of α_k as the coefficients for design variables generated by the K levels of the stratum variable. These design variables may be created using any method but the most frequent choice is either referent cell or deviation from means coding. There are $K - 1$ parameters or degrees of freedom associated with the stratification variable. The model in (1) has a stratum-specific intercept and constant slopes. Thus the effect of the covariates is the same for all strata. The covariate vector, $\mathbf{x}$, may contain both main effects as well as higher-order terms such as interactions and squared terms, but may not contain terms that indicate the stratum.

An extension of the model in (1) is possible when the vector $\mathbf{z}$ contains covariates that measure stratum characteristics, e.g. gender and race as noted above. The vector may also contain continuous covariates. Age is often used as a stratification variable. In this setting one may add interactions to (1), which yield a model with stratum-specific slopes. Suppose strata are defined by gender and $z_k = 0$ or $1(1 = \text{male})$ records the gender of the subject. The logit for an extended model is

$$g(\mathbf{x}_{kj}, z_k) = \beta_0 + \alpha_k z_k + \boldsymbol{\beta}' \mathbf{x}_{kj} + z_k \times \boldsymbol{\gamma}' \mathbf{x}_{kj}. \quad (2)$$

The model for females is

$$g(\mathbf{x}_{kj}, z_k = 0) = \beta_0 + \boldsymbol{\beta}' \mathbf{x}_{kj},$$

and the model for males is

$$g(\mathbf{x}_{kj}, z_k = 1) = \beta_0 + \alpha_1 + (\boldsymbol{\beta} + \boldsymbol{\gamma})' \mathbf{x}_{kj}.$$

The model in (2) allows for stratum-specific intercepts as well as stratum-specific slopes. Maximum likelihood estimators of the parameters in (1) or (2) are obtained by extending the likelihood function (*see* **Logistic Regression**) to include a product over strata. The **likelihood** function for the model in (1) is

$$l(\alpha, \beta,) = \prod_{k=1}^{K} \prod_{j=1}^{n_k} \zeta(\mathbf{x}_{kj}, z_k), \quad (3)$$

where $\zeta(\mathbf{x}_{kj}, z_k) = \pi(\mathbf{x}_{kj}, z_k)^{y_{kj}} [1 - \pi(\mathbf{x}_{kj}, z_k)]^{1-y_{kj}}$. Application of the likelihood function in (3) to the model in (2) is accomplished by adding the requisite additional terms to the logit. Estimators of the parameters may be obtained from logistic regression software (*see* **Software, Biostatistical**) by inclusion of the variables recording stratum-specific data into the model.

Thus the model as shown in (1) or (2) does not represent anything particularly new or difficult for the investigator familiar with the logistic regression model. The model-building issues and details are identical to those of the ordinary logistic model, or for that matter any regression model.

Problems begin to arise which require a different approach when the number of strata becomes large and, at the same time, the number of observations within each stratum remains fixed. Application of the logistic regression model to this setting will be described in the remainder of this article.

Logistic Regression with Highly Stratified Data

A convenient setting to illustrate the use of logistic regression with highly stratified data is the matched case–control study design. In this study design subjects are stratified on the basis of covariates believed to be associated with the outcome. Age and gender are examples of commonly used stratification variables. Within each stratum a sample of subjects with the outcome present, called cases ($y = 1$), and a sample of subjects without the outcome, called controls ($y = 0$), is chosen. The number of cases and controls need not be constant across strata, but the most common matched design is one where each stratum includes one case and one control. Study variables are collected on all subjects. We develop the methods for analysis of highly stratified data for the general case. Greater detail is provided for the one-to-one matched design because it can be analyzed using standard logistic regression software.

The methods to be described may be used in settings other than matched case–control studies. For example, suppose that, in a study of student performance, data were collected from 1000 different schools and a fixed number of students was selected from each school. The outcome variable is whether the student "passed" a particular course or standardized test. In this example there are 1000 strata defined by school. The conditional likelihood approach described below is the same for both the case–control study and the general highly stratified design. More stringent sampling assumptions are required in the case–control study, see [3, Chapter 6].

We begin by providing some motivation for the need for special methods for the highly stratified study. We noted in (1) that we could handle the stratified sample by including variables created from the stratification variables in the model. This approach works well when the number of subjects in each stratum is large and strata are few. However, matched studies have few subjects per stratum. For example, in the one-to-one matched design with K case–control pairs we have only two subjects per stratum. A fully stratified analysis of the model in (1) with p covariates would require estimation of $(K + p)$ parameters, the $p + 1$ slope coefficients for the covariates, and the $K - 1$ coefficients for the stratum-specific design variables, using a sample of size $2K$. The optimality properties of the method of maximum likelihood, derived by letting the sample size, K, become large, hold only when the number of parameters remains fixed. In any matched study this is not the case, as the number of parameters increases at the same rate as the sample size. For example, when analyzing a matched one-to-one design via the fully stratified likelihood in (3) using a logistic regression model containing one dichotomous covariate and the $K - 1$ design variables for strata, it can be shown (see [1, p. 250]) that the bias in the estimate of the coefficient is 100%. If we regard the stratum-specific parameters as (nuisance) parameters whose values are neither of great interest to us nor are essential for the inferences required in the study, and we are willing to forgo their estimation, then we can create a conditional likelihood which will yield maximum likelihood estimators of the slope coefficients in the logistic regression model that are consistent and asymptotically normally distributed. The mathematical details of conditional likelihood analysis may be found in [2] (*see* **Likelihood**). We summarize its application to the matched design. Liang [6], in related work, considers a general approach to the analysis of highly stratified data.

The Conditional Logistic Regression Model

Suppose that there are K strata with n_{k1} cases (subjects with $y = 1$) and n_{k0} controls (subjects with $y = 0$) in stratum k, $k = 1, 2, \ldots, K$. The conditional likelihood for the kth stratum is obtained as the probability of the observed data conditional on the stratum total sample size (fixed by the sampling design) and the total number of cases, the **sufficient statistic** for the stratum-specific **nuisance parameter**. This probability is the ratio of the probability of the observed outcome to the probability for all possible assignments of n_{k1} subjects with $y = 1$ and n_{k0} subjects with $y = 0$ to $n_k = n_{k0} + n_{k1}$ subjects. The number

of possible assignments is the n_k choose n_{k1} combinations. Let the subscript j denote any one of these assignments. For any assignment we let subjects 1 to n_{k1} correspond to the subjects with $y = 1$ and subjects $n_{k1} + 1$ to n_k to the subjects with $y = 0$. This will be indexed by i for the observed data and by i_j for the jth possible assignment. The contribution to the conditional likelihood for the kth stratum is

$$
l_k(\boldsymbol{\beta})
= \frac{\displaystyle\prod_{i=1}^{n_{k1}} \Pr(y_{ki} = 1|\mathbf{x}_{ki}) \prod_{i=n_{k1}+1}^{n_k} \Pr(y_{ki} = 0|\mathbf{x}_{ki})}{\displaystyle\sum_j \left[\prod_{i_j=1}^{n_{k1}} \Pr(y_{ki_j} = 1|\mathbf{x}_{ki_j}) \times \prod_{i_j=n_{k1}+1}^{n_k} \Pr(y_{ki_j} = 0|\mathbf{x}_{ki_j}) \right]}, \quad (4)
$$

where the summation over j in the denominator is over the n_k choose n_{k1} combinations. The full conditional likelihood is the product of the $l_k(\boldsymbol{\beta})$ over the K strata,

$$
l(\boldsymbol{\beta}) = \prod_{k=1}^{K} l_k(\boldsymbol{\beta}). \quad (5)
$$

If we substitute the logistic regression model with the logit defined in (1), $\pi(\mathbf{x}_{ki}) = \Pr(y_{ki} = 1|\mathbf{x}_{ki})$, into (4), then (5) simplifies to

$$
l_k(\boldsymbol{\beta}) = \frac{\displaystyle\prod_{i=1}^{n_{k1}} \pi(\mathbf{x}_{ki}) \prod_{i=n_{k1}+1}^{n_k} [1 - \pi(\mathbf{x}_{ki})]}{\displaystyle\sum_j \left\{ \prod_{i_j=1}^{n_{k1}} \pi(\mathbf{x}_{ki_j}) \prod_{i_j=n_{k1}+1}^{n_k} [1 - \pi(\mathbf{x}_{ki_j})] \right\}}. \quad (6)
$$

Since the terms of the form $\exp(\beta_0 + \alpha_k)/[1 + \exp(\beta_0 + \alpha_k + \mathbf{x}'_{ki}\boldsymbol{\beta})]$ appear equally in both the numerator and denominator of (6) they cancel out, and (6) simplifies to

$$
l_k(\boldsymbol{\beta}) = \frac{\displaystyle\prod_{i=1}^{n_{k1}} \exp(\boldsymbol{\beta}'\mathbf{x}_{ki})}{\displaystyle\sum_j \left(\prod_{i_j=1}^{n_{k1}} \exp(\boldsymbol{\beta}'\mathbf{x}_{ki_j}) \right)}, \quad (7)
$$

which depends only on the unknown parameter vector β. The conditional maximum likelihood estimator for β is that value which maximizes (5) when the expression in (7) is used for $l_k(\beta)$. Most software packages performing logistic regression have the capability to fit this conditional logistic regression model (*see* **Software, Biostatistical**).

The argument leading to expression (7) is more complicated for a case–control study and requires assumptions about sampling of cases and controls and applications of **Bayes' theorem**. The details will not be presented here but may be found in [3, Chapters 6 and 7].

One must always keep in mind when using the conditional likelihood in (7) that it was obtained by beginning with the usual logistic regression model. Thus, one still interprets the coefficients as "log-odds ratios". The original logistic regression model (1) or (2) tends to become lost in the arithmetic process of re-expressing the likelihood in (7). This point can be especially confusing to those analyzing data from a one-to-one matched case–control study.

The one-to-one matched design is probably the most frequent example of the use of a conditional logistic regression model. We show how one may analyze this design using standard logistic regression software, since not all packages have the capability to perform conditional logistic regression. More general software must be used in other matched designs and in the general highly stratified setting.

Logistic Regression Analysis for the One-to-One Matched Study

In the one-to-one matched study there are two subjects within each stratum. To simplify the notation, let $\mathbf{x}_{k1}$ denote the covariate vector for the case and $\mathbf{x}_{k0}$ the covariate vector for the control in the kth stratum. Using this notation, the conditional likelihood, (7), for the kth stratum is

$$l_k(\beta) = \frac{\exp(\beta' \mathbf{x}_{k1})}{\exp(\beta' \mathbf{x}_{k1}) + \exp(\beta' \mathbf{x}_{k0})}. \quad (8)$$

Further simplification is obtained by dividing the numerator and denominator of (8) by $\exp(\beta' \mathbf{x}_{k0})$, yielding

$$l_k(\beta) = \frac{\exp[\beta'(\mathbf{x}_{k1} - \mathbf{x}_{k0})]}{1 + \exp[\beta'(\mathbf{x}_{k1} - \mathbf{x}_{k0})]}. \quad (9)$$

The expression on the right-hand side of (9) is identical to a logistic regression model with the constant term set equal to zero, $\beta_0 = 0$, and covariate vector equal to the value of the case minus the value of the control, $\mathbf{x}_k^* = \mathbf{x}_{k1} - \mathbf{x}_{k0}$. This algebraic simplification allows one to use standard logistic regression software to compute the conditional maximum likelihood estimators of the coefficients and their standard errors. To accomplish this, one performs the following data modifications: define the sample size as the number of case–control pairs, compute the difference vector $\mathbf{x}_k^*$, compute a *pseudo*-response variable equal to 1, $y_k^* = 1$, and exclude the constant term from the model, e.g. force its value to be equal to zero. Thus, from a computational point of view, the one-to-one matched design presents no new challenges.

We have found that in the process of creating the differences and setting the "outcome" equal to 1, one can lose sight of the model. It is important to distinguish between the logistic regression model being fit to the data and the computational manipulations required to fit this model with standard logistic regression software. The process is less confusing if one focuses on the logistic regression model first and then considers the computations needed to obtain the parameter estimates. A few examples should help to illustrate this point.

Suppose we have a dichotomous independent variable coded zero or one. This variable is correctly modeled via a single coefficient in the logit, irrespective of whether we enter the variable via a design variable or treat it as continuous. The difference variable which we obtain by subtracting the value of the case from that of the control may take on one of three possible values: $(-1, 0$ or $1)$. If we had mistakenly thought of the difference variable as being the actual data, then we would have incorrectly modeled the variable by including two design variables in the model. The correct method is to create a difference variable and treat it as if it were continuous.

As a second example, suppose we have a variable such as race, coded at three levels. To model this variable correctly in the one-to-one matched design, we create, for each case and control in a pair, the values of the two design variables representing race. We compute the difference between these two design variables for the case and control and model each of these differences as if it were continuous. The same process is followed for any categorical scaled covariate. Note that the computer software may not recognize the differences in design variables as being created from the same variable, so one has to be sure that all design variables are included in the model. Another point to keep in mind is that differences between variables used to form strata are equal to zero for all strata and thus will not be useful as main effects. However, one may include interaction terms between stratification variables and other covariates, because differences in these interaction variables will likely not be zero.

In summary, the conceptual process for modeling matched or highly stratified data is identical to that of the usual logistic regression model. If one develops the modeling strategy for highly stratified data as if one had unstratified data, and then uses the conditional likelihood, then one will always be proceeding correctly.

Examples of the Use of the Conditional Logistic Regression Model

For illustrative purposes we use a small one-to-one matched data set obtained from a study of factors associated with the birth of a low birthweight baby (less than 2500 g). These data are in [3, Appendix 3]. These data, as well as the other data sets used in [3], may be obtained in the logistic regression menu at **internet** address http://www-unix.oit.umass.edu/~statdata. A one-to-one matched data set was obtained from an unmatched study of 189 births of which 59 were low weight. The matched data were obtained by randomly selecting, for each woman who gave birth to a low birthweight baby, a mother of the same age who did not give birth to a low birthweight baby. For three of the young mothers (age less than 17) it was not possible to identify a match since there were no mothers of normal weight babies of that age. The data consist of 56 age-matched case–control pairs. Variables selected for use in this example are a prior pre-term delivery (ptd, $1 = $ yes, $0 = $ no), smoking status (during pregnancy) of the mother (smoke, $1 = $ yes, $0 = $ no), history of hypertension (ht, $1 = $ yes, $0 = $ no), presence of uterine irritability (ui, $1 = $ yes, $0 = $ no), and the weight of the mother at the last menstrual period (lwt, pounds).

In ordinary logistic regression the coefficient for a model containing only one dichotomous variable is equal to the log of the cross-product ratio (odds ratio) from the **two-by-two table** of outcome by

the dichotomous variable. The same result is true when the conditional logistic model is used with a one-to-one matched study and the model contains a single dichotomous variable. The estimator of the odds ratio in a one-to-one matched study is the ratio of the frequencies of the discordant pairs. These are the frequencies in the off main diagonal cells of a 2×2 table cross-classifying the dichotomous variable for the case by the control. For example, consider the smoking status of the mother. The 2×2 table is shown in Table 1 and the results from fitting the conditional logistic regression model containing this variable are shown in Table 2. The odds ratio computed from Table 1 is $\hat{\psi} = 22/8 = 2.75$ and its log is $\ln \hat{\psi} = 1.012$. The results presented in Table 2 show that the coefficient for smoke is identically equal to the log of the odds ratio from Table 1. A confidence interval for the odds ratio may be obtained by exponentiating the end points of the confidence interval for the coefficient shown in Table 2. The resulting interval is (1.22, 6.18) indicating that, in these data, smoking during pregnancy is a risk factor for giving birth to a low birthweight baby. The significance of the coefficient may be tested using the Wald statistic (*see* **Likelihood**), labeled as z in Table 2, and whose two-tailed **P value** is 0.014. The appropriateness of both the confidence interval and test depend on an assumption that the sample size, 56 in this case, is large enough to employ the large-sample distributional properties (normality) of maximum likelihood estimators.

If one did not have available software specifically to perform conditional logistic regression, then

Table 1 Cross-classification of the smoking status of the case by the control

Case	Control		Total
	No	Yes	
No	18	8	26
Yes	22	8	30
Total	40	16	56

Table 2 Results from fitting a conditional logistic regression model containing the dichotomous variable, smoking status of the mother

Variable	Coeff.	Std. error	z	P	95% CIE
Smoke	1.012	0.413	2.45	0.014	(0.202, 1.821)

the previously described method of creating difference variables could be used before beginning full-scale modeling of the data. This technique is not as important as it once was as most of the commonly available packages either have specific conditional logistic regression routines, or methods for adapting other routines are explained in their manuals. Again we wish to reinforce the point that the method of creating difference variables will only work for the one-to-one matched study. Any other design must be modeled through specific conditional logistic regression software.

We present in Table 3 the results of fitting a more complex model. The purpose of this model is to illustrate the use and interpretation of results from a multivariable conditional logistic regression model. See [3, Chapter 7] for a discussion of the issues involved in developing a model within the context of the current example and conditional logistic regression.

We obtain estimates of the odds ratios and their confidence intervals by exponentiating the estimated coefficients and end points of their confidence intervals in Table 3. These are shown in Table 4. The odds ratio and confidence interval presented for the weight of the mother at the last menstrual period is for a 10 pound increase in weight. The results for last menstrual period (lwt) are obtained from Table 3 by multiplying the coefficient and end points of the confidence interval by 10 before exponentiating. This is done since lwt is measured in pounds, and an odds ratio for a one pound weight difference is likely not to be clinically meaningful.

The odds ratios in Table 4 suggest an important increase in risk of delivering of a low birthweight baby for prior pre-term deliveries, smoking during pregnancy, presence of hypertension, and presence of uterine irritability. The odds ratio for the weight of the mother at the last menstrual period suggests

Table 3 Results from fitting a conditional logistic regression model containing prior pre-term delivery, smoking status of the mother, presence of hypertension, presence of uterine irritability, and the weight of the mother at the last menstrual period to 56 matched pairs

Variable	Coeff.	Std. error	z	P	95% CIE
ptd	1.671	0.747	2.24	0.025	(0.207, 3.135)
smoke	1.480	0.562	2.63	0.009	(0.378, 2.582)
ht	2.330	1.003	2.32	0.020	(0.364, 4.296)
ui	1.345	0.694	1.94	0.052	(−0.015, 2.705)
lwt	−0.015	0.008	−1.88	0.060	(−0.031, 0.001)

Table 4 Estimated odds ratios and 95% confidence intervals for prior pre-term deliveries, smoking status of the mother, presence of hypertension, presence of uterine irritability, and the weight of the mother at the last menstrual period (10 lb increase)

Variable	Odds ratio	95% CIE
ptd	5.32	(1.23, 22.99)
smoke	4.39	(1.46, 13.22)
ht	10.28	(1.44, 73.41)
ui	3.84	(0.99, 14.95)
lwt	0.86	(0.73, 1.01)

an approximate 14% decrease in risk per 10 pound increase in weight. This interpretation assumes that the logit is linear in lwt. One should always check the scale of all continuous variables in any regression model. We did this using a method based on design variables for the quartiles of lwt (see [3, p. 194]), which supported the linearity assumption for lwt.

The confidence interval estimates in Table 4 are quite wide for the dichotomous variables. This instability is due to the fact that the variance estimator is inversely related to the number of discordant pairs. The analysis presented in Tables 2 and 3 is based on 56 pairs and the numbers of discordant pairs are 19, 30, 10, and 16, respectively, for the dichotomous variables. The widths of the confidence intervals in Table 4 are a result of the relatively few discordant pairs. This points out an important consideration that must be kept in mind at the design stage of a study. The gain in precision obtained from matching and using conditional logistic regression may be offset by a loss owing to few discordant pairs for dichotomous covariates. In general, the variance estimator of the slope coefficient is a function of how different the subjects with $y = 1$ are from those with $y = 0$ within each stratum.

Likelihood ratio tests may be used for model testing and refinement in a manner similar to that discussed in the article on logistic regression. In the case of conditional logistic regression the likelihood for model zero, "the no data model", is obtained by setting the coefficient vector equal to zero in (7). This model is essentially a coin toss with stratum specific probability $\Pr(Y_{kj} = 1) = n_{k1}/n_k$.

Application of the conditional logistic regression model to other, more complicated, matched or highly stratified designs is, for all intents and purposes, identical to the one-to-one matched study discussed. The essential point to keep in mind is that one uses and interprets the estimated coefficients in a manner identical to ordinary logistic regression. Although not illustrated in the example, because of relatively few matched pairs, one may use matching or stratification variables to form interactions with variables in the model but one may not include them as main effect terms. Much of the content of this article is based on [3].

References

[1] Breslow, N.E. & Day, N.E. (1980). *Statistical Methods in Cancer Research*. Vol. 1. *The Analysis of Case–Control Studies*. Oxford University Press, New York.

[2] Cox, D.R. & Hinkley, D.V. (1974). *Theoretical Statistics*. Chapman & Hall, New York.

[3] Hosmer, D.W. & Lemeshow, S. (1989). *Applied Logistic Regression*. Wiley, New York.

[4] Kelsey, J.L., Thompson, W.D. & Evans, A.S. (1986). *Methods in Observational Epidemiology*. Oxford University Press, New York.

[5] Kleinbaum, D.G., Kupper, L.L. & Morgenstern, H. (1982). *Epidemiologic Research: Principles and Quantitative Methods*. Van Nostrand Reinhold, New York.

[6] Liang, K.Y. (1987). Extended Mantel–Haenszel estimating procedure for multivariate logistic regressions, *Biometrics* **43**, 289–300.

[7] Rothman, K.J. (1986). *Modern Epidemiology*. Little, Brown & Company, Boston.

[8] Schlesselman, J.J. (1982). *Case–Control Studies*. Oxford University Press, New York.

(*See also* **Binary Data; Correlated Binary Data**)

DAVID W. HOSMER & STANLEY LEMESHOW

Logistic-Normal Model *see* Quantal Response Models

Logit *see* Logistic Regression

Loglinear Models

Multivariate analysis has occupied a prominent place in the classical development of statistical theory and methodology. The analysis of cross classified **categorical data**, or **contingency table** analysis as it is often called, represents the *discrete* multivariate analog of **analysis of variance** for continuous response variables, and now plays an important role in biostatistical practice. This article provides an introduction to some of the more widely used techniques for the analysis of contingency table data using loglinear models and to the statistical theory that underlies them, revising and extending an earlier review article [25] (for additional material on this topic, and related methods, *see* **Categorical Data Analysis; Contingency Table**).

The term *contingency*, used in connection with tables of cross classified categorical data, seems to have originated with **Karl Pearson** [56], who for an $s \times t$ table defined contingency to be any measure of the total deviation from "independent probability". The term is now used to refer to the table of counts itself. Prior to this formal use of the term, statisticians going back at least to Quetelet [59] worked with cross classifications of counts to summarize the association between variables. Pearson [54] had laid the groundwork for his approach to contingency tables when he developed his **chi-square test** for comparing observed and expected (theoretic) frequencies. Yet Pearson preferred to view contingency tables involving the cross classification of two or more polytomies as arising from a partition of a set of **multivariate, normal** data, with an underlying continuum for each polytomy. This view led Pearson [55] to develop his tetrachoric correlation coefficient for **2 × 2 tables**, and this work in turn spawned an extensive literature well chronicled by Lancaster [50] (*see* **Association, Measures of**).

The most serious problems with Pearson's approach were (i) the complicated infinite series linking the tetrachoric correlation coefficient with the frequencies in a 2×2 table, and (ii) his insistence that it always made sense to assume an underlying continuum, even when the dichotomy of interest was dead–alive or employed–unemployed, and that it was reasonable to assume that the probability distribution over such a continuum was normal. In contradistinction, Yule [67] chose to view the categories of a cross classification as fixed, and he set out to consider the structural relationship between or among the discrete variables represented by the cross classification, via various functions of the cross product ratio. Especially impressive in this,

Yule's first paper on the topic, is his notational structure for n attributes or 2^n tables, and his attention to the concept of partial and joint association of dichotomous variables.

The debate between Pearson and Yule over whose approach was more appropriate for contingency table analysis raged for many years (see, for example, Pearson & Heron [58]), and the acrimony it engendered was exceeded only by that associated with Pearson's dispute with R.A. Fisher over the adjustment in the **degrees of freedom** (df) for the **chi-square test** of independence in the $s \times t$ table. [In this latter case Pearson was simply incorrect; as Fisher [30] first noted, $\mathrm{df} = (s - 1)(t - 1)$.]

Although much work on two-dimensional contingency tables followed the pioneering efforts by Pearson and Yule, it was not until 1935 that Bartlett, as a result of a suggestion by Fisher, utilized Yule's cross product ratio to define the notion of second-order **interaction** in a $2 \times 2 \times 2$ table, and to develop an appropriate test for the absence of such an interaction [6]. The multivariate generalizations of Bartlett's work, beginning with the work of Roy & Kastenbaum [62], form the basis of the loglinear model approach to contingency tables, which is described in detail below.

The past 40 years have seen a burgeoning literature on the analysis of contingency tables. Some of this literature emphasizes the use of the minimum modified chi-square approach (e.g. Grizzle et al. [43]) or the use of the minimum discrimination information approach (e.g. Gokhale & Kullback [K]), but the bulk of it follows Fisher in the use of **maximum likelihood**. For most contingency table problems, the minimum discrimination information approach yields maximum likelihood estimates. More recently, attention has turned to the development of hierarchical **Bayesian** approaches, which lead to the computation of *posterior distributions* (rather than point estimates) for quantities of interest (see, for example, Leonard [51], Albert & Gupta [3], Epstein & Fienberg [21], and Gelman et al. [33]).

Except for a few attempts at the use of additive (linear) models (see, for example, Bhapkar & Koch [7]), almost all of the papers written on the topic emphasize the use of loglinear or logit models. Key papers by Birch [8], Darroch [12], Good [34], and Goodman [37, 38], plus the availability of high-speed computers, served to spur renewed interest in the problems of categorical data analysis, and

culminated in a series of books first published in the 1970s and which focused in large part on the use of loglinear models for both two-dimensional and multidimensional tables (see, for example, [E], [H], [K], [L], [M], [N], [Q]). The past decade has seen an even greater flourishing of this expository literature, only some of which we reference here.

The subsequent sections of this presentation deal primarily with the analysis of contingency table data using loglinear models. The next section describes three examples that will serve to illustrate some of the methods of analysis, and the third section discusses briefly sampling models and estimation methods used in conjunction with categorical data analysis. The fourth section outlines the basic statistical theory associated with maximum likelihood estimation and loglinear models, including brief descriptions of the family of graphical loglinear models emanating from the work of Darroch et al. [17], and related work on the collapsing of contingency tables, as well as brief discussions of **capture–recapture** methods and latent trait (*see* **Latent Class Analysis**) and **Rasch models**, and their linkage to loglinear models. The fifth section contains examples of analysis to illustrate the basic theoretic results. The sixth section presents a brief introduction to Bayesian hierarchical approaches to loglinear models. We end with a guide to some computer programs for loglinear model analysis.

Three Examples

In this article we use three examples to illustrate the models and methods described. Two of these are classic examples, from Bartlett [6] and Waite [66], which have been analyzed repeatedly in the literature and have been used in many texts. The third, due to Edwards & Havranek [20], appears in the more recent texts by Edwards [I] and by Whitaker [S].

The data reported by Bartlett [6] in his pioneering article, and included here in Table 1, are from an *experiment* giving the response (alive or dead) of 240 plants for each combination of two explanatory variables, time of planting (early or late), and length of cutting (high or low).

The questions to be answered are as follows: (i) What are the effects of time of planting and length of cutting on survival? (ii) Do they interact in their effect on survival?

Table 1 $2 \times 2 \times 2$ table

| Time of planting: | | Early | | Late | |
Length of cutting:		High	Low	High	Low
Response	Alive	156	107	84	31
	Dead	84	133	156	209
Total		240	240	240	240

Source: Bartlett [6].

Table 2   Fingerprints of the right hand classified by the number of whorls and small loops

| | | | Small loops | | | | |
Whorls	0	1	2	3	4	5	Total
0	78	144	204	211	179	45	861
1	106	153	126	80	32		497
2	130	92	55	15			292
3	125	38	7				170
4	104	26					130
5	50						50
Total	593	453	392	306	211	45	2000

Source: Waite [66].

The data in Table 2, from Waite [66], give the cross classification of right-hand fingerprints according to the number of whorls and small loops. The total number of whorls and small loops is at most five, and the resulting table is triangular. There the question of interest is more complicated because, as a result of the constraint forcing the data into the triangular structure, the number of whorls is "related to" the number of small loops. Such an array of counts is referred to as an *incomplete contingency table*, and the incomplete structure, in the case of the Waite data, was the cause of yet another controversy involving Pearson [57], this time with J.A. Harris (see Harris & Treloar [44]). The fit of a relatively simple model to these data is explored below. (See also [63], for a re-examination of Pearson's introduction of the methods used by Waite.)

The data in Table 3 come from a prospective epidemiologic study of 1841 workers in a Czechoslovakian car factory, intended to investigate the potential risk factors for coronary thrombosis (see Edwards & Havranek [20]). There are six variables corresponding to prognostic factors in the table:

A   (smoking: yes, no)
B   (strenuous mental work: yes, no)

Table 3   Prognostic factors in coronary heart disease

| | | | | B | No | | Yes | |
F	E	D	C	A	No	Yes	No	Yes
Negative	<3	<140	No		44	40	112	67
			Yes		129	145	12	23
		≥140	No		35	12	80	33
			Yes		109	67	7	9
	≥3	<140	No		23	32	70	66
			Yes		50	80	7	13
		≥140	No		24	25	73	57
			Yes		51	63	7	16
Positive	<3	<140	No		5	7	21	9
			Yes		9	17	1	4
		≥140	No		4	3	11	8
			Yes		14	17	5	2
	≥3	<140	No		7	3	14	14
			Yes		9	16	2	3
		≥140	No		4	0	13	11
			Yes		5	14	4	4

Source: Edwards & Havranek [20].

C   (strenuous physical work: yes, no)
D   (systolic blood pressure: <140, ≥140)
E   (ratio of beta and alpha lipoproteins: <3, ≥3)
F   (family anamnesis of coronary heart disease: yes, no).

Sampling Models and Estimation for Contingency Tables

Let $\mathbf{x}' = (x_1, x_2, \ldots, x_t)$ be a vector of observed counts for t cells, structured in the form of a cross classification such as in Tables 1 and 2, where $t = 2^3 = 8$ and $t = 21$, respectively. Now let $\mathbf{m}' = (m_1, m_2, \ldots, m_t)$ be the vector of expected values that are assumed to be functions of unknown parameters $\boldsymbol{\theta}' = (\theta_1, \theta_2, \ldots, \theta_s)$, where $s < t$. Thus one can write $\mathbf{m} = \mathbf{m}(\boldsymbol{\theta})$.

There are three standard sampling models for the observed counts in contingency tables.

1. *Poisson model.* The $\{x_i\}$ are observations from independent **Poisson** random variables with means $\{m_i\}$ and **likelihood** function

$$\prod_{i=1}^{t} [m_i^{x_i} \exp(-m_i)/x_i!]. \tag{1}$$

2. *Multinomial model.* The total count $N = \sum_{i=1}^{t} x_i$ is a random sample from an infinite population,

where the underlying cell probabilities are $\{m_i/N\}$, and the likelihood is

$$N! \cdot N^{-N} \prod_{i=1}^{t} (m_i^{x_i}/x_i!) \qquad (2)$$

(*see* **Multinomial Distribution**).

3. *Product-multinomial model*. The cells are partitioned into sets, and each set has an independent multinomial structure, as in the multinomial model.

For the Bartlett data in the preceding section, the sampling model is product-multinomial – there are actually four independent binomials, one for each of the four experimental conditions corresponding to the two factors, time of planting and length of cutting.

For each of these sampling models the estimation problem can typically be structured in terms of a "distance" function, $K(\mathbf{x}, \mathbf{m})$, where parameter estimates $\hat{\theta}$ are chosen so that the distance between $\mathbf{x}$ and $\mathbf{m} = \mathbf{m}(\theta)$, as measured by $K(\mathbf{x}, \mathbf{m})$, is minimized. The *minimum chi-square method* uses the distance function

$$X^2(\mathbf{x}, \mathbf{m}) = \sum_{i=1} (x_i - m_i)^2/m_i, \qquad (3)$$

and the *minimum discrimination information method* uses

$$G^2(\mathbf{x}, \mathbf{m}) = 2 \sum_{i=1}^{t} x_i \log(x_i/m_i). \qquad (4)$$

For the three basic sampling models for contingency tables, choosing $\hat{\theta}$ to minimize $G^2(\mathbf{x}, \mathbf{m})$ in (4) is equivalent to maximizing the likelihood function provided that

$$\sum_{i=1}^{t} m_i(\hat{\theta}) = \sum_{i=1}^{t} x_i \qquad (5)$$

(and that constraints similar to (5) hold for each of the sets of cells under product-multinomial sampling). Moreover, the estimators that minimize each of (3) to (5) in such circumstances belong to the class of *best asymptotic normal* (**BAN**) *estimates* for $\mathbf{m}$ (see Bishop et al. [E] for further discussion of asymptotic equivalence). Because of various additional asymptotic properties, and because of the smoothness of maximum likelihood estimates in relatively sparse tables, many authors have preferred to work with maximum likelihood estimates (MLEs), which minimize (4). We restrict our attention to MLEs, except for the "related" material on Bayesian estimation in a later section.

Basic Theory for Loglinear Models

Set-up for Two- and Three-way Tables

For expected values $\{m_{ij}\}$ for a 2×2 table,

		B	
A		1	2
	1	m_{11}	m_{12}
	2	m_{21}	m_{22}

a standard measure of association for the row and column variables, A and B, respectively, is the *cross product ratio* (also referred to as the **odds ratio**) proposed by Yule [67]:

$$\alpha = m_{11}m_{22}/m_{12}m_{21}. \qquad (6)$$

Independence of A and B is equivalent to setting $\alpha = 1$, and can also be expressed in loglinear form:

$$\log m_{ij} = u + u_{1(i)} + u_{2(j)}, \qquad (7)$$

where

$$\sum_{i=1}^{2} u_{1(i)} = \sum_{j=1}^{2} u_{2(j)} = 0. \qquad (8)$$

Note that the choice of notation here parallels that for analysis of variance models.

Bartlett's [6] no-second-order interaction model for the expected values in a $2 \times 2 \times 2$ table,

m_{111}	m_{121}		m_{112}	m_{122}
m_{211}	m_{221}		m_{212}	m_{222}

is based on equating the values of α in each layer of the table; that is

$$m_{111}m_{221}/m_{121}m_{211} = m_{112}m_{222}/m_{122}m_{212}. \qquad (9)$$

The expression given in (9) can be represented in loglinear form as

$$\log m_{ijk} = u + u_{1(i)} + u_{2(j)} + u_{3(k)} + u_{12(ij)}$$
$$+ u_{13(ik)} + u_{23(jk)}, \qquad (10)$$

where, as in (8), each subscripted u-term sums to zero over any subscript; for example,

$$\sum_i u_{12(ij)} = \sum_j u_{12(ij)} = 0. \qquad (11)$$

All of the parameters in (10) can be written as functions of cross product ratios (see Bishop et al. [E]). Our u-term notation follows that in Bishop et al. [E] and Fienberg [J], and differs somewhat from the λ notation adopted for example by Goodman [39, 40, 42] and by Agresti [B, C]. Furthermore, we have used symmetric linear constraints in (11), whereas other authors often choose to set selected u-terms equal to zero. The following results hold independent of the choice of parameterization and constraints.

For the sampling schemes described in the preceding section, the minimal **sufficient statistics** (msss) are the two-dimensional marginal totals, $\{x_{ij+}\}, \{x_{i+k}\}$, and $\{x_{+jk}\}$ (except for linearly redundant statistics included for purposes of symmetry), where a "+" indicates summation over the corresponding subscript. The MLEs of the $\{m_{ijk}\}$ under the model given in (10) must satisfy the likelihood equations,

$$\hat{m}_{ij+} = x_{ij+}, \quad i, j = 1, 2,$$

$$\hat{m}_{i+k} = x_{i+k}, \quad i, k = 1, 2,$$

$$\hat{m}_{+jk} = x_{+jk}, \quad j, k = 1, 2, \qquad (12)$$

usually solved by some form of iterative procedure (*see* **Iterative Proportional Fitting**). For the Bartlett data, the third set of equations in (12) corresponds to the binomial sampling constraints.

General Results

The results described in the preceding section generalize directly to ones that are applicable to any form of cross classification, and to a variety of models that are linear in the logarithmic scale for the expected cell values. It is helpful to have these results available in this general form so that we can adapt them to specific models for specific circumstances. Four results are described here: (i) the form of the data summaries or sufficient statistics for a model, which take the form of linear combinations of counts, often sums as in the preceding section; (ii) the form of the equations that produce maximum likelihoods, setting these data summaries equal to their expected values;

(iii) the equivalence of MLEs under different sampling models; and (iv) the large-sample chi-square distribution for the usual **goodness-of-fit** statistics. The technical details follow, and some readers may wish to skip the remainder of the section until they have seen additional special cases.

Suppose that we have a collection of counts organized in the form of a vector, **x**, with a corresponding vector of expected values, **m**. We are interested in models for **m** such that we can represent the log expectations $\lambda' = (\log m_1, \ldots, \log m_t)$ as linear combinations of the parameters θ. Then the following results hold under the Poisson and multinomial sampling schemes:

1. Corresponding to each parameter in θ is an MSS that is expressible as a linear combination of the $\{x_i\}$. (More formally, if $\mathcal{M}$ is used to denote the loglinear model specified by $\mathbf{m} = \mathbf{m}(\theta)$, then the MSSs are given by the projection of **x** on to $\mathcal{M}$, $P_{\mathcal{M}}\mathbf{x}$. For a more detailed discussion, see Haberman [N].)

2. The MLE, $\hat{\mathbf{m}}$, of **m**, if it exists, is unique and satisfies the likelihood equations

$$P_{\mathcal{M}}\hat{\mathbf{m}} = P_{\mathcal{M}}\mathbf{x}. \qquad (13)$$

(Note that the equations in (12) are a special case of those given by (13).)

Necessary and sufficient conditions for the existence of a solution to the likelihood equations, (13), are relatively complex (see Haberman [L]). A sufficient condition is that all cell counts be positive – that is, $x > \mathbf{0}$ – but MLEs for loglinear models exist in many sparse situations in which a large fraction of the cells have zero counts.

For product-multinomial sampling situations, the basic multinomial constraints (i.e. that the counts must add up to the multinomial sample sizes) must be taken into account. Typically, some of the parameters in θ that specify the loglinear model $\mathcal{M}$, such as $\mathbf{m} = \mathbf{m}(\theta)$, are fixed by these constraints.

More formally, let $\mathcal{M}$ be a loglinear model for **m** under product-multinomial sampling which corresponds to a loglinear model $\mathcal{M}$ under Poisson sampling such that the multinomial constraints "fix" a subset of the parameters, θ, used to specify $\mathcal{M}$. Then:

3. The MLE of **m** under product-multinomial sampling for the model $\mathcal{M}$ is the same as the

MLE of **m** under Poisson sampling for the model $\mathcal{M}$.

As a consequence of result 3, the expressions given in (12) are the likelihood equations for the $2 \times 2 \times 2$ table under the no-second-order interaction model for Poisson or multinomial sampling, as well as for product-multinomial sampling when any set of one-way or two-way marginal totals is fixed (i.e. these correspond to the multinomial constraints).

A final result, which is used to assess the fit of loglinear models, can be stated in the following informal manner:

4. If $\hat{\mathbf{m}}$ is the MLE of **m** under a loglinear model, and if the model is correct, then the statistics

$$X^2 = \sum_{i=1}^{t} (x_i - \hat{m}_i)^2 / \hat{m}_i \qquad (14)$$

and

$$G^2 = 2 \sum_{i=1}^{t} x_i \log(x_i / \hat{m}_i) \qquad (15)$$

have asymptotic χ^2 distributions with $t - s$ degrees of freedom, where s is the total number of independent constraints implied by the loglinear model and the multinomial sampling constraints (if any). If the model is not correct, then X^2 and G^2, in (14) and (15), are stochastically larger than χ^2_{t-s}.

Expression 15) is the minimizing value of the distance function, (5), but (14) is not the minimizing chi-square value for the function given in (3). Both χ^2 and G^2 are special cases of the family of *power-divergence statistics*, the distance function of which takes the form

$$K(\mathbf{x}, \hat{\mathbf{m}}) = \frac{2}{\phi(\phi+1)} \sum_{i=1}^{t} x_i \left[\left(\frac{x_i}{\hat{m}_i} \right)^{\phi} - 1 \right], \quad (16)$$

where ϕ is a real-valued parameter in the interval $-\infty < \phi < \infty$. The statistic χ^2 corresponds to $\phi = 1$, and the statistic G^2 corresponds to the limit as $\phi \to 0$. For further details on the properties of the general family of power divergence statistics, see Read & Cressie [61].

In the next section, these basic results are applied in the context of three data sets presented in the previous section.

Loglinear Models for High-dimensional Tables

The same ideas and ANOVA-like models in the logarithmic scale are useful for multiway tables. For such models, the minimal sufficient statistics are sets of marginal totals of the full table. Furthermore, all independence or conditional independence relationships are representable as loglinear models, and these models have estimated expected values that can be computed directly. There is a somewhat larger class of loglinear models with this direct or *decomposable* representation described below. For all loglinear models that are not decomposable, we require an iterative solution of likelihood equations.

Not all applications of loglinear models involve such simple structures as 2^3 tables or incomplete 6×6 arrays. Indeed, much of the methodology was developed in the mid-1960s to deal with very large, highly multidimensional tables. For example, in the National Halothane Study [10], investigators considered data on the use of (i) five anesthetic agents in operations involving (ii) four levels of risk, and patients of (iii) two sexes, (iv) ten age groups, with (v) seven differing physical statuses (levels of anesthetic risk) and (vi) previous operations (yes, no) for (vii) three different years, from (viii) 34 different institutions. Two sets of data were collected, the first consisting of all deaths within six weeks of surgery, and the second consisting of a sample (of comparable size) of all those exposed to surgery. Thus the data consisted of two very sparse $5 \times 4 \times 2 \times 10 \times 7 \times 2 \times 3 \times 34$ tables, each containing in excess of $57\,000$ cells. One of the more successful approaches used in the analysis of the data in these tables was based on loglinear models and the generalizations of the methods illustrated in this section.

One of the key reasons why loglinear models have become so popular in such analyses is that they lead to a simplified description of the data in terms of marginal totals – the minimal sufficient statistics of result 1 of the section "Basic theory for loglinear models". This is especially important when the table of data is large and sparse. For more details on the halothane study analyses, see Bishop et al. [E].

The doubly subscripted u-term notation introduced in the previous sections generalizes immediately to multiway tables. As in the previous section, we restrict attention to hierarchical models, in which if any u-term is set equal to zero, all of its higher order relatives must be set equal to zero; for example, setting $u_{12(ij)} = 0$ for all i, j implies setting $u_{123(ijk)} = 0$ for all i, j, k.

We need to think of parameters in loglinear models as deviations from lower-order parameters; they can also be represented and interpreted as a function of generalized odds ratios or cross product ratios; for example, see Fienberg [J] or Agresti [A, B].

In a multiway contingency table, the model that results from setting exactly one two-factor term (and all its higher-order relatives) equal to zero is called a *partial association* model. For example, in four dimensions, if we set $u_{12(ij)} = 0$ for all i, j, then the minimal sufficient statistics are $\{x_{i+kl}\}$ and $\{x_{+jkl}\}$, and the resulting partial association model corresponds to the conditional independence of variables 1 and 2 given 3 and 4. The corresponding maximum likelihood estimates for the expected cell frequencies are

$$\hat{m}_{ijkl} = \frac{x_{i+kl}x_{+jkl}}{x_{++kl}} \quad \text{for all } i, j, k, l. \quad (17)$$

For more details on partial association models and their uses, see Bishop et al. [E].

Loglinear Models and Graphical Representations

One of the major innovations of the past 15 years has been the development of methods associated with a subfamily of loglinear models known as *graphical loglinear models*. The formulation of graphical models is due originally to Darroch et al. [17], and has now found its way into several introductory textbooks on loglinear models (e.g. [F], [I], [R]), and serves as the basis for several monographs [O, S].

We begin with some special notation and then define the class of graphical models. We denote the situation in which F and G are conditionally independent given H by $F \perp G|H$. Thus, in a three-way table, if variables 1 and 2 are conditionally independent given 3, we denote this by

$$1 \perp 2|3.$$

Similarly, in a four-way table, if variables 1 and 2 are conditionally independent given 3 and 4, we denote this by $1 \perp 2|\{3, 4\}$.

In formal mathematics, a *graph* $G = (K, E)$ is based on a set of vertices, K, and a set of edges, E, which consists of pairs of elements from K. We depict such a graph using a picture

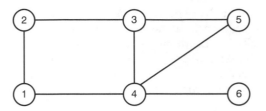

Figure 1 An illustrative graph with six vertices and seven edges, and a 4-cycle

with vertices linked by edges. For example, the graph $G = (K, E)$ with $K = \{1, 2, 3, 4, 5, 6\}$ and $E = \{(1, 2), (1, 4), (2, 3), (3, 4), (3, 5), (4, 5), (4, 6)\}$ corresponds to Figure 1.

The following definition links partial association models to the absence of edges in a graph. Let $\mathbf{X} = (X_1, X_2, \ldots, X_k)$ be a vector of random variables, and $K = \{1, 2, \ldots, k\}$. Furthermore, let $K\backslash\{i, j\}$ be the set of vertices in K excluding i and j. An undirected graph is an independence graph if there is no edge between two vertices whenever the variables they represent are conditionally independent given all remaining variables, that is $i \perp j|K\backslash\{i, j\}$ for all $(i, j) \notin E$, which corresponds to the partial association model discussed in the preceding subsection. This simply means that we can represent all possible conditional independence relationships in terms of the absence of edges in an undirected graph.

In the above example with $K = \{1, 2, 3, 4, 5, 6\}$ and $E = \{(1, 2), (1, 4), (2, 3), (3, 4), (3, 5), (4, 5), (4, 6)\}$, there are $\binom{6}{2} = 15$ possible edges that could have connected the six vertices, nine of which are absent and each of which corresponds to a conditional independence statement of the form $1 \perp 3|\{2, 4, 5, 6\}$. Some of these conditional independence relationships can be combined and expressed in a more succinct form that is intuitive from the graph. For example, the single conditional relationship, $\{1, 2\} \perp \{5, 6\}|\{3, 4\}$, which can be seen from the "separation" of $\{1, 2\}$ from $\{5, 6\}$ by $\{3, 4\}$ in the graph, summarizes four different conditional independence relationships.

Independence graphs can be used in connection with all random variables with positive density (continuous or discrete), and many of the results for independence graphs discussed in Lauritzen [O] and Whittaker [S] are applicable to such random variables. For the purposes of this article, however, we can think in terms of categorical variables, and the models that have independence graph representations are said to be *graphical models*. For categorical variables, all graphical models are loglinear. (For further details, see Lauritzen [O] and Whittaker [S].)

For three-way tables, the models of complete independence (no edges), joint independence (two absent edges), and conditional independence (one absent edge) are graphical, but the no-second-order interaction model is not, because the graph with all three edges present corresponds to the saturated model. Thus, all graphical models for three-way tables are *decomposable*; that is, the expected values can be written *explicitly* as a product and/or ratio of the expected marginal totals corresponding to the sufficient statistics. In this sense, the expected values can be *directly decomposed* in terms of the corresponding margins. In such circumstances, the MLEs can be written out directly and have a simple interpretation. There are also a number of especially interesting technical results that apply to decomposable loglinear models [O].

For four-way tables, the graph with four edges in a cycle; that is, corresponding to the joint occurrence of $2 \perp 3 | \{1, 4\}$ and $1 \perp 4 | \{2, 3\}$ and with $E = \{(1, 2), (2, 3), (3, 4), (1, 4)\}$, is graphical but also *nondecomposable*. This means that the model is not decomposable and thus the expected values under the model cannot be expressed as an explicit function of the marginal totals corresponding to the sufficient statistics $\{x_{ij++}\}$, $\{x_{+jk+}\}$, $\{x_{++kl}\}$, and $\{x_{i++l}\}$.

As we saw above, all graphical models for three-way tables are decomposable. For higher-way tables, a graphical model is nondecomposable whenever its independence graph includes a cycle involving four or more vertices. Thus in the above example involving six variables where $K = \{1, 2, 3, 4, 5, 6\}$ and $E = \{(1, 2), (1, 4), (2, 3), (3, 4), (3, 5), (4, 5), (4, 6)\}$, there is a four-cycle involving the edges linking $\{1, 2, 3, 4\}$ and thus the corresponding graphical loglinear model is nondecomposable.

In general, we have the following relationship among classes of loglinear models:

hierarchical models

$\cup$

graphical models

$\cup$

decomposable models

$\cup$

conditional independence models.

Model Selection and Collapsing

Many authors have devised techniques for selecting among the class of loglinear models applicable for contingency table structures. These typically (although not always) resemble corresponding model selection procedures for analysis of variance and regression models (*see* **Variable Selection**). See, for example, the discussions in Agresti [B], Bishop et al. [E], and Fienberg [J]. Edwards [I] and Whitaker [S] have special sections on model selection that take special advantage of the form of graphical models and the link between edges and two-factor effects.

A special aspect of model selection relates to the issue of when is it possible to work with and report loglinear model effects from a reduced table, collapsing over one or more variables of initial interest. The problem of collapsing was first taken up in Bishop [9] and Bishop et al. [E], who defined the concept in terms of the parameters of the loglinear model itself, now referred to as *parametric collapsibility*. Their discussion led to an extensive literature, in which differing definitions of collapsibility were proposed, including *model collapsibility* in which MLEs for the probabilities associated with a subset of variables, say A, can be performed directly in the A-margin of the table (see Asmussen & Edwards [4] and Lauritzen [O] for further details and references).

When a contingency table is not collapsible with respect to a subset of variables, inferences about the relationships among the remaining variables drawn from the corresponding marginal table are inevitably misleading. The best known example of this problem is referred to as **Simpson's paradox** or Yule's paradox. It is usually described as a situation involving three binary variables A, B, and C, such that the cross product ratio between A and B is greater than 1 for each level of C (i.e. there is a positive conditional relationship) but the cross product ratio in the marginal table for A and B is less than 1 (i.e. there is a negative marginal relationship).

Capture Multiple Recapture Analyses

This type of analysis estimates the size of a nonchanging population (see, for example, Bishop et al. [E] and Fienberg [24]). If the members of nonchanging populations are sampled k successive times (possibly dependent), the resulting recapture history data can be displayed in the form of a 2^k table with one missing cell, corresponding to those never sampled. Such an array is amenable to loglinear analysis, the results of which can be used to project a value for the missing cell.

In recent years there have been a number of major applications of the capture–recapture methodology ($k = 2$), especially in the context of the US decennial **census**; for example, see Zaslavsky & Wolfgang [68] and Fienberg [26], and in a variety of epidemiologic settings. For a detailed description of the history of the methodology and its potential for use in the context of epidemiology and public health, see Hook & Regal [45], and the International Working Group for Disease Monitoring and Forecasting [46, 47].

A key assumption in the use of standard loglinear models for capture–recapture and multiple-recapture population estimation is that of constant capture probabilities, or homogeneity. A traditional approach to allow for heterogeneity has been stratification, with separate models used for individual homogeneous strata. The problem with stratification as a strategy is that it often leads to very sparse cross classifications, and a substantial increase in the variability associated with population estimates. Recent developments linked to a variation of the Rasch model have led to extensions of the standard models that allow for special multiplicative forms of heterogeneity; for example see Agresti [1] and Darroch et al. [18].

(For further details on these and related models for population size estimation, *see* **Capture–Recapture; Rasch Models**.)

Latent Trait and Rasch Models

In psychologic tests or attitude studies, we are often interested in quantifying the value of an unobservable *latent trait*, such as mathematic ability or manual dexterity, on a sample of individuals. While latent traits are not directly measurable, we can either assume something about the way in which the latent trait relates to the observable or *manifest* variables or assume that we can assess indirectly a person's value for the latent trait from his/her responses to a set of well chosen items on a test (see, for example [5]).

In the 1970s, Goodman [40] and Haberman [N] developed a special representation for the analysis of contingency tables for manifest variables using loglinear models in the presence of latent variables, beginning with the traditional model in which the manifest variables are conditionally independent given the latent variables.

The second approach is prevalent in educational testing and has recently found its way into a wide variety of applications. The simplest model in this domain was introduced by Rasch [60], and is known as the Rasch model. Given responses from n individuals to k items in a test, the Rasch model permits the estimation of parameters associated with individuals and with items, as well as prediction of the person's behavior when confronted with a different set of items from the same domain. In the 1980s, an important relationship between the Rasch model and loglinear models was recognized by Tjur [65], Cressie & Holland [11], and Duncan [19]. The representation of these models in terms of symmetry and **quasi-symmetry** was presented in Fienberg & Meyer [29], Darroch [14] and Darroch & McCleod [15]. See also Anderson [D] and the article on **Rasch Models** for a presentation of this topic.

Association Models for Ordinal Variables

Loglinear models as described in this article ignore any structure linking the categories of variables, yet biostatistical problems often involve variables with ordered categories; for example, differing dosage levels for a drug or the severity of symptoms or side effects. Beginning in the late 1970s, methods for a special class of models, known as *association* models, moved to the forefront of methodological research. Goodman [41] provided a framework for association models that builds on extensions to standard loglinear models and utilizes multiplicative interaction terms. For a detailed description of these and other methods for ordinal variables, see Agresti [A] and Clogg & Shidadeh [G]. Etzioni et al. [23] provide a useful review of association models for ordinal variables in medical research using notation compatible with this article.

Loglinear Model Analyses

Bartlett's Data and No-Second-Order Interaction

For the 2^3 table of Bartlett, variables 2 (time of planting) and 3 (length of cutting) are fixed by design, so that $\hat{m}_{+jk} = 240$, and the estimated expected values under the no-second-order interaction model of the expressions given in (12) are shown in Table 4. These

Table 4 Observed and expected values for the Bartlett data, including the no-second-order interaction model

Cell	Observed x	Estimated expected $\hat{m}$
1,1,1	156	161.1
2,1,1	84	78.9
1,2,1	84	78.9
2,2,1	156	161.1
1,1,2	107	101.9
2,1,2	133	138.1
1,2,2	31	36.1
2,2,2	209	203.9

values were computed by Bishop et al. [E] using the method of *iterative proportional fitting* (IPF). Bartlett originally found the solution to (14) by noting that the constraints in his specification (11), reduced (14) to a single cubic equation for the discrepancy $\Delta = \hat{m}_{111} - x_{111}$. Note that the expected values satisfy (14), e.g., $\hat{m}_{12+} = 78.9 + 36.1 = 115 = 84 + 31 = x_{12+}$. The goodness-of-fit statistics for this model are $X^2 = 2.27$ and $G^2 = 2.29$. Using result 4 of the preceding section, one compares these values to tail values of the chi-square distribution with 1 df, for example $\chi_1^2(0.10) = 2.71$, and this suggests that the no-second-order interaction model provides an acceptable fit to the data.

Since the parameters u, $\{u_{2(j)}\}$, $\{u_{3(k)}\}$, and $\{u_{23(jk)}\}$ are fixed by the binomial sampling constraints for these data, the model given by (12) is often rewritten as

$$\log(m_{1jk}/m_{2jk}) = 2[u_{1(1)} + u_{12(1j)} + u_{13(2k)}]$$
$$= w + w_{2(j)} + w_{3(k)}, \qquad (18)$$

where

$$\sum_j w_{2(j)} = \sum_k w_{3(k)} = 0.$$

Expression (18) is referred to as a *logit* model for the log odds for alive versus dead (*see* **Logistic Regression**). The simple additive structure corresponds to Bartlett's notion of no-second-order interaction.

Waite's Fingerprint Data and Quasi-independence

For the Waite fingerprint data of Table 2, one model that has been considered is the simple additive log-linear model of (9), but only for those cells where

positive counts are possible; that is, in the upper triangular section. For cells with $i > j$, $m_{ij} = 0$ a priori. This restricted version of the independence model is referred to as a **quasi-independence** model, and the results of the preceding section can be used in connection with it. The MSSs are still the row and column totals (result 1). The likelihood equations under multinomial sampling are (applying results 1 and 2):

$$\hat{m}_{i+} = x_{i+}, \quad i = 0, 1, 2, \ldots, 5,$$
$$\hat{m}_{+j} = x_{+j}, \quad j = 0, 1, 2, \ldots, 5, \qquad (19)$$

where $m_{ij} = 0$ for $i > j$. A solution of (19) satisfying the model can be found directly, or by using a standard iterative procedure. The estimated expected values for the fingerprint data under the model of quasi-independence are given in Table 5, and they satisfy the marginal constraints in (19).

The goodness-of-fit statistics for this model are $X^2 = 399.8$ and $G^2 = 450.4$, which correspond to values in the very extreme right-hand tail of the χ_{10}^2 distribution. Thus the model of quasi-independence seems inappropriate. Darroch [13] describes the loglinear model of F-independence (with more parameters than the quasi-independence model), which takes into account the way in which the constraint – that the number of small loops plus the number of whorls cannot exceed 5 – makes the usual definition of independence inappropriate. This model in loglinear form is

$$\log m_{ij} = u + u_{1(i)} + u_{2(j)} + u_{3(5-i-j)}, \qquad (20)$$

where the u_3 parameters correspond to diagonals along which the sum of the numbers of whorls and small loops is constant. Darroch & Ratcliff [16] illustrate the fit of the F-independence model to a

Table 5 Estimated expected values for fingerprint data under quasi-independence

Whorls	Small loops 0	1	2	3	4	5	Total
0	200.6	167.4	166.6	150.3	131.1	45.0	861
1	122.2	101.9	101.4	91.6	79.9		497
2	85.5	71.4	71.0	64.1			292
3	63.8	53.2	53.0				170
4	70.9	59.1					130
5	50.0						50
Total	93	453	392	306	211	45	2000

Table 6 Goodness of fit of partial association models for coronary heart disease data

A	*					
B	22.65	*				
C	42.80	689.99	*			
D	28.72	12.23	14.81	*		
E	40.02	17.24	18.63	31.06	*	
F	21.31	22.79	22.15	18.35	18.32	*
	A	B	C	D	E	F

related set of fingerprint data involving large rather than small loops.

Application of Graphical Loglinear Models: Prognostic Factors for Coronary Disease

To illustrate some of the features of graphical models, we now analyze the data in Table 3 on prognostic factors for coronary heart disease among 1841 men in a Czech car factory. Our analysis follows closely that in Whittaker [S]. We begin by examining all partial association models and computing G^2 for each of the 15 partial association models found by setting one two-factor term equal to zero (see Table 6).

There are 16 df associated with each G^2 value. If we drop edges in a graph using the 0.05 P value for a χ^2 variable with 16 df, that is 26.30, then we end up with the graph shown in Figure 2.

The likelihood ratio statistic for the loglinear model corresponding to this graph is $G^2 = 83.75$ with 51 df. This corresponds to a P value of 0.0026, and suggests that we have deleted too many edges. A few additional steps of addition and deletion yield the model

$$[ABCE][ADE][BF],$$

for which the likelihood ratio statistic $G^2 = 44.59$ with 42 df suggests a well fitting model. The corresponding independence graph is shown in Figure 3.

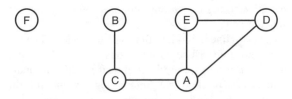

Figure 2 A preliminary graphical model for the prognostic factors example based on partial association models

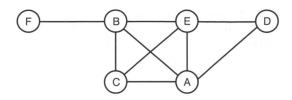

Figure 3 An intermediate graphical model for the prognostic factors example

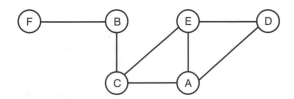

Figure 4 The final graphical model for the prognostic factors example

The alternative graphical model shown in Figure 4, with two fewer edges, is somewhat simpler than the preferred model reported by Edwards [I] and fits the data well.

In Figure 4, F (family history) is conditionally independent of {D, E} (the physical symptoms), given {A,B,C} (the behavioral conditions). For further details on the analysis of this data set using graphical models, see Edwards [I] and Whitaker [S].

Bayesian Approaches

Background

In recent years, much attention has been directed to the development of Bayesian approaches for contingency tables and loglinear models. Early references include Good [35, 36] and Fienberg & Holland [28]. Initial attempts at formulating a Bayesian approach to estimation in contingency tables concentrated on the problem of incorporating *prior knowledge* about unobservable cell proportions or about expected cell counts. Those early efforts resulted in the derivation of the Dirichlet family of distributions as the *conjugate* family of **prior distributions** for cell proportions and expected counts. More recently, emphasis has been placed on formulation of more complex prior distributions that permit incorporating information about the underlying structure in a contingency table (e.g. Albert & Gupta [2, 3], Knuiman & Speed

[48], and Epstein & Fienberg [21, 22]), and on computational issues (e.g. Gelman & Rubin [32], Epstein & Fienberg [21], and Gelman et al. [33]).

The general approach adopted by most of these authors has been as follows: using either the multinomial or the Poisson sampling models, incorporate uncertainty about the expected cell proportions (or expected cell counts) via the Dirichlet conjugate family of prior distributions, with variations to account for more or less structure in the expected cell means. **Markov chain Monte Carlo** methods (see, for example, Gelfand & Smith [31]) can then be used to approximate the marginal posterior distributions of the expected cell values or of any continuous functions of m.

A different, but parallel line of development is described in the work of, for example, Leonard [51], Laird [49], and Nazaret [53]. These authors address the problem of estimation in contingency tables from a loglinear model approach, and attempt to use Bayesian results similar to those developed by Lindley & Smith [52] for the linear model. Except where convenient for computations, we will describe the Bayesian methods that address contingency tables directly, without resorting to results from the linear models literature.

To introduce the Bayesian approach to estimation, we consider the counts $\{x_i\}$, $i = 1, \ldots, t$ (t equals the number of cells), to be observations from independent Poisson random variables, with means or expected values $\{m_i\}$. In the Bayesian framework, the $\{m_i\}$ are random variables having some prior distribution, and the statistician's task is to update the prior to a *posterior distribution* by incorporating the information about the $\{m_i\}$ provided by the observed counts $\{x_i\}$. For the multinomial sampling model, we are interested in the marginal posterior distributions of parameters of a loglinear model, $\{\theta_i\}$, or the posterior distribution of the expected cell values, $\{m_j\}$. For the Poisson and the multinomial sampling models, likelihood functions are given in (1) and (2).

Estimation and Computation

Here we refer to the Poisson sampling model. Results, however, also apply to the multinomial model after appropriate normalization (see, for example, Gelman et al. [33]).

The simplest way to incorporate prior information about the value of the expected cell counts $\{m_i\}$ is via

the Dirichlet conjugate family of prior distributions. If $\{m_i\}$ are jointly distributed a priori as independent Dirichlet random variables with parameters k and $\{\eta_i\}$, then the joint prior distribution has density function

$$p(\mathbf{m}|k, \boldsymbol{\eta}) \propto \prod_{i=1}^{t} m_i^{k\eta_i - 1}, \qquad (21)$$

where $k > 0$ and $\eta_i > 0$. For $\boldsymbol{\eta} = \{\eta_i\}$, parameters η_i can be thought of as our prior "guess" about the value of $\{m_i\}$, while the *flattening constant* k [27, 35] represents our prior certainty about those guesses.

For the likelihood corresponding to the Poisson sampling model in (1), and for $p(\mathbf{m}|k, \boldsymbol{\eta})$ as in (21), the posterior distribution of the expected cell counts $\mathbf{m}$ is proportional to the product of the likelihood function and the prior distribution

$$p(\mathbf{m}|\mathbf{x}, k, \boldsymbol{\eta}) \propto \prod_{i} p(x_i|m_i) \times p(m_i|k, \eta_i)$$

$$\propto \prod_{i} \exp\{-m_i\} m_i^{x_i + k\eta_i - 1}. \qquad (22)$$

Gelman & Rubin [32] and Gelman et al. [33] have developed a Bayesian version of IPF (BIPF) starting from (22) and using the multiplicative version of the loglinear model. Their algorithm produces estimates of marginal posterior distributions of the $\{m_i\}$ (or of continuous functions of the $\{m_i\}$) rather than point estimates (as does the standard IPF). In this sense, BIPF is a misnomer, since it incorrectly suggests that the Bayes estimates obtained are, as in the frequentist case, just point estimates of the $\{m_i\}$. For some details on the derivation of BIPF, the reader is referred to Gelman & Rubin [32].

Examples

In the previous section, we applied the BIPF to the Bartlett 2^3 table and to Edwards & Havraneck's [20] six-way table on prognostic factors for heart disease. In both examples we used a multinomial sampling model with the constraints imposed by the sampling scheme.

The loglinear models that we fit to each data set were those described earlier. Thus, for the $2 \times 2 \times 2$ table of Bartlett, we used a loglinear model with main effects and all two-way interactions, while for the six-way table we used a model corresponding to

$$[ABC][ACE][ADE][BF].$$

Table 7 Observed values, posterior means of expected values, and percentiles of posterior distribution of expected values for the Bartlett data, including the no-second-order interaction model

Cell	Observed x	Posterior mean	Posterior percentiles				
			5th	25th	50th	75th	90th
1,1,1	156	161.13	150.67	156.82	161.31	165.37	170.97
2,1,1	84	78.87	69.03	74.63	78.69	83.18	89.33
1,2,1	84	78.75	68.67	74.45	78.43	82.78	89.67
2,2,1	156	161.25	150.33	157.22	161.57	165.55	171.33
1,1,2	107	101.89	91.06	97.36	101.87	106.43	112.83
2,1,2	133	138.11	127.17	133.57	138.13	142.64	148.94
1,2,2	31	36.01	29.56	32.89	35.81	38.91	43.67
2,2,2	209	203.99	196.33	201.09	204.19	207.11	210.44

Table 8 Prognostic factors in coronary heart disease: posterior means of expected counts

F	E	D	C	B A	No No	Yes	Yes No	Yes
Negative	<3	<140	No		41.2	33.6	104.7	68.2
			Yes		122.1	139.0	15.0	24.6
		≥140	No		32.9	16.5	83.5	33.4
			Yes		97.4	68.1	12.0	12.0
	≥3	<140	No		27.0	31.7	68.6	64.3
			Yes		52.7	83.4	6.5	14.8
		≥140	No		26.9	26.5	68.4	53.9
			Yes		52.6	69.8	6.5	12.4
Positive	<3	<140	No		6.3	5.1	21.2	13.8
			Yes		18.5	21.1	3.0	5.0
		≥140	No		5.0	2.5	16.9	6.8
			Yes		14.8	10.3	2.4	2.4
	≥3	<140	No		4.1	4.8	13.9	13.0
			Yes		8.0	12.6	1.3	3.0
		≥140	No		4.1	4.0	13.8	10.9
			Yes		8.0	10.6	1.3	2.5

We incorporated prior information via the Dirichlet conjugate family (see (21)), with $k\eta_i = 0.5$ for all i, that results is noninformative prior densities for the expected cell counts $\{m_i\}$.

Our Bayesian results for the Bartlett data are given in Table 7. To highlight the differences between results obtained from the frequentist and the Bayesian approaches (see Table 4 for the former), we provide not only a point estimate for the expected counts $\{m_i\}$ (we chose the means of the marginal posterior distributions as our point estimates) but also the posterior 5th, 25th, 50th, 75th, and 95th percentiles of the distributions of each $\{m_i\}$.

Note that, as required by the sampling scheme, $\hat{m}_{12+} = 78.75 + 36.01 = 114.8 = 84 + 31 = x_{12+}$ (within numerical error), and that the same holds true for $\hat{m}_{11+}$, $\hat{m}_{21+}$, and $\hat{m}_{22+}$.

We give results obtained for the prognostic factors for heart disease data in Table 8, which shows the means of the marginal posterior distributions of the expected cell counts $\{m_i\}$. Note that, as required, the sum of the estimated expected counts equals N, the total number of individuals in the study.

Brief Guide to Computer Programs for Loglinear Model Analysis

As with other forms of multivariate analysis, the analysis of multidimensional contingency tables relies heavily on computer programs. A large number of these have been written to compute estimated parameter values for loglinear models and associated test statistics, and most computer installations at major universities have one or more programs available for users (*see* **Software, Biostatistical**).

The most widely used numerical procedure for the calculation of maximum likelihood estimates for loglinear models a decade ago was IPF, which iteratively adjusts the entries of a contingency table to have marginal totals equal to those used in specifying the likelihood equations. The IPF approach has been implemented in the BMDP 4F Program and in SPSS. The major advantage of the IPF method is that it requires limited computer memory capabilities since it does not require matrix inversion or equivalent computations, and thus can be used in connection with the analysis of very high-dimensional tables. Its major disadvantage is that it does not provide, in an easily accessible form, estimates of the basic loglinear model parameters (and an estimate of their asymptotic covariance matrix); it provides only estimated expected values.

The other numerical approaches suggested for the computation of maximum likelihood estimates are typically based on classical procedures for solving nonlinear equations, such as modifications of Newton's method or the Newton–Raphson method (*see* **Optimization and Nonlinear Equations**). Since such approaches can be implemented as part of the methods for the broader class of **generalized linear models** of which loglinear and logit models are special cases (see, for example, McCullagh & Nelder [P]), a common approach in several computer packages is to embed loglinear and logit models approaches as part of GLM routines, see; for example **S-PLUS** GLIM, SAS (PROC GENMOD), STATA, and SYSTAT. The virtue of these programs is that they produce both estimated expected values and estimated parameter values, and an estimate of the asymptotic covariance matrix. The user of a GLM package should be sure to check the specific parameterization used, as the constraints on the loglinear models typically vary from package to package. No matter what the choice of parametrization for the loglinear model parameters, the estimates of the expected values and the goodness of fit statistic values should agree with those computed using the IPF algorithm. Some packages such as BMDP and SPSS also have separate subroutines for logit and logistic regression models. SAS's JMP has only a logistic regression routine.

Agresti [C] includes an especially nice appendix with a guide to SAS and SPSS programming, and Agresti [B] includes examples from GLIM and

BMDP. Stokes et al. [64] provide a detailed guide with examples for the SAS PROC CATMOD, which can be used for loglinear models as well as a number of other approaches to the analysis of categorical data.

Before running any of the loglinear model or generalized linear model routines referred to above on sparse multiway tables with one or more zero entries, users should read the package documentation with care, since some packages may treat zeros in an unexpected fashion.

Textbook References

[A]   Agresti, A. (1984). *Analysis of Ordinal Categorical Data*. Wiley, New York. (An introduction to the analysis of categorical data with special emphasis on loglinear models and their variants for ordinal data. It emphasizes the use of cross product ratios to describe association in different ways.)

[B]   Agresti, A. (1990). *Categorical Data Analysis*. Wiley, New York. (A second generation introduction to loglinear models for the analysis of categorical data. It includes a mix of theory and methods, as well as many examples.)

[C]   Agresti, A. (1996). *An Introduction to Categorical Data Analysis*. Wiley, New York. (A second generation non-mathematical introduction to loglinear models for the analysis of categorical data. It includes many examples and a guide to computing in SAS and SPSS.)

[D]   Anderson, E.B. (1990). *The Statistical Analysis of Categorical Data*. Springer-Verlag, Heidelberg. (A second generation introduction to loglinear models, including such topics as association models for ordinal data, **correspondence analysis**, graphical models, and the Rasch model.)

[E]   Bishop, Y.M.M., Fienberg, S.E. & Holland, P. (1975). *Discrete Multivariate Analysis: Theory and Practice*. MIT Press, Cambridge, Mass. (A systematic exposition and development of the loglinear model for the analysis of contingency tables through the early 1970s, primarily using maximum likelihood estimation, and focusing on the use of iterative proportional fitting. It includes chapters on measures of association, and others on special related topics. It contains both theory and numerous examples from many disciplines with detailed analyses.)

[F]   Christensen, R. (1990). *Loglinear Models*. Springer-Verlag, New York. (An intermediate introduction to loglinear models, with special emphasis on interpretation including graphical models. It also contains chapters on logistic regression and logistic discrimination (*see* **Discriminant Analysis, Linear**.)

[G]   Clogg, C.C. & Shidadeh, E.S. (1994). *Statistical Models for Ordinal Variables*. Sage, Thousand Oaks. (An introduction to association models logit-type regression models for ordinal variables.)

[H]   Cox, D.R. & Snell, E.J. (1989). *Analysis of Binary Data*, 2nd Ed. Chapman & Hall, New York. (The second edition of an early guide to the analysis of categorical data by D.R. Cox, including basic results for loglinear and logit models. It contains numerous examples and references.)

[I]   Edwards, D. (1995). *Introduction to Graphical Modeling*. Springer-Verlag, New York. (A detailed introduction to graphical models and their estimation with special attention to applications. Material on categorical variables is often integrated with that for continuous variables. It includes specifically developed computer programs.)

[J]   Fienberg, S.E. (1980). *The Analysis of Cross-classified Categorical Data*, 2nd Ed. MIT Press, Cambridge, Mass. (A comprehensive introduction, for those with some training in statistical methodology, to the analysis of categorical data using loglinear models and maximum likelihood estimation. The emphasis is on methodology, with numerous examples and problems.)

[K]   Gokhale, D.V. & Kullback, S. (1978). *The Information in Contingency Tables*. Marcel Dekker, New York. (A development of minimum discrimination information procedures for linear and loglinear models. It contains a succinct theoretical presentation, followed by numerous examples.)

[L]   Haberman, S.J. (1974). *The Analysis of Frequency Data*. University of Chicago Press, Chicago. (A highly mathematical, advanced presentation of statistical theory associated with loglinear models and of related statistical and computational methods. It contains examples, but is suitable only for mathematical statisticians who are familiar with the topic.)

[M]   Haberman, S.J. (1978). *Analysis of Qualitative Data*, Vol. 1: *Introductory Topics*. Academic Press, New York. (See next entry.)

[N]   Haberman, S.J. (1979). *Analysis of Qualitative Data*, Vol. 2: *New Developments*. Academic Press, New York. (An intermediate-level, two-volume introduction to the analysis of categorical data via loglinear models, emphasizing maximum likelihood estimates computed via the Newton–Raphson algorithm. Volume 1 examines complete cross classifications, and Volume 2 considers multinomial response models, incomplete tables, and related topics. The volumes contain many examples, problems, and solutions, and a computer program listing (for two-way tables) is included in Volume 2.)

[O]   Lauritzen, S.L. (1996). *Graphical Models*. Oxford University Press, Oxford. (An advanced mathematical treatment of graphical models and their analysis, for both continuous and categorical variables, with emphasis on topics such as decomposability and exact tests.)

[P]   McCullagh, P. & Nelder, J.A. (1989). *Generalized Linear Models*, 2nd Ed. Chapman & Hall, London. (The definitive introduction to generalized linear models and their properties, including loglinear and logit models as special cases. It includes many examples.)

[Q]   Plackett, R.L. (1974). *The Analysis of Categorical Data*. Griffin, London. (A concise introduction to statistical theory and methods for the analysis of categorical data. It assumes a thorough grasp of basic principles of statistical inference. There is considerable emphasis on two-way tables. It contains many examples and exercises.)

[R]   Santner, T.J. & Duffy, D.E. (1989). *The Statistical Analysis of Discrete Data*. Springer-Verlag, New York. (A graduate level introduction to loglinear models and other methods for the analysis of discrete data. It includes discussions of Bayesian methods, graphical models, and logistic regression.)

[S]   Whitaker, J. (1990). *Graphical Models in Applied Multivariate Statistics*. Wiley, New York. (A somewhat mathematical introduction to graphical loglinear models with extensive examples and applications. It deals with both directed and undirected graphs.)

Other References

[1]   Agresti, A. (1994). Simple capture–recapture models permitting unequal catchability and variable sampling effort, *Biometrics* **50**, 494–500.

[2]   Albert, J.H. & Gupta, A.K. (1982). Mixtures of Dirichlet distributions and estimation in contingency tables, *Annals of Statistics* **10**, 61–68.

[3]   Albert, J.H. & Gupta, A.K. (1983). Estimation in contingency tables using prior information, *Journal of the Royal Statistical Society, Series B* **45**, 60–69.

[4]   Asmussen, S. & Edwards, D. (1983). Collapsibility and response variables in contingency tables, *Biometrika* **70**, 567–578.

[5]   Baker, F.B. (1992). *Item Response Theory. Parameter Estimation Techniques*. Marcel Dekker, New York.

[6]   Bartlett, M.S. (1935). Contingency table interactions, *Journal of the Royal Statistical Society, Supplement* **2**, 248–252.

[7]   Bhapkar, V.P. & Koch, G. (1968). On the hypotheses of "no interaction" in contingency tables, *Biometrics* **24**, 567–594.

[8]   Birch, M.W. (1963). Maximum likelihood in three-way contingency tables, *Journal of the Royal Statistical Society, Series B* **25**, 229–233.

[9]   Bishop, Y.M.M. (1971). Effects of collapsing multidimensional contingency tables, *Biometrics* **27**, 545–562.

[10]   Bunker, J.P., Forrest, W.H. Jr, Mosteller, F. & Vandam, L. (1969). *The National Halothane Study*, Report of the Subcommittee on the National Halothane Study of the Committee on Anesthesia, Division of Medical Sciences, National Academy of Sciences - National Research Council, National Institutes of Health, National Institute of General Medical Sciences, Bethesda, US Government Printing Office, Washington.

[11] Cressie, N.E. & Holland, P.W. (1983). Characterizing the manifest probabilities of latent trait models, *Psychometrika* **48**, 129–141.

[12] Darroch, J.N. (1962). Interaction in multi-factor contingency tables, *Journal of the Royal Statistical Society, Series B* **24**, 251–263.

[13] Darroch, J.N. (1971). A definition of independence for bounded-sum, nonnegative, integer-valued variables, *Biometrika* **58**, 357–368.

[14] Darroch, J.N. (1986). Quasi-symmetry, in *Encyclopedia of Statistical Sciences*, Vol. 7, S. Kotz & N.L. Johnson, eds. Wiley, New York, pp. 469–473.

[15] Darroch, J.N. & McCloud, P.I. (1990). Separating two sources of dependence in repeated influenza outbreaks, *Biometrika* **77**, 237–243.

[16] Darroch, J.N. & Ratcliff, D. (1973). Tests of F-independence with reference to quasi-independence and Waite's fingerprint data, *Biometrika* **60**, 395–402.

[17] Darroch, J.N., Lauritzen, S.L. & Speed, T.P. (1980). Markov fields and log-linear interaction models for contingency tables, *Annals of Statistics* **8**, 522–539.

[18] Darroch, J.N., Fienberg, S.E., Glonek, G. & Junker, B. (1993). A three-sample multiple-recapture approach to census population estimation with heterogeneous catchability, *Journal of the American Statistical Association* **88**, 1137–1148.

[19] Duncan, O.D. (1983). Rasch measurement: further examples and discussion, in *Survey Measurement of Subjective Phenomena*, Vol. 2, C.F. Turner & E. Martin, eds. Russell Sage, New York, Chapter 12, pp. 367–403.

[20] Edwards, D.E. & Havranek, T. (1985). A fast procedure for model search in multidimensional contingency tables, *Biometrika* **72**, 339–351.

[21] Epstein, L.D. & Fienberg, S.E. (1991). Using Gibbs sampling for Bayesian inference in multidimensional contingency tables, in *Computing Science and Statistics: Proceedings of the 23rd Symposium on the Interface*, E.M. Keramidas & S.M. Kaufman, eds. pp. 215–223.

[22] Epstein, L.D. & Fienberg, S.E. (1992). Bayesian estimation in multidimensional contingency tables, in *Bayesian Analysis in Statistics and Econometrics*, P.K. Goel, & N.S. Iyengar, eds. Lecture Notes in Statistics, Vol. 75, Springer-Verlag, New York, pp. 27–41.

[23] Etzioni, R.D., Fienberg, S.E., Gilula, Z. & Haberman, S.J. (1994). Statistical models for the analysis of ordered categorical data in public health and medical research, *Statistical Methods in Medical Research* **3**, 179–204.

[24] Fienberg, S.E. (1972). The multiple recapture census for closed populations and incomplete 2^k contingency tables, *Biometrika* **59**, 591–603.

[25] Fienberg, S.E. (1982). Contingency tables, in *Encyclopedia of Statistical Sciences*, Vol. 2, S. Kotz & N.L. Johnson, eds. Wiley, New York, pp. 161–170.

[26] Fienberg, S.E. (1992). Bibliography on capture–recapture modeling with application to census undercount adjustment, *Survey Methodology* **18**, 143–154.

[27] Fienberg, S.E. & Holland, P.W. (1972). On the choice of flattening constants for estimating multinomial probabilities, *Journal of Multivariate Analysis* **2**, 127–134.

[28] Fienberg, S.E. & Holland, P.W. (1973). Simultaneous estimation of multinomial cell probabilities, *Journal of the American Statistical Association* **68**, 683–691.

[29] Fienberg, S.E. & Meyer, M.M. (1983). Loglinear models and categorical data analysis with psychometric and econometric applications, *Journal of Econometrics* **22**, 191–214.

[30] Fisher, R.A. (1922). On the interpretation of chi-square from contingency tables, and the calculation of P, *Journal of the Royal Statistical Society* **85**, 87–94.

[31] Gelfand, A.E. & Smith, A.F.M. (1990). Sampling-based approaches to calculating marginal densities, *Journal of the American Statistical Association* **85**, 398–409.

[32] Gelman, A. & Rubin, D.B. (1991). Simulating the posterior distribution of loglinear contingency tables, *Unpublished Technical Report*, Department of Statistics, Harvard University.

[33] Gelman, A., Carlin, J.B., Stern, H.S. & Rubin, D.B. (1995). *Bayesian Data Analysis*. Chapman & Hall, London.

[34] Good, I.J. (1963). Maximum entropy for hypothesis formulation, especially for multidimensional contingency tables, *Annals of Mathematical Statistics* **34**, 911–934.

[35] Good, I.J. (1965). *The Estimation of Probabilities: An Essay in Modern Bayesian Methods*. MIT Press, Cambridge, Mass.

[36] Good, I.J. (1967). A Bayesian significance test for multinomial distributions (with discussion), *Journal of the Royal Statistical Society, Series B* **29**, 399–431.

[37] Goodman, L.A. (1963). On methods for comparing contingency tables, *Journal of the Royal Statistical Society, Series A* **126**, 94–108.

[38] Goodman, L.A. (1964). Simultaneous confidence limits for cross-product ratios in contingency tables, *Journal of the Royal Statistical Society, Series B* **26**, 86–102.

[39] Goodman, L.A. (1971). The analysis of multidimensional contingency tables: stepwise procedures and direct estimation methods for building models for multiple classifications, *Technometrics* **13**, 33–61.

[40] Goodman, L.A. (1978). *Analyzing Quantitative/Categorical Data*. Abt Books, Cambridge, Mass. (a collection of papers).

[41] Goodman, L.A. (1979). Simple models for the analysis of association in cross-classification having ordered categories, *Journal of the American Statistical Association* **74**, 537–552.

[42] Goodman, L.A. (1984). *Analysis of Cross-classified Data Having Ordered Categories*. Harvard University Press, Cambridge, Mass. (a collection of papers).

[43] Grizzle, J.E., Starmer, C.F. & Koch, G.G. (1969). Analysis of categorical data by linear models, *Biometrics* **25**, 489–504.

[44] Harris, J.A. & Treloar, A.E. (1927). On a limitation in the applicability of the contingency coefficient, *Journal of the American Statistical Association* **22**, 460–472.

[45] Hook, E.B. & Regal, R.R. (1995). Capture–recapture methods in epidemiology: methods and limitations, *Epidemiological Reviews* **17**, 243–264.

[46] International Working Group for Disease Monitoring and Forecasting (1995) Capture–recapture and multiple-record systems estimation I: history and theoretical development, *American Journal of Epidemiology* **142**, 1047–1058.

[47] International Working Group for Disease Monitoring and Forecasting (1995). Capture–recapture and multiple-record systems estimation II: applications in human diseases, *American Journal of Epidemiology* **142**, 1059–1068.

[48] Knuiman, M.W. & Speed, T.P. (1988). Incorporating prior information into the analysis of contingency tables, *Biometrics* **44**, 1061–1071.

[49] Laird, N.M. (1978). Empirical Bayes methods for two-way contingency tables. *Biometrika* **65**, 581–590.

[50] Lancaster, H.O. (1969). *The Chi-Squared Distribution*, Wiley, New York, Chapters 11 and 12.

[51] Leonard, T. (1975). Bayesian estimation methods for two-way contingency tables, *Journal of the Royal Statistical Society, Series B* **37**, 23–37.

[52] Lindley, D.V. & Smith, A.F.M. (1972). Bayes estimates for the linear model (with discussion), *Journal of the Royal Statistical Society, Series B* **34**, 1–42.

[53] Nazaret, A. (1987). Bayesian log linear estimates for three-way contingency tables, *Biometrika* **74**, 401–410.

[54] Pearson, K. (1900). On a criterion that a given system of deviations from the probable in the case of a correlated system of variables is such that it can be reasonably supposed to have arisen from random sampling, *Philosophical Magazine, 5th Series* **50**, 157–175.

[55] Pearson, K. (1900). Mathematical contributions to the theory of evolution in the inheritance of characters not capable of exact quantitative measurement, VIII, *Philosophical Transactions of the Royal Society of London, Series A* **195**, 79–150.

[56] Pearson, K. (1904). On the theory of contingency and its relation to association and normal correlation, *Draper's Company Research Memoirs, Biometric Series I*, 1–35.

[57] Pearson, K. (1930). On the theory of contingency. Note on Professor J. Arthur Harris' papers on the limitation in the applicability of the contingency coefficient, *Journal of the American Statistical Association* **25**, 320–323.

[58] Pearson, K. & Heron, D. (1913). On theories of association, *Biometrika* **9**, 159–315.

[59] Quetelet, M.A. (1849). *Letters Addressed to H.R.H. the Grand Duke of Saxe Coburg and Gotha on the Theory of Probabilities as Applied to the Moral and Political Sciences* (translated from the French by Olinthus Gregory Downs). Charles and Edwin Layton, London.

[60] Rasch, G. (1960). *Probabilistic Models for Some Intelligence and Attainment Tests*. The Danish Institute of Educational Research; expanded Ed. (1980), The University of Chicago Press, Chicago.

[61] Read, T.R.C. & Cressie, N.A.C. (1988). *Goodness-of-Fit Statistics for Discrete Multivariate Data*. Springer-Verlag, New York.

[62] Roy, S.N. & Kastenbaum, M.A. (1956). On the hypothesis of no "interaction" in a multiway contingency table, *Annals of Mathematical Statistics* **27**, 749–757.

[63] Stigler, S. (1992). Studies in the history of probability and statistics XLIII. Karl Pearson and quasi-independence, *Biometrika* **79**, 563–575.

[64] Stokes, M.E., Davis, C.S. & Koch, G.G. (1995). *Categorical Data Analysis Using the SAS System*. SAS Institute, Cary.

[65] Tjur, T. (1982). A connection between Rasch's item analysis model and a multiplicative Poisson model, *Scandinavian Journal of Statistics* **9**, 23–30.

[66] Waite, H. (1915). Association of fingerprints, *Biometrika* **10**, 421–478.

[67] Yule, G.U. (1900). On the association of attributes in statistics: with illustration from the material of the childhood society, &c., *Philosophical Transactions of the Royal Society of London, Series A* **194**, 257–319.

[68] Zaslavsky, A.M. & Wolfgang, G.S. (1993). Triple-system modeling of census, post-enumeration survey, and administrative-list data, *Journal of Business Economics and Statistics* **11**, 279–288.

A.L. CARRIQUIRY & S.E. FIENBERG

Lognormal Distribution

The lognormal distribution is one of the most commonly used distributions for modeling the data arising in biostatistical studies.

The **random variable** X has a two-parameter lognormal distribution with parameters μ and σ^2 if $Y = \ln X$ has a **normal distribution** with mean μ and variance σ^2. The probability density function of the lognormal distribution is

$$f(x) = \frac{1}{x\sigma(2\pi)^{1/2}} \exp\left[-\frac{(\ln x - \mu)^2}{2\sigma^2}\right],$$
$$x > 0, -\infty < \mu < \infty, \quad \sigma > 0,$$

where σ is called the shape parameter.

The three-parameter lognormal distribution, a generalization of the two-parameter lognormal distribution, is obtained when X in the above definition is replaced by $(X - c)$ with $x > c$, where c is any real number (see [10] for further details). c is called the location parameter.

Properties

The properties of the two-parameter lognormal distribution are:

1. Mean $= \exp(\mu + \sigma^2/2)$.
2. Variance $= \exp(2\mu + \sigma^2)[\exp(\sigma^2) - 1]$.
3. Median $= \exp(\mu)$.
4. Mode $= \exp(\mu - \sigma^2)$.
5. The 100 pth percentile (**quantile**) $= \exp(\mu + z_p\sigma^2)$, where z_p is the pth percentile of the standard normal distribution.
6. The standardized lognormal distribution tends to the standard normal distribution as σ tends to zero.
7. The **moment generating function** of the lognormal distribution does not exist.

For more properties of the two- and three-parameter lognormal distributions, see [6] and [10].

Estimation of Parameters

The estimation of parameters μ and σ^2 of the two-parameter lognormal distribution, in general, follows from the above logarithmic transformation (of the data) and related estimation methods for the normal distribution. We refer the reader to [19] and [13] for an extensive discussion of statistical inference for the two-parameter lognormal distribution. The methods of estimation for the three-parameter lognormal and the truncated lognormal distributions are more complicated [4, 5]. The estimation in the presence of **censored data** is discussed in [4].

Applications

Aitchison & Brown [1] provide an extensive discussion of early history, the geneses and applications of lognormal distributions. Koch [11, 12] has discussed the geneses of lognormal distributions arising from biological and pharmacological mechanisms; for example, he considered the lognormal distribution for modeling the metabolic turnover. Many applications of the lognormal distributions in biochemistry are discussed in [15] and its references.

The lognormal distributions are useful for modeling data arising in many medical studies. The *hazard* function of the lognormal distribution first increases and then decreases. In many cancer studies the lognormal distribution is used as a survival distribution [2, 8, 9, 20] (*see* **Parametric Models in Survival Analysis**).

Lawrence [14] and the references cited in his paper provide an extensive review of the applications of the lognormal distribution in medical studies such as the incubation period of disease, the time to recovery, and duration of survival.

The delta–lognormal distribution, a variant of a lognormal distribution, appears in the analysis of ichthyoplankton data [17]. The **Poisson** mixture using the lognormal distribution arises in many ecologic studies such as the analyses of species frequency data [3, 8] (*see* **Contagious Distributions**). For more applications of the lognormal distribution arising in ecologic studies, see [7].

Mosimann & Campbell [16] discuss the lognormal distribution as a model for tissue growth. In the same paper, they also discuss the uses of the multivariate lognormal distribution for size and shape analyses arising in **allometry** studies.

References

[1]   Aitchison, J. & Brown, J.A.C. (1957). *The Lognormal Distribution*. Cambridge University Press, Cambridge.

[2]   Bennett, S. (1983). Log-logistic regression models for survival data, *Applied Statistics* **32**, 165–171.

[3]   Bliss, C.I. (1966). An analysis of some insect trap records, *Sankhyā, Series A* **28**, 123–136.

[4]   Cohen, A.C. (1988). Censored, truncated, and grouped estimation, in *Lognormal Distributions, Theory and Applications*, E.L. Crow & K. Shimizu, eds. Marcel Dekker, New York, pp. 139–172.

[5]   Cohen, A.C. (1988). Three-parameter estimation, in *Lognormal Distributions, Theory and Applications*, E.L. Crow & K. Shimizu, eds. Marcel Dekker, New York, pp. 113–137.

[6]   Crow, E.L. & Shimizu, K. eds (1988). *Lognormal Distributions, Theory and Applications*. Marcel Dekker, New York.

[7]   Dennis, B. & Patil, G.P. (1988). Applications in ecology, in *Lognormal Distributions, Theory and Applications*, E.L. Crow & K. Shimizu, eds. Marcel Dekker, New York, pp. 303–330.

[8]   Farewell, V.T. & Prentice, R.L. (1979). A study of distributional shape in life testing, *Technometrics* **19**, 69–75.

[9]   Feinleib, M. (1960). A method for analysing log-normally distributed survival data with incomplete follow-up, *Journal of the American Statistical Association* **55**, 534–545.

[10] Johnson, N.L. & Kotz, S. (1970). *Distributions in Statistics: Continuous Univariate Distributions*, Vol. 1. Wiley, New York, Chapter 14.

[11] Koch, A.L. (1966). The logarithm in biology: I. Mechanisms generating the log-normal distribution, *Journal of Theoretical Biology* **12**, 276–290.

[12] Koch, A.L. (1969). The logarithm in biology: II. Distributions simulating the log-normal, *Journal of Theoretical Biology* **23**, 251–268.

[13] Land, C.E. (1988). Hypothesis tests and interval estimates, in *Lognormal Distributions, Theory and Applications*, E.L. Crow & K. Shimizu, eds. Marcel Dekker, New York, pp. 87–112.

[14] Lawrence, R.J. (1988). The lognormal as event-time distribution, in *Lognormal Distributions, Theory and Applications*, E.L. Crow & K. Shimizu, eds. Marcel Dekker, New York, pp. 211–266.

[15] Masuyama, M. (1984). A measure of biochemical individual variability, *Biomedical Journal* **26**, 337–346.

[16] Mosimann, J.E. & Campbell, G. (1988). Applications in biology: simple growth models, in *Lognormal Distributions, Theory and Applications*, E.L. Crow & K. Shimizu, eds. Marcel Dekker, New York, pp. 287–302.

[17] Pennington, M. (1983). Efficient estimators of abundance, for fish and plankton surveys, *Biometrics* **39**, 281–286.

[18] Preston, F.W. (1948). The commonness, and rarity, of species, *Ecology* **29**, 254–283.

[19] Shimizu, K. (1988). Point estimation, in *Lognormal Distributions, Theory and Applications*, E.L. Crow & K. Shimizu, eds. Marcel Dekker, New York, pp. 27–86.

[20] Whittemore, A. & Altshuler, B. (1976). Lung cancer incidence in cigarette smokers: further analysis of Doll and Hill's data for British physicians, *Biometrics* **32**, 805–816.

M. RATNAPARKHI

Logrank Test

The *logrank test* (so named by Peto & Peto [1]) is a rank test for comparing two samples of right-censored survival data. A careful description of its several origins, history, and connection to other tests for one-, two- and k-sample problems in censored survival data is given in the article **Linear Rank Tests in Survival Analysis**. Here we merely define the test in the simplest situation.

Let $\tilde{X}_{hi}$, for $i = 1, \ldots, n_h, h = 1, 2$, be independent nonnegative **random variables** with absolutely continuous distribution function F_h and **hazard rate** α_h. We do not observe the $\tilde{X}_{hi}$ but rather the right-censored samples $(X_{hi}, D_{hi}), X_{hi} = \tilde{X}_{hi} \wedge U_{hi}$, and $D_{hi} = I\{X_{hi} = \tilde{X}_{hi}\}$ for some censoring times $U_{hi}, i = 1, \ldots, n_h, h = 1, 2$. It is assumed that there is *independent censoring* (*see* **Censored Data**), which would be true if the U_{hi} were independent random variables, independent of the $\tilde{X}_{hi}$. In accordance with the assumption of absolutely continuous distributions, we assume that all $\tilde{X}_{hi}$ are distinct (no ties). *See* **Tied Survival Times** for further generalization.

The (two-sample) logrank test tests the hypothesis $H_0 : F_1 = F_2$ (or equivalently $\alpha_1 = \alpha_2$) by comparing the observed number of events in group 1,

$$O_1 = \sum_{i=1}^{n_1} D_{hi},$$

with the so-called expected number of events in group 1 under H_0 (*see* **Expected Number of Deaths**). The latter is estimated as

$$E_1 = \sum_{h=1}^{2} \sum_{i=1}^{n_h} D_{hi} \frac{Y_1(X_{hi})}{Y_1(X_{hi}) + Y_2(X_{hi})},$$

where $Y_h(t) = \sum_{k=1}^{n_h} I\{X_{hk} \geq t\}$ is the *number at risk* in group h at time t (*see* **Risk Set**). Indeed, it may be shown (still assuming no ties) that in large samples, $(O_1 - E_1)/\sqrt{V_1}$ is asymptotically **standard normal**, with

$$V_1 = \sum_{h=1}^{2} \sum_{i=1}^{n_h} D_{hi} \frac{Y_1(X_{hi})Y_2(X_{hi})}{(Y_1(X_{hi}) + Y_2(X_{hi}))^2}.$$

Reference

[1] Peto, R. & Peto, J. (1972). Asymptotically efficient rank invariant test procedures (with discussion), *Journal of the Royal Statistical Society, Series A* **135**, 195–206.

(*See also* **Survival Analysis, Overview**)

NIELS KEIDING

Long-Term Care *see* Health Services Organization in the US

Longitudinal Data Analysis, Overview

Longitudinal data arise when each member of one or more *cohorts* or *panels* of subjects provides a measurement on a number of occasions [21]. The cohort may be defined, for example, in terms of the date of birth of its members, the time of onset of a disease or, in the case of a clinical trial, the beginning of treatment or time of randomization. The *repeated (serial) measures* might be quantitative or qualitative, and may also be multivariate. For simplicity, however, the present discussion will be limited to univariate measures. Together, the results of these measurements will form a *response profile* (particular examples being *growth curves* (*see* **Nonlinear Growth Curve**) and time *trends* arising from **pharmacokinetic experiments**). Typically, longitudinal or repeated measures data are collected prospectively, but it is also possible to collect them retrospectively through the use of medical records, for example.

Time series data are similar to those described in this section but, on the whole, they can be distinguished from the latter because they usually arise from a single or, at most, a few extended sequences of observations as opposed to a larger number of shorter sequences. **Survival data**, *event history data* (*see* **Repeated Events**) *multistate* (e.g. states of well-being, morbidity, and death) *transition data* (*see*, **Fix–Neyman Process**) and **competing risks data** are also similar to repeated measures data in that they all involve observation over time. However, instead of enquiring about the state of a patient at each of a series of discrete times, investigators interested in survival times, for example, usually aim to record the exact date of death of each of the patients (i.e. the time of death is, in theory, a continuous rather than a discrete variable). The methods of analysis required for such data are distinctive, often involving time as an explicit response variable, and are covered for example, in **Survival Analysis, Overview**. In practice, many event recording systems do not record continuously but only to within discrete intervals of time, and continuously recorded data can be well approximated by grouping over short intervals of time. Such discrete event history or survival data

can then be considered as a series of repeated qualitative measurements on each subject and analyzed using the methods of this article in which time is a covariate or design factor [44].

Studies may involve more than one timescale. For example, treatment studies often consider both time under treatment and subject's age, and multistate transition processes may involve effects due to time since entry to the current state and the cumulative time spent in that and other states. Care may be required to insure that effects on each scale are all **identifiable**. The difficulties posed by **age–period–cohort** effects are a well known example.

Longitudinal studies may be observational (e.g. **cohort studies** epidemiologic surveys) or experimental (e.g. controlled **clinical trials**). In a clinical trial, the treatment might remain constant for any particular cohort or group of patients (with random allocation of patients to the competing treatments) or vary from one occasion to another (with random allocation to groups defined by the order in which the treatments are received). In the case of the latter, the trial is an example of the use of a **crossover design**.

The simplest kind of longitudinal study involves taking measurements on all subjects at the same times: that is, each patient provides exactly the same set of measures. It is possible, however, for both the number and spacing of the repeated measures to vary from one subject to another. The latter may arise from the design of the study, but in addition may be due to unintentionally missing observations. Patients might, for example, fail to keep an appointment on a given date, might be too ill to be interviewed, or might permanently drop out of or be lost from the study through a variety of causes (e.g. death, emigration, or refusal to continue treatment). The various approaches to the statistical analysis of longitudinal data differ in their ability to cope with missing data and in the assumptions made concerning the mechanism by which the missing data might arise. Missing data are a challenge to valid inference from longitudinal studies (*see* **Diggle–Kenward Model for Dropouts; Nonignorable Dropout in Longitudinal Studies**). (For details of modeling missing data mechanisms, see, for example, Little [45] or Diggle & Kenward [14].) Investigators should minimize the occurrence of missing values, avoiding them altogether wherever possible. If missing values are inevitable, then investigators should collect as much information as possible about the reasons for the missing data and to try to incorporate this information in their analysis.

Examples of Longitudinal Studies

First, let us consider experimental studies. Frison & Pocock [26] describe a clinical trial in which 152 patients with heart disease were randomly allocated to treatment using an active drug or a placebo during a 12-month follow-up period. The concentration of the liver enzyme creatine phosphokinase (CPK) in the patients' serum was measured as an indicator of liver damage arising as a side effect of the treatment. Each patient had three pretreatment measurements which were taken at 2 months before, 1 month before, and at the time of randomization. They also had eight posttreatment measurements taken every 1.5 months after randomization. An example of a simple crossover trial is provided by Hills & Armitage [32]. The experiment was a comparison of the effects of an active drug and a placebo in the treatment of enuresis. One group of patients received 14 consecutive days of treatment with the active treatment, followed by a similar period of treatment using the placebo. A second group received the treatment combinations in the reverse order: placebo followed by active drug. The response variable was the number of dry nights out of 14: that is, each patient provided two measures – one corresponding to each of the two periods of treatment.

Longitudinal surveys are also common in medical research. Here we describe three longitudinal studies of lung function. Laird & Ware [39], for example, describe a survey in which pulmonary function in about 200 schoolchildren was examined under normal conditions, then during an air pollution alert and on three successive weeks following the alert. The main aim of the study was to determine whether the volume of air exhaled in the first second of a forced exhalation (FEV_1) was depressed during the alert. The analysis of repeated **categorical** measures has been illustrated by Ware et al. [55]. Children were assessed annually at ages 9–12 to evaluate the potential effects of air pollution on persistent wheeze. Parents were asked about wheezing by their children during the previous year and responses were grouped into three mutually exclusive categories or states: no wheeze, wheeze with colds, or wheeze apart from colds. Our final example concerns a survey

with many missing observations. Lavange & Helms [41] analyzed data from a study of 72 children aged from 3 to 12 years. These data are also discussed by Little [45]. A measure of maximum expiratory flow rate was obtained annually, and differences in the resulting growth curve were related to the sex and race of the children. The number of actual measurements recorded on each child ranged from 1 to 8 (with an average of 4.2). Some values were missing because the child was either older than 3 at the beginning of the study, or younger than 12 at the end of it.

In the analysis of longitudinal data, the critical feature to recognize is that, since sets of measures are obtained from the same subjects, these measures are likely to be **correlated**, and can rarely be considered as independent even after conditioning upon known predictors or **explanatory variables**. How that dependence is dealt with is a principal distinguishing feature of different methods of analysis. However, before outlining these, we now consider more preliminary examination of the data.

Graphical Displays and Data Exploration

Diggle et al. [15] give the following simple guidelines for the exploration of longitudinal data using **graphical displays**:

1. show as much of the relevant data as possible rather than data summaries;
2. highlight aggregate patterns of potential scientific interest;
3. identify both **cross-sectional** and longitudinal patterns in the data;
4. make easy the identification of unusual individuals or unusual observations.

Here we produce a few simple plots for data on salsolinol levels (Table 1). These data were collected during an investigation into the role that the alkaloid salsolinol plays in bodily dependence on alcohol [30]. Fourteen individuals attending an alcohol treatment unit were observed over a period of four days immediately after being admitted to the unit, measurement of salsolinol being made from urine samples taken daily throughout the study period. The individuals were categorized as being in one of two groups: those considered to be severely dependent

Table 1 Salsolinol concentrations on four successive days

Obs.	Group	Day 1	Day 2	Day 3	Day 4
1	2	0.64	0.70	1.00	1.40
2	1	0.33	0.70	2.33	3.20
3	2	0.73	1.85	3.60	2.60
4	2	0.70	4.20	7.30	5.40
5	2	0.40	1.60	1.40	7.10
6	2	2.60	1.30	0.70	0.70
7	2	7.80	1.20	2.60	1.80
8	1	5.30	0.90	1.80	0.70
9	1	2.50	2.10	1.12	1.01
10	2	1.90	1.30	4.40	2.80
11	1	0.98	0.32	3.91	0.66
12	1	0.39	0.69	0.73	2.45
13	1	0.31	6.34	0.63	3.86
14	2	0.50	0.40	1.10	8.10

Source: Hand & Taylor [30].

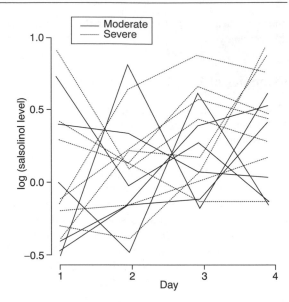

Figure 2 Salsolinol data – individual profiles after log transformation

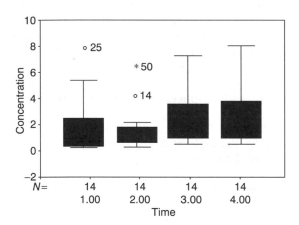

Figure 1 Salsolinol concentrations over time

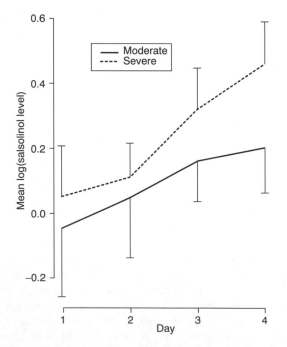

Figure 3 Mean profiles of salsolinol levels after log transformation for severe and moderate alcohol dependent groups

and those judged to be only moderately dependent. The response variables for the study are the four repeated measurements of urine concentrations of salsolinol. First, box plots (*see* **Graphical Displays**) of the distributions of the measurements at any one time point (see Figure 1) indicates **skewness**. A logarithmic **transformation** (base ten) of the salsolinol concentrations was therefore carried out prior to any further analysis. We next plot the time course for each individual subject, distinguishing the subjects from each of the two alcohol dependency groups (Figure 2).

In Figure 3 is shown a plot of the mean values of the logged salsolinol levels for the two groups,

together with their **standard errors**. An alternative would have been to plot a series of box plots, perhaps revealing more information about between-subject differences at each of the time points. Figure 3 highlights the difference between the two groups in rates of change over time, although the main message appears to be that the groups are, in fact, very similar. Although graphs of means such as that found in Figure 3 (and, less often, box plots) are much more commonly seen than those for the response profiles for individual subjects, great care must be taken in their interpretation. Figure 3 hides the pattern of *within-subject* changes. A graph of the latter type might also be very misleading if there were increasing numbers of dropouts over time, with the plotted means being calculated from the survivors at each time. If the dropping out is any way dependent on the present or previous state of the subject then the later means will be **biased**. One way of avoiding this bias is to plot means derived from cases with complete data, but the latter approach might be very inefficient if there are lots of dropouts.

Plots such as those provided in Figures 2 and 3 might indicate how one might extract suitable summary measures for each subject for a subsequent simple analyses of these response features. Visualizing the patterns in the data, and the subsequent extraction of the required response features, might be aided by smoothing each of the individual time courses. A search for the time of maximum response in a pharmacokinetic experiment, for example, might be quite difficult in the presence of considerable within-subject "noise". An example of smoothing in a pharmacokinetic experiment using a **moving average** prior to response feature extraction (the time of maximal response) is provided in Durcan et al. [18]. Other applications of smoothing methods, together with examples of their use, are described in Diggle et al. [15].

Another possibility is a simple multiple scatter plot (ignoring group differences) for the logged salsolinol concentrations. This sort of plot is ideal for the exploration of the correlation structure of repeated measures, although in a more complex data set with greater group differences, it would be preferable to remove the effects of explanatory variables and produce plots using the **residuals**. The results are not presented here, because there seems to be very little evidence of **serial correlation**. Finally, a plot that can be helpful in revealing the relative magnitudes of the sources of variance that give rise to correlations in continuous measures over time is the **variogram**.

Methods of Analysis for Continuous Responses

This section will be concerned with a few of the more commonly used strategies for the analysis of longitudinal data, with particular reference to continuous (usually **normally distributed**) outcome measures. We assume that the primary interest lies in changes in the average response over time at different levels of various explanatory factors, taking into account possible dependencies during **hypothesis testing** and **estimation**. The technical aspects of the methods will not be discussed in any detail but will be covered elsewhere. Methods for the analysis of categorical responses, transitions, and responses in the form of counts will be covered briefly in the next section.

Multivariate Generalizations of Paired t Tests

The **paired t test** is one of the basic methods for analyzing a simple two period, pretest/posttest study, comparing an estimate of the simple time 1 − time 2 difference contrast with the variance of this estimate. For greater numbers of measurement occasions, the multivariate generalization of this test is **multivariate analysis of variance** (MANOVA), that extends this approach to various linear contrasts relating to different aspects of change. As the paired t test can be generalized to an analysis of change scores, in which differences are regressed against factors and covariates, so too can this be done within MANOVA, in the form of *multivariate analysis of covariance (MANCOVA)*. These procedures enable one to test the differences between vectors of means with an entirely arbitrary pattern of correlations between the repeated measures. This method is therefore not dependent on any unrealistic assumptions concerning the patterns of serial dependencies, but is also likely to be less powerful than more refined methods that explicitly acknowledge the serial nature of the observations and correctly model the dependencies between them. These methods fail altogether when there are more design cells than subjects, a common occurrence where there are numerous measurement occasions.

Autoregression and Ante-Dependence

Another standard method for dealing with the correlation in the responses from a simple two-period study is **analysis of covariance** – analyzing the time-2 response conditional upon the time-1 response and predictors of change. This approach too can be generalized to larger numbers of measurement occasions. The **autocorrelation** or *autocovariance* between responses can either be considered as a nuisance to be allowed for in an analysis or, in some applications, it can be regarded as the property of particular interest. Consider a possible model for serial dependencies between repeated quantitative measurements. Let $e_1, e_2, \ldots, e_T$ be uncorrelated random variables, where e_t has a mean of zero and variance σ_t^2 for $t = 1, 2, \ldots, T$. Now define a series of measurements $Y_1, Y_2, \ldots, Y_T$ by

$$Y_1 = e_1,$$
$$Y_t = \gamma_t Y_{t-1} + e_t, \quad t = 2, 3, \ldots, T.$$

If the γs are all equal ($\gamma_t = \gamma$ for all t) and so the variance terms ($\sigma_t^2 = \sigma^2$ for all t), then these equations describe a stationary first-order *autoregressive process* (*see* **ARMA and ARIMA Models**). If, however, these parameters are permitted to vary with time then the equations describe first-order **ante-dependence**. A measurement at time t (that is Y_t) is dependent on the value of Y_{t-1} but, conditional on the value of Y_{t-1}, it is independent of all previous measurements. In general, a set of ordered measurements $Y_1, Y_2, \ldots, Y_T$ is said to have an independence structure of order r if the measurement at time t (with t greater than r), given the preceding r measurements, is independent of all further preceding measurements. Kenward [35] describes a method of assessing the order of a sequence of observations.

A simple unrestricted autoregressive model will involve $T(T + 1)/2$ variance and covariance parameters, as would the equivalent MANOVA. An advantage of the ante-dependence approach is that it provides a simple but flexible path for specifying more restrictive dependencies, increasing efficiency for the testing of contrasts of interest and giving the capability of analyzing studies with few subjects and numerous measurement occasions.

In the analysis of a longitudinal data set, one can approach the problem of serial depencies from several points of view. If we ignore their possible existence the analysis will be simpler, but the resulting inferences are likely to be invalid. If we can replace the response profile for each subject by one

or possibly more summary statistics (*derived variables*) which extract the distinct features of interest then the problem is side-stepped. Any resulting analysis of these extracted *response features* will be unaffected by the serial dependencies in the original observations. Again, we might also choose to modify our original approach to analyze the data as if there were no serial dependencies (as in the traditional **analysis of variance** for a *nested* or **split-plot** experiment – the repeated measures being nested within subjects) but then to make adjustments to the resulting test statistics (or their degrees of freedom) to allow for them. This is the rationale for the well-known *Greenhouse–Geisser adjustment* (see [29]) (*see* **Analysis of Variance for Longitudinal Data**).

The more refined methods will be more difficult to carry out and interpret and, more importantly, will not necessarily be robust to an incorrect specification of these serial dependencies. Great care must be exercised in their use.

A related problem concerning the analysis of data from crossover studies is the possible presence of *carryover effects*. In the simplest design – the two-period, two-treatment crossover experiment – this is completely confounded with the treatment by period interaction or order effect. A carryover effect arises when an effect of an early treatment persists in later periods of the trial. This might be due to an inadequate washout period between two periods of chemotherapy, for example, or because the first treatment has induced some permanent change in the patient. Many authors have suggested that this design should only be used when it can be assumed a priori that such carryover effects are absent. Crossover designs should only be used when the short-term relief of chronic symptoms, rather than a cure, is the goal of the trial (examples being the use of lithium in the control of manic symptoms, or the use of insulin to control blood sugar levels).

Time-by-Time Analysis

Following the common practice of plotting of group means for each separate time point, it comes as no surprise to find that investigators very frequently carry out separate statistical analyses at each of the time points. If there are n time points being considered, then there will be n separate analyses. On the whole, this is not a method of analysis that should be encouraged – it lacks power and the repeated tests are not statistically independent – although Finney [24] has advocated this **time-by-time analysis** when the number of times is small and the intervals between them large. Quite often, the researcher is interested in the question "At what time do the groups become significantly different?" and this is frequently the motivation for time-by-time analyses. If the latter is the case, then a modification of the approach by Kenward [35] might be preferred. This is essentially a series of analyses of covariance looking at group differences at any given time point, typically using the previous one or two values as covariates. The method is based on assumptions concerning the ante-dependence structure of the data and the reader is referred to Kenward [35] for technical details. Examples of the use of Kenward's method under the assumption of second-order ante-dependence can be found in Crowder & Hand [13], and for the analysis of the salsolinol data under the assumption of first order ante-dependence in Everitt & Dunn [22].

Derived Variables

Inspection of the individual time courses in Figure 3 leads naturally to two related ideas. The first is to ask what summary statistic or derived variable might be extracted for each case which best describes the main feature of interest in the serial measurements. There may, however, be more than one feature of interest in a series of repeated measures. For our salsolinol data, for example, the two which immediately come to mind are the average of the four measurements for each individual and an overall rate of change (linear trend) for that individual. The second idea is based on fitting a separate **regression** model (growth curve) to each case. One might, for instance, use ordinary **least squares** to fit a straight line to each individual's data. The resulting estimates for the intercept term and slope parameter would, of course, convey the same information as the derived variables from the first approach, but they do suggest that one might extend the idea to the fitting of some sort of **multilevel** or **random effects** model to the data. This will be developed in the following subsection. Here we deal with the analysis of derived variables.

Having obtained the derived variables, we then enter them into a second stage of analysis to estimate their mean for two or more groups and to test for possible differences between these groups. Returning to the salsolinol data, it is in fact possible to

derive a mean for the concentrations at the four times and three orthogonal polynomial trends (that is, linear, quadratic, and cubic trends) (*see* **Orthogonality; Polynomial Regression**). Differences in the means and trends across groups can be tested using simple t tests (or, in general, using ANOVA models) – each of the four derived variables being analyzed separately. Alternatively, we might wish to test for differences in all three trends simultaneously using **Hotelling's T^2 statistic** or, more generally, through the use of multivariate analysis of variance (MANOVA) procedures. One could, of course, include the average over time in this multivariate test, but this is usually analyzed separately so that one carries out separate analyses for the overall level and for the pattern of temporal change.

Random Effects Models

Returning once more to the salsolinol measurements, let Y_{ijk} represent the logarithm of the salsolinol concentration for the jth subject in the ith group on the kth day. Note that subjects are nested within groups. A possible regression model to describe the whole data set is

$$Y_{ijk} = \beta_0 + \alpha_i + \omega_{ij} + (\beta_i + \beta_{ij})t_k + \varepsilon_{ijk},$$

where t_k is the time to the kth measurement, and the parameters β_0, α_i, and β_i (the so-called fixed effects) correspond to the intercept term, the effect of being in the ith group on the intercept ($i = 1, 2$) and the linear effect of time in the ith group, respectively. The random effects are ω_{ij}, the effect on the intercept of subject j within group i, β_{ij}, the variation of the linear effect of time which is characteristic of subject j within the ith group, and the residual "error" term ε_{ijk}. In terms of the derived variables described above, the linear trend for the ijth individual is equivalent to the estimate of $\beta_i + \beta_{ij}$, but note that we are not now interested in estimating it explicitly – only its variance and possibly covariance with other effects. The random effects are all assumed to have zero expectation and the effects of real interest to the investigator are the β_is and possibly the α_is. Assuming that the responses are conditionally **multivariate normal**, we can then use **maximum likelihood** to estimate the fixed effects and the variances and covariances of the random effects, together with their respective standard errors [39].

Structural Equation and Latent Variable Models

Consider the observed variable, Y, which is now acknowledged to be measured with error. Typically,

$$Y = F + E,$$

where F is a latent variable or factor and E is the corresponding measurement error. If we now consider a series of repeated measures, Y_t, $t = 1, 2, \ldots, T$, with $Y_t = F_t + E_t$, it might be realistic to assume that the Fs are serially correlated, but that the Es are statistically independent. We also usually assume that the Fs and Es are independent. A latent first-order autoregressive model, for example, would have the form

$$Y_1 = F_1 + E_1$$
$$Y_t = \gamma F_{t-1} + E_t, \quad t = 2, 3, \ldots, T.$$

This simple latent variable model might well provide a **parsimonious** description of a series of measures when a similar first-order autoregressive model for the observed measurements would be hopeless. By acknowledging measurement error in this way, we can often considerably simplify the interpretation of the relationships within a set of serial measures. The above model (and any other) implies a particular structure for the covariance matrix of the repeated measures, and the model can therefore be fitted and its **goodness of fit** tested using covariance structure or **structural equation modeling** software (see [17], for example).

Another possibility is a random walk or Wiener model (*see* **Brownian Motion and Diffusion Processes**). Here

$$Y_1 = F_1 + E_1,$$
$$Y_t = F_1 + F_2 + \cdots + F_t + E_t, \quad t = 2, 3, \ldots, T.$$

Here the F_ts are random increments (or decrements) in the response variable Y_t which are "frozen in", accumulating over time. A third possibility is a latent growth curve model of the following form:

$$Y_1 = F_1 + E_1,$$
$$Y_2 = F_1 + F_2 + E_2,$$
$$Y_t = F_1 + \gamma_t F_2 + E_t, \quad t = 3, 4, \ldots, T.$$

In this case the two factors, F_1 and F_2, represent a baseline and a rate of growth (or decline), respectively, and it is quite usual to see that they are

correlated; a relatively large child at the start of a longitudinal study, for example, also growing at a rate greater than most of the other children. The reader will note the similarity of this and the random effects model of a previous section.

Quite often, it is of interest to compare growth curves of two or more cohorts of subjects. The covariance structure software can easily deal with this by simultaneously fitting growth curve models to two or more observed **covariance** (or moments) **matrices**. One can then test for the equality of parameters of interest across the groups.

Robust Parameter Covariance Estimates

It will have become apparent that for analyzing longitudinal data, although the main interest may lie in estimating the effects of risk factors and exposures on the expected value of the response, it often seems necessary to expend more effort to ensure that the model for the variances and covariances among the response is correct. Huber [34], and subsequently White [57] and Royall [51], proposed a heteroscedastic consistent "sandwich" estimator for the parameter covariance matrix (*see* **Generalized Estimating Equations**). Variants of this covariance estimator are available among many of the software implementations of procedures described above (e.g. EQS). At the cost of reduced efficiency – often trivial but sometimes large – the use of this method provides some relief from an excessive concern that the random part need be correctly specified in every detail (*see* **Robustness**).

Methods for Responses in the Form of Counts and Categorical Responses

Multivariate distributions for categorical and count data lack the flexibility of the multivariate normal distribution that underlies many of the methods for analyzing repeated continuous responses. In general, choices of distribution that have simple expressions for marginal distributions yield unpleasant expressions for joint or conditional distributions. The statistical literature is awash with models based on various distributions and parameterizations that may cleverly fit the particular needs of the problem illustrated by the authors, but that lack generality. We consider here only methods that we believe have wide scope for application. The principal styles of analysis of repeated count and categorical data tend to focus upon one of two rather different aspects of the overall process. The methods of *survival analysis* tend to focus on issues of timing and on problems, where the observation scheme is – at least nominally – continuous in time (*see* **Survival Analysis, Overview**). The remaining methods tend to focus rather more on *state occupancy* and *transition*, and often assume a discrete (and often equally spaced) observation scheme shared by all subjects and an analysis in which the treatment of the timescale is often implicit or simply another within subjects factor. These latter are the methods discussed here. This separation in styles of analysis is not always desirable, hampering our ability to generalize conclusions across observation and sample design schemes [4]. Methods that combine these two styles, such as *competing risk models*, are available but are typically cumbersome in use.

Contingency Tables and Loglinear Models

There is an extensive literature examining cross tabulated data from longitudinal studies of discrete outcomes, in particular making use of **loglinear models**. While in general useful as a preliminary tool, for scientific analysis of repeated measures data the interpretation of the parameters presents problems [6]. Kenward & Jones [36], for example, argue that the approach is more suited to "correlation rather than regression analysis". Discrete time Markov transition models (*see* **Markov Chains**) have received considerable attention, even though exactly how results relate to the process measured on a continuous timescale often remains open. Transition tables relating to social and economic mobility have been much studied [5]. Typically, all such tables show strong temporal associations among categories, often largely due to a tendency for simple persistence within the current class (*spurious contagion* [23]; *cumulative inertia* [47]). This has generated more specific forms of **contingency table** test for **quasi-independence** and **quasi-symmetry** (see Everitt [20]).

Latent Class Models

These inertia effects led to the exploration of *mover–stayer* models, a simple form of **latent class model** [42], in which attempts are made to explain

a complex temporal association among categories by the admixture of populations each following a more simple temporal process. In this instance, the "stayer" population simply persists in the same category, while the movers might all share a uniform transition rate. Of course, latent class methods have also been applied to longitudinal data to tackle problems of misclassification. The estimation of so-called **hidden Markov chains** is a more recent interest, whether for transitions between states of psychopathology and estimated by maximum likelihood [60], or for repeated screenings for cervical cancer and estimated by Gibbs sampling [52, 58] (*see* **Markov Chain Monte Carlo**). An approach using continuous latent variables for categorical data is discussed below under GEE estimation.

Conditional or Fixed Effects Models

Although the inclusion of subject specific fixed effects as dummy variables into **logistic regression** models for repeated binary measures does not lead directly to a satisfactory form of analysis (due to the *incidental parameter* problem [50]; *see* **Estimating Functions**), an analysis conditioning on the **sufficient statistic** for such a subject-specific effect does. In the simple two-period case without covariates, this corresponds to the **McNemar test** [48]. More generally, it corresponds to a form of **conditional logistic regression** [2, 9, 10], a method familiar to those analyzing matched **case–control studies**. This approach yields estimates only of risk factors or exposures that are time-varying, and can be inefficient where there is substantial use between subject information on effects of interest.

Random Effects or Integrated Likelihood Models

At the cost of assuming subject effects to be uncorrelated with included explanatory variables, a random effects approach provides estimation of time-constant effects and more efficient estimates of time-varying effects. Assuming some distribution for subject-specific effects provides a likelihood for a sequence of discrete outcomes of the form

$$L_i = \int \prod_{j=1}^{T} h^{-1}(Y_{ij}|X_{ij}; \boldsymbol{\beta}, \tau_i) \mathrm{d}G(\tau).$$

In general, however, most choices of link function $h(\cdot)$ and parametric distribution $G(\cdot)$ for the subject-specific effects do not lead to an analytically tractable expression, even when the problem is simplified to one of time-constant subjects effects (the so-called "one factor" model). Choice of the complementary log–log link together with a distribution of subject effects from the Hougaard family [33], for example the **gamma distribution**, offers some possibilities and can be combined with discrete latent classes [53]. Recourse to computational brute force – for example, using quadrature [27] or Monte Carlo methods [52] – allows the use of the potentially more flexible multivariate normal distribution for subject effects. Somewhat curiously, the computational burden becomes little greater if parametric restrictions are eased and instead the **nonparametric maximum likelihood estimator** of the random effects distribution is used [38]. In this case the distribution is represented by mass points with both weights and locations as free parameters, reducing the integration of the above equation to a summation (and almost always over fewer points than that required for "parametric quadrature"). The relationship between the nonparametric and conditional estimators is discussed in Lindsay et al. [43].

Penalized or Predictive Quasi-likelihood and Generalized Linear Mixed Models

An alternative approach to the computation of L_i is through some linearizing approximation, described as *penalized quasi-likelihood* (PQL) by Breslow & Clayton [7]. Essentially, this involves the iteratively reweighted least squares equations of standard GLM estimation [46] being extended to include current estimates of the random effects as well as those for fixed effects. For binary response data and few measurement occasions, this approach does not perform well [8, 16], particularly with respect to estimation of the random effects parameters. However, in many other circumstances it performs much better and offers a flexible and simple approach that yields satisfactory estimates for covariate effects of interest. A similar approach can be used to estimate the parameters of **marginal models** [28] that are considered in more detail in the next two sections.

Empirical Generalized Least Squares

All the preceding approaches have involved specifying some model for the covariance among observations due to the impact of subject-specific effects and past history, and estimating effects of interest conditional upon these effects. An alternative approach is to specify functional forms for the relationships of primary interest – say, the marginal relationship between outcomes and features of the study design – with the rest of the model that deals with covariances being saturated. In the *empirical generalized least squares* approach of Koch et al. [37], implemented in the SAS procedure CATMOD (*see* **Categorical Data Analysis**), the marginal expected proportions are replaced directly by their observed values to provide empirical logits, limiting this method to design matrices involving only discrete variables. These are then linearly related to explanatory variables. Since these proportions are neither independent nor equally variable, ordinary least squares estimation is not appropriate. However, the covariance matrix for these empirical logits will typically be block diagonal with one block for each unique combination of between subjects factors. The ith block is then estimated by $\mathbf{D}_i\mathbf{V}_i\mathbf{D}_i^{\mathrm{T}}$, where $\mathbf{D}_i$ is the matrix of partial derivatives of the logits with respect to the marginal proportions and $\mathbf{V}_i$ is their covariance matrix. With the need to avoid undefined empirical logits and singularities in the estimated covariance matrix, this approach has trouble with sparse data. Kenward & Jones [36] suggest 25–30 responses for each response function for reliable results, typically limiting this method to very few repeated measures. The general approach has been extended to tackle incomplete data and other response functions [40].

Estimation Using a "Working Covariance Matrix" and Generalized Estimating Equations

This powerful and flexible approach is described in the article on **Generalized Estimating Equations**. The approach represents a multivariate generalization of **quasi-likelihood** estimation, allowing a Fisher-scoring method of estimation for models for which a full likelihood may not be known. Although more commonly used to estimate marginal or population-average models, the generalized estimating equations (GEE) approach can also be used to estimate models including subject specific random effects [59].

Muthén [49] presented a related general approach that fits mixed effects and latent variable models to categorical data using a two-stage estimation method.

This was based on first estimating fixed effects (thresholds and coefficients), their covariance matrix, a conditional covariance matrix of errors and their covariance matrix, all based on pairwise bivariate probit. The second stage then fits models to these first-stage estimates. For large samples without complex patterns of missing data and with response measures of mixed type, this is a flexible and powerful method.

Marginal Maximum Likelihood Models

In fact, there are a number of parameterizations that include the marginal means as parameters and that allow closed form likelihood representations for binary sequences. Bahadur [3] described how the joint distribution of a binary sequence could be parameterized in terms of the marginal means and the marginal correlations. Estimation is, however, nonstandard in that the marginal correlations are subject to a reasonably complex set of linear inequality constraints. Fitzmaurice & Laird [25] provided a "mixed" parameterization, one involving the marginal means but parameterizing the association in terms of conditional odds ratios. These latter are unconstrained, and this parameterization also provides orthogonality between the regression and association parameters. It has the disadvantage of conditional parameterizations in that the association measures are specific to a fixed sequence length, and thus this model is not suitable in circumstances involving missing data (or variable length sequences) without further adaptation. Ekholm et al. [19] have provided a third parameterization, this time using the marginal means and the dependence ratio, the first-order dependence ratios being of the form $E[Y_{ij} = 1,\ Y_{ik} = 1]/(E[Y_{ij} = 1]E[Y_{ik} = 1])$. Within this parameterization, the dependence ratios are subject to relatively simple constraints, the mean and association parameters are not orthogonal, and the model is asymmetric; different results will be obtained depending upon which response is coded 1 or 0.

Time-by-Time Analysis

A structured approach to time-by-time analysis, one that provides a rather straightforward method for dealing with missing data, has been provided by Wei & Stram [56]. They provided an estimator for the covariance matrix of the sets of parameters estimated at each time and a method for tackling the problem of multiple testing.

Derived Variable Analysis

The summary measures method can be applied as for continuous data but with the obvious modification of changes in the form and estimation of the derived variables.

Ordinal Data

Extensions from binary to ordinal responses (*see* **Ordered Categorical Data**) are possible for most, though not all, of the methods described [1]. Among random effects approaches, the log-gamma mixed complementary-log–log link models extend directly to ordinal data [12]. The **proportional odds** generalization of the logistic model [11] with random effects can be estimated directly by ML [28] or, if the ordinal response is transformed into a set of binary responses each indicating a response above or below each threshold, then PQL or GEE estimation become easily implemented [7]. In principle, the empirical generalized least squares approach may be applied, but the problems associated with sparse data become still more pressing than with binary data. The multivariate probit-based latent variable approach of Muthén [49] generalizes naturally to the ordinal case.

Count Data

Where the response measure represents an accumulation of discrete events over an interval of time, the **Poisson** likelihood offers a natural starting point. Variable interval lengths are straightforwardly dealt with by means of an *offset*. Extra-variation between subjects beyond that due to the included explanatory variables of the model may be accounted for either by a random effect or by *quasi-likelihood* or robust parameter covariance estimation. Assuming a gamma distribution for the subject-specific variation in rate leads to the well known **negative binomial** model.

Where there have been repeated observation intervals with explanatory variables that vary between intervals, then the approaches available are essentially parallel to those described for repeated binary outcomes. Conditional and parametric random effects estimation are both feasible [31]. Thall & Vail [54] describe a GEE approach. Little progress has been made with latent variable models for count data.

References

[1]   Agresti, A. (1989). A survey of models for repeated ordered categorical response data, *Statistics in Medicine* **8**, 1209–1224.

[2]   Andersen, E.B. (1980). *Discrete Statistical Models with Social Science Applications.* North-Holland, Amsterdam.

[3]   Bahadur, R.R. (1961). A representation of the joint distribution of responses to *n* dichotomous items, in *Studies in Item Analysis and Prediction*, H. Solomon, ed. Stanford University Press, Stanford, pp. 118–168.

[4]   Bartholomew, D.J. (1973). *Stochastic Models for Social Processes.* Wiley, New York.

[5]   Blumen, J., Koggan, M. & McCarthy, D.J. (1955). *The Industrial Mobility of Labour as a Probability Process.* Cornell University Press, Ithaca, New York.

[6]   Bonney, G.E. (1987). Logistic regression for dependent binary observations, *Biometrics* **43**, 951–973.

[7]   Breslow, N.E. & Clayton, D.G. (1993). Approximate inference in generalized linear mixed models, *Journal of the American Statistical Association* **88**, 9–25.

[8]   Breslow, N.E. & Lin, X. (1995). Bias correction in generalized linear mixed models with a single component of dispersion, *Biometrika* **82**, 81–92.

[9]   Conoway, M.R. (1989). Analysis of repeated categorical measurements with conditional likelihood methods, *Journal of the American Statistical Association* **84**, 53–62.

[10]   Conoway, M.R. (1990). A random effects model for binary data, *Biometrics* **46**, 317–328.

[11]   Cox, D.R. & Snell, E.J. (1989). *Analysis of Binary Data*, 2nd Ed. Chapman & Hall, London.

[12]   Crouchley, R. (1995). A random effects model for ordered categorical data, *Journal of the American Statistical Association* **90**, 489–498.

[13]   Crowder, M.J. & Hand, D.J. (1990). *Analysis of Repeated Measures.* Chapman & Hall, London.

[14]   Diggle, P.J. & Kenward, M.G. (1994). Informative drop-outs in longitudinal data analysis, *Applied Statistics* **43**, 49–93.

[15]   Diggle, P.J., Liang, K.-L. & Zeger, S.L. (1994). *Analysis of Longitudinal Data.* Oxford University Press, Oxford.

[16]   Drum, O. & McCullagh, P. (1993). Comment to Fitzmaurice, G.M., Laird, N. and Rotnitsky, A. Regression models for discrete longitudinal responses, *Statistical Science* **8**, 284–309.

[17]   Dunn, G., Everitt, B. & Pickles, A. (1993). *Modelling Covariances and Latent Variables Using EQS.* Chapman & Hall, London.

[18]   Durcan, M.J., McWilliam, J.R., Campbell, I.C., Neale, M.C. & Dunn, G. (1988). Chronic antidepressant drug regimes and food and water intake in rats, *Pharmacology Biochemistry & Behavior* **30**, 299–302.

[19]   Eckholm, A., Smith, P.W.F. & MacDonald, J.W. (1995). Marginal regression analysis of a multivariate binary response, *Biometrika* **82**, 847–854.

[20]   Everitt, B.S. (1992). *The Analysis of Contingency Tables,* 2nd Ed. Chapman & Hall, London.

[21]   Everitt, B.S. (1995). The analysis of repeated measures: a practical review with examples, *Statistician* **44**, 113–136.

[22]   Everitt, B.S. & Dunn, G. (1993). *Applied Multivariate Data Analysis.* Edward Arnold, London.

[23]   Feller, W. (1966). *An Introduction to Probability Theory and Its Applications.* Wiley, New York.

[24]   Finney, D.J. (1990). Repeated measurements: what is measured and what repeats?, *Statistics in Medicine* **9**, 639–644.

[25]   Fitzmaurice, G.M. & Laird, N.M. (1993). A likelihood based method for analysing longitudinal binary responses, *Biometrika* **80**, 141–151.

[26]   Frison, I. & Pocock, S.J. (1992). Repeated measures in clinical trials: analysis using mean summary statistics and its implications for design, *Statistics in Medicine* **11**, 1685–1704.

[27]   Gibbons, R.D. & Hedeker, D.R. (1992). Full information item bi-factor analysis, *Psychometrika* **57**, 423–436.

[28]   Goldstein, H. (1991). Nonlinear multilevel models, with an application to discrete response data, *Biometrika* **78**, 45–52.

[29]   Hand, D.J. & Crowder, M. (1996). *Practical Longitudinal Data Analysis.* Chapman & Hall, London.

[30]   Hand, D.J. & Taylor, C.C. (1987). *Multivariate Analysis of Variance and Repeated Measures.* Chapman & Hall, London.

[31]   Hausmann, J., Hall, B. & Grilliches, Z. (1981) Econometric models for count data with an application to the patent–R&D relationship. Mimeo, MIT Press, Cambridge, Mass.

[32]   Hills, M. & Armitage, P. (1979). The two-period crossover clinical trial, *British Journal of Clinical Pharmacology* **8**, 7–20.

[33]   Hougaard, P. (1986). A class of multivariate failure time distributions, *Biometrika* **73**, 671–678 (correction: **75** (1988) 395).

[34]   Huber, P.J. (1967). The behavior of maximum likelihood estimators under non-standard conditions, *Proceedings of the Fifth Berkeley Symposium on Mathematical Statistics and Probability*, Vol. 1. University of California Press, Berkeley, pp. 221–233.

[35]   Kenward, M.G. (1987). A method for comparing profiles of repeated measurements, *Applied Statistics* **36**, 296–308.

[36]   Kenward, M.G. & Jones, B. (1992). Alternative approaches to the analysis of binary and categorical repeated measurements, *Journal of Biopharmaceutical Statistics* **2**, 137–170.

[37]   Koch, G.G., Landis, J.R., Freeman, D.H. & Lehnen, R.G. (1977). A general methodology for the analysis of repeated measurement of categorical data, *Biometrics* **33**, 133–158.

[38]   Laird, N.M. (1978). Non-parametric maximum likelihood estimation of a mixing distribution, *Journal of the American Statistical Association* **73**, 805–811.

[39]   Laird, N.M. & Ware, J.H. (1982). Random effects models for longitudinal data, *Biometrics* **38**, 963–974.

[40]   Landis, J.R., Miller, M.E., Davis, C.S. & Koch, G.G. (1988). Some general methods for the analysis of categorical data in longitudinal studies, *Statistics in Medicine* **7**, 109–137.

[41]   Lavange, L.M. & Helms, R.W. (1983). The analysis of incomplete data with modeled covariance structures. Mimeo 1449, University of North Carolina, Institute of Statistics.

[42]   Lazarsfeld, P.F. & Henry, N.W. (1968). *Latent Structure Analysis*. Houghton Mifflin, Boston.

[43]   Lindsay, B.G., Clogg, C.C. & Grego, J. (1991). Semiparametric estimation in the Rasch model and related experimental response models including a simple latent class model for item analysis, *Journal of the American Statistical Association* **86**, 96–107.

[44]   Lindsey, J.K. (1993). *Models for Repeated Measurements*. Oxford University Press, Oxford.

[45]   Little, R.J. (1995). Modelling the drop-out mechanism in repeated-measures studies, *Journal of the American Statistical Association* **90**, 1112–1121.

[46]   McCullagh, P. & Nelder, J.A. (1989) *Generalized Linear Models*, 2nd Ed. Chapman & Hall, London.

[47]   McGinnis, R. (1968). A stochastic model of social mobility, *American Sociological Review* **23**, 712–722.

[48]   McNemar, Q. (1947). A note on the sampling error of the difference between correlated proportions or percentages, *Psychometrika* **12**, 153–157.

[49]   Muthén, B. (1984). A general structural equation model with dichotomous ordered categorical and continuous latent variable indicators, *Psychometrika* **49**, 115–132.

[50]   Neyman, J. & Scott, E. (1948). Consistent estimates based on partially consistent observations, *Econometrica* **16**, 1–32.

[51]   Royall, R.M. (1986). Model robust confidence intervals using maximum likelihood estimation, *International Statistical Review* **54**, 221–226.

[52]   Spiegelhalter, D.J., Thomas, A., Best, N.G. & Gilks, W.R. (1995). *BUGS: Bayesian Inference Using Gibbs Sampling, Version 5.0*. MRC Biostatistics Unit, Cambridge.

[53]   Spilerman, S. (1972). Extensions to the mover–stayer model, *American Journal of Sociology* **78**, 599–626.

[54]   Thall, P.F. & Vail, S.C. (1990). Some covariance models for longitudinal count data with overdispersion, *Biometrics* **46**, 657–671.

[55]   Ware, J.H., Lipsitz, S. & Speizer, F.E. (1988). Issues in the analysis of repeated categorical outcomes, *Statistics in Medicine* **7**, 95–107.

[56]   Wei, L.J. & Stram, D.O. (1988). Analysing repeated measurements with possibly missing observations by modelling marginal distributions, *Statistics in Medicine* **7**, 139–148.

[57]   White, H. (1980). Maximum likelihood estimation of misspecified models, *Econometrica* **50**, 1–25.

[58]   Zeger, S.L. & Karim, M.R. (1991). Generalized linear models with random effects: a Gibbs sampling approach, *Journal of the American Statistical Association* **86**, 79–86.

[59]   Zeger, S.L., Liang, K.-Y. & Albert, P.S. (1988). Models for longitudinal data: a generalized estimating equation approach, *Biometrics* **44**, 1049–1060.

[60]   Zoccolillo, M., Pickles, A., Quinton, D. & Rutter, M. (1992). The outcome of childhood conduct disorder: implications for defining adult personality disorder and conduct disorder, *Psychological Medicine* **22**, 971–986.

GRAHAM DUNN & ANDREW PICKLES

Lorenz Curve *see* Gini, Corrado

Loss Function

The consequences of any decision will depend on the true state of nature, which determines whether the action corresponding to that decision is beneficial or harmful. The statistical formalization of this concept (*see* **Decision Theory**) has the following components:

Θ is the set of all possible states of nature θ.

D is the set of all possible decisions (actions) d.

$L(\theta, d)$ is the loss function that expresses the consequences of decision d when the state of nature θ holds.

By convention, the loss function is usually taken to be nonnegative, and is to be minimized. Since losses are to be compared or minimized, only the relative values of the losses of different decisions are important. Some synonyms for loss are "regret" and "cost". Alternatively, consequences are sometimes described in terms of "gain" or **"utility"**, and then maximization is the objective.

The loss function is useful in both statistical theory and in practical applications. A decision theoretic formulation of an existing procedure can clarify its interpretation by identifying its implicit loss function, and suggest generalizations. Practical applications include setting criteria to determine decisions related to disease for **screening**, setting treatment policy, **quality of life** issues, and study design.

Theoretical Uses of Loss Functions

A statistical decision procedure $\delta(X)$ yields a decision $d \in D$ based on the data X. Members of a set Δ of statistical procedures $\delta(X)$ are compared based on the loss function $L[\theta, \delta(X)]$ which, being a function of X, is a **random variable**. The risk of a decision procedure $\delta(X)$ is the **expectation** of the loss function, $R(\theta, \delta) = \mathrm{E}\{L[\theta, \delta(X)]|\theta\}$. Frequentist approaches (*see* **Inference**) compare procedures $\delta_1(X)$ and $\delta_2(X)$ by comparing the **risk** functions $R(\theta, \delta_1)$ and $R(\theta, \delta_2)$. In general, no procedure will minimize $R(\theta, \cdot)$ for all θ, so additional conditions are usually imposed. In ideal cases, the set Δ can be restricted according to a criterion such as **unbiasedness** (*see* **Minimum Variance Unbiased (MVU) Estimator; Most Powerful Test**), symmetry, or invariance [4], so that the risk function of some $\delta \in \Delta$ is dominated by all others, making the choice clear. Another approach, **minimax**, chooses the procedure which minimizes the maximum possible expected loss for any θ. **Bayesian** solutions minimize the expectation of $R(\theta, \delta)$ taken with respect to the **prior distribution** of θ.

Hypothesis testing can be viewed in terms of loss functions. Consider a hypothesis test of a **null hypothesis** H_0: $\theta = \theta_0$ vs. an **alternative hypothesis** H_1: $\theta = \theta_1$. Defining our loss to be 0 for a correct conclusion and 1 for an incorrect one gives the loss function shown in Table 1. The test is a decision function defined so that $\delta(x) = 1$ leads to rejection of the null hypothesis and $\delta(x) = 0$ leads to acceptance. The corresponding expected loss is shown in Table 2.

Thus 0–1 loss leads to expected losses which are type I and type II errors in hypothesis testing. The traditional approach to hypothesis testing restricts Δ

Table 1 Loss function for a hypothesis test

True parameter value	Decide $\theta = \theta_0$	Decide $\theta = \theta_1$
	Losses	
H_0: θ_0	0	1
H_1: θ_1	1	0

so that all tests considered have a fixed type II error. Minimizing the risk then amounts to maximizing the **power** of the test. Structuring the problem in this way aids in formulating more complex problems. For example, Emerson & Tritchler [3] elaborate the decision problem to incorporate a third type of error (Type III error) for a two-sided testing strategy (*see* **Alternative Hypothesis**), concluding that a treatment is beneficial when the null hypothesis is false, but the treatment is actually harmful.

Parameter **estimation** can also be expressed in terms of an underlying loss function. Consider the decision procedure to be the parameter estimate $\hat{\theta}(X)$, which asserts the decision that the true parameter has value $\hat{\theta}(x)$. If $L[\theta, \hat{\theta}(X)] = [\hat{\theta}(X) - \theta]^2$, then $R(\theta, \hat{\theta})$ is **mean square error**.

Practical Applications of Loss Functions

Besides illuminating and guiding statistical theory, loss functions are of use in specific applications. Often the initial step of posing a problem in a decision theoretic framework will help to clarify aspects of a problem, even if the full decision theoretic solution is not required. Formulating loss functions will enable us to incorporate practical considerations into methodology which are ignored in standard techniques. Some examples follow.

Suppose that the cost of the estimation error can be quantified in monetary units by the loss function $L(\mu, \overline{X}) = \lambda(\overline{X} - \mu)^2$. Then $R(\mu, \overline{x}) = \lambda\sigma_x^2/n$ is a function of only the sample size n, where the risk falls as n grows. We can add a term $C(n)$ to the loss function which states the cost of obtaining a sample

Table 2 Expected losses for a hypothesis test

True parameter value	Risk
θ_0	$0 + 1 \times \Pr(\text{decide } \theta = \theta_1|\theta_0)$
θ_1	$1 \times \Pr(\text{decide } \theta = \theta_0|\theta_1) + 0$

of that size, and determine the n which minimizes the resulting loss given assumptions about σ_x^2 [1] (*see* **Sample Size Determination**).

Colton [2] proposed a loss function to guide the design of **clinical trials**. A treatment to be studied will affect two populations of patients: the $2n$ subjects on the two arms of the trial, and the "patient horizon", which consists of the N future patients who will be treated based on the results of that trial until future research provides an even newer treatment. Colton assigns a loss of λ to receiving the inferior treatment and 0 for the better treatment. Then, if the trial results are erroneous and lead to the adoption of the inferior treatment, the loss is $\lambda[n + (N - 2n)]$, since one arm of the trial and the patient horizon will receive the inferior treatment. If the correct treatment is chosen, a loss of λn is incurred by the arm on the inferior treatment. The relevant state of nature is the true treatment difference; a value for this is assumed and λ is taken to be proportional to it. Thus, the risk is $\lambda[n + (N - 2n)\text{Pr(choose inferior)}]$ for an assumed value of λ. This risk is a function of the sample size n; the first term of the above sum increases as n, but both factors of the second term decrease. This expresses the tradeoff between the welfare of the trial subjects and the patient horizon. Colton's loss formulation provides an interesting perspective on the impact of clinical trials.

Shannon et al. [6] consider the screening of patients for clinical trial eligibility. An initial screening of potential trial participants is done to select patients for further evaluation to determine eligibility. Table 3 shows the losses incurred by screening. The cost of evaluation is taken to be 1, and the loss due to discarding an eligible subject is ϕ times that, where $\phi > 1$ is specified subjectively.

In the examples, numerical losses were assigned to outcomes such as losing a trial participant or administering an inferior treatment. Losses of such a nature can be very difficult to quantify. Also, even if only monetary costs are involved, their direct interpretation as loss may be inadequate, especially after expectations are taken. These assessment and representation problems are addressed by utility theory, which derives techniques for quantifying perceptions of losses associated with complex outcomes having many incommensurate attributes [5]. If certain axioms hold, such loss functions accurately reflect preference when expectations are taken.

References

[1]   Cochran, W.G. (1977). *Sampling Techniques*. Wiley, New York.

[2]   Colton, T. (1963). A model for selecting one of two medical treatments, *Journal of the American Statistical Association* **58**, 388–400.

[3]   Emerson, J.D. & Tritchler, D. (1987). The three-decision problem in medical decision making, *Statistics in Medicine* **6**, 101–112.

[4]   Ferguson, T.S. (1967). *Mathematical Statistics: A Decision Theoretic Approach*. Academic Press, New York.

[5]   Keeney, R.L. & Raiffa, H. (1976). *Decisions with Multiple Objectives: Preferences and Value Tradeoffs*. Wiley, New York.

[6]   Shannon, W.D., Bryant, J., Logan, T.F. & Day, R. (1995). An application of decision theory to patient screening for an autologous tumour vaccine trial, *Statistics in Medicine* **14**, 2099–2110.

D. TRITCHLER

Table 3 Loss function for eligibility screening

True state	Decision	
	Evaluate	Discard
	Losses	
Eligible	1	ϕ
Ineligible	1	0

Loss to Follow-Up Bias *see* Bias, Nondifferential

Louis, Pierre-Charles-Alexandre

Born: 1787, in Aï, France.
Died: June 9, 1872, in France.

P.-C.-A. Louis initially studied to be a lawyer; however, he abandoned law for medicine at the age of 20. After completing his initial medical training in Paris in 1813, he traveled throughout Russia for a period of seven years, eventually settling in Odessa. When

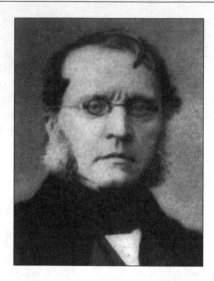

Louis's medical training proved inadequate to combat an epidemic of diphtheria that occurred in Odessa in 1820, he resolved to return to Paris for additional study; however, he did not find much of use in the lectures of contemporary Parisian physicians.

With his appointment to the hospital, La Charité, in the early 1820s, Louis hoped to forge a more scientific foundation for medicine by collecting extensive records about the patients in the hospital, e.g. their ages, length of residence in Paris, the number who died and recovered from each disease, and the number of days duration of the disease. Louis used these records to determine the **mean** (or average) value for each analytical category and published his findings. In his study of typhoid fever, for example, Louis determined that it was primarily a disease of the young since the mean age of the 50 fatal cases was 23 and the mean age of the 88 who recovered was 21. In his 1835 treatise, *Recherches sur les effets de la saignée*, Louis provided the most famous example of his so-called "numerical method"; he demonstrated that the then common therapeutic practice of bloodletting was not as efficacious as its advocates believed, since 18 patients died out of 47 who had been bled (i.e. 38%) whereas only nine died out of the 36 patients who were not bled (i.e. 25%).

Louis's impact on the Parisian medical scene was most pronounced during the second quarter of the nineteenth century. In 1832, his followers founded the Société Médicale d'Observation to publish findings based on the numerical method. Although the society published three memoirs in 1837, 1844, and 1856, it did not survive after the retirement of Louis from public life in the mid 1850s following the premature death of his only son. Nevertheless, Louis had a long-term impact through the many students that he trained, including such prominent contributors to nineteenth century medicine and public health as the English physician and vital statistician **William Farr** and the American physician, Oliver Wendell Holmes.

J. ROSSER MATTHEWS

Lowest Adverse Effect Level *see* Risk Assessment for Environmental Chemicals

Luria–Delbrück Distribution *see* Bacterial Growth, Division, and Mutation

Lyapunov Exponent *see* Chaos Theory

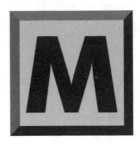

M-Estimator *see* Robustness

Magic Square Designs

A *magic square* of size n is a set of integers in an $n \times n$ square such that each of the n rows, n columns, and the two main diagonals have the same sum m. A magic square is called *pandiagonal* if all the $2(n-1)$ wrap-around diagonals (the combined diagonals that are $+g$ and $-(n-g)$ from a main diagonal, for $g = 1, \ldots, n-1$) also sum to m, and *symmetrical* if all pairs of cells that are symmetrically opposite the center of the square sum to $2m/n$. In the usual case of a *magic square of order n*, the integers used are 1 to n^2, and $m = n(n^2 + 1)/2$. A pandiagonal and a symmetric magic square of order 4 ($m = 34$, $2m/n = 17$) are, respectively,

15	10	3	6
4	5	16	9
14	11	2	7
1	8	13	12

16	2	3	13
5	11	10	8
9	7	6	12
4	14	15	1

For further discussion and methods of construction, see Dénes & Keedwell [6] and Freeman [8], and the references therein.

Phillips [10] showed how the entries of a magic square of size n with distinct integers can be used to give the times at which the n^2 runs for a **factorial experiment** are made so that the main effects are *linear-trend-free*; that is, **orthogonal** to a straight line trend over time. If n has k factors, $n = n_1 n_2 \ldots n_k, n_i > 1$, then a design for (up to) $2k$ factors with levels $n_1, n_2, \ldots, n_k$ (each twice) can be obtained for which the main effects and at least some of the two-factor **interactions** are linear-trend-free (more if the magic square is symmetrical). For example, consider the $n = 4$ pandiagonal magic square above. Letting rows 1 to 4 represent $a_0 b_0, a_0 b_1, a_1 b_0$, and $a_1 b_1$, respectively, and columns 1 to 4 represent $c_0 d_0, c_0 d_1, c_1 d_0$, and $c_1 d_1$, respectively, gives, in the usual notation, the following run order for a 2^4 design for which all two-factor interactions are linear-trend-free:

$$(a, abcd, cd, b, bd, c, abc, ad, bc,$$
$$d, abd, ac, acd, ab, 1, bcd).$$

Fewer factors can be used with levels that are products of the n_i, and some n_i can be omitted. For example, a magic square of size 6 can be used for a complete replicate $2^2 \times 3^2$, $2 \times 3 \times 6$ or 6^2 design, or for two replicates of a 2×3^2 or a 3×6 design, or three replicates of a $2^2 \times 3$ or a 2×6 design, etc. If there is more than 1 replicate, then it may be possible to measure order effects within each replicate. A pandiagonal magic square of order n can be used to obtain an n^{3-1} **Latin square** (three factors each at n levels) or, for n odd, an n^{4-2} **Graeco-Latin square** (four factors each at n levels) for which main effects are linear-trend-free. There has been considerable further progress made on trend-free and trend-**robust** designs; see, for example, Bailey et al. [1], Bradley & Yeh [5], and Lin & Dean [9].

There are many connections between magic squares and *Latin squares*; see, for example, Dénes & Keedwell [6]. Amongst these are that if the integers $\{1, \ldots, n\}$ are used n times, then the magic square is a *diagonal Latin square*, and a pandiagonal magic square is a *Knut Vik design*. The Knut Vik design, which generalizes the well-known 5×5 knight's move Latin square, has five orthogonal constraints (block or treatment structures) of size n: rows, columns, the two sets of wrap-around diagonals, and the labels.

Another Latin square design, intended for n treatments in a spatial row–column layout, with one further block structure is the *Magic Latin square* (attributed to **G.M. Cox** – see Federer [7]). This requires a composite $n = n_1 \times n_2$, and forms spatially compact blocks using congruent $n_1 \times n_2$ rectangular blocks formed by the intersection of n_1 adjoining rows and n_2 adjoining columns. The extra set of blocks is not orthogonal to rows and columns, and care is needed in the analysis – see Bailey et al. [2, 3]. An example with $n = 4 = 2 \times 2$, showing the extra block boundaries, is

1	2	3	4
3	4	1	2
2	1	4	3
4	3	2	1

When $n_1 \neq n_2$, a *super magic Latin square* uses both $n_1 \times n_2$ blocks, and $n_2 \times n_1$ blocks to form two extra sets of blocks. An example with $n = 6 = 2 \times 3 = 3 \times 2$ (with the two blocking structures to the right) is

1	2	3	4	5	6
6	4	5	2	3	1
3	5	1	6	2	4
4	6	2	5	1	3
5	3	6	1	4	2
2	1	4	3	6	5

The nonaliased contrasts in the two extra sets of blocks are not orthogonal – see Bailey et al. [2].

The *gerechte designs* introduced by Behrens [4] can be regarded as a generalization of magic Latin squares which use any convenient spatially compact blocks of size n. The block shapes do not need to be congruent, so that gerechte Latin square designs can be obtained for any n. Gerechte designs also exist for rectangular arrays. Careful analysis is required – see Bailey et al. [2, 3].

References

[1]   Bailey, R.A., Cheng, C.-S. & Kipnis, P. (1992). Construction of trend-resistant factorial designs, *Statistica Sinica* **2**, 393–411.

[2]   Bailey, R.A., Kunert, J. & Martin, R.J. (1990). Some comments on gerechte designs. I. Analysis for uncorrelated errors, *Journal of Agronomy and Crop Science* **165**, 121–130.

[3]   Bailey, R.A., Kunert, J. & Martin, R.J. (1991). Some comments on gerechte designs. II. Randomization analysis, and other methods that allow for inter-plot dependence, *Journal of Agronomy and Crop Science* **166**, 101–111.

[4]   Behrens, W.U. (1956). Die Eignung verschiedener Feldversuchs-anordnungen zum Ausgleich der Bodenunterschiede, *Zeitschrift für Acker-und Pflanzenbau* **101**, 243–278.

[5]   Bradley, R.A. & Yeh, C.-M. (1988). Trend-free block designs, in *Encyclopedia of Statistical Sciences*, Vol. 9, S. Kotz & N.L. Johnson, eds. Wiley, New York, pp. 324–328.

[6]   Dénes, J. & Keedwell, A.D. (1974). *Latin Squares and Their Applications*. English Universities Press, London, Sections 6.1–6.3.

[7]   Federer, W.T. (1955). *Experimental Design–Theory and Applications*. Macmillan, New York, Section XV-3.

[8]   Freeman, G.H. (1985). Magic square designs, in *Encyclopedia of Statistical Sciences*, Vol. 5, S. Kotz & N.L. Johnson, eds. Wiley, New York, pp. 173–174.

[9]   Lin, M. & Dean, A.M. (1991). Trend-free block designs for varietal and factorial experiments, *Annals of Statistics* **19**, 1582–1596.

[10] Phillips, J.P.N. (1964). The use of magic squares for balancing and assessing order effects in some analysis of variance designs, *Applied Statistics* **13**, 67–73.

(*See also* **Factorial Designs in Clinical Trials; Youden Squares and Row–Column Designs**)

R.J. MARTIN

Mahalanobis Distance

In 1936, **P.C. Mahalanobis** [22] proposed a measure, known as the generalized distance, or Mahalanobis distance, to assess the divergence between two populations based on observations on p characters or variates; the square of this distance is given by

$$\Delta^2 = \frac{1}{p}(\mu_1 - \mu_2)' \Sigma^{-1}(\mu_1 - \mu_2),$$

where μ_1 and μ_2 are the mean vectors of the p variates in the two populations, and Σ is the common **covariance matrix**.

Historical Background

In the 1920s, **Karl Pearson** and his associates considered the problem of "asserting significant resemblance or divergence" between racial groups based on anthropological observations (*see* **Anthropometry**). Following Pearson's suggestion, Tildesley [45] considered a measure, known as the "Coefficient of Racial Likeness" (CRL), given by

$$\frac{1}{p}\sum_{i=1}^{p} \frac{(m_{i1} - m_{i2})^2}{\sigma_{i1}^2/n_{i1} + \sigma_{i2}^2/n_{i2}} - 1,$$

where m_{i1}, σ_{i1}^2, and n_{i1} denote the mean, the variance, and the sample size, respectively, corresponding to the ith variate in the first population, and m_{i2}, σ_{i2}^2, and n_{i2} similarly correspond to the second population. In 1926, Pearson [29] considered only the first term of the above expression. Romanovsky [39] also considered some similar criteria.

Mahalanobis, during his study on caste-groups in India, observed that the coefficient of racial likeness was influenced by sample sizes and it failed to measure the divergence [14]. He [21] suggested a general class of measures, and, in particular, considered the following when homoscedasticity holds:

$$D_0^2 = \frac{1}{p}\sum_{i=1}^{p} \frac{(m_{i1} - m_{i2})^2}{\overline{\sigma}_i^2} - \frac{1}{p}\sum_{i=1}^{p} \left(\frac{1}{n_{i1}} + \frac{1}{n_{i2}} \right),$$

where $\overline{\sigma}_i^2$ is a "reliable" value for the common variance of the ith variate. Mahalanobis cited a number of comparisons in which the coefficient of racial

likeness and his D_0^2 measure gave widely different results, but he claimed that the values of D_0^2 gave better representation of known anthropological facts. Furthermore, Mahalanobis also proposes measures to assess divergence in variance, **skewness**, and **kurtosis**.

Later, Mahalanobis [22] introduced the correlations among the variates in defining such a measure, and proposed the measure Δ^2 given above. The sample version of Δ^2 for known Σ is given by

$$D_1^2 = \frac{1}{p}(\overline{\mathbf{x}_1} - \overline{\mathbf{x}_2})' \Sigma^{-1}(\overline{\mathbf{x}_1} - \overline{\mathbf{x}_2}),$$

as well as by

$$D_2^2 = \frac{1}{p}(\overline{\mathbf{x}_1} - \overline{\mathbf{x}_2})' \Sigma^{-1}(\overline{\mathbf{x}_1} - \overline{\mathbf{x}_2}) - \left(\frac{1}{n_1} + \frac{1}{n_2} \right),$$

where $\overline{\mathbf{x}_1}$ and $\overline{\mathbf{x}_2}$ are the sample mean vectors based on samples of sizes n_1 and n_2, respectively. It may be noted that D_2^2 is **unbiased** for estimating Δ^2. For unknown Σ, the sample version of Δ^2 is given by

$$D^2 = \frac{1}{p}(\overline{\mathbf{x}_1} - \overline{\mathbf{x}_2})' \mathbf{S}^{-1}(\overline{\mathbf{x}_1} - \overline{\mathbf{x}_2}),$$

where $\mathbf{S}$ is the pooled within-group sample covariance matrix with degrees of freedom (df) $n_1 + n_2 - 2$.

Under the assumption that the p variates are distributed as a normal distribution in each of the two populations, the distribution of $pD_1^2 n_1 n_2/(n_1 + n_2)$ is noncentral **chi-square** with p df and noncentrality parameter $p\Delta^2 n_1 n_2/(n_1 + n_2)$. R.C. Bose [3, 4] obtained this result along with the **moments** of D_1^2. S.N. Bose [6, 7] also obtained the moments of D_1^2, but without using its distribution explicitly.

For the problem of testing equality of mean vectors of two p-variate normal distributions with common but unknown covariance matrix Σ, Hotelling [19] suggested the **Hotelling's** T^2 statistic, given by

$$T^2 = n_1 n_2 (n_1 + n_2)^{-1} pD^2,$$

as the test statistic and also as a modified form of the Coefficient of Racial Likeness. It was shown by Hotelling [19] that the null distribution of

$$\frac{T^2}{n_1 + n_2 - 2} \frac{n_1 + n_2 - p - 1}{p}$$

is the **F distribution** with p and $n_1 + n_2 - p - 1$ df. This result was also obtained by Fisher [17, 18] in his pioneering papers on **discriminant analysis**; however, Fisher's derivation is not rigorous. Mahalanobis [22] obtained the first four moments of D^2, assuming Σ to be a diagonal matrix. The nonnull distribution of the above statistic is F with df p and $n_1 + n_2 - p - 1$, and noncentrality parameter $n_1 n_2 (n_1 + n_2)^{-1} p\Delta^2$; this was first obtained by Bose & Roy [5]. For a review of the evolution of the D^2-statistic, see DasGupta [14].

Mahalanobis Δ as a Distance

The frame of reference for the work of Mahalanobis was the p-variate normal distribution for the variates under study. It is now known that many standard distance measures, such as Kolmogorov's variational distance, the Hellinger distance, Rao's distance, and so on, are increasing functions of Δ when the two distributions are p-variate normal distributions with mean vectors μ_1 and μ_2, and common covariance matrix Σ [27]. This result also holds for a variety of distance measures for elliptic distributions with different locations but common shape parameters [28]. For other related developments on distance functions, see Rao [31, 33, 37], Matusita [26], and Burbea & Rao [8].

Role of Mahalanobis Distance in Discriminatory Analysis

In order to discriminate between two populations based on observations on p characters X, Fisher [17, 18] considered a linear discriminant function $l'X$ to maximize $[l'(\overline{X_1} - \overline{X_2})]^2/(l'Sl)$. The optimal l turns out to be proportional to $S^{-1}(\overline{X_1} - \overline{X_2})$ and correspondingly, the above ratio becomes pD^2. Fisher then suggested to consider pD^2 as the test statistic to test "significance of the discriminant function", which means testing the equality of the population mean vectors. In this development, Fisher's frame of reference was of course two p-variate normal distributions with common covariance matrix. For the problem of discrimination between two p-variate normal distributions with different covariance matrices, see Anderson [2] and McLachlan [27].

For detailed developments on discriminatory analysis, see Cacoullos [9]. For discrimination of Gaussian processes, see Rao & Varadarajan [38].

Test on Distance

As discussed earlier, Hotelling [19] first proposed a test for $\Delta^2 = 0$ when the underlying distributions are normal with common but unknown covariance matrix. Rao [30, 32] proposed a test for "additional distance", which may be posed as $p\Delta_p^2 = q\Delta_q^2 (q < p)$, where Δ_p^2 denotes the value of Δ^2 based on p variates. DasGupta & Perlman [16] have shown that the power of Hotelling's T^2-test based on p variates may be smaller than the power of the test based on a subset of q variates unless the increase $p\Delta_p^2 - q\Delta_q^2$ is sufficiently large; they have suggested a test based on a preliminary sample so that the effectiveness of inclusion of additional variates could be ascertained.

Rao [35] considered tests for assigned (linear) discriminant functions, as well as for specifications of the ratios of discriminant function coefficients. All of these, in principle, fall into the realm of testing additional distance.

The null distribution of D^2 can be used to obtain simultaneous confidence intervals for $l'(\mu_1 - \mu_2)$; see Anderson [2].

Role of Mahalanobis Distance in Classificatory Analysis

The problem of classifying an observation vector X into one of two p-variate distributions with mean vectors μ_1 and μ_2, and common covariance matrix Σ, was first posed by Fisher [17] and developed later by Wald [47], Rao [34, 36], and Anderson [1], among many others; see McLachlan [27] for an extensive collection of results on this topic. For reviews of earlier work, see DasGupta [11, 13], Cacoullos [9], and Krishnaiah & Kanal [20].

When the parameters are known, the class of Bayes rules is given by the following: classify X into the first population if

$$(\mu_1 - \mu_2)'\Sigma^{-1}\{X - (\mu_1 + \mu_2)/2\} \geq C;$$

otherwise classify into the second population. The probabilities of misclassification of any such rule are functions of Δ; in particular, if $C = 0$, the probabilities of misclassification are equal and the common value decreases as Δ increases. This result also holds when the parameters μ_1, μ_2, and Σ are unknown and they are respectively replaced by $\overline{X_1}$, $\overline{X_2}$, and

S in the above rule, and $n_1 = n_2$; for more detailed results, see DasGupta [12].

DasGupta & Kinderman [15] posed the concept of classifiability which sought condition on the structure of the populations in order to control probabilities of misclassification arbitrarily; for a related development, see Schaafsma & Steerneman [41]. For bounds, approximations, and asymptotic expansions relating to probabilities of misclassification, see McLachlan [27] and DasGupta [12]. For the problem of classification into one of two p-variate normal distributions with different covariance matrices, and the related role of Mahalanobis distance, see McLachlan [27]. Statistical methods for selecting variables in relation to the problem of classification and discriminatory analysis have been discussed in McLachlan [27] and Seber [44] (*see* **Variable Selection**).

Asymptotic Distribution of Δ

For the case of normal distributions, it follows from DasGupta [10] that

$$E(pD^2) = f(f - p - 1)^{-1} p\Delta^2$$
$$+ (n_1^{-1} + n_2^{-1}) f(f - p - 1)^{-1} p,$$

where $f = n_1 + n_2 - 2$. Hence

$$\hat{\Delta}^2 = (f - p - 1)f^{-1}D^2 - (n_1^{-1} + n_2^{-1})$$

is unbiased for estimating Δ^2. Moreover, the variance of $\hat{\Delta}^2$ is given by

$$(f - p - 3)^{-1} \left\{ 2(p\Delta^2)^2 \right.$$
$$+ 4n_1^{-1}n_2^{-1}(n_1 + n_2)(f - 1)p\Delta^2$$
$$\left. + 2p(f - 1)(n_1 + n_2)^2 n_1^{-2} n_2^{-2} \right\}$$

(see Schaafsma [40]).

It has been shown by Schaafsma & Van Verk [42, 43] that

$$E(\sqrt{p}D) = \sqrt{p}\Delta + (4f)^{-1}(2p + 1)(\sqrt{p}\Delta)$$
$$+ (2f)^{-1}(p - 1)\kappa(\sqrt{p}\Delta)^{-1} + O(f^{-2}),$$

and

$$\mathcal{L}\left[f^{1/2}(\sqrt{p}D - \sqrt{p}\Delta) \right] \rightarrow N\left(0, \kappa + \tfrac{1}{2} p\Delta^2 \right),$$

as $n_1, n_2 \rightarrow \infty$, where $f(n_1 + n_2)n_1^{-1}n_2^{-1} \rightarrow \kappa \in (0, \infty)$.

Other Applications

The domain of applications of Mahalanobis distance is quite extensive. In particular, the role of Mahalanobis distance in profile analysis (*see* **Summary Measures Analysis of Longitudinal Data**) and cluster analysis is significant (*see* **Cluster Analysis of Subjects, Nonhierarchical Methods**). See Mardia et al. [25], Van Ryzin [46], and Rao [36], in particular. The first application of Mahalanobis distance in cluster analysis is given in Mahalanobis et al. [23]. It may be noted that Mardia [24] has introduced a concept called "Mahalanobis angle", and illustrated its usefulness.

References

[1]   Anderson, T.W. (1951). Classification by multivariate analysis, *Psychometrika* **16**, 31–50.

[2]   Anderson, T.W. (1984). *An Introduction to Multivariate Statistical Analysis*, 2nd Ed. Wiley, New York.

[3]   Bose, R.C. (1936). On the exact distribution and moment coefficients of the D^2-statistic, *Sankhyā* **2**, 143–154.

[4]   Bose, R.C. (1936). A note on the distribution of differences in mean values of two samples drawn from two multivariate normally distributed populations and the definition of the D^2-statistic, *Sankhyā* **2**, 379–384.

[5]   Bose, R.C. & Roy, S.N. (1938). The distribution of studentized D^2-statistic, *Sankhyā* **4**, 19–38.

[6]   Bose, S.N. (1936). On the complete moment coefficients of the D^2-statistic, *Sankhyā* **2**, 385–396.

[7]   Bose, S.N. (1937). On the moment coefficients of the D^2-statistic, and certain integral and differential equations connected with the multivariate normal populations, *Sankhyā* **3**, 105–124.

[8]   Burbea, J. & Rao, C.R. (1982). Entropy differential metric, distance and divergence measures in probability spaces: a unified approach, *Journal of Multivariate Analysis* **12**, 575–596.

[9]   Cacoullos, T., ed. (1973). *Discriminant Analysis and Applications*. Academic Press, New York.

[10]   DasGupta, S. (1968). Some aspects of discrimination function coefficients, *Sankhyā; Series A* **30**, 387–400.

[11]   DasGupta, S. (1973). Theories and methods in classification: a review, in *Discriminant Analysis and Applications*, T. Cacoullos, ed. Academic Press, New York, pp. 77–137.

[12]   DasGupta, S. (1974). Probability inequalities and errors in classification, *Annals of Statistics* **2**, 751–762.

[13]   DasGupta, S. (1982). Optimum rules for classification into two multivariate normal populations with the same covariance matrix, in *Handbook of Statistics*, Vol. 2, P.R. Krishnaiah & L. Kanal, eds. North-Holland, New York, pp. 47–60.

[14] DasGupta, S. (1993). The evolution of the D^2-statistic of Mahalanobis, *Sankhyā, Series A* **55**, 442–459.

[15] DasGupta, S. & Kinderman, A. (1974). Classifiability and designs for sampling, *Sankhyā* **36**, 237–250.

[16] DasGupta, S. & Perlman, M.D. (1974). Power of the noncentral F-test: effect of additional variates on Hotelling's T^2 test, *Journal of the American Statistical Association* **69**, 174–180.

[17] Fisher, R.A. (1936). The use of multiple measurements in taxonomic problems, *Annals of Eugenics* **7**, 179–188.

[18] Fisher, R.A. (1938). The statistical utilization of multiple measurements, *Annals of Eugenics* **8**, 376–386.

[19] Hotelling, H. (1931). The generalization of Student's ratio, *Annals of Mathematical Statistics* **2**, 360–368.

[20] Krishnaiah, P.R. & Kanal, L., eds (1982). *Handbook of Statistics*, Vol. 2. North-Holland, New York.

[21] Mahalanobis, P.C. (1930). On tests and measures of group divergence, *Journal of the Asiatic Society of Bengal* **26**, 541–588.

[22] Mahalanobis, P.C. (1936). On the generalized distance in statistics, *Proceedings of the National Institute of Sciences of India* **2**, 49–55.

[23] Mahalanobis, P.C., Majumder, D.N. & Rao, C.R. (1949). Anthropometric survey of the United Provinces, 1941: a statistical study, *Sankhyā* **9**, 90–234.

[24] Mardia, K.V. (1977). Mahalanobis distance and angles, in *Multivariate Analysis*, Vol. IV, P.R. Krishnaiah, ed. North-Holland, New York pp. 495–511.

[25] Mardia, K.V., Kent, T. & Bibby, M. (1979). *Multivariate Analysis*. Academic Press, New York.

[26] Matusita, K. (1952). Decision rule based on the distance for the classification problem, *Annals of the Institute of Statistical Mathematics* **8**, 67–77.

[27] McLachlan, G.J. (1992). *Discriminant Analysis and Statistical Pattern Recognition*. Wiley, New York.

[28] Mitchell, A.F.S. & Krzanowski, W.J. (1985). The Mahalanobis distance and elliptic distributions, *Biometrika* **72**, 464–467.

[29] Pearson, K. (1926). On the coefficient of racial likeness, *Biometrika* **18**, 105–117.

[30] Rao, C.R. (1946). Tests on discriminant functions in multivariate analysis, *Sankhyā* **7**, 407–414.

[31] Rao, C.R. (1949). On the distance between two populations, *Sankhyā* **9**, 246–248.

[32] Rao, C.R. (1949). On the problems arising out of discrimination with multiple characters, *Sankhyā* **9**, 343–366.

[33] Rao, C.R. (1954). On the use and interpretation of distance functions in statistics, *Bulletin of the International Statistical Institute* **34**, 90–97.

[34] Rao, C.R. (1950). Statistical inference applied to classificatory problems, *Sankhyā* **10**, 229–256.

[35] R.C. Bose, Chakravarti, I.M., Mahalanobis, P.C., Rao, C.R. & Smith, J.C. (1970). Inference on discriminant function coefficients, in *Essays in Probability and Statistics*. R.C. Bose et al., eds. University of North Carolina Press, Chapel Hill.

[36] Rao, C.R. (1973). *Linear Statistical Inference and Its Applications*, 2nd Ed. Wiley, New York.

[37] Rao, C.R. (1982). Diversity and dissimilarity coefficients: a unified approach, *Journal of Theoretical Population Biology* **21**, 24–43.

[38] Rao, C.R. & Varadarajan, V.S. (1963). Discrimination of Gaussian process, *Sankhyā* A **25**, 303–350.

[39] Romanovsky, V. (1928). On the criteria that two given samples belong to the same normal population (on the different coefficients of racial likeness), *Metron* **7**, 3–46.

[40] Schaafsma, W. (1982). Selecting variables in discriminant analysis for improving upon classical procedures, in *Handbook of Statistics*, Vol. 2, P.R. Krishnaiah & L.N. Kanal, eds. North-Holland, New York, pp. 857–881.

[41] Schaafsma, W. & Steerneman, T. (1981). Discriminant analysis when the number of features is unbounded, *IEEE Transactions on Systems, Man and Cybernetics* **SMC-11**(2), 144–151.

[42] Schaafsma, W. & Van Verk, G.N. (1977). Classification and discrimination problems with applications, part I, *Statistica Neerlandica* **31**, 25–45.

[43] Schaafsma, W. & Van Verk, G.N. (1979). Classification and discrimination problems with applications, part II, *Statistica Neerlandica* **33**, 91–126.

[44] Seber, G.A.F. (1984). *Multivariate Observations*. Wiley, New York.

[45] Tildesley, M.L. (1921). A first study of the Burnese skull, *Biometrika* **13**, 247–251.

[46] Van Ryzin, J., ed. (1977). *Classification and Clustering*. Academic Press, New York.

[47] Wald, A. (1944). On a statistical problem arising in the classification of an individual into one of two groups, *Annals of Mathematical Statistics* **15**, 145–162.

(*See also* **Classification, Overview; Multivariate Analysis, Overview**)

SOMESH DASGUPTA

Mahalanobis, Prasanta Chandra

Born: June 29, 1893, in Calcutta, India.
Died: 1972, in India.

Prasanta Chandra Mahalanobis was educated at Presidency College, Calcutta, and King's College, Cambridge, where he completed the Tripos in Mathematics and Natural Science (Physics). In Part II of the Tripos, he was the only candidate to receive a first class in physics. Cambridge University awarded him a research scholarship. Before starting his research, he traveled to Calcutta for a short vacation, but never returned to England. The war intervened. Also, he had found a teaching job and plenty of other interesting things to do in Calcutta.

Just before Mahalanobis left England for this vacation, his tutor, W.H. Macaulay, drew his attention to the journal **Biometrika**. Mahalanobis found the articles interesting and purchased an entire set of available volumes and brought these back to Calcutta. A window was opened to a new area of science, permanently changing the direction of his life.

Early on, one of his mentors, Acharya Brojendranath Seal, a philosopher and an encyclopedist who was also interested in statistics, said to him "Prasanta, . . . you have to do work in India similar to that of Karl Pearson in England. In today's world, whether it is science or social service, without statistical methods there is no way. This is your job." (Translated from a note in Bengali by P.C. Mahalanobis dated April 17, 1945.) Mahalanobis, who had already begun to read **Karl Pearson's** papers in *Biometrika*, took this challenge seriously. He thus developed an interest in statistical analysis of biological data, which was to last throughout his life and to which he was to make profound contributions.

In 1920, Mahalanobis met the Director of the Zoological and Anthropological Survey of India, Nelson Annandale, who requested Mahalanobis to analyze some **anthropometric** data on a group of Anglo-Indians of Calcutta. Mahalanobis analyzed the data and published his first paper on statistics [1]. He continued to analyze the other anthropometric data in this sample, and presented a synthesis of results in his Presidential Address to the anthropology section of the Indian Science Congress in 1925. In the address, "Analysis of race-mixture in Bengal", Mahalanobis sought to provide answers to several anthropological questions by using statistical methods. (An expanded version of this address was later published by him in 1927 [3].) For example, do Anglo-Indians show a greater affinity with the higher castes of Bengal or with the lower castes? Or, is there any appreciable admixture with aboriginal tribes? To answer such questions, a measure of distance between population groups based on anthropometric measurements was necessary. The only available statistic for comparing resemblance between populations was Pearson's coefficient of racial likeness (CRL) [11, 13].

Mahalanobis realized that the CRL provided a test of divergence between samples drawn from two populations rather than a measure of the actual magnitude of the divergence, because the magnitude of the CRL was dependent on sample sizes. In the study on Anglo-Indians, Mahalanobis proposed and used a measure of the actual magnitude of divergence that he called the "first (provisional) measure of caste distance", D. The resulting inferences derived by Mahalanobis have been found to be largely valid from his own work conducted later in the United Provinces [10] and in Bengal, as well as in later studies of others using more extensive data and more sophisticated statistical techniques.

During the period 1926–1927, Mahalanobis spent about six months in Karl Pearson's laboratory in the University College, London. During this period, he undertook an extensive analysis of anthropometric data of various European population groups, and closely examined the utility of the CRL for measuring population relationships. In the process, the statistical shortcomings of the CRL became clearer. Upon returning to India, Mahalanobis's ideas on the problem of incorporating the observed **correlations** among anthropometric measurements used in measuring distance took a more concrete form. He published a seminal paper, "On tests and measures of Group Divergence" in 1930, in which the famous D^2-statistic was proposed (*see* **Mahalanobis Distance**) [4]. Based primarily on work done by him in Pearson's laboratory, Mahalanobis published a paper in *Biometrika* in the same year [5]. This paper was the "first application of CRL to the discrimination of racial differences to be ascertained from measurements on the living" (p. 94). It dealt with the populations of Sweden, and Mahalanobis presented an innovative graphical display of anthropometric interrelationships among the populations, taking two additional extrinsic variables into account, geographical location of habitat and occupation. Thus, the concept of forming clusters of populations began to take shape (*see* **Cluster Analysis, Variables**).

Mahalanobis subsequently proposed the "natural" generalized distance D^2 for correlated variates, as well as its Studentized form using sample values of parameters [8]. In retrospect, it is clear that both measures play a fundamental, important role in statistics and data analysis. The practical impact of the D^2 statistic has been enormous, and continues to be used in many branches of science.

Mahalanobis was apparently not satisfied with simply providing a valuable tool (D^2) for cluster analysis. He began to raise fundamental issues about the application of the D^2 statistic, and argued that inferences on affinities among populations may depend on the number of measurements chosen for assessing distances between populations; in which case, conclusions would not have the desired practical significance. Affinity configurations may change if one set of measurements is replaced by another. Mahalanobis thus laid down an important axiom for the validity of cluster analysis, "dimensional convergence of D^2" [9]. Suppose D_p^2 and D_∞^2 denote, respectively, the distance between a pair of populations based on a set of p measurements and the distance based on all of the measurements. Since it is not possible practically to study all possible measurements, biometrical studies must rely on a finite number, p, of measurements. For affinity relationships to be stable, the distance based on p characters should be a good approximation of that based on the set of all possible characters. For Mahalanobis's distance measure, it can be shown that $D_p^2 \leq D_\infty^2$ and $D_p^2 \to D_\infty^2$ as $p \to \infty$. Mahalanobis's axiom of dimensional convergence states that a suitable choice of p can be made if and only if D^2 is finite. Unfortunately, this important axiom is not mentioned in most textbooks on numerical taxonomy or cluster analysis.

The formulation of the D^2 statistic, derivation of its properties, and its applications are undoubtedly the most profound contributions of Mahalanobis to biostatistics. However, Mahalanobis made many other interesting contributions. Some of the early statistical studies he undertook were on **experimental designs** in agriculture. In 1924, he made some important discoveries pertaining to the probable error of results of agricultural experiments, which put him in touch with **R.A. Fisher**. Later, in 1926, he met Fisher at the Rothamsted Experimental Station and a close personal relationship was immediately established that lasted until Fisher's death. He possessed an uncanny sense of numbers and could quickly point out recording mistakes in data. In two papers entitled, "Revision of Risley's anthropometric data", Mahalanobis [6, 7] reconstructed the large series of anthropometric data, which were earlier condemned as faulty and unsuitable for statistical analysis. This work was highly praised by Sir Ronald Fisher [12]. He also conducted studies on dextrality of snail shells, correlates of disease prevalence in humans and plants,

demography, and so on. In most of these studies, Mahalanobis developed novel statistical methods or made innovative applications of known methods. For example, in one of his early statistical studies on the **prevalence** of dysentery and its correlates, Mahalanobis [2] developed some useful smoothing techniques for **time-series** data using Fourier series (*see* **Fast Fourier Transform (FFT)**). Such techniques are now commonly used.

Mahalanobis's contributions to large-scale **sample surveys**, which are among his most significant and lasting gifts to statistics, began with problems of the estimation of area and yield of the jute crop in Bengal in 1937. He was able to demonstrate that estimates based on sample surveys were often more accurate than those based on complete enumeration, and that sample surveys could yield estimates with small margins of error within a short time and at a smaller cost than complete enumeration. He made many methodological contributions to survey sampling that included optimal choice of sampling design (*see* **Optimal Design**) using **variance** and cost functions, and the technique of an **interpenetrating** network of subsamples for assessment and control of errors, especially **nonsampling errors**, in surveys. The concept of pilot surveys was a forerunner of **sequential analysis** developed by **Abraham Wald**, as acknowledged by Wald. In addition to introducing these concepts, Mahalanobis raised important and difficult philosophical questions on the **randomness** and representativeness of a sample, which remain relevant and challenging even today. He was elected Chairman of the United Nations Sub-Commission on Statistical Sampling in 1947, and held this post till 1951. His tireless advocacy of the usefulness of sample surveys resulted in the final recommendation of this Sub-Commission that sampling methods should be extended to all parts of the world. Mahalanobis received the Weldon Medal from Oxford University in 1944 and was elected a Fellow of The Royal Society, London, in 1945, for his fundamental contributions to statistics, particularly in the area of large-scale sample surveys.

As a scientist, Mahalanobis was, above all, a great applied statistician. Statistics were to be used for a better understanding of scientific data, and for decision-making for the welfare of society. Innovation, systematization and concrete applications are the hallmarks of the applied statistics practiced by Mahalanobis.

References

[1] Mahalanobis, P.C. (1922). Anthropological observations on the Anglo-Indians of Calcutta. Part I: Analysis of male stature, *Records of the Indian Museum* **23**, 1–96.

[2] Mahalanobis, P.C. (1926). Appendicitis, rainfall and bowel complaints. Part II. Scope of the enquiry, *Calcutta Medical Journal* **21**, 151–187.

[3] Mahalanobis, P.C. (1927). Analysis of race-mixture in Bengal, *Journal of Asiatic Society of Bengal* **23**, 301–333.

[4] Mahalanobis, P.C. (1930). On tests and measures of group divergence, *Journal of Asiatic Society of Bengal* **26**, 541–588.

[5] Mahalanobis, P.C. (1930). A statistical study of certain anthropometric measurements from Sweden, *Biometrika* **22**, 94–108.

[6] Mahalanobis, P.C. (1933). Revision of Risley's anthropometric data relating to tribes and castes of Bengal, *Sankhyā* **1**, 76–105.

[7] Mahalanobis, P.C. (1934). Revision of Risley's data relating to Chittagong hill tribes, *Sankhyā* **1**, 267–276.

[8] Mahalanobis, P.C. (1936). On the generalized distance in statistics, *Proceedings of the National Institute of Science* **2**, 49–55.

[9] Mahalanobis, P.C., Bose, R.C. & Roy, S.N. (1937). Normalization of statistical variates and the use of rectangular coordinates in the theory of sampling distributions (appendix), *Sankhyā* **3**, 35–40.

[10] Mahalanobis, P.C., Majumder, D.N. & Rao, C.R. (1949). Anthropometric survey of the United Provinces, 1941: a statistical study, *Sankhyā* **9**, 90–324.

[11] Pearson, K. (1936). On the coefficient of racial likeness, *Biometrika* **13**, 105–117.

[12] Rao, C.R. (1974). Prasanta Chandra Mahalanobis, 1893–1972. *Biographical Memories of Fellows of the Royal Society* **19**, 455–492.

[13] Tildesley, M.L. (1921). A first study of the Burmese skull, *Biometrika* **13**, 247–251.

J.K. GHOSH & PARTHA P. MAJUMDER

Main Effects Contrast *see* Contrasts

Mainland, Donald

Born: April 5, 1902.
Died: July 1985 in Kent, Connecticut.

Donald Mainland graduated in medicine at Edinburgh. He later taught anatomy in Edinburgh and received a Doctor of Science degree there for his research in embryology and histology. He moved to Manitoba, Canada, in 1927 and in 1930 became Professor and Chairman of the Department of Anatomy at Dalhousie University.

His early publications showed a concern about measurement issues, and foreshadowed an increasing interest in statistics. In 1936 he wrote on problems of chance in clinical work [2] and the following year he published his first book on statistics in medicine [3]. In 1950 he became Professor of Medical Statistics at New York University and shortly afterwards published his best known book, *Elementary Medical Statistics* [4]. Thereafter, Mainland was a prolific and influential writer on statistical topics.

In addition to his books, Mainland's notable contributions included several series of short essays on statistical topics, most of which were not published in journals but circulated to those "who were lucky enough to learn about 'the Notes', and to satisfy Mainland's hardy standards for the mailing list" [1]. From August 1959 to September 1966 he produced 145 items in the series, *Notes from a Laboratory of Medical Statistics* [5], a further 104 items in the series, *Notes on Biometry in Medical Research* [7], and 16 longer articles as "statistical ward rounds" from 1967 to 1969 in *Clinical Pharmacology and Therapeutics* [6].

After his retirement, Mainland continued to publish occasionally on statistical issues, with two typical outspoken and readable papers published in the *British Medical Journal* when he was in his eighties [8, 9].

The common sense consistently displayed in his writings was undoubtedly greatly aided by his extensive research and teaching in biology – he had also published a textbook on anatomy – and active participation in clinical research.

In 1970, when Mainland ceased writing his series in *Clinical Pharmacology and Therapeutics*, his successor in that role, Alvan Feinstein, described Mainland's contributions to improving the understanding and practice of statistics in medicine [1]. Among his generous comments Feinstein observed, "With his textbook . . . and his many other writings, he has probably contributed as much as any single person to the statistical sensibility of clinical investigators in North America" [1].

References

[1] Feinstein, A.R. (1970). Clinical biostatistics – 1. A new name – and some other changes of the guard, *Clinical Pharmacology and Therapeutics* **11**, 135–148 (reprinted in Feinstein, A.R. (1977). *Clinical Biostatistics.* C.V. Mosby Co., Saint Louis, pp. 1–14).

[2] Mainland, D. (1936). Problems of chance in clinical work, *British Medical Journal* **2**, 221–224.

[3] Mainland, D. (1938). *The Treatment of Clinical and Laboratory Data: An Introduction to Statistical Ideas and Methods for Medical and Dental Workers.* Oliver & Boyd, Edinburgh.

[4] Mainland, D. (1950). *Elementary Medical Statistics: the Principles of Quantitative Medicine* (2nd Ed., 1963). W.B. Saunders, Philadelphia.

[5] Mainland, D. (1959–1966) *Notes from a Laboratory of Medical Statistics* (a series of 145 mimeographed notes distributed by the author).

[6] Mainland, D. (1967–1969) Statistical ward rounds, *Clinical Pharmacology and Therapeutics* **8**, 139–146 to **10**, 576–586 (a series of 16 articles).

[7] Mainland, D. (1967–1970) *Notes on Biometry in Medical Research.* Veterans, Administration Monographs, Washington.

[8] Mainland, D. (1984). Statistical ritual in clinical journals: is there a cure? – I, *British Medical Journal* **288**, 841–843.

[9] Mainland, D. (1984). Statistical ritual in clinical journals: is there a cure? – II, *British Medical Journal* **288**, 920–922.

DOUGLAS G. ALTMAN

Major Histocompatibility Complex
see HLA System

Malaria *see* Epidemic Models, Deterministic

Mallows' C_p Statistic

This criterion can be helpful in selecting a biased linear model with fewer parameters and lower **mean square error** (MSE) than one with more parameters and their associated estimation errors. If a p-parameter linear model is fitted by unweighted **least squares** to n observations $y_1, \ldots, y_n$ (supposed uncorrelated and homoscedastic with variance σ^2) giving a residual sum of squares RSS_p (*see* **Analysis of Variance**), then C_p is defined by

$$C_p = (\text{RSS}_p/s^2) - (n - 2p),$$

where s^2 is a trustworthy estimate of σ^2.

This criterion was introduced by Jones [2] in the equivalent form

$$JC_p(\text{say}) = [\text{RSS}_p - (n - 2p)s^2]/n.$$

Under the conditions stated and if $\text{E}(s^2) = \sigma^2$, JC_p is an **unbiased** estimate of the MSE, $\text{E}\{\sum \hat{y}_i - \text{E}(y_i)]^2/n\}$, of the model's fitted values as estimates of the true expectations of the observations. (A model with low MSE, as thus defined, may have good performance only for values of the independent variables in the region already observed.)

In order to guide the delicate practical choice of linear model from a number of alternatives, Mallows [3] developed his independent discovery of C_p into a graphical plot of C_p against p on which the line $C_p = p$ is drawn. In this plot the value of p is (roughly) the contribution to C_p from the variance of the estimated parameters, while the remainder $C_p - p$ is (roughly) the contribution from the **bias** of the model. This feature makes the plot a useful device for a broad assessment of the C_p values of a range of models. Its use does not (or at least should not) in itself inhibit choice of the model with the minimum value of C_p. Moreover, if that choice is made, the plot gives no obvious quantitative indication of the extent to which that minimum value, converted to JC_p, underestimates, as a consequence of selection bias, the actually operative MSE. (In [4], Mallows uses asymptotics in which, realistically, p goes to infinity with n – to provide such a quantitative indication, for a range of applications of the plot.)

The numerical comparisons in Burman [1] suggest that the use of just a "one-deep", leave-one-out cross-validatory criterion (*see* **Cross-Validation**) may be more **robust** than C_p with respect to that selection bias. However, suggestions like this should be treated cautiously: the whole area abounds in competing and only partially substantiated claims.

For the relationship between C_p and Akaike's AIC, *see* **Akaike's Criteria**.

References

[1]   Burman, P. (1996). Model fitting via testing, *Statistica Sinica* **6**, 589–601.
[2]   Jones, H.L. (1946). Linear regression functions with neglected variables, *Journal of the American Statistical Association* **41**, 356–369.
[3]   Mallows, C.L. (1973). Some comments on C_p, *Technometrics* **15**, 661–675.
[4]   Mallows, C.L. (1995). More comments on C_p, *Technometrics* **37**, 362–372.

(*See also* **Diagnostics; Goodness of Fit; Model, Choice of; Multiple Linear Regression; Variable Selection**)

M. STONE

Malthus, Thomas Robert

Born: February 17, 1766, in Guildford, UK.
Died: December 23, 1834, in Bath, UK.

After an early education by private tutors, Malthus went to Jesus College, Cambridge, where he studied history, poetry, modern languages, classics, and mathematics. He was elected to a Fellowship at Jesus in 1793, and became a curate in a small town, Albury, in 1798. In that year he published the first version of his celebrated *Essay on the Principle of Population as it affects the Future Improvement of Society*, to be followed in his lifetime by five further editions. Malthus argued that a population would tend to increase geometrically, whereas the means of subsistence would increase only linearly. The consequent pressure caused by increasingly inadequate means of support would be a major determinant of political events and structures. The task of government was to counteract this dire prognosis by measures of population control, such as the encouragement of later marriage, rather than relying on increased poverty and mortality. Malthus's gloomy views ran counter to those of many progressive thinkers, but influenced Darwin's thought.

Malthus was a strong advocate of statistical investigation, and was a founder member of the Statistical Society of London (later the **Royal Statistical Society**) in 1834. His death, only nine months later, led the Society's Council to lament the loss of one "so celebrated in every part of the world where the science of Statistics is cultivated", describing him as "an ardent lover of truth, ... a sedulous investigator of facts, and a generous encourager of all who have followed in the same laborious path" [2] (see also [1, 3]).

The "Malthusian parameter" denotes the rate of increase that would ultimately be achieved by a population with observed age-specific birth and death-rates (*see* **Demography**).

References

[1]   Keyfitz, N. (1985). Malthus, Thomas Robert, in *Encyclopedia of Statistical Sciences*, Vol. 5, S. Kotz & N.L. Johnson, eds. Wiley, New York, pp. 189–190.
[2]   Royal Statistical Society (1934). *Annals of the Royal Statistical Society, 1834–1934*. Royal Statistical Society, London.
[3]   Stephen, L. (1896). Malthus, Thomas Robert, *Dictionary of National Biography* **36**, 1–5.

P. ARMITAGE

Malthusian Parameter *see* **Branching Processes**

Managed Care *see* **Health Services Organization in the US**

Manhattan Metric *see* **Genetic Distance**

Mann–Whitney Test *see* **Wilcoxon–Mann–Whitney Test**

Manski–Lerman Sampling *see* Case–Control Study, Two-Phase

Mantel's Test for Clustering *see* Clustering

Mantel–Haenszel Methods

Biomedical, clinical, patient-oriented, and public health research investigations frequently focus on the relationship between a primary **factor**, such as an exposure, a new therapy, or an intervention, and a **response variable** such as disease classification, functional status, or degree of improvement. When both of these variables are reported on categorical data scales, the resulting data typically are summarized as observed frequencies in a two-way **contingency table**. However, this *factor–response* relationship may be influenced by other *covariables* or **covariates**, such as clinical centers or baseline characteristics. Consequently, appropriate adjustments for these covariables must be incorporated into the data analysis.

The historical review of Mantel–Haenszel methods outlined in this article is drawn heavily from the extensive review article by Kuritz et al. [34]. In a classic paper, Cochran [13] proposed a test for several **two-by-two tables** based on **binomial** model assumptions. Five years later, Mantel & Haenszel (MH) [46] approached this same problem using a **hypergeometric** probability model, which permits either exact tests or requires only the overall sample size to be large for asymptotic results to hold. The resulting test statistics from these two procedures are nearly identical, except for applications in which the within-table sample sizes are sparse. In particular, the MH test statistic is entirely appropriate for within-table sample sizes as small as two, provided that there are enough tables. Birch [5] demonstrated that when within-table **odds ratios** are homogeneous, the MH test statistic is the uniformly **most powerful** unbiased (UMPU) test. Also, it is asymptotically equivalent to specific likelihood ratio (LR) tests from unconditional

logistic regression when within-table sample sizes are large, and to specific LR tests from **conditional logistic regression** when within-table sample sizes are small [9].

Mantel–Haenszel (MH) procedures are most useful to test H_0: "no partial association" against alternatives encompassing an average effect of the *factor* on the *response* across strata based on the set of *covariables*. In many situations, the sample sizes for some tables may be sparse, the magnitude of the partial association may vary across tables, and the association may be small within subtables. However, if the association is slight, but consistent across the tables, MH procedures will be effective in detecting that association.

Perhaps the most important distinguishing feature of the MH procedures are their connections to randomization model considerations. Quite frequently, health research data are collected under observational study designs such as **case–control studies**, or convenience sampling for a randomized, **multicenter** efficacy trial. For such situations, MH procedures provide a randomization, design-based approach to **hypothesis testing**. These methods require no assumptions other than the **randomization** of subjects to factor levels, either explicitly as in randomized controlled **clinical trials**, or implicitly by hypothesis or from conditional distribution arguments for observational data from restrictive populations such as **retrospective studies**, nonrandomized **cohort** studies or case–control studies [30, 35].

In a strict statistical sense, the conclusions from an MH analysis might apply only to the study sample. Consequently, generalizations to a target population require nonstatistical arguments concerning the representativeness of the study subjects to the individuals in the target population. These issues of "extended inference," in contrast to "local inference," are discussed in more detail in Koch et al. [30, 31].

The MH methods for hypothesis testing and estimation of an average odds ratio for a set of 2×2 tables are reviewed in this article, both for factor-response and repeated measures study designs. Extensive details on the variance formulae for this average odds ratio are provided in [34], using a unified set of notation. The applications of these methods for investigating treatment differences and within-treatment change over time are illustrated using data from two different randomized, controlled **clinical trials**.

For the sake of brevity, the extensions of this MH methodology to a set of $s \times r$ contingency tables are summarized, but are illustrated only once using repeated measures ordinal data. The matrix formulations for these generalized MH methods are outlined in the Appendix.

The extent to which the factor–response partial association varies across tables is of critical concern to the interpretation of final results. For a set of 2×2 tables, methods assessing the variation of stratum-specific odds ratios are reviewed in Gart [24], and a popular method to test for homogeneity of the odds ratios across strata under minimal assumptions is described in Breslow & Day [9] (*see* **Breslow–Day Test**). In settings in which sample sizes are adequate within each table, additive **loglinear models** can be fitted to the data and interaction evaluated through tests for their goodness of fit [2, 7]. Otherwise, an exact procedure based on the extended hypergeometric distribution is described in [40] and [50], and has been implemented in the **StatXact** software of Mehta & Patel [50] (*see* **Exact Inference for Categorical Data**).

Notation and General Methodology

Let $h = 1, 2, \ldots, t$ index strata and let n_{hij} denote the number of sample subjects jointly classified as belonging to the ith factor level, the jth level of response, and the hth stratum. The resulting $s \times r$ contingency table for the hth stratum can be summarized as in Table 1.

For hypotheses involving the *factor–response* association, h indexes the t levels of stratification determined by the cross-classification of the covariables. However, for repeated measurement designs, the primary hypothesis involves homogeneity of the response distribution across levels of the repeated

Table 1   The observed contingency table for stratum h

Factor levels	Response variable categories				
	1	2	...	r	Total
1	n_{h11}	n_{h12}	...	n_{h1r}	$n_{h1.}$
2	n_{h21}	n_{h22}	...	n_{h2r}	$n_{h2.}$
$\vdots$	$\vdots$	$\vdots$		$\vdots$	$\vdots$
s	n_{hs1}	n_{hs2}	...	n_{hsr}	$n_{hs.}$
Total	$n_{h.1}$	$n_{h.2}$	...	$n_{h.r}$	n_h

measurement dimension, so that h indexes the t subjects or unique matched sets.

If the row marginal totals $\{n_{hi.}\}$ and column marginal totals $\{n_{h.j}\}$ in Table 1 are assumed fixed, the overall H_0: "no partial association" can be stated as

H_0: For each of the stratum levels indexed by $h = 1, 2, \ldots, t$, the response variable is distributed at random with respect to the factor levels   (1)

In other words, from a finite population sampling perspective, H_0 assumes that the observed data in each row of the hth stratum can be regarded as a successive set of simple random samples of sizes $\{n_{hi.}\}$ from a fixed population corresponding to the column marginal totals $\{n_{h.j}\}$.

Under H_0 in (1), the observed frequencies, $\{n_{hij}\}$, follow the multiple hypergeometric probability model,

$$\Pr(\mathbf{n}_h | H_0) = \frac{\displaystyle\prod_{i=1}^{s} n_{hi.}! \prod_{j=1}^{r} n_{h.j}!}{n_h! \displaystyle\prod_{i=1}^{s} \prod_{j=1}^{r} n_{hij}!}. \quad (2)$$

The expression in (2) simplifies to the familiar Fisher's exact probability for a single 2×2 table (*see* **Fisher's Exact Test**). In general, under H_0 in (1), we can compute expected values for each frequency and the covariance of each frequency with each of the other frequencies in Table 1 as outlined in the Appendix. Using these quantities, we can investigate a series of alternative hypotheses involving "average effects" of the primary factor on the distribution of the response variable, adjusted for the strata effects, depending on the measurement scales of each.

Alternative Hypothesis: General Association

When both row and column variables are measured on nominal scales (*see* **Nominal Data**), H_0 can be rejected in favor of the response variable differing in nonspecific patterns across factor levels, adjusted for the covariates. As noted in the Appendix, the generalized MH **chi-square test** statistic in (A3), with $(s-1)(r-1)$ **degrees of freedom** (df) is based on the sums of the differences between the observed and expected frequencies, relative to the sum of the covariance matrices over the t tables.

In unmatched studies, for the special case in which $s = r = 2$, the resulting data can be summarized in a set of t 2×2 tables. Here $Q_{\text{MH}(1)}$ is identical to the test statistic proposed in Birch [5], is identical (except for the lack of a continuity correction) to the statistic recommended in Mantel & Haenszel [46], and differs from the test statistic proposed in Cochran [13] only by a factor of $(n_h - 1)/n_h$ in the variance term for each table.

In repeated measurement or matched design, $Q_{\text{MH}(1)}$ simplifies to a number of familiar test statistics as noted in White et al. [62] and Somes [58]. In particular, if the response variable is dichotomous $r = 2$, $Q_{\text{MH}(1)}$ is equivalent to **McNemar's test** [48] when $s = 2$ and to Cochran's Q criterion [12] when $s > 2$. Furthermore, for $r > 2$ and $s > 2$, this result is identical to the "Lagrange multiplier" test derived in Birch [6], the test of interchangeability due to Madansky [41], and the extended Mantel–Haenszel criterion described in Darroch [14], Mantel & Byar [44], and White et al. [62].

Alternative Hypothesis: Mean Responses Differ

If the response variable is ordinal (*see* **Ordered Categorical Data**), the average response for each factor level can be estimated by assigning column **scores**, say $a_{h1}, a_{h2}, \ldots, a_{hr}$, and forming the mean score,

$$\overline{f}_{hi} = \sum_{j=1}^{r} \frac{a_{hj} n_{hij}}{n_{hi\cdot}}, \tag{3}$$

for the ith row within the hth stratum. The specific choice of the scores is not discussed here; further details are available in Landis et al. [36], Koch & Edwards [29], and Koch et al. [32].

As summarized in the Appendix, differences of these s mean scores from their corresponding expected values across the subtables, relative to their covariances, can be used to create a test statistic, $Q_{\text{MH}(2)}$ in (A4), that reflects the extent to which the mean scores for certain levels of the factor consistently exceed (or are exceeded by) the mean scores for other levels of the factor. In

particular, for $s = 2$ this test is identical to the extended MH test statistic proposed in Mantel [42]. Moreover, if marginal **rank** or ridit-type scores are obtained from each table, with midranks assigned for ties, $Q_{\text{MH}(2)}$ is equivalent to an extension of the Kruskal–Wallis **analysis of variance** (ANOVA) test on ranks, conditioning on the levels of the strata (*see* **Nonparametric Methods**); for $s = 2$, this is the van Elteren [61] test, for which additional discussion is given in Lehmann & Dabrerd [38]. More recent evaluation of the MH mean score statistic is found in Davis & Chung [15].

Within repeated measures designs, $Q_{\text{MH}(2)}$ is equivalent to the MH statistic provided in Breslow & Day [9] for matched case–control data with an ordinal risk factor. Where marginal rank scores are assigned within each stratum, $Q_{\text{MH}(2)}$ simplifies to the Friedman [20] chi-square criterion from a two-way rank ANOVA within blocks for subjects (*see* **Nonparametric Methods**). In both designs, $Q_{\text{MH}(2)}$ with df $= (s - 1)$ provides increased statistical **power** to detect departures from homogeneity across factor levels for an ordered response variable, relative to $Q_{\text{MH}(1)}$ with df $= (s - 1)(r - 1)$, although more complex patterns of association will not necessarily be detected.

Alternative Hypothesis: Linear Trend in Mean Responses

When both rows and columns are measured on an ordinal scale, we can assign row scores, say $c_{h1}, c_{h2}, \ldots, c_{hs}$, to the rows, as well as $a_{h1}, a_{h2}, \ldots, a_{hr}$ assigned to the columns. Then, as outlined in the Appendix, the generalized MH test statistic with df $= 1$ investigates the extent to which there is a consistent positive (or negative) association between the response scores and the factor level scores in the respective strata. Specifically, $Q_{\text{MH}(3)}$ in (A5) is directed at the extent to which H_0 is contradicted in favor of a linear progression in the average response across the levels of the factor relative to the assigned scores.

This statistic, $Q_{\text{MH}(3)}$, is identical to the correlation statistic proposed by Mantel [42] and Birch [6]. If marginal rank or ridit-type scores are assigned to both the rows and columns of each table, with midranks assigned for ties, this statistic is equivalent to an extension of the **Spearman rank correlation** test, conditioning on the levels of the covariates. With only one degree of freedom, this statistic has increased power relative to either $Q_{\mathrm{MH}(1)}$ or $Q_{\mathrm{MH}(2)}$ for linear correlation alternatives relative to the assigned scores.

Factor–Response Designs

The MH methods for the standard *factor–response* designs will be described, first beginning with the familiar 2×2 table layout.

2×2 Tables

In this simplest case, the data can be arranged in a series of t 2×2 tables. All three test statistics outlined in the Appendix are identical, having df $= 1$, and simplify (except for the lack of a continuity correction) to the familiar MH statistic,

$$
Q_{\mathrm{MH}(1)} = \frac{\left[\displaystyle\sum_{h=1}^{t} n_{h11} - \sum_{h=1}^{t} \frac{n_{h1.} n_{h.1}}{n_h} \right]^2}{\displaystyle\sum_{h=1}^{t} \frac{n_{h1.} n_{h2.} n_{h.1} n_{h.2}}{n_h^2 (n_h - 1)}}. \quad (4)
$$

Guidelines concerning sample size requirements in order for the chi-square approximation for $Q_{\mathrm{MH}(1)}$ to be appropriate are provided by Mantel & Fleiss [45]; briefly, the sum across the t strata of the observed frequency for each cell of the 2×2 table should have an expected value exceeding 5 and an allowable range of 5 on each side of the expected value. Further sample size discussions are available in Breslow & Day [9], Fleiss [19], and Koch et al. [32].

This MH statistic in (4) can be viewed as a test directed at the alternative hypothesis that a weighted average of the stratum-specific odds ratios, say $\bar{\psi} = \sum_h w_h \psi_h / \sum_h w_h$, differs from 1, the expected value under H_0. Having rejected H_0, the most widely accepted estimator for $\bar{\psi}$ is

$$
\hat{\bar{\psi}}_{\mathrm{MH}} = \frac{\displaystyle\sum_{h=1}^{t} n_{h11} n_{h22} / n_h}{\displaystyle\sum_{h=1}^{t} n_{h12} n_{h21} / n_h}, \quad (5)
$$

as proposed in the original MH paper [46]. In addition, many estimators have been proposed for the common odds ratio, ψ, under the assumption of homogeneity of the stratum-specific odds ratios. Among these are the unconditional maximum likelihood [21, 24], Woolf [63], and the modified Woolf [22, 25] estimator. These estimators require large within-stratum sample sizes, assuming that the number of strata t remains fixed, but the total number of subjects increases without bound. In contrast, the conditional maximum likelihood estimator [5, 23] is appropriate with as few as $n_h = 2$ observations per stratum, provided that t is sufficiently large.

All of these estimators are **consistent**, asymptotically normal, and (at $\psi = 1$ for $\hat{\bar{\psi}}_{\mathrm{MH}}$) asymptotically efficient [8, 60]. Simulation work by McKinlay [47] and Hauck et al. [28] has demonstrated that there is little difference among the estimators in terms of bias and precision for the unmatched design with large numbers of subjects in each stratum. The Woolf and modified Woolf statistics have been shown to have a large bias problem as stratum sample sizes become more moderate. When considering ease of computation together with statistical properties, McKinlay [47] has recommended using the MH estimator in (5).

A number of variance formulas for the average odds ratio in (5) have been proposed over the years, as summarized in Kuritz et al. [34]. Based on theoretical considerations, as well as simulation studies [10, 18, 53], the estimator of choice for computing the asymptotic variance of the MH average odds ratio in (5) is

$$
\mathrm{var}_{\mathrm{RBG}}(\hat{\bar{\psi}}_{\mathrm{MH}})
$$

$$
= \frac{(\hat{\bar{\psi}}_{\mathrm{MH}}^2) \displaystyle\sum_{h=1}^{t} \left\{ \frac{S_h}{n_h} \left[\frac{n_{h22}}{\hat{\bar{\psi}}_{\mathrm{MH}}} + n_{h12} \right] + \frac{R_h}{n_h} \left[\frac{n_{h21}}{\hat{\bar{\psi}}_{\mathrm{MH}}} + \frac{n_{h11}}{\hat{\bar{\psi}}_{\mathrm{MH}}^2} \right] \right\}}{\left(\displaystyle\sum_{h=1}^{t} S_h \right)^{-2}}
$$

$$
(6)
$$

where $R_h = n_{h11} n_{h22} / n_h$, $S_h = n_{h12} n_{h21} / n_h$, and the subscript "RBG" denotes "Robins, Breslow and Greenland". This variance estimator has been selected for the asymptotic method of choice in the StatXact software system [50].

When there is only one stratum ($t = 1$), this RBG variance estimator simplifies to the usual large-sample variance for the odds ratio from a single 2×2 table, as presented in Fleiss [19], which is

$$
\mathrm{var}(\hat{\psi}) = \hat{\psi}^2 \left(\frac{1}{n_{11}} + \frac{1}{n_{12}} + \frac{1}{n_{21}} + \frac{1}{n_{22}} \right). \quad (7)
$$

Unlike the alternative model-based estimates of "partial association", the MH estimate in (5) was intended to be a weighted average of the individual odds ratios [43], where the weights are related to the precision of $\hat{\psi}_h$ [9, 17]. In fact, Mantel & Haenszel [46] indicated their disbelief in the constancy of the underlying odds ratio, stating that the assumption of a constant relative risk is usually untenable. McKinlay [47] interpreted (5) as representing the constant component of an association across strata; whereas Landis et al. [35] and others refer to this quantity as "average partial association". Even though the stratum-specific odds ratios may be heterogeneous, one often is interested in a summary measure [26]. However, most investigators generally agree that a combined odds ratio, which is based on individual odds ratios that differ substantially in direction, some being less than unity and others greater than unity, can be difficult to interpret and perhaps should not be used.

Formal statistical tests for this hypothesis of homogeneous odds ratios across strata can be conducted within the context of fitting an additive logit-linear model with either maximum likelihood or weighted least squares methods, provided that the within-stratum sample sizes are adequate. Details of these methods are provided in Koch et al. [32] and Agresti [2]. Otherwise, under an extension of the hypergeometric probability model in (2), Breslow & Day [9] proposed a test statistic directed at the potential lack of homogeneity of odds ratios (*see* **Breslow–Day Test**),

$$Q_{\mathrm{BD}} = \sum_{h=1}^{t} \frac{\left[n_{h11} - \mathrm{E}(n_{h11}|\widehat{\overline{\psi}}_{MH})\right]^2}{\mathrm{var}(n_{h11}|\widehat{\overline{\psi}}_{MH})}, \quad (8)$$

where $\mathrm{E}(n_{h11}|\widehat{\overline{\psi}}_{\mathrm{MH}})$ is the expected value of n_{h11} under the hypothesis of homogeneity of odds ratios,

$\mathrm{var}(n_{h11}|\widehat{\overline{\psi}}_{\mathrm{MH}})$ is the variance of n_{h11} under the same hypothesis, and $\widehat{\overline{\psi}}_{\mathrm{MH}}$ is the estimate of the average odds ratio under this homogeneity hypothesis. Assuming acceptably large sample sizes in each subtable, Q_{BD} can be compared to the chi-square distribution with df $= t - 1$ for assessing statistical significance. This test statistic and p value is produced within the FREQ procedure in SAS [54]. Further work has recently been done evaluating tests of association and homogeneity, along with estimators of common odds ratios and risk ratios, in sparse data situations [51, 56, 57].

The data in Table 2 were obtained from a randomized, controlled clinical trial conducted at each of eight clinics, as reported in Beitler & Landis [4]. The purpose of the study was to investigate the effect of a topical cream drug therapy in curing nonspecific gynecologic infections. The binary response variable was classified as favorable or unfavorable response to treatment.

The data displayed in Table 2, collapsed over the eight clinics, indicate that 42.3% of women receiving the active drug reported a favorable response, compared to 32.9% of women receiving the control, resulting in an (unadjusted) odds ratio of 1.50, and a relative risk of 1.29. By applying the MH method for 2×2 tables in (4) to a single table, we note that the observed "pivot cell" frequency is $\sum_{h=1}^{t} n_{h11} = 55$, with expected value under H_0 of 48.57, and variance of 15.99, yielding a test statistic of $Q_{\mathrm{MH}(1)} = 2.59$, with $p = 0.11$. Consequently, at the standard 5% level of statistical significance, we would conclude that this drug is not different from the control therapy.

However, the same data from Table 2 are shown again in Table 3, stratified by clinic, sorted by largest sample size ($n_1 = 73$) to smallest sample size ($n_8 = 13$).

Table 2 The distribution of favorable response to active drug and control treatments in the multicenter randomized clinical trial: collapsed over clinics

Clinic no.	Treatment	Response Favorable	Unfavorable	Total	Proportion favorable	Relative risk	Odds ratio
Collapsed	Drug	55	75	130	0.423	1.29	1.50
	Control	47	96	143	0.329		
	Subtotal	102	171	273	0.374		

Source: Beitler & Landis [4].

Table 3 The distribution of favorable response to active drug and control treatments in the multicenter randomized clinical trial

Clinic no.	Treatment	Response		Total	Proportion favorable	Risk estimates	
		Favorable	Unfavorable			Relative risk	Odds ratio
1	Drug	11	25	36	0.306	1.13	1.19
	Control	10	27	37	0.270		
	Subtotal	21	52	73	0.288		
2	Drug	16	4	20	0.800	1.16	1.82
	Control	22	10	32	0.688		
	Subtotal	38	14	52	0.731		
3	Drug	14	5	19	0.737	2.00	4.80
	Control	7	12	19	0.368		
	Subtotal	21	17	38	0.553		
4	Drug	2	14	16	0.125	2.13	2.29
	Control	1	16	17	0.059		
	Subtotal	3	30	33	0.091		
5	Drug	6	11	17	0.353	9.29	14.13
	Control	0	12	12	0.000		
	Subtotal	6	23	29	0.207		
6	Drug	1	10	11	0.091	2.74	3.00
	Control	0	10	10	0.000		
	Subtotal	1	20	21	0.048		
7	Drug	1	4	5	0.200	1.80	2.00
	Control	1	8	9	0.111		
	Subtotal	2	12	14	0.143		
8	Drug	4	2	6	0.667	0.78	0.33
	Control	6	1	7	0.857		
	Subtotal	10	3	13	0.769		

Source: Beitler & Landis [4].

Now the MH test in (4), with df $= 1$, for the statistical significance of the treatment effect is $Q_{MH(1)} = 6.38$, with $p = 0.01$. Thus, in contrast to the test on the data collapsed over the eight clinics ($p = 0.11$), we reject the null hypothesis of "no partial association", in favor of the alternative hypothesis suggesting that the treatments (drug vs. control) on average are not homogeneous across the eight clinics.

Note that although seven of the eight odds ratios from the eight clinics indicate that drug therapy constitutes a more effective treatment for curing nonspecific gynecologic infections than the control treatment, they differ in magnitude from a low of 1.2 (stratum 1) to a high of 14.1 (stratum 5). Also note that these individual table estimates of the odds ratio for strata 5 and 6 were obtained after adding 0.5 to each cell of the 2×2 table due to the observed zero frequency [19]. The only stratum showing an inverse relationship was clinic 8. Using the Breslow–Day test in (8) for homogeneity of odds ratios, we obtain $Q_{BD} = 7.80$ with df $= 7$, ($p = 0.33$). Thus, despite this wide range in the magnitude of the stratum-specific odds ratios, these data do not provide sufficient evidence to reject the hypothesis of homogeneous odds ratios.

The MH average odds ratio in (5), adjusting for these strata effects, is $\widehat{\psi}_{MH} = 2.14$, somewhat larger than the unadjusted estimate of 1.50. Furthermore, the 95% confidence interval for the MH average odds ratio, using the RBG variance in (6), is (1.197,

3.807). This confidence interval, by not containing 1.0, suggests that after adjustments for the variability in the response by clinic, the drug is significantly associated with a favorable response.

General s × r Tables

In general, there are *s* levels of the row factor and *r* levels of the response variable, giving rise to *t s × r* contingency tables, as in Table 1. For these settings, the generalized MH methods outlined in the Appendix are illustrated in Kuritz et al. [34] and Landis et al. [35, 37]. For purposes of brevity in this article, we will defer the application of these generalized MH hypothesis testing methods until Example 3 in the subsequent section.

Estimation of treatment effects is much more complex for the general *s × r* table situation, particularly if one or both of the dimensions of the tables are not ordinally scaled. Investigators have been developing some extensions of the MH estimating procedure, including variance and covariance estimators and in sparse data situations [15, 16, 27, 39, 49, 55], although none appears to be fully generalizable to a series of *s × r* tables. Ordinal models provide summary measures [1, 11], but the sample size requirements and structural model assumptions, such as **proportional odds**, are much more restrictive than required for the MH methods to be applied.

Repeated Measures Designs

The use of MH methods for the analysis of categorical data obtained from repeated measures designs was described in the early papers by Mantel & Haenszel [46], and by Birch [5, 6] and Gart [24]. Breslow & Day [9] illustrated the use of these methods for matched case–control data, including the incorporation of scores for an ordinal risk factor. Otherwise, Agresti [2], Darroch [14], Kuritz et al. [34], Landis et al. [37], Mantel & Byar [44], White et al. [62] and others [3, 33, 52] described the use of these methods for a variety of repeated measures and longitudinal designs (*see* **Longitudinal Data Analysis, Overview**).

The hypotheses within these designs involve the extent to which the response variable varies across the repeated measures factor (within-subject conditions, case–control status), on average, across the strata (subjects, matched sets). For example, all the matched analyses illustrated in Breslow & Day [9] can be formulated within this framework utilizing the MH methods.

2 × 2 Tables

Researchers are frequently interested in comparing the prevalence of a condition under two different circumstances or time periods for the same set of subjects, or in comparing the risk factor prevalence in a matched-pair set of subjects (*see* **Matched Pairs with Categorical Data**). In such applications, a 2×2 table is constructed, in which the row and column dimensions correspond to the level of the condition or risk factor for each dimension of the repeated measure. To illustrate these methods, consider the data in Table 4, summarizing the binary level of obstetrical post-partum pain [Some/More (2–4) vs. None/Little (0–1)] at 4 hours and subsequently at 8 hours after delivery, for each mother from the subgroup of 185 women receiving a combination drug labeled (A and B). More extensive descriptions

Table 4 The general layout for the cross-classification of two binary repeated measures using post-partum pain[a] at 4 and 8 hours after delivery for all patients assigned to the combination drugs A and B

Treatment subgroup	Initial pain	Pain at 4 hours	Pain at 8 hours		Totals
			Some/More	None/Little	
A and B	Combined	Some/More	19 (*a*)	31 (*b*)	50
		None/Little	6 (*c*)	129 (*d*)	135
		Total	25	160	185
			(*a* + *c*)	(*b* + *d*)	

[a]Pain level reported as 0 = None, 1 = Little, 2 = Some, 3 = Lots, 4 = Terrible, at each hour of follow-up; Some/More pain obtained by combining levels 2–4.
Source: Kuritz et al. [34].

and analyses of these data are provided in Koch et al. [32] and Kuritz et al. [34].

We can utilize the same MH test statistic in (4) to test the null hypothesis that the prevalence of pain (Some/More) is the same at 4 and 8 hours after delivery. In order to implement this test, with appropriate adjustments for the paired data structure within subjects, the data for each woman must be summarized in a 2×2 frequency table with entries of 1s and 0s, as displayed in Table 5. Note that the frequency of women reporting Some/More pain at both 4 and 8 hours ($a = 19$) in Table 4 gives rise to 19 2×2 tables of profile type 1 in Table 5. In total, there are $n = 185$ subtables in Table 5, although those of profile type 1 ($a = 19$) and type 4 ($d = 129$) do not contribute to the test statistic in (4), due to the equality of observed and expected frequencies and a variance term of zero in the denominator.

In summarizing these data in Tables 4 and 5, it should also be noted that this layout is identical to the format used to summarize the frequencies for case–control data from epidemiologic investigations involving matched pairs, where the rows in Table 4 represent the exposure categories for the cases, and the columns represent the exposure categories for the controls.

In this context, the randomization model test statistic in (4) simplifies to $Q_{MH(1)} = (b - c)^2/(b + c)$, which is identical to the McNemar [48] statistic for repeated measures data from 2×2 tables. This test statistic asymptotically follows the chi-square distribution with df = 1. Note, however, that it is completely determined by the off-diagonal cells "b" and "c", and thus the asymptotics for this statistic are linked directly to the number of discordant pairs of observations, $b + c$, rather than the total sample size n. When $b + c$ does not exceed 20, it is preferable to perform an exact conditional test based on the binomial distribution, as implemented within StatXact [40, 50].

The usual MH average odds ratio as defined in (5) simplifies to $\widehat{\psi}_{MH} = b/c$, using the notation for 2×2 tables from repeated measures designs as in Table 4. Furthermore, the preferred confidence interval approach for this estimator is to use either the RBG variance in (6) or the exact procedure based on the binomial distribution, which applies to b given $b + c$. Both the RBG and the exact procedure are computed easily within the StatXact [50] package.

These odds ratio and confidence interval procedures are illustrated for nine subsets of the post-partum data from the multicenter study described in Kuritz et al. [34]. In particular, for each combination of treatment (Placebo, A only, and A and B) subgroup and initial pain status (Some, Lots, and Combined), these MH average odds ratios, and their RBG 95% confidence intervals were computed and are presented in Table 6. Note that the MH odds ratios for women reporting "Some" initial pain are similar across treatments, ranging from 2.3 for those receiving Placebo to 3.0 for those receiving both A and B. However, due to the small sample sizes of $b + c$, the RBG 95% confidence intervals around each of these odds ratios barely include 1, suggesting only slight evidence that the level of pain at 8 hours differs from that at 4 hours.

In contrast, among women who reported "Lots" of initial pain, the MH average odds ratio ranged from ($\widehat{\psi}_{MH} = 1.38$) in the Placebo subgroup, to ($\widehat{\psi}_{MH} = 9.50$) among women randomized to the A and B combination drug. Furthermore, the RBG 95% confidence intervals suggest that the levels of pain at 4 and 8 hours are different (improved at 8 hours) for those on Drug A only (1.34, 8.30), and particularly so for

Table 5 The binary level of post-partum pain[a] at 4 and 8 hours after delivery by individual patient profiles for a representative subgroup in the multicenter randomized clinical trial

Profile type	No. of tables (patients)	No. of hours	Level of post-partum pain Some/More (2–4)	None/Little (0–1)	Total
1	$a = 19$	4	1	0	1
		8	1	0	1
		Subtotal	2	0	2
2	$b = 31$	4	1	0	1
		8	0	1	1
		Subtotal	1	1	2
3	$c = 6$	4	0	1	1
		8	1	0	1
		Subtotal	1	1	2
4	$d = 129$	4	0	1	1
		8	0	1	1
		Subtotal	0	2	2

[a]Pain level reported as 0 = None, 1 = Little, 2 = Some, 3 = Lots, and 4 = Terrible, at each hour of follow-up; Some/More pain obtained by combining levels 2–4.
Source: Kuritz et al. [34].

Table 6 A cross-classification of two binary repeated measures using post-partum pain[a] at 4 and 8 hours after delivery: patients stratified by treatment and initial pain

Treatment subgroup	Initial pain	Response profile at hours 4 and 8				Total	MH average odds ratio	RBG 95% CIs
		SS (a)	SN (b)	NS (c)	NN (d)			
Placebo	Some	17	16	7	40	80	2.29	(0.94, 5.56)
	Lots	41	11	8	30	90	1.38	(0.55, 3.42)
	Combined	58	27	15	70	170	1.80	(0.96, 3.38)
A only	Some	11	15	6	46	78	2.50	(0.97, 6.44)
	Lots	31	20	6	41	98	3.33	(1.34, 8.30)
	Combined	42	35	12	87	176	2.92	(1.51, 5.62)
A and B	Some	5	12	4	64	85	3.00	(0.97, 9.30)
	Lots	14	19	2	65	100	9.50	(2.21, 40.79)
	Combined	19	31	6	129	185	5.17	(2.16, 12.38)

[a]Pain level reported as 0 = None, 1 = Little, 2 = Some, 3 = Lots, and 4 = Terrible, at each hour of follow-up; Some/More pain obtained by combining levels 2–4.
Source: Kuritz et al. [34].

those receiving the combination A and B drugs (2.21, 40.79).

When initial pain status (Some or Lots) is ignored, by combining the strata within treatment, the odds ratios again demonstrate a clear gradient across treatment subgroups, with the least evidence for a difference in level of pain at 4 and 8 hours among women receiving Placebo ($\widehat{\psi}_{MH} = 1.80$) and the strongest evidence for such a difference among women receiving both A and B ($\widehat{\psi}_{MH} = 5.17$). For each treatment subgroup, these measures of association are somewhat smaller for the combined group of women than for the subset with "Lots" of initial pain.

General d × L Tables

In the most general case, a repeated measures design involves d measurement conditions (within-subject treatments, time points, and matched-set members) and L levels of the response variable. To illustrate this situation, consider the data displayed in Table 7 from a pediatric cardiology study conducted at the C.S. Mott Children's Hospital, Ann Arbor, Michigan. As described further in Landis et al. [37], each of 14 puppies was administered each of five variable pulse duration treatments, delivered at a separate site in the esophagus for 30 minutes. The purpose of the study was to investigate the effect of variable pulse duration

Table 7 Lesion severity[a] of acute electrical injury by variable pulse duration for each of 14 puppies

Puppy no.	Pulse duration (ms)					Mean response
	2	4	6	8	10	
6	0	0	5	0	3	1.60
7	0	3	3	4	5	3.00
8	0	3	4	3	2	2.40
9	2	2	3	0	4	2.20
10	0	0	4	4	3	2.20
12	0	0	0	4	4	1.60
13	0	4	4	4	0	2.40
15	0	4	0	0	0	0.80
16	0	3	0	1	1	1.00
17	–	–	0	1	0	0.33
19	0	0	1	1	0	0.40
20	–	0	0	2	2	1.00
21	0	0	2	3	3	1.60
22	–	0	0	3	0	0.75

[a]Lesion severity graded as 0 = no lesion to 5 = acute inflammation of extraesophageal fascia: – denotes missing data.
Source: data provided by Dr C.L. Webb, and C.S. Mott, Children's Hospital, Ann Arbor.

on the development of acute electrical injury during transesophageal atrial pacing.

Each of the five treatments, distinguished by pulse durations of either 2, 4, 6, 8, or 10 ms, was applied at a separate site of the esophagus. At the conclusion of the experiment, the electrical injury lesion at each site was classified according to the depth of injury

Table 8 Distribution of severity of lesion[a] by pulse duration: collapsed across 14 puppies

Pulse duration (ms)	Severity of lesion						Total	Mean response
	0	1	2	3	4	5		
2	10	0	1	0	0	0	11	0.18
4	7	0	1	3	2	0	13	1.46
6	6	1	1	2	3	1	14	1.86
8	3	3	1	3	4	0	14	2.14
10	5	1	2	3	2	1	14	1.93
Total	31	5	6	11	11	2	66	1.58

[a]Lesion severity graded as 0 = no lesion to 5 = acute inflammation of extraesophageal fascia.

by histologic examination using an ordinal staging scale from 0 (no lesion) to 5 (acute inflammation of the fascia). These lesion severity data are displayed in Table 7, showing the response at each pulse duration, together with the mean response across pulse durations, for each puppy.

The primary hypothesis under investigation in this experiment is whether the mean lesion severity differs by pulse duration (mean responses differ), and in particular, whether mean lesion severity increases with increasing pulse duration (linear trend in mean responses). By collapsing these responses over individual puppies, the overall response profiles of lesion severity for each condition (pulse duration) are displayed in Table 8. In particular, note that the mean lesion severity increases from 0.18 (due to 10 of 11 puppies having a response of "0") at 2 ms to 1.93 at 10 ms.

To incorporate the appropriate adjustments for the repeated measures (within puppy) across measurement conditions (pulse duration levels), the data for each puppy must be structured in a separate table which displays the response of the puppy at each of the measurement conditions. Let $h = 1, \ldots, N$ index subjects, $k = 1, \ldots, L$ index the response categories, and $g = 1, \ldots, d$ index the measurement conditions. Then, in the cells of each table, $y_{hgk} = 1$ if the hth subject is classified into the kth response category at the gth repeated measure, and is equal to 0 otherwise.

This general $d \times L$ table is illustrated using the data for puppy number 7 from Table 7, as displayed in Table 9. In particular, the response pattern for this puppy was no lesion (severity 0) at pulse duration of 2 ms, a lesion severity of 3 measured at both 4 and 6 ms, a lesion of severity 4 at 8 ms, and an acute inflammation of extraesophageal fascia (severity 5) was measured at the pulse duration of 10 ms.

Table 9 Distribution of severity of lesion[a] by pulse duration for puppy number 7

Pulse duration (ms)	Severity of lesion						Total
	0	1	2	3	4	5	
2	1	0	0	0	0	0	1
4	0	0	0	1	0	0	1
6	0	0	0	1	0	0	1
8	0	0	0	0	1	0	1
10	0	0	0	0	0	1	1
Total	1	0	0	2	1	1	5

[a]Lesion severity graded as 0 = no lesion to 5 = acute inflammation of extraesophageal fascia.

These data in Table 7, restructured according to the format in Table 9, permit investigation of all three alternative hypotheses relative to the null hypothesis of "no partial association". For comparative purposes, we present each of these three test statistics in Table 10, first of all unadjusted for the 14 strata (puppies), assuming simple random sampling (SRS) and labeled "SRS Sample Covariance Structure". Secondly, each of these three alternative hypotheses is investigated within the MH framework adjusted for the 14 strata (puppies) and labeled "Repeated Measures Covariance Structure".

By treating both the factor levels (pulse duration) and response levels (severity of lesion) as nominal scale variables, the randomization model test statistic in (A3) in the Appendix provides a test of the null hypothesis given in (1) relative to the alternative that there is a general, nonspecific association between pulse duration and severity of lesion. As shown in Table 10, the adjusted test statistic is $Q_{MH(1)} = 22.85$, in contrast to the unadjusted SRS test, $Q_{MH(1)} = 21.20$. In this case, this nonspecific test for general association with df $= 20$ shows only

Table 10 Randomization model test statistics for association between pulse duration and lesion severity under simple random sample (SRS) and repeated measurement sample assumptions: 14 puppies

Alternative hypothesis	Equation number in Appendix	df	SRS sample covariance structure		Repeated measures covariance structure	
			Test statistic	Significance level	Test statistic	Significance level
General association	(A3)	20	21.20	0.39	22.85	0.30
Row mean scores differ	(A4)	4	9.88	0.04	12.35	0.02
Nonzero correlation	(A5)	1	6.76	0.01	8.80	<0.01

minimal effects due to adjusting for the within-puppy correlation. Furthermore, without incorporating the ordinal nature of both of these variables, there is no evidence of an association between pulse duration and severity of the lesions ($p = 0.30$). However, the sample size is not large enough for $Q_{MH(1)}$ to follow a chi-square distribution with df = 20, or to detect general association departures from H_0.

On the other hand, if we do incorporate the ordinal nature of lesion severity, assigning scores of $0, 1, \ldots, 5$, but still consider pulse duration as a nominal variable, we can compute an observed mean lesion severity score as in (3), which is summarized for the unadjusted data (collapsed over the 14 puppies) in the last column of Table 8. Consequently, the randomization model test statistic in (A4) of the Appendix can be used to test the null hypothesis of "no partial association" in (1) against the more specific alternative hypothesis that the mean scores for the five pulse durations are different, adjusting for the strata. As displayed in Table 10, the adjusted test statistic is $Q_{MH(2)} = 12.35$, in contrast to the unadjusted test statistic of $Q_{MH(2)} = 9.88$. Since these tests compare the five mean lesion severity scores (in a fashion equivalent to a two-way ANOVA), the degrees of freedom have been reduced from 20 to 4, resulting in increased statistical power to reject H_0. In fact, not only does the significance level for the adjusted statistic decrease from $p = 0.30$ to $p = 0.02$, indicating that the five pulse durations do not give rise to the same mean levels of lesion severity, but the significance level for the unadjusted test (ignoring within-puppy correlation) is only $p = 0.04$, twice as large as for the adjusted test statistic. This increase in power due to adjustments for within-puppy correlation is already noticeable with only 14 puppies, and small $d = 5$ repeated measures within puppy.

Finally, we can investigate the alternative hypothesis of a linear progression in mean lesion severity scores by computing the test statistic in (A5) in the Appendix using equally spaced row scores of 1, 2, 3, 4, and 5 for the pulse duration levels. The resulting adjusted test statistic is $Q_{MH(3)} = 8.80$, in contrast to the unadjusted test statistic, $Q_{MH(3)} = 6.76$. With one degree of freedom, these test statistics for "nonzero correlation" are highly significant ($p < 0.01$). Thus, when incorporating the ordinal nature of both variables, these data provide strong evidence that increasing the pulse duration (from 2 ms to 10 ms) is associated with a linear increase in the mean lesion severity. Not only does this df = 1 test for linear trend in mean severity most closely address the clinical research question, but it is also most justified in terms of sample size adequacy.

References

[1] Agresti, A. (1980). Generalized odds ratios for ordinal data, *Biometrics* **36**, 59–67.

[2] Agresti, A. (1990). *Categorical Data Analysis*. Wiley, New York.

[3] Arndt, S., Davis, C.S., Miller, D.D. & Andreasen, N.C. (1993). Effect of antipsychotic withdrawal on extrapyramidal symptoms: statistical methods for analyzing single-sample repeated-measures data, *Neuropsychopharmacology* **8**, 67–75.

[4] Beitler, P.J. & Landis, J.R. (1985). A mixed-effects model for categorical data, *Biometrics* **41**, 991–1000.

[5] Birch, M.M. (1964). The detection of partial association, I: the 2×2 case, *Journal of the Royal Statistical Society, Series B* **26**, 313–324.

[6] Birch, M.W. (1965). The detection of partial association, II: the general case, *Journal of the Royal Statistical Society, Series B* **27**, 111–124.

[7] Bishop, Y.M.M., Fienberg, S.E. & Holland, P.W. (1975). *Discrete Multivariate Analysis*. MIT Press, Cambridge, Mass.

[8] Breslow, N.E. (1981). Odds ratio estimators when the data are sparse, *Biometrika* **68**, 73–84.

[9] Breslow, N.E. & Day, N.E. (1980). *Statistical Methods in Cancer Research*, Vol. 1, IARC Science Publication No. 32. International Agency for Research on Cancer, Lyon.

[10] Breslow, N.E. & Liang, K.Y. (1982). The variance of the Mantel–Haenszel estimator, *Biometrics* **38**, 943–952.

[11] Clayton, D.G. (1974). Some odds ratio statistics for the analysis of ordered categorical data, *Biometrika* **61**, 525–531.

[12] Cochran, W.G. (1950). The comparison of percentages in matched samples, *Biometrika* **37**, 256–266.

[13] Cochran, W.G. (1954). Some methods for strengthening the χ^2 test, *Biometrics* **10**, 417–457.

[14] Darroch, J.N. (1981). The Mantel–Haenszel test and tests of marginal symmetry: fixed effects and mixed models for a categorical response, *International Statistical Review* **49**, 285–307.

[15] Davis, C.S. & Chung, Y. (1995). Randomization model methods for evaluating treatment efficacy in multicenter clinical trials, *Biometrics* **51**, 1163–1174.

[16] Davis, L.J. (1985). Generalization of the Mantel–Haenszel estimator to nonconstant odds ratios, *Biometrics* **41**, 487–495.

[17] Dayal, H.H. (1978). On the desirability of the Mantel–Haenszel summary measure in case-control studies of multi-factor etiology of disease, *American Journal of Epidemiology* **108**, 506–511.

[18] Flanders, W.D. (1985). A new variance estimator for the Mantel–Haenszel odds ratio, *Biometrics* **41**, 637–642.

[19] Fleiss, J.L. (1981). *Statistical Methods for Rates and Proportions*, 2nd Ed. Wiley, New York.

[20] Friedman, M. (1937). The use of ranks to avoid the assumption of normality implicit in the analysis of variance, *Journal of the American Statistical Association* **32**, 675–701.

[21] Gart, J.J. (1962). On the combination of relative risks, *Biometrics* **18**, 601–610.

[22] Gart, J.J. (1966). Alternative analyses of contingency tables, *Journal of the Royal Statistical Society, Series B* **28**, 164–179.

[23] Gart, J.J. (1970). Point and interval estimation of the common odds ratio in the combination of 2×2 tables with fixed marginals, *Biometrics* **57**, 471–475.

[24] Gart, J.J. (1971). The comparison of proportions: a review of significance tests, confidence intervals and adjustment for stratification, *Review of the International Statistical Institute* **39**, 48–61.

[25] Gart, J.J. & Zweifel, J.R. (1967). On the bias of various estimators of the logit and its variance with application to quantal bioassay, *Biometrika* **54**, 181–187.

[26] Greenland, S. (1982). Interpretation and estimation of summary ratios under heterogeneity, *Statistics in Medicine* **1**, 217–227.

[27] Greenland, S. (1989). Generalized Mantel–Haenszel estimators for $K\, 2 \times J$ tables, *Biometrics* **45**, 183–191.

[28] Hauck, W.W., Anderson, S. & Leahy, F.J. (1982). Finite-sample properties of some old and some new estimators of a common odds ratio from multiple 2×2 tables, *Journal of the American Statistical Association* **77**, 145–152.

[29] Koch, G.G. & Edwards, S. (1987). Clinical efficacy trials with categorical data, in *Statistical Methods in the Pharmaceutical Industry*, K. Peace, ed. Marcel Dekker, New York, see Chapter 9.

[30] Koch, G.G., Gillings, D.B. & Stokes, M.E. (1980). Biostatistical implications of design, sampling, and measurement to health science data analysis, *Annual Review of Public Health* **1**, 163–225.

[31] Koch, G.G., Amara, I.A., Davis, G.W. & Gillings, D.B. (1982). A review of some statistical methods for covariance analysis of categorical data, *Biometrics* **38**, 563–595.

[32] Koch, G.G., Imrey, P.B., Singer, J.M., Atkinson, S.S. & Stokes, M.E. (1985). *Analysis of Categorical Data*. Presses de l'Université Montreal, Montreal.

[33] Kuritz, S.J. & Landis, J.R. (1988). Attributable risk estimation from matched case–control data, *Biometrics* **44**, 355–367.

[34] Kuritz, S.J., Landis, J.R. & Koch, G.G. (1988). A general overview of Mantel–Haenszel methods: applications and recent developments, *Annual Review of Public Health* **9**, 123–160.

[35] Landis, J.R., Heyman, E.R. & Koch, G.G. (1978). Average partial association in three way contingency tables: a review and discussion of alternative tests, *International Statistical Review* **46**, 237–254.

[36] Landis, J.R., Cooper, M.M., Kennedy, T. & Koch, G.G. (1979). A computer program for testing average partial association in three-way contingency tables (PARCAT), *Computer Programs in Biomedicine* **9**, 223–246.

[37] Landis, J.R., Miller, M.E., Davis, C.S. & Koch, G.G. (1988). Some general methods for the analysis of categorical data in longitudinal studies, *Statistics in Medicine* **7**, 109–137.

[38] Lehmann, E.L. & Dabrerd, H.J.M. (1975). *Nonparametrics: Statistical Methods Based on Ranks*. Holden–Day, San Francisco.

[39] Liang, K.Y. (1987). Extended Mantel–Haenszel estimating procedure for multivariate logistic regression models, *Biometrics* **43**, 289–299.

[40] Lynch, J.C., Landis, J.R. & Localio, A.R. (1991). StatXact. *American Statistician* **45**, 151–154.

[41] Madansky, A. (1963). Tests of homogeneity for correlated samples, *Journal of the American Statistical Association* **58**, 97–119.

[42] Mantel, N. (1963). Chi-square tests with one degree of freedom: extensions of the Mantel–Haenszel procedure, *Journal of the American Statistical Association* **58**, 690–700.

[43] Mantel, N. (1977). Tests and limits for the common odds ratio of several 2×2 contingency tables: methods

in analogy with the Mantel–Haenszel procedure, *Journal of Statistical Planning and Inference* **1**, 179–189.

[44] Mantel, N. & Byar, D.P. (1978). Marginal homogeneity, symmetry and independence, *Communications in Statistics – Theory and Methods A* **7**, 953–976.

[45] Mantel, N. & Fleiss, J.L. (1980). Minimum expected cell size requirements for the Mantel–Haenszel one degree of freedom chi-square test and a related rapid procedure, *American Journal of Epidemiology* **112**, 129–134.

[46] Mantel, N. & Haenszel, W. (1959). Statistical aspects of the analysis of data from retrospective studies of disease, *Journal of the National Cancer Institute* **22**, 719–748.

[47] McKinlay, S.M. (1978). The effect of nonzero second-order interaction on combined estimators of the odds ratio, *Biometrika* **65**, 191–202.

[48] McNemar, Q. (1947). Note on the sampling error of the difference between correlated proportions or percentages, *Psychometrika* **12**, 153–157.

[49] Mickey, R.M. & Elashoff, R.M. (1985). A generalization of the Mantel–Haenszel estimator of partial association for $2 \times J \times K$ tables, *Biometrics* **41**, 623–635.

[50] Mehta, C. & Patel, N. (1995). *StatXact*. CYTEL Software Corporation, Cambridge.

[51] O'Gorman, T.W., Woolson, R.F., Jones, M.P. & Lemke, J.H. (1990). Statistical analysis of $K\, 2 \times 2$ tables: a comparative study of estimators/test statistics for association and homogeneity, *Environmental Health Perspectives* **87**, 103–107.

[52] Ramakrishnan, V., Goldberg, J., Henderson, W.G., Eisen, S.A., True, W., Lyons, M.J. & Tsuang, M.T. (1992). Elementary methods for the analysis of dichotomous outcomes in unselected samples of twins, *Genetic Epidemiology* **9**, 273–287.

[53] Robins, J., Breslow, N. & Greenland, S. (1986). Estimators of the Mantel–Haenszel variance consistent in both sparse data and large strata limiting models, *Biometrics* **42**, 311–324.

[54] SAS Institute Inc. (1989). *SAS/STAT User's Guide, Version 6*, 4th Ed., Vol. 1. SAS Institute Inc., Cary.

[55] Sato, T. (1991). An estimating equation approach for the analysis of case-control studies with exposure measured at several levels, *Statistics in Medicine* **10**, 1037–1042.

[56] Sato, T. (1992). Estimation of a common risk ratio in stratified case–cohort studies, *Statistics in Medicine* **11**, 1599–1605.

[57] Sato, T. (1994). Risk ratio estimation in case–cohort studies, *Environmental Health Perspectives* **102**, Supplement 8, 53–56.

[58] Somes, G.W. (1986). The generalized Mantel–Haenszel statistic, *American Statistician* **40**, 106–108.

[59] Stokes, M., Davis, C.S. & Koch, G.G. (1995). *SAS for Categorical Data Analysis*. SAS Institute Inc., Cary.

[60] Tarone, R.E., Gatt, J.J. & Hauck, W.W. (1983). On the asymptotic inefficiency of certain noniterative estimators of a common relative risk or odds ratio, *Biometrika* **70**, 519–522.

[61] van Elteren, P.H. (1960). On the combination of independent two-sample tests of Wilcoxon, *Bulletin of the International Statistical Institute* **37**, 351–361.

[62] White, A.A., Landis, J.R. & Cooper, M.M. (1982). A note on the equivalence of several marginal homogeneity test criteria for categorical data, *International Statistical Review* **50**, 27–34.

[63] Woolf, B. (1955). On estimating the relation between blood group and disease, *Annals of Human Genetics* **19**, 251–253.

Appendix

Under H_0 in (1), the observed frequencies in Table 1 have expected values,

$$E\{\mathbf{n}_h | H_0\} = n_h[\mathbf{p}_{h.*} \otimes \mathbf{p}_{h*.}] = \mathbf{m}_h, \qquad \text{(A1)}$$

where $\mathbf{p}_{h.*}$ contains the marginal column proportions $(n_{h.j}/n_h)$ in the hth stratum, $\mathbf{p}_{h*.}$ contains the marginal row proportions $(n_{hi.}/n_h)$ in the hth stratum, and $\otimes$ denotes left-hand Kronecker product multiplication, where the matrix on the left multiplies each element in the matrix on the right.

Furthermore, the covariance matrix for these observed frequencies under the null hypothesis of randomness in (1) is

$$V\{\mathbf{n}_h | H_0\} = \frac{n_h^2}{n_h - 1}(\mathbf{D}_{\mathbf{p}_{h.*}} - \mathbf{p}_{h.*}\mathbf{p}'_{h.*})$$

$$\otimes (\mathbf{D}_{\mathbf{p}_{h*.}} - \mathbf{p}_{h*.}\mathbf{p}'_{h*.}) = \mathbf{V}_h, \quad \text{(A2)}$$

where $\mathbf{D}_{\mathbf{p}_h}$ is a diagonal matrix with elements of the vector $\mathbf{p}_h$ on the main diagonal.

Without loss of generality, let $\mathbf{A}_{1h} = [(\mathbf{I}_{(r-1)}, \mathbf{0}_{(r-1)}) \otimes (\mathbf{I}_{(s-1)}, \mathbf{0}_{(s-1)})]$ be a linear operator matrix, which eliminates the last row and last column frequencies from each stratum. Then the generalized Mantel–Haenszel test for H_0 against the nonspecific alternative that the distributions of the response variable are not homogeneous across the s factor levels is

$$Q_{\text{MH}(1)} = \left\{\sum_{h=1}^{t}(\mathbf{n}_h - \mathbf{m}_h)'\mathbf{A}'_{1h}\right\}\left\{\sum_{h=1}^{t}\mathbf{A}_{1h}\mathbf{V}_h\mathbf{A}'_{1h}\right\}^{-1}$$

$$\times \left\{\sum_{h=1}^{t}\mathbf{A}_{1h}(\mathbf{n}_h - \mathbf{m}_h)\right\}, \qquad \text{(A3)}$$

which follows a chi-square distribution with df $= (s-1)(r-1)$ under H_0 for large $n_{.ij}$.

If the response variable is reported on an ordinal scale, scores can be assigned to the response levels to compute row mean scores. In this case, the alternative hypothesis to "no partial association" is that there are location shifts for these mean scores across factor levels of the row variable. Let $\mathbf{A}_{2h} = \mathbf{a}'_h \otimes [\mathbf{I}_{(s-1)}, \mathbf{0}_{(s-1)}]$ be an $(s-1) \times sr$ matrix with $\mathbf{a}'_h = (a_{h1}, \ldots, a_{hr})$, where a_{hj} is the score chosen to reflect the ordinal nature of the jth level of response for the hth stratum. Then the Mantel–Haenszel test for equality among the mean responses for the s subpopulations relative to the response variable score vectors $\{\mathbf{a}_h\}$ is

$$Q_{\mathrm{MH}(2)} = \left\{ \sum_{h=1}^{t}(\mathbf{n}_h - \mathbf{m}_h)'\mathbf{A}'_{2h} \right\} \left\{ \sum_{h=1}^{t}\mathbf{A}_{2h}\mathbf{V}_h\mathbf{A}'_{2h} \right\}^{-1}$$
$$\times \left\{ \sum_{h=1}^{t}\mathbf{A}_{2h}(\mathbf{n}_h - \mathbf{m}_h) \right\}, \tag{A4}$$

which follows a chi-square distribution with df = $(s - 1)$ under H$_0$ for large $n_{.i.}$.

When both the response variable and the row variable are ordinally scaled, scores can be assigned to both the response levels and the factor levels in the hth stratum. In this situation, the test is directed at the extent to which there is a linear trend on the mean scores across the levels of the row variable, or equivalently, a nonzero correlation between the row and column variables. For this case, let $\mathbf{A}_{3h} = [\mathbf{a}'_h \otimes \mathbf{c}'_h]$, where the $\{\mathbf{a}_h\}$ are defined as before and the $\{\mathbf{c}_h\} = (c_{h1}, c_{h2}, \ldots, c_{hs})$ specify a set of scores for the ith level of the row variable in the hth stratum. The resulting test statistic

$$Q_{\mathrm{MH}(3)} = \left\{ \sum_{h=1}^{t}(\mathbf{n}_h - \mathbf{m}_h)'\mathbf{A}'_{3h} \right\} \left\{ \sum_{h=1}^{t}\mathbf{A}_{3h}\mathbf{V}_h\mathbf{A}'_{3h} \right\}^{-1}$$
$$\times \left\{ \sum_{h=1}^{t}\mathbf{A}_{3h}(\mathbf{n}_h - \mathbf{m}_h) \right\}, \tag{A5}$$

follows a chi-square distribution with df = 1 under H$_0$ for large $N = \sum_{h=1}^{t} n_h$. Further discussion of these three expressions of the Mantel–Haenszel statistic and their implementation using SAS [54] can be found in Stokes et al. [59].

J. RICHARD LANDIS, TONYA J. SHARP,
STEPHEN J. KURITZ & GARY G. KOCH

Manual of Operations *see* Clinical Trials Protocols

Map Distance *see* Genetic Map Functions

Map, Statistical *see* Statistical Map

Mapping Disease Patterns

For as long as disease patterns have been mapped there has been skepticism over the value of the pictures which are drawn. For instance, a map of the geography of the 1832 influenza epidemic in Glasgow (Scotland) was produced by the inmates of a lunatic asylum, mainly to occupy their time [1]. Later, in the nineteenth century, the value of mapping disease patterns was recognized as specific epidemiologic breakthroughs were attributed to the insight gained from mapping. Often cited is a map of the distribution of deaths from the 1848 cholera epidemic in London (England) which, so the tale goes, inspired the removal of the handle of the water pump at the center of a cluster of dots on the map, resulting in the curtailing of the epidemic [12].

Maps of diseases are like news pictures of crowd trouble. Viewers should always ask themselves what is not being shown in the map while looking at what is there. In particular, look around the edge of the map. Ask why it ends where it does. For instance, maps of diseases are often centered on the point the author thinks is most important. Figure 1 shows the central section of John Snow's map of deaths from cholera in Soho. Note how the eye is drawn to the pump in the center, particularly by the very high number of deaths at the intersection of Cambridge and Broad Streets. Had Snow drawn his map of all of London he would have discovered a greater density of deaths just south of the river Thames, as shown in Figure 2. This concentration would have changed location again had Snow had recourse to an isodemographic base map, as shown in Figure 3. As our picture of a disease pans out, as we include more cases and as we change the way

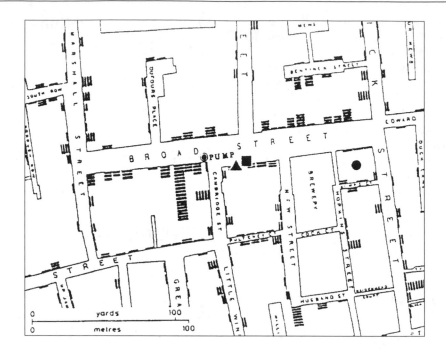

Figure 1 John Snow's map of cholera deaths in Soho, London, 1854 – taken from Cliff & Haggett [1, Figure 1.15D]

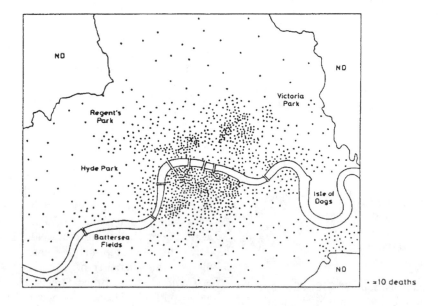

Figure 2 Cholera deaths in London in 1849 – taken from Cliff & Haggett [1, Figure 1.3B]

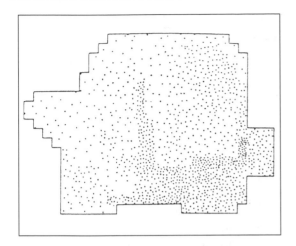

Figure 3 Figure 2 on a population cartogram – taken from Cliff & Haggett [1, Figure 1.18D]

we view the picture, the patterns on our maps show change too.

Disease mapping has been most strongly influenced by the history of diseases. Figure 4 shows the prevalence of 12 major causes of death in England and Wales since the publication of Snow's map of cholera. Infectious diseases now account for a tiny fraction of deaths in developed countries (which can afford most disease mapping and research). It is causes of death which are not declining, such as suicide, and those which are rising in importance, such as cancers, which increasingly interest researchers.

For these causes of illness and death the analysis of point patterns around particular sites is still a major issue, but the patterns are usually far less clearly spatially defined than were outbreaks of cholera. More importantly, it is increasingly being accepted that more abstract factors, such as social inequality, can lie behind particular patterns of disease, and these require more abstract mappings for their study.

There are many different ways of mapping disease but here there is only space to explore one alternative. The alternatives include traditional choropleth mapping, where areas on a map are shaded according to statistics about the population. Most common in epidemiology is the mapping of areas colored by their standardized mortality ratios (*see* **Standardization Methods**). Another common form of mapping is to map points or the incidences of disease, and often color is also used here to highlight different types of disease. Various different point symbols can be used in mapping, particularly common is the use of proportional circles which are colored or segmented to highlight different features of a disease. The size of the circles is often made proportional to the population at risk of contracting a disease, at which point this type of cartography begins to merge into iso-demographic mapping [4, 5].

Diseases occur across a population as much as across land. That is not to say that geographic distributions are not important, but that we should take account of the distribution of the population at risk

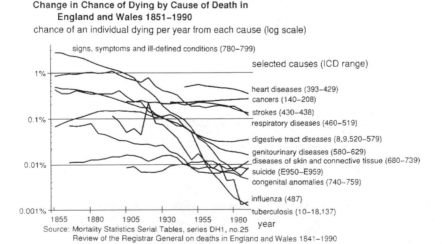

Figure 4 Cause of death 1855–1990 – taken from Dorling [3, Figure 5.21]

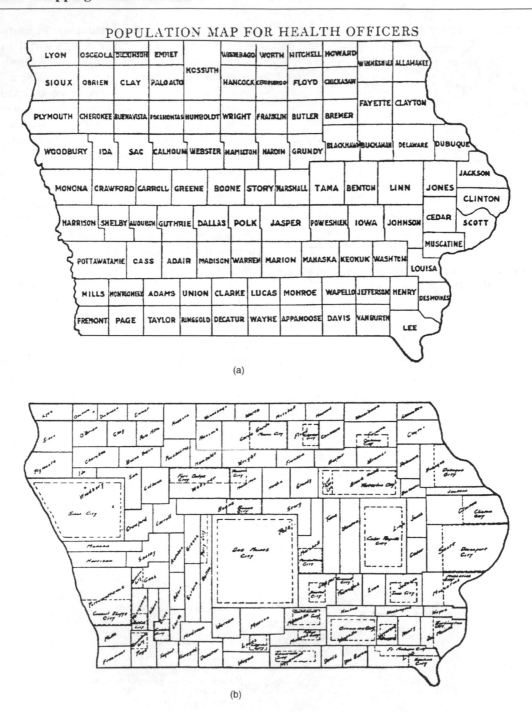

(a)

(b)

Figure 5   The use of cold vaccine in Iowa County Area, 1926 – taken from Wallace [15, p. 1023]

to a particular disease, or cause, before mapping its pattern. One way in which this can be done is to use a map projection which draws every area in proportion to the number of people at risk living in that area – hence the term isodemographic ("equal people"). Isodemographic maps, more commonly called cartograms, are used for many purposes, mostly obviously in mapping the geography of elections. However, their most established use has been in disease mapping. Figure 5 shows one of the earliest examples of a cartogram designed for epidemiologic purposes [15, p. 1023]. Figure 5(a) is the conventional map of the counties of Iowa State, and Figure 5(b) is an equal population cartogram upon which colored pins were placed to show the locations of reportable diseases.

The square in the middle of the cartogram is Des Moines city in Polk County.

The designer of the Iowa cartogram was a doctor working in the state department of health. Many researchers have been struck by the idea that they could learn more about disease through mapping it in unconventional ways. The first cartogram of London was an "epidemiologic map" produced by a doctor working for the then London County Council Department of Public Health [14]. The cartogram (Figure 6) contained crosses drawn in the borough rectangles to show the incidence of polio during the 1947 epidemic. Because the rectangles were each drawn with the same height, their widths are proportional to population as well as their areas. The borough

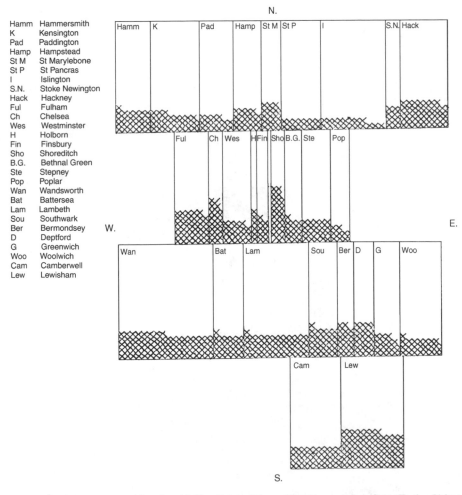

Figure 6 London borough cartogram showing 1947 poliomyelitis notifications – taken from Taylor [14, p. 201]

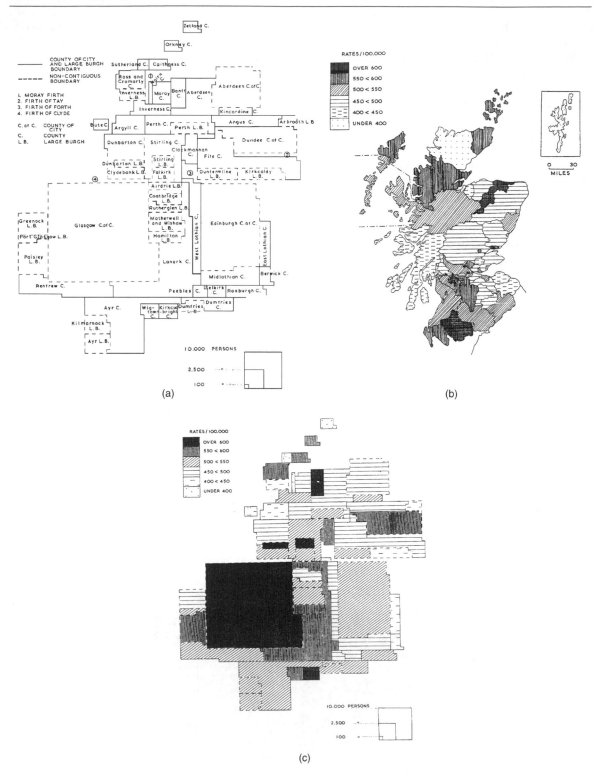

Figure 7 Cartogram and map of Scottish health districts – taken from Forster [6]. (a) Cartogram of females aged 45–54 in 1961 by Scottish health districts; (b) map of 1959–63 mortality rates of females aged 45–54 by district; (c) 1959–63 mortality rates of females aged 45–54 shown in (a)

with the highest rate of polio and hence the tallest column of crosses in the Figure was Shoreditch. Almost exactly 100 years separates the two London epidemics, which were first drawn on a map and cartogram, respectively. Cartograms showing distributions within countries came later.

A claim was made to have produced the first cartograms showing national disease distributions only a decade after the crude cartogram of London was first drawn [6]. The nation was Scotland, and a separate cartogram was constructed by hand for each of eight age–sex groups. Figure 7 shows the cartogram being used to study the 1959–1963 mortality of women in Scotland aged 45–54. The author of this cartogram concluded that a national series of cartograms should be produced for each age–sex group for use in epidemiologic studies in Britain. This was never done, and it is debatable whether such an exact mapping base is needed in most studies. A single isodemographic base map of the whole population will usually suffice to uncover all but the most subtle of patterns.

A National Atlas of Disease Mortality in the UK was published in 1963 under the auspices of the Royal Geographical Society; the atlas contained no cartograms. However, a revised edition was published a few years later which made copious use of a "demographic base map" [7]. It is interesting to note that, when the revised edition was being prepared, the president of the Society was Dudley Stamp, who believed that "The fundamental tool for the geographical analysis is undoubtedly the map or, perhaps more correctly, the cartogram" [13, p. 135]. In the cartogram which was used in the revised national atlas (Figure 8), squares were used to represent urban areas, while diamonds were used to show statistics for rural districts. No attempt was made to maintain contiguity, but a stylized coastline was placed around the symbols, which were all drawn with their areas in proportion to the populations at risk from the disease being shown on each particular cartogram.

In the *National Atlas of Disease Mortality in the United Kingdom*, Howe used a national cartogram to display the distribution of standardized mortality between 1959 and 1963 from separate as well as all causes of death for both men and women. High rates were seen in northern districts and some Inner London boroughs (including Shoreditch, which is also highlighted on one of the earliest cartograms of London; see above). Extremely high rates in central Scotland were particularly noticeable, as were the

low rates in districts which surround London. At the extremes the average man living in Salford was 50% more likely to die each year than his counterpart in Bournemouth [7]. Both these areas are shrunk on a "normal" map. The pattern for women was very similar to that for men although, in general, it was less pronounced. However, women did have the highest mortality rate of any area on the map in rural Dunbartonshire, where they were more than twice as likely to die each year than were women nationally (allowing for local age structure). The cartogram highlights this area, but also puts it in the perspective of the populations at risk from the high mortality rates for women in and around the Glasgow area. Questions for investigation are immediately generated by comparing the maps in Howe's atlases with those produced by Forster for a decade earlier (see Figure 7).

Isodemographic mapping is also used to study the prevalence of disease – individual cases of a disease or death which together might possibly be connected. Figure 9 shows the distribution of cases of Wilm's tumor, a childhood cancer, identified in New York State between 1958 and 1962, drawn upon an equal land area map. Apparent clusters of cases have been marked on the map [8]. In the second diagram in Figure 9, the same cases are drawn upon an equal population cartogram and the apparent clusters can be seen to have been quite evenly dispersed across the population. The same process has been used in Figure 10 to illustrate how cases of Salmonella food poisoning occurring in Arkansas in 1974 were not unduly clustered in Pulaski county [2].

In recent years researchers have turned their attention to trying to develop cartograms upon which actual, rather than illusory, clusters of disease can be identified (*see* **Clustering**). The major problem with using population cartograms to identify clusters of disease is that the choice of which areas are closest to which on a cartogram can be quite arbitrary. For instance, if the same set of incidences of one particular disease were plotted on three different cartograms, then different parts of the country may appear to have dense clusters of cases depending on which cartogram was chosen. This would be true regardless of whether the clusters were to be identified by eye or by statistical procedures; the different base maps would result in different patterns emerging. The proposition that there is no single "true answer" as to whether a disease is clustered does not go down

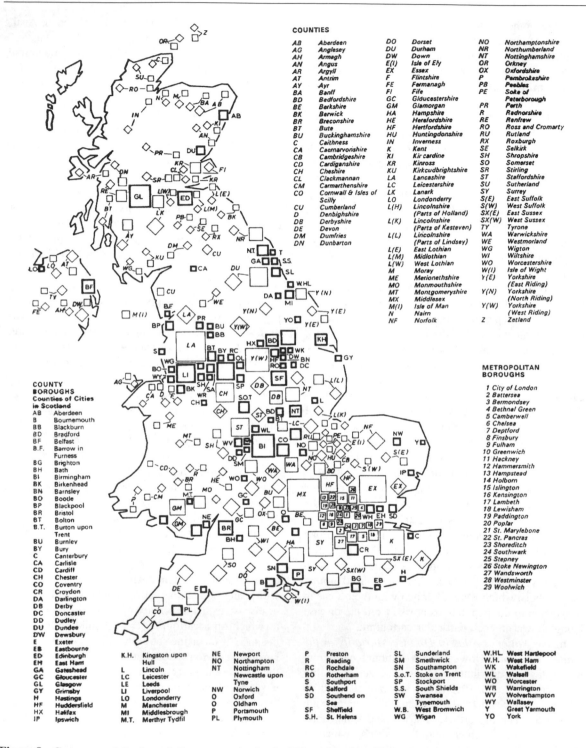

Figure 8   Cartogram of districts of disease mapping in the UK – taken from Howe [7]

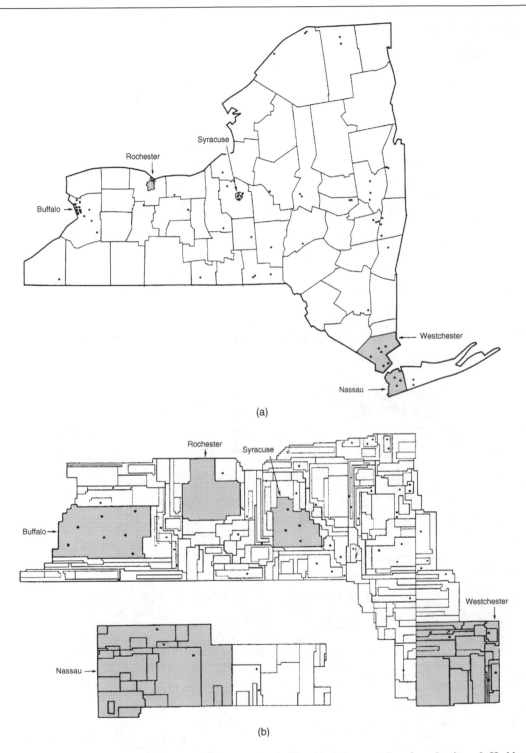

Figure 9 Wilm's tumour cases on (a) map and (b) cartogram in New York State – taken from Levison & Haddon [8]

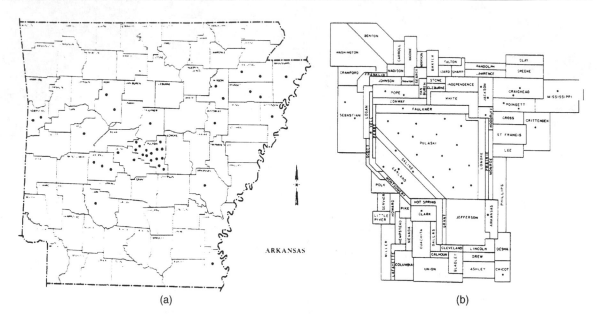

Figure 10   Salmonella Newport cases on (a) map and (b) cartogram in Arkansas State – taken from Dean [2]

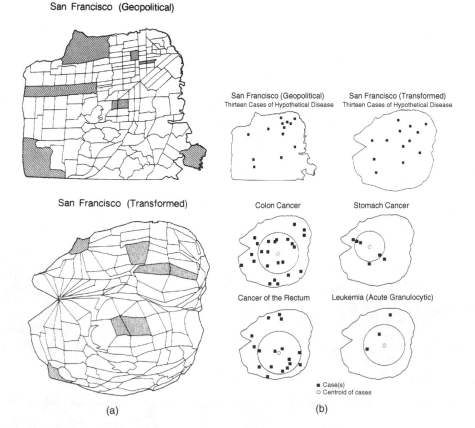

Figure 11   San Francisco map (a) for 1980 census, and cartogram (b) of hypothetical and actual diseases – taken from Selvin et al. [11]

too well in some circles. Because of this problem a group of researchers at Berkeley developed a computer algorithm for identifying incidences of disease [9]. The algorithm was used to produce the cartogram in Figure 11 of San Francisco county, upon which apparent clusters of disease were shown to be false [11]. However, application of the method to another California county did provide evidence of some clustering of high cancer rates near oil refineries [10].

Mapping of disease patterns is becoming increasingly common due to the proliferation of computer mapping. However, many of these programs were designed to produce general maps of any subject and are often most appropriate to show land use or the distribution of points in physical space. Over most of the course of the last century, doctors, public health officials, and researchers have discovered and rediscovered that traditional maps often do not provide the most appropriate projection to look for patterns of disease. Here, a few alternatives have been shown of just one different form of disease mapping to try to explain why it involves more than just sticking pins in paper.

Acknowledgments

The author is grateful to Robert Israel for commenting on a draft of this article and to the following people for permission to reproduce the copyright material shown here: Peter Haggett (*Atlas of Disease Distributions*) for Figures 1–3; Pam Beckley (Her Majesty's Stationery Office) for Figure 5; Michael Plommer (Office for National Statistics) for Figure 6; Carol Torselli (*British Medical Journal*) for Figure 7; Marian Tebben (*Public Health Reports*) for Figure 9; and Mina Chung (American Public Health Association) for Figure 10.

References

[1]   Cliff, A.D. & Haggett, P. (1988). *Atlas of Disease Distributions. Analytical Approaches to Epidemiological Data*. Blackwell, Oxford.

[2]   Dean, A.G. (1976). Population-based spot maps: an epidemiologic technique, *American Journal of Public Health* **66**, 988–989.

[3]   Dorling, D. (1995). *A New Social Atlas of Britain*. Wiley, Chichester.

[4]   Dorling, D. (1996). *Area Cartograms: Their Use and Creation*, Concepts and Techniques in Modern Geography (CATMOG) no. 59. School of Environmental Sciences, University of East Anglia, Norwich.

[5]   Dorling, D. & Fairbairn, D. (1997). *Mapping: Ways of Representing the World*. Longman, London.

[6]   Forster, F. (1966). Use of a demographic base map for the presentation of areal data in epidemiology, *British Journal of Preventive and Social Medicine* **20**, 165–171.

[7]   Howe, G.M. (1970). *National Atlas of Disease Mortality in the United Kingdom*, Revised and Enlarged Edition. Nelson, London.

[8]   Levison, M.E. & Haddon, W. (1965). The area adjusted map: an epidemiological device, *Public Health Reports* **80**, 55–59.

[9]   Selvin, S., Merrill, D., Sacks, S., Wong, L., Bedell, L. & Schulman, J. (1984). *Transformations of Maps to Investigate Clusters of Disease*. Laboratory Report, LBL-18550, Lawrence, Berkeley.

[10]   Selvin, S., Shaw, G., Schulman, J. & Merrill, D. (1987). Spatial distribution of disease: three case studies, *Journal of the National Cancer Institute* **79**, 417–423.

[11]   Selvin, S., Merrill, D., Schulman, J., Sacks, S., Bedell, L. & Wong, L. (1988). Transformations of maps to investigate clusters of disease, *Social Science and Medicine* **26**, 215–221.

[12]   Snow, J. (1854). *On the Mode of Communication of Cholera*. Churchill Livingstone, London.

[13]   Stamp, L.D. (1962). A geographer's postscript, in *Taxonomy and Geography*, D. Nichols, ed. The Systematics Association, London, pp. 153–158.

[14]   Taylor, I. (1955). An epidemiology map, *Ministry of Health Monthly Bulletin* **14**, 200–201.

[15]   Wallace, J.M. (1926). Population map for health officers, *American Journal of Public Health* **16**, 1023.

(*See also* **Geographic Patterns of Disease; Geographical Analysis**)

DANIEL DORLING

Marginal Cost–Effectiveness Ratio
see Health Economics

Marginal Homogeneity *see* Square Contingency Table

Marginal Likelihood

Suppose that $\mathbf{X} = (X_1, \ldots, X_n)'$ is a vector of random variables whose distribution depends on parameter vectors $\boldsymbol{\beta}$ and $\boldsymbol{\lambda}$. We suppose that $\boldsymbol{\beta}$ is of primary interest, whereas $\boldsymbol{\lambda}$ is a **nuisance parameter** and typically is of very high dimension. Our aim is to define a derived **likelihood** that would be suitable for inference about $\boldsymbol{\beta}$ when $\boldsymbol{\lambda}$ is unknown.

Let $f(\mathbf{x}; \boldsymbol{\beta}, \boldsymbol{\lambda})$ be the probability density function (pdf) of $\mathbf{X}$; on data $\mathbf{X} = \mathbf{x}$, it defines the joint likelihood function

$$L(\boldsymbol{\beta}, \boldsymbol{\lambda}; \mathbf{x}) \propto f(\mathbf{x}; \boldsymbol{\beta}, \boldsymbol{\lambda}),$$

which can be used for inference. However, when $\boldsymbol{\lambda}$ is of high dimension, it becomes difficult to interpret the information about $\boldsymbol{\beta}$. In fact, the **maximum likelihood** estimator (MLE) of $\boldsymbol{\beta}$ can have very poor properties, even asymptotically, if the dimension of $\boldsymbol{\lambda}$ increases with that of $\mathbf{X}$. To make inferences about $\boldsymbol{\beta}$ itself without regard to $\boldsymbol{\lambda}$, it is useful to define a derived likelihood which, by some method, eliminates $\boldsymbol{\lambda}$. Marginal likelihood provides one way of doing this.

Suppose that there exists a one-to-one transformation of $\mathbf{X}$ into $(\mathbf{A}, \mathbf{T})$ and that the joint pdf of $(\mathbf{A}, \mathbf{T})$ factors as

$$f(\mathbf{a}, \mathbf{t}; \boldsymbol{\beta}, \boldsymbol{\lambda}) = f(\mathbf{a}; \boldsymbol{\beta}) f(\mathbf{t}|\mathbf{a}; \boldsymbol{\beta}, \boldsymbol{\lambda}), \qquad (1)$$

where the marginal density of $\mathbf{A}$ does not depend on $\boldsymbol{\lambda}$.

The *marginal likelihood* of $\boldsymbol{\beta}$ based on $\mathbf{A}$ is

$$L_{\mathrm{m}}(\boldsymbol{\beta}; \mathbf{a}) \propto f(\mathbf{a}; \boldsymbol{\beta}), \qquad (2)$$

and this could be used for inference about $\boldsymbol{\beta}$. In general, there is a loss of information in restricting attention to (2) for inference; sometimes, however, invariance or other arguments suggest that A contains the whole of the available information about $\boldsymbol{\beta}$. Even when such arguments do not apply, however, there may still be advantage to using (2) as the basis of inference since it conveniently eliminates $\boldsymbol{\lambda}$.

Two examples serve to illustrate the ideas.

Example 1

Suppose that variability in the measurement of blood glucose is of interest and that pairs of measurements are taken on n independent individuals. Thus, we might assume that X_{1i}, X_{2i} are independent $\mathrm{N}(\lambda_i, \beta^2)$ variates, where λ_i represents the true glucose level for the ith individual and β^2, the variance of the

measurement error, is of interest. The maximum likelihood estimate of β^2 is

$$\hat{\beta}^2 = \sum (x_{1i} - x_{2i})^2/(4n),$$

which converges to $\beta^2/2$ in probability as $n \to \infty$. This is an instance in which the mle is inconsistent.

A marginal likelihood, in this problem, is naturally based on the statistics, $A_i = X_{1i} - X_{2i}$, $i = 1, \ldots, n$, which are independent $\mathrm{N}(0, 2\beta^2)$ variates. This gives rise to the marginal likelihood

$$L_{\mathrm{m}}(\beta^2; a) = \beta^{-n} \exp\left[-\sum a_i^2/(4\beta^2)\right].$$

The corresponding marginal mle, $\hat{\beta}_{\mathrm{m}}^2 = \sum a_i^2/(2n)$ converges in probability to the correct value β^2 as $n \to \infty$. The choice of the A_is as the basis for inference about β^2 is a natural one; the difference in the measurements for each individual provides the information about β^2 intuitively.

Example 2

A second example arises in Cox's **proportional hazards** model [3] (*see* **Cox Regression Model**). The hazard function for the time to failure T is

$$\lambda(t; z) = \lambda_0(t) \exp(\mathbf{z}'\boldsymbol{\beta}), \qquad (3)$$

where $\mathbf{z} = (z_1, \ldots, z_p)'$ is a vector of fixed covariates. In this model, the baseline hazard rate $\lambda_0(t)$ is left arbitrary and the covariates z are assumed to act multiplicatively on the baseline rate with $\boldsymbol{\beta} = (\beta_1, \ldots \beta_p)'$, the vector of regression parameters being of primary interest.

Suppose that $T_1, \ldots, T_n$ is a sample with covariates $\mathbf{z}_1, \ldots, \mathbf{z}_n$. Let $T_{(1)}, \ldots, T_{(n)}$ be the **order statistic** from $T_1, \ldots, T_n$ with corresponding covariates $\mathbf{z}_{(1)}, \ldots, \mathbf{z}_{(n)}$ and let $\mathbf{R} = (R_1, \ldots, R_n)$ be the rank vector. Thus, R_i is the **rank** of the variate T_i among $(T_1, \ldots, T_n)$. The distribution of $\mathbf{R}$ can be shown to be

$$f(\mathbf{r}; \boldsymbol{\beta}) = \Pr(\mathbf{R} = \mathbf{r})$$

$$= \prod_{i=1}^{n}\left[\exp(\mathbf{z}_{(i)}'\boldsymbol{\beta}) \Big/ \sum_{j=1}^{n} \exp(\mathbf{z}_{(j)}'\boldsymbol{\beta})\right], \quad (4)$$

and this defines a marginal likelihood for $\boldsymbol{\beta}$. This likelihood (4) is identical to Cox's **partial likelihood**

[3]. These arguments can be extended to allow right **censoring** in the data [6].

We conclude with a number of remarks.

1. Marginal likelihood was first introduced by Fraser [4, 5] in the context of the structural model. In his work and in the related work of Kalbfleisch & Sprott [8], the A_is are allowed to depend on the parameter β.

2. Group invariance arguments can be used in both of the examples given here to justify the use of **A** or **R** as the basis of inference for β. Barnard [1] describes these arguments in general, and Kalbfleisch & Prentice [6, 7] apply them to the proportional hazards model (3). Other approaches to assessing the "**sufficiency**" of **A** for inference have been discussed by Sprott [9] and Barndorff-Nielsen [2], among others.

3. Marginal likelihood is one of several methods for obtaining derived likelihoods about a parameter of interest. Conditional likelihood (*see* **Conditional Probability**), partial likelihood and **profile likelihood** are other approaches which can apply, depending upon the structure of the statistical problem.

References

[1]   Barnard, G.A. (1963). Some aspects of the fiducial argument, *Journal of the Royal Statistical Society, Series B* **25**, 111–114.

[2]   Barndorff-Nielsen, O. (1976). Nonformation, *Biometrika* **63**, 567–571.

[3]   Cox, D.R. (1972). Regression models and life tables (with discussion), *Journal of the Royal Statistical Society, Series B* **34**, 187–220.

[4]   Fraser, D.A.S. (1967). Data transformations and the linear model, *Annals of Mathematical Statistics* **38**, 1456–1465.

[5]   Fraser, D.A.S. (1968). *The Structure of Inference*. Wiley, New York.

[6]   Kalbfleisch, J.D. & Prentice, R.L. (1973). Marginal likelihoods based on Cox's regression and life model, *Biometrika* **60**, 267–278.

[7]   Kalbfleisch, J.D. & Prentice, R.L. (1980). *The Statistical Analysis of Failure Time Data*, Wiley, New York.

[8]   Kalbfleisch, J.D. & Sprott, D.A. (1970). Application of likelihood methods to models involving large number of parameters (with discussion), *Journal of the Royal Statistical Society, Series B* **32**, 175–208.

[9]   Sprott, D.A. (1975). Marginal and conditional sufficiency, *Biometrika* **62**, 599–605.

JOHN D. KALBFLEISCH

Marginal Models

Marginal models are important when several response variables are simultaneously of interest on each subject in a study. We may expect these responses to be interdependent simply because the same subject is involved for all observations. Because of this dependence among the observations, a multivariate distribution will be required to model them adequately. Marginal regression models are based on the corresponding marginal distributions. In most cases repeated measurements will be involved; therefore we restrict our examples to such studies. In other words, the *same* response variable will be measured several times on subjects, either because they are found in clusters or because they are observed longitudinally over time [8] (*see* **Longitudinal Data Analysis, Overview**).

The full multivariate distribution describes the dependence among the responses on each subject. In certain situations, such as in the experimentation of a **clinical trial**, the dependence relations among responses will be of direct interest. Thus, for example, in a longitudinal setting, we may be concerned with how a response depends on the previous history of a subject, including dependence on previous responses. Then, a conditional distribution will be appropriate. However, in other situations, such as epidemiologic population studies of prevalence, we may be interested in the marginal distribution of responses within the population at each point in time or for each member of a cluster or matched group (*see* **Clustering**). The term *marginal* means that we are concerned with each distribution response separately, conditional on covariates but not on any of the other responses.

A special kind of conditional distribution involves **random effects**. By conditioning on one or more latent variables accounting for heterogeneity among subjects, a multivariate distribution is induced. In the simplest case it has uniform dependence among all responses within a cluster. In what follows the term "conditional distribution" refers to conditioning directly on the other responses of a subject, and not to random effects.

Clustered and longitudinal studies pose fairly distinct problems. The observations on a cluster are generally not ordered, so they are interchangeable. The same marginal model will often apply to any member of the cluster, although, in some cases, responses will depend on cluster size. However, in a longitudinal study, observations are ordered in time, so that early observations cannot be made to depend on more recent ones. A model at any point in time should be constructed in ignorance of future observations. In most situations the marginal distribution may be expected to change over time.

To see the relationships between multivariate, conditional, and marginal distributions, consider the simplest example of a repeated categorical response. If we have two observations of the response, then the joint or multivariate (here bivariate) distribution can be represented by the probabilities π_{ij}, where the two indices indicate the combination of categories observed (*see* **Square Contingency Table**). The marginal distributions are given by the probabilities, $\pi_{i.} = \sum_j \pi_{ij}$ and $\pi_{.j} = \sum_i \pi_{ij}$, and the conditional distributions by $\pi^1_{i|j} = \pi_{ij}/\pi_{.j}$ and $\pi^2_{j|i} = \pi_{ij}/\pi_{i.}$.

To take a concrete example, consider first a clustered, rather than a longitudinal, response. Suppose that we have a sample of subjects for whom we classify each eye as having either good or poor vision. Observations can be represented as a simple **2 × 2 contingency table** with entries being the frequencies, n_{ij}, where the indices refer to the responses on the two eyes. Information on the bivariate distribution, π_{ij}, is contained in the body of the table. A conditional distribution corresponds to fixing the value of one of the two responses, so that information is obtained from the corresponding row or column. We can reconstruct the complete multivariate distribution from a pair of conditional distributions. Finally, information on the marginal distributions is contained in the marginal totals. This pair of marginal distributions, by itself, does not allow us to reconstruct the complete multivariate distribution. Attempts to do so involve what is called the **ecologic fallacy**.

Marginal distributions inform us about the average state of a population. They tell us nothing about the relationships among the responses for individual members of the population. Two responses may have identical marginal distributions without there being a similar dependence between the responses for many, or indeed any, individual subjects. Consider two rather extreme fictitious examples of the joint distributions that might correspond to results under two treatments (Table 1). In the left table there is a large probability that only one eye of any given individual will be good; the treatment helps only one

Table 1

Right eye	Left eye		Right eye	Left eye	
	Good	Poor		Good	Poor
Good	0.01	0.47	Good	0.46	0.02
Poor	0.47	0.05	Poor	0.02	0.50

eye, but for almost all individuals. In the right table the probability is high that both eyes will be similar; this treatment helps both eyes of half of the individuals. Thus, in the first case the conditional probability is $0.02 (= 0.01/0.48)$ that one eye will be good, given that the other is, while in the second case it is $0.96 (= 0.46/0.48)$. However, marginally, under both treatments, both eyes have exactly the same distribution, known as marginal homogeneity, with a probability of 0.48 for a good left eye and the same for a good right eye. Thus, the fact that the marginal probabilities of both left and right eyes being good are the same tells us nothing about whether both eyes of a given subject will be good. Conversely, if the relationship between marginal distributions were different under two treatments, then this would not exclude the individual response relationships between eyes being the same for both treatments [1] (*see* **Matched Pairs with Categorical Data**).

For the cluster of two eyes, a reasonable bivariate distribution that allows for interchangeability would set $\pi_{12} = \pi_{21}$, or equivalently, the conditional probabilities, $\pi^1_{1|1} = \pi^2_{1|1}$, to yield a trinomial distribution. From this, the marginal probabilities are easily obtained as $\pi_{1.} = \pi_{.1} = \pi_{11} + (\pi_{12} + \pi_{21})/2$.

Consider now a slightly more complex example with a binary response, this time in a longitudinal context [11]. Subjects are followed over time, all beginning in one state, but at some point switching to a second state. This may be represented by a horizontal line, running through time on a graph, starting at level one but jumping vertically down to level zero at the switch point, then continuing horizontally at that level. Each subject may change state at a different time, so that the vertical lines do not coincide. The average or typical individual will have the vertical line situated at the mean of all jump times. However, the marginal model will be a sigmoid curve dropping slowly from one and flattening off at zero. No individual can follow such a curve because they must be in one state or the other, not part way between. The marginal curve gives the average number of subjects in each state at each point in time, but tells us nothing about the trajectory of a typical individual.

From these examples, we can see why marginal models are sometimes called *population-averaged models*, whereas conditional models are *subject-specific* [12]. The choice between the two types will depend on the question being asked. For example, if the response is presence or absence of repeated infections under two treatments, the population-averaged model describes the global difference in infection rates between the treatments, while the subject-specific model looks at the probability of infection of a typical individual, given treatment. Population-averaged models depend on the degree of heterogeneity in the population; the same process in two populations with different heterogeneity will yield different population-averaged models. The dependence of marginal response on an explanatory variable will be smaller than the corresponding individual average dependence in a random effects model, this difference increasing with heterogeneity.

Care must be taken that a marginal model does correspond to the population of interest. For example, in the setting of a clinical trial, the "population" is rather artificial, for a number of reasons, including the facts that the subjects are volunteers and that all are started on treatments at arbitrary points in time. In such a context, marginal statements would appear to have limited value.

A marginal model can be constructed in two opposing ways. We may start with some known multivariate distribution (or set of conditional distributions) and determine the marginal distributions. Or we may specify directly the marginal distributions. We have already seen that, in the latter case, the multivariate distribution will not be uniquely defined, so that additional relationships will have to be specified. Each approach has certain advantages and disadvantages.

First, we should note that the multivariate normal distribution is quite exceptional and should not be taken as a general example for model construction. Both the conditional and the marginal distributions are easy to derive, and both are also normal. This is a unique case.

Generally, if the conditional distributions are of a simple known form, the marginal distributions will be complex, usually analytically intractable, and vice

versa. This means that if we start with some reasonable conditional distributions that might be appropriate to describe the dependence at the individual level in the phenomenon under study, the marginal distributions will be complex and difficult to handle. But if we start with some simple and well-known marginal distribution that we find easy to understand at the population level, then we are implicitly imposing one of a number of possible conditional distributions, implying a complex relationship at the individual level. For example, if we took the conditional distribution, say for the left eye given the condition of the right eye, to be Bernoulli, then we would only be assuming that members under the same condition of the right eye had the same probability of response for the left eye. The marginal distribution would not be Bernoulli but a weighted average of the two Bernoulli distributions. However, if we took the marginal to be Bernoulli, again for the left eye, then we would be assuming that *all* members of the population had the same probability.

Scientifically, it should be clear that the first approach is more reasonable. Marginal or population descriptions do not generally have a meaning on their own, but only as built upon acceptable underlying individual dependence relationships. Nevertheless, certain statisticians have argued that the second is justifiable to answer some population questions.

A conditional model depends on the number of other responses upon which a given response is made to depend (think of a cluster of teeth instead of eyes), while a marginal model does not. The latter is said to be reproducible [7]. Thus, a marginal model has the same interpretation for clusters of all sizes, while a conditional model does not. Random effects models also have this characteristic. Hence, as might be expected, direct conditioning often is not appropriate for clustered data. However, reproducibility is generally not a desirable property for longitudinal data. Unequal sized longitudinal "clusters" have histories of different lengths.

For simple categorical data, such as two-way tables, both conditional and marginal models can be constructed fairly easily. Suppose that we want to study the influence of some explanatory variable, x_k, on the two binary responses, $i = 1, 2$ and $j = 1, 2$. The state of two eyes, used above, would be one example, but the study could also be longitudinal. We can construct a model based on a series of multinomial distributions such that $\sum_i \sum_j \pi_{ijk} = 1$ for all k.

Then, the (conditional) **loglinear regression model**, based on a conditional bivariate Bernoulli distribution, is

$$\log\left(\frac{\pi_{11k}\pi_{12k}}{\pi_{21k}\pi_{22k}}\right) = \log\left(\frac{\pi_{1|1,k}^1 \pi_{1|2,k}^1}{\pi_{2|1,k}^1 \pi_{2|2,k}^1}\right)$$

$$= 2\log\left(\frac{\dot{\pi}_{1\cdot k}}{\dot{\pi}_{2\cdot k}}\right)$$

$$= \beta_{10} + \beta_{11}x_k$$

$$\log\left(\frac{\pi_{11k}\pi_{21k}}{\pi_{12k}\pi_{22k}}\right) = \log\left(\frac{\pi_{1|1,k}^2 \pi_{1|2,k}^2}{\pi_{2|1,k}^2 \pi_{2|2,k}^2}\right)$$

$$= 2\log\left(\frac{\dot{\pi}_{\cdot 1k}}{\dot{\pi}_{\cdot 2k}}\right)$$

$$= \beta_{20} + \beta_{21}x_k$$

$$\log\left(\frac{\pi_{11k}\pi_{22k}}{\pi_{12k}\pi_{21k}}\right) = \beta_{30} + \beta_{31}x_k,$$

where $\dot{\pi}_{\cdot jk}$ and $\dot{\pi}_{i\cdot k}$ are the geometric means. Although the conditional probabilities must be adjusted to follow the linear regression across tables, indexed by k, this allows the marginal frequencies, upon which they are conditioned, to be held constant at their observed values. Inferences are then independent of these observed marginal totals, and of wide applicability. Although the conditional probability distributions are Bernoulli, the same for all subjects with a given value of x_k, the corresponding marginal distributions are not, being again weighted averages over all values of x_k.

Consider now the following corresponding marginal regression model:

$$\log\left(\frac{\pi_{11k} + \pi_{12k}}{\pi_{21k} + \pi_{22k}}\right) = \log\left(\frac{\pi_{1\cdot k}}{\pi_{2\cdot k}}\right)$$

$$= \beta_{10} + \beta_{11}x_k$$

$$\log\left(\frac{\pi_{11k} + \pi_{21k}}{\pi_{12k} + \pi_{22k}}\right) = \log\left(\frac{\pi_{\cdot 1k}}{\pi_{\cdot 2k}}\right)$$

$$= \beta_{20} + \beta_{21}x_k$$

$$\log\left(\frac{\pi_{11k}\pi_{22k}}{\pi_{12k}\pi_{21k}}\right) = \beta_{30} + \beta_{31}x_k.$$

Here, we have chosen the log **odds ratio** to describe the dependence between the two binary responses (a less elegant solution being to use the correlation). In this model the marginal probabilities are Bernoulli, the same for all subjects with a given value of x_k,

while the joint and conditional ones are not: they vary in some complex unexplained (by the model) way among subjects with the same x_k. In addition, the observed marginal frequencies are not held fixed, unless a saturated model is fitted, because those in individual tables, indexed by k, must be estimated so as to follow the linear regression model. Because inference is not made conditional on the observed marginal frequencies, this limits the applicability of any empirical conclusions concerning dependence, drawn from this model, to tables with the same marginal frequencies.

These models have several interesting contrasting characteristics. The first, loglinear regression, is a **generalized linear model**, whereas the second is not. This means that the parameter estimates are considerably more difficult to obtain in the latter case. This is further complicated if correlations are used (for more than two responses), because inequality constraints must be applied. At the same time, the conditional model, but not the marginal one, fixes the marginal totals at their observed values, something that is often considered to be a prerequisite for analyzing a contingency table. Finally, from the general properties of the **exponential family**, the dependence parameters, β_{30} and β_{31}, in the above marginal model are information orthogonal to the marginal regression parameters, β_{10}, β_{11}, β_{20}, and β_{21}. In other words, the elements of the information matrix relating these parameters together are zero so that their estimates are asymptotically uncorrelated. This is not true in the conditional model.

To avoid the complexities of the specification of dependence relationships when marginal distributions are the primary point of interest, one widely used approach has been to set up regression equations only describing how the marginal responses are believed to depend on the explanatory variables (similar to the first two of the three equations for the marginal model above). As members of the generalized linear model family, the score equations for estimating the parameters are well understood. But because responses are not independent, some matrix of "working" correlations is introduced into these equations, yielding **generalized estimating equations** (GEE); see [4] and [12].

Such equations have the property that, if the regression is correctly specified, the point estimates of the regression coefficients will be asymptotically consistent no matter what "working" matrix is chosen (although there is no simple empirical way of checking correctness). However, this is accompanied by at least two major inconveniences. Except in special cases, the GEE corresponds to no statistical model in the accepted sense of the term, i.e. no model that allows us to calculate the probability of the observed or any future data. Thus, no likelihood function is available, singularly complicating the tasks of obtaining useful measures of precision of the point estimates and of comparing "models". Generally only quasi-standard errors and a quasi-score function are available for making inferences and there is considerable debate about the choice of the former. Standard errors are well known to be unreliable in small samples of categorical data.

Although the examples given here have only involved simple binary responses, extensions to more complex **polytomous**, including ordinal, responses (*see* **Ordered Categorical Data**) are available. For more complex models, see, for example, [2], [3], [5], [6], and [9]. The reader may also wish to consult the review paper [10].

References

[1]   Agresti, A. (1989). A survey of models for repeated ordered categorical response data, *Statistics in Medicine* **8**, 1209–1224.

[2]   Azzalini, A. (1994). Logistic regression for autocorrelated data with application to repeated measures, *Biometrika* **81**, 767–775.

[3]   Balagtas, C.C., Becker, M.P. & Lang, J.B. (1995). Marginal modelling of categorical data from crossover experiments, *Applied Statistics* **44**, 63–77.

[4]   Gilmour, A.R., Anderson, R.D. & Rae, A.L. (1985). The analysis of binomial data by a generalized linear mixed model, *Biometrika* **72**, 593–599.

[5]   Glonek, G.F.V. (1996). A class of regression models for multivariate categorical responses, *Biometrika* **83**, 15–28.

[6]   Lang, J.B. & Agresti, A. (1994). Simultaneously modeling joint and marginal distributions of multivariate categorical responses, *Journal of the American Statistical Association* **89**, 625–632.

[7]   Liang, K.Y., Zeger, S.L. & Qaquish, B. (1992). Multivariate regression for categorical data, *Journal of the Royal Statistical Society, Series B* **54**, 3–40.

[8]   Lindsey, J.K. (1993). *Models for Repeated Measurements*. Oxford University Press, Oxford.

[9]   Molenberghs, G. & Lesaffre, E. (1994). Marginal modelling of correlated ordinal data using a multivariate Plackett distribution, *Journal of the American Statistical Association* **89**, 633–644.

[10]   Pendergast, J.F., Gange, S.J., Newton, M.A., Lindstrom, M.J., Palta, M. & Fisher, M.R. (1996). A survey of methods for analyzing clustered binary response data, *International Statistical Review* **64**, 89–118.

[11]   Sheiner, L.B., Beal, S.L. & Sambol, N.C. (1989). Study designs for dose-ranging, *Clinical Pharmacology and Therapeutics* **46**, 63–77.

[12]   Zeger, S.L., Liang, K.Y. & Albert, P.S. (1988). Models for longitudinal data: a generalized estimating equation approach, *Biometrics* **44**, 1049–1060.

(*See also* **Binary Data; Correlated Binary Data; McNemar Test**)

J.K. LINDSEY

Marginal Models for Multivariate Survival Data

Multivariate survival or failure-time data arise when each study subject may experience several events or when there exists some natural or artificial grouping of subjects which induces dependence among failure times of the same group. Biomedical examples include the sequence of tumor recurrences or infection episodes, the development of physical symptoms or diseases in several organ systems, the occurrence of blindness in the left and right eyes, the onset of a disease among family members, the initiation of cigarette smoking by classmates, and the appearance of tumor in litter-mates exposed to a carcinogen.

Suppose that there are n independent units each of which can potentially experience K types of failures. Let T_{ik} be the time when the kth type of failure occurs on the ith unit, and let C_{ik} be the corresponding **censoring** time. Define $X_{ik} = \min(T_{ik}, C_{ik})$ and $\Delta_{ik} = I(T_{ik} \leq C_{ik})$, where $I(\cdot)$ is the indicator function (*see* **Dummy Variables**). Also, let $\mathbf{Z}_{ik}(\cdot) = [Z_{1ik}(\cdot), \ldots, Z_{pik}(\cdot)]'$ denote a p-vector of possibly **time-dependent covariates** for the ith unit with respect to the kth type of failure. The failure time vector $\mathbf{T}_i = (T_{i1}, \ldots, T_{iK})$ and the censoring time vector $\mathbf{C}_i = (C_{i1}, \ldots, C_{iK})$ are assumed to be independent, conditional on the covariate vector $\mathbf{Z}_i = (\mathbf{Z}'_{i1}, \ldots, \mathbf{Z}'_{iK})$, $i = 1, \ldots, n$. The units are allowed to have unequal numbers of failures, which is achieved by setting C_{ik} to zero whenever T_{ik} is missing.

It is natural and convenient to formulate the marginal distribution for each type of failure with a **proportional hazards model**. Depending on whether the baseline hazard functions are different or identical among the K types of failures, the marginal hazard function for the kth type of failure on the ith unit is

$$\lambda_k(t; \mathbf{Z}_{ik}) = \lambda_{0k}(t) \exp[\boldsymbol{\beta}' \mathbf{Z}_{ik}(t)], \tag{1}$$

or

$$\lambda_k(t; \mathbf{Z}_{ik}) = \lambda_0(t) \exp[\boldsymbol{\beta}' \mathbf{Z}_{ik}(t)], \tag{2}$$

where $\lambda_{0k}(t), k = 1, \ldots, K$, and $\lambda_0(t)$ are unspecified baseline hazard functions, and $\boldsymbol{\beta}$ is a p-vector of unknown regression parameters. In some applications it is necessary to allow $\lambda_{0k}(t), k = 1, \ldots, K$, to be different, whereas in others it suffices to assume a common baseline hazard function. In both models (1) and (2), we set $\boldsymbol{\beta}$ to be the same among the K submodels, which entails no loss of generality since this structure can always be achieved by introducing appropriate type-specific covariates.

Inference Procedures

If all the failure times were independent, then the **partial likelihood** functions for $\boldsymbol{\beta}$ would be

$$L(\boldsymbol{\beta}) = \prod_{i=1}^{n} \prod_{k=1}^{K} \left\{ \frac{\exp[\boldsymbol{\beta}' \mathbf{Z}_{ik}(X_{ik})]}{\sum_{j=1}^{n} Y_{jk}(X_{ik}) \exp[\boldsymbol{\beta}' \mathbf{Z}_{jk}(X_{ik})]} \right\}^{\Delta_{ik}}$$

under model (1) and

$$L(\boldsymbol{\beta}) =$$

$$\prod_{i=1}^{n} \prod_{k=1}^{K} \left\{ \frac{\exp[\boldsymbol{\beta}' \mathbf{Z}_{ik}(X_{ik})]}{\sum_{j=1}^{n} \sum_{l=1}^{K} Y_{jl}(X_{ik}) \exp[\boldsymbol{\beta}' \mathbf{Z}_{jl}(X_{ik})]} \right\}^{\Delta_{ik}}$$

under model (2), where $Y_{ik}(t) = I(X_{ik} \geq t)$. The corresponding score functions would be

$$\mathbf{U}(\boldsymbol{\beta}) = \sum_{i=1}^{n} \sum_{k=1}^{K} \Delta_{ik} \left[\mathbf{Z}_{ik}(X_{ik}) - \frac{\mathbf{S}_k^{(1)}(\boldsymbol{\beta}, X_{ik})}{S_k^{(0)}(\boldsymbol{\beta}, X_{ik})} \right] \tag{3}$$

and

$$\mathbf{U}(\boldsymbol{\beta}) = \sum_{i=1}^{n} \sum_{k=1}^{K} \Delta_{ik} \left[\mathbf{Z}_{ik}(X_{ik}) - \frac{\overline{\mathbf{S}}^{(1)}(\boldsymbol{\beta}, X_{ik})}{\overline{S}^{(0)}(\boldsymbol{\beta}, X_{ik})} \right], \tag{4}$$

where

$$\mathbf{S}_k^{(0)}(\boldsymbol{\beta}, t) = \sum_{j=1}^{n} Y_{jk}(t) \exp\left[\boldsymbol{\beta}' \mathbf{Z}_{jk}(t)\right],$$

$$\mathbf{S}_k^{(1)}(\boldsymbol{\beta}, t) = \sum_{j=1}^{n} Y_{jk}(t) \exp\left[\boldsymbol{\beta}' \mathbf{Z}_{jk}(t)\right] \mathbf{Z}_{jk}(t),$$
$$k = 1, \ldots, K,$$

and

$$\overline{\mathbf{S}}^{(r)}(\boldsymbol{\beta}, t) = \sum_{k=1}^{K} \mathbf{S}_k^{(r)}(\boldsymbol{\beta}, t), r = 0, 1.$$

In both cases, the solution to $[\mathbf{U}(\boldsymbol{\beta}) = \mathbf{0}]$ is denoted by $\hat{\boldsymbol{\beta}}$.

Although the failure times within the same unit tend to be **correlated**, the estimator $\hat{\boldsymbol{\beta}}$ can be shown to be consistent for $\boldsymbol{\beta}$ and asymptotically p-variate normal provided that the marginal models are correctly specified. However, the conventional **covariance matrix** estimator $\mathcal{I}^{-1}(\hat{\boldsymbol{\beta}})$, where $\mathcal{I}(\boldsymbol{\beta}) = -\partial^2 \log L(\boldsymbol{\beta})/\partial \boldsymbol{\beta}^2$, is no longer valid, the reason being that $\mathcal{I}(\boldsymbol{\beta})$ is not the covariance matrix of $\mathbf{U}(\boldsymbol{\beta})$ in the presence of intraclass dependence. By approximating $\mathbf{U}(\boldsymbol{\beta})$ with a sum of independent and identically distributed zero-mean random vectors, one can show that, for large n and relatively small K, the random vector $\mathbf{U}(\boldsymbol{\beta})$ is approximately zero-mean normal with covariance matrix estimator

$$\mathbf{V}(\boldsymbol{\beta}) = \sum_{i=1}^{n} \sum_{k=1}^{K} \sum_{l=1}^{K} \mathbf{W}_{ik}(\hat{\boldsymbol{\beta}}) \mathbf{W}_{il}(\hat{\boldsymbol{\beta}})',$$

where

$$\mathbf{W}_{ik}(\boldsymbol{\beta}) = \Delta_{ik} \left[\mathbf{Z}_{ik}(X_{ik}) - \frac{\mathbf{S}_k^{(1)}(\boldsymbol{\beta}, X_{ik})}{S_k^{(0)}(\boldsymbol{\beta}, X_{ik})} \right]$$

$$- \sum_{j=1}^{n} \frac{\Delta_{jk} Y_{ik}(X_{jk}) \exp[\boldsymbol{\beta}' \mathbf{Z}_{ik}(X_{jk})]}{S_k^{(0)}(\boldsymbol{\beta}, X_{jk})}$$

$$\times \left[\mathbf{Z}_{ik}(X_{jk}) - \frac{\mathbf{S}_k^{(1)}(\boldsymbol{\beta}, X_{jk})}{S_k^{(0)}(\boldsymbol{\beta}, X_{jk})} \right]$$

and

$$
\mathbf{W}_{ik}(\boldsymbol{\beta}) = \Delta_{ik}\left[\mathbf{Z}_{ik}(X_{ik}) - \frac{\overline{\mathbf{S}}^{(1)}(\boldsymbol{\beta}, X_{ik})}{\overline{S}^{(0)}(\boldsymbol{\beta}, X_{ik})}\right]
$$

$$
- \sum_{j=1}^{n}\sum_{l=1}^{K}\frac{\Delta_{jl}Y_{ik}(X_{jl})\exp[\boldsymbol{\beta}'\mathbf{Z}_{ik}(X_{jl})]}{\overline{S}^{(0)}(\boldsymbol{\beta}, X_{jl})}
$$

$$
\times\left[\mathbf{Z}_{ik}(X_{jl}) - \frac{\overline{\mathbf{S}}^{(1)}(\boldsymbol{\beta}, X_{jl})}{\overline{S}^{(0)}(\boldsymbol{\beta}, X_{jl})}\right]
$$

under models (1) and (2), respectively. Consequently, $\hat{\boldsymbol{\beta}}$ is approximately normal with covariance matrix estimator $\mathbf{D}(\hat{\boldsymbol{\beta}}) = \mathcal{I}^{-1}(\hat{\boldsymbol{\beta}})\mathbf{V}(\hat{\boldsymbol{\beta}})\mathcal{I}^{-1}(\hat{\boldsymbol{\beta}})$. We call $\mathcal{I}^{-1}(\hat{\boldsymbol{\beta}})$ and $\mathbf{D}(\hat{\boldsymbol{\beta}})$ the naive and robust estimators, respectively. In the case of $K = 1$, the matrix $\mathbf{D}(\hat{\boldsymbol{\beta}})$ reduces to the Lin–Wei [14] robust covariance matrix estimator for the maximum partial likelihood estimator under **misspecified** proportional hazards models. To test the global hypothesis that $\boldsymbol{\beta} = \boldsymbol{\beta}_0$, one may use the chi-square statistic $\mathbf{U}'(\boldsymbol{\beta}_0)\mathbf{V}^{-1}(\boldsymbol{\beta}_0)\mathbf{U}(\boldsymbol{\beta}_0)$ or $(\hat{\boldsymbol{\beta}} - \boldsymbol{\beta}_0)'\mathbf{D}^{-1}(\hat{\boldsymbol{\beta}})(\hat{\boldsymbol{\beta}} - \boldsymbol{\beta}_0)$; to test the general linear hypothesis H_0: $\mathbf{L}\boldsymbol{\beta} = \mathbf{d}$, where $\mathbf{L}$ is an $r \times p$ matrix of constants and $\mathbf{d}$ is an $r \times 1$ vector of constants, one refers $(\mathbf{L}\hat{\boldsymbol{\beta}} - \mathbf{d})'\{\mathbf{L}\mathbf{D}(\hat{\boldsymbol{\beta}})\mathbf{L}'\}^{-1}(\mathbf{L}\hat{\boldsymbol{\beta}} - \mathbf{d})$ to the **chi-square distribution** with r **degrees of freedom**.

The above results are analogous to those of the **generalized estimation equations** (GEE) for the analysis of **marginal models** for **longitudinal data** with an independence working assumption. A similar idea can be used to estimate the cumulative baseline hazard functions $\Lambda_{0k}(t) = \int_0^t \lambda_{0k}(u)\mathrm{d}u$, $k = 1, \dots, K$, and $\Lambda_0(t) = \int_0^t \lambda_0(u)\mathrm{d}u$ for models (1) and (2). Specifically, under the independence working assumption, the Aalen–Breslow type estimators for $\Lambda_{0k}(t)$ and $\Lambda_0(t)$ are

$$
\hat{\Lambda}_{0k}(t) = \sum_{i=1}^{n}\frac{I(X_{ik} \leq t)\Delta_{ik}}{S_k^{(0)}(\hat{\boldsymbol{\beta}}, X_{ik})}, \quad k = 1, \dots, K, \quad (5)
$$

and

$$
\hat{\Lambda}_0(t) = \sum_{i=1}^{n}\sum_{k=1}^{K}\frac{I(X_{ik} \leq t)\Delta_{ik}}{\overline{S}^{(0)}(\hat{\boldsymbol{\beta}}, X_{ik})}. \quad (6)
$$

These estimators are consistent and asymptotically normal. In fact, the p-vector of random processes,

$$
n^{1/2}[\hat{\Lambda}_{01}(t) - \Lambda_{01}(t), \dots, \hat{\Lambda}_{0K}(t) - \Lambda_{0K}(t)]',
$$

converges weakly to a p-dimensional zero-mean Gaussian random field, and the covariance between $\hat{\Lambda}_{0k}(t)$ and $\hat{\Lambda}_{0l}(s)$ can be estimated by $\sum_{i=1}^{n}\xi_{ik}(t; \hat{\boldsymbol{\beta}})\xi_{il}(s; \hat{\boldsymbol{\beta}})$, where

$$
\xi_{ik}(t; \boldsymbol{\beta})
$$
$$
= \frac{I(X_{ik} \leq t)\Delta_{ik}}{S_k^{(0)}(\boldsymbol{\beta}, X_{ik})}
$$
$$
- \sum_{j=1}^{n}\frac{I(X_{jk} \leq t)\Delta_{jk}Y_{ik}(X_{jk})\exp[\boldsymbol{\beta}'\mathbf{Z}_{ik}(X_{jk})]}{S_k^{(0)}(\boldsymbol{\beta}, X_{jk})^2}
$$
$$
- \left[\sum_{j=1}^{n}\frac{I(X_{jk} \leq t)\Delta_{jk}S_k^{(1)}(\boldsymbol{\beta}, X_{jk})}{S_k^{(0)}(\boldsymbol{\beta}, X_{jk})^2}\right]'
$$
$$
\times \mathcal{I}^{-1}(\boldsymbol{\beta})\sum_{l=1}^{K}\mathbf{W}_{il}(\boldsymbol{\beta}).
$$

In addition, $n^{1/2}[\hat{\Lambda}_0(t) - \Lambda_0(t)]$ converges weakly to a zero-mean Gaussian process, and the covariance between $\hat{\Lambda}_0(t)$ and $\hat{\Lambda}_0(s)$ can be estimated by $\sum_{i=1}^{n}\sum_{k=1}^{K}\sum_{l=1}^{K}\xi_{ik}(t; \hat{\boldsymbol{\beta}})\xi_{il}(s; \hat{\boldsymbol{\beta}})$, where

$$
\xi_{ik}(t; \boldsymbol{\beta})
$$
$$
= \frac{I(X_{ik} \leq t)\Delta_{ik}}{\overline{S}^{(0)}(\boldsymbol{\beta}, X_{ik})}
$$
$$
- \sum_{j=1}^{n}\sum_{l=1}^{K}\frac{I(X_{jl} \leq t)\Delta_{jl}Y_{ik}(X_{jl})\exp[\boldsymbol{\beta}'\mathbf{Z}_{ik}(X_{jl})]}{\overline{S}^{(0)}(\boldsymbol{\beta}, X_{jl})^2}
$$
$$
- \left[\sum_{j=1}^{n}\sum_{l=1}^{K}\frac{I(X_{jl} \leq t)\Delta_{jl}\overline{\mathbf{S}}^{(1)}(\boldsymbol{\beta}, X_{jl})}{\overline{S}^{(0)}(\boldsymbol{\beta}, X_{jl})^2}\right]'
$$
$$
\times \mathcal{I}^{-1}(\boldsymbol{\beta})\mathbf{W}_{ik}(\boldsymbol{\beta}).
$$

The large-sample properties for the corresponding baseline survival function estimators $\exp[-\hat{\Lambda}_{0k}(t)]$, $k = 1, \dots, K$, and $\exp[-\hat{\Lambda}_0(t)]$ follow from the **delta method**. Furthermore, simple modifications can be made to estimate the survival functions associated with specific covariate values.

Software Availability

The estimators $\hat{\boldsymbol{\beta}}$, $\hat{\Lambda}_{0k}$, $k = 1, \dots, K$, and $\hat{\Lambda}_0$ are constructed under the independence working assumption, and therefore can be obtained from any existing software for the **Cox regression**. The robust covariance matrix estimator for $\hat{\beta}$ is available in **S-PLUS**, SAS, and STATA packages, as well as in a special FORTRAN program [12]. The robust variance–covariance estimators for $\hat{\Lambda}_{0k}, k = 1, \ldots, K$, and $\hat{\Lambda}_0$ have not been implemented in commercially available software packages.

An Example

We now provide an illustration with the well-known Diabetic Retinopathy Study [4], which was conducted by the National Eye Institute to evaluate the effectiveness of laser photocoagulation in delaying the onset of blindness in patients with diabetic retinopathy. The study enrolled 1742 patients. One eye of each patient was randomly selected for photocoagulation and the other eye was observed without treatment. The patients were followed over several years for the occurrence of blindness in their left and right eyes.

We confine our attention to a subset of the data with 197 high-risk patients previously analyzed by Huster et al. [7] and Lin [13]. By the end of the study, 54 treated eyes and 101 control eyes in this subsample had developed blindness. In this example, each patient could potentially experience blindness in both eyes; therefore, there are two failure types with $k = 1$ and 2, denoting the left and right eyes, respectively. Since there are no biological differences between the left and right eyes, it is natural to assume a common baseline hazard function for the two failure types.

As mentioned above, the primary objective of this study was to assess whether laser photocoagulation delays the occurrence of blindness. Because juvenile and adult diabetes have very different courses, it is desirable to examine how the age at onset of diabetes may affect the time to blindness. Thus, we consider model (2) with $\mathbf{Z}_{ik} = (Z_{1ik}, Z_{2ik}, Z_{3ik})'$, $i = 1, \ldots, 197; k = 1, 2$, where

$$Z_{1ik} = \begin{cases} 1, & \text{if the } k\text{th eye of the } i\text{th patient} \\ & \text{was on treatment,} \\ 0, & \text{otherwise;} \end{cases}$$

$$Z_{2ik} = \begin{cases} 1, & \text{if the } i\text{th patient had adult} \\ & \text{onset diabetes,} \\ 0, & \text{if the } i\text{th patient had juvenile} \\ & \text{onset diabetes;} \end{cases}$$

Table 1

Variable	Parameter estimate	Stand. error estimate	
		Naive	Robust
Treatment (Z_1)	−0.425	0.218	0.185
Diabetic type (Z_2)	0.341	0.199	0.196
Interaction ($Z_1 \times Z_2$)	−0.846	0.351	0.304

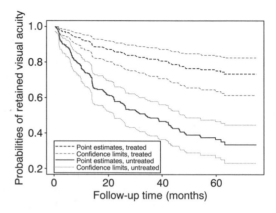

Figure 1 Estimates and pointwise 95% confidence intervals for survival functions

and $Z_{3ik} = Z_{1ik} \times Z_{2ik}$. The results for the estimation of the regression parameters are shown in Table 1. The robust standard error estimates are appreciably smaller than the naive estimates, the latter ignoring the dependence between the left and right eyes. The treatment appears to be effective, and this effect is much stronger for adult-onset diabetes than for juvenile-onset diabetes.

Figure 1 displays the estimates and pointwise 95% confidence intervals for the survival functions, namely, the probabilities of retained visual acuity, for adult-onset diabetes, separated by treatment groups. As expected, these probabilities are much higher for the treated eyes than for the untreated ones.

Further Results

The estimation of β under models (1) and (2) was first studied by Wei et al. [23] and Lee et al. [9], respectively, and further developed by Lin [13], while the estimation of $\Lambda_{0k}, k = 1, \ldots, K$, and Λ_0 was investigated by Spiekerman & Lin [22]. The latter authors established a rigorous asymptotic theory for the estimation of both the regression parameters and baseline hazard functions under a general marginal model which allows M, $1 \le M \le K$, different baseline hazard functions among the K types of failures. In a separate paper, they [21] developed a class of graphical and numerical techniques for checking the adequacy of models (1) and (2). The readers are referred to the aforementioned papers for further theoretical details as well as additional numerical examples. Incidentally, Huster et al. [7] studied model (2) with a parametric baseline hazard function, while Guo & Lin [6] deal with discrete-time versions of models (1) and (2).

Liang et al. [11] proposed a different procedure for analyzing model (2). Their estimating function is similar to (4), but they replaced $\overline{\mathbf{S}}^{(1)}/\overline{S}^{(0)}$ by an analog which exploits pairwise comparisons of independent observations. The actual form of their **estimating function** is

$$\sum_{i=1}^{n}\sum_{k=1}^{K} I[n_i(X_{ik}) > 0]\Delta_{ik}$$

$$\times \left[\mathbf{Z}_{ik}(X_{ik}) - n_i^{-1}(X_{ik})\sum_{j\neq i}\sum_{l} \mathbf{e}_{ik,jl}(\boldsymbol{\beta}, X_{ik})\right],$$

where $n_i(t) = \sum_{j\neq i}\sum_{l} Y_{jl}(t)$ and

$$\mathbf{e}_{ik,jl}(\boldsymbol{\beta}, t) = \frac{\begin{aligned}&Y_{ik}(t)\mathbf{Z}_{ik}(t)\exp[\boldsymbol{\beta}'\mathbf{Z}_{ik}(t)]\\ &+Y_{jl}(t)\mathbf{Z}_{jl}(t)\exp[\boldsymbol{\beta}'\mathbf{Z}_{jl}(t)]\end{aligned}}{\begin{aligned}&Y_{ik}(t)\exp[\boldsymbol{\beta}'\mathbf{Z}_{ik}(t)]\\ &+Y_{jl}(t)\exp[\boldsymbol{\beta}'\mathbf{Z}_{jl}(t)]\end{aligned}}.$$

The resultant estimator is **consistent** and asymptotically normal. The relative efficiency of $\hat{\boldsymbol{\beta}}$ vs. the Liang et al. estimator has not been investigated.

Estimating functions (3) and (4) were derived under the independence working assumption. As in the case of **longitudinal data**, it may be more efficient to use estimating functions that take into account the nature of dependence explicitly. This amounts to incorporating certain weight functions into estimating functions (3) and (4). The resultant estimators remain consistent and asymptotically normal with a sandwich-type variance estimator under mild regularity conditions on the weight function. Due to censoring and the nonlinear nature of the proportional hazards model, it is difficult to construct optimal weight functions. Cai & Prentice [2] investigated a weight function that is the inverse of the

covariance matrix of the marginal martingales associated with the T_{ik}s. Their theoretical calculations and simulation studies indicated that the efficiency gains in using such weighted estimating functions over estimating functions (3) and (4) are small unless the correlations of failure times are unusually high.

There has been considerable research on semiparametric multivariate failure time distributions which characterize the strength of association among failure time components by a limited number of parameters while leaving the forms of the marginal distributions unspecified (e.g. [3], [18], [1]). One may extend these multivariate distributions by formulating their marginal distributions with model (1) or (2). One may then estimate the marginal regression parameters and baseline hazard functions by (3) and (5) or (4) and (6) and proceed to estimate the association parameters by the pseudo-**maximum likelihood** method [5]. This approach was mentioned by Bandeen-Roche & Liang [1], but its inferential properties have yet to be investigated.

Prentice & Hsu [19] studied simultaneous regression on the marginal hazard ratios and pairwise dependencies, which is analogous to the regression on the means and covariances of noncensored multivariate responses [20]. They used the estimating function of Cai & Prentice [2] for the marginal hazard ratio parameters and developed a similar *ad hoc* estimating function for the dependence parameters. They showed that the solutions to this pair of estimating functions are consistent and asymptotically normal, with a sandwich-type covariance matrix estimator.

The **accelerated failure-time** and **additive hazards models** are two important alternatives to the proportional hazards model. The former relates the logarithm of the failure time linearly to the covariates [8], while the latter relates the conditional hazard function linearly to the covariates [16]. One may formulate the marginal distributions of multivariate failure time data with accelerated failure time models or additive hazards models rather than proportional hazards models. The corresponding inference procedures were studied, respectively, by Lin & Wei [15] and Lee et al. [10], and by Lin & Ying [17].

References

[1]   Bandeen-Roche, K.J. & Liang, K.-Y. (1996). Modelling failure time associations in data with multiple levels of clustering, *Biometrika* **83**, 29–39.

[2] Cai, J. & Prentice, R.L. (1995). Estimating equations for hazard ratio parameters based on correlated failure time data, *Biometrika* **82**, 151-164.

[3] Clayton, D.G. (1978). A model for association in bivariate life tables and its applications in epidemiological studies of familial tendency in chronic disease incidence, *Biometrika* **65**, 141-151.

[4] Diabetic Retinopathy Study Research Group (1981). Diabetic retinopathy study, *Investigative Ophthalmology and Visual Science* **21**, 149-226.

[5] Gong, G. & Samaniego, F.J. (1981). Pseudo maximum likelihood, *Annals of Statistics* **9**, 861-869.

[6] Guo, S.W. & Lin, D.Y. (1994). Regression analysis of multivariate grouped survival data, *Biometrics* **50**, 632-639.

[7] Huster, W.J., Brookmeyer, R. & Self, S.G. (1989). Modelling paired survival data with covariates, *Biometrics* **45**, 145-156.

[8] Kalbfleisch, J.D. & Prentice, R.L. (1980). *The Statistical Analysis of Failure Time Data.* Wiley, New York.

[9] Lee, E.W., Wei, L.J. & Amato, D.A. (1992). Cox-type regression analysis for large numbers of small groups of correlated failure time observations, in *Survival Analysis: State of the Art*, J.P. Klein & P.K. Goel, eds. Kluwer, Dordrecht, pp. 237-247.

[10] Lee, E.W., Wei, L.J. & Ying, Z. (1993). Linear regression analysis for highly stratified failure time data, *Journal of the American Statistical Association* **88**, 557-565.

[11] Liang, K.-Y., Self, S.G. & Chang, Y.-C. (1993). Modeling marginal hazards in multivariate failure-time data, *Journal of the Royal Statistical Society, Series B* **55**, 441-453.

[12] Lin, D.Y. (1993). MULCOX2: a general computer program for the Cox regression analysis of multivariate failure time data, *Computer Methods and Programs in Biomedicine* **40**, 279-293.

[13] Lin, D.Y. (1994). Cox regression analysis of multivariate failure time data: the marginal approach, *Statistics in Medicine* **13**, 2233-2247.

[14] Lin, D.Y. & Wei, L.J. (1989). The robust inference for the Cox proportional hazards model, *Journal of the American Statistical Association* **84**, 1074-1078.

[15] Lin, J.S. & Wei, L.J. (1992). Linear regression analysis for multivariate failure time observations, *Journal of the American Statistical Association* **87**, 1071-1097.

[16] Lin, D.Y. & Ying, Z. (1994). Semiparametric analysis of the additive risk model, *Biometrika* **81**, 61-71.

[17] Lin, D.Y. & Ying, Z. (1997). Additive hazards regression models for survival data, in *Proceedings of the First Seattle Symposium in Biostatistics: Survival Analysis*, D.Y. Lin & T.R. Fleming, eds. Springer-Verlag, New York, pp. 185-198.

[18] Oakes, D. (1989). Bivariate survival models induced by frailties, *Journal of the American Statistical Association* **84**, 487-493.

[19] Prentice, R.L. & Hsu, L. (1997). Regression on hazard ratios and cross-ratios in multivariate failure time analysis, *Biometrika*, **84**, 349-363.

[20] Prentice, R.L. & Zhao, L.P. (1991). Estimating equations for parameters in means and covariances of multivariate discrete and continuous responses, *Biometrics* **47**, 825-839.

[21] Spiekerman, C.F. & Lin, D.Y. (1996). Checking the marginal Cox model for correlated failure time data, *Biometrika* **83**, 143-156.

[22] Spiekerman, C.F. & Lin, D.Y. (1996). Marginal Regression Models for Multivariate Failure Time Data, *Technical Report 144*. Department of Biostatistics, University of Washington.

[23] Wei, L.J., Lin, D.Y. & Weissfeld, L. (1989). Regression analysis of multivariate incomplete failure time data by modeling marginal distributions, *Journal of the American Statistical Association* **84**, 1065-1073.

D.Y. LIN

Marginal Probability

In many situations, interest focuses on probability distributions for multiple random variables. For example, one may be studying height, weight, blood pressure, and cholesterol levels in a population, variables likely to be **correlated** with one another. Knowledge of the joint distribution of these variables allows one to calculate the probabilities associated with any particular outcome of interest. Marginal probabilities relate to the univariate distribution, or marginal distribution, associated with any of the variables under consideration.

To fix notation, first consider a **bivariate** model for two random variables X and Y. Let $f_{X,Y}(x, y)$ denote the joint probability mass function if X and Y are discrete or the joint probability density function if X and Y are continuous. If X and Y are discrete, the marginal probability mass functions of X and Y are given by

$$f_X(x) = \sum_y f_{X,Y}(x, y)$$

and

$$f_Y(y) = \sum_x f_{X,Y}(x, y),$$

where the summations are taken over all of the values of Y or X. In this case, the joint probability mass function can be written in tabular form, with the columns corresponding to the possible values of X and the rows to the values of Y. Then the marginal distribution of X corresponds to the column sums of the table, and the marginal distribution of Y corresponds to the row sums of the table.

When X and Y are continuous, the marginal probability density functions of X and Y are given by

$$f_X(x) = \int_{-\infty}^{\infty} f_{X,Y}(x, y) \, dy$$

and

$$f_Y(y) = \int_{-\infty}^{\infty} f_{X,Y}(x, y) \, dx.$$

As a special case, when (X, Y) follows a **bivariate normal distribution** with means (μ_X, μ_Y) and **covariance matrix**

$$\begin{pmatrix} \sigma_X^2 & \sigma_{XY} \\ \sigma_{XY} & \sigma_Y^2 \end{pmatrix},$$

then the marginal probability density function of X follows a univariate **normal distribution** with mean μ_X and variance σ_X^2, and similarly for Y.

These marginal distributions can be used to compute probabilities or expectations that involve only X or Y. However, the marginal distributions do not completely describe the joint distribution of X and Y. In fact, many different joint distributions can yield the same marginal distributions. The variables X and Y are independent if and only if the joint distribution of (X, Y) is given by the product of the marginal distributions of X and Y. **Conditional probability** distributions refer to the distribution of one variable for a given value of the other variable.

For multivariate distributions with more than two variables, the corresponding summations or integrals are carried out over the complete range of the other variables under consideration. Extensions to mixtures of discrete and continuous variables are straightforward. For further information, see Casella & Berger [1, Chapter 4]. Regression modeling of multivariate responses sometimes focuses on modeling the marginal mean responses of the observations as a function of covariates, with the correlations between responses possibly being viewed as **nuisance parameters**. Diggle et al. [2, Chapter 8] review marginal modeling of multivariate discrete and continuous responses.

References

[1]   Casella, G. & Berger, R.L. (1990). *Statistical Inference*. Wadsworth, Belmont.

[2]   Diggle, P.J., Liang, K.-Y. & Zeger, S.L. (1994). *Analysis of Longitudinal Data*. Clarendon Press, Oxford.

(*See also* **Longitudinal Data Analysis, Overview; Marginal Models; Marginal Models for Multivariate Survival Data**)

DAVID WYPIJ

Mark–Recapture *see* Capture–Recapture

Marked Point Process *see* Point Processes

Marker Association Segregation Chi-Square (MASC) *see* Disease–Marker Association

Marker Processes

In many survival studies, individuals give rise to **stochastic processes**, called *marker processes*, that in some way measure the state of "health" of the individuals. Thus, the observed path of the marker process provides information on the propensity of the individual to fail. Such covariates have the potential to be useful in various ways and, in this brief introductory article, we attempt to identify some of these and to give entry points to the developing literature in this area.

Many examples of marker processes arise in survival studies (*see* **Survival Analysis, Overview**). In **clinical trials**, for example, it is common at each follow-up visit to take repeated measures of general health status or of the stage or severity of the disease. In equipment reliability studies, there are often repeated measures of the wear or degradation of the item under study. In the study of the time to breakdown of automobiles, for example, a simple and highly informative marker process is total kilometers traveled. In the study of infection with the Human Immunodeficiency Virus (HIV), much attention has been focused on the estimation of the distribution of "incubation time"; that is, the time from infection with HIV until the diagnosis of AIDS (*see* **AIDS and HIV**). Various marker processes, such as CD4-lymphocyte counts, have been studied and used to provide information both on the time since infection began and on the probability of developing AIDS.

Jewell & Kalbfleisch [5] outline some potential uses of marker processes and their classification forms the basis of the following summary:

1. *Improving estimation of a survival distribution.* In many instances the observed path of the marker provides information on the residual life of the individual under study. The basic idea is that the marker can be utilized to provide an estimate of the residual life for an individual who is **censored**. This can provide more and better information for the estimation of the survivor function (*see* **Survival Distributions and Their Characteristics**). In some instances this allows for adjustment for dependent or informative censoring mechanisms. Taylor et al. [14] and Robins & Rotnitzky [12] give good discussion and examples.

2. *Serving as a surrogate for survival in a comparative trial.* If the time to failure is typically long, then a full survival study may be prohibitively expensive or else require too long for completion. In such instances there may be substantial advantage to using marker processes as **surrogates** for the failure time in investigating the existence and size of treatment effects. In this approach it is required that the survival time be directly related to the marker so that a treatment effect on the marker will have a consequent effect on survival. This potential use of markers was the motivation of Cox [3] in his original paper in this area. Prentice [10] gives a detailed and comprehensive discussion of surrogate endpoints, potential uses, and caveats.

3. *Estimating the time of onset of a disease.* Sometimes the time of onset of a disease is not or cannot be observed. In such instances a marker measured on an affected individual may provide information on the elapsed time since onset. For example, in HIV the time of infection is typically unknown and markers may assist in estimating the time of onset. In a comparative trial, **confounding** of the time of onset with treatment or other comparison has the potential to introduce **bias** into the estimation of effects. The marker's information on time of onset can be used to adjust comparisons in this context and so help to compensate for the onset of confounding. Applications involving unknown onset have been considered by several authors. In the estimation of the incubation period in AIDS, Berman [1] and Muñoz et al. [8] provide examples. Rai & Matthews [11] consider the use of tumor size at death in animal carcinogenicity trials (*see* **Tumor Incidence Experiments**) to estimate the unobserved time since tumor onset. Brookmeyer & Gail [2] and Muñoz et al. [7] consider some theoretical issues associated with the onset of confounding.

In modeling the relationship between the marker process and the survival probabilities, it is convenient to utilize the hazard function. Let $\{X(t) : t > 0\}$ represent the marker process and let $T > 0$ be the time to failure. Conditionally upon the current and past values of the marker, the **hazard** function or failure rate is naturally specified as

$$\lambda(t|X(s), 0 \le s \le t)$$
$$= \lim_{\Delta t \to 0} \Pr\{T \in [t, t + \Delta t)|T \ge t, X(s),$$
$$0 \le s \le t\}/\Delta t. \tag{1}$$

Various more specific parametric and nonparametric models based on (1) could be specified and considered. In applications, other covariates, either fixed or **time-dependent**, may also be present and one may wish to extend (1) to incorporate them into the model. In a comparative trial, for example, (1) could be extended to include treatment effects.

To utilize the marker to estimate residual life or time since onset, as discussed above, the stochastic laws governing $X(t)$ as well as the relationship between $X(t)$ and the failure rate must both be considered. Jewell & Kalbfleisch [4, 5] have provided one example. They consider an additive model for (1),

$$\lambda(t|X(s) : 0 \le s \le t) = h_0(t) + \beta X(t),$$

where $h_0(t)$ is a baseline hazard and β is a regression parameter relating the nonnegative valued marker $X(t)$ to the failure rate. To complete the model, they make various assumptions about $h_0(t)$ and specify simple Markov models for $X(t)$ (*see* **Markov Processes**). From these specifications the dependence of the distribution of residual and past life on current marker values is investigated. Other approaches to jointly modeling the marker process and the failure mechanism are given in Pawitan & Self [9], Shi et al. [13], Jewell & Nielson [6], and Tsiatis et al. [15].

References

[1]   Berman, S.M. (1990). A stochastic model for the distribution of HIV latency time based on T4 counts, *Biometrika* **77**, 733–741.

[2]   Brookmeyer, R. & Gail, M. (1987). Biases in prevalent cohorts, *Biometrics* **43**, 739–749.

[3]   Cox, D.R. (1983). A remark on censoring and surrogate response variables, *Journal of the Royal Statistical Society, Series B* **45**, 391–393.

[4]   Jewell, N.P. & Kalbfleisch, J.D. (1992). Marker processes and applications to AIDS, in *AIDS Epidemiology: Methodological Issues*, N.P. Jewell, K. Dietz & V. Farewell, eds. Birkhauser, Boston.

[5]   Jewell, N.P. & Kalbfleisch, J.D. (1996). Marker processes in survival analysis, *Lifetime Data Analysis* **2**, 15–29.

[6]   Jewell, N.P. & Nielsen, J.P. (1993). A framework for consistent prediction rules based on markers, *Biometrika* **80**, 153–164.

[7]   Munõz, A., Carey, V., Taylor, J.M.G., Chmiel, J.S., Kingsley, L., Raden, M.V. & Hoover, D.R. (1992). Estimation of time since exposure for a prevalent cohort, *Statistics in Medicine* **11**, 939–952.

[8]   Munõz, A., Wang, M.-C., Bass, S., Taylor, J.M.G., Kingsley, L.A., Chmiel, J.S., Polk, B.F. & the Multicenter AIDS Cohort Study Group (1989). Acquired immunodeficiency syndrome (AIDS)-free time after human immunodeficiency virus type 1 (HIV-1) seroconversion in homosexual men, *American Journal of Epidemiology* **130**, 530–539.

[9]   Pawitan, Y. & Self, S. (1993). Modelling disease marker processes in AIDS, *Journal of the American Statistical Association* **88**, 719–726.

[10]   Prentice, R.L. (1989). Surrogate endpoints in clinical trials: definition and operational criteria, *Statistics in Medicine* **8**, 431–440.

[11]   Rai, S. & Matthews, D.E. (1995). The analysis of incomplete data using stochastic covariates, *Canadian Journal of Statistics* **23**, 29–42.

[12]   Robins, J.M. & Rotnitzky, A. (1992). Recovery of information and adjustment for dependent censoring using surrogate markers, in *AIDS Epidemiology: Methodological Issues*, N.P. Jewell, K. Dietz & V. Farewell, eds. Birkhauser, Boston.

[13]   Shi, M., Taylor, J.M.G. & Muñoz, A. (1996). Models for residual time to AIDS, *Lifetime Data Analysis* **2**, 1–14.

[14]   Taylor, J.M.G., Munõz, A., Bass, S.M., Saah, A.J., Chmiel, J.S., Kingsley, L.A. & the Multicentre AIDS Cohort Study (1990). Estimating the distribution of times from HIV seroconversion to AIDS using multiple imputation, *Statistics in Medicine* **9**, 505–514.

[15]   Tsiatis, A.A., DeGruttola, V. & Wulfsohn, M.S. (1995). Modelling the relationship of survival to longitudinal data measured with error. Applications to survival and CD4 counts in patients with AIDS, *Journal of the American Statistical Association* **90**, 27–37.

JOHN D. KALBFLEISCH

Markers *see* Biased Sampling of Cohorts in Epidemiology

Markov Chain Monte Carlo

Markov chain Monte Carlo (MCMC) is a powerful technique for performing integration by **simulation**. In recent years, MCMC has revolutionized the application of **Bayesian** statistics. Many high-dimensional, complex models which were formerly intractable can now be handled routinely. MCMC has also been used in specialized non-Bayesian problems. Introductory material on MCMC methods and biostatistical applications can be found in Gilks et al. [20] and Gelman & Rubin [13].

Suppose that we wish to evaluate the expected value (**expectation**) of some function $g(\theta)$ over a probability density function $f(\theta): E_f[g(\theta)] = \int g(\theta)f(\theta)d\theta$. If we could draw samples $\theta^{(1)}, \theta^{(2)}, \ldots, \theta^{(n)}$ independently from $f(\theta)$, then we could estimate

$$\hat{E}_f[g(\theta)] = \frac{1}{n}\sum_{i=1}^{n}g(\theta^{(i)}). \quad (1)$$

This technique is called **Monte Carlo** *integration*. We have $\text{var}\{\hat{E}_f[g(\theta)]\} = \text{var}_f[g(\theta)]/n$, so the estimate

$\hat{E}_f[g(\theta)]$ can be made as accurate as desired by increasing the sample size n. In Bayesian applications, our density $f(\theta)$ is a posterior distribution $f(\theta|\mathbf{x})$, where θ is a collection of model unknowns (parameters and missing data), and $\mathbf{x}$ denotes observed data. The function $g(\theta)$ might be the kth element of the vector θ, for example, in which case $E_f[g(\theta)]$ would be the posterior expectation of θ_k. Other forms for $g(\cdot)$ could be used to evaluate posterior **variances, correlations, quantiles**, etc. Note that the accuracy of $\hat{E}_f[g(\theta)]$ is not limited by the amount of data in $\mathbf{x}$.

Typically in Bayesian applications, θ is high-dimensional and $f(\theta|\mathbf{x})$ has a complicated, nonstandard form. Sampling independently from $f(\theta|\mathbf{x})$ is generally not possible. Therefore we could try to devise sampling schemes which generate *dependent* samples $\theta^{(1)}, \theta^{(2)}, \ldots, \theta^{(n)}$, but for which (1) is still a **consistent** estimator of $E_f[g(\theta)]$. One possibility is to use a **Markov chain**: this is then *Markov chain* Monte Carlo. A Markov chain generates each iterate $\theta^{(i)}$, taking into account only the previous value $\theta^{(i-1)}$. Subject to some regularity conditions, a Markov chain will generate samples $\theta^{(i)}$ from its *stationary* distribution, for large i.

In general, it is surprisingly easy to construct a Markov chain the stationary distribution of which is our target distribution $f(\theta|\mathbf{x})$, and for which (1) is a consistent estimator of $E_f[g(\theta)]$. The method was first proposed in 1953 by Metropolis et al. [24], and was generalized in 1970 by Hastings [23]. For many years, the **algorithm** was used mainly in the field of statistical mechanics. In 1984 the *Gibbs sampling* algorithm (later recognized as a special case of the Metropolis–Hastings algorithm) was proposed by Geman & Geman [15] as a tool for image reconstruction (*see* **Image Analysis and Tomography**). In 1990, the considerable potential of the Gibbs sampler was brought to the attention of the wider statistical community by Gelfand & Smith [8]. A generalization of the Metropolis–Hastings algorithm was proposed by Green [22] in 1995.

The Metropolis–Hastings Algorithm

We now describe the Metropolis–Hastings algorithm. For notational convenience we suppress dependence on data $\mathbf{x}$, and for the moment we continue to assume that θ is a continuous random vector. We begin the chain with an arbitrary starting value, $\theta^{(0)}$, and then

produce the chain $\theta^{(1)}, \theta^{(2)}, \ldots$ by iterating around the following two steps. At each iteration $i + 1$:

Step 1: generate a *candidate* value θ' from a *proposal distribution* $q(\cdot|\theta^{(i)})$;

Step 2: with probability

$$\alpha(\theta^{(i)}, \theta') = \min\left[1, \frac{f(\theta')q(\theta^{(i)}|\theta')}{f(\theta^{(i)})q(\theta'|\theta^{(i)})}\right] \tag{2}$$

accept the candidate (i.e. set $\theta^{(i+1)}$ equal to θ'); otherwise reject the candidate (i.e. set $\theta^{(i+1)}$ equal to $\theta^{(i)}$).

Heuristically, we aim to generate dependent samples from $f(\cdot)$ by sampling from a more convenient distribution at Step 1, and then correcting for this in a rather unintuitive but appropriate way at Step 2. To implement Step 2, generate a **pseudo-random number** u from a **uniform** $(0, 1)$ **distribution**. If $u \leq \alpha(\theta^{(i)}, \theta')$ accept θ'; otherwise reject it. The choice of the proposal density $q(\cdot|\cdot)$ is largely up to the user, the prime considerations being computational convenience and rapid mixing (see below). Note that the target density $f(\cdot)$ need not be normalized to integrate to one, since the normalization constant cancels in (2). This is particularly convenient for Bayesian analyses, where the posterior distribution $f(\theta|\mathbf{x})$ is proportional to the **likelihood** $p(\mathbf{x}|\theta)$ times the **prior** $p(\theta)$. Thus $p(\mathbf{x}|\theta)p(\theta)$ can be used in place of $f(\cdot)$ in (2), and there is no need to evaluate the normalization constant $\int p(\mathbf{x}|\theta)p(\theta)\mathrm{d}\theta$.

For the Metropolis–Hastings chain to be useful, it must be *irreducible*. Informally, irreducibility means that the chain is able to reach anywhere within the domain of $f(\cdot)$ within a finite number of iterations (see [37] for a more careful definition). If the chain is irreducible, it will eventually settle down to produce samples $\theta^{(i)}$ from its *stationary* distribution, which can be shown to be $f(\cdot)$. Thus the choice of starting value $\theta^{(0)}$ is not important, although it is generally advisable to avoid starting values well into the tails of $f(\theta)$, which could delay convergence to $f(\cdot)$. There is no particular advantage in starting the chain at the mode of $f(\cdot)$, since the chain must still be run long enough for it to "forget" its starting value. If the chain is reducible, it will never forget its starting value, since the starting value will determine which parts of the space can be reached. Irreducibility is generally easily verified by inspecting the form of

$q(\cdot|\cdot)$, although in some genetics applications involving complex pedigrees, establishing irreducibility can be difficult (see [30]).

When applied to output from an irreducible Metropolis–Hastings chain, (1) is a consistent estimator of $E_f[g(\theta)]$. In calculating (1) it is usual to discard the first m iterates of the chain (the *burn-in*), during which the chain exhibits dependence on the starting value $\theta^{(0)}$. Several methods have been developed for diagnosing *convergence* (i.e. determining m) and for determining the run length n. Most are approximate in some way, and the most popular [12, 25] monitor the sample path of only univariate quantities, such as a single element of θ. Some methods rely on output from a single chain, and others require multiple chains to be run. For a recent review of convergence diagnostics, see Cowles & Carlin [5]. There is some debate in the literature regarding the number of chains to run: Gelman & Rubin [11, 12] advocate several long chains, while Geyer [16] recommends one very long chain. There is no justification for running a large number of short chains.

There is no justification for attempting to create pseudo-independent samples for input into (1) by *thinning* the output (i.e. using only every jth iterate from the chain) or, even worse, by running a large number of short chains and using only the last iterate from each. The theory of ergodic Markov chains guarantees the consistency of (1), despite the obvious lack of independence within the chain. The only justification for thinning is to reduce computer storage requirements.

Besides being irreducible, it is also important that the chain is *geometrically ergodic*; in other words, that convergence towards the stationary distribution $f(\cdot)$ proceeds at a geometric rate (see [37]). Unless the chain is geometrically ergodic, it is not possible to say anything useful about the variance of (1), and the chain may be very badly behaved, producing long meanders and erratic behavior. Nongeometrically ergodic chains are therefore effectively useless. Unfortunately, establishing geometric ergodicity in any particular context is not trivial, and theory tends to lag somewhat behind practice, although useful results have been obtained (see [28] and references therein). If the chain is geometrically ergodic, the variance of (1) can be estimated. A popular method is the method of *batch means*: the output is divided into n_1 consecutive batches of size n_2, and the sample mean $\bar{g}_j$ of $g(\cdot)$ within each batch j is calculated.

If n_2 is large enough, the batch means will be approximately independent, and the variance of (1) can be estimated as n_1^{-1} times the usual sample variance of $\bar{g}_1, \bar{g}_2, \ldots, \bar{g}_{n_1}$. Often, n_1 is set to about 20. Other methods of variance estimation are given by Geyer [16]. An estimate of the variance of (1) can be used to calculate how much longer to run the chain.

The Metropolis–Hastings algorithm is not limited to situations in which θ is a continuous random vector, although this is the usual situation in biostatistical applications. Discrete variables occur in genetics applications, where some elements of θ are unobserved genotypes, and in applications where discrete-valued covariates are missing. The same form of acceptance probability (2) applies regardless of whether $f(\cdot)$ is a probability, a probability density, a product of probabilities and densities, or a density with respect to an arbitrary measure.

Proposal Distributions

Considerable freedom can be exercised in the choice of proposal distribution $q(\theta'|\theta^{(i)})$, provided that the resulting chain is both irreducible and geometrically ergodic. In a Bayesian context, $q(\theta'|\theta^{(i)})$ may also depend on the data **x**. A *symmetric* proposal, for which $q(\theta'|\theta^{(i)}) = q(\theta^{(i)}|\theta')$ for all θ' and $\theta^{(i)}$, results in an acceptance probability (2) which does not depend on $q(\cdot|\cdot)$. This is the form described in the original algorithm of Metropolis et al. [24]. An *independence* proposal is one which does not depend on $\theta^{(i)}$, so $q(\theta'|\theta^{(i)}) = q(\theta')$. Independence proposals can be either very good (trivially, setting $q(\theta') = f(\theta')$ results in an acceptance probability of 1.0 and independent sampling from $f(\cdot)$), or very bad (if the tails of $q(\cdot)$ are lighter than those of $f(\cdot)$, then the chain will not even be geometrically ergodic [28]).

Many other forms of proposal are possible; see Tierney [36]. Different choices will result in different rates of *mixing*. A rapidly mixing chain will move about the domain of $f(\cdot)$ fluidly, and will quickly converge to $f(\cdot)$. A slow-mixing chain will exhibit significant long-lag **autocorrelations**, and will require a very long run to obtain adequate precision in (1). It is difficult in general to predict the behavior of any particular choice of proposal. A proposal distribution which nearly always results in rejection at Step 2 will be slow-mixing, since the chain will only occasionally move. However, a proposal distribution which nearly always results in acceptance may also be slow mixing, if the high acceptance rate is achieved by proposing only very small steps. Gelman et al. [14] show, for a large class of problems using a symmetric proposal, that one should aim for acceptance rates in the range 0.15–0.5.

Hybrid chains [36] employ a set of proposal distributions $q_1(\cdot|\cdot)$, $q_2(\cdot|\cdot)$, ..., at each iteration choosing one proposal either randomly, or deterministically by cycling through the set. For example q_1 could be a symmetric proposal, and q_2 an independence proposal. A hybrid chain is often better than the sum of its parts; for example, it may be irreducible and geometrically ergodic even if none of the constituent single-proposal chains are.

Single-component Metropolis–Hastings is a special case of a hybrid chain. Vector θ is partitioned into k components $\theta = (\theta_1, \theta_2, \ldots, \theta_k)$; for example, each component could be just one element of θ. For each component j, a proposal $q_j(\theta'_j|\theta^{(i)})$ is defined which updates only component j, generating a candidate point $\theta' = (\theta_1^{(i)}, \ldots, \theta_{j-1}^{(i)}, \theta'_j, \theta_{j+1}^{(i)}, \ldots, \theta_k^{(i)})$. The acceptance probability (2) then becomes

$$\alpha(\theta^{(i)}, \theta') = \min\left[1, \frac{f(\theta')q_j(\theta_j^{(i)}|\theta')}{f(\theta^{(i)})q_j(\theta'_j|\theta^{(i)})}\right], \quad (3)$$

assuming that the choice of proposal q_j does not depend on the current θ. Most applications of Metropolis–Hastings use single-component updating, since it is much easier to construct proposals in low dimensions. However, when $f(\cdot)$ specifies high correlations between elements of θ, single-component updating can produce very slow mixing, unless highly correlated elements are blocked into the same component.

The *Gibbs sampler* is a special case of single-component Metropolis–Hastings, in which

$$q_j(\theta'_j|\theta^{(i)}) = f(\theta'_j|\theta_1^{(i)}, \ldots, \theta_{j-1}^{(i)}, \theta_{j+1}^{(i)}, \ldots, \theta_k^{(i)}), \quad (4)$$

where the conditional distribution $f(\theta_j|\cdot)$ is derived from the target joint distribution $f(\theta)$, and is called the *full conditional distribution* of θ_j. When $f(\theta)$ is a product of terms, as in the applications described below, the full conditional distribution for θ_j is proportional to the product of those terms containing θ_j. With proposal distributions of the form of (4), the acceptance probability (3) is equal to 1.0, so the chain never rejects. As for generic single-component Metropolis–Hastings, an iteration of the

Gibbs sampler involves updating only one θ_j; subsequent iterations may choose j at random, or deterministically by cycling through $j = 1, \ldots, k$. Thus the Gibbs sampler consists entirely in sampling from full conditional distributions, at each iteration updating one parameter, conditioning on the current values of all the other parameters (and data). Note that, in other articles, a Gibbs iteration is sometimes defined as one complete cycle of updating. Below we use $f(\theta'_j|\cdot)$ to denote (4).

Sampling from full conditional distributions can be difficult, but if they are univariate and log-concave (which they often are), *adaptive rejection sampling (ARS)* can be used [19]. See Gilks [17] for further details on constructing and sampling from full conditional distributions. Gibbs sampling and ARS are implemented in the BUGS **software** [33], for general-purpose Bayesian modeling.

Slow mixing in the Gibbs sampler, or any other single-component updating method, can sometimes be resolved by reparameterization. An important example occurs in Bayesian linear models. The linear predictor $\alpha_0 + \alpha_1 x_{1\ell} + \cdots + \alpha_p x_{p\ell}$, where $x_{1\ell}, \ldots x_{p\ell}$ denote **covariates** for individual ℓ, should be reparameterized as $\beta_0 + \alpha_1(x_{1\ell} - \bar{x}_1) + \cdots + \alpha_p(x_{p\ell} - \bar{x}_p)$, where $\bar{x}_j$ denotes the sample mean of $\{x_{j\ell}, \ell = 1, 2, \ldots\}$. Centering the covariates in this way will reduce posterior correlations between the intercept α_0 and the regression coefficients α_j. Another important example of reparameterization occurs in **hierarchical models**. Consider the Bayesian **random effects model**

$$y_{j\ell} \sim N(\mu + \alpha_j, \sigma_1^2), \qquad \alpha_j \sim N(0, \sigma_2^2),$$
$$\mu \sim N(0, \sigma_3^2), \quad (5)$$

where $j = 1, \ldots, m$, $\ell = 1, \ldots, n$, and the $y_{j\ell}$ are observed data. Gelfand et al. [9] show that the Gibbs sampler mixes poorly for this problem if n is large in relation to m. Thus the mixing rate deteriorates as information on the random effects increases, contradicting a common supposition that mixing is worst when information is scarce. Gelfand et al. [9] suggest a simple reparameterization, which they call *hierarchical centering*:

$$y_{j\ell} \sim N(\beta_j, \sigma_1^2), \qquad \beta_j \sim N(\mu, \sigma_2^2).$$

With this parameterization, the mixing rate increases with both m and n. The idea extends to more complex hierarchical models with nested random effects. See Roberts & Sahu [29] for a rigorous theoretical evaluation of reparameterization strategies in hierarchical models.

Various other strategies have been devised for improving mixing: see Gilks & Roberts [18] for a review.

Reversible-Jump MCMC

The preceding discussion implicitly assumes that the length of vector θ is fixed and known. However, Green [22] has recently demonstrated that important classes of models contain a variable number of parameters, and that the Metropolis–Hastings algorithm extends naturally to these situations. Examples of such models include mixture models [27] where the number of mixture components is unknown, and **change-point problems** with an unknown number of changepoints. Such models allow an essentially nonparametric approach to curve-fitting. Another important example concerns model choice or model averaging, where several models must be entertained, possibly varying in number of parameters. From a Bayesian perspective, the individual models can be thought of as components of an encompassing model.

The general problem is best conveyed with a toy example. Assume that survival times $\mathbf{x}$ in a clinical trial are **exponentially** distributed, and let θ_1 and θ_2 denote log-mortality rates for each arm of the trial. We consider two models: Model 1 asserts that $\theta_1 = \theta_2$; and Model 2 that $\theta_1 \neq \theta_2$. Let $k = 1, 2$ index the models. We place **priors** on k; on θ_1 given $k = 1$; and on θ_1 and θ_2 given $k = 2$. These ingredients define the posterior distribution $f(k, \theta|\mathbf{x})$, where the length of θ is equal to k. We can consider various types of proposal distribution. For example, proposal type A could change θ without changing k, and since this does not affect the dimensionality, the usual acceptance formula (2) applies. Proposal type B could change k. For example, if $k^{(i)} = 1$, type B1 could set $k' = 2$, $\theta_1' = \theta_1^{(i)}$ and sample $\theta_2' \sim N(\theta_1^{(i)}, \sigma^2)$, where σ^2 is fixed. If $k^{(i)} = 2$, type B2 could set $k' = 1$, $\theta_2' = \theta_1' = \theta_1^{(i)}$. Note that, in this example, proposal B2 involves no sampling. Assume that, at any iteration, a type B proposal is chosen with probability 0.5. Then the acceptance probability of a B1 move is, from (2),

$$\min\left[1, \frac{f(2, \theta_1', \theta_2'|(\mathbf{x})\mathrm{d}\theta_1'\mathrm{d}\theta_2' \times I(\theta_1' = \theta_1^{(i)})}{\left\{\begin{array}{l} f(1, \theta_1^{(i)}|\mathbf{x})\mathrm{d}\theta_1^{(i)} \times (2\pi)^{-1/2}\sigma^{-1} \\ \times \exp\{-[1/(2\sigma^2)](\theta_2' - \theta_1^{(i)})^2\}\mathrm{d}\theta_2' \end{array}\right\}}\right] \quad (6)$$

where $I(\cdot)$ denotes the indicator function (*see* **Dummy Variables**). Notice that each density in (6) is converted into a probability through postmultiplication by dimensional terms $\mathrm{d}\theta_1^{(i)}$, etc. However, these dimensional terms cancel in the numerator and denominator, and so they can be ignored. This is a consequence of *dimension matching* in the proposal distributions. Dimension matching is not automatic. For example, suppose that the B1 proposal samples both $\theta_1' \sim N(\theta_1^{(i)}, \sigma^2)$ and $\theta_2' \sim N(\theta_1^{(i)}, \sigma^2)$, but the B2 proposal is as before; then the denominator in (6) would become

$$f(1, \theta_1^{(i)}|\mathbf{x})\mathrm{d}\theta_1^{(i)} \times (2\pi)^{-1/2}\sigma^{-1}\exp\{-[1/(2\sigma^2)]$$
$$\times [(\theta_1' - \theta_1^{(i)})^2 + (\theta_2' - \theta_1^{(i)})^2]\}\mathrm{d}\theta_1'\mathrm{d}\theta_2'.$$

Now the dimensional terms no longer cancel, so the algorithm is not well-defined.

This example illustrates that the usual Metropolis–Hastings algorithm can be used when the dimensionality of θ is unknown. Proposal distributions may propose changes to the dimension, but for each such proposal it must be checked that the reverse proposal satisfies the dimension-matching requirement. Of course, all the usual problems of mixing still apply to this more general framework.

Applications

By now, Markov chain Monte Carlo techniques have been applied in most areas of statistics, in particular biostatistics. For example, the book edited by Gilks et al. [20] contains applications in vaccine efficacy (*see* **Vaccine Studies**), clinical monitoring (*see* **Data and Safety Monitoring,**) **pharmacokinetics**, disease **mapping**, medical imaging (*see* **Image Analysis and Tomography**), genetics (*see* **Human Genetics, Overview**), and epidemiologic **measurement error**. Also, the book edited by Berry & Stangl [2] includes applications in medical **decision analysis, clinical trial** design, **crossover trials, meta-analysis** and change-point analysis of randomized trials, pharmacokinetics, tumor hemodynamics (*see*

Tumor Growth) and perinatal mortality (*see* **Infant and Perinatal Mortality**). Rather than attempting to review biostatistical applications of MCMC *per se*, we focus on applications of MCMC in modeling situations familiar to biostatisticians; specifically hierarchical models, **missing data, censored data**, measurement error, and temporally or spatially correlated data (*see* **Geographical Analysis; Time Series**).

Hierarchical Models

By far the most common area of application of MCMC has been to hierarchical models, such as (5) (see, for example, [7], [8], and [10]). Most applications employ the Gibbs sampler, since full conditional distributions for the random effect parameters involve only a small subset of the data, and are generally log concave. For example, in the simple hierarchical model (5), assuming for convenience that variance parameters are known, the full conditional distributions are:

$$p(\alpha_j|\cdot) = N\left(\frac{\overline{y}_{j.} - \mu}{1 + n^{-1}\sigma_1^2\sigma_2^{-2}}, \frac{1}{n\sigma_1^{-2} + \sigma_2^{-2}}\right), \quad (7)$$

$$p(\mu|\cdot) = N\left(\frac{\overline{y}_{..} - \overline{\alpha}}{1 + m^{-1}n^{-1}\sigma_1^2\sigma_3^{-2}}, \frac{1}{mn\sigma_1^{-2} + \sigma_3^{-2}}\right), \quad (8)$$

where $\overline{y}_{j.} = \sum_{\ell=1}^{n} y_{j\ell}/n$, $\overline{y}_{..} = \sum_{j=1}^{m}\sum_{\ell=1}^{n} y_{i\ell}/(mn)$, and $\overline{\alpha}_. = \sum_{j=1}^{m}\alpha_j/m$. Running the Gibbs sampler corresponds to sampling from (7) for each j, and from (8), where all variables being conditioned upon take on their most recently sampled values.

Much more elaborate hierarchical models, with covariates, multivariate responses, and more levels in the hierarchy, can also be handled straight forwardly using Gibbs sampling; see for example, Gilks et al. [21]. In most applications, the Gibbs sampler mixes well, and when it does not, reparameterization strategies can be tried (see above). The current popularity of MCMC owes much to its successful application to hierarchical models, which are ubiquitous in biostatistics. In particular, Smith et al. [31] have applied such models to meta-analysis problems.

Imperfect Data

Most, if not all, biostatistical data sets contain imperfections due to missing, censored, or inaccurately measured data. In the pre-Gibbs era, such imperfections were often difficult to handle, and required problem-specific solutions. Here we show that a wide class of data-imperfection problems can be handled in a generic framework, using the Gibbs sampler.

Suppose that a dependent variable, y_ℓ, and a covariate, x_ℓ, have been recorded for each individual $\ell = 1, \ldots, n$. Assuming that the y_ℓ are conditionally independent, with probability density specified by $p(y_\ell|x_\ell, \theta)$, the posterior distribution of the model parameters θ is proportional to

$$\prod_{\ell}^{n} p(y_\ell|x_\ell, \theta) \cdot p(\theta), \quad (9)$$

where $p(\theta)$ denotes the prior density for θ.

Now suppose that the data are imperfect in some way. Let z_ℓ denote the observations on individual ℓ, and let $p(z_\ell|x_\ell, y_\ell, \phi)$ be a model describing the relationship between the observed, imperfect, data and the ideal data. Assuming that covariates are conditionally independent in the population, with probability specified by $p(x_\ell|\psi)$, the joint posterior distribution of θ, ϕ, ψ and $\{x_\ell, y_\ell\}$ is proportional to

$$\prod_{\ell}^{n} p(x_\ell|\psi) \times p(y_\ell|x_\ell, \theta) \times p(z_\ell|x_\ell, y_\ell, \phi)$$
$$\times p(\psi)p(\theta)p(\phi), \quad (10)$$

assuming independent priors.

For example, if the covariates x_ℓ are measured with error, then z_ℓ represents the measured value of x_ℓ and ϕ will include parameters specifying the bias and precision of the measurement process (*see* **Errors in Variables**). In many applications, the dependence of z_ℓ on y_ℓ in the measurement model will be dropped. Similarly, if the dependent variable is measured with error, then z_ℓ represents the measured value of y_ℓ, and the measurement model may drop the dependence on x_ℓ. If the covariates are error-free, the first term in (10) may be omitted, as it will not affect inference for the other variables. See Spiegelhalter et al. [32] for an application in which both dependent and independent variables are measured with error. In studies containing substantial measurement error, external validation studies may be performed, which will introduce further multiplicative terms in (10): see Richardson & Gilks [26] for details.

The above set-up also includes missing data as a special case. Suppose that x_ℓ is not recorded for some individuals. Then z_ℓ records whether x_ℓ has been recorded (for example, $z_\ell = 1$ if x_ℓ is missing; $z_\ell = 0$ otherwise), and $p(z_\ell | x_\ell, y_\ell, \phi)$ describes the probability that x_ℓ is missing. The set-up allows for the possibility that the missingness of x_ℓ may depend on x_ℓ itself, or on y_ℓ, or both. If z_ℓ does not depend on x_ℓ, the term $p(z_\ell | x_\ell, y_\ell, \phi)$ in (10) may be omitted. However, it is important that this term is retained if it does depend on x_ℓ, as this will affect the posterior distribution of x_ℓ, and hence of θ (i.e. the missingness is informative; *see* **Nonignorable Dropout in Longitudinal Studies**). Similar considerations apply if y_ℓ is missing for some individuals: here z_ℓ indicates the missingness of y_ℓ, which is informative if it depends on y_ℓ. The above set-up also accommodates situations in which both x_ℓ and y_ℓ can be missing. An important class of missing data problems occurs in the field of genetics, where the missing covariate data x_ℓ are unobserved genotypes in a pedigree, and the observed data y_ℓ are phenotypes or marker genotypes. In such problems, the x_ℓ are not conditionally independent given ψ, so the analysis framework described here would need to be adapted; see, for example, Thompson & Guo [35] or Thomas & Gauderman [34].

Censored data can also be accommodated in the above framework. If the dependent variable is right-censored at y_ℓ^*, then $z_\ell = (y_\ell^{**}, c_\ell)$, where $y_\ell^{**} = \min(y_\ell, y_\ell^*)$ and $c_\ell = 1$ if $y_\ell > y_\ell^*$, $c_\ell = 0$ otherwise. The model allows for informative censoring; noninformative censoring obtains when y_ℓ^* does not depend on y_ℓ, given x_ℓ. Similarly, censored covariates can also be accommodated; see Gilks et al. [21] for an example.

The Gibbs sampler, applied to the posterior (10), involves the following full conditional distributions:

$$p(\theta | \cdot) \propto \prod_\ell^n p(y_\ell | x_\ell, \theta) p(\theta), \qquad (11)$$

$$p(\psi | \cdot) \propto \prod_\ell^n p(x_\ell | \psi) p(\psi), \qquad (12)$$

$$p(\phi | \cdot) \propto \prod_\ell^n p(z_\ell | x_\ell, y_\ell, \phi) p(\phi), \qquad (13)$$

$$p(x_\ell | \cdot) \propto p(x_\ell | \psi) \times p(y_\ell | x_\ell, \theta)$$
$$\times p(z_\ell | x_\ell, y_\ell, \phi), \qquad (14)$$

$$p(y_\ell | \cdot) \propto p(y_\ell | x_\ell, \theta) \times p(z_\ell | x_\ell, y_\ell, \phi). \qquad (15)$$

Running the Gibbs sampler corresponds to sampling from (11)–(13) and, for each ℓ, from (14) and (15), where all variables being conditioned upon take on their most recently sampled values. If any of these full conditional distributions is awkward to sample from directly, it can be replaced by a set of lower-dimensional full conditional distributions, or by a single Metropolis–Hastings step. The point to note about (11) is that it has the same form as the posterior distribution of θ given full, accurately measured data, as in (9), so the sampling involved in this part of the Markov chain presents no new difficulties. The full conditionals (14) and (15) should be easy to sample from, since they involve only a small subset of the data and would typically be low-dimensional.

A special problem arises when n itself is unknown, due to an unknown number of individuals being selectively lost from the study (for whom, of course, x_ℓ and y_ℓ are unknown). Thus the posterior distribution is variably dimensioned, since it involves an unknown number of missing x_ℓ and y_ℓ variables. For this problem, a reversible-jump Metropolis–Hastings step would need to be included in the sampling, in which missing individuals are added or removed. De Angelis et al. [6] consider such a problem in AIDS epidemiology, where the missing individuals are those who have not yet been diagnosed with AIDS, but who are infected with the HIV virus (*see* **AIDS and HIV**).

Temporally or Spatially Correlated Data

In many biostatistical applications, it is useful to be able to specify relatedness between data items without attempting to model the causal connections between them. For example, in disease maps (*see* **Mapping Disease Patterns**), disease incidence in one county might be expected to be similar to disease incidence in neighboring counties, but direct causal links between them might not be realistic. Similarly, disease incidence in one calendar year might be expected to be similar to disease incidence in adjacent years, or changes in disease incidence might be similar to changes in adjacent years. Markov random field (MRF) models allow such dependence to be expressed purely descriptively, without causal implications. Four example, suppose that μ_ℓ is the disease incidence rate at time ℓ: then a MRF model might specify

$$p(\mu_\ell|\mu_{-\ell},\theta) = p(\mu_\ell|\mu_{\ell-1},\mu_{\ell+1},\theta), \qquad (16)$$

for $\ell = 2, \ldots, n-1$, with some related form for $\ell = 1, n$, where $\mu_{-\ell}$ denotes $\{\mu_1, \ldots, \mu_{\ell-1}, \mu_{\ell+1}, \ldots, \mu_n\}$, and θ is a set of parameters specifying the similarity of disease rates in adjacent years. Equation (16) says that μ_ℓ is conditionally independent of $\mu_1, \ldots, \mu_{\ell-2}, \mu_{\ell+2}, \ldots, \mu_n$, given $\mu_{\ell-1}, \mu_{\ell+1}$, and θ. This structure could be used to induce some smoothness in the time series. Note that a MRF model is nondirected, since, for example, the distribution of μ_ℓ is specified in terms of $\mu_{\ell-1}$, and vice versa. A second-order MRF model might specify

$$p(\delta_\ell|\delta_{-\ell},\theta) = p(\delta_\ell|\delta_{\ell-1},\delta_{\ell+1},\theta), \qquad (17)$$

where $\delta_\ell = \mu_\ell - \mu_{\ell-1}$. This structure could be used to induce smoothness in the gradient of the time series.

Eq. (16) or (17) defines a MRF prior distribution on the unobserved, underlying, rates of disease incidence. For a noncontagious disease, observed disease incidence y_ℓ for each ℓ might be assumed to be independently **Poisson** (μ_ℓ). Bayesian inference for this problem, for known θ, is straightforward using Gibbs sampling, despite the nondirected structure of the MRF prior. Under (16), the full conditional distribution for μ_ℓ is simply

$$p(\mu_\ell|\cdot) \propto p(\mu_\ell|\mu_{-\ell},\theta) \times p(y_\ell|\mu_\ell), \qquad (18)$$

where $p(y_\ell|\mu_\ell)$ is Poisson (μ_ℓ). The Gibbs sampler simply involves sampling from (18) for each ℓ, always conditioning upon the most recently sampled values in $\mu_{-\ell}$. If θ is unknown, it should be sampled from its full conditional distribution, but this is generally difficult to derive from (18). Besag et al. [4] discuss MRF prior models which are specified through joint "pairwise-difference" distributions, from which derivations of all full conditional distributions is straightforward. Besag et al. [3] and Bernardinelli & Montomoli [1] discuss Gibbs sampling for disease maps using MRF priors.

References

[1]   Bernardinelli, L. & Montomoli, C. (1992). Empirical Bayes versus fully Bayesian analysis of geographical variation in disease risk, *Statistics in Medicine* **11**, 983-1007.

[2]   Berry, D.A. & Stangl, D.K. (1996). *Bayesian Biostatistics*. Marcel Dekker, New York.

[3]   Besag, J., York, J. & Mollié, A. (1991). Bayesian image restoration, with two applications in spatial statistics, *Annals of the Institute of Statistical Mathematics* **43**, 1-21.

[4]   Besag, J., Green, P.J., Higdon, D. & Mengersen, K. (1995). Bayesian computation and stochastic systems, *Statistical Science* **10**, 3-41.

[5]   Cowles, M.K. & Carlin, B.P. (1996). Markov chain Monte Carlo convergence diagnostics: a comparative review, *Journal of the American Statistical Association* **91**, 883-904.

[6]   De Angelis, D., Gilks, W.R. & Day, N.E. (1998). Bayesian projection of the acquired immune deficiency epidemic, (with discussion), *Applied Statistics* **47**, 449-498.

[7]   Dellaportas, P. & Smith, A.F.M. (1993). Bayesian inference for generalized linear and proportional hazards models via Gibbs sampling, *Applied Statistics* **42**, 443-460.

[8]   Gelfand, A.E. & Smith, A.F.M. (1990). Sampling-based approaches to calculating marginal densities, *Journal of the American Statistical Association* **85**, 398-409.

[9]   Gelfand, A.E., Sahu, S.K. & Carlin, B.P. (1995). Efficient parameterisations for normal linear mixed models, *Biometrika* **82**, 479-488.

[10] Gelfand, A.E., Hills, S.E., Racine-Poon, A. & Smith, A.F.M. (1990). Illustration of Bayesian inference in normal data models using Gibbs sampling, *Journal of the American Statistical Association* **85**, 972-985.

[11] Gelman, A. (1996). Inference and monitoring convergence, in *Markov Chain Monte Carlo in Practice*, W.R. Gilks, S. Richardson & D.J. Spiegelhalter, eds. Chapman & Hall, London, pp. 131-143.

[12] Gelman, A. & Rubin, D.B. (1992). Inference from iterative simulation using multiple sequences (with discussion), *Statistical Science* **7**, 457-511.

[13] Gelman, A. & Rubin, D.B. (1996). Markov chain Monte Carlo methods in biostatistics, *Statistical Methods in Medical Research* **5**, 339-355.

[14] Gelman, A., Roberts, G.O. & Gilks, W.R. (1996). Efficient Metropolis jumping rules, in *Bayesian Statistics 5*, J.M. Bernardo, J.O. Berger, A.P. Dawid & A.F.M. Smith, eds. Oxford University Press, Oxford, pp. 599-607.

[15] Geman, S. & Geman, D. (1984). Stochastic relaxation, Gibbs distributions and the Bayesian restoration of images, *IEEE Transactions on Pattern Analysis and Machine Intelligence* **6**, 721-741.

[16] Geyer, C.J. (1992). Practical Markov chain Monte Carlo, *Statistical Science* **7**, 473-511.

[17] Gilks, W.R. (1996). Full conditional distributions, in *Markov Chain Monte Carlo in Practice*, W.R. Gilks, S. Richardson & D.J. Spiegelhalter, eds. Chapman & Hall, London, pp. 75-88.

[18] Gilks, W.R. & Roberts, G.O. (1996). Strategies for improving MCMC, in *Markov Chain Monte Carlo in Practice*, W.R. Gilks, S. Richardson & D.J. Spiegelhalter, eds. Chapman & Hall, London, pp. 89-114.

[19] Gilks, W.R. & Wild, P. (1992). Adaptive rejection sampling for Gibbs sampling, *Applied Statistics* **41**, 337–348.

[20] Gilks, W.R., Richardson, S. & Spiegelhalter, D.J., eds. (1996). *Markov Chain Monte Carlo in Practice*. Chapman & Hall, London.

[21] Gilks, W.R., Wang, C.C., Yvonnet, B. & Coursaget, P. (1993). Random-effects models for longitudinal data using Gibbs sampling, *Biometrics* **49**, 441–453.

[22] Green, P.J. (1995). Reversible jump MCMC computation and Bayesian model determination, *Biometrika* **82**, 711–732.

[23] Hastings, W.K. (1970). Monte Carlo sampling methods using Markov chains and their applications, *Biometrika* **57**, 97–109.

[24] Metropolis, N., Rosenbluth, A.W., Rosenbluth, M.N., Teller, A.H. & Teller, E. (1953). Equations of state calculations by fast computing machine, *Journal of Chemical Physics* **21**, 1087–1091.

[25] Raftery, A.E. & Lewis, S.M. (1996). Implementing MCMC, in *Markov Chain Monte Carlo in Practice*, W.R. Gilks, S. Richardson & D.J. Spiegelhalter, eds. Chapman & Hall, London, pp. 115–130.

[26] Richardson, S. & Gilks, W.R. (1993). Conditional independence models for epidemiological studies with covariate measurement error, *Statistics in Medicine* **12**, 1703–1722.

[27] Richardson, S. & Green, P.J. (1997). On Bayesian analysis of mixtures with an unknown number of components, (with discussion) *Journal of the Royal Statistical Society, Series B* **59**, 731–792.

[28] Roberts, G.O. (1996). Markov chain concepts related to sampling algorithms, in *Markov Chain Monte Carlo in Practice*, W.R. Gilks, S. Richardson & D.J. Spiegelhalter, eds. Chapman & Hall, London, pp. 45–57.

[29] Roberts, G.O. & Sahu, S.K. (1997). Updating schemes, correlation structure, blocking and parameterization for the Gibbs sampler, *Journal of the Royal Statistical Society, Series B* **59**, 291–317.

[30] Sheehan, N. & Thomas, A. (1993). On the irreducibility of a Markov chain defined on a space of genotypic configurations by a sampling scheme, *Biometrics* **49**, 163–175.

[31] Smith, T.C., Spiegelhalter, D.J. & Thomas, A. (1995). Bayesian approaches to random-effects meta-analysis: a comparative study, *Statistics in Medicine* **14**, 2685–2699.

[32] Spiegelhalter, D.J., Best, N.G., Gilks, W.R. & Inskip, H. (1996). Hepatitis B: a case study in MCMC methods, in *Markov Chain Monte Carlo in Practice*, W.R. Gilks, S. Richardson & D.J. Spiegelhalter, eds. Chapman & Hall, London, pp. 21–43.

[33] Spiegelhalter, D.J., Thomas, A., Best, N.G. & Gilks, W.R. (1995). *BUGS: Bayesian Inference using Gibbs Sampling*, Version 0.30. Medical Research Council Biostatistics Unit, Cambridge.

[34] Thomas, D.C. & Gauderman, W.J. (1996). Gibbs sampling methods in genetics, in *Markov Chain Monte Carlo in Practice*, W.R. Gilks, S. Richardson & D.J. Spiegelhalter, eds. Chapman & Hall, London, pp. 420–440.

[35] Thompson, E.A. & Guo, S.W. (1991). Evaluation of likelihood ratios for complex genetic models, *IMA Journal of Mathematical Applications in Medicine and Biology* **8**, 149–169.

[36] Tierney, L. (1994). Markov chains for exploring posterior distributions (with discussion), *Annals of Statistics* **22**, 1701–1762.

[37] Tierney, L. (1996). Introduction to general state-space Markov chain theory, in *Markov Chain Monte Carlo in Practice*, W.R. Gilks, S. Richardson & D.J. Spiegelhalter, eds. Chapman & Hall, London, pp. 59–74.

(*See also* **Computer-Intensive Methods**)

W.R. GILKS

Markov Chains

Markov chains refer to a collection of **random variables** with a special dependency structure. We begin by discussing discrete time Markov chains which are sequences of random variables, denoted by $\{X_n, 0 \leq n < \infty\}$. These stochastic processes are a generalization of a sequence of independent discrete random variables. The random variables, X_n, assume a common discrete set of possible values, $\mathcal{S}$, called the *state space*. Since $\mathcal{S}$ is countable, we can, by relabeling the states, assume that they are labeled by the positive integers. For a finite state space, $\mathcal{S} = \{0, 1, \ldots, K\}$ for some K, while for a countably infinite state space $\mathcal{S} = \{0, 1, \ldots\}$. The dependency structure is defined by the *Markov property*, which is defined by:

$$\Pr(X_{n+1} = j | X_1 = i_1, \ldots, X_{n-1} = i_{n-1}, X_n = i)$$
$$= \Pr(X_{n+1} = j | X_n = i).$$

If we allow the index n to represent the present time and $\{1, \ldots, n-1\}$ to represent the past, then the Markov property can be interpreted to imply that future events are conditionally independent of the past given the present. The Markov property implies that the chain, upon entering state i, will stay in that state for a random period governed by a **geometric** probability distribution.

The probability $\Pr(X_{n+1} = j | X_n = i)$ is called a *one-step transition probability*, a transition from state i to state j in one time unit. This probability depends upon three quantities: i, j, and n. If the transition probability is independent of n, then we say the transitions are *time homogeneous* or *stationary*. If, in addition, the transition probabilities are independent of i, then the Markov chain is a sequence of independent, identically distributed (iid) random variables. For the rest of this article, we assume time homogeneous transitions, the most commonly considered case.

It is convenient to represent the transition probabilities $p_{ij} = \Pr(X_1 = j | X_0 = i)$ in matrix form, $\mathbf{P} = (p_{ij})$, a square matrix the dimension of which equals that of S. Each row of $\mathbf{P}$ is a discrete probability distribution, so the rows must satisfy two conditions; (i) $p_{ij} \geq 0$ and (ii) $\sum_{j \in S} p_{ij} = 1$. A matrix $\mathbf{P}$ satisfying (i) and (ii) is called a one-step transition probability matrix. Such matrices include the case of identical rows where the underlying random variables are independent.

To give a complete description of a time homogeneous Markov chain, one needs to specify three components: (i) the state space S; (ii) the transition probability matrix $\mathbf{P}$; and (iii) the initial probability distribution, $\Pr(X_0 = i), i \in S$. Given those three quantities, the entire evolution of the Markov chain can be characterized. Often that evolution is described in two ways, the n-step transition probabilities; that is, $\Pr(X_{n+m} = j | X_m = i) = p_{ij}^{(n)}$, and the marginal probability distribution at time n, $\Pr(X_n = j)$. Both can be derived from the *Chapman–Kolmogorov equations*. For n-step transitions write $\Pr(X_{n+m} = j | X_0 = i) = \sum_{k \in S} \Pr(\{X_m = k\} \cap \{X_{n+m} = j\} | X_0 = i) = \Pr(X_m = k | X_0 = i) \cdot \Pr(X_{m+n} = j | X_m = k) = \sum_{k \in S} p_{ik}^{(m)} p_{kj}^{(n)}$. These equations can be most conveniently expressed in matrix form: $\mathbf{P}^{(m+n)} = \mathbf{P}^{(m)} \mathbf{P}^{(n)}$, where $\mathbf{P}^{(n)} = (p_{ij}^{(n)})$, the n-step transition probability matrix. By iterating this expression, it is easy to show that $\mathbf{P}^{(n)} = \mathbf{P}^n$; that is, the n-step transition probability matrix is the nth power of the one-step transition matrix.

If the Markov chain is initiated at time 0 with a probability distribution, $\pi^{(0)}$, then it follows that the marginal probability distribution at time n, $\pi^{(n)} = \pi^{(0)} P^{(n)} = \pi^{(0)} P^n$, the product of the initial probability distribution vector with the n-step transition matrix.

An important consideration is the limiting behavior of the Markov chain. Does it **converge** to a single state or does it continue to move through all the states in the state space? To answer this question, a classification of each state and a partitioning of the state space is introduced. This is done by first defining a relation between two states:

Definition.   State $i \in S$ communicates with state $j \in S$ if and only if there exists an $n \geq 0$ such that $p_{ij}^{(n)} > 0$.

So state i communicates with state j if there is a positive probability that a chain starting in i will reach j in finite time.

Definition.   States $i, j \in S$ intercommunicate if i communicates with j and j communicates with i.

The relation defined by state intercommunication is an equivalence relation and it partitions the state space S into equivalence classes of intercommunicating states. When a Markov chain has a single equivalence class of states, that chain is said to be *irreducible*.

The long-run behavior of the Markov chain can be deduced from a very simple idea, whether a Markov chain which starts in a state i is certain to eventually return to that state. If $\Pr(X_n = i$ for some $n > 0 | X_0 = i) = 1$, then eventual return is certain. However, because of the Markov property, if we are guaranteed of returning a single time, then once we return, we are guaranteed of a second return, and so on. Consequently, if one return is certain, then an infinite number of returns is also certain, and we say that state i is *recurrent*. However, if the probability of eventual return to i is less than 1, then with each return to i, there is a positive probability of this being the final visit to i. Eventually, no further returns will occur. In this case, the state i is called *transient*, and the number of visits to state i will be a random variable with a geometric distribution. One important result is that for any single equivalence class of states, all of those states are recurrent or all are transient.

If we are interested in the long-run fraction of time that the Markov chain spends in state i, we can restrict attention to recurrent states, because this relative frequency must converge to 0 for the transient states. For an irreducible Markov chain, the vector $\boldsymbol{\alpha} = (\alpha_1, \alpha_2, \ldots)$, where α_i represents the long-run fraction of time spent in state i, satisfies the system of linear equations

$$\boldsymbol{\alpha} = \boldsymbol{\alpha}\mathbf{P}, \qquad \sum_{i \in \mathcal{S}} \alpha_i = 1.$$

The vector $\boldsymbol{\alpha}$ represents a probability distribution. According to the theory of Markov chains, for an irreducible Markov chain these equations will have a unique solution giving a probability distribution or no solution at all. In the former case, the states of the Markov chain are *positive recurrent*, and the mean value of the time to return to state i is $1/\alpha_i$. In the latter case, either all the states are transient, or all the states are recurrent, but the mean value of the time to return to a state is infinite, in which case, the states are said to be *null recurrent*.

In the positive recurrent case, this distribution $\boldsymbol{\alpha}$ is referred to by a variety of names: the "equilibrium", "stationary", or "invariant" distribution; even the "steady state" distribution. The latter is often subject to misinterpretation, since the Markov chain continues to sojourn throughout the state space. The vector $\boldsymbol{\alpha}$ gives the long-run fraction of time spent in any state. It is also the invariant distribution in that if the chain is initiated according to the distribution $\boldsymbol{\alpha}$, then the marginal distribution of the chain at all future times is also $\boldsymbol{\alpha}$.

One can also look at the limiting behavior of the n-step transition probabilities, $\lim_{n \to \infty} p_{ij}^{(n)}$. Of course, this limit will be 0 if i does not communicate with j or if j is transient. However, even if $\alpha_j > 0$, this still does not guarantee that the limit exists. The phenomenon that must be considered is called *periodicity*.

Definition.   A state $i \in \mathcal{S}$ is periodic with period k if $p_{ii}^{(n)} > 0$ only for $n = jk$, $j = 1, 2, \ldots$.

In words, a state i is periodic with period k implies that if the Markov chain is initially in state i, it can return to that state only in even multiples of k units of time. A chain with period 1 is *aperiodic*. Periodicity is also a class property; that is, all states in an equivalence class of states have the same period.

Theorem.   For an aperiodic, irreducible, positive recurrent Markov chain, $\lim_{n \to \infty} p_{ij}^{(n)} = \alpha_j$.

Thus, for an aperiodic, irreducible, positive recurrent (also called an *ergodic*) Markov chain, the probability vector solution to the system of equilibrium equations $\boldsymbol{\alpha} = \boldsymbol{\alpha}\mathbf{P}$ gives the long-run average fraction of time that the chain spends in each state and is the limiting probability that the chain will be found in each state of $\mathcal{S}$ at a time far in the future. Notice that in the ergodic case, $\lim_{n \to \infty} p_{ij}^{(n)} = \alpha_j$, independent of i, the initial state. In this case, the long-run behavior of the chain is independent of its starting location.

A final concept that is useful in biostatistical applications is that of an *absorbing state*, a state i satisfying $p_{ii} = 1$. Once the chain enters i, it can never leave that state. Such states arise, for example, in cell metastasis models (*see* **Cell-Cycle Models**). Starting with a normal cell, the cell may transition through a series of reversible states; however, if it reaches a cancerous state, then it continues to be cancerous for ever after. One can also use the concept as a method to determine the expected amount of time required for the chain, starting in state i, to first reach j. If we let e_{ij} represent the expected value of the first time the chain reaches j, then these quantities satisfy the system of equations: $e_{ij} = 1 + \sum_{k \in \mathcal{S}} p_{ik} e_{kj}$ for $j \neq i$, while $e_{ii} = 0$.

It is straightforward to estimate the elements of the transition matrix, $\mathbf{P}$, by **maximum likelihood**. Assume that we are given a single path of a Markov chain that is observed over the time interval $[0, N]$. Each time the chain enters state i, the next transition is independent of the entire transition history, and that step is given by a discrete probability distribution on $\mathcal{S}$ given by $\{p_{ij}, j \in \mathcal{S}\}$. If we observe transitions over N steps, and N_{ij} gives the number of transitions from state i to j, then the maximum likelihood estimator of p_{ij} is given by N_{ij}/N_i, where $N_i = \sum_{j \in \mathcal{S}} N_{ij}$. In some models, the transition probabilities are constrained to have a special form which is a parametric function of some variable θ; that is, $p_{ij} = p_{ij}(\theta)$. Here, one must write the **likelihood** function of θ, an expression which will have the following **multinomial** form: $L(\theta | N_{ij}, i, j \in \mathcal{S}) = p_{X_0}(\theta) \prod_{i \in \mathcal{S}} \prod_{j \in \mathcal{S}} (p_{ij}(\theta))^{N_{ij}}$, where $p_{X_0}(\theta)$ represents the likelihood of the initial state of the Markov chain. This multinomial-like expression must be maximized over θ. The resulting estimators are asymptotically normally distributed, and the methodology is similar to what would be done with data from a **contingency table**. The seminal work on estimation of Markov chains was done by Anderson & Goodman [1]. The reader should also consult Billingsley [2].

Continuous Time Markov Chains

Many Markov chain models are formulated in continuous time, rather than discrete time. In this situation, the Markov chain is represented by $\{X_t, t \geq 0\}$. The state space, S is also discrete and is again taken to be $\{1, 2, \ldots, N\}$ for a finite Markov chain or $\{1, 2, \ldots, \}$ for the countable state space case.

The Markov property for the continuous time case is expressed by the relation

$$\Pr(X_{t+s} = j | X_s = i, X_u = i_u, 0 \leq u < s)$$
$$= \Pr(X_{t+s} = j | X_s = i).$$

We consider only the time homogeneous case; that is, $\Pr(X_{t+s} = j | X_s = i) = p_{ij}(t)$, a transition from i to j over t time units which does not depend upon s. Again, the future evolution of the chain is conditionally independent of the past given the present state. Suppose at some time t, the chain is in state i, and we are interested in how much longer it will stay in state i before it jumps to a different state. The Markov property indicates that the remaining sojourn time in i must be independent of the past; hence it must be independent of the amount of time it has already sojourned in state i. This "memoryless" property implies that the sojourn time in each state is governed by an **exponential** distribution.

The basic ideas developed earlier for discrete time Markov chains carry over directly to continuous time Markov chains. For example, the state space can be decomposed into equivalence classes of intercommunicating states, and those classes contain states which are all recurrent or all transient. There is, however, a major difference between the discrete time and continuous time Markov chains. In the discrete time case, there is a smallest increment of time, one time unit. In the continuous time case, there is no smallest unit of time, so one can consider state transitions over arbitrarily small periods of time. Consequently, the concept of a one-step transition probability matrix, $\mathbf{P}$, does not apply to the continuous time case. In its place, a *transition rate* matrix, $\mathbf{Q} = (q_{ij})$, is introduced. The individual transition rates are defined by

$q_{ij} = p'_{ij}(0)$. Since $\sum_{j \in S} p_{ij}(t) = 1$ for all t, it follows that $\sum_{j \in S} q_{ij} = 0$. Consequently, each row of $\mathbf{Q}$ must sum to 0. The diagonal elements of $\mathbf{Q}$ are nonpositive, while the off-diagonal elements are nonnegative, since

$$q_{ij} = \begin{cases} \lim_{h \to 0} \dfrac{p_{ii}(h) - 1}{h} \leq 0, & \text{if } i = j, \\[2ex] \lim_{h \to 0} \dfrac{p_{ij}(h)}{h} \geq 0, & \text{if } i \neq j. \end{cases}$$

The elements of the $\mathbf{Q}$ matrix have direct interpretations concerning the behavior of the Markov chain. Recall that the holding time in each state is governed by an exponential distribution. The parameter of that distribution for state i is given by $-q_{ii} = \sum_{j \neq i} q_{ij}$. Once the chain leaves state i, it must jump to another state $j \neq i$. The probability that it jumps to j is given by $q_{ij} / \sum_{k \neq i} q_{ik}$. One could also associate each $\{q_{ij}, j \neq i\}$ with an independent exponential (q_{ij}) random variable, T_{ij}. Suppose that $T_i = \min_{j \neq i} T_{ij}$ and $T_{ij} < T_{ik}, k \neq i, j$. Then, upon entering state i, the chain will stay in state i for T_i time units, then jump to j.

The Chapman–Kolmogorov equations for the continuous time case are $\mathbf{P}(s + t) = \mathbf{P}(s)\mathbf{P}(t)$. These can be rewritten, $\mathbf{P}(t + h) = \mathbf{P}(t)\mathbf{P}(h)$. By subtracting $\mathbf{P}(h)$ from both sides and taking the limit as $h \to 0$, we obtain the Kolmogorov forward equations,

$$\mathbf{P}'(t) = \mathbf{P}(t)\mathbf{Q}, \qquad \mathbf{P}(0) = \mathbf{I},$$

a system of first-order differential equations with constant coefficients. These equations have a solution,

$$\mathbf{P}(t) = \exp(\mathbf{Q}t) = \mathbf{I} + t\mathbf{Q} + \frac{t^2}{2!}\mathbf{Q}^2 + \cdots.$$

Suppose that one introduces the **eigenvalue** decomposition of $\mathbf{Q}$, $\mathbf{Q} = \mathbf{USV}$, where $\mathbf{U}$ and $\mathbf{V}$ are orthogonal matrices of **eigenvectors**, and $\mathbf{S}$ is a diagonal matrix of eigenvalues of $\mathbf{Q}$. Using this representation of $\mathbf{Q}$, one can write $\mathbf{P}(t) = \mathbf{UD}(t)\mathbf{V}$, where $\mathbf{D}(t)$ is the diagonal matrix $\exp(t\mathbf{S})$. In the case of a positive recurrent, irreducible Markov chain, the transition probabilities converge to a limiting probability distribution, $\boldsymbol{\alpha}$, and this distribution is characterized by the equations

$$\mathbf{O} = \boldsymbol{\alpha}\mathbf{Q}, \sum_{i \in S} \alpha_i = 1.$$

This equilibrium or stationary vector is the eigenvector corresponding to the eigenvalue 0 of $\mathbf{Q}$. For continuous time Markov chains, the concept of periodicity does not appear; hence, in the positive recurrent case, α represents the long-run fraction of time the Markov chain spends in each of the states in the state space. In addition, $\alpha_j = \lim_{t \to \infty} p_{ij}(t)$.

The most common continuous time Markov chain is the birth–death process (*see* **Stochastic Processes**), a process in which transitions take place only to adjacent states in $\mathcal{S}$; $q_{ij} = 0$ if $j \neq i - 1, i$ or $i + 1$. Often, one uses the notation $\lambda_i = q_{ii+1}$ and $\mu_i = q_{ii-1}$, which denote the birth and death rates in state i. In the positive recurrent case, the stationary distribution of the chain is given by

$$\alpha_i = k \prod_{j=1}^{i} \frac{\lambda_{j-1}}{\mu_j},$$

where k is a normalization constant to insure that this gives a probability distribution.

The estimation of the parameters of a continuous time Markov chain is similar to estimation in discrete time. We consider the case in which $\mathcal{S} = \{1, \ldots, K\}$. Assume that we are given a single sample path that is observed over the time interval $[0,T]$, and that the initial state is chosen at random. From this sample path, we can reduce to the **sufficient statistics** $\{N_{ij}, 1 \leq i, j, \leq K, i \neq j\}$, the total number of transitions from state i to state j and $\{\tau_i, 1 \leq i \leq K\}$, where τ_i represents the total amount of time spent in state i. The likelihood function is given by

$$L = \left[\prod_{i=1}^{K} \prod_{j=1, j \neq i}^{K} \left(\frac{q_{ij}}{-q_{ii}}\right)^{N_{ij}}\right] \left[\prod_{i=1}^{K} \exp(q_{ii}\tau_i)\right].$$

By taking logarithms, recalling that $q_{ii} = -\sum_{j \neq i} q_{ij}$ and maximizing this expression over q_{ij}, we find the maximum likelihood estimates of q_{ij} to be given by $\hat{q}_{ij} = N_{ij}/\tau_i$, provided that the denominator is positive. If $I_i = 0$, then state i was never entered, and we have no data from which to estimate the transition rates departing from state i. One can also use **Bayesian methods** in this problem. It is possible that a particular model might impose a parametric structure on the transition rates, a situation requiring a different estimation procedure.

Examples of Markov Chains in Biostatistics

We now illustrate the basic concepts discussed above using two classical examples in biostatistics.

Example 1. Radiation Damage

Reid & Landau [4] introduced a Markov chain to model the increase in or recovery from **radiation** damage to an organism. There are $K + 1$ states, $\{0, \ldots, K\}$, where 0 denotes no radiation damage, K denotes an absorbing state with perceptible damage, and $\{1, \ldots, K - 1\}$ denote intermediate states with increasingly severe states of damage. In discrete time, the one step transition probability matrix is given by the following $(K + 1) \times (K + 1)$ matrix in which $q_i + p_i = 1, 1 \leq i < K$,

$$\mathbf{P} = \begin{pmatrix} 1 & 0 & 0 & 0 & \ldots & 0 \\ q_1 & 0 & p_1 & 0 & \ldots & 0 \\ 0 & q_2 & 0 & p_2 & \ldots & 0 \\ \ldots & \ldots & \ldots & \ldots & \ldots & \ldots \\ 0 & \ldots & 0 & q_{K-1} & 0 & p_{K-1} \\ 0 & 0 & \ldots & 0 & 0 & 1 \end{pmatrix}.$$

In this model, the states 0 and K are absorbing states. If the chain is any intermediate state, $1 \leq i < K$, then it will move to an adjacent state. Once the chain hits an absorbing state, it stays there forever, hence the equivalence classes are $\{0\}, \{K\}, \{1, \ldots, K - 1\}$. The single state classes are recurrent, while the intermediate class is transient. One might ask for the probability, given the chain is initiated in state $i, 1 \leq i \leq K - 1$, that it will reach the healthy state 0 before it reaches the permanently damaged state K. Reid & Landau studied this model under the assumption that $p_i = i/K$ and $q_i = 1 - i/K$. For this particular set of transitions, they showed that if the chain is in state i, then the probability of the chain hitting state K before it returns to the normal state 0 is given by

$$\frac{1}{2^{K-1}} \sum_{j=0}^{i-1} \binom{K-1}{j}, \quad \text{for } 1 \leq i \leq K.$$

Example 2. Compartment Models

Compartment models are a very large class of models used in **pharmacokinetics** and pharmacodynamics, tracking the flow of substances in the body. The compartments refer to containers such as organs or the blood stream itself. Jacquez [3] gives a comprehensive treatment of these models. While the number of particles of drug or pollutant will be very large, these models often assume independence of movement within the compartments. Thus, these models give the transition structure for one particle, and the behavior of the aggregate can be predicted using the **central limit theorem** and the **law of large numbers**.

A typical compartment model is formulated in continuous time. Consider, for example, a three-state model given by the **Q** matrix

$$\mathbf{Q} = \begin{pmatrix} q_{11} & q_{12} & q_{13} \\ q_{21} & q_{22} & 0 \\ 0 & 0 & 0 \end{pmatrix}.$$

Recall that $q_{11} = -(q_{12} + q_{13})$ and $q_{22} = -q_{21}$. State 1 refers to the bloodstream, 2 refers to the liver, while 3 refers to the bladder, from which the pollutant will be expelled. The drug will reside in the bloodstream for an exponential period, then move either to the bladder or to the liver. The drug will stay in the liver for an exponential period, then move back to the bloodstream. Finally, any drug that reaches the bladder will be removed from the system, so this represents an absorbing state. Again, the bloodstream state and the liver state are transient, while state 3 is absorbing. Consequently, it is of interest to calculate the total amount of time that the pollutant will spend in the liver where damage can occur, and the time it spends in the system before it is removed.

Consider the following numerical example. Suppose that

$$\mathbf{Q} = \begin{pmatrix} -2 & 1 & 1 \\ 1 & -1 & 0 \\ 0 & 0 & 0 \end{pmatrix}.$$

The eigenvalues of **Q** are $(0, -0.382, -2.618)$. If we assume that there is a bolus injection of pollutant at time 0 into the bloodstream, then the transition probabilities for a single particle can be found from the Kolmogorov forward equations. Specifically, we find that

$$p_{11}(t) = 0.276 \exp(-0.382t) + 0.724 \exp(-2.618t),$$

$$p_{12}(t) = 0.448 \exp(-0.382t) - 0.448 \exp(-2.618t),$$

$$p_{13}(t) = -0.724 \exp(-0.382t)$$
$$-0.276 \exp(-2.618t) + 1.$$

Thus, the pollutant concentration decreases in the bloodstream according to a mixture of exponentials. It increases, then decreases in the liver, and eventually it all resides in the bladder.

References

[1]   Anderson, T.W. & Goodman, L. (1957). Statistical inference for Markov chains, *Annals of Mathematical Statistics* **28**, 89–109.

[2]   Billingsley, P. (1981). *Statistical Inference for Markov Processes*. Chicago University Press, Chicago.

[3]   Jacquez, J.A. (1972). *Compartmental Analysis in Biology and Medicine*. Elsevier, Amsterdam.

[4]   Reid, A.T. & Landau, H.G. (1951). A suggested chain process for radiation damage, *Bulletin of Mathematical Biophysics* **13**, 153–163.

J. LEHOCZKY

Markov Processes

A Markov process is often described as a "process without memory": our estimate of the probability of a future event concerning its behavior *given (complete)* information about its present state will not change if we are given in addition any information about its past behavior. See the first section for an illustration of this.

The concept of a "Markov process" is so general as to embrace most models of random systems evolving in time (*see* **Stochastic Processes**): from "classical" *random walks*, **Markov chains**, **branching processes**, *birth-and-death processes, diffusions* and their associated *stochastic differential equations*, to the "postclassical" *branching diffusions, measure-valued diffusions, interacting systems* (which include *contact processes* etc.), which are destined to play an ever more important part in **mathematical biology**. Each of the italicized topics has a huge literature and its own special methods; and it is often better to search the literature for *these* "keywords" rather than the all-embracing "Markov processes". However, Markov-process theory has, of course, unifying themes and methods (*martingale theory, large-deviation theory*, etc.) which pervade all of its branches.

We take a brief tour through the subject, designed to allow glimpses of several topics italicized above.

Simple Random Walk

Suppose that we toss a fair coin just before times 1, 2, 3, ..., and regard the state of our system at time n (which can be 0, 1, 2, ...) as the number of heads minus the number of tails obtained by that time. (We have $X_0 = 0$.) For illustration, regard time 100 as the "present". Suppose that we know that $X_{100} = 6$. *Given* this information and any additional information about the "past" results of the first 99 tosses, X_{101} is either 5 or 7 with probability 1/2 each. The Markov property is obvious here.

We can prove, for example, that the distribution of X_n at time n is approximated by the **normal distribution** of mean 0 and variance n (hence standard deviation $n^{1/2}$), and that, "almost surely" (that is, with probability exactly 1), X_n will fluctuate infinitely, taking every integer (whole-number) value infinitely often.

Markov Chain in Discrete Time

For a Markov chain in discrete time with stationary probabilities, X_n, $n = 0, 1, 2, ...$, is a random integer describing the state of the system at time n. The probabilistic law of the system is described by the ("initial") distribution of X_0 and by a "matrix" (or array) of transition probabilities p_{ij}: for each n, the (conditional) probability of the "future" event that $X_{n+1} = j$, given the "present" information that $X_n = i$ and any extra information about the "past" $X_0, X_1, ..., X_{n-1}$, is p_{ij}. [Our random walk has $p_{ij} = 1/2$ if $j = i + 1$ or $j = i - 1$, and $p_{ij} = 0$ otherwise.] The sort of questions in which we are interested are the following. Is the system "ergodic" in that, over the long term, it will almost surely share out its time amongst the various states in a predetermined way? At the other extreme, if there is an absorbing state a for which $p_{aa} = 1$, will the system almost surely eventually end up in state a? (For example, is some population almost surely destined to die out?)

Markov Chain in Continuous Time

We modify things so that our system can jump at *any* time, not just at integer-valued times, and this requires us to define *jump-rates* q_{ij} rather than "jump probabilities" p_{ij}. We denote the integer-valued state of our system at time t, where $t \geq 0$, by X_t. Suppose that $j \neq i$. Given the "present" information that $X_t = i$ and any information about the past values X_s for $s < t$, the probability that the system will jump from i to j between times t and $t + h$, where h is a small number, will be $q_{ij}h + o(h)$, where $o(h)$ is a term negligibly small *compared with* h when h tends to 0.

Generalized Birth-and-Death (GBD) Process

This has the property that $q_{ij} = a_i$ for some a_i if $j = i + 1$, $q_{ij} = b_i$ for some b_i if $j = i - 1$, and $q_{ij} = 0$ for other pairs (i, j), where $j \neq i$. Thus X can only jump to a neighboring state. We can answer the analogues of the questions raised in the section "Markov chain in discrete time".

Continuous-Time Random Walk (CTRW)

This is a GBD process with $a_i = b_i = 1/2$ for every i. It will behave rather like the random walk in the first section.

(Standard) Birth-and-Death (BD) Process

This (the simplest type of continuous-time *branching process*) is a GBD process in which only nonnegative integer states 0, 1, 2, ... are allowed, and we have $a_i = \lambda i$, $b_i = \mu i$ for some constants λ (the "birth rate" per individual) and μ (the "death rate" per individual). Here, we think of X_t as the size of a population at time t. If $X_t = i$, then there are i animals alive at time t, each of which can give birth (to one child) "at rate λ", resulting in a jump rate of $a_i = \lambda i$ for X from i to $i + 1$; if $i > 0$, then each of the i animals can die "at rate μ", resulting in a jump rate of $b_i = \mu i$ for X from i to $i - 1$. State 0 is absorbing. Here are some unsurprising results. In the subcritical case when $\mu > \lambda$, so the death rate exceeds the birth rate, and then the population will almost surely die out. In the supercritical case when $\lambda > \mu$, then, almost surely, the population will either die out or will grow "exponentially" in a sense which can be made precise. In the critical case when $\lambda = \mu$, the population will almost surely die out.

(Mathematical) Brownian Motion (BM) B

We now take the first of several steps in building more complex processes from the processes already introduced. If we renormalize CTRW suitably, then we obtain as a limit the most important of all stochastic processes: **Brownian motion**. We take a large number N, and let X be a GBD process with $a_i = N/2$ and $b_i = N/2$. This process is jumping very fast. Consider $Y_t = X_t/N^{1/2}$. Then Y is jumping just as fast as X, but is making only small jumps of size $1/N^{1/2}$. We choose $N^{1/2}$ because of the fact that a standard deviation of $n^{1/2}$ appeared in our discussion in the first section. What happens is that the law of the rescaled process Y converges as N tends to infinity to the law of Brownian motion B. The process B takes real values, not integer values. The Markov property of B is conveyed by the fact that conditional on the "present" information that $B_t = x$ and any information about the past $(B_s : s < t)$, the "future" random variable B_{t+s} has exactly the normal distribution of mean x and variance s. (The fact that the mean value of B_{t+s} given the values $(B_s : s \leq t)$ is the value of B_t signifies that B is a *martingale*.)

It is no accident that, if $p(t, x)$ is the density function at x of the law of B_t if $B_0 = 0$, i.e. of the normal distribution with mean 0 and variance t, then

$$p(t, x) = \frac{1}{(2\pi t)^{1/2}} \exp\left(-\frac{x^2}{2t}\right)$$

solves the heat equation

$$\frac{\partial p}{\partial t} = \frac{1}{2}\frac{\partial^2 p}{\partial x^2}.$$

This explains the frequent occurrence of second-derivative "diffusion terms" in books on mathematical biology. The function $p(s; x, y) = p(s, y - x)$ is now the transition probability density for B from x to y in an interval of duration s: it plays a role analogous to that of the one-step transition probability p_{ij} for a Markov chain in discrete time.

Brownian motion B is quite remarkable. It approximates many processes. It is amazingly rich and we can "find within B" many other processes including all those we have so far studied. This gives a very illuminating way of proving (rigorously) the celebrated **Central Limit Theorem** on the ubiquitous nature of the normal distribution. We can even "find within B" seemingly much more complicated processes such as

the Dawson–Watanabe process described later. We can use B to describe "white-noise perturbations" of ordinary differential equations, turning them into the stochastic differential equations which describe diffusions, and so on.

Diffusions

Brownian motion is the most important diffusion process. We can think of a more general diffusion process on the real line in two ways: either as the limit of a GBD process produced in a way analogous to that in which we obtained BM from CTRW; or as the solution of a *stochastic differential equation (SDE)* of the form

$$\frac{dX}{dt} = b(X_t) + \sigma(X_t)\frac{dB}{dt},$$

where σ and b are functions. This SDE can be thought of as a random perturbation of the ordinary differential equation (ODE) $dX/dt = b(X_t)$. (The b here has a quite different connotation from that of the b_i in GBDs.) The Brownian path is nowhere differentiable, so dB/dt is completely meaningless in Newtonian terms. Even so, the great Japanese mathematician, K. Itô, constructed the *stochastic calculus* (nowadays based on *martingale theory*), which allows rigorous formulation and analysis of SDEs. Solutions of SDEs inherit the Markov property from the (particularly strong version of the) Markov property possessed by Brownian motion. Conversely, any (real-valued) Markov process X which fluctuates continuously in time (and which satisfies very mild regularity conditions) is the solution of an SDE as above.

The transition density function $p(s; x, y)$ of the solution X of our *first*-order SDE solves the *second*-order partial differential equation (PDE)

$$\frac{\partial p}{\partial s} = \frac{1}{2}\sigma(x)^2\frac{\partial^2 p}{\partial x^2} + b(x)\frac{\partial p}{\partial x},$$

which amazing fact allows us to prove even the deepest known theorems on these and certain other PDEs of importance in mathematical biology by probabilistic methods (see below).

Diffusion theory has seen truly spectacular development over the last 40 years. One important way in which diffusions are used is again in approximating other processes: choosing a diffusion with the same "infinitesimal characteristics" as a more complex process can often give a good guide to how that process behaves.

Branching Brownian Motion and the FKPP Equation

The FKPP equation for $u(t, x)$ studied by Fisher and independently by Kolmogorov, Petrovskii, and Piskunov,

$$\frac{\partial u}{\partial t} = \frac{1}{2}\frac{\partial^2 u}{\partial x^2} + u(1 - u),$$

$$u(0, x) = \begin{cases} 1, & \text{if } x < 0, \\ 0, & \text{if } x > 0, \end{cases} \tag{1}$$

is perhaps the most famous in mathematical biology: it is the simplest *reaction–diffusion equation*. Here, $u(t, x)$ is thought of as describing the density at time t and position x of a population of animals, where there is a logistic constraint on population growth and where the animals diffuse around. (This statement does not in itself specify any random model!) Strange to say: by far the deepest analytic results on the equation have been obtained by H.P. McKean, M. Bramson, J. Neveu, and B. Chauvin & A. Rouault, using probabilistic methods on a stochastic model, branching Brownian motion (BBM), with "free" (rather than logistic) growth. The birthing is exactly as for the pure-birth process, which is a BD process with $\lambda = 1$ and $\mu = 0$. Each child is born at its parent's current position. Once born, animals perform independent Brownian motions. The whole system is Markov, the state of the system at time t summarizing both how many animals are then alive and exactly where they all are. McKean showed that the unique solution $u(t, x)$ of (1) is given by the probability that if we start with one animal born at position x at time 0, then at least one animal is to the left of 0 at time t. If $l(t)$ denotes the leftmost particle position at time t and we start with one animal born at time 0 at position 0, then we have, almost surely, as $t \to \infty$,

$$\frac{l(t)}{t} \to -2^{1/2},$$

and this explains the celebrated "approximate traveling-wave" nature of the solution to (1). If we simulate the situation when at time 0 there is just one animal at position 0, we see that the tracks of the animals almost exactly fill a triangle. All the exact traveling-wave solutions of the FKPP equation have explicit probabilistic representations, even though BBM is the wrong model in biological terms (see the section "MVDs with interaction; improving on FKPP" below).

Measure-Valued Diffusions (MVDs)

The simulation mentioned above is enough to convince one of the good sense of thinking of the random flows of measures ("mass distributions"). Let me explain the most fundamental MVD: the *Dawson–Watanabe (D–W) process*. We take a large number N. We think of each animal as having mass $1/N$, and start with N animals at position 0. Births and deaths are according to a BD process with $\lambda = N/2$ and $\mu = N/2$. Note that this is a critical situation, in which the process will eventually die out. Each particle performs BM, independently of all others. As N tends to infinity, the law of evolution converges to that of the Dawson–Watanabe process. In one dimension, but only in one dimension, we can think of the value of the (D–W) process at time $t > 0$ as being a positive density function u of a mass distribution. This evolves as the solution of a *stochastic partial differential equation (SPDE)*, a perturbed heat equation

$$\frac{\partial u}{\partial t} = \frac{1}{2}\frac{\partial^2 u}{\partial x^2} + [u(t, x)]^{1/2}W,$$

where W now denotes a space–time white-noise process derived from a "Brownian motion" (the "Brownian sheet") with two-dimensional "time". Leading experts in this field include D.A. Dawson, E.B. Dynkin, S.N. Evans, J.F. le Gall, E. Perkins, and J.B. Walsh. Important biological applications, especially to genetics, have been given by D.A. Dawson, P. Donnelly, S.N. Ethier, and T.G. Kurtz.

Interacting Systems

Complicated as they are, the above-mentioned models are not complicated enough. Their particles perform their Brownian motions independently of one another: no account is taken of overcrowding or of the interaction between different particles. By contrast, the theory of interacting systems allows more or less anything. One has to be aware of the scope of this theory, even if only a handful of people can currently claim deep understanding. Leading experts include R. Durrett, G. Grimmett, H. Kesten, R. Holley, and T.M. Liggett.

One of the simplest interacting systems is the three-dimensional *contact-process* model for the spread of disease through cells which are considered to be cubes stacked together, and occupying the whole of space. A healthy cell becomes infected at "jump-rate" (a constant) I times the number of infected neighbors while an infected cell recovers at constant "jump-rate" R. (This system is too complicated to be a Markov chain – its state-space is "uncountable" – but it is a Markov process.) We suppose that at time 0 only a finite number of cells are infected. The system exhibits phase transition: if I/R is less than some critical number c (the precise value of which is currently unknown), then the disease will almost surely die out; while if I/R is greater than c, then the disease can (with positive probability) persist for ever, infecting ever more cells. The *time-dependent Ising model* from magnetism, now much used by statisticians in *image processing*, (*see* **Image Analysis and Tomography**), is closely related.

MVDs with Interaction; Improving on FKPP

Some extremely interesting work has been done by C. Mueller, R.B. Sowers and R. Tribe on an interacting system with "logistic" inhibition of **population growth**: an MVD with density satisfying the FKPP equation with an extra term $[u(1-u)]^{1/2}W$ on the right-hand side, with W as before. The system possesses a "coherence" not present in the deterministic model, and can be regarded as superior to it in many respects. Mueller, Sowers, and Tribe study "traveling-wave" aspects.

Self-Organization; Adapting to the Environment

A striking feature of (naturally occurring and man-made) interacting systems is their ability to behave in a pseudo-intelligent way. Brilliant use of this was made in the *Dynamic Alternative Routing* strategy for telephone networks developed by F.P. Kelly and

R. Gibbens along with British Telecom. Similar use is made in **neural nets**. Biological "networks" in fungi, ant colonies, anastomosis of blood vessels near tumours (bad!), or in wound healing (good!), are complex interacting systems; at present, models of such systems can only be studied by **simulation**, which can certainly identify bad models even if it cannot conclusively validate good ones.

A Plea

There is a great need to make the more modern material described in this article a lot more accessible to applied workers – and to mathematicians too!

A Few References

The literature is truly vast. Most of it can be discovered via the key names given, in the various databases now available, and in the following. For the first five sections, see, for example, Feller [6, 7], Grimmett & Stirzacker [8], and Karlin & Taylor [9, 10]. For the next two sections, see, for example, Breiman [1], Ethier & Kurtz [5], and Øksendal [12]. For the following two sections – and things are getting much harder now – see, for example, Dawson [2], Donnelly & Kurtz [3], Durrett & Levin [4], and Mueller & Sowers [11].

References

[1]   Breiman, L. (1968). *Probability*. Addison-Wesley, Reading, Mass.
[2]   Dawson, D.A. (1993). Measure-Valued Markov Processes, in *Ecole d'Eté de Probabilités de Saint-Flour XXI*, P.L. Henniquin, ed., *Lecture Notes in Mathematics* 1541, Springer-Verlag, Berlin, pp. 2–260.
[3]   Donnelly, P. & Kurtz, T.G. (1996). A countable representation of the Fleming–Viot measure-valued diffusion, *Annals of Probability* **24**, 698–742.
[4]   Durrett, R. & Levin, S.A. (1994). Stochastic spatial models – a user's guide to ecological applications, *Philosophical Transactions of the Royal Society of London* **343**, 329–350.
[5]   Ethier, S.N. & Kurtz, T.G. (1986). *Markov Processes: Characterization and Convergence*. Wiley, New York.
[6]   Feller, W. (1957). *Introduction to Probability Theory and its Applications*, Vol. 1, 2nd Ed. Wiley, New York.
[7]   Feller, W. (1966). *Introduction to Probability Theory and its Applications*, Vol. 2, Wiley, New York.

[8]   Grimmett, G. & Stirzacker, D. (1992). *Probability and Random Processes*, 2nd Ed. Oxford University Press, Oxford.

[9]   Karlin, S. & Taylor, H.M. (1975). *A First Course in Stochastic Processes*. Academic Press, New York.

[10]   Karlin, S. & Taylor, H.M. (1981). *A Second Course in Stochastic Processes*. Academic Press, New York.

[11]   Mueller, C. & Sowers, R.B. (1995). Random traveling waves for the KPP equation with noise, *Journal of Functional Analysis* **128**, 439–498.

[12]   Øksendal, B. (1992). *Stochastic Differential Equations*, 3rd Ed. Springer-Verlag, Berlin.

(*See also* **Counting Process Methods in Survival Analysis; Epidemic Models, Spatial; Epidemic Models, Stochastic; Migration Processes; Queuing Processes; Semi-Markov Processes**)

DAVID WILLIAMS

Martingale *see* Counting Process Methods in Survival Analysis

Martingale Difference Arrays *see* Central Limit Theory

Martingale Residual *see* Residuals for Survival Analysis

Martini, Paul

Born: January 25, 1889, in Frankenthal, Germany.
Died: September 8, 1964, near Bonn, Germany.

Paul Martini was born in Frankenthal (Palatinate) in the southwestern region of Germany. He studied medicine at the universities of Munich and Kiel. He worked on his thesis in the Institute of Physiology in Munich and obtained his doctorate in medicine in 1917.

He was an assistant in the II. Medizinische Universitätsklinik in Munich which was at that time headed by one of the famous German internists, Friedrich von Mueller. In 1926 he become "extraordinary" professor of medicine. He left the university when he was appointed head physician in the St Hedwigskrankenhaus in Berlin, a large community hospital. In 1932 Martini returned to university life. From that time until he retired he held the chair of internal medicine at the University of Bonn and was director of the Universitätsklinik für Innere Medizin und Nervenkrankheiten.

Among his scientific work, his 1932 Monograph *Methodenlehre der therapeutischen Forschung* [1] is of particular importance. This book contains all the elements of the controlled **clinical trial** and is the first in modern times addressing the problem of a scientific methodology as regards therapeutic research. It is evident that the use of placebo (*see* **Blinding or Masking**) is meant even when this word is not used. Martini wrote: "the medicines have to be given to the patient in a form or in a galenic preparation that their special character or their purpose can not be recognized, they have to be camouflaged. The results have to be evaluated by means of statistics and probability calculus". **Randomization** is not clearly addressed, but subsequent publications make it likely that alternating procedures, for example based on day of birth, were used.

In an article published in 1934, Martini again explained his methodology of therapeutic trials and defended himself against the arguments that had been raised against his ideas [2].

In 1957 he published in the Deutsche Medizinische Wochenschrift his ideas about double-blind trials [3]. He rejected the method of double-blindness as he was not convinced that the results of such trials were superior to the single-blind trials. In 1961 Martini was chairman of an international seminar in the field of drug trials in Berlin.

Martini was a highly esteemed physician and had among his patients many personalities of the political scene in Bonn. During the time of national socialism he was able to avoid involvement. In 1948 he was president of the first postwar "Internistenkongress" (annual meeting of the German Society of Internal Medicine) in Wiesbaden. In 1964 he died in his country house in the Eifel near Bonn.

References

[1]   Martini, P. (1932). *Methodenlehre der therapeutischen Forschung*. Julius Springer, Berlin. (Second edition

published in 1947 under the title *Methodenlehre der therapeutisch klinischen Forschung.*)

[2]   Martini, P. (1934). Rationelle Medizin (Rational medicine), *Muenchner Medizinische Wochenschrift* **81**, 1411–1416.

[3]   Martini, P. (1957). Die unwissentliche Versuchsanordnung und der sogenannte doppelte Blindversuch (The unknown experimental design and the so-called double-blind trial), *Deutsche Medizinische Wochenschrift* **82**, 597–602.

(*See also* **History of Clinical Trials**)

H.J. DENGLER

Mass Action *see* Epidemic Models, Deterministic

Matched Analysis

On grounds of both validity and efficiency, the appropriate analysis of data involving category matching mandates the use of stratified analysis methods based on the strata used in the matching process [6] (*see* **Stratification**). Two important methods for analyzing category matched (or, more generally, stratified) data are the **Mantel–Haenszel** procedure [9] and **conditional logistic regression** (see [1, Chapter 7], and [5, Chapter 20]).

The Mantel–Haenszel (MH) test statistic [9] is the most widely used and recommended method for testing for overall association in a stratified analysis. And, as we will see, the MH test statistic for stratified data analysis is based on the (central) **hypergeometric distribution**. For dichotomous disease and exposure variables (the setting for this presentation), the MH testing procedure involves a one **degree-of-freedom** (continuity-corrected) **chi-squared statistic** of the general form

$$\chi^2_{\text{MH}} = [|A - \text{E}_0(A)| - 1/2]^2 / \text{var}_0(A), \quad (1)$$

where A is the random variable denoting the total number (over all strata) of diseased subjects in

each stratum who are exposed (i.e. the total number of "exposed cases"), $\text{E}_0(A)$ is the expected total number of exposed cases under the **null hypothesis** of no **association** between exposure and disease, and $\text{var}_0(A)$ is the **variance** of the total number of exposed cases under the same null hypothesis.

Suppose that there are G strata defined by the matching process, with the gth stratum having the structure given in Table 1.

Table 1   Data layout for the gth stratum ($g = 1, 2, \ldots, G$)

	E	$\overline{E}$	
D	A_g	B_g	m_{1g}
$\overline{D}$	C_g	D_g	m_{0g}
	n_{1g}	n_{0g}	n_g

The four marginal frequencies n_{1g}, n_{0g}, m_{1g}, and m_{0g} in the gth stratum convey no information about the strength of the association between exposure and disease in that stratum, but rather indicate only the "amount of information" in that stratum. Consequently, the four marginal frequencies within each stratum may be assumed (with no compromise to validity) to be "fixed" for analysis purposes, even though the sampling scheme actually used may not have imposed such constraints on the margins of these G **2 × 2 tables**.

Conditional on these fixed margins for all strata, it is sufficient to focus entirely on the "A_g cell", namely, the number of exposed cases in the gth stratum, $g = 1, 2, \ldots, G$. The test statistic (1) is then a conditional test since properties of the **random variable** $A = \sum_{g=1}^{G} A_g$ are based on the condition that the four margins in each stratum are fixed. More specifically, assuming fixed margins and no exposure-disease association, A_g is a (central) hypergeometric random variable, so that

$$\text{E}_0(A) = \sum_{g=1}^{G} (n_{1g} m_{1g}) / n_g \quad \text{and}$$

$$\text{var}_0(A) = \sum_{g=1}^{G} (n_{1g} n_{0g} m_{1g} m_{0g}) / (n_g - 1) n_g^2.$$

Finally, some algebra can be used to write expression (1) in the form

$$\chi^2_{\mathrm{MH}} = \frac{\left[\left|\sum_{g=1}^{G}(A_gD_g - B_gC_g)/n_g\right| - 1/2\right]^2}{\sum_{g=1}^{G}(n_{1g}n_{0g}m_{1g}m_{0g})/(n_g - 1)n_g^2}; \quad (2)$$

under the null hypothesis of no exposure–disease association, it can be shown that the test statistic (2) has, for "large samples", an approximate chi-square distribution with 1 df.

It is very important to stress that the "large samples" assumption for the test statistic (2) pertains to the pooled information over all G strata, rather than to stratum-specific numbers. Consequently, in the use of the Mantel–Haenszel test statistic (2), it is permissible to have relatively small numbers in each stratum as long as the total number of subjects on the margins over all strata is sufficiently large. Without going into detail, this form of **robustness** to sparse stratum-specific data accrues due to the assumption of fixed stratum-specific margins, an assumption that maintains validity at only a slight cost in efficiency. Specific criteria for appropriate sample sizes to maintain the validity of the chi-squared approximation for (2) have been proposed by Mantel & Fleiss [8]. They recommend using (2) provided that the quantities

$$E_0(A) - \left[\sum_{g=1}^{G}\max(0, m_{1g} - n_{0g})\right] \quad \text{and}$$

$$\left[\sum_{g=1}^{G}\min(n_{1g}, m_{1g})\right] - E_0(A)$$

both exceed 5 in value.

It is important to mention that the use of the Mantel–Haenszel test statistic (2) should be avoided when there is evidence of strong **effect modification** in the data, as would be reflected by widely varying stratum-specific estimated **odds ratios** $\widehat{OR}_g = A_gD_g/B_gC_g, g = 1, 2, \ldots, G$. Because of the structure of the numerator in (2), the value of (2) can be very small (suggesting no exposure–disease association) when, in fact, some stratum-specific estimated odds ratios are significantly greater than 1 and some are significantly less than 1. Indeed, claims of optimal statistical properties for the Mantel–Haenszel test [11] are valid only in the situation where stratum-specific population odds ratios all have the same

value. Tests for lack of uniformity of stratum-specific odds ratios are discussed in Chapter 4 of [1].

Given the assumption of a common population odds ratio for all strata, it makes sense to compute a summary estimator of this common odds ratio; such an estimator is typically a weighted average of the G stratum-specific estimated odds ratios. Mantel & Haenszel [9] proposed several such summary estimators for use in **case–control studies**. The most notable of these is the $\widehat{mOR}$, which is defined as

$$\widehat{mOR} = \left[\sum_{g=1}^{G}(A_gD_g)/n_g\right] \Big/ \left[\sum_{g=1}^{G}(B_gC_g/n_g)\right]$$

$$= \sum_{g=1}^{G} W_g(\widehat{OR}_g) \Big/ \sum_{g=1}^{G} W_g, \quad (3)$$

where $W_g = B_gC_g/n_g$. An interesting property of $\widehat{mOR}$ is that it equals unity only when expression (2) is zero, a property that is not shared by other summary estimators (see [5, Chapter 17]). Another advantage of the $\widehat{mOR}$ over other summary estimators is that it can be used without alteration when there are zero frequencies within the body of some of the stratum-specific tables.

For certain types of matched data, expressions (2) and (3) have simple structures. As one example, for a matched pairs case–control study where each stratum (or pair) consists of one case and one control, then expression (2) reduces to $(b - c)^2/(b + c)$ apart from continuity correction, and expression (3) equals b/c, where b is the number of strata where the case is exposed and the control is not, and c is the number of strata where the control is exposed and the case is not. For the special case of R-to-1 matching, see either Chapter 5 in [1] or Chapter 18 in [5]. For **confidence interval** methods based on (3) in case–control studies with multiple matching, see [3], [12], and [13]. Finally, some generalizations of the Mantel–Haenszel test have been developed for situations where the exposure variable is **nominal** with several categories [9] and where the exposure variable is ordinal (*see* **Measurement Scale**) in nature [2, 7].

A more general and flexible method for the analysis of matched (or, in general, stratified) data is conditional logistic regression (*see* **Logistic Regression, Conditional**). This multivariable modeling procedure is specifically designed to be used when there are small stratum-specific sample sizes. Hence, it is ideally suited for the analysis of matched study designs or to similar situations involving very fine stratification; in fact, its use in these situations is mandatory to avoid **biased** estimates of important odds ratio parameters. In contrast to stratified data analysis methods, conditional logistic regression methods do not require all variables to be categorized; for example, continuous exposure, **confounding**, and effect-modifying variables can be treated as such. In addition, it is theoretically possible to consider simultaneously in one model several exposure variables and to examine potential confounding and effect modification effects due to **covariates** not involved in the matching process.

Suppose we consider the case–control format, with $\mathbf{x}_{1g}, \mathbf{x}_{2g}, \ldots, \mathbf{x}_{m_g g}$ denoting the observed data vectors for the total of $m_g = (m_{1g} + m_{0g})$ cases and controls in the gth stratum, $g = 1, 2, \ldots, G$. Without loss of generality, we arrange these data vectors so that the first m_{1g} vectors belong to the m_{1g} cases in the gth stratum. For a dichotomous response variable D with $D = 1$ signifying a case and $D = 0$ signifying a control, consider fitting by conditional logistic regression the logistic model

$$\text{logit}[\Pr(D_{lg} = 1)] = \alpha_g + \boldsymbol{\beta}' \mathbf{x}_{lg},$$

$$l = 1, 2, \ldots, m_g \quad \text{and} \quad g = 1, 2, \ldots, G.$$

Then, the contribution from the gth stratum to the full conditional **likelihood** has the structure

$$\text{CL}_g = \prod_{l=1}^{m_{1g}} \exp(\boldsymbol{\beta}' \mathbf{x}_{lg}) \Bigg/ \sum_u \left[\prod_{l=1}^{m_{1g}} \exp(\boldsymbol{\beta}' \mathbf{x}_{ulg}) \right], \tag{4}$$

where the sum $\sum_u$ in the denominator is over all partitions of the set of integers $\{1, 2, \ldots, m_g\}$ into two subsets, the first of which contains m_{1g} elements; there are $m_g!/m_{1g}!m_{0g}!$ such partitions. Thus, CL_g is the conditional probability that the first m_{1g} of the m_g data vectors $\mathbf{x}_{1g}, \mathbf{x}_{2g}, \ldots, \mathbf{x}_{m_g g}$ go with the cases (as they actually do) considering all possible arrangements of these m_g data vectors; in other words, CL_g is the conditional probability of the observed data. The full conditional likelihood CL is then equal to $\text{CL} = \prod_{g=1}^{G} \text{CL}_g$, and standard **maximum likelihood methods** can be used to estimate and to make **inferences** about the elements of $\boldsymbol{\beta}$.

It is important to note that the conditional likelihood CL based on (4) depends only on $\boldsymbol{\beta}$, the parameter vector of interest. The **nuisance parameters** $\alpha_1, \alpha_2, \ldots, \alpha_G$ indexing the matching strata have been eliminated via this permutation procedure, thus precluding the need to estimate unnecessarily an often large number of parameters that provide no information about important exposure–disease odds ratio parameters of interest. In addition, precisely the same likelihood CL is obtained regardless of whether we consider the data to have arisen from a follow-up study or from a case–control study. Also, CL has precisely the structure of Cox's **partial likelihood** [4], based on the **proportional hazards model**, for analyzing follow-up study data. However, an important distinction is that each stratum-specific set in the denominator of CL, instead of involving *all* persons in the study who are disease-free at the time each incident case is identified, consists only of the m_{0g} controls specifically associated with (e.g. sampled at the same time as) the m_{1g} cases.

As an illustration of the conditional likelihood approach for matched data, consider a matched case–control study involving G cases, where the gth case is individually matched to R_g controls on one or more variables. Then, $m_{1g} = 1$, $m_{0g} = R_g$, $m_g = (R_g + 1)$, and the conditional likelihood CL takes the specific form

$$\prod_{g=1}^{G} \left[1 + \sum_{l=2}^{R_g+1} \exp[\boldsymbol{\beta}'(\mathbf{x}_{lg} - \mathbf{x}_{1g})] \right]^{-1}. \tag{5}$$

Given the structure of this expression, if any of the elements of $\mathbf{x}$ are matching variables, taking the same value for each member of a matched set, then their contribution to the likelihood is zero and the corresponding elements of $\boldsymbol{\beta}$ cannot be estimated. However, by incorporating such matching variables in the model as **interaction** terms with exposure factors, one can model the variation in odds ratios across matched sets.

Finally, to appreciate that these conditional likelihood methods do, in fact, yield recognizable results in well-known special cases, consider the simple matched pairs case–control study considered earlier, where $R_g = 1$ for all g and where there is a single dichotomous exposure variable. With $e^\beta = \text{EOR}$, the exposure odds ratio parameter, it can be shown that (5) is proportional to

$$[\text{EOR}/(1 + \text{EOR})]^b [1/(1 + \text{EOR})]^c.$$

By differentiating the logarithm of the above expression with respect to EOR, equating it to zero, and solving, one finds that the conditional maximum likelihood estimator of EOR is $\widehat{mOR} = b/c$, the ratio of discordant pairs. In contrast, the unconditional maximum likelihood estimator of EOR is $(b/c)^2$, which dramatically illustrates the potential bias associated with the use of unconditional likelihood methods for finely stratified data. While not as extreme as illustrated here, the bias of unconditional likelihood methods is found in many other sparse data situations [10]. These findings emphasize the need to consider the use of conditional likelihood methods when fitting logistic models involving many strata and/or other nuisance parameters to data sets of limited size.

References

[1] Breslow, N.E. & Day, N.E. (1980). *Statistical Methods in Cancer Research*, Vol. 1: *The Analysis of Case-Control Studies*. International Agency for Research on Cancer, Lyon.

[2] Clayton, D.G. (1974). Some odds ratio statistics for the analysis of ordered categorical data, *Biometrika* **61**, 525–531.

[3] Connett, J., Ejigou, A., McHugh, R. & Breslow, N.E. (1982). The precision of the Mantel–Haenszel odds ratio estimator in case–control studies with multiple matching, *American Journal of Epidemiology* **116**, 875–877.

[4] Cox, D.R. (1975). *The Analysis of Binary Data*. Methuen, London.

[5] Kleinbaum, D.G., Kupper, L.L. & Morgenstern, H. (1982). *Epidemiologic Research: Principles and Quantitative Methods*. Lifetime Learning Publications, Belmont.

[6] Kupper, L.L., Karon, J.M., Kleinbaum, D.G., Morgenstern, H. & Lewis, D.K. (1981). Matching in epidemiologic studies: Validity and efficiency considerations, *Biometrics* **37**, 293–302.

[7] Mantel, N. (1963). Chi-square tests with one degree of freedom: extensions of the Mantel–Haenszel procedure, *Journal of the American Statistical Association* **58**, 690–700.

[8] Mantel, N. & Fleiss, J.L. (1980). Minimum expected cell size requirements for the Mantel–Haenszel one-degree of freedom chi-square test and a related rapid procedure, *American Journal of Epidemiology* **112**, 129–134.

[9] Mantel, N. & Haenszel, W. (1959). Statistical aspects of the analysis of data from retrospective studies of disease, *Journal of the National Cancer Institute* **22**, 719–748.

[10] Pike, M.C., Hill, A.P. & Smith, P.G. (1980). Bias and efficiency in logistic analysis of stratified case–control studies, *International Journal of Epidemiology* **9**, 89–95.

[11] Radhakrishna, S. (1965). Combination of results from several 2 × 2 contingency tables, *Biometrics* **21**, 86–98.

[12] Robins, J., Breslow, N. & Greenland, S. (1986). Estimators of the Mantel–Haenszel variance consistent in both sparse data and large-strata limiting models, *Biometrics* **42**, 311–323.

[13] Sato, T. (1990). Confidence limits for the common odds ratio based on the asymptotic distribution of the Mantel–Haenszel estimator, *Biometrics* **46**, 71–80.

(*See also* **Confounder; Confounder Summary Score; Matching**)

LAWRENCE L. KUPPER

Matched Pairs with Categorical Data

Matched pairs with categorical data arise when two measurements of the same categorical variable are obtained from each independent experimental unit. The repeated measurements might be obtained at two time points, for example, if a patient's condition is categorized as "good" or "poor" at diagnosis and then again six months after diagnosis. In other applications, the variable of interest might be measured under two different conditions. As an example, a patient's response to treatment, categorized as satisfactory or unsatisfactory, might be evaluated following treatment with the standard therapy and then again following treatment with a new therapy. The repeated measurements could also be obtained from each member of a matched set. In a matched **case–control study**, for example, each independent experimental unit consists of a case (individual with a specified disease or condition) and a control (individual without the disease or condition) individually matched to the case by factors such as age, sex, residence, employer, etc.

Such data can be displayed in a two-way **contingency table**. Table 1 shows the general layout when two measurements of a categorical response with I categories are obtained from each experimental unit. In this table, n_{ij} is the observed frequency

Table 1 Two-way contingency table for matched pairs with categorical data

First measurement of response	Second measurement of response					
	1	...	j	...	I	Total
1	n_{11}	...	n_{1j}	...	n_{1I}	n_{1+}
⋮	⋮	⋱	⋮	⋱	⋮	⋮
i	n_{i1}	...	n_{ij}	...	n_{iI}	n_{i+}
⋮	⋮	⋱	⋮	⋱	⋮	⋮
I	n_{I1}	...	n_{Ij}	...	n_{II}	n_{I+}
Total	n_{+1}	...	n_{+j}	...	n_{+I}	n

in the ith row and jth column of the table, n_{i+} and n_{+j} denote the row and column marginal frequencies, respectively, and n is the total number of independent experimental units. The data layout displayed in Table 1 is one example of a **square contingency table**. The possible types of response variables include **polytomous data**, **ordered categorical data**, and, for the special case of $I = 2$, **binary data**.

Statistical Inference

Statistical inference for matched pairs with categorical data focuses generally on comparing the marginal distributions of the two correlated responses (*see* **Marginal Models**). Let π_{ij} denote the probability of being in the ith row and jth column, for $i, j = 1, \ldots, I$, and let π_{i+} and π_{+j} denote the corresponding row and column marginal probabilities. The hypothesis of marginal homogeneity is

$$\pi_{i+} = \pi_{+i}, \quad i = 1, \ldots, I.$$

The hypothesis of symmetry,

$$\pi_{ij} = \pi_{ji}, \quad i \neq j,$$

is also sometimes of interest. Other hypotheses include **quasi-symmetry** and **quasi-independence**.

Binary Response

When $I = 2$, the hypothesis of symmetry implies marginal homogeneity, and vice versa. In this situation marginal homogeneity is assessed using the **McNemar test**. This test is a special case of the general class of **Mantel–Haenszel methods**. If the

sample size n is small, **exact tests for categorical data**, specifically, the exact one-sample test for the success probability of the **binomial distribution**, should be used.

Polytomous Response (see **Polytomous Data**)

Let $d_i = n_{i+} - n_{+i}$ and let $\mathbf{d}' = (d_1, \ldots, d_{I-1})$. Stuart [25] proposed a test of marginal homogeneity using the statistic

$$W_0 = \mathbf{d}' \mathbf{V}_0^{-1} \mathbf{d},$$

where $\mathbf{V}_0$, the sample **covariance matrix** under the null hypothesis of marginal homogeneity, has diagonal elements $n_{i+} + n_{+i} - 2n_{ii}$ and offdiagonal elements $-(n_{ij} + n_{ji})$. The asymptotic null distribution of W_0 is χ^2 with $I - 1$ df (χ_{I-1}^2). For **2 × 2 tables**, the test based on W_0 is identical to McNemar's test. For $I \times I$ tables, Stuart's statistic is the $I - 1$ df general association statistic from the class of Mantel–Haenszel methods.

Bhapkar [4] considered the statistic $W = \mathbf{d}' \mathbf{V}^{-1} \mathbf{d}$, where $\mathbf{V}_0$ is replaced with the unrestricted sample covariance matrix estimator $\mathbf{V}$, which has diagonal elements $n_{i+} + n_{+i} - 2n_{ii} - (n_{i+} - n_{+i})^2$ and offdiagonal elements $-(n_{ij} + n_{ji}) - (n_{i+} - n_{+i})(n_{j+} - n_{+j})$. The statistic W is asymptotically optimal, as shown by Wald [26], and can be computed using weighted **least squares** methodology for the analysis of categorical data [10] (*see* **Categorical Data Analysis**). Ireland et al. [11] noted that $W = W_0 / (1 - W_0/n)$.

Although maximum likelihood estimators of the cell probabilities under the hypothesis of marginal homogeneity cannot be expressed in closed form, likelihood methods can also be used to test marginal homogeneity. Madansky [19] gave the generalized maximum **likelihood ratio test** comparing the likelihood maximized under the hypothesis of marginal homogeneity to the likelihood maximized in the unrestricted case. The likelihood ratio test is also presented by Plackett [22, pp. 79–80], who uses the approach of Wedderburn [27]. Firth & Treat [8] and Lipsitz [16] describe how to conduct this test using standard statistical software.

An alternative likelihood-based approach tests marginal homogeneity in the context of the model for quasi symmetry by comparing the maximized likelihoods for the symmetry and quasi-symmetry models (see, for example, Agresti [2, pp. 358–359]). While this test can be carried out using standard software for fitting a **loglinear model**, it is conditional on the model of quasi-symmetry holding.

For polytomous responses ($I > 2$), the hypotheses of marginal homogeneity and symmetry are not equivalent. Under the null hypothesis of symmetry, the expected count in the (i, j) cell, with $i \neq j$, is estimated by $(n_{ij} + n_{ji})/2$. Substituting the estimated expected cell counts into the usual formula for the Pearson χ^2 test, Bowker [5] derived the statistic

$$X^2 = \sum_{i<j} \frac{(n_{ij} - n_{ji})^2}{n_{ij} + n_{ji}}.$$

Under the null hypothesis of symmetry, X^2 is approximately $\chi^2_{I(I-1)/2}$. When $I = 2$, this test is identical to McNemar's test.

A likelihood-ratio test can also be used. The test statistic is

$$G^2 = 2 \sum_{i \neq j} n_{ij} \log \left(\frac{2n_{ij}}{n_{ij} + n_{ji}} \right).$$

Since the hypothesis of symmetry has a loglinear model representation, G^2 can be computed using standard software for fitting loglinear models.

Ordered Categorical Response (see **Ordered Categorical Data***)*

The tests of marginal homogeneity described in the previous section use $I - 1$ df to compare the I pairs of marginal proportions. For ordered categorical variables, alternative tests that use the additional information provided in the ordering of the categories are more powerful for certain types of departures from the null hypothesis.

One approach is to compare marginal mean scores instead of marginal distributions. Given a set of scores that are appropriately assigned to the categories according to the alternative one wishes to detect, 1 df tests of marginal homogeneity analogous to the Stuart and Bhapkar tests can be carried out. The corresponding Stuart-type statistic (using the null covariance matrix estimator $\mathbf{V}_0$) is the Mantel–Haenszel mean score statistic; this test is discussed in White et al. [28]. If marginal rank scores are assigned, the statistic is equivalent to the Friedman [9] test obtained from a two-way

rank analysis of variance with subjects as blocks (*see* **Ranks**). Agresti [1, Section 2.3] discusses the corresponding Bhapkar-type statistic (using the unrestricted covariance matrix estimator $\mathbf{V}$) and gives additional references; this test can be computed using weighted least squares methodology for the analysis of categorical data (*see* **Categorical Data Analysis**).

Another approach to testing marginal homogeneity for ordered classifications is based on the conditional symmetry model [20; 2, pp. 361–364]. This loglinear model has only one more parameter than the symmetry model. When conditional symmetry holds, a 1 df chi-square statistic for testing marginal homogeneity is the difference between the likelihood-ratio lack-of-fit statistics for the symmetry and conditional symmetry models. Agresti [1] mentions additional methods useful in the analysis of ordered categorical responses.

Example

Table 2 displays the cross-classification of right eye and left eye unaided distant vision grade in 7477 women employees, aged 30–39 years, in British Royal Ordnance factories during 1943–1946. The outcome variable of interest is an ordered categorical variable with four levels. These data, first quoted by Stuart [24], have been analyzed by numerous authors.

First, treating the categories as nominal rather than ordered, the tests of marginal homogeneity give χ^2 statistics of 11.957, 11.976, and 11.986 for Stuart's W_0, Bhapkar's W, and Madansky's likelihood-ratio statistic, respectively. With respect to the χ^2_3 null distribution, all are significant at $\alpha = 0.01$. The alternative likelihood-based approach of testing marginal homogeneity in the context of the quasi-symmetry model gives a likelihood-ratio statistic of $19.250 - 7.274 = 11.976$, also with 3 df. The values 19.250

Table 2 Right eye and left eye unaided distance vision of 7477 women

Grade of right eye	Grade of left eye				Total
	Highest	Second	Third	Lowest	
Highest	1520	266	124	66	1976
Second	234	1512	432	78	2256
Third	117	362	1772	205	2456
Lowest	36	82	179	492	789
Total	1907	2222	2507	841	7477

and 7.274 are the likelihood-ratio statistics for symmetry (6 df) and quasi-symmetry (3 df), respectively. Bowker's test for symmetry gives $X^2 = 19.107$, which agrees closely with the corresponding value from the likelihood-ratio test.

If one treats the categories as ordered, the use of equally-spaced scores for the levels gives χ^2 statistics of 11.947 (Mantel–Haenszel mean score) and 11.97 (weighted least squares). The Friedman statistic (Mantel–Haenszel mean score test using rank scores) is 11.885. With respect to their asymptotic χ_1^2 null distributions, all three of these criteria are significant at $\alpha = 0.001$.

The likelihood-ratio lack-of-fit statistic from the conditional symmetry model is 7.35 with 5 df. Since this model provides a satisfactory fit to the data ($P = 0.2$), the difference between the likelihood-ratio statistics from the symmetry and conditional symmetry models also tests marginal homogeneity. The value of the statistic is $19.250 - 7.35 = 11.9$, which is also significant at $\alpha = 0.001$.

Related Topics

The above methods are useful in analyzing matched pairs from a single population. In some situations there may be multiple populations defined by additional covariates of interest. If all covariates are categorical with a sufficiently large sample size in each covariate strata, a wide variety of types of regression models can be fitted using the general weighted least squares approach [10], which is described specifically for correlated responses by Koch et al. [13] and others. This methodology is applicable for binary, polytomous, and ordered categorical variables. A major shortcoming, however, is that this method fails if there are continuous covariates and/or small stratum-specific sample sizes.

Maximum likelihood regression models for matched pairs with binary data are discussed by Cox & Snell [7], Lipsitz et al. [18], and other authors. Breslow & Day [6] focus specifically on the use of conditional logistic regression (*see* **Logistic Regression, Conditional**), in the analysis of matched case–control studies. The **generalized estimating equations** (GEE) procedure of Liang & Zeger [14] and its extensions can also be used to analyze matched binary outcomes with covariates. Generalizations of the GEE methodology to polytomous and

ordered categorical outcomes have also been studied [23, 15, 3, 12, 21, 17].

References

[1]   Agresti, A. (1983). Testing marginal homogeneity for ordinal categorical variables, *Biometrics* **39**, 505–510.

[2]   Agresti, A. (1990). *Categorical Data Analysis*. Wiley, New York.

[3]   Agresti, A., Lipsitz, S. & Lang, J.B. (1992). Comparing marginal distributions of large, sparse contingency tables, *Computational Statistics and Data Analysis* **14**, 55–73.

[4]   Bhapkar, V.P. (1966). A note on the equivalence of two test criteria for hypotheses in categorical data, *Journal of the American Statistical Association* **61**, 228–235.

[5]   Bowker, A.H. (1948). A test for symmetry in contingency tables, *Journal of the American Statistical Association* **43**, 572–574.

[6]   Breslow, N.E. & Day, N.E. (1980). *Statistical Methods in Cancer Research*. Vol. 1: *The Analysis of Case–Control, Studies*. International Agency for Research on Cancer, Lyon.

[7]   Cox, D.R. & Snell, E.J. (1989). *Analysis of Binary Data*. Chapman & Hall, London.

[8]   Firth, D. & Treat, B.R. (1988). Square contingency tables and GLIM, *GLIM Newsletter* **16**, 16–20.

[9]   Friedman, M. (1937). The use of ranks to avoid the assumption of normality implicit in the analysis of variance, *Journal of the American Statistical Association* **32**, 675–701.

[10] Grizzle, J.E., Starmer, C.F. & Koch, G.G. (1969). Analysis of categorical data by linear models, *Biometrics* **25**, 489–504.

[11] Ireland, C.T., Ku, H.H. & Kullback, S. (1969). Symmetry and marginal homogeneity of an $r \times r$ contingency table, *Journal of the American Statistical Association* **64**, 1323–1341.

[12] Kenward, M.G. & Jones, B. (1992). Alternative approaches to the analysis of binary and categorical repeated measurements, *Journal of Biopharmaceutical Statistics* **2**, 137–170.

[13] Koch, G.G., Landis, J.R., Freeman, J.L., Freeman, D.H. & Lehnen, R.G. (1977). A general methodology for the analysis of experiments with repeated measurement of categorical data, *Biometrics* **33**, 133–158.

[14] Liang, K.Y. & Zeger, S.L. (1986). Longitudinal data analysis using generalized linear models, *Biometrika* **73**, 13–22.

[15] Liang, K.Y., Zeger, S.L. & Qaqish, B. (1992). Multivariate regression analyses for categorical data (with discussion), *Journal of the Royal Statistical Society, Series B* **54**, 3–40.

[16] Lipsitz, S.R. (1988). Methods for analyzing repeated categorical outcomes, *Unpublished PhD Dissertation*. Department of Biostatistics, Harvard University.

[17]   Lipsitz, S.R., Kim, K. & Zhao, L. (1994). Analysis of repeated categorical data using generalized estimating equations, *Statistics in Medicine* **13**, 1149-1163.

[18]   Lipsitz, S.R., Laird, N.M. & Harrington, D.P. (1990). Maximum likelihood regression methods for paired binary data, *Statistics in Medicine* **9**, 1517-1525.

[19]   Madansky, A. (1963). Tests of homogeneity for correlated samples, *Journal of the American Statistical Association* **58**, 97-119.

[20]   McCullagh, P. (1978). A class of parametric models for the analysis of square contingency tables with ordered categories, *Biometrika* **65**, 413-418.

[21]   Miller, M.E., Davis, C.S. & Landis, J.R. (1993). The analysis of longitudinal polytomous data: generalized estimating equations and connections with weighted least squares, *Biometrics* **49**, 1033-1044.

[22]   Plackett, R.L. (1981). *The Analysis of Categorical Data*. Griffin, London.

[23]   Stram, D.O., Wei, L.J. & Ware, J.H. (1988). Analysis of repeated ordered categorical outcomes with possibly missing observations and time-dependent covariates, *Journal of the American Statistical Association* **83**, 631-637.

[24]   Stuart, A. (1953). The estimation and comparison of strengths of association in contingency tables, *Biometrika* **40**, 105-110.

[25]   Stuart, A. (1955). A test for homogeneity of the marginal distributions in a two-way classification, *Biometrika* **42**, 412-416.

[26]   Wald, A. (1943). Tests of statistical hypotheses concerning several parameters when the number of observations is large, *Transactions of the American Mathematical Society* **54**, 426-482.

[27]   Wedderburn, R.W.M. (1974). Generalized linear models specified in terms of constraints, *Journal of the Royal Statistical Society, Series B* **36**, 449-454.

[28]   White, A.A., Landis, J.R. & Cooper, M.M. (1982). A note on the equivalence of several marginal homogeneity test criteria for categorical data, *International Statistical Review* **50**, 27-34.

CHARLES S. DAVIS

Matching

Before discussing the procedure known as matching, it is necessary to provide some background and motivation for its use. In epidemiologic studies, it is typically the situation that valid **estimation** of the strength of the relationship between a response variable D of interest (e.g. the presence, $D = 1$, or not, $D = 0$, of some particular disease) and an independent variable E of interest (e.g. the presence, $E = 1$, or not, $E = 0$, of some exposure) necessitates the consideration of so-called **confounding** factors (*see* **Confounder**). Ignoring or inappropriately accounting for the effects of confounding factors can often lead to invalid (i.e. statistically inconsistent) and inefficient estimation of the true exposure–disease association of interest.

As a simple example, suppose that the dichotomous response (or disease) variable D of interest is the presence or absence of lung cancer and that the dichotomous independent (or exposure) variable E of interest is the presence or absence of a history of occupational exposure to asbestos. Then, a dichotomous variable C such as cigarette smoking status (e.g. evidence, $C = 1$, or not, $C = 0$, of a history of smoking), which is an established risk factor for the development of lung cancer, will be a confounder if, *in the data under consideration*, its distribution among the group of study subjects with a history of occupational exposure to asbestos (the "exposed group") is different from its distribution among the group of study subjects who do not have a history of occupationally related asbestos exposure (the "unexposed group"). If C is, in fact, a confounder in the data under consideration, then appropriate adjustment for C *at the analysis stage* (e.g. by **stratification** methods or, equivalently, by multivariable modeling) would be needed. In our particular example involving the three dichotomous variables D, E, and C, one could fit the **logistic regression** model logit $[\Pr(D = 1)] = \beta_0 + \beta_1 E + \gamma_1 C$ by appropriate **likelihood** methods to obtain an adjusted (for C) estimated **odds ratio** $\exp(\hat{\beta}_1)$ and to obtain a corresponding **interval estimator** for the population E–D odds ratio $\exp(\beta_1)$. Here, we are assuming that C is not an **effect modifier** (i.e. there is no **interaction** between E and C), so that it is not necessary to include the product term EC in the above model; we will make this no interaction assumption in our discussion to follow.

However, adjustment for C at the analysis stage can be problematic. For example, if almost all of the study subjects with a history of smoking have lung cancer (i.e. are "cases"), and if a large proportion of the study subjects with no smoking history are "noncases", then such stratum-specific imbalances can lead to poor statistical efficiency in the point and interval estimation of the odds ratio parameter $\exp(\beta_1)$. In more realistic situations where there are typically several confounders to consider simultaneously, distributional imbalances in strata defined by combinations of levels of these confounders can severely compromise the reliability of multivariable modeling analyses.

Design Options: Restriction and Matching

By using appropriate strategies at the *design stage* of a study, it is often possible to avoid many of the confounder-related distributional imbalance problems mentioned earlier. For example, consider a potentially confounding variable such as gender. One way to avoid completely any possible problems associated with an analysis stage adjustment for the variable gender is to decide, at the design stage, to restrict the study so that it involves either only males or only females. This simple study design option is called (*total*) *restriction* because the potential confounder is completely restricted to have exactly the same value for every study subject. Clearly, the disadvantage of (total) restriction is the lack of generalizability of the study results; in our example, by employing (total) restriction with respect to gender, the study conclusions would necessarily only pertain either to males or to females.

Matching, in contrast to total restriction, is a form of *partial restriction* on study subject selection, partial in the sense that only the so-called "referent (or comparison) group", and not the "index group", is chosen subject to certain restrictions. More specifically, for follow-up studies (*see* **Cohort Study**), once the index group of exposed ($E = 1$) subjects is randomly selected from the population of interest, the referent group of unexposed ($E = 0$) subjects is then chosen to be similar to the exposed group with respect to the distributions of one or more potentially confounding factors. For **case–control studies**, once the index group of diseased ($D = 1$) subjects is chosen at random from the population of interest, the referent group of nondiseased ($D = 0$) subjects is picked to be similar to the cases with respect to the distributions of one or more potentially confounding factors. We use the word "similar", rather than "identical", because the index and matched referent groups will generally not have exactly the same confounder distributions after matching; the degree of similarity will depend on the type and the extent of matching employed.

To discuss types of matching schemes, we need to distinguish between matching on continuous variables (e.g. age, weight, cholesterol level) and matching on categorical variables (e.g. gender, race). Matching on a continuous variable (say, X) necessitates the specification of a rule for deciding when an index subject's value (say, X_1) and a referent subject's value (say, X_0) are "close enough" to declare that the two subjects are "matched" on X. In so-called "caliper matching", one specifies a caliper (or tolerance) value C and declares the index and referent subjects to be matched if $|X_1 - X_0| \leq C$.

The smaller is C, the tighter will be the match on X, but, correspondingly, the harder it will be to find index–referent pairs to satisfy such a stringent matching criterion [8, 9].

Since, in standard epidemiologic practice, variables are generally categorized for matching purposes (e.g. note that caliper matching defines categories of width C), we will henceforth focus on so called *category (or frequency) matching*. In particular, index and referent subjects are said to be matched on a categorized potential confounder if they are in the same category of that variable. In the realistic situation where category matching involves several potential confounding variables, index and referent subjects are said to be matched when they are in the same category for each and every one of the categorized matching variables under consideration. For example, suppose that there are three categorized matching variables of interest: age in four categories (30–39, 40–49, 50–59, and 60–69), race (black, white, and other), and gender (male and female). Then, there will be 24 strata defined by the various combinations of these three matching variables, with, for example, one stratum consisting of black females between the ages of 40 and 49.

In general, then, matching can be considered to be pre (or design stage)-stratification, as opposed to **post** (or analysis stage)-**stratification**, with the goal of such matching being to form strata that are sufficiently balanced to permit valid, stable, and efficient statistical analyses. Once matching is employed at the design stage, it is mandatory at the analysis stage to take the matching into account via the use of appropriate stratified analysis methods [5]. Such **categorical data analysis** procedures include the approach of **Mantel & Haenszel** [6] and the use of conditional logistic regression methods [1, 4] (*see* **Logistic Regression, Conditional; Matched Analysis**).

Types of Matching Schemes

There are various types of matching schemes that can be used. One of the more popular matching schemes, especially in case–control studies, is known as *pair matching*. Pair matching refers to the special situation when each stratum is assumed, for analysis purposes, to contain exactly one index subject and one referent subject. However, this assumption will generally lead to an inefficient stratified analysis when the pairing is artificial and unnecessary. For example, for a stratum of cases and controls consisting of black females between the ages of 40 and 49, any case in that stratum could theoretically be paired with any control without altering the basic within-stratum structure. Retaining this "random" pairing in the analysis is clearly unwarranted, and such an "overmatched analysis" generally leads to some loss in statistical efficiency [2]. In contrast, the term "**overmatching**" commonly refers to an undesirable design-stage strategy of matching on variables that make the cases and controls too much alike with respect to exposure status. Such variables are generally of two types, namely, so-called "intervening variables" that are intermediate in the causal pathway between exposure and disease and variables that are (at best) very weak risk factors for the disease in question but are nevertheless highly correlated with exposure status [10]. Such overmatching can sometimes lead to a meaningful loss in statistical efficiency, especially in case–control studies (see "Discussion" below).

A generalization of pair matching is a procedure known as R-to-1 matching, where each stratum is considered to contain one index subject and exactly R referent subjects. Miettinen [7] and others have shown that there is little to gain statistically by taking $R > 4$. For example, when comparing R-to-1 matching with pair matching ($R = 1$) in case–control studies, Ury [11] has shown that the **Pitman efficiency** of the Mantel–Haenszel test for stratified data is $2R/(R + 1)$, so that the Pitman efficiency only increases from 1.600 for $R = 4$ to 1.667 when $R = 5$.

In the most general category matching situation, a particular stratum (say, the gth of G strata) may contain R_g referent subjects and S_g index subjects, giving a *matching ratio* of R_g/S_g (which is not necessarily an integer). If this matching ratio varies with g, then we have a *variable matching ratio plan*. If the matching ratio does not vary over the strata (e.g. as with R-to-1 matching), then we have a *fixed*

matching ratio plan. With either plan, the appropriate data analysis would still appropriately accumulate stratum-specific information; and, in terms of statistical efficiency, a fixed matching ratio plan is usually somewhat better.

Advantages and Disadvantages of Category Matching

Some of the *positive aspects* of category matching in epidemiologic studies are as follows:

1. Category matching a set of referent subjects to a **random sample** of index subjects can often lead to a more statistically efficient analysis than can be obtained by choosing the same number of referent subjects by random sampling. This efficiency advantage will tend to occur when the matching variables are well-established determinants of the response variable (e.g. are important risk factors for the disease under study) and are expected to be quite differentially distributed between the exposed and unexposed groups in the observed data (i.e. are anticipated to be strong confounders). For more detailed discussion, see Kupper et al. [5] and Karon & Kupper [3].
2. Matching on a variable like neighborhood of residence can lead to efficient adjustment for the potentially confounding effects of a wide range of social and economic factors that would be difficult, if not impossible, to measure and hence to control.
3. Matching can often lead to savings in time and money. For example, when the cases in a case–control study are chosen from records in different hospitals or in different companies within some industry, it is preferable, for reasons of simplicity and convenience in data collection (and also possibly on validity and efficiency grounds), to choose controls for each case from that same set of hospital or company records.
4. Matching in the selection of the referent group with respect to a given set of potential confounders does not preclude controlling for other nonmatched confounders at the analysis stage via multivariable modeling procedures like conditional logistic regression. In this regard, a recommended strategy would be to match only on important risk factors considered a priori to be highly likely to manifest themselves as strong

confounders in the data, and to adjust (if necessary) for other factors at the analysis stage.

Some possible *negative aspects* of category matching in epidemiologic studies are the following:

1. Category matching can be a costly enterprise, both with regard to the *direct* costs of time and labor required to find the appropriate matches and the *indirect* costs (in terms of information loss) owing to the discarding of available referents not able to satisfy possibly stringent matching criteria.

2. When employing category matching, simultaneous recruitment of cases and controls can be problematic since there is no way to know in advance exactly how many controls will be needed to meet sample size requirements in different matching strata defined by the sample of cases. To circumvent this problem, a new "randomized recruitment" method for matching has been developed [12, 13].

3. The referent group chosen by category matching ends up being more like the index group than like the underlying population of referents being sampled. In particular, matching generally precludes the evaluation of the underlying population relationships between the matching variables and exposure status in follow-up studies or between the matching factors and disease status in case–control studies.

4. If the strata defined by the category matching process are wide (so that there is room for the matching factors each to vary sufficiently in value within particular strata), it is possible that stratum-specific residual confounding due to the matching factors can still be present. Appropriate adjustment for such stratum-specific residual confounding at the analysis stage can be accomplished using multivariable modeling procedures.

Discussion

In summary, category matching on potential confounders can be a fruitful design-based strategy in both follow-up and case–control studies when reliable information, based on knowledge of the disease process under study and previous research findings, indicates that such variables are well-established disease determinants (i.e. are strong risk factors) expected to be quite differentially distributed between exposed and unexposed groups if matching is not employed (e.g. under random sampling of the referent group).

As a word of caution, the use of matching requires more care in case–control studies than in follow-up studies. Since exposure information is collected *after* the occurrence of disease in case–control studies, indiscriminate *overmatching* of controls to cases simultaneously on several factors can lead to a substantial loss in efficiency relative to random sampling of the control group. For example, consider a pair-matched case–control study involving n case–control pairs, where a is the number of pairs where both the case and control are exposed, b is the number of pairs where the case is exposed and the control is not, c is the number of pairs where the control is exposed and the case is not, and d is the number of pairs where neither the case nor the control is exposed. Then, the Mantel–Haenszel test statistic [6] takes the form $(b-c)^2/(b+c)$, and the appropriate odds ratio estimator is b/c (namely, the ratio of discordant pairs). Hence, the effective sample size in such a study is the total number of discordant pairs $(b+c)$, not n. If the matching variables are each correlated with the exposure variable, then overmatching generally increases the number of uninformative pairs in the observed data, namely $(a+d)$, thus leading to a (possibly substantial) loss in efficiency. Thus, in case–control studies especially, the best policy is to consider as candidate matching variables only well-established strong risk factors for the disease in question. As mentioned earlier, matching either on intervening variables or on very weak risk factors highly correlated with exposure status should be avoided.

References

[1]   Breslow, N.E. & Day, N.E. (1980). *Statistical Methods in Cancer Research*, Vol. 1: *The Analysis of Case–Control Studies*. International Agency for Research on Cancer, Lyon.

[2]   Brookmeyer, R., Liang, K.Y. & Linet, M. (1986). Matched case–control designs and overmatched analyses, *American Journal of Epidemiology* **124**, 693–701.

[3]   Karon, J.M. & Kupper, L.L. (1982). In defense of matching, *American Journal of Epidemiology* **116**, 852–866.

[4]   Kleinbaum, D.G., Kupper, L.L. & Morgenstern, H. (1982). *Epidemiologic Research: Principles and Quantitative Methods*. Lifetime Learning Publications, Belmont.

[5] Kupper, L.L., Karon, J.M., Kleinbaum, D.G., Morgenstern, H. & Lewis, D.K. (1981). Matching in epidemiologic studies: validity and efficiency considerations, *Biometrics* **37**, 293–302.

[6] Mantel, N. & Haenszel, W. (1959). Statistical aspects of the analysis of data from retrospective studies of disease, *Journal of the National Cancer Institute* **22**, 719–748.

[7] Miettinen, O.S. (1969). Individual matching with multiple controls in the case of all-or-none responses, *Biometrics* **22**, 339–355.

[8] Raynor, W.J. & Kupper, L.L. (1981). Category matching of continuous variables in case–control studies, *Biometrics* **37**, 811–817.

[9] Rubin, D.R. (1973). Matching to remove bias in observational studies, *Biometrics* **29**, 159–183.

[10] Schlesselman, J.J. (1982). *Case–Control Studies: Design, Conduct, Analysis.* Oxford University Press, New York.

[11] Ury, H.K. (1975). Efficiency of case–control studies with multiple controls per case: continuous or dichotomous data, *Biometrics* **31**, 643–649.

[12] Weinberg, C.R. & Wacholder, S. (1990). The design and analysis of case–control studies with biased sampling, *Biometrics* **46**, 963–975.

[13] Weinberg, C.R. & Sandler, D.P. (1991). Randomized recruitment in case–control studies, *American Journal of Epidemiology* **134**, 421–431.

LAWRENCE L. KUPPER

Matching Coefficient of Numerical Taxonomy *see* Agreement, Measurement of

Maternal Mortality

Maternal mortality claims the lives of some 585 000 women a year, 99% of them in the developing world. It is the main cause of death among young women aged 15–19, and the third or fourth most common cause in women of childbearing age, generally defined as 15–49. The differences between the developed and the developing world in levels of maternal mortality are greater than for any other indicator of public health: in developed countries a woman has a lifetime risk of maternal death of 1 in 1800: in developing countries this risk is 1 in 48. However,

the risks range from 1 in 4000 in the industrialized of countries of northern Europe, to 1 in 12 in eastern and western Africa [1]. Maternal mortality also has severe consequences for the health of children: in developing countries the baby born to a woman who dies in childbirth rarely survives, and her older children face much greater risks of death [7].

Definition of Maternal Mortality

A maternal death is the death of a woman while pregnant, or within 42 days of the termination of pregnancy, irrespective of the duration and site of the pregnancy, from any cause related to or aggravated by the pregnancy or its management, but not from accidental or incidental causes [9]. This classification therefore includes deaths from abortion, spontaneous or induced, or from an ectopic pregnancy, but not deaths in pregnancy or the postpartum period caused by violence or accidents.

The distinction between causes related to, or aggravated by, pregnancy or its management gives rise to two other definitions: "direct" and "indirect" obstetric deaths. Direct obstetric deaths are those related to complications of pregnancy, labor or in the 42-day postpartum period (the puerperium), from interventions, or from incorrect treatment or omissions in treatment. Indirect obstetric deaths are those resulting from a pre-existing disease, or one that developed during pregnancy, and that is aggravated by pregnancy. Before 1975, deaths from indirect causes were not classified as maternal deaths.

Causes of Maternal Deaths

On the evidence of a few good community-based studies, direct causes account for the majority–80%–of maternal deaths. In turn, five major causes account for 80% of these direct maternal deaths. Although there is some variation in their relative importance among regions, the distribution of the five causes at global level is as follows: hemorrhage (25%); sepsis (15%); unsafe abortion (13%); eclampsia (8%) and obstructed labor (7%). Indirect causes of maternal death, such as anemia, malaria, cardiovascular disease, hepatitis, and diabetes, account for the remaining 20% of all maternal deaths [1] (*see* **Cause of Death, Underlying and Multiple**).

Sources of Data on Maternal Mortality

Gathering data on maternal mortality is difficult and expensive – and often beyond the resources of the very countries in which the problem is greatest. The chief sources of information are vital registration systems, health services data, and population-based surveys (*see* **Administrative Databases; Surveys, Health and Morbidity; Vital Statistics, Overview**).

Few developing countries have registration systems to provide information on the numbers of deaths (*see* **Death Certification**). Those that do can rarely provide information on the cause of death, or require that death certificates note pregnancy status. Moreover, in countries where induced abortion is illegal, official statistics seldom fully reflect deaths from this cause. Health service statistics suffer from **selection bias**: women who die in pregnancy or childbirth in health facilities often differ in important health and socioeconomic characteristics from pregnant women in the broader community. It is also difficult to define the appropriate catchment area of a hospital (*see* **Hospital Market Area**) for the derivation of ratios and rates. **Population-based studies**, therefore, have been used increasingly to gather information. Their most important drawback is expense: maternal mortality is a rare event compared with **infant mortality**, for example, and sample sizes need to be very large to obtain reliable estimates. Costs are somewhat lower where questions are added to **censuses** or surveys: the "sisterhood method", for example, has yielded useful information on maternal mortality by asking adult respondents whether any sisters have died in their childbearing years. The most reliable data, however, where vital registration is incomplete or lacking, are obtained from studies that identify all deaths to women of reproductive age (reproductive age mortality surveys, or RAMOS). Interviewers consult many community sources and then, on the basis of symptoms described by family members and health care providers, classify the deaths as maternal or otherwise. Very few countries have been able to afford these studies.

Given these problems, but faced with the need to measure progress in reducing maternal mortality, the **World Health Organization** (WHO) and the United Nations International Children's Emergency Fund (UNICEF) have recently developed new estimates of maternal mortality [10]. They used country data where available, adjusted for undercount and

misclassification, and developed a model to predict values for countries with no reliable national data. At the global level, the new estimates represent a significant upward revision of the annual number of maternal deaths – an increase of 80 000 over the figure of just over 500 000 in use for the past 10 years.

Measuring Maternal Mortality

The three most common measures of maternal mortality are the lifetime risk, the maternal mortality rate, and the maternal mortality ratio. The ratio is the number of maternal deaths per 100 000 live births during a certain time period, and is, therefore, a measure of the risks women face when they are pregnant, generally called obstetric risk. However, in order to run this risk, women must be pregnant. The lifetime risk and the maternal mortality rate take account of fertility: they measure both obstetric risk, and the frequency with which women are exposed to that risk through pregnancy. This is seen most easily in the maternal mortality rate: the number of maternal deaths per 100 000 women of reproductive age during a certain time period. The following equation demonstrates the relationship [2]:

$$\text{maternal mortality rate} = \text{maternal mortality ratio}$$
$$\times \text{ general fertility rate}$$
$$\frac{\text{maternal deaths}}{\text{women 15-49}} = \frac{\text{maternal deaths}}{\text{live births}}$$
$$\times \frac{\text{live births}}{\text{women 15-49}}.$$

In using data on maternal mortality it is important to note how the maternal mortality rate is defined. Historically, it was defined as the number of maternal deaths per 100 000 live births, i.e. the definition of the ratio given above, and this is still the definition used in the tenth revision of the **International Classification of Diseases** published by WHO in 1992 in order to provide consistency with previous editions [9]. However, in its analytical work on maternal mortality WHO also distinguishes between the rate and the ratio using the definitions given above [1, 10], as exemplified in Table 1. The distinction is important for directing attention to appropriate interventions.

Table 1 Measures of maternal mortality in developed and developing countries, 1990

	Maternal mortality ratio (maternal deaths per 100 000 live births)	Number of maternal deaths	Lifetime risk[a] of maternal death (1 in:)
World	430	585 000	60
More developed regions	27	4000	1800
Less developed regions	480	582 000	48

Sources: [1, Table 2; 10].
[a]Lifetime risk devised by Roger Rochat, Emory University School of Medicine, USA. Calculated as $1 - (1 - MMR)^{(1.2TFR)}$], where the maternal mortality ratio (MMR) is expressed as a decimal and the total fertility rate (TFR) is adjusted by 1.2 to allow for pregnancies not ending in live births.

The other measure of maternal mortality that also takes into account both the risks within pregnancy and the risks of pregnancy is lifetime risk. In fact, this is the more commonly used indicator of international disparity, conveying graphically the risks of pregnancy in countries with high fertility. Table 1 presents the regional differences in maternal mortality ratios and lifetime risk by region.

Wide though the differences in maternal mortality ratios are, they are much less than the differences in lifetime risk: the risks women face in pregnancy and childbirth are compounded by the frequency with which they face those risks.

Actions to Reduce Maternal Mortality

It follows that maternal mortality can be reduced by interventions that reduce fertility, and that reduce obstetric risk (*see* **Reproduction**). Reductions in the total number of pregnancies result in fewer women at risk of a maternal death: a comparison of maternal mortality in Bali, Indonesia, and Menoufia, Egypt in the 1980s provides a telling example. The maternal mortality ratio in Bali was 718: in Menoufia it was 190–3.8 times as high. Yet the maternal mortality rate of 69 in Bali was only 1.5 times as high as the rate of 45 in Menoufia – because fertility was lower in Bali [3]. Changes in fertility, closely associated with the adoption of family planning, therefore have an important impact on the maternal mortality rate (and on lifetime risk).

Changes in fertility can also affect the maternal mortality ratio by reducing the number of high-risk

pregnancies – pregnancies that are unwanted and that may lead women to run the risk of unsafe abortion, or pregnancies in women of older age, or who have had four or more previous births, or whose last birth occurred less than two years previously. These women are often the first to use family planning services, when available. In Bali, contraceptive use was higher, and fertility rates lower among older women than in Menoufia. However, since, in general, most births occur to women at "safe" ages and parities, the majority of maternal deaths do too. Thus, the chief reductions in the maternal mortality ratio are to be achieved by reducing the risks in pregnancy.

Underlying the immediate medical causes of maternal death are many factors contributing to the risk of maternal death. Women's socioeconomic status is a powerful determinant of their health status–and of their access to health services. Socioeconomic status also affects fertility, and the risk of maternal death: women with no, or little, primary education have more children than women with secondary and higher education (*see* **Social Classifications**). Raising women's status is necessary to improving maternal health, but is a long-term objective. In the short term, interventions to reduce the number of obstetric complications, and the number of deaths among women who develop complications, are essential.

Basic Maternal Care

Women need care throughout pregnancy, delivery, and in the postpartum period. Antenatal care is necessary to inform women on how to take care of themselves throughout pregnancy and childbirth, how to recognize danger signals, and what to do should complications arise. It is also necessary to treat conditions that can lead to complications, such as anemia, or which are aggravated by pregnancy, such as malaria and viral hepatitis. Health facilities providing antenatal care, however, need to be linked closely with facilities able to deal with complications that may arise: it is doubtful whether antenatal care that is not part of a more comprehensive system contributes to maternal mortality reduction [6]. Care in delivery should include attendance by trained personnel, in clean conditions to prevent sepsis, and, again, with access to health facilities and providers with the skills, equipment, and drugs to prevent, detect, and manage complications during birth, and during the postpartum period. A recent review and **meta-analysis** (synthesis of findings) of studies of maternal mortality in developing countries indicates that care in the postpartum period is essential: 60% of maternal deaths occurred in the postpartum period [5]. Almost half of postpartum deaths – 45% – occurred in the first 24 hours after delivery, and nearly three-quarters within the first week. The time of death varied according to cause: most postpartum deaths from hemorrhage and pregnancy-induced hypertension (eclampsia) occurred during the first day and week after delivery: most postpartum deaths from sepsis occurred in the second week and later.

Essential Obstetric Care and Emergency Obstetric Care

While basic maternal care meets the needs of all women whose pregnancies, labor, or delivery are uncomplicated, or who are able to return to this care when a complication has been successfully treated, an estimated one-third to one-half of pregnant women develop obstetric complications, and an estimated 15% develop complications that require emergency care. Both essential obstetric care for all complications, and emergency care, have been known by the acronym EOC, giving rise to some confusion. The Inter-Agency Group (IAG) on safe motherhood, comprised of representatives of several of the UN agencies and nongovernmental organizations active in

the field of reproductive health, recommends differentiating between these terms by use of the acronym ECOC for Essential Care of Obstetric Complications, and EMCOC for Emergency Care for Obstetric Complications. The obstetric functions provided by ECOC include the functions necessary for EMCOC and, according to the IAG, should be available to all pregnant women with problems, including complications of unsafe abortion. ECOC comprises: surgical obstetrics; anesthesia and medical treatment; blood replacement and manual procedures; labor monitoring, management of problem pregnancies, and neonatal special care (statement developed at the IAG meeting, February 1996).

Maternal Health

Reductions in maternal mortality cannot be equated with improvements in maternal health. They may even be associated with increases in maternal morbidity – the disabilities suffered by women as a result of pregnancy, childbirth, and abortion, or the exacerbation of existing health problems by pregnancy. It has been estimated that for every woman who dies in pregnancy, another 15 survive but suffer long-term consequences [8]. It is also important to recognize that maternal health is part of women's health more broadly defined: this might seem a truism, but some are concerned that emphasis on maternal mortality has stressed women's maternal roles to the exclusion of recognition of other influences on women's health that also, though more indirectly, would improve maternal health [6]. In a slightly different vein, others worry that the drive to measure mortality, and the impact of programs on mortality, may divert resources that would be better deployed in strengthening implementation of those programs. They argue for developing indicators that measure progress in increasing the availability, quality and utilization of maternity services, thus contributing to improved maternal health more generally [4]. The new estimates and methodology developed by WHO and UNICEF, should help to reduce this pressure to produce ratios and **rates**. It is generally agreed, however, that investments in maternal health services, including family planning, provide significant health benefits to women at low cost and are essential components of basic health care. Work [11] on the burden of death and disability caused by various diseases, and on the health benefits and costs of interventions, found prenatal and delivery care and family planning to be among the most cost-effective of health interventions (*see* **Health Economics**).

References

[1] Abou Zahr, C., Wardlaw, T., Stanton, C. & Hill, K. (1996). Maternal mortality, *World Health Statistics Quarterly* **49**, 77–87.
[2] Fortney, J.A. (1987). The importance of family planning in reducing maternal mortality, *Studies in Family Planning* **18**, 109–114.
[3] Fortney, J.A., Susanti, I., Gadalia, S., Saleh, S., Feldblum, P.J. & Potts, M. (1988). Maternal mortality in Indonesia and Egypt, *International Journal of Gynecology and Obstetrics* **26**, 21–32.
[4] Graham, W., Filippi, V.G.A. & Ronsmans, C. (1996). Demonstrating programme impact on maternal mortality, *Health Policy and Planning* **11**, 16–20.
[5] Li, X.F., Fortney, J.A., Kotelchuck, M. & Glover, L.H. (1996). The postpartum period: the key to maternal mortality, *International Journal of Gynecology and Obstetrics* **54**, 1–10.
[6] McDonagh, M. (1996). Is antenatal care effective in reducing maternal morbidity and mortality? *Health Policy and Planning* **11**, 1–15.
[7] Over, M., Ellis, R.P., Huber, J.H. & Solon, O. (1992). The consequences of adult ill-health, in *The Health of Adults in the Developing World*, R.G.A. Feachem, T. Kjellstrom, C.J.L. Murray, M. Over & M.A. Phillips, eds. Oxford University Press for the World Bank, New York, pp. 161–207.
[8] Starrs, A. (1987). Preventing the tragedy of maternal deaths, *Report on the Safe Motherhood Conference 1987*.
[9] WHO (1992). *International Statistical Classification of Diseases and Related Health Problems*, 10th revision. World Health Organization, Geneva.
[10] WHO and UNICEF (1996). Revised 1990 estimates of maternal mortality. A new approach by WHO and UNICEF, *WHO/FRH/MSM96.11* and *UNICEF/PLN/96.1*.
[11] World Bank (1993). Investing in health, *World Development Report*. Published for the World Bank by Oxford University Press, Washington.

(*See also* **Health Services Data Sources in Canada; Health Services Data Sources in Europe; Health Services Data Sources in the US**)

J. NASSIM

Mathematical Biology, Overview

Mathematical biology has become a flourishing field in which real mathematics combines with real biology. The field is represented by numerous refereed journals, including *Journal of Mathematical Biology, Bulletin of Mathematical Biology, Biomathematics, IMA Journal of Mathematics Applied in Medicine and Biology, Journal of Theoretical Biology, Mathematical Biosciences, Biological Cybernetics*, and *Theoretical Population Biology*. In addition, there are frequent biological articles in *Biophysical Journal* and *SIAM Journal of Applied Mathematics*, and occasional mathematical articles in *Journal of Neurophysiology*, and even *Journal of Molecular Biology*. Lecture note series include *Lecture Notes in Biomathematics* and *Lectures on Mathematics in the Life Sciences*. There are also a number of good recent general textbooks [4, 8, 14], an excellent collection of mathematically sophisticated research papers [12], a survey of applications and unsolved problems in biomedical imaging [3], and important monographs on computational biology [23], stochastic models of carcinogenesis [22], and cardiac arrhythmias [25]. Medical applications include tomographic imaging, genetic linkage analysis, cardiac arrhythmias, epidemic diseases and control strategies, carcinogenesis, and tumor chemotherapy. A recent conference was reviewed in *Science* [6]. This list is necessarily incomplete, but it may be useful for beginning reading in the field.

Mathematical biology consists, not of the mathematics of living things, but of the mathematics of *models* of living things; and choosing the level of simplification and the nature of the abstraction is perhaps the modeler's most distinctive contribution. Mathematical skill and biological knowledge are necessary conditions for success in modeling, but the art of selecting the essential ingredients of complex and elusive phenomena goes beyond them.

> Simplification in mathematical modeling is both a blessing and a curse. The curse is the partial loss of predictive power that comes from whatever lack of correspondence there may be between the model and the real world. The blessing is the insight that comes from the process of pruning away unnecessary detail and leaving behind only what is essential.
> ... The models presented here are in the nature of

metaphors, and these metaphors will have served their purpose if they have helped the reader to see through the bewildering complexity of living systems to the underlying simplicity of certain biological processes and functions (Hoppensteadt and Peskin [8, p. 3]).

It is natural, in this era of fast computation, to want to build as much realism as possible into biological models, and rely on the power of the computer to approximate the complex systems of equations that result and make quantitative predictions that can be tested against experimental data. While not minimizing the practical utility of computer **simulation**, e.g. in cardiac pacemaker design or in predicting the course of epidemics, it may be that the most distinctive contribution of mathematics to biology lies in the opposite direction: simplifying to the point where it is possible to prove *theorems* about the model, and not only to compute with it. The computational route may yield a model that gives good predictions, but is just as impenetrable to understanding as the original biological system, whereas, when one proves a theorem about a model, that theorem is likely to give insight into the underlying biology. Proving nontrivial theorems about models that are adequate "metaphors," to use Hoppensteadt & Peskin's term, is the summit of mathematical biology, but it is ascended only occasionally, and such achievements are worthy to be celebrated. This article delves into the reasoning processes of five good examples, and shows, through them, several different ways that mathematical reasoning can enhance our understanding of biological systems. The five papers are selected as illustrations, without any attempt at a historical review of the place of each in its field.

Neurons with Excitatory Interactions can Oscillate in Phase Opposition

It is well known that neurons with excitatory interactions can synchronize each other, and that neurons with *inhibitory* interactions can entrain each other to oscillate with opposite phases, but what Kopell & Somers show is that excitatory coupling can lead to phase opposition as well [11]. They use singular perturbation theory to study a neuronal model of the relaxation oscillator type (but quite general in form), in which there is a fast-activating current x and a slow-activating current y, governed by the equations

$\varepsilon \dot{x} = F(x, y)$, $\dot{y} = G(x, y)$, the singular limit being taken as $\varepsilon \to 0$. The *nullclines* (loci in the x,y plane of $F = 0$ and $G = 0$) are assumed to be sigmoidal (for the slow current) and cubic (for the fast current). With x on the horizontal axis and y on the vertical axis, the cubic nullcline has three branches: left (descending), middle (ascending), and right (descending), and the two nullclines intersect along the middle branch of the cubic. When ε is small, the neuron's periodic trajectory descends the left branch to its minimum, jumps horizontally to the right branch, ascends the left branch to its maximum, and jumps horizontally back to the left branch. Mutual excitatory coupling between a pair of neurons is modeled by assuming that, when neuron 1 is on its right branch (high x), neuron 2's cubic nullcline is shifted upward on the y axis, and vice versa.

The fundamental condition that must be met for an antiphase solution is that the time to *ascend* the original cubic nullcline is less than the time to *descend* the shifted cubic nullcline. Kopell & Somers reparameterize the slow current (substituting z for y) in such a way that $\mathrm{d}z/\mathrm{d}t$ is constant and positive on the left branch of the unshifted cubic nullcline, $z = 0$ corresponding to the leftward jump point, and $z = 1$ to the minimum. Now suppose that neuron 1 starts just at the point of a jump to the right branch, while neuron 2 is at some $z \in (0, 1)$. Neuron 2 will immediately follow in jumping to the left branch of the shifted cubic nullcline, because neuron 1 is on its right branch. If the fundamental condition is satisfied, then there are z close enough to 0 that neuron 1 will jump back to the left branch before neuron 2 has completed its descent to the minimum, so neuron 2 will end up, after this pair of jumps, back on its original nullcline at a new position $E(z)$. Kopell & Somers prove that, if the fundamental condition holds, and in addition $E(0) > 0$ and $0 \le E'(z) < 1$, then there is a stable antiphase solution. Furthermore, the antiphase solution persists in the nonsingular case $\varepsilon > 0$.

Kopell & Somers then show that the hypotheses of the theorem hold for several commonly used models of neuronal firing, including the Morris–Lecar equations. This system, which was first analyzed from a qualitative dynamics point of view by Rinzel & Ermentrout [17], is a simplified model of excitable membranes that captures many of their important features. It postulates voltage-gated Ca^{2+} (fast) and K^+ (slow) channels, and has nullclines on the (x, y)

phase plane of the cubic and sigmoid types described above. The model has three equilibria [5]: a stable rest point, an unstable node, and a saddle point. The unstable manifold of the saddle point, which contains the rest point, forms an attracting invariant loop. The system generates action potentials in a realistic manner.

It turns out that it is possible for both antiphase and the more typical in-phase oscillations to be stable under the same excitatory coupling conditions. Arrays of bistable oscillators with nearest-neighbor coupling may show "fractured synchrony", i.e. domains within which activity is synchronous, while neighboring domains are in phase opposition [19, Figure 14].

Mutation Rates can be Estimated from Gene Polymorphisms

Mutation rates refer to the history of a population over an extended time, whereas gene **polymorphisms** refer to a cross-section at one time. Using the method of "coalescence", Kimmel & Chakraborty are able to make inferences about genetic history from the present state of the population [9]. Short segments of DNA are often repeated in the genome, and when the units of these "tandem repeats" are 2–6 nucleotides long, they are called "microsatellites". Mutations occur relatively frequently in the repeat length; they can cause expansion or contraction. Kimmel & Chakraborty use the Wright–Fisher model (*see* **Population Genetics**) for genetic evolution without selection in a population of constant size N, a model that ignores diploidy, and treats the $2N$ chromosomes of the $(k+1)$th generation as if they were sampled uniformly and independently, with replacement, from the $2N$ chromosomes of the kth generation. That is equivalent to the number of copies of each chromosome in the $(k+1)$th generation having a symmetric **multinomial distribution** [10]. Let each chromosome have a probability ν per generation of a mutation at a given locus (regarded as a **Poisson process**), and let the size U of that mutation (replacing an allele of size X by an allele of size $X + U$) be a **random variable** independent of the time of the mutation. Under the Wright–Fisher model, any two chromosomes selected from the current generation, if followed backward in their parentage, eventually "coalesce", i.e. have a common parent, and the time to

T (going backward from the current generation) when coalescence occurs is approximately **exponentially distributed** with parameter $1/2N$, if N is large [10, p. 36].

Now imagine that two chromosomes are drawn at random from the current population, with repeat lengths X_i and X_j at a given locus. Since mutations can occur on either branch of the coalescence tree, the number n of mutations since the two chromosomes had a common ancestor is Poisson-distributed with parameter $2\nu T$. Since the probability **generating function** (pgf) for the **Poisson distribution** with parameter $2\nu t$ is $\exp[2\nu t(s-1)]$ and the exponential density at $T = t$ is $(1/2N)\exp(-t/2N)$, the pgf $\mu(s) = \mathrm{E}(s^n)$ for the number of mutation events is

$$\mu(s) = \frac{1}{2N}\int_0^\infty \exp(-t/2N)\exp[2\nu t(s-1)]\mathrm{d}t$$
$$= \frac{1}{1 - 4N\nu(s-1)}.$$

So far, we have taken into account the random processes determining the time to coalescence and the number of mutations since coalescence, but not the random size of the mutation $X \to X + U$. Kimmel & Chakraborty [9] allow an arbitrary function $\varphi(s)$ for the pgf of the mutation size, since its probability distribution is currently an active area of research [18]. Since any mutation has an equal probability of affecting X_i or X_j, its effect on $X_i - X_j$ has pgf $\psi(s) = \frac{1}{2}[\varphi(s) + \varphi(1/s)]$. We now have a compound distribution for $X_i - X_j$, i.e. a random number n of mutations with pgf $\mu(s)$, each step contributing a random amount to the size difference with pgf $\psi(s)$. The pgf of $X_i - X_j$ is, therefore, found by composition:

$$\lambda(s) = \mu \circ \psi = \frac{1}{1 - 4N\nu[\psi(s) - 1]}.$$

The variance of $X_i - X_j$ is found by differentiating $\lambda(s)$ twice and setting $s = 1$; it is $4\nu N\psi''$. This quantity may also be expressed as $4\nu N\mathrm{E}(\hat{U}^2)$, by introducing the symmetrized random variable $\hat{U}$, with the probability distribution $\Pr(\hat{U} = n, n \in \mathbb{Z}) = \frac{1}{2}(p_n + p_{-n})$, where $p_n = \Pr(U = n)$. An empirically convenient measure of variability is the probability of homozygosity $\Pr(X_i = X_j)$, which is p_0 in the Laurent expansion of $\lambda(s) = \sum_{k \in \mathbb{Z}} p_k s^k$. p_0 can be evaluated by means of the Cauchy integral formula,

$$p_0 = \frac{1}{2\pi i} \oint_{|s|=1} \frac{\lambda(s)}{s} \mathrm{d}s.$$

The SIR Model for Epidemics has Chaotic Solutions

The existence of **chaos** in models for epidemics has been debated many times, and found in some computer simulations [15], but Glendinning & Perry [7] are able to give a definitive answer, at least in a simple case (the SIR model), using Melnikov's method. The SIR model for the spread of diseases is highly simplified, but captures important features of epidemics (*see* **Epidemic Models, Deterministic**). S stands for the proportion of *susceptible* individuals, I for *infected*, and R for *recovered*. The equations of the model are:

$$\dot{S} = -B(I, t)S + \mu - \mu S,$$

$$\dot{I} = B(I, t)S - (\gamma + \mu)I,$$

$$\dot{R} = \gamma I - \mu R,$$

where $S + I + R$, representing the total population, is set equal to 1. μ is the birth (= death) rate (all newborns are assumed susceptible); γ is the rate of recovery (transition to a permanently immune state). Glendinning & Perry [7] take $B(I, t) = \beta(t)I^2$, and assume that $\beta(t)$ has the form $\beta_0(1 + \beta_1 \sin \omega t)$. The sinusoidal term might arise from the annual school calendar, or from long-term cyclical variation in social or environmental factors. Choosing an exponent of $I > 1$ is not implausible, because there might be a threshold for the concentration of viruses in the environment to become infectious, or individuals could harbor low-level infections that increase susceptibility, without becoming infectious [13, p. 200]. The dynamics may be thought of as taking place on the cylinder $(I, R, t) \in \mathbb{R} \times \mathbb{R} \times S^1$, since the forcing term is periodic in t. Consider a Poincaré section at a fixed time (modulo $2\pi/\omega$). If S and R are given at a certain time in one period, then the equations predict what S and R will be at that time in the next period. Thus we have a map f of the (S, R) plane into itself. "Chaos" can be defined in this way [24, Section 4.11 and Proposition 4.2.7]: there exists a compact and invariant set Λ in the Poincaré section such that:

1. Λ contains periodic points of all orders, and the periodic points are dense in Λ
2. there also exist, in Λ, an uncountably infinite number of points (S, R) such that an orbit started at (S, R) never repeats itself
3. there exists at least one starting point (S', R') in Λ from which the orbit comes arbitrarily close to every point in Λ
4. the Poincaré map has "sensitive dependence on initial conditions" on Λ, which means that $\exists \varepsilon > 0$ such that, for every $(S, R) \in \Lambda$, there are points arbitrarily close to (S, R) that eventually separate from (S, R) by at least ε.

This harvest of dynamics is reaped simply by proving that the map f has a saddle point y whose stable and unstable manifolds intersect transversely (i.e. they cross, other than at y) [24, Section 4.4]. (By the *stable manifold* is meant the set of points that approach y under successive iteration by f; by the *unstable manifold* is meant the set of points that approach y under backwards iteration by f. These will both be smooth curves.)

The key step is demonstrating that the stable and unstable manifolds cross. Melnikov's method [24, Section 4.5] deals with the case where the flow is governed by an arbitrarily small periodic perturbation of a Hamiltonian system: $\dot{q} = \partial H/\partial p$, $\dot{p} = -\partial H/\partial q$. The unperturbed system is assumed to have a *homoclinic orbit* $[q^0(t), p^0(t)](-\infty < t < \infty)$ such that $\lim_{t \to \infty} q^0(t) = y$ and $\lim_{t \to \infty} q^0(t) = y$. The interior of the homoclinic orbit is assumed to be filled with a continuous family of periodic orbits. Let $\vec{F}(q, p)$ be the unperturbed flow, and $\vec{G}(q, p, t, \varepsilon)$ be the perturbation, both smoothly varying in all their arguments. The Melnikov function is defined as

$$M(t) = \int_{-\infty}^{\infty} \vec{F}[q^0(s-t), p^0(s-t)] \times \vec{G}[q^0(s-t),$$

$$p^0(s-t), t]\mathrm{d}s,$$

$\times$ standing for the vector cross-product. If $M(t_0) = 0$ for some t_0, and $\mathrm{d}M/\mathrm{d}t|_{t_0} \neq 0$, then the stable and unstable manifolds of y will intersect transversely for sufficiently small ε. Conversely, if $M(t)$ is always $\neq 0$, the stable and unstable manifolds will not intersect. The computational utility of Melnikov's formula is that the integral is carried out on the unperturbed orbits. After elaborate transformations, Glendinning

& Perry are able to cast the equations of the SIR model into the form of a Hamiltonian unperturbed system and a perturbation. The Melnikov conditions are indeed satisfied, but only if the periodic term is on a very long time scale, not, for example, the annual scale that we expect in epidemics.

Hydrostatic Forces Determine the Geometry of the Aortic Valve

The objective of this theory was to derive the geometric form of the aortic valve of the heart from the hydrostatic forces acting on it when it balloons out to block the retrograde flow of blood into the heart [16]. The valve consists of three pockets, arranged as $120°$ sectors of a circle, meeting in the middle when the valve closes under retrograde flow. The fibers of each leaflet are suspended from the two points where the sector boundary meets the circumference, called *commissural points*. The intrinsic coordinates of the valve surface, (u, v), are defined so that the curves $v = $ const. are the fibers, $v = 0$ being the free edge. u measures arc length along the fibers, $u = 0$ marking the midline. The Cartesian coordinates in space, $\mathbf{X} = (x, y, z)$, are chosen so that the $z = 0$ plane contains the three commissural points (each pair suspending one of the valve leaflets), and $x = y = z = 0$ is the center of the circle through the three points. The equation of the leaflet surface, $\mathbf{X}(u, v)$, is regarded as unknown, to be determined by mechanical equilibrium under hydrostatic forces. $T(u, v)$ is the tension in the fibers, and p_0 is the pressure load applied to the leaflet, assumed uniform. The equations of equilibrium are

$$\frac{\partial}{\partial u}\left(T\frac{\partial \mathbf{X}}{\partial u}\right) + p_0\left(\frac{\partial \mathbf{X}}{\partial u} \times \frac{\partial \mathbf{X}}{\partial v}\right) = 0. \quad (1)$$

Peskin & McQueen [16] prove that: (i) $T(u, v)$ is independent of u (the tension is constant along each fiber); (ii) the fibers are geodesics on the surface of the valve leaflet; and (iii) the u, v coordinate curves are orthogonal. By a change of variables $dV/dv = T(v)/p_0$, equalizing the force per unit of V, (1) transforms into

$$\frac{\partial \mathbf{X}}{\partial V} = \frac{\partial \mathbf{X}}{\partial u} \times \frac{\partial^2 \mathbf{X}}{\partial u^2}. \quad (2)$$

Peskin & McQueen make use of a remarkable analogy between (2) and the equations of vortex

dynamics in moving fluids. They think of V as a *time* variable, so that (2) can be regarded as describing the filling-out of the leaflet by a single fiber, sweeping across the leaflet as V increases, moving in the direction of its binormal at each point. Eq. (2) is the same as the "self-induction approximation" in hydrodynamics for the motion of a line vortex, i.e. its motion under the influence of the velocity field it itself generates. The geometry problem becomes an initial-value problem: starting with $\mathbf{X}(u, 0)$, defined at the free edge of the leaflet, propagate $\mathbf{X}(u, V)$ forward in the "time" variable V, toward the circumference where the leaflet is suspended. The free edge $\mathbf{X}(u, 0)$ looks like a hyperbola when projected onto the x, y plane, and like a cubic when projected onto the x, z plane. To carry out the computations, they use a method developed by Buttke [2] for approximating the motion of a line vortex in a three-dimensional incompressible, isentropic fluid. According to the numerical solution, the fibers are not uniformly spread over the leaflet, but are gathered in bundles formed by the rolling up of the leaflet surface, just as vortex lines tend to kink as they move in a fluid. This result was unexpected, but it agrees very well with the observed anatomy of the aortic valve leaflet. Peskin & McQueen describe their surprise at the degree of agreement between theory and observation:

> When this work was undertaken, our goal was to produce a smooth array of fibers that would function as an aortic valve ... We were aware of the complicated branching structure of the collagen fibers that support the actual valve, but we thought of such a structure as being "too biologic" to be modeled within the present framework...Imagine our astonishment, then, when the result first appeared on the workstation screen! These results show that considerations of mechanical equilibrium determine the anatomy of the aortic valve in a much more detailed way than we had dared to hope [16, p. H326].

Knot Topology Establishes the Mechanism of Tn3 Resolvase

Tn3 resolvase is an enzyme that catalyzes recombination of duplex DNA at specific sites, i.e. the cutting of both strands of two DNA molecules and reattachment of the cut ends of the first molecule to the cut ends of the second, and vice versa [20]. DNA-binding proteins form the template, or *synaptosome*, to which the recombining partners attach. The Tn3 resolvase, a representative example of a major family of these recombinases, acts on closed circular DNA. Its function is in DNA transposition, moving a segment of DNA from one position to another. It is called a *topoisomerase*, because its action changes the topology of the molecule. From the topologic changes it induces, Sumners was able, in a brilliant analysis, to deduce its mechanism of action [21]. He treated the DNA attached to the synaptosome according to Conway's theory of *rational tangles* [1, Section 2.3]. A tangle is a circular region in the projection plane of a knot or link, such that the knot or link crosses the circumference at exactly four points (called NW, NE, SW, SE). A few examples will clarify the idea. The (∞) tangle is just two vertical strings, and the (0) tangle is two horizontal strings. The (3) tangle is made by winding two horizontal strings around each other so that they make three left-handed twists. (In the case of DNA, such twists are "supercoiled", since the primary structure is already coiled.) To make a (3, 2) tangle out of a (3) tangle, first reflect the (3) tangle along the NW–SE diagonal, than make two twists of the free horizontal ends. The process can be continued to make tangles with more indices. The *sum* of two tangles is formed simply by joining the NE end of the first to the NW end of the second, and the SE end of the first to the SW end of the second. From a tangle, a knot or link can be formed by the "numerator construction", which consists of connecting the NW end to the NE end, and the SW end to the SE end. Conway proves that the *continued fraction* derived from a tangle, for example $n + 1/[m + (1/l)]$ from the tangle (l, m, n), characterizes the knot formed by the numerator construction, in the sense that two knots formed from tangles are equivalent if and only if their continued fractions have the same value.

Closely following the biology of the recombination process, Sumners assumes that the DNA strands on the synaptosome form a tangle in Conway's sense, and furthermore that the synaptosome tangle is the sum of two tangles, O_b and P, P representing the two "parental" segments, lying parallel on the synaptosome, that are to be cut and recombined, and O_b representing the rest of the (possibly twisted) DNA that is bound to the synaptosome, but not involved directly in recombination. The actual DNA molecule, before and after recombination, is assumed to be derived by the numerator construction $N(\cdot)$ from the

tangle. The original substrate, in Conway's notation, is $N(O_b + P)$, and it is topologically just a circle. After recombination, the product is $N(O_b + R)$. Whereas P is the (0) tangle (two parallel horizontal strands), R is either the (1) tangle or the (−1) tangle (one twist, formed when the strands are cut and recombine). Sumners takes advantage of the fact that occasionally two or three recombination events occur. Then, according to this model, the products should be $N(O_b + 2R)$ and $N(O_b + 3R)$, respectively. Since the topology of the products in each case is known experimentally, the equations can be solved for the tangles O_b and R. $N(O_b + R)$ is known to be a Hopf link (the simplest two-component link, two circles passed through one another), $N(O_b + 2R)$ is a figure of eight knot, and $N(O_b + 3R)$ is a Whitehead link (two circles joined so that one becomes a figure eight). Sumners proves, on the basis of this information, that R must consist of one left-handed twist, and O_b must consist of three left-handed twists in the vertical direction. In other words, the DNA is supercoiled on the synaptosome, in addition to being prepared for cutting. The *pièce de résistance* of this work is being able to predict, on the basis of the model derived from $N(O_b + jR)$, $j = 1, 2, 3$, what kind of knot $N(O_b + 4R)$ will be. Quadruple recombination is rare, but it does occur; the prediction is a knot called 6_2, a six-crossing composite knot, which agrees with experiment.

Conclusion

Each of these five studies illuminates one of the values of proving theorems in mathematical biology. Kopell & Somers [11] (first section) achieve two things. They predict a new phenomenon – oscillation in phase opposition by neurons coupled through excitatory interactions. They also exhibit the mechanism of that effect, through their analysis of the singular solution. Kimmel & Chakraborty's work [9] on estimation of mutation rate from microsatellite polymorphisms (second section) shows how mathematical reasoning can connect two qualitatively distinct phenomena, in this case one stretched out over the history of the population, and the other observed in a cross-section at a single time. Glendinning & Perry's study [7] of chaos in the SIR model for epidemics (third section) is important, not because the chaotic regime is expected to occur under typical circumstances, but because it resolves a question about dynamics that no amount of computer simulation could ever settle, being necessarily confined to a finite time period, a finite number of starting points, and finite precision. Peskin & McQueen's demonstration [16] that equilibrium under hydrostatic forces can account for the geometry of the aortic valve (fourth section), apart from the fascination of its reasoning, shows how isomorphism in formal structure sometimes makes it possible for a large body of mathematical knowledge to be translated and applied in a new area. In this case, methods from vortex hydrodynamics could be used to study the equations of shape of a body in equilibrium. Finally, Sumners' elegant application [21] of knot theory in DNA biochemistry (fifth section) illustrates how mathematical proof can, at least occasionally, give a definitive answer to a question of mechanism. Each of the selected papers also illustrates the crucial step of formulating a model rich enough to capture the phenomena, yet simple enough to be tractable. Mathematical analysis in biology will remain a subtle art, but when theorems can be proved about realistic models, they are likely to shed valuable light on biologic mechanisms.

References

[1]   Adams, C.C. (1994). *The Knot Book*. W.H. Freeman, New York.

[2]   Buttke, T.F. (1988). A numerical study of superfluid turbulence in the self-induction approximation, *Journal of Computational Physics* **76**, 301–326.

[3]   Committee on the Mathematics and Physics of Emerging Dynamic Biomedical Imaging. (1996). *Mathematics and Physics of Emerging Biomedical Imaging*. National Academy Press, Washington.

[4]   Edelstein-Keshet, L. (1988). *Mathematical Models in Biology*. Random House, New York.

[5]   Ermentrout, G.B. & Rinzel, J. (1996). Reflected waves in an inhomogeneous excitable medium, *SIAM Journal of Applied Mathematics* **56**, 1107–1128.

[6]   Fagerström, T., Jagers, P., Shuster, P. & Szathmáry, E. (1996). Biologists put on mathematical glasses, *Science* **274**, 2039–2040.

[7]   Glendinning, P. & Perry, L.P. (1997). Melnikov analysis of chaos in a simple epidemiological model, *Journal of Mathematical Biology* **35**, 359–373.

[8]   Hoppensteadt, F.C. & Peskin, C.S. (1992). *Mathematics in Medicine and the Life Sciences*. Springer-Verlag, New York.

[9]   Kimmel, M. & Chakraborty, R. (1996). Measures of variation at DNA repeat loci under a general stepwise mutation model, *Theoretical Population Biology* **50**, 345–367.

[10] Kingman, J.F.C. (1982). On the genealogy of large populations, *Journal of Applied Probability* **19A**, 27–43.

[11] Kopell, N. & Somers, D. (1995). Anti-phase solutions in relaxation oscillators coupled through excitatory interactions, *Journal of Mathematical Biology* **33**, 261–280.

[12] Lander, E.S. & Waterman, M.S., eds. (1995). *Calculating the Secrets of Life*. National Academy Press, Washington.

[13] Liu, W-M., Levin, S.A. & Iwasa, Y. (1986). Influence of nonlinear incidence rates upon the behavior of SIRS epidemiological models, *Journal of Mathematical Biology* **23**, 187–204.

[14] Murray, J.D. (1993). *Mathematical Biology*, 2nd Ed. Springer-Verlag, Berlin.

[15] Olsen, L.T. & Schaffer, W.M. (1990). Chaos versus noisy periodicity: alternative hypotheses for childhood epidemics, *Science* **249**, 499–504.

[16] Peskin, C.S. & McQueen, D.M. (1994). Mechanical equilibrium determines the fractal fiber architecture of aortic heart valve leaflets, *American Journal of Physiology* **266**, H319–H328.

[17] Rinzel, J. & Ermentrout, G.B. (1989). Analysis of neural excitability and oscillations, in *Methods in Neuronal Modeling: From Synapses to Networks*, C. Koch & I. Seger, eds. MIT Press, Cambridge, Mass., pp. 135–169.

[18] Rubinsztein, D.C., Amos, W., Leggo, J., Goodburn, S., Jain, S., Li, S-H., Margolis, R.L., Ross, C.A. & Ferguson-Smith, M.A. (1995). Microsatellite evolution – evidence for directionality and variation in rate between species, *Nature Genetics* **10**, 337–343.

[19] Somers, D. & Kopell, N. (1995). Waves and synchrony in networks of oscillators of relaxation and non-relaxation type, *Physica D* **89**, 169–183.

[20] Stark, W.M., Boocock, M.R. & Sherratt, D.J. (1992). Catalysis by site-specific recombinases, *Trends in Genetics* **8**, 432–439.

[21] Sumners, D.L. (1992). Knot theory and DNA, *Proceedings of Symposia in Applied Mathematics* **45**, 39–72.

[22] Tan, W-Y. (1991). *Stochastic Models of Carcinogenesis*. Marcel Dekker, New York.

[23] Waterman, M.S. (1995). *Introduction to Computational Biology: Maps, Sequences and Genomes*. Chapman & Hall, London.

[24] Wiggins, S. (1990). *Introduction to Applied Nonlinear Dynamical Systems and Chaos*. Springer-Verlag, New York.

[25] Winfree, A.T. (1987). *When Time Breaks Down*. Princeton University Press, Princeton.

STEVEN MATTHYSSE

Matlab *see* Software, Biostatistical

Matrix Algebra

The algebra that we learn when teenagers has letters of the alphabet, each representing a number. For example: a father and son are x and y years old, respectively, and their total age is 70. In a decade the father will be twice as old as the son. Hence $x + y = 70$ and $x + 10 = 2(y + 10)$, and so $x = 50$ and $y = 20$.

In contrast, matrix algebra is the algebra of letters each representing many numbers, with those numbers always arrayed in the form of a rectangle (or square). An example is

$$\mathbf{X} = \begin{bmatrix} 9 & 0 & 7 & t \\ u^2 + v & -3 & 6.1 & 5^3 \end{bmatrix}.$$

General Description

A *matrix* is a rectangular array of numbers, which can be any mixture of numbers that are complex, real, zero, positive, negative, decimal, fractions, or algebraic expressions. When none of them is complex (i.e. involving $\sqrt{-1}$), the matrix is said to be *real*. And because statistics deals with data, which are real numbers (especially biological data), almost all of this article applies to real matrices. Each number in a matrix is called an *element*: in being some representation of a single number it is called a *scalar*, to contrast with matrix which represents many numbers.

Elements are always set out in rows and columns with the number of rows and columns being called the *order* (or *dimension*) of the matrix. Thus, the illustrated $\mathbf{X}$ has order 2×4 ("two by four") with the number of rows being mentioned first. Sometimes the order is used as a subscript to the matrix symbol; for example, $\mathbf{X}_{2 \times 4}$. In this encyclopedia the widespread custom is used of denoting matrices by bold face, capital, roman letters.

Elements of a matrix can be represented by letters, having subscripts to denote location (row and column) in the matrix. Thus, a matrix $\mathbf{A}$ might be represented as

$$\mathbf{A} = \begin{bmatrix} a_{11} & a_{12} & a_{13} \\ a_{21} & a_{22} & a_{23} \\ a_{31} & a_{32} & a_{33} \end{bmatrix}.$$

The first subscript indicates row, and the second column; for example, a_{23} is in row 2 and column 3. More briefly, we can write

$$\mathbf{A} = \{a_{ij}\} \quad \text{for } i = 1, 2, 3 \text{ and } j = 1, 2, 3.$$

When $\mathbf{B}$ has r rows and c columns,

$$\mathbf{B} = \{b_{ij}\} \quad \text{for } i = 1, 2, \ldots, r \text{ and } j = 1, 2, \ldots, c.$$

A more compact form is

$$\mathbf{B} \left\{_{\mathrm{m}} b_{ij}\right\}_{i=1, \, j=1}^{r \quad c},$$

the m indicating that it is a matrix. The element in the first row and first column (e.g. a_{11} in $\mathbf{A}$ and the 9 in $\mathbf{X}$) is called the *leading element*.

By virtue of a matrix being a rectangular array there are many special forms, the first two of which are square matrices and vectors.

Square Matrices

1. Square matrices have the same number of rows as columns. $\mathbf{A}$ is an example.
2. Elements on the diagonal from upper left to lower right, those with both subscripts the same, are *diagonal elements*; they constitute *the diagonal of the matrix*.
3. Elements immediately below the diagonal constitute the *sub-diagonal*.
4. Elements not on the diagonal are *off-diagonal elements*.
5. When all off-diagonal elements are zero, and at least some diagonal elements are nonzero, the matrix is a *diagonal matrix*.
6. When all elements below (above) the diagonal are zero the matrix is said to be *upper (lower) triangular*.

Vectors

When a matrix has only one column it is a *column vector* or, more usually, just *vector*; and it shall here be denoted by a bold face, lower case, roman letter, usually from the last part of the alphabet; for example,

$$\mathbf{x} = \begin{bmatrix} 1 \\ 7 \\ -4 \\ 0 \end{bmatrix}.$$

When a matrix has only one row it is called a *row vector*. The notation is similar to that for a column vector, except for a superscript prime:

$$\mathbf{y}' = [0 \quad -4 \quad 9 \quad 12 \quad 37].$$

A column vector is a matrix of order $r \times 1$ when it has r elements; its transpose, a row vector, has order $1 \times r$. For both vectors, r is often called the *order* of the vector.

Basic Operations

A minimal requirement for matrix algebra is to define the arithmetic operations. Moreover, the rectangular nature of matrices begets numerous operations that do not exist for scalars; for example, changing rows into columns, and columns into rows.

The Transpose of a Matrix

Changing $\mathbf{A}$ so that its rows become columns (and hence its columns become rows) gives a matrix called the *transpose* of $\mathbf{A}$, traditionally written as $\mathbf{A}'$ (and sometimes today as $\mathbf{A}^T$). Thus for

$$\mathbf{A} = \begin{bmatrix} 1 & 2 & 3 & 4 \\ 6 & 1 & -2 & 5 \end{bmatrix}, \qquad \mathbf{A}' = \begin{bmatrix} 1 & 6 \\ 2 & 1 \\ 3 & -2 \\ 4 & 5 \end{bmatrix}.$$

Note that the transpose of $\mathbf{A}'$ is $\mathbf{A}$: $(\mathbf{A}')' = \mathbf{A}$. Also, the transpose of a column vector is a row vector (and vice versa):

$$[1 \quad 2 \quad 3]' = \begin{bmatrix} 1 \\ 2 \\ 3 \end{bmatrix}.$$

This explains the use of $\mathbf{y}'$ at the end of the preceding section.

Partitioned Matrices

The rows and columns of a matrix can be partitioned into a representation that is a matrix of matrices of smaller orders:

$$\mathbf{K} = \begin{bmatrix} 1 & 2 & \vdots & 3 & 4 \\ 6 & 8 & \vdots & 4 & 0 \\ 9 & 8 & \vdots & 1 & 2 \\ \hdashline 6 & 8 & \vdots & 3 & 9 \\ 4 & 1 & \vdots & 6 & 1 \end{bmatrix} = \begin{bmatrix} \mathbf{K}_{11} & \mathbf{K}_{12} \\ \mathbf{K}_{21} & \mathbf{K}_{22} \end{bmatrix}, \quad \text{for}$$

$$\mathbf{K}_{11} = \begin{bmatrix} 1 & 2 \\ 6 & 8 \\ 9 & 8 \end{bmatrix},$$

and so on. $\mathbf{K}$ is a *partitioned* matrix; the $\mathbf{K}$s with subscripts are *submatrices* of $\mathbf{K}$.

In transposing a partitioned matrix, not only is the matrix of submatrices transposed, but each submatrix is also transposed. Thus

$$\begin{bmatrix} \mathbf{A} & \mathbf{B} \\ \mathbf{C} & \mathbf{D} \end{bmatrix}' = \begin{bmatrix} \mathbf{A}' & \mathbf{C}' \\ \mathbf{B}' & \mathbf{D}' \end{bmatrix}.$$

A matrix can also be partitioned into its columns (or its rows); for example,

$$\mathbf{K} = [\mathbf{k}_1 \quad \mathbf{k}_2 \quad \mathbf{k}_3 \quad \mathbf{k}_4],$$

where each of the subscripted $\mathbf{k}$s is a column of $\mathbf{K}$.

The Trace of a Matrix

The trace of a matrix is defined only for a square matrix; and *trace* of $\mathbf{A}$ is the sum of the diagonal elements of $\mathbf{A}$, often written as $\text{tr}(\mathbf{A})$. Note that $\text{tr}(\mathbf{A}) = \text{tr}(\mathbf{A}')$, and $\text{tr}(\text{scalar}) = \text{scalar}$.

Addition and Subtraction

Addition and subtraction are defined only for matrices of the same order, whereupon the matrices are said to be *conformable* for addition and subtraction. Then, for $\mathbf{A} = \{a_{ij}\}$ and $\mathbf{B} = \{b_{ij}\}$,

$$\mathbf{A} + \mathbf{B} = \{a_{ij} + b_{ij}\}.$$

If two matrices do not have the same order their sum and difference do not exist. Note the properties

$$(\mathbf{A} \pm \mathbf{B})' = \mathbf{A}' \pm \mathbf{B}'$$

and

$$\text{tr}(\mathbf{A} \pm \mathbf{B}) = \text{tr}(\mathbf{A}) \pm \text{tr}(\mathbf{B}).$$

Scalar Multiplication

For λ being a scalar, $\lambda\mathbf{A}$ is $\mathbf{A}$ with every element multiplied by λ. Thus, for $\mathbf{A} = \{a_{ij}\}$, $\lambda\mathbf{A} = \{\lambda a_{ij}\}$.

Equality and Null Matrices

Two matrices are equal only when they are equal element by element. Thus, for

$$\mathbf{A} = \begin{bmatrix} 1 & 2 \\ 6 & 8 \end{bmatrix}, \qquad \mathbf{B} = \begin{bmatrix} 1 & 2 \\ 6 & 8 \end{bmatrix} \quad \text{and}$$

$$\mathbf{C} = \begin{bmatrix} 1 & 2 \\ 5 & 8 \end{bmatrix},$$

$\mathbf{A} = \mathbf{B}$, but $\mathbf{A} \neq \mathbf{C}$. Furthermore,

$$\mathbf{A} - \mathbf{B} = \begin{bmatrix} 1-1 & 2-2 \\ 6-6 & 8-8 \end{bmatrix} = \begin{bmatrix} 0 & 0 \\ 0 & 0 \end{bmatrix} = \mathbf{0}.$$

Any matrix having every element zero is a *null matrix*. It is a zero of matrix algebra: note that it is *a* zero not *the* zero, because null matrices can be of any order.

Multiplication

Multiplication of matrices differs greatly from that of scalars. First of all, $\mathbf{AB}$ and $\mathbf{BA}$ can, and often do, differ. To distinguish between the two, $\mathbf{AB}$ is described as $\mathbf{B}$ *pre-multiplied* by $\mathbf{A}$ (or as $\mathbf{A}$ *post-multiplied* by $\mathbf{B}$).

The *inner product* of two vectors is a row vector post-multiplied by a column vector, with both vectors having the same number of elements; for example,

$$[1 \quad 7 \quad 2]\begin{bmatrix} 3 \\ 5 \\ 9 \end{bmatrix} = 1(3) + 7(5) + 2(9) = 56.$$

Thus for $\mathbf{x}' = \{x_i\}_{i=1}^n$ and $y' = \{y_i\}_{i=1}^n$,

$$\mathbf{x}'y = \sum_{i=1}^n x_i y_i.$$

In contrast, an *outer product* is a column vector post-multiplied by a row vector

$$\mathbf{xy}' = \{x_i y_j\}.$$

In this case, the vectors can be of different orders. Note that an inner product is a scalar, whereas an outer product is a matrix.

The product $\mathbf{AB}$ exists only when $\mathbf{A}$ has as many columns as $\mathbf{B}$ has rows; and then $\mathbf{A}$ and $\mathbf{B}$ are described as being *conformable for the product* $\mathbf{AB}$, whereupon

$$\mathbf{A}_{r \times c}\mathbf{B}_{c \times t} = \mathbf{P}_{r \times t}.$$

In $\mathbf{P}$, the element in row i and column j is the inner product of row i of $\mathbf{A}$ and column j of $\mathbf{B}$:

$$\mathbf{P}_{r \times t} = \{p_{ij}\} = \left\{ \sum_{k=1}^c a_{ik}b_{kj} \right\} \quad \text{for } i = 1, \ldots, r$$

$$\text{and } j = 1, \ldots, t.$$

A simple numerical example of this is

$$\begin{bmatrix} 1 & 0 \\ 2 & -1 \end{bmatrix}\begin{bmatrix} 3 & 4 & 7 \\ -5 & 6 & 8 \end{bmatrix}$$

$$= \begin{bmatrix} [1 \quad 0]\begin{bmatrix} 3 \\ -5 \end{bmatrix} & [1 \quad 0]\begin{bmatrix} 4 \\ 6 \end{bmatrix} & [1 \quad 0]\begin{bmatrix} 7 \\ 8 \end{bmatrix} \\ [2 \quad -1]\begin{bmatrix} 3 \\ -5 \end{bmatrix} & [2 \quad -1]\begin{bmatrix} 4 \\ 6 \end{bmatrix} & [2 \quad -1]\begin{bmatrix} 7 \\ 8 \end{bmatrix} \end{bmatrix}$$

$$= \begin{bmatrix} 1(3)+0(-5) & 1(4)+0(6) & 1(7)+0(8) \\ 2(3)+(-1)(-5) & 2(4)+(-1)6 & 2(7)+(-1)8 \end{bmatrix}$$

$$= \begin{bmatrix} 3 & 4 & 7 \\ 11 & 2 & 6 \end{bmatrix}.$$

Important consequences of this definition of multiplication are that $\mathbf{AB}$ exists only for $\mathbf{A}_{r \times c}$ and $\mathbf{B}_{c \times t}$; both $\mathbf{AB}$ and $\mathbf{BA}$ exist only for $\mathbf{A}_{r \times c}$ and $\mathbf{B}_{c \times r}$, but they will be of different orders (and so not equal) unless $r = c$. Even then, $\mathbf{AB}$ and $\mathbf{BA}$ are not necessarily equal. For example,

$$\begin{bmatrix} 1 & 0 \\ 2 & -1 \end{bmatrix}\begin{bmatrix} 3 & 4 \\ -5 & 6 \end{bmatrix} = \begin{bmatrix} 3 & 4 \\ 11 & 2 \end{bmatrix}, \quad \text{but}$$

$$\begin{bmatrix} 3 & 4 \\ -5 & 6 \end{bmatrix}\begin{bmatrix} 1 & 0 \\ 2 & -1 \end{bmatrix} = \begin{bmatrix} 11 & -4 \\ 7 & -6 \end{bmatrix}.$$

Products with Null Matrices

Every product of a matrix with a null matrix is a null matrix: but those null matrices are not necessarily of the same order. Thus, $\mathbf{0}_{3 \times 2}\mathbf{A}_{2 \times 5} = \mathbf{0}_{3 \times 5}$ and $\mathbf{A}_{2 \times 5}\mathbf{0}_{5 \times 6} = \mathbf{0}_{2 \times 6}$.

Products with Diagonal Matrices

Pre-(post-)multiplying $\mathbf{A}$ by a diagonal matrix $\mathbf{D}$ multiplies each row (column) of $\mathbf{A}$ by the corresponding diagonal element of $\mathbf{D}$.

Identity Matrices

If every diagonal element of a diagonal matrix is a one the matrix is called an *identity* matrix, $\mathbf{I}$; pre- or post-multiplication of $\mathbf{A}$ by an identity matrix yields $\mathbf{A}$. Thus $\mathbf{I}$-matrices are the unities of matrix algebra.

Transposing a Product

The transpose of a product is the product of the transposed matrices in reverse order. Thus

$$(\mathbf{AB})' = \mathbf{B}'\mathbf{A}' \quad \text{and} \quad (\mathbf{XAY})' = \mathbf{Y}'\mathbf{A}'\mathbf{X}'.$$

Trace of a Product

The trace of a product equals the trace of cyclic permutations of that product: $\text{tr}(\mathbf{AB}) = \text{tr}(\mathbf{BA})$ and $\text{tr}(\mathbf{ABC}) = \text{tr}(\mathbf{CAB}) = \text{tr}(\mathbf{BCA})$, but these three do not equal the trace of $\mathbf{ACB}$.

Powers of Matrices

Only square matrices have powers: $\mathbf{A}_{2\times 4}\mathbf{A}_{2\times 4}$ does not exist. $\mathbf{A}_{4\times 4}\mathbf{A}_{4\times 4}$ written as $\mathbf{A}_{4\times 4}^2$ does.

Hadamard Products

The (i, j)th element of $\mathbf{AB}$ is $\sum_k a_{ik}b_{kj}$. But there are other ways of defining a product. One is the *Hadamard product*, defined as

$$\mathbf{A} \cdot \mathbf{B} = \{a_{ij}b_{ij}\}.$$

Thus, the (i, j)th element of the Hadamard product is the product of the (i, j)th elements of $\mathbf{A}$ and $\mathbf{B}$ – which must have the same order.

Direct Products

There is also the direct product

$$\mathbf{A} \otimes \mathbf{B} = \{a_{ij}\mathbf{B}\}.$$

When $\mathbf{A}$ has order $p \times q$ and $\mathbf{B}$ has order $r \times s$, $\mathbf{A} \otimes \mathbf{B}$ has order $pr \times qs$. For example,

$$\begin{bmatrix} 3 & 4 \\ 2 & 1 \end{bmatrix} \otimes [6 \quad 7 \quad 8] = \begin{bmatrix} 3[6 & 7 & 8] & 4[6 & 7 & 8] \\ 2[6 & 7 & 8] & 1[6 & 7 & 8] \end{bmatrix}$$

$$= \begin{bmatrix} 18 & 21 & 24 & 24 & 28 & 32 \\ 12 & 14 & 16 & 6 & 7 & 8 \end{bmatrix}.$$

Laws of Algebra

Provided that conformability requirements are met, the following equalities hold:

$$(\mathbf{A} + \mathbf{B}) + \mathbf{C} = \mathbf{A} + \mathbf{B} + \mathbf{C},$$

$$(\mathbf{AB})\mathbf{C} = \mathbf{A}(\mathbf{BC}) = \mathbf{ABC},$$

$$\mathbf{A}(\mathbf{B} + \mathbf{C}) = \mathbf{AB} + \mathbf{AC},$$

$$\mathbf{A} + \mathbf{B} = \mathbf{B} + \mathbf{A}.$$

This last equality is the commutative law of addition. In contrast, its mate, the commutative law of multiplication, does not generally hold for matrices; that is, $\mathbf{AB}$ and $\mathbf{BA}$ are not usually equal. Indeed, there are situations in which one exists and the other does not; and when they do both exist they can be of different orders; and even when they both exist and are of the same order (for which $\mathbf{A}$ and $\mathbf{B}$ must be the square and of the same order) they are not necessarily equal.

Contrasts with Scalar Algebra

The following results illustrate differences in the algebra of matrices compared with that of scalars:

1. $\mathbf{AX} + \mathbf{BX} = (\mathbf{A} + \mathbf{B})\mathbf{X} \neq \mathbf{X}(\mathbf{A} + \mathbf{B})$;
2. $\mathbf{XP} + \mathbf{QX}$ does *not* have $\mathbf{X}$ as a factor;
3. $\mathbf{AB} = \mathbf{0}$ does not imply that $\mathbf{A}$ or $\mathbf{B}$ are $\mathbf{0}$, nor does it imply that $\mathbf{BA}$ is $\mathbf{0}$;
4. $\mathbf{Y}^2 = \mathbf{0}$ defines $\mathbf{Y}$ as *nilpotent* and does *not* imply that $\mathbf{Y}$ is $\mathbf{0}$:
5. $\mathbf{Z}^2 = \mathbf{I}$ does *not* imply that $\mathbf{Z}$ is $\pm \mathbf{I}$;
6. $\mathbf{Q}^2 = \mathbf{Q}$ defines $\mathbf{Q}$ as *idempotent* but does not imply that $\mathbf{Q}$ is $\mathbf{0}$ or $\mathbf{I}$.

Examples of these last four features are as follows:

$$\mathbf{AB} = \begin{bmatrix} 1 & 1 \\ 1 & 1 \end{bmatrix}\begin{bmatrix} 1 & 1 \\ -1 & -1 \end{bmatrix} = \mathbf{0},$$

$$\mathbf{BA} = \begin{bmatrix} 1 & 1 \\ -1 & -1 \end{bmatrix}\begin{bmatrix} 1 & 1 \\ 1 & 1 \end{bmatrix} = \begin{bmatrix} 2 & 2 \\ -2 & -2 \end{bmatrix},$$

$$\mathbf{Y}^2 = \begin{bmatrix} 1 & 1 \\ -1 & -1 \end{bmatrix}^2 = \mathbf{0},$$

$$\mathbf{Z}^2 = \begin{bmatrix} 1 & 0 \\ 4 & -1 \end{bmatrix}^2 = \mathbf{I},$$

and

$$\mathbf{Q}^2 = \begin{bmatrix} 3 & -2 \\ 3 & -2 \end{bmatrix}^2 = \mathbf{Q}.$$

One may be tempted to think of these examples as pathologic cases. To some extent they are, born of the need to have illustrations that occupy minimum space; but they serve as stern warnings that what can be done in scalar algebra does not always carry over to matrix algebra.

Special Matrices

Square matrices and vectors have already been mentioned as special forms of matrices. There are many others, some arising from their intrinsic properties, and others from the applications in which they arose. Just a few of the more commonly occurring ones are mentioned here.

Symmetric Matrices

A is defined as being symmetric when

$$\mathbf{A}' = \mathbf{A}.$$

That can occur only when **A** is square. Its rows are then mirror images of its columns:

$$\begin{bmatrix} 1 & 7 & 0 \\ 7 & 2 & -3 \\ 0 & -3 & 9 \end{bmatrix}' = \begin{bmatrix} 1 & 7 & 0 \\ 7 & 2 & -3 \\ 0 & -3 & 9 \end{bmatrix};$$

and $a_{ij} = a_{ji}$.

BB′ and **B′B** are both symmetric. This is true for any **B**. Then **BB′** (and **B′B**) have diagonal elements that are sums of squares of elements of rows (columns) of **B**: and

$$\mathrm{tr}(\mathbf{BB}') = \mathrm{tr}(\mathbf{B}'\mathbf{B}) = \sum_i \sum_j b_{ij}^2.$$

When **B** is real, $\mathbf{BB}' = \mathbf{0}$ and $\mathrm{tr}(\mathbf{BB}') = 0$ each imply that $\mathbf{B} = \mathbf{0}$.

Elementary Vectors

Columns of identity matrices are *elementary vectors*, represented as $e_i^{(n)}$, the ith column in **I** of order n.

Skew-Symmetric Matrices

$\mathbf{A}' = -\mathbf{A}$ defines **A** as *skew-symmetric*.

Summing Vectors

A vector having every element a one (1.0) is a *summing vector*, often denoted as **1**. It is so named because $\mathbf{1}'\mathbf{x}$ is the sum of all elements in **x**.

Matrices having Every Element Unity

$\mathbf{J}_{p \times k} = \mathbf{1}_p \mathbf{1}_k'$ is a matrix having every element being 1.0. Its most frequent occurrence in statistics is when it is square: $\mathbf{J}_n = \mathbf{1}_n \mathbf{1}_n'$. A useful variant is $\bar{\mathbf{J}}_{\mathbf{n}} = (1/n)\mathbf{J}_n$. Then,

$$\mathbf{C}_n = \mathbf{I}_n - \bar{\mathbf{J}}_n$$

is a *centering matrix*, with

$$\mathbf{C}_n \mathbf{x} = \{x_i - \bar{x}\} \quad \text{and} \quad \mathbf{x}' \mathbf{C}_n \mathbf{x} = \sum_{i=1}^n (x_i - \bar{x})^2,$$

for $\bar{x} = \sum_{i=1}^n x_i / n = \mathbf{1}'\mathbf{x}/n$.

Probability Transition Matrices

When elements of a matrix **P** are probabilities that add to unity over each row, $\mathbf{P1} = \mathbf{1}$. Then $\mathbf{P}^k \mathbf{1} = \mathbf{1}$ for any positive integer k, and **P** is called a *probability transition matrix*. It is *doubly stochastic* if $\mathbf{1}'\mathbf{P} = \mathbf{1}'$ (or, equivalently, $\mathbf{P}'\mathbf{1} = \mathbf{1}$), meaning that column sums are also unity.

Idempotent Matrices

A is *idempotent* when $\mathbf{A}^2 = \mathbf{A}$; then $\mathbf{I} - \mathbf{A}$ is also idempotent (but $\mathbf{A} - \mathbf{I}$ is not).

Orthogonality

1. The *norm* of a real vector **x** is $(\mathbf{x}'\mathbf{x})^{1/2}$.
2. **x** is a *unit vector* when $\mathbf{x}'\mathbf{x} = 1$.
3. $\mathbf{u} = \mathbf{x}/(\mathbf{x}'\mathbf{x})^{1/2}$, known as normalized **x**, is always a unit vector when **x** is real.

Nonnull vectors **x** and **y** are *orthogonal vectors* when $\mathbf{x}'\mathbf{y} = 0$ ($= \mathbf{y}'\mathbf{x}$) (*see* **Orthogonality**).

Vectors **v** and **w** are *orthonormal vectors* when they are orthogonal ($\mathbf{v}'\mathbf{w} = 0$) and each is a unit vector ($\mathbf{v}'\mathbf{v} = 1$ and $\mathbf{w}'\mathbf{w} = 1$).

A collection of vectors of the same order is said to be an *orthogonal set of vectors* when they are pairwise orthonormal.

When $\mathbf{P}_{r \times c}$ has rows that are an orthonormal set, $\mathbf{PP}' = \mathbf{I}$. If $\mathbf{P}$ is square with orthonormal rows (columns), then its columns (rows) are also orthonormal, $\mathbf{PP}' = \mathbf{I} = \mathbf{P}'\mathbf{P}$ and $\mathbf{P}$ is an *orthogonal matrix*.

Certain special forms of orthogonal matrices go by the names Helmert, Givens, and Householder. The latter, for example, is $\mathbf{I} - 2\mathbf{hh}'$ when $\mathbf{h}'\mathbf{h} = 1$.

Quadratic Forms

$\mathbf{x}'\mathbf{Ax}$ is a *quadratic form*, in which $\mathbf{A}$ can always be (taken as) symmetric. $\mathbf{x}'\mathbf{Ax}$ is a homogeneous second-order function of the elements of $\mathbf{x}$:

$$\mathbf{x}'\mathbf{Ax} = \sum_i x_i^2 a_{ii} + \sum x_i x_j a_{ij} = \sum_i x_i^2 a_{ii}$$
$$+ \sum_{j \neq i} x_i x_j (a_{ij} + a_{ji}),$$

and on taking $\mathbf{A} = \mathbf{A}'$, that is, $a_{ij} = a_{ji}$,

$$\mathbf{x}'\mathbf{Ax} = \sum_i x_i^2 a_{ii} + 2 \sum_{j>i} x_i x_j a_{ij}.$$

If $\mathbf{x}'\mathbf{Ax} > 0$ for all $\mathbf{x} \neq \mathbf{0}$, $\mathbf{x}'\mathbf{Ax}$ is called a *positive definite (p.d.) quadratic form*, and $\mathbf{A}\ (= \mathbf{A}')$ is a *p.d. matrix*. If $\mathbf{x}'\mathbf{Ax} \geq 0$ for all $\mathbf{x} \neq \mathbf{0}$ *and* $\mathbf{x}'\mathbf{Ax} = \mathbf{0}$ for some $\mathbf{x} \neq \mathbf{0}$, then $\mathbf{x}'\mathbf{Ax}$ and $\mathbf{A}$ are *positive semidefinite* (p.s.d.). The classes of quadratic forms and matrices that include those which are p.d. and p.s.d. are called *nonnegative definite* (n.n.d.).

Determinants

Definition

Associated with any square matrix $\mathbf{A}_{n \times n}$ is its determinant $|\mathbf{A}|$. It is a scalar, an n-order, homogeneous polynomial function of the elements. Two easy examples are for $\mathbf{A}$ of order 2 and 3:

$$|\mathbf{X}| = \begin{vmatrix} a_1 & a_2 \\ b_1 & b_2 \end{vmatrix} = a_1 b_2 - a_2 b_1$$

and

$$|\mathbf{Y}| = \begin{vmatrix} a_1 & a_2 & a_3 \\ b_1 & b_2 & b_3 \\ c_1 & c_2 & c_3 \end{vmatrix} = a_1 b_2 c_3 + a_2 b_3 c_1$$
$$+ a_3 b_1 c_2 - a_3 b_2 c_1 - a_1 b_3 c_2 - a_2 b_1 c_3.$$

For $\mathbf{A}$ of order n, the definition is more difficult: $|\mathbf{A}|$ is the sum of the n different terms that are each a signed product of one element from every row and column of $\mathbf{A}$. In writing $|\mathbf{A}|$ with the rows being $\mathbf{a}', \mathbf{b}', \mathbf{c}', \ldots$, a product written in alphabetic order has sign equal to $(-1)^p$, with p being the sum of the number of reverse sequences of the subscripts. For example, $a_2 b_3 c_1$ in the preceding $|\mathbf{Y}|$ has $p = 2$ because 2, 1 and 3, 1 are reverse sequences; hence, the sign for $a_2 b_3 c_1$ is $(-1)^2 = +1$. For $a_3 b_2 c_1$ there are three reverse sequences, 3, 2 and 3, 1 and 2, 1 and so the sign is $(-1)^3 = -1$.

Minors and Cofactors

Deleting from $|\mathbf{A}|$ the row and column containing a_{ij} leaves a determinant of order $n - 1$ that is called the *minor*, $|\mathbf{M}_{ij}|$, of a_{ij} in $|\mathbf{A}|$. Also $(-1)^{i+j}|\mathbf{M}_{ij}|$, the *signed minor*, is called the *cofactor* of a_{ij} in $|\mathbf{A}| : c_{ij} = (-1)^{i+j}|\mathbf{M}_{ij}|$. Then

$$|\mathbf{A}| = \sum_{i=1}^n a_{ij} c_{ij} \quad \text{for all } j \quad \text{and}$$

$$|\mathbf{A}| = \sum_{j=1}^n a_{ij} c_{ij} \quad \text{for all } i,$$

but

$$0 = \sum_{i=1}^n a_{ij} c_{ij'} \quad \text{for all } j \neq j' \quad \text{and}$$

$$0 = \sum_{j=1}^n a_{ij} c_{i'j} \quad \text{for all } i \neq i'.$$

Calculation

Computers now handle the calculation of determinants. Numerous available shortcuts and associated properties of determinants are detailed in the literature, which was especially rich on this subject up through the 1930s. Searle [4] deals with a few of these topics.

Some Properties Useful for Statistics

1. $|\mathbf{A}'| = |\mathbf{A}|$.
2. $|\mathbf{A}^k| = (|\mathbf{A}|)^k$, for integer k.
3. $|\mathbf{AB}| = |\mathbf{A}||\mathbf{B}|$.

4. $|\mathbf{A}| = +1$, for orthogonal $\mathbf{A}$ (i.e. $\mathbf{A}'\mathbf{A} = \mathbf{I} = \mathbf{A}\mathbf{A}'$).
5. $|\mathbf{A}| = 0$, for idempotent $\mathbf{A}$ (i.e. $\mathbf{A}^2 = \mathbf{A}$), except for $\mathbf{A} = \mathbf{I}$.
6. $|\mathbf{I}| = 1$.
7. $|\lambda\mathbf{A}_{n \times n}| = \lambda^n|\mathbf{A}|$, for scalar λ.

Inverse Matrices

Existence

In matrix arithmetic, the very definition of multiplication precludes any obvious definition of division. Indeed, there is no such thing as matrix division; *division by a matrix does not exist*. Instead, multiplication by an inverse matrix is used, similar to the scalar equivalence of dividing by six (for example) being identical to multiplying by $1/6 = 6^{-1}$, the inverse of six: and

$$(6^{-1})6 = 1 = 6(6^{-1}).$$

There is one big difference: whereas every scalar different from zero has an inverse, not every nonnull matrix does.

Suppose that $\mathbf{A}$ has an inverse. Denote it by $\mathbf{A}^{-1}$, as is customary. Then with $\mathbf{I}$ being a "one" of matrix algebra, the matrix analogy of scalars is $(\mathbf{A}^{-1})\mathbf{A} = \mathbf{I} = \mathbf{A}(\mathbf{A}^{-1})$, where the parentheses are solely for emphasis, the usual writing being

$$\mathbf{A}^{-1}\mathbf{A} = \mathbf{I} = \mathbf{A}\mathbf{A}^{-1}.$$

This requirement demands that two conditions must be satisfied in order for $\mathbf{A}^{-1}$ to exist:

(i) $\mathbf{A}$ must be square;
(ii) $|\mathbf{A}| \neq 0$.

If either or both (i) and (ii) are not satisfied, $\mathbf{A}$ has no inverse; note, particularly, that every nonsquare matrix has no inverse.

When, for $\mathbf{A}$ square, $|\mathbf{A}| \neq 0$, $\mathbf{A}$ is called *nonsingular*, and if $|\mathbf{A}| = 0$ then $\mathbf{A}$ is called *singular*.

Form

The general form of $\mathbf{A}^{-1}$ is

$$\mathbf{A}^{-1} = \frac{1}{|\mathbf{A}|} \begin{bmatrix} \text{the matrix that is } \mathbf{A} \\ \text{with every element} \\ \text{replaced by its cofactor} \end{bmatrix}^{\text{transposed}}$$

and $|\mathbf{A}|\mathbf{A}^{-1}$ is called the *adjugate* or *adjoint* of $\mathbf{A}$.

Some Basic Properties

1. $\mathbf{A}^{-1}$ is unique (for given $\mathbf{A}$).
2. $|\mathbf{A}^{-1}| = 1/|\mathbf{A}|$.
3. $\mathbf{A}^{-1}$ is nonsingular.
4. $(\mathbf{A}^{-1})^{-1} = \mathbf{A}$.
5. $(\mathbf{A}')^{-1} = (\mathbf{A}^{-1})'$.
6. $\mathbf{A}' = \mathbf{A} \Rightarrow (\mathbf{A}^{-1})' = \mathbf{A}^{-1}$.
7. $(\mathbf{AB})^{-1} = \mathbf{B}^{-1}\mathbf{A}^{-1}$.

In all of these results, and whenever an inverse is used, one must always be certain that the matrix satisfies (i) and (ii) above; namely, squareness and nonzero determinant.

Four Special Cases

Denote a diagonal matrix having all its diagonal elements $\lambda_1, \ldots, \lambda_n$ nonzero by

$$\mathbf{D} = \{{}_{\text{d}}\lambda_i\}_{i=1}^n \,;$$

then,

$$\mathbf{D}^{-1} = \{{}_{\text{d}}1/\lambda_i\}_{i=1}^n \,, \quad \mathbf{I}^{-1} = \mathbf{I},$$

$$(a\mathbf{I}_n + b\mathbf{J}_n)^{-1} = \frac{1}{a}\left(\mathbf{I}_n - \frac{b}{a+nb}\mathbf{J}_n\right),$$

$$\mathbf{P}\mathbf{P}' = \mathbf{I} = \mathbf{P}'\mathbf{P} \quad \text{implies} \quad \mathbf{P}^{-1} = \mathbf{P}'.$$

Algebra with Inverses

Compared with using division in scalar algebra, one has to be much more careful in using inverses in matrix algebra. This is because one never divides by a matrix; instead, in dealing with equations, one multiplies by an inverse. For example, given $\mathbf{A}$, $\mathbf{B}$ and $\mathbf{AX} = \mathbf{B}$, the equation can be pre-multiplied, on both sides, by $\mathbf{A}^{-1}$ (provided that it exists) to obtain $\mathbf{A}^{-1}\mathbf{AX} = \mathbf{A}^{-1}\mathbf{B}$ and thus $\mathbf{IX} = \mathbf{A}^{-1}\mathbf{B}$ or $\mathbf{X} = \mathbf{A}^{-1}\mathbf{B}$. Note that $\mathbf{X}$ does not equal $\mathbf{BA}^{-1}$. Provided that conformability is satisfied, one could post-multiply $\mathbf{AX} = \mathbf{B}$ by $\mathbf{A}^{-1}$ and obtain $\mathbf{AXA}^{-1} = \mathbf{BA}^{-1}$; but that is it. No further simplification occurs.

Suppose that we have $\mathbf{P}$, $\mathbf{Q}$ and $\mathbf{K}$ such that $\mathbf{PK} = \mathbf{QK}$. This leads to $\mathbf{P} = \mathbf{Q}$ *only* if $\mathbf{K}^{-1}$ exists.

Inverses can also be used in factoring; for example, $\mathbf{R} + \mathbf{RST} = \mathbf{R}(\mathbf{I} + \mathbf{ST}) = \mathbf{R}(\mathbf{T}^{-1} + \mathbf{S})\mathbf{T}$, provided that $\mathbf{T}^{-1}$ exists.

Verifying the form of a particular inverse is often achieved by the following argument. Suppose that it is postulated that $\mathbf{A}$ inverse is $\mathbf{Q}$. Verifying this can be achieved by considering the product $\mathbf{AQ}$. If that can be shown to be equal to $\mathbf{I}$, thus $\mathbf{AQ} = \mathbf{I}$, then $\mathbf{A}^{-1}\mathbf{AQ} = \mathbf{A}^{-1}\mathbf{I}$; that is, $\mathbf{Q} = \mathbf{A}^{-1}$. For example, suppose that $\mathbf{A}$ is $(\mathbf{I} + \mathbf{XY})$ and $\mathbf{Q}$ is $\mathbf{I} - \mathbf{X}(\mathbf{I} + \mathbf{YX})^{-1}\mathbf{Y}$. Then $\mathbf{A}^{-1}$ is shown to be $\mathbf{Q}$ by considering $\mathbf{AQ}$:

$$\begin{aligned}
\mathbf{AQ} &= (\mathbf{I} + \mathbf{XY})[\mathbf{I} - \mathbf{X}(\mathbf{I} + \mathbf{YX})^{-1}\mathbf{Y}] \\
&= \mathbf{I} + \mathbf{XY} - (\mathbf{I} + \mathbf{XY})\mathbf{X}(\mathbf{I} + \mathbf{YX})^{-1}\mathbf{Y} \\
&= \mathbf{I} + \mathbf{XY} - (\mathbf{X} + \mathbf{XYX})(\mathbf{I} + \mathbf{YX})^{-1}\mathbf{Y} \\
&= \mathbf{I} + \mathbf{XY} - \mathbf{X}(\mathbf{I} + \mathbf{YX})(\mathbf{I} + \mathbf{YX})^{-1}\mathbf{Y} \\
&= \mathbf{I} + \mathbf{XY} - \mathbf{XY} \\
&= \mathbf{I},
\end{aligned}$$

and so $\mathbf{A}^{-1} = \mathbf{Q}$.

Computers and Inverses

The arithmetic required for calculating an inverse matrix can be voluminous. Fortunately, computers have eased this situation enormously and many **software** packages include reliable routines for doing the arithmetic. Nevertheless, there are cases in which rounding error can lead to erroneous results; thankfully, this occurs very seldom, and software often handles it satisfactorily.

Rank

Linear Dependence and Independence of Vectors

$$\mathbf{Xa} = [\mathbf{x}_1 \quad \mathbf{x}_2 \quad \ldots \quad \mathbf{x}_c] \begin{bmatrix} a_1 \\ a_2 \\ \vdots \\ a_i \\ \vdots \\ a_c \end{bmatrix} = \sum_{i=1}^{c} a_i \mathbf{x}_i$$

is a vector. It is a *linear combination* of the vectors $\mathbf{x}_1, \mathbf{x}_2, \ldots, \mathbf{x}_c$.

If, for a given $\mathbf{X}$ (with all columns nonnull), a nonnull vector $\mathbf{a}$ exists such that $\mathbf{Xa} = \mathbf{0}$, then the columns of $\mathbf{X}$ are said to be a set of *linearly dependent vectors*. If no such $\mathbf{a}$ exists, the columns are *linearly independent vectors*. These definitions exclude null vectors.

A Definition of Rank

If c columns are linearly dependent, there is always a smaller number of them that are linearly independent. In fact, there may be several sets of less than c columns that are linearly independent, with those sets not necessarily all having the same number of columns. The greatest number of columns in such a set is called the *rank of* $\mathbf{A}$, often denoted $r(\mathbf{A})$. Thus, $r(\mathbf{A})$ is the largest number of linearly independent columns available from $\mathbf{A}$. The "largest" is usually omitted. Thus, $r(\mathbf{A})$ is the number of linearly independent columns in $\mathbf{A}$.

Some Properties and Consequences

Rank is an important and exceedingly useful concept in matrix algebra, with widespread applications. A list of some of the properties of rank follows:

1. The numbers of linearly independent rows and columns in a matrix are the same, $r(\mathbf{A})$.
2. $r(\mathbf{0}) = 0$.
3. $r(\mathbf{A}_{p \times q}) \leq p$ and $r(\mathbf{A}_{p \times q}) \leq q$.
4. $r(\mathbf{A}_{n \times n}) \leq n$.
5. $r(\mathbf{A}_{n \times n}) < n \Leftrightarrow \mathbf{A}$ is singular, $|\mathbf{A}| = \mathbf{0}$, with $\mathbf{A}^{-1}$ not existing.
6. $r(\mathbf{A}_{n \times n}) = n \Leftrightarrow \mathbf{A}$ is nonsingular, $|\mathbf{A}| \neq \mathbf{0}$, with $\mathbf{A}^{-1}$ existing: $\mathbf{A}$ is said to be of *full rank*.
7. $r(\mathbf{A}_{p \times q}) = p < q$ means that $\mathbf{A}$ has *full row rank*.
8. $r(\mathbf{A}_{p \times q}) = q < p$ means that $\mathbf{A}$ has *full column rank*.
9. $\mathbf{A}_{p \times q}$ having rank r can always be expressed as $\mathbf{A}_{p \times q} = \mathbf{K}_{p \times r}\mathbf{L}_{r \times q}$, where $\mathbf{K}$ has full column rank r and $\mathbf{L}$ has full row rank r.
10. $r(\mathbf{AB}) \leq$ lesser of $r(\mathbf{A})$ and $r(\mathbf{B})$.
11. $r(\mathbf{A}) = tr(\mathbf{A})$ for idempotent $\mathbf{A}$.
12. $r(\mathbf{A}) = r(\mathbf{A}')$.
13. $r(\mathbf{A}) = r(\mathbf{AA}')$.
14. $r(\mathbf{A}) = r(\mathbf{TA})$ for nonsingular $\mathbf{T}$.
15. $r(\mathbf{A}^{-1}) = r(\mathbf{A}) = n$ for $\mathbf{A}_{n \times n}$.

Left and Right Inverses

For given $\mathbf{A}_{r \times c}$, there exists:

1. $\mathbf{A}^{-1}$, the inverse of $\mathbf{A}$, such that $\mathbf{A}^{-1}\mathbf{A} = \mathbf{I} = \mathbf{AA}^{-1}$ if and only if $\mathbf{A}$ is square, with $|\mathbf{A}| \neq 0$; or
2. $\mathbf{L}_{c \times r}$, a *left inverse* of $\mathbf{A}$, such that $\mathbf{LA} = \mathbf{I}_c$ (and $\mathbf{AL} \neq \mathbf{I}_r$) only if $\mathbf{A}$ has full column rank; or

3. $\mathbf{R}_{c\times r}$, a *right inverse* of $\mathbf{A}$, such that $\mathbf{AR} = \mathbf{I}_r$ (and $\mathbf{RA} \neq \mathbf{I}_c$) only if $\mathbf{A}$ has full row rank; or
4. neither an $\mathbf{A}^{-1}$, $\mathbf{L}$, *nor* $\mathbf{R}$ of (1), (2), or (3) – for example, any matrix having at least one null row and one null column.

Only when $\mathbf{A}^{-1}$ exists does $\mathbf{A}$ have both an $\mathbf{L}$ and an $\mathbf{R}$; and they both equal $\mathbf{A}^{-1}$. Otherwise, if $\mathbf{A}$ has full column (row) rank it has left (right) inverses of many values.

Vector Spaces

Since a vector of order n has n elements, it can be considered as a point in n-space, which is denoted R^n. Consider a set of vectors S, in R^n. Suppose, for every pair of vectors $\mathbf{x}_i$ and $\mathbf{x}_j$ in S, that both the sum $\mathbf{x}_i + \mathbf{x}_j$ and the vectors $a\mathbf{x}_i$ and $b\mathbf{x}_i$ for any scalars a and b are in S; then S is a *vector space*.

Suppose that every vector in the vector space S can be expressed as a linear combination of the set of t vectors, $\mathbf{x}_1, \mathbf{x}_2, \ldots, \mathbf{x}_t$. Then that set *spans*, or *generates*, S and is called a *spanning* set of S. If those t vectors are also linearly independent, they are said to be a *basis* for S, and the number of such vectors is the *dimension* of S, dim(S).

There are many vector spaces of order n; and each of them usually has several bases.

Range and Null Spaces

$\mathbf{A}$ of rank r has r linearly independent columns. All vectors that are linear combinations of those columns form a vector space. It is known as the *column space* of $\mathbf{A}$, the *range* of $\mathbf{A}$, or the *manifold* of $\mathbf{A}$, often denoted by $\mathcal{R}(\mathbf{A})$. Clearly, $r = \mathrm{r}(\mathbf{A}) = \dim[\mathcal{R}(\mathbf{A})]$.

The space defined by the many vectors $\mathbf{x}$ for which $\mathbf{Ax} = \mathbf{0}$ (with $\mathbf{A}$ being rectangular or square and singular) is the *null space* of $\mathbf{A}$, denoted $\mathcal{N}(\mathbf{A})$. Its dimension is the *nullity* of $\mathbf{A}$: nullity($\mathbf{A}$) = dim$[\mathcal{N}(\mathbf{A})]$.

Equivalent and Congruent Canonical Forms

Elementary Operators

Three particular adaptations of identity matrices are *elementary operators; each is an identity matrix* with

(i) two rows (or columns) interchanged, or (ii) λ in place of a one in the diagonal, or (iii) λ in place of a zero in an off-diagonal element. These and all products of any numbers of them are nonsingular.

Equivalent Canonical Form

For any $\mathbf{A}_{p\times q}$, of rank r, there always exists a $\mathbf{P}$ and a $\mathbf{Q}$, each a product of elementary operators, such that

$$\mathbf{P}_{p\times p}\mathbf{A}_{p\times q}\mathbf{Q}_{q\times q} = \begin{bmatrix} \mathbf{I}_{r\times r} & \mathbf{0} \\ \mathbf{0} & \mathbf{0} \end{bmatrix} = \mathbf{K}, \text{ say.}$$

$\mathbf{K}$ is the *equivalent canonical form* of $\mathbf{A}$; or the *canonical form under equivalence* of $\mathbf{A}$. Because $\mathbf{P}$ and $\mathbf{Q}$ are products of elementary operators, they are nonsingular, and so the equation $\mathbf{PAQ} = \mathbf{K}$ leads to $\mathbf{A} = \mathbf{P}^{-1}\mathbf{KQ}^{-1}$. If $\mathbf{A}$ is nonsingular, $\mathbf{K} = \mathbf{I}$ and $\mathbf{A}^{-1} = \mathbf{QP}$.

Congruent Canonical Form

When $\mathbf{A}$ is symmetric (and hence square), the $\mathbf{Q}$ of $\mathbf{PAQ}$ can be $\mathbf{P}'$, giving

$$\mathbf{PAP}' = \begin{pmatrix} \mathbf{I}_r & \mathbf{0} \\ \mathbf{0} & \mathbf{0} \end{pmatrix} = \mathbf{C},$$

known as the *congruent canonical form* of $\mathbf{A}$ or the *canonical form under congruence*.

En route to deriving $\mathbf{C}$, one can obtain the form

$$\mathbf{P}_*\mathbf{AP}'_* = \begin{pmatrix} \mathbf{D}_r & \mathbf{0} \\ \mathbf{0} & \mathbf{0} \end{pmatrix} = \mathbf{C},$$

where $\mathbf{D}_r$ is a diagonal matrix of order and rank r. For $\mathbf{A}$ being real, $\mathbf{P}_*$ will be real; but if $\mathbf{D}_r$ has negative elements, $\mathbf{P}$ in obtaining $\mathbf{C}$ will be complex. For $\mathbf{A}$ being nonnegative definite, elements of $\mathbf{D}_r$ are always positive and $\mathbf{P}$ is always real.

Utility: Sums of Squares

The utility of these canonical forms is their existence. For each $\mathbf{A}$ there are many values of $\mathbf{P}$ (and $\mathbf{Q}$) but usually not any one of them is of particular interest. It is the fact that they exist that is important, and that provides the means for establishing other useful results. For example, consider the quadratic form $q = \mathbf{x}'\mathbf{Ax}$ with $\mathbf{A} = \mathbf{A}'$ of rank r. Then there is a $\mathbf{P}$ such that $\mathbf{PAP}' = \mathbf{C}$. Thus, $q = \mathbf{x}'\mathbf{P}^{-1}\mathbf{PAP}'(\mathbf{P}')^{-1}\mathbf{x}$, and letting $\mathbf{y} = (\mathbf{P}')^{-1}\mathbf{x}$ gives $q = \mathbf{y}'\mathbf{C}\mathbf{y}$ which, because

$$\mathbf{C} = \begin{pmatrix} \mathbf{I}_r & \mathbf{0} \\ \mathbf{0} & \mathbf{0} \end{pmatrix},$$

becomes $q = \sum_{i=1}^{r} y_i^2$. Thus, without knowing $\mathbf{P}$ except for its existence and nonsingularity, we can show that a quadratic form can always be expressed as a sum of r squared terms, where r is the rank of the (symmetric) matrix $\mathbf{A}$ of the quadratic form. That is a result of great importance in considering the distribution of quadratic forms of normally distributed random variables.

Generalized Inverses

Definition

For any nonnull matrix $\mathbf{A}$, there is a unique matrix $\mathbf{M}$ satisfying:

  (i) $\mathbf{AMA} = \mathbf{A}$;
  (ii) $\mathbf{MAM} = \mathbf{M}$;
  (iii) $(\mathbf{AM})' = \mathbf{AM}$; and
  (iv) $(\mathbf{MA})' = \mathbf{MA}$.

These are the *Penrose* conditions and $\mathbf{M}$ is the *Moore–Penrose inverse*. Whereas $\mathbf{M}$ is unique, there are (with one exception) many matrices $\mathbf{G}$ satisfying

$$\mathbf{AGA} = \mathbf{A},$$

which is condition (i). Each matrix $\mathbf{G}$ satisfying $\mathbf{AGA} = \mathbf{A}$ is called a *generalized inverse* of $\mathbf{A}$, and if it also satisfies $\mathbf{GAG} = \mathbf{G}$ it is a *reflexive generalized inverse*. The exception is when $\mathbf{A}$ is nonsingular: there is then only one $\mathbf{G}$; namely, $\mathbf{G} = \mathbf{A}^{-1}$.

Arbitrariness

That there are many matrices $\mathbf{G}$ can be illustrated by showing ways in which from one $\mathbf{G}$ others can be obtained. Thus, if $\mathbf{A}$ is partitioned as

$$\mathbf{A} = \begin{bmatrix} \mathbf{A}_{11} & \mathbf{A}_{12} \\ \mathbf{A}_{21} & \mathbf{A}_{22} \end{bmatrix},$$

where $\mathbf{A}_{11}$ is nonsingular with the same rank as $\mathbf{A}$, then

$$\mathbf{G} =$$
$$\begin{bmatrix} \mathbf{A}_{11}^{-1} - \mathbf{U}\mathbf{A}_{21}\mathbf{A}_{11}^{-1} - \mathbf{A}_{11}^{-1}\mathbf{A}_{12}\mathbf{V} - \mathbf{A}_{11}^{-1}\mathbf{A}_{12}\mathbf{W}\mathbf{A}_{21}\mathbf{A}_{11}^{-1} & \mathbf{U} \\ \mathbf{V} & \mathbf{W} \end{bmatrix}$$

is a generalized inverse of $\mathbf{A}$ for any values of $\mathbf{U}$, $\mathbf{V}$ and $\mathbf{W}$. This can be used to show that a generalized inverse of a symmetric matrix is not necessarily symmetric; and that of a singular matrix is not necessarily singular [4, p. 219].

A simpler illustration of arbitrariness is that if $\mathbf{G}$ is a generalized inverse of $\mathbf{A}$ then so is

$$\mathbf{G}^* = \mathbf{GAG} + (\mathbf{I} - \mathbf{GA})\mathbf{S} + \mathbf{T}(\mathbf{I} - \mathbf{AG}),$$

for any values of $\mathbf{S}$ and $\mathbf{T}$.

Generalized Inverses of $X'X$

The matrix $\mathbf{X}'\mathbf{X}$ plays an important role in statistics, usually involving a generalized inverse thereof, which has several useful properties. Thus, for $\mathbf{G}$ satisfying

$$\mathbf{X}'\mathbf{X}\mathbf{G}\mathbf{X}'\mathbf{X} = \mathbf{X}'\mathbf{X},$$

$\mathbf{G}'$ is also a generalized inverse of $\mathbf{X}'\mathbf{X}$ (and $\mathbf{G}$ is not necessarily symmetric). Also,

1. $\mathbf{X}\mathbf{G}\mathbf{X}'\mathbf{X} = \mathbf{X}$;
2. $\mathbf{X}\mathbf{G}\mathbf{X}'$ is invariant to $\mathbf{G}$;
3. $\mathbf{X}\mathbf{G}\mathbf{X}'$ is symmetric, whether or not $\mathbf{G}$ is;
4. $\mathbf{X}\mathbf{G}\mathbf{X}' = \mathbf{X}\mathbf{X}^+$ for $\mathbf{X}^+$ being the Moore–Penrose inverse of $\mathbf{X}$.

Solving Linear Equations

A Single Solution

Given $\mathbf{A}$ and $\mathbf{y}$, the equations $\mathbf{A}\mathbf{x} = \mathbf{y}$ are linear in the unknowns, the elements of $\mathbf{x}$. When $\mathbf{A}$ is nonsingular, the equations are solved uniquely, as $\mathbf{x} = \mathbf{A}^{-1}\mathbf{y}$. But for singular or rectangular $\mathbf{A}$, solutions involve using a generalized inverse of $\mathbf{A}$. The following results apply.

First, equations $\mathbf{A}\mathbf{x} = \mathbf{y}$ are said to be *consistent* when any linear relationships existing among rows of $\mathbf{A}$ also exist among elements of $\mathbf{y}$. Only then do solutions exist. Secondly, for singular or rectangular $\mathbf{A}$ there will be many solutions for $\mathbf{x}$, except when $\mathbf{A}$ has full column rank, whereupon there is only one solution, $\mathbf{x} = (\mathbf{A}'\mathbf{A})^{-1}\mathbf{A}'\mathbf{y}$: and this includes, of course, the case of nonsingular $\mathbf{A}$.

Many Solutions

When $\mathbf{A}$ has less than full column rank, there are many solutions. They are characterized as follows, with $\mathbf{G}$ being a generalized inverse satisfying $\mathbf{AGA} = \mathbf{A}$:

1. $\tilde{\mathbf{x}} = \mathbf{G}\mathbf{y}$ is a solution if and only if $\mathbf{AGA} = \mathbf{A}$.
2. Letting $\mathbf{G}$ take all its possible values in $\tilde{\mathbf{x}} = \mathbf{G}\mathbf{y}$ (for $\mathbf{y} \neq \mathbf{0}$) generates all possible solutions.
3. $\tilde{\mathbf{x}} = \mathbf{G}\mathbf{y} + (\mathbf{I} - \mathbf{GA})\mathbf{z}$ is a solution for any arbitrary $\mathbf{z}$ of the same order as $\mathbf{x}$.
4. For a given $\mathbf{G}$, letting $\mathbf{z}$ take all possible values in $\tilde{\mathbf{x}} = \mathbf{G}\mathbf{y} + (\mathbf{I} - \mathbf{GA})\mathbf{z}$ generates all possible solutions.
5. When $\tilde{\mathbf{x}}_1, \tilde{\mathbf{x}}_2, \ldots, \tilde{\mathbf{x}}_t$ are any solutions, $\sum_{i=1}^{t} \lambda_i \tilde{\mathbf{x}}_i$ is a solution (with $\mathbf{y} \neq \mathbf{0}$) if and only if $\sum_{i=1}^{t} \lambda_i = 1$; this condition is not needed when $\mathbf{y} = \mathbf{0}$.
6. For $\mathbf{A}_{p \times q}$ and $\mathbf{y} \neq \mathbf{0}$ there are $q - r(\mathbf{A}) + 1 - \delta_{\mathbf{y},\mathbf{0}}$ linearly independent solutions, where $\delta_{\mathbf{y},\mathbf{0}} = 1$ when $\mathbf{y} = \mathbf{0}$ and zero otherwise.
7. The value of $\mathbf{k}'\tilde{\mathbf{x}}$ is invariant to $\tilde{\mathbf{x}}$ if and only if $\mathbf{k}' = \mathbf{k}'\mathbf{GA}$.
8. When $\mathbf{y} = \mathbf{0}$, solutions are orthogonal to rows of $\mathbf{A}$; and solutions orthogonal to each other can always be derived. The vector space spanned by the solutions, sometimes called the *solution space*, is the *orthogonal complement* of the row space of $\mathbf{A}$.

Partitioned Matrices

Some results for partitioned matrices used in statistics are as follows.

Orthogonality

If $\mathbf{P} = [\mathbf{A} \quad \mathbf{B}]$ is orthogonal,

$$\mathbf{PP}' = \mathbf{I} \Rightarrow [\mathbf{A} \quad \mathbf{B}] \begin{bmatrix} \mathbf{A}' \\ \mathbf{B}' \end{bmatrix} = \mathbf{I} \Rightarrow \mathbf{AA}' + \mathbf{BB}' = \mathbf{I},$$

$$\mathbf{P}'\mathbf{P} = \mathbf{I} \Rightarrow \begin{bmatrix} \mathbf{A}' \\ \mathbf{B}' \end{bmatrix} [\mathbf{A} \quad \mathbf{B}] = \mathbf{I} \Rightarrow \begin{bmatrix} \mathbf{A}'\mathbf{A} & \mathbf{A}'\mathbf{B} \\ \mathbf{B}'\mathbf{A} & \mathbf{B}'\mathbf{B} \end{bmatrix}$$

$$= \begin{bmatrix} \mathbf{I} & \mathbf{0} \\ \mathbf{0} & \mathbf{I} \end{bmatrix} \Rightarrow \mathbf{A}'\mathbf{A} = \mathbf{I}, \qquad \mathbf{A}'\mathbf{B} = \mathbf{0}$$

and $\mathbf{B}'\mathbf{B} = \mathbf{I}$.

Note that $\mathbf{AA}'$ and $\mathbf{BB}'$ are not identity matrices.

Determinants

$$\begin{vmatrix} \mathbf{A} & \mathbf{B} \\ \mathbf{C} & \mathbf{D} \end{vmatrix} = |\mathbf{A}||\mathbf{D} - \mathbf{CA}^{-1}\mathbf{B}| = |\mathbf{D}||\mathbf{A} - \mathbf{BD}^{-1}\mathbf{C}|,$$

provided that $\mathbf{A}^{-1}$ and $\mathbf{D}^{-1}$ exist, where needed.

Inverses

$$\begin{bmatrix} \mathbf{A} & \mathbf{B} \\ \mathbf{C} & \mathbf{D} \end{bmatrix}^{-1} = \begin{bmatrix} \mathbf{A}^{-1} & \mathbf{0} \\ \mathbf{0} & \mathbf{0} \end{bmatrix} + \begin{bmatrix} -\mathbf{A}^{-1}\mathbf{B} \\ \mathbf{I} \end{bmatrix}$$

$$\times (\mathbf{D} - \mathbf{CA}^{-1}\mathbf{B})^{-1}[-\mathbf{CA}^{-1} \quad \mathbf{I}]$$

$$= \begin{bmatrix} \mathbf{0} & \mathbf{0} \\ \mathbf{0} & \mathbf{D}^{-1} \end{bmatrix} + \begin{bmatrix} \mathbf{I} \\ -\mathbf{D}^{-1}\mathbf{C} \end{bmatrix}$$

$$\times (\mathbf{A} - \mathbf{BD}^{-1}\mathbf{C})^{-1}[\mathbf{I} \quad -\mathbf{BD}^{-1}],$$

again provided that $\mathbf{A}^{-1}$ and $\mathbf{D}^{-1}$ exist as needed.

Schur Complements

In

$$\begin{bmatrix} \mathbf{A} & \mathbf{B} \\ \mathbf{C} & \mathbf{D} \end{bmatrix}$$

the *Schur complement* of $\mathbf{A}$ is $\mathbf{D} - \mathbf{CA}^{-1}\mathbf{B}$ and that of $\mathbf{D}$ is $\mathbf{A} - \mathbf{BD}^{-1}\mathbf{C}$. The inverse of one involves that of the other:

$$(\mathbf{D} - \mathbf{CA}^{-1}\mathbf{B})^{-1} = \mathbf{D}^{-1} + \mathbf{D}^{-1}\mathbf{C}$$

$$\times (\mathbf{A} - \mathbf{BD}^{-1}\mathbf{C})^{-1}\mathbf{BD}^{-1}.$$

This result also applies when the two minus signs are changed to plus, and the plus to minus. It also has some useful special cases; for example,

$$(\mathbf{D} \pm \lambda \mathbf{t}\mathbf{t}')^{-1} = \mathbf{D}^{-1} \mp \frac{\mathbf{D}^{-1}\mathbf{t}\mathbf{t}'\mathbf{D}^{-1}}{(\lambda^{-1} \pm \mathbf{t}'\mathbf{D}^{-1}\mathbf{t})}.$$

Generalized Inverses

By analogy with expressions for the inverse, one might expect (with $\mathbf{A}^-$ being a generalized inverse of $\mathbf{A}$)

$$\tilde{\mathbf{Q}} = \begin{bmatrix} \mathbf{A}^- & \mathbf{0} \\ \mathbf{0} & \mathbf{0} \end{bmatrix} + \begin{bmatrix} -\mathbf{A}^- & \mathbf{B} \\ \mathbf{I} \end{bmatrix}$$

$$\times (\mathbf{D} - \mathbf{CA}^-\mathbf{B})^-[-\mathbf{CA}^- \quad \mathbf{I}]$$

to be a generalized inverse of

$$\mathbf{Q} = \begin{bmatrix} \mathbf{A} & \mathbf{B} \\ \mathbf{C} & \mathbf{D} \end{bmatrix}.$$

It is, if and only if $r(\mathbf{Q}) = r(\mathbf{A}) + r(\mathbf{D} - \mathbf{CA}^-\mathbf{B})$. Satisfying this rank condition depends upon $\mathbf{A}^-$. For some values of $\mathbf{A}^-$ the condition will be satisfied and for others it will not. Only when it is satisfied will $\tilde{\mathbf{Q}}$ be a generalized inverse of $\mathbf{Q}$.

Direct Sums

The direct sum of matrices $\mathbf{A}$ and $\mathbf{B}$, each of any order, is defined as

$$\mathbf{A} \oplus \mathbf{B} = \begin{bmatrix} \mathbf{A} & \mathbf{0} \\ \mathbf{0} & \mathbf{B} \end{bmatrix}.$$

Extension to the direct sum of more than two matrices is straightforward.

Provided that the needed conformability requirements are met,

$$(\mathbf{A} \oplus \mathbf{B}) + (\mathbf{C} \oplus \mathbf{D}) = (\mathbf{A} + \mathbf{C}) \oplus (\mathbf{B} + \mathbf{D}),$$

$$(\mathbf{P} \oplus \mathbf{Q})(\mathbf{L} \oplus \mathbf{M}) = \mathbf{PL} \oplus \mathbf{QM},$$

and

$$(\mathbf{X} \oplus \mathbf{Y})^{-1} = \mathbf{X}^{-1} \oplus \mathbf{Y}^{-1}.$$

Direct Products

The *direct product* of two matrices, each of any order, is defined as

$$\mathbf{A}_{p \times q} \otimes \mathbf{B}_{m \times n} = \begin{bmatrix} a_{11}\mathbf{B} & \cdots & a_{1q}\mathbf{B} \\ \vdots & & \\ a_{p1}\mathbf{B} & \cdots & a_{pq}\mathbf{B} \end{bmatrix}_{pm \times qn}$$
$$= \{a_{ij}\mathbf{B}\}_{i=1, j=1}^{p \quad q}.$$

It is sometimes called the *Kronecker product*. Some properties follow – assuming that conformability requirements are met:

1. $\mathbf{x}' \otimes \mathbf{y} = \mathbf{yx}' = \mathbf{y} \otimes \mathbf{x}'$;
2. $\lambda \otimes \mathbf{A} = \lambda \mathbf{A} = \mathbf{A} \otimes \lambda$;
3. $(\mathbf{A} \otimes \mathbf{B})' = \mathbf{A}' \otimes \mathbf{B}'$, *not* $\mathbf{B}' \otimes \mathbf{A}'$;
4. $(\mathbf{A} \otimes \mathbf{B})(\mathbf{X} \otimes \mathbf{Y}) = \mathbf{AX} \otimes \mathbf{BY}$;
5. $(\mathbf{P} \otimes \mathbf{Q})^{-1} = \mathbf{P}^{-1} \otimes \mathbf{Q}^{-1}$, *not* $\mathbf{Q}^{-1} \otimes \mathbf{P}^{-1}$;
6. $[\mathbf{A}_1 \quad \mathbf{A}_2] \otimes \mathbf{B} = [\mathbf{A}_1 \otimes \mathbf{B} \quad \mathbf{A}_2 \otimes \mathbf{B}]$,
    $\mathbf{A} \otimes [\mathbf{B}_1 \quad \mathbf{B}_2] \neq [\mathbf{A} \otimes \mathbf{B}_1 \quad \mathbf{A} \otimes \mathbf{B}_2]$;
7. $r(\mathbf{A} \otimes \mathbf{B}) = r(\mathbf{A})r(\mathbf{B})$;
8. $\text{tr}(\mathbf{A} \otimes \mathbf{B}) = \text{tr}(\mathbf{A})\text{tr}(\mathbf{B})$;
9. $|\mathbf{A}_{p \times p} \otimes \mathbf{B}_{m \times m}| = |\mathbf{A}|^m |\mathbf{B}|^p$.

Sometimes $\mathbf{A} \otimes \mathbf{B} = \{a_{ij}\mathbf{B}\}$ as defined above is called the *right direct product*, to distinguish it from $\mathbf{B} \otimes \mathbf{A}$,

which is then called the *left direct product*; and on rare occasions $\{a_{ij}\mathbf{B}\}$ will be found defined as $\mathbf{B} \otimes \mathbf{A}$.

Eigenvalues and Eigenvectors

The equation

$$\mathbf{Au} = \lambda \mathbf{u}, \text{ i.e. } (\mathbf{A} - \lambda \mathbf{I})\mathbf{u} = \mathbf{0},$$

has solutions for $\mathbf{u}$ provided that $\mathbf{A} - \lambda \mathbf{I}$ is singular. This occurs when

$$|\mathbf{A} - \lambda \mathbf{I}| = \mathbf{0}.$$

This is called the *characteristic equation* of $\mathbf{A}$; for $\mathbf{A}_{n \times n}$ it is a polynomial of order n and therefore has n solutions for λ. Those solutions are the **eigenvalues** (or *eigenroots*) of $\mathbf{A}$. They can be real or complex, positive or negative, or zero. For each eigenvalue, λ_* say, a corresponding value of $\mathbf{u}$ can be obtained from solving the equations $(\mathbf{A} - \lambda_* \mathbf{I})\mathbf{u} = \mathbf{0}$, as

$$\mathbf{u}_* = [\mathbf{I} - (\mathbf{A} - \lambda_* \mathbf{I})^-(\mathbf{A} - \lambda_* \mathbf{I})]\mathbf{z}$$

for arbitrary $\mathbf{z}$. (Searle [4, Section 11.4] has details.) $\mathbf{u}_*$ is the **eigenvector** corresponding to λ_*.

Numerical Example

For

$$\mathbf{A} = \begin{bmatrix} 2 & 2 & 0 \\ 2 & 1 & 1 \\ -7 & 2 & -3 \end{bmatrix},$$

the characteristic equation $|\mathbf{A} - \lambda \mathbf{I}| = 0$ reduces to $(\lambda - 1)(\lambda - 3)(\lambda + 4) = 0$, so that the eigenvalues are 1, 3, and -4. For $\lambda_* = 1$ the eigenvector, from the equation for $\mathbf{u}_*$,

$$\mathbf{u}_* = \left[\mathbf{I} - \begin{pmatrix} 1 & 2 & 0 \\ 2 & 0 & 1 \\ -7 & 2 & -4 \end{pmatrix}^- \begin{pmatrix} 1 & 2 & 0 \\ 2 & 0 & 1 \\ -7 & 2 & -4 \end{pmatrix} \right] \begin{bmatrix} z_1 \\ z_2 \\ z_3 \end{bmatrix}$$

$$= \left[\mathbf{I} + \tfrac{1}{4} \begin{pmatrix} 0 & -2 & 0 \\ -2 & 1 & 0 \\ 0 & 0 & 0 \end{pmatrix} \begin{pmatrix} 1 & 2 & 0 \\ 2 & 0 & 1 \\ -7 & 2 & -4 \end{pmatrix} \right] \begin{bmatrix} z_1 \\ z_2 \\ z_3 \end{bmatrix}$$

$$= \left[\mathbf{I} + \tfrac{1}{4} \begin{pmatrix} -4 & 0 & -2 \\ 0 & -4 & 1 \\ 0 & 0 & 0 \end{pmatrix} \right] \begin{bmatrix} z_1 \\ z_2 \\ z_3 \end{bmatrix}$$

$$= \begin{bmatrix} 0 & 0 & -\tfrac{1}{2} \\ 0 & 0 & \tfrac{1}{4} \\ 0 & 0 & 1 \end{bmatrix} \begin{bmatrix} z_1 \\ z_2 \\ z_3 \end{bmatrix} = \begin{bmatrix} -\tfrac{1}{2}z_3 \\ \tfrac{1}{4}z_3 \\ z_3 \end{bmatrix} \text{ for any } z_3 \neq 0.$$

Similarly, for $\lambda_* = 3$,

$$\mathbf{u}_* = \left[\mathbf{I} - \begin{pmatrix} -1 & 2 & 0 \\ 2 & -2 & 1 \\ -7 & 2 & -3 \end{pmatrix}^{-} \begin{pmatrix} -1 & 2 & 0 \\ 2 & -2 & 1 \\ -7 & 2 & -3 \end{pmatrix}\right]\mathbf{z}$$

$$= \left[\mathbf{I} - \frac{1}{2}\begin{pmatrix} -2 & -2 & 0 \\ -2 & -1 & 0 \\ 0 & 0 & 0 \end{pmatrix}\begin{pmatrix} -1 & 2 & 0 \\ 2 & -2 & 1 \\ -7 & 2 & -3 \end{pmatrix}\right]\mathbf{z}$$

$$= \left[\mathbf{I} - \frac{1}{2}\begin{pmatrix} -2 & 0 & -2 \\ 0 & -2 & -1 \\ 0 & 0 & 0 \end{pmatrix}\right]\mathbf{z} = \begin{bmatrix} 0 & 0 & -1 \\ 0 & 0 & -\frac{1}{2} \\ 0 & 0 & 1 \end{bmatrix}\mathbf{z}$$

$$= \begin{bmatrix} -z_3 \\ -\frac{1}{2}z_3 \\ z_3 \end{bmatrix}.$$

The case of $\lambda_* = -4$ is left to the reader.

Properties of Eigenvalues

See **Eigenvalue**.

Properties of Eigenvectors

See **Eigenvector**.

Some Summaries

Orthogonal Matrices

Any two of (i) $\mathbf{A}$ being square, (ii) $\mathbf{AA}' = \mathbf{I}$, and (iii) $\mathbf{A}'\mathbf{A} = \mathbf{I}$ imply the third; and define $\mathbf{A}$ as being orthogonal. The properties of orthogonal $\mathbf{A}$ include the following:

1. rows (columns) are orthonormal;
2. $|\mathbf{A}| = \pm 1$;
3. λ being an eigenroot of $\mathbf{A}$ implies that $1/\lambda$ is also;
4. $\mathbf{AB}$ is orthogonal when $\mathbf{A}$ and $\mathbf{B}$ are.

Idempotent Matrices

Idempotent $\mathbf{A}$ of order n has the following properties:

1. $\mathbf{A}^2 = \mathbf{A}$;
2. $\mathbf{A}$ is singular, unless $\mathbf{A} = \mathbf{I}$;
3. $r(\mathbf{A}) = tr(\mathbf{A})$;
4. $\mathbf{I} - \mathbf{A}$ is idempotent, with $r(\mathbf{I} - \mathbf{A}) = n - r(\mathbf{A})$;

5. If $\mathbf{A}$ is also symmetric (but not $\mathbf{I}$) it is positive semidefinite, and can be expressed as $\mathbf{A} = \mathbf{LL}'$ for $\mathbf{L}'\mathbf{L} = \mathbf{I}$;
6. for idempotent $\mathbf{A}$ and $\mathbf{B}$, $\mathbf{AB}$ is idempotent if $\mathbf{AB} = \mathbf{BA}$;
7. $r(\mathbf{A})$ eigenroots of $\mathbf{A}$ are 1.0, and $n - r(\mathbf{A})$ are 0;
8. there is a $\mathbf{U}$ such that

$$\mathbf{U}^{-1}\mathbf{AU} = \begin{bmatrix} \mathbf{I}_{r(\mathbf{A})} & \mathbf{0} \\ \mathbf{0} & \mathbf{0} \end{bmatrix};$$

9. $\mathbf{P} = \mathbf{I} - \mathbf{X}(\mathbf{X}'\mathbf{X})^{-}\mathbf{X}'$ is idempotent, and is very useful in statistics.

Matrices $a\mathbf{I} + b\mathbf{J}$

The matrix $a\mathbf{I} + b\mathbf{J}$ for $\mathbf{J} = \mathbf{11}'$ occurs in a number of analysis of variance situations in statistics. When of order n it has the following properties:

$$(a_1\mathbf{I} + b_1\mathbf{J})(a_2\mathbf{I} + b_2\mathbf{J}) = a_1a_2\mathbf{I} + (a_1b_2 + a_2b_1$$
$$+ nb_1b_2)\mathbf{J},$$
$$(a\mathbf{I} + b\mathbf{J})^{-1} = \frac{1}{a}\left(\mathbf{I} - \frac{b}{a + nb}\mathbf{J}\right),$$
$$|a\mathbf{I} + b\mathbf{J}| = a^{n-1}(a + nb).$$

Eigenroots are a, $n - 1$ times, and $a + nb$ once.

Nonnegative Definite Matrices

If $\mathbf{A}$ is nonnegative definite (n.n.d.):

1. $\mathbf{x}'\mathbf{Ax} \geq 0$, for all $\mathbf{x} \neq 0$;
2. $\mathbf{A}$ is assumed to be symmetric, because otherwise it can be replaced by $\frac{1}{2}(\mathbf{A} + \mathbf{A}')$;
3. $|\mathbf{A}| \geq 0$;
4. diagonal elements of $\mathbf{A}$ are ≥ 0;
5. principal leading minors are ≥ 0;
6. eigenroots are ≥ 0;
7. if $\mathbf{A}$ is positive definite (p.d.), all of the above $\geq$ 0 symbols become > 0;
8. for real $\mathbf{X}$, $\mathbf{X}'\mathbf{X}$ is n.n.d.

For real $\mathbf{X}$ of full column rank:

1. $\mathbf{X}'\mathbf{X}$ is p.d.;
2. $(\mathbf{X}'\mathbf{X})^{-1}$ exists;
3. $\mathbf{XX}'$ has Moore–Penrose inverse $\mathbf{X}(\mathbf{X}'\mathbf{X})^{-2}\mathbf{X}'$.

Canonical and Other Forms

For any matrix $\mathbf{A}_{p \times q}$ of rank r:

1. Equivalent canonical form:

$$\mathbf{PAQ} = \begin{bmatrix} \mathbf{I}_r & \mathbf{0} \\ \mathbf{0} & \mathbf{0} \end{bmatrix}, \quad \mathbf{P} \text{ and } \mathbf{Q} \text{ nonsingular.}$$

2. Similar canonical form:

$$\mathbf{AU} = \mathbf{UD}\{\lambda\},$$

where $\mathbf{D}\{\lambda\}$ is the diagonal matrix of eigenroots; and $\mathbf{U}$ is the matrix of corresponding eigenvectors. $\mathbf{U}^{-1}$ exists when the diagonability theorem is satisfied (*see* **Eigenvector**), and then

$$\mathbf{U}^{-1}\mathbf{AU} = \mathbf{D}\{\lambda\}.$$

3. Singular-valued decomposition:

$$\mathbf{A} = \mathbf{L} \begin{bmatrix} \Delta_r & \mathbf{0} \\ \mathbf{0} & \mathbf{0} \end{bmatrix} \mathbf{M}',$$

where $\mathbf{L}$ and $\mathbf{M}$ are each orthogonal, and $\Delta_r = (\Delta^2)^{1/2}$, where

$$\mathbf{L}'\mathbf{AA}'\mathbf{L} = \begin{bmatrix} \Delta^2 & \mathbf{0} \\ \mathbf{0} & \mathbf{0} \end{bmatrix} \quad \text{and}$$

$$\mathbf{M}'\mathbf{A}'\mathbf{AM} = \begin{bmatrix} \Delta^2 & \mathbf{0} \\ \mathbf{0} & \mathbf{0} \end{bmatrix},$$

with Δ^2 being the diagonal matrix of the (positive) eigenroots of $\mathbf{A}'\mathbf{A}$ (or, equivalently, of $\mathbf{AA}'$).

For symmetric $\mathbf{A}$ of order p and rank r:
4. Diagonal form:

$$\mathbf{PAP}' = \begin{bmatrix} \mathbf{D}_r & \mathbf{0} \\ \mathbf{0} & \mathbf{0} \end{bmatrix}, \quad \text{with } \mathbf{D}_r \text{ diagonal, order } r.$$

When $\mathbf{A}$ is n.n.d., elements of $\mathbf{D}_r$ are positive.
5. Congruent canonical form:

$$\mathbf{RAR}' = \begin{bmatrix} \mathbf{I}_r & \mathbf{0} \\ \mathbf{0} & \mathbf{0} \end{bmatrix}, \quad \text{for } \mathbf{R} \text{ possibly complex.}$$

When $\mathbf{A}$ is n.n.d., $\mathbf{R}$ is real.
6. Orthogonal similar canonical form:

$$\mathbf{U}'\mathbf{AU} = \mathbf{D}\{\lambda\},$$

with $\mathbf{U}$ being orthogonal and $\mathbf{U}^{-1} = \mathbf{U}'$.

7. Spectral decomposition:

$$\mathbf{A} = \sum_i \lambda_i \mathbf{u}_i \mathbf{u}_i',$$

for λ_i being an eigenroot and $\mathbf{u}_i$ its corresponding eigenvector.

Solving Equations by Iteration

Current computing facilities provide numerous methods of arithmetically solving equations which cannot be solved algebraically. Matrix notation permits succinct description of one of these methods.

For n equations in n unknowns, represented by $\mathbf{x}$, let the equations be

$$\mathbf{f}(\mathbf{x}) = \mathbf{0}, \tag{1}$$

and define

$$\mathbf{G}(\mathbf{x}) = \{g_{ij}(\mathbf{x})\} = \left\{ \frac{\partial}{\partial x_j} f_i(\mathbf{x}) \right\} \quad \text{for}$$
$$i, j = 1, \ldots, n. \tag{2}$$

Suppose that $\mathbf{x}_r$ is an approximate solution for $\mathbf{x}$ to $\mathbf{f}(\mathbf{x}) = \mathbf{0}$. Then an improved approximation is $\mathbf{x}_{r+1}$ for

$$\mathbf{f}(\mathbf{x}_{r+1}) = \mathbf{f}(\mathbf{x}_r) + \mathbf{G}(\mathbf{x}_r)\Delta_r, \tag{3}$$

where

$$\Delta_r = \mathbf{x}_{r+1} - \mathbf{x}_r. \tag{4}$$

Were $\mathbf{x}_{r+1}$ to be a solution to (1) then $\mathbf{f}(\mathbf{x}_{r+1})$ would be $\mathbf{0}$ and (3) would yield

$$\Delta_r = -[\mathbf{G}(\mathbf{x}_r)]^{-1}\mathbf{f}(\mathbf{x}_r), \tag{5}$$

and with this, (4) gives

$$\mathbf{x}_{r+1} = \Delta_r + \mathbf{x}_r. \tag{6}$$

In this way, (5) and (6) provide an iterative procedure for calculating a solution: for some initial value $\mathbf{x}_0$, use (5) to obtain Δ_0 and then (6) to obtain $\mathbf{x}_1$; and back to (5) to obtain Δ_1, and so on.

Differential Calculus with Matrices

A number of situations in statistics involve maximizing or minimizing a function: for example, maximum likelihood estimation, least squares estimation, minimum variance procedures, minimizing loss functions, and so on. In many cases, differentiation of matrix expressions is involved, for which the following results are often useful.

Differentiating with Respect to a Scalar

Suppose that the elements of $\mathbf{A} = \{a_{ij}\}$ are functions of a scalar x. Then

$$\frac{\partial \mathbf{A}}{\partial x} = \left\{ \frac{\partial a_{ij}}{\partial x} \right\},$$

$$\frac{\partial \mathbf{A}^{-1}}{\partial x} = -\mathbf{A}^{-1} \frac{\partial \mathbf{A}}{\partial x} \mathbf{A}^{-1},$$

$$\mathbf{A} \frac{\partial \mathbf{A}^-}{\partial x} \mathbf{A} = -\mathbf{A}\mathbf{A}^- \frac{\partial \mathbf{A}}{\partial x} \mathbf{A}^-\mathbf{A},$$

where $\mathbf{A}^-$ is a generalized inverse of $\mathbf{A}$, satisfying $\mathbf{A}\mathbf{A}^-\mathbf{A} = \mathbf{A}$. Also,

$$\mathbf{A} \frac{\partial (\mathbf{A}'\mathbf{A})^-}{\partial x} \mathbf{A}' = -\mathbf{A}(\mathbf{A}'\mathbf{A})^- \frac{\partial (\mathbf{A}'\mathbf{A})}{\partial x} (\mathbf{A}'\mathbf{A})^-\mathbf{A}'.$$

Also, for $\mathbf{A} = \mathbf{A}'$ and elements of $\mathbf{T}$ not involving x,

$$\mathbf{P} = \mathbf{T}(\mathbf{T}'\mathbf{A}\mathbf{T})^{-1}\mathbf{T}' \text{ has } \frac{\partial \mathbf{P}}{\partial x} = -\mathbf{P}\frac{\partial \mathbf{A}}{\partial x}\mathbf{P}.$$

Differentiating with Respect to Elements of a Vector

The basis of differentiating with respect to elements of $\mathbf{x}$ is defining what is meant by $\partial/\partial\mathbf{x}$. This is important, because the definition determines the form of its various applications, and because not all writers use the same definition. Any presentation of this topic should therefore start by defining $\partial/\partial\mathbf{x}$.

A widely used convention is that, for $\mathbf{x}$ being a column vector, $\partial/\partial\mathbf{x}$ is also: thus, for $\mathbf{x} = [x_1 \ldots x_n]'$, we define

$$\mathbf{x} = \{_c x_i\}_{i=1}^n \quad \text{and} \quad \frac{\partial}{\partial \mathbf{x}} = \left\{_c \frac{\partial}{\partial x_i} \right\}_{i=1}^n.$$

Thus $\partial/\partial\mathbf{x}$ is a vector of differential operators. With this definition come the following basic results:

$$\frac{\partial}{\partial \mathbf{x}}(\mathbf{a}'\mathbf{x}) = \frac{\partial}{\partial \mathbf{x}}(\mathbf{x}'\mathbf{a}) = \mathbf{a} \quad \text{and} \quad \frac{\partial}{\partial \mathbf{x}}(\mathbf{x}'\mathbf{A}) = \mathbf{A}.$$

Then, in order to maintain feasible matrix dimensions, the convention is adopted that

$$\frac{\partial}{\partial \mathbf{x}}(\mathbf{A}\mathbf{x}) = \frac{\partial}{\partial \mathbf{x}}(\mathbf{x}'\mathbf{A}'),$$

and so

$$\frac{\partial}{\partial \mathbf{x}}(\mathbf{A}\mathbf{x}) = \mathbf{A}'.$$

This leads to

$$\frac{\partial}{\partial \mathbf{x}}(\mathbf{x}'\mathbf{A}\mathbf{x}) = \mathbf{A}\mathbf{x} + \mathbf{A}'\mathbf{x} \quad \text{for } \mathbf{A} \text{ not symmetric,}$$

$$= 2\mathbf{A}\mathbf{x} \qquad \text{for } \mathbf{A} \text{ symmetric.}$$

Differentiating with Respect to Elements of a Matrix

Again, the basic definition is important: for scalar θ and $\mathbf{X}_{p \times q}$,

$$\frac{\partial \theta}{\partial \mathbf{X}} = \left\{_m \frac{\partial \theta}{\partial x_{ij}} \right\}_{i=1 \ j=1}^{p \quad q}.$$

For $\mathbf{X}$ having functionally unrelated elements,

$$\frac{\partial}{\partial \mathbf{X}}[\text{tr}(\mathbf{X}\mathbf{A})] = \mathbf{A}'.$$

But for symmetric $\mathbf{X}$,

$$\frac{\partial}{\partial \mathbf{X}}[\text{tr}(\mathbf{X}\mathbf{A})] = \mathbf{A} + \mathbf{A}' - \text{diag}(\mathbf{A}),$$

where $\text{diag}(\mathbf{A})$ is the diagonal matrix of the diagonal elements of $\mathbf{A}$. Of course, these results also apply to $\text{tr}(\mathbf{A}\mathbf{X}) = \text{tr}(\mathbf{X}\mathbf{A})$.

Differentiating Determinants

Let x_{ij} be the (i, j)th element of $\mathbf{X}$, and let $|\mathbf{X}_{ij}|$ be its cofactor in $|\mathbf{X}|$. Then, for $\mathbf{X}$ having functionally unrelated elements:

$$\frac{\partial |\mathbf{X}|}{\partial x_{ij}} = |\mathbf{X}_{ij}|, \qquad \frac{\partial |\mathbf{X}|}{\partial \mathbf{X}} = |\mathbf{X}|(\mathbf{X}^{-1})',$$

and

$$\frac{\partial}{\partial \mathbf{X}} \log |\mathbf{X}| = (\mathbf{X}^{-1})'.$$

For symmetric $\mathbf{X}$, comparable results are

$$\frac{\partial |\mathbf{X}|}{\partial x_{ij}} = (2 - \delta_{ij})|\mathbf{X}_{ij}|,$$

where $\delta_{ij} = 0$ except when $i = j$, and then $\delta_{ii} = 1$,

$$\frac{\partial |\mathbf{X}|}{\partial \mathbf{X}} = |\mathbf{X}|[2\mathbf{X}^{-1} - \mathrm{diag}(\mathbf{X}^{-1})],$$

and

$$\frac{\partial}{\partial \mathbf{X}} \log |\mathbf{X}| = 2\mathbf{X}^{-1} - \mathrm{diag}(\mathbf{X}^{-1}).$$

Finally, for any nonsingular $\mathbf{X}$, symmetric or not,

$$\frac{\partial}{\partial \mathbf{y}} \log |\mathbf{X}| = \mathrm{tr}\left(\mathbf{X}^{-1}\frac{\partial \mathbf{X}}{\partial \mathbf{y}}\right).$$

Jacobians

When $\mathbf{y}$ is a vector of n differentiable functions of the n elements of $\mathbf{x}$, such that the transformation of $\mathbf{x}$ to $\mathbf{y}$, to be denoted $\mathbf{x} \to \mathbf{y}$, is 1-to-1, then the matrix

$$\mathbf{J}_{\mathbf{x}\to\mathbf{y}} = \left(\frac{\partial \mathbf{x}}{\partial \mathbf{y}}\right) = \left\{{}_{\mathrm{m}}\frac{\partial x_j}{\partial y_i}\right\}_{i=1\ j=1}^{n\quad n}$$

is the *Jacobian matrix* of $\mathbf{x} \to \mathbf{y}$. For example, if $\mathbf{y} = \mathbf{Ax}$,

$$\mathbf{J}_{\mathbf{x}\to\mathbf{y}} = \left[\frac{\partial(\mathbf{A}^{-1}\mathbf{y})'}{\partial \mathbf{y}}\right] = (\mathbf{A}^{-1})'.$$

$||\mathbf{J}_{\mathbf{x}\to\mathbf{y}}||$, the positive value of the determinant of $\mathbf{J}_{\mathbf{x}\to\mathbf{y}}$, is called the *Jacobian* of $\mathbf{x} \to \mathbf{y}$. It is needed when using $\mathbf{x} \to \mathbf{y}$ on an integral such as

$$\varphi = \int f(\mathbf{x}) \mathrm{d}\mathbf{x},$$

where $f(\mathbf{x})$ is a scalar function of elements of $\mathbf{x}$. If $\mathbf{x} \to \mathbf{y}$ is $\mathbf{y} = g(\mathbf{x})$, then

$$\varphi = \int f(g^{-1}[y]) ||\mathbf{J}_{\mathbf{x}\to\mathbf{y}}|| \mathrm{d}\mathbf{y}.$$

With the identity $||\mathbf{J}_{\mathbf{x}\to\mathbf{y}}|| \equiv 1/||\mathbf{J}_{\mathbf{y}\to\mathbf{x}}||$, with elements of $\mathbf{J}_{\mathbf{y}\to\mathbf{x}}$ sometimes being easier to derive than those of $\mathbf{J}_{\mathbf{x}\to\mathbf{y}}$, and when notation other than $\mathbf{x}$ and $\mathbf{y}$ is the context, confusion easily arises as to whether φ involves $\mathbf{J}_{\mathbf{x}\to\mathbf{y}}$ or $\mathbf{J}_{\mathbf{y}\to\mathbf{x}}$. Fortunately, there is a mnemonic that clarifies the situation. Defining the transformation as old $\to$ new, one always uses $\mathbf{J}_{\mathrm{old}\to\mathrm{new}}$, abbreviated to $\mathbf{J}_{\mathrm{o}\to\mathrm{n}}$. In the latter the subscripts are always in the sequence "on", not "no". This always works.

Vec and Vech Operators

Vec and vech are operators that vectorize a matrix. It can be done in various ways, the most useful of which is stacking the columns of a matrix one under the other. For $\mathbf{X}_{p\times q}$, the resulting column is denoted vec $\mathbf{X}$, a column of order pq. For example,

$$\mathbf{X} = \begin{bmatrix} 1 & 2 & 3 \\ a & b & c \end{bmatrix} \text{ gives } \mathrm{vec}\,\mathbf{X} = \begin{bmatrix} 1 \\ a \\ 2 \\ b \\ 3 \\ c \end{bmatrix}.$$

Three useful properties are as follows:

$$\mathrm{vec}(\mathbf{ABC}) = (\mathbf{C}' \otimes \mathbf{A})\mathrm{vec}\,\mathbf{B},$$

$$\mathrm{tr}(\mathbf{AB}) = (\mathrm{vec}\,\mathbf{A}')'\mathrm{vec}\,\mathbf{B},$$

$$\mathrm{tr}(\mathbf{AZ}'\mathbf{BZC}) = \mathrm{tr}[\mathbf{Z}'(\mathbf{BZCA})]$$

$$= (\mathrm{vec}\,\mathbf{Z})'\mathrm{vec}(\mathbf{BZCA})$$

$$= (\mathrm{vec}\,\mathbf{Z})'(\mathbf{A}'\mathbf{C}' \otimes \mathbf{B})\mathrm{vec}\,\mathbf{Z}.$$

The operator vech $\mathbf{X}$ is defined for $\mathbf{X}$ being symmetric. It has the columns of $\mathbf{X}$, starting at the diagonal elements, stacked one under the other. For example,

$$\mathbf{X} = \begin{bmatrix} 1 & 2 & 3 \\ 2 & x & y \\ 3 & y & \alpha \end{bmatrix} \text{ has } \mathrm{vech}\,\mathbf{X} = \begin{bmatrix} 1 \\ 2 \\ 3 \\ x \\ y \\ \alpha \end{bmatrix}.$$

Henderson & Searle [1, 2] give some history and numerous details.

A particular use of vec and vech is in calculating $||\mathbf{J}_{\mathbf{X}\to\mathbf{Y}}||$. This is the positive value of the determinant of

$$\mathbf{J}_{\mathbf{X}\to\mathbf{Y}} = \frac{\partial(\mathrm{vec}\,\mathbf{X})'}{\partial(\mathrm{vec}\,\mathbf{Y})'},$$

and if $\mathbf{X}$ and $\mathbf{Y}$ are both symmetric, vec is replaced by vech.

Matrices having Complex Numbers as Elements

Because statistics almost always deals with real numbers (e.g. data) and not complex numbers that involve $i = \sqrt{-1}$, most of this article deals with real matrices, those having no complex numbers as elements. Nevertheless, since many texts do deal with matrices of complex numbers, a few basic definitions are given here.

In scalar arithmetic the complex number $a - ib$ is called the *complex conjugate* of $a + ib$, and the two numbers are a *conjugate pair*. Likewise with matrices, $\overline{\mathbf{M}} = \mathbf{A} - i\mathbf{B}$ is the *complex conjugate* of $\mathbf{M} = \mathbf{A} + i\mathbf{B}$, with $\mathbf{M}$ and $\overline{\mathbf{M}}$ being a *conjugate pair*. $\mathbf{M}$ is said to be *Hermitian* when $\overline{\mathbf{M}}' = \mathbf{M}$; and $\mathbf{M}$ is *unitary* if $\overline{\mathbf{M}}'\mathbf{M} = \mathbf{I}$. Thus, being Hermitian is the complex counterpart of being symmetric, as is unitary of orthogonal.

Some Matrix Usage in Statistics

The development and description of statistical methodology benefits enormously from the use of matrices. The following examples briefly illustrate some of the widely used situations in which matrix notation so efficiently encapsulates a multitude of results.

Means and Variances

$\mathbf{x}$ being a vector of random variables with mean $\boldsymbol{\mu}$ implies that $\mathrm{E}(\mathbf{x}) = \boldsymbol{\mu}$, where E represents expectation. Then, because the ith element of $\mathbf{x}$ has a variance, σ_i^2, and each pair of elements, the ith and jth say, have a covariance, σ_{ij}, these variances and covariances can be arrayed in a symmetric matrix, called the variance–**covariance matrix**, for which we use the symbol $\boldsymbol{\Sigma}$. For example, for $\mathbf{x}$ of order 3,

$$\boldsymbol{\Sigma} = \mathrm{var}(\mathbf{x}) = \begin{bmatrix} \sigma_1^2 & \sigma_{12} & \sigma_{13} \\ \sigma_{12} & \sigma_2^2 & \sigma_{23} \\ \sigma_{13} & \sigma_{23} & \sigma_3^2 \end{bmatrix}.$$

A more general expression is

$$\boldsymbol{\Sigma} = \mathrm{var}(\mathbf{x}) = \mathrm{E}(\mathbf{x} - \boldsymbol{\mu})(\mathbf{x} - \boldsymbol{\mu})'.$$

For a linear change of variables, from $\mathbf{x}$ to $\mathbf{y} = \mathbf{T}\mathbf{x}$, the mean vector and the variance–covariance matrix are easily established as

$$\mathrm{E}(\mathbf{y}) = \mathrm{E}(\mathbf{T}\mathbf{x}) = \mathbf{T}\mathrm{E}(\mathbf{x}) = \mathbf{T}\boldsymbol{\mu}$$

and

$$\mathrm{var}(\mathbf{y}) = \mathrm{var}(\mathbf{T}\mathbf{x}) = \mathrm{E}(\mathbf{T}\mathbf{x} - \mathbf{T}\boldsymbol{\mu})(\mathbf{T}\mathbf{x} - \mathbf{T}\boldsymbol{\mu})'$$
$$= \mathrm{E}\mathbf{T}(\mathbf{x} - \boldsymbol{\mu})(\mathbf{x} - \boldsymbol{\mu})'\mathbf{T}' = \mathbf{T}\boldsymbol{\Sigma}\mathbf{T}'.$$

Suppose that $\mathbf{T}$ is a row vector, $\mathbf{t}'$. Then, because a variance is never negative, $\mathrm{var}(\mathbf{t}'\mathbf{y}) = \mathbf{t}'\boldsymbol{\Sigma}\mathbf{t} \geq 0$ and so $\boldsymbol{\Sigma}$ is n.n.d.

Correlation

A **correlation** matrix, $\mathbf{P}$ say, is a matrix with 1.0 as its diagonal elements and correlations $\rho_{ij} = \sigma_{ij}/(\sigma_i^2\sigma_j^2)^{1/2}$ (for $i \neq j$) as its off-diagonal elements. Define $\mathbf{D}$ as the diagonal matrix of the σ_i^2 terms. Then $\mathbf{P} = \mathbf{D}^{-1/2}\boldsymbol{\Sigma}\mathbf{D}^{-1/2}$.

A frequently used form of $\boldsymbol{\Sigma}$ is one which has σ^2 for all diagonal elements (variances) and $\rho\sigma^2$ for all off-diagonal elements (covariances). Then,

$$\boldsymbol{\Sigma} = \sigma^2\mathbf{P} \quad \text{for} \quad \mathbf{P} = (1 - \rho)\mathbf{I} + \rho\mathbf{J},$$

and, for order k,

$$|\boldsymbol{\Sigma}| = \sigma^{2k}(1 - \rho)^{k-1}(1 - \rho + k\rho).$$

Since $\boldsymbol{\Sigma}$ is n.n.d., $|\boldsymbol{\Sigma}| \geq 0$, which implies that $1 + (k - 1)\rho \geq 0$; that is, $\rho \geq -1/(k - 1)$. This is a consequence that one would not be inclined to anticipate on assuming the same covariance, $\rho\sigma^2$, between each pair of variables.

Sums of Squares and Products

For a column vector $\mathbf{x}_j$, the jth column of $\mathbf{X}$, the sum of squares of its elements x_{ij} is $\sum_i x_{ij}^2 = \mathbf{x}_j'\mathbf{x}_j$; and $\sum_i x_{ij}x_{ij'} = \mathbf{x}_j'\mathbf{x}_{j'}$. Thus, $\mathbf{X}'\mathbf{X} = \{_m \mathbf{x}_j'\mathbf{x}_{j'}\}$ is a matrix of these sums of squares and products.

For $\mathbf{x}_j$ having n elements, define $\mathbf{C}_n = \mathbf{I}_n - \overline{\mathbf{J}}_n$, the centering matrix of order n. Then, $\mathbf{X}'\mathbf{C}_n\mathbf{X}$ has terms $\sum_i(x_{ij} - \overline{x}_{.j})^2$ in its diagonal and terms $\sum_i(x_{ij} - \overline{x}_{.j})(x_{ij'} - \overline{x}_{.j'})$ as its off-diagonal elements, with $\overline{x}_{.j} = \mathbf{1}_n'\mathbf{x}_j/n$. It is the matrix of sums of squares and products corrected for the mean.

If $\boldsymbol{\Delta}$ is defined as the diagonal matrix of the diagonal elements of $\mathbf{X}'\mathbf{C}\mathbf{X}$, then the correlation matrix $\mathbf{P} = \mathbf{D}^{-1/2}\boldsymbol{\Sigma}\mathbf{D}^{-1/2}$ described earlier is estimated by $\mathbf{R} = \boldsymbol{\Delta}^{-1/2}\mathbf{X}'\mathbf{C}\mathbf{X}\boldsymbol{\Delta}^{-1/2}$.

The Multivariate Normal Distribution

The density function of a normally distributed random variable x having mean μ and variance σ^2 is $\{\exp[-\frac{1}{2}(x - \mu)^2/\sigma^2]\}/(2\pi\sigma^2)^{1/2}$. The counterpart of this for a vector $\mathbf{x}$ of random variables distributed $\mathrm{N}(\boldsymbol{\mu}, \boldsymbol{\Sigma})$, meaning that it has mean $\boldsymbol{\mu}$ and variance–covariance matrix $\boldsymbol{\Sigma}$, and having a **multivariate normal distribution**, is $\{\exp[-\frac{1}{2}(\mathbf{x} - \boldsymbol{\mu})'\boldsymbol{\Sigma}^{-1}(\mathbf{x} - \boldsymbol{\mu})]\}/(|2\pi\boldsymbol{\Sigma}|)^{1/2}$. The **moment generating function** of linear combinations $\mathbf{Kx}$ of $\mathbf{x}$ is $\exp(\mathbf{t}'\mathbf{K}\boldsymbol{\mu} + \frac{1}{2}\mathbf{t}'\mathbf{K}\boldsymbol{\Sigma}\mathbf{K}'\mathbf{t})$.

A very neat consequence of using matrices is the derivation of marginal and conditional distributions in the multivariate normal distribution $\mathbf{x} \sim N(\boldsymbol{\mu}, \boldsymbol{\Sigma})$. It stems from partitioning $\mathbf{x}$, $\boldsymbol{\mu}$, and $\boldsymbol{\Sigma}$ as

$$\mathbf{x} = \begin{bmatrix} \mathbf{x}_1 \\ \mathbf{x}_2 \end{bmatrix}, \qquad \boldsymbol{\mu} = \begin{bmatrix} \boldsymbol{\mu}_1 \\ \boldsymbol{\mu}_2 \end{bmatrix} \quad \text{and}$$

$$\boldsymbol{\Sigma} = \begin{bmatrix} \boldsymbol{\Sigma}_{11} & \boldsymbol{\Sigma}_{12} \\ \boldsymbol{\Sigma}_{21} & \boldsymbol{\Sigma}_{22} \end{bmatrix}$$

with $\boldsymbol{\Sigma}_{21} = (\boldsymbol{\Sigma}_{12})'$. Then a marginal distribution is

$$\mathbf{x}_1 \sim N(\boldsymbol{\mu}_1, \boldsymbol{\Sigma}_{11})$$

and a conditional distribution is

$$\mathbf{x}_1|\mathbf{x}_2 \sim N[\boldsymbol{\mu}_1 + \boldsymbol{\Sigma}_{12}\boldsymbol{\Sigma}_{22}^{-1}(\mathbf{x}_2 - \boldsymbol{\mu}_2),$$

$$\boldsymbol{\Sigma}_{11} - \boldsymbol{\Sigma}_{12}\boldsymbol{\Sigma}_{22}^{-1}\boldsymbol{\Sigma}_{21}].$$

Details are available in Searle [3, Section 2.4f].

Quadratic Forms

Every sum of squares is a homogeneous second-degree function of data. It can therefore be represented as a quadratic form $\mathbf{x}'\mathbf{Ax}$ for $\mathbf{x}$ being the vector of data and $\mathbf{A}$ being symmetric. A variety of properties pertaining to $\mathbf{x}'\mathbf{Ax}$ are then available for whatever sums of squares one is interested in. Some of these properties for $\mathbf{x} \sim N(\boldsymbol{\mu}, \boldsymbol{\Sigma})$ are as follows:

1. $E(\mathbf{x}'\mathbf{Ax}) = \text{tr}(\mathbf{A}\boldsymbol{\Sigma}) + \boldsymbol{\mu}'\mathbf{A}\boldsymbol{\mu}$ (normality is not needed for this result);
2. $\text{var}(\mathbf{x}'\mathbf{Ax}) = 2\text{tr}(\mathbf{A}\boldsymbol{\Sigma})^2 + 4\boldsymbol{\mu}'\mathbf{A}\boldsymbol{\Sigma}\mathbf{A}\boldsymbol{\mu}$;
3. $\mathbf{x}'\mathbf{Ax}$ has a (noncentral) **chi-square distribution** if and only if $\mathbf{A}\boldsymbol{\Sigma}$ is idempotent;
4. $\mathbf{x}'\mathbf{Ax}$ and $\mathbf{Lx}$ are stochastically independent if and only if $\mathbf{L}\boldsymbol{\Sigma}\mathbf{A} = \mathbf{0}$;
5. $\mathbf{x}'\mathbf{Ax}$ and $\mathbf{x}'\mathbf{Bx}$ are stochastically independent if and only if $\mathbf{B}\boldsymbol{\Sigma}\mathbf{A} = \mathbf{0}$ or, equivalently, $\mathbf{A}\boldsymbol{\Sigma}\mathbf{B} = \mathbf{0}$.

Regression and Linear Models

There is an enormous volume of literature on these topics, most of it using matrix algebra. Only a minute sampling of it is given here.

Consider a vector of data $\mathbf{y}$, modeled as having expected value $E(\mathbf{y}) = \mathbf{X}\boldsymbol{\beta}$ with $\mathbf{X}$ being known and $\boldsymbol{\beta}$ being a vector of unknown parameters. Defining $\boldsymbol{\varepsilon}$ as $\mathbf{y} - E(\mathbf{y})$, a vector of residuals leads to modeling $\mathbf{y}$ as $\mathbf{y} = \mathbf{X}\boldsymbol{\beta} + \boldsymbol{\varepsilon}$. **Least squares** estimation of $\boldsymbol{\beta}$ dictates minimizing $(\mathbf{y} - \mathbf{X}\boldsymbol{\beta})'(\mathbf{y} - \mathbf{X}\boldsymbol{\beta})$ with respect to $\boldsymbol{\beta}$ and taking the resulting value of $\boldsymbol{\beta}$, say $\hat{\boldsymbol{\beta}}$, as the estimator of $\boldsymbol{\beta}$. This leads to the equations $\mathbf{X}'\mathbf{X}\hat{\boldsymbol{\beta}} = \mathbf{X}'\mathbf{y}$. In regression (*see* **Multiple Linear Regression**) $\mathbf{X}$ almost always has full column rank, so that $\mathbf{X}'\mathbf{X}$ is nonsingular and hence $\hat{\boldsymbol{\beta}} = (\mathbf{X}'\mathbf{X})^{-1}\mathbf{X}'\mathbf{y}$. But with many more **general linear models** $(\mathbf{X}'\mathbf{X})^{-1}$ does not exist and a generalized inverse $(\mathbf{X}'\mathbf{X})^-$ has to be used. In that case there are many solutions for $\hat{\boldsymbol{\beta}}$, and to indicate this they can be denoted by $\boldsymbol{\beta}^o$. Thus, $\boldsymbol{\beta}^o = (\mathbf{X}'\mathbf{X})^-\mathbf{X}'\mathbf{y}$.

Since $\boldsymbol{\beta}^o$ becomes $\hat{\boldsymbol{\beta}}$ when $(\mathbf{X}'\mathbf{X})^{-1}$ exists, the properties of $\hat{\boldsymbol{\beta}}$ are included among those of $\boldsymbol{\beta}^o$, just a few of which are as follows:

1. There are many solutions, $\boldsymbol{\beta}^o$, but for each of them $\hat{\mathbf{y}} = \mathbf{X}\boldsymbol{\beta}^o = \mathbf{X}(\mathbf{X}'\mathbf{X})^-\mathbf{X}'\mathbf{y}$ is the same, because $\mathbf{X}(\mathbf{X}'\mathbf{X})^-\mathbf{X}'$ is invariant to $(\mathbf{X}'\mathbf{X})^-$.
2. $E(\boldsymbol{\beta}^o) \neq \boldsymbol{\beta}$, but $E(\mathbf{X}\boldsymbol{\beta}^o) = \mathbf{X}\boldsymbol{\beta}$.
3. The residual sum of squares

$$\text{SSE} = (\mathbf{y} - \hat{\mathbf{y}})'(\mathbf{y} - \hat{\mathbf{y}}) = \mathbf{y}'\mathbf{y} - \mathbf{y}'\mathbf{X}(\mathbf{X}'\mathbf{X})^-\mathbf{X}'\mathbf{y}$$

is invariant to $(\mathbf{X}'\mathbf{X})^-$. Because it can be expressed as $\text{SSE} = \mathbf{y}'[\mathbf{I} - \mathbf{X}(\mathbf{X}'\mathbf{X})^-\mathbf{X}']\mathbf{y}$, with the matrix being idempotent, the expected value of SSE for $\mathbf{y} \sim N(\mathbf{X}\boldsymbol{\beta}, \sigma^2\mathbf{I}_N)$ is $E(\text{SSE}) = [N - r(\mathbf{X})]\sigma^2$. Also, SSE/σ^2 has a chi-square distribution. Moreover, the sum of squares due to fitting the model is $\mathbf{y}'\mathbf{X}(\mathbf{X}'\mathbf{X})^-\mathbf{X}'\mathbf{y}$; it too has a (noncentral) chi-square distribution, and it is stochastically independent of SSE.

Readers whose appetite has been whetted by this introduction to regression and linear models will find plenty of books and papers to satiate their hunger.

References

[1]   Henderson, H.V. & Searle, S.R. (1979). Vec and vech operators for matrices, with some uses in Jacobians and multivariate statistics, *Canadian Journal of Statistics* **7**, 65–81.

[2]   Henderson, H.V. & Searle, S.R. (1981). The vec permutation matrix, the vec operator and Kronecker

products: a review, *Linear and Multilinear Algebra* **9**, 271–288.

[3] Searle, S.R. (1971). *Linear Models*. Wiley, New York.

[4] Searle, S.R. (1982). *Matrix Algebra Useful for Statistics*. Wiley, New York.

(*See also* **Matrix Computations**)

SHAYLE R. SEARLE

Matrix Computations

Much of the development and formulation of the mathematical and statistical models that biostatisticians use relies heavily on matrix notation (*see* **Matrix Algebra**). For example, matrix notation is often the preferred way to describe the mathematics underlying many of the procedures in statistical packages (*see* **Software, Biostatistical**). Routines are now widely available that implement standard matrix operations including matrix multiplication and the solution of systems of linear equations, facilitating computer implementation of matrix formulas presented in the literature. Some knowledge of the alternative available **algorithms** is helpful both for implementers of matrix formulas and for users of existing statistical package implementations. In the following we comment on some alternative widely used approaches to linear **least squares** and related calculations.

Areas where matrix computations have a large place include **regression** methods, **multivariate analysis, maximum likelihood** estimation, **robust** estimation, smoothing, and **optimization**. Linear matrix computational methods are more generally important because nonlinear problems are frequently handled by solving a sequence of linearized problems. Numerical linear algebra is, effectively, another name for matrix computations.

Modern numerical matrix algebra gains much of its power from the use of a relatively small number of matrix decompositions, whose numerical properties are well understood. Major aims are guaranteed accuracy, speed of computation (efficiency), and the ability to handle all inputs [6, 7, 9]. The article [9] discusses several topics that we omit or only mention in passing.

Implementing Matrix Computations

Matrix computations must reckon with the finite precision of computer arithmetic. Most common computers now implement the IEEE standard for **floating point arithmetic**, which has around seven decimal digits single-precision and around 16 decimal digit double-precision arithmetic. The double-precision standard is a sound basis on which to build accurate and reliable algorithms.

Technical accuracy and efficiency issues are reasons for providing expert "black box" implementations of what might appear simple calculations such as $||\mathbf{x}|| = (\mathbf{x}'\mathbf{x})^{1/2}$ and matrix multiplication. Specifications for sets of lower-level routines have been established in the **numerical analysis** literature, where they are known as BLAS (basic linear algebra subroutines) [1]. The BLAS, or other such lower-level routines, then make effective building blocks in the creation of higher-level routines.

Understanding Matrix Methods

There are often, in matrix computations just as elsewhere, several different ways to solve the same problem. Knowledge of matrix algorithms may allow the substitution of one algorithm for another when required. For example, a published formula may involve a matrix operation not found in available software. Additional information that is required from a routine may be available, for someone who understands the algorithm, as an adaptation of existing output.

Often it is helpful to know what accuracy can reasonably be expected from a calculation. When results from different algorithms for the same problem differ numerically (perhaps in decimal places after the third or fourth), which is more accurate? What characteristics of input data may lead to such differences in accuracy? Knowledge of the algorithm may be even more important when a calculation fails.

Matrix Inversion

The use of matrix inverses is a convenience in writing down matrix formulas. However, direct implementation of such formulas rarely leads to algorithms that are optimal for practical computation. For example, solving $\mathbf{Sb} = \mathbf{c}$ for $\mathbf{b}$ is preferable to forming $\mathbf{S}^{-1}$ and computing $\mathbf{b} = \mathbf{S}^{-1}\mathbf{c}$. Avoiding unnecessary matrix inversion reduces computational effort, leading to a small improvement in precision. There is a choice of default actions where the inverse does not exist. Later in this article we illustrate approaches which avoid the explicit calculations of matrix inverses.

Linear Least Squares

Linear **least squares** has been the context for much of the discussion of statistical matrix computations. As well as being important for linear least squares, the matrix computations we describe are important building blocks for many other statistical computations.

We consider the contrived example

$$(\mathbf{X}|\mathbf{y}) = \begin{bmatrix} 1 & 7 & 8 & 6 \\ 1 & -3 & 4 & 4 \\ 1 & 2 & 2 & 0 \\ 1 & 2 & 2 & 6 \\ 1 & 7 & 6 & 5 \\ 1 & 2 & 4 & 7 \\ 1 & -3 & 2 & 3 \\ 1 & 2 & 4 & 1 \\ 1 & 2 & 4 & 4 \end{bmatrix}.$$

Given $\mathbf{X}(n \times p)$ and $\mathbf{y}(n \times 1)$, least squares calculations determine $\mathbf{b}(p \times 1)$ such that

$$(\mathbf{y} - \mathbf{Xb})'(\mathbf{y} - \mathbf{Xb}) = ||\mathbf{y} - \mathbf{Xb}||^2 \qquad (1)$$

is a minimum. In the example above one minimizes the sum of squares $[6 - (b_1 + 7b_2 + 8b_3)]^2 + [4 - (b_1 - 3b_2 + 4b_3)]^2 + \cdots$

Algebraically, the linear least squares problem (1) is equivalent to solving what are called the normal equations, i.e.

$$\mathbf{X'Xb} = \mathbf{X'y}. \qquad (2)$$

If $\mathbf{S} = \mathbf{X'X}$ is singular, theoretical arguments show that the normal equations are consistent, but rather than just one solution there are an infinity of solutions. An example appears below in the section on linear dependencies.

We describe and contrast two approaches to the linear least squares problem, one of which forms and solves the normal equations, while the other (the QR method) avoids formation of the normal equations.

A Normal Equation Approach

An effective way to solve the normal equations is to use the Cholesky algorithm, which modifies Gaussian elimination to take advantage of the symmetry of the normal equation matrix of coefficients. Diagrammatically, the steps are

$$(\mathbf{X}|\mathbf{y}) \rightarrow \begin{pmatrix} \mathbf{X'X} & \mathbf{X'y} \\ (\mathbf{X'y})' & \mathbf{y'y} \end{pmatrix} \rightarrow \begin{pmatrix} \mathbf{R} & \mathbf{d} \\ \mathbf{0'} & r_{yy} \end{pmatrix}. \qquad (3)$$

The normal equations $\mathbf{X'Xb} = \mathbf{X'y}$ reduce to $\mathbf{Rb} = \mathbf{d}$, where $\mathbf{R}$ is $p \times p$ upper triangular, i.e. below diagonal elements are zero. (It might also be described as right triangular, which perhaps justifies the symbol $\mathbf{R}$.) It is convenient to take $\mathbf{R}$ to be the upper triangular matrix which is formed by the Cholesky decomposition of $\mathbf{X'X}$, i.e. $\mathbf{R'R} = \mathbf{X'X}$. On the right-hand side of (3), $\mathbf{R}$ is augmented with an additional row and column, to form an array which is the Cholesky decomposition of $(\mathbf{X}|\mathbf{y})'(\mathbf{X}|\mathbf{y})$.

For our numerical example the system of equations $\mathbf{Rb} = \mathbf{d}$ is

$$\begin{pmatrix} 3 & 6 & 12 \\ 0 & 10 & 4 \\ 0 & 0 & 4 \end{pmatrix} \begin{pmatrix} b_1 \\ b_2 \\ b_3 \end{pmatrix} = \begin{pmatrix} 12 \\ 2 \\ 2 \end{pmatrix}.$$

Calculations are completed by solving first for $b_3 \left(= \frac{1}{2} \right)$, then for $b_2 (= 0)$ in terms of b_3, and finally for $b_1 (= 2)$ in terms of b_2 and b_3.

The QR Method for Linear Least Squares

Our description will emphasize points of contact with the normal equations approach. The QR method omits the intermediate step in (3). It determines

$$\mathbf{Q}(\mathbf{X}|\mathbf{y}) = \begin{pmatrix} \mathbf{R} & \mathbf{d} \\ \mathbf{0} & \mathbf{z} \end{pmatrix}, \qquad (4)$$

where $\mathbf{Q}(n \times n)$ is a product of orthogonal matrices and is hence orthogonal, i.e. $\mathbf{Q'Q} = \mathbf{QQ'} = \mathbf{I} = \mathrm{diag}(1, \dots, 1)$. The vector $\mathbf{z}$ is $(n - p) \times 1$. If we insist that $\mathbf{R}$ have positive diagonal elements, then it is algebraically identical to the matrix $\mathbf{R}$ formed by the Cholesky decomposition of $\mathbf{X'X}$. The quantity $\mathbf{z'z}$ is the sum of squares of residuals from the regression, and equals r_{yy}^2.

Other Methods for Least Squares

Other methods for least squares include the once popular Gauss–Jordan scheme, which calculates $(\mathbf{X}'\mathbf{X})^{-1}$ as well as $\mathbf{b}$. There are in addition a range of iterative methods for least squares, which have found particular application in large sparse problems [3, 6, 9].

Linear Dependencies

In the data set

$$(\mathbf{X}|\mathbf{y}) = \begin{bmatrix} 1 & -2 & -4 & -1 \\ 1 & 1 & -1 & 0 \\ 1 & 2 & 0 & 4 \\ 1 & 5 & 3 & 7 \end{bmatrix},$$

the third column is the difference between the second column and twice the first column. Linear dependencies, of which this is a trivial example, arise in least squares problems when one or more variables are a linear combination of earlier variables. The normal equations are

$$\begin{pmatrix} 4 & 6 & -2 \\ 6 & 34 & 22 \\ -2 & 22 & 26 \end{pmatrix} \begin{pmatrix} b_1 \\ b_2 \\ b_3 \end{pmatrix} = \begin{pmatrix} 10 \\ 45 \\ 25 \end{pmatrix}.$$

The matrix of coefficients $\mathbf{S} = \mathbf{X}'\mathbf{X}$ is, because the coefficients in row 3 are the difference between row 2 and twice row 1, *singular*. Hence $\mathbf{S}^{-1}$ does not exist. Nevertheless the coefficients are, because from normal equations, consistent. With b_3 chosen arbitrarily, $b_2 = 1.2 - b_3$ and $b_1 = 0.7 + 2b_3$. Such nonunique solutions occur when one variable or term in a model is a linear combination of other terms.

In **analysis of variance** applications, dependencies may arise because there are inadequate data to allow the estimation of one or more parameters associated with main effects or interactions. Alternately, one or more **explanatory** variables may be an exact linear combination of other terms in the model, and a decision is needed on which terms to include. Dependencies may be a result of an unanticipated feature of the input data, or of a mistake in the data.

Dependencies are, when working with observational data on a large number of variables, surprisingly common. They may be a huge source of frustration, especially if the program responds by exiting with an uninformative error message. Sensible

default actions, and information on the coefficients of the linear relation, may be a huge help. Where column i of $\mathbf{X}$ is a linear combination of earlier columns, an easy device which will allow calculations to continue is to set b_i to zero, effectively deleting column i of $\mathbf{X}$. It would be useful to have criteria for detecting instances where a near singularity may make results nonsensical or hard to interpret. Regrettably, there are no effective simple criteria that will cover all circumstances.

Normal Equations vs. QR

At a fixed level of numerical precision the QR decomposition will solve a wider range of problems than normal equation methods. The difference is marked when there are strong dependencies between the columns of $\mathbf{X}$, leading to a large **standard error** for one or more elements of $\mathbf{b}$. A consequence of large standard error(s) is that the additional numerical precision is unlikely to be statistically meaningful.

The solution of the normal equations retains very nearly the accuracy of $\mathbf{X}'\mathbf{X}$ and $\mathbf{X}'\mathbf{y}$. Where $\mathbf{X}$ has an initial column of ones, precision may be assisted by expressing values in remaining columns as differences from the column mean, prior to forming $\mathbf{X}'\mathbf{X}$ and $\mathbf{X}'\mathbf{y}$. Careful implementations of normal equation methods take this precaution. The precision of $\mathbf{X}'\mathbf{X}$ and $\mathbf{X}'\mathbf{y}$ is then equivalent to that of an accurately formed correlation matrix. In applications in the biological and social sciences, where differences from the mean are rarely accurate to more than two or three significant digits, this seems adequate precision.

Caution may nevertheless advise use of the QR method except in those applications – unbalanced analysis of variance, for example – where columns of $\mathbf{X}$ are unlikely to be highly correlated. There is a helpful discussion in [5] which compares the normal equation method with QR (see also [6]).

QR Algorithms

Another name for the QR method is orthogonal reduction to upper triangular form. Available algorithms for QR include Householder and modified Gram–Schmidt (MGS), which proceed columnwise, and the Givens algorithm, which operates on new rows one at a time to incorporate them into the current version of $\mathbf{R}$. We discuss these in more detail below.

Elements of $\mathbf{Q}$ are unlikely to be stored explicitly; instead, key quantities are stored from which $\mathbf{Q}$ can be reconstructed as required.

Algorithms for QR factorization effectively form rows of $\mathbf{R}$ as linear combinations of rows of $\mathbf{X}$ rather than as linear combinations of rows of $\mathbf{X}'\mathbf{X}$. They avoid the loss of accuracy which, in normal equation methods, may occur in the formation of $\mathbf{X}'\mathbf{X}$ and $\mathbf{X}'\mathbf{y}$. There is some additional computational cost. When p is much smaller than n, use of QR approximately doubles the number of multiplications and divisions compared with using the normal equations.

Various diagnostic and other information that may be required for least squares modeling may be computed straightforwardly from submatrices of $\mathbf{Q}$. Examples include leverage statistics (*see* **Diagnostics**), and the variance–**covariance matrix** of **residuals**. Brief details appear in a later section.

Some Key Matrix Methods

Here we discuss in more detail several algorithms that have major importance in statistical computation, including algorithms mentioned above. We emphasize the connections between algorithms which, to first appearance, are quite different.

Cholesky Decomposition

Given a positive definite matrix $\mathbf{S}$, perhaps formed as $\mathbf{X}'\mathbf{X}$, the Cholesky decomposition determines an upper triangular matrix $\mathbf{R}$ such that $\mathbf{S} = \mathbf{R}'\mathbf{R}$. Equivalently, one may form $\mathbf{S} = \mathbf{U}'\mathbf{D}\mathbf{U}$, where $\mathbf{D}$ is diagonal and $\mathbf{U}$ is upper triangular with unit diagonal.

Several algorithms are available, which differ in the order in which they form elements of $\mathbf{R}$. In the version we now describe, elements in the first row of $\mathbf{R}$ are formed as

$$r_{11} = \sqrt{s_{11}}, \qquad r_{1j} = r_{11}^{-1} s_{1j}, \quad j = 1, \ldots, p.$$

Then, for $i = 2, \ldots, p$, calculate

$$s_{ij}^{(i-1)} = s_{ij} - \sum_{k=1}^{i-1} r_{ki} r_{kj}, \quad j = i, \ldots, p,$$

and

$$r_{ii} = [s_{ii}^{(i-1)}]^{1/2}, \quad \text{if } (i < p) \; r_{ij} = r_{ii}^{-1} s_{ij}^{(i-1)},$$
$$j = i+1, \ldots, p.$$

Note that if $\mathbf{X}$ has an initial column of ones and remaining columns are centered by expressing values as differences from the column mean, then $1 - s_{ii}^{-1} s_{ii}^{(i-1)}$ is the squared multiple correlation measuring the dependence of column k of $\mathbf{X}$ on earlier columns. Where $r_{ii} = 0$, all elements in that row may be set to zero.

The Cholesky decomposition may be used in solving the generalized weighted least squares problem, where $\mathbf{W}$ is a positive-definite symmetric weighting matrix. Observe that if $\mathbf{U}$ is upper triangular such that $\mathbf{U}'\mathbf{U} = \mathbf{W}$, then

$$(\mathbf{y} - \mathbf{X}\mathbf{b})'\mathbf{W}(\mathbf{y} - \mathbf{X}\mathbf{b}) = (\mathbf{y}^* - \mathbf{X}^*\mathbf{b})'(\mathbf{y}^* - \mathbf{X}^*\mathbf{b}),$$

where $\mathbf{y}^* = \mathbf{U}\mathbf{y}, \mathbf{X}^* = \mathbf{U}\mathbf{X}$. This is now in the form of (1).

Simulation from a **multivariate normal distribution** with $p \times p$ variance–covariance matrix $\Sigma = \mathbf{R}'\mathbf{R}$ may be handled by setting $\mathbf{u} = \mathbf{R}'\mathbf{x}$, where elements of $\mathbf{x}$ are independent normal random deviates each with mean 0 and variance 1.

The Householder QR Algorithm

The Householder QR algorithm has wide application apart from least squares. It is, for example, used in forming the singular value decomposition, which we describe below. It is usually motivated by describing the matrix $\mathbf{Q}$ of (4) as a product of Householder *reflections*

$$\mathbf{I} - \frac{2\mathbf{w}_i\mathbf{w}_i'}{\tau_i}, \quad i = 1, \ldots, p,$$

where $\tau_i = ||\mathbf{w}_i||^2$. The first reflection reduces to zero elements all elements except the first in the initial column of $\mathbf{X}$, replacing the first row of $\mathbf{X}$ by the first row of $\mathbf{R}$. The second takes the matrix so formed and reduces to zero all elements below the second row in its second column, replacing the second row of this matrix with the second row of $\mathbf{R}$. In the adaptation of the Householder method, for which we give algebraic details, one or more rows of $\mathbf{R}$ may differ from the result of applying Householder reflections by a change of sign of all elements in the row [8]. This simplifies the detailed algebraic description and simplifies the algorithm.

Let $\mathbf{x}_j^{(k-1)}$ ($j \geq k$) be the result of applying rotations $1, \ldots, k-1$ to column j of $\mathbf{X}$, but with elements $1, \ldots, k-1$ set to zero when $k > 1$. Then

$$r_{kk} = \left\| \mathbf{x}_k^{(k-1)} \right\|, \qquad r_{kj} = r_{kk}^{-1} \left(\mathbf{x}_k^{(k-1)} \right)' \mathbf{x}_j^{(k-1)},$$
$$j > k. \qquad (5)$$

For elements in rows after the kth we use

$$\mathbf{x}_j^{(k)} = \mathbf{x}_j^{(k-1)} - \alpha_k^{-1} \left(x_{kj}^{(k-1)} \mathrm{sgn} \left(x_{kk}^{(k-1)} \right) \right.$$
$$\left. + r_{kj} \right) \mathbf{x}_k^{(k-1)}, \quad j > k,$$

where $\alpha_k = |x_{kk}| + r_{kk}$.

Where a column is a linear combination of earlier columns, this leads to $r_{ii} = 0$. The easiest way to deal with this is to move any such column to the final column position. More generally, the columns of $\mathbf{X}$ may be permuted so that columns which are highly dependent on earlier columns are taken last – a device known as *pivoting*. The initial order of columns can, if this is required, be restored when calculations are complete. Additional orthogonal rotations may be required to recover the matrix $\mathbf{R}$ that corresponds to the original ordering.

The Modified Gram–Schmidt QR Algorithm

If the variant of Householder just described is applied to a matrix $\mathbf{X}$ which is augmented with p initial rows of zeros, this leads, essentially, to the modified **Gram–Schmidt** (MGS) algorithm [8]. The MGS algorithm may be described in terms of residuals from repeated regressions. This statistical interpretation is a main reason for mentioning it here.

Let $\mathbf{e}_j^{(k-1)}$ be the vector of residuals when the column $j, j \geq k$, of $\mathbf{X}$ is regressed on columns $1, \ldots, k-1$. Then the MGS algorithm forms

$$r_{kk} = \left\| \mathbf{e}_k^{(k-1)} \right\|, \qquad r_{kj} = r_{kk}^{-1} \left(\mathbf{e}_k^{(k-1)} \right)' \mathbf{e}_j^{(k-1)}.$$

Thus the MGS algorithm uses least squares vectors of residuals to form elements of $\mathbf{R}$. For details see [3], [6], [7], [8], [10], and [11].

The Givens QR Algorithm

This algorithm operates on $\mathbf{X}$ one row at a time, where Householder and modified Gram–Schmidt operate on columns. It is useful where the QR decomposition must from time to time be updated as new data become available.

The matrix $\mathbf{R}$ is filled initially with zeros. Planar rotations,

$$\begin{pmatrix} \cos\theta & \sin\theta \\ -\sin\theta & \cos\theta \end{pmatrix}, \qquad (6)$$

then rotate rows of $\mathbf{X}$, one at a time, into the upper triangular array. Thus $\mathbf{R}$ is sequentially updated as each new row of $\mathbf{X}$ is rotated into the upper triangular scheme. The rotations which operate on row k ($k > p$) of $\mathbf{X}$ replace y_k with z_k, where z_k^2 is the increase in the residual sum of squares when row k is included. The planar rotations in the Givens QR algorithm are often called Givens rotations.

Another use for planar rotations is to remove rows that were earlier included, i.e. to *downdate* $\mathbf{R}$. A stable algorithm requires access to the matrix $\mathbf{Q}$ [3, 6]. The algorithm in [4] is as stable as possible when $\mathbf{Q}$ is not available.

Orthogonalization of the Columns of X

One way to view the QR method is that it reduces the problem of minimizing $\|\mathbf{y} - \mathbf{Xb}\|$ to that of minimizing $\|\mathbf{y} - \mathbf{X}^*\mathbf{b}^*\|$, where $\mathbf{X}^* = \mathbf{X}\mathbf{R}^{-1}$ and $\mathbf{b}^* = \mathbf{Rb}$. It replaces $\mathbf{X}$ by a matrix $\mathbf{X}^*$ the columns of which are orthogonal, i.e. $(\mathbf{X}^*)'\mathbf{X}^*$ is the matrix $\mathbf{I} = \mathrm{diag}(1, \ldots, 1)$.

Let

$$\mathbf{Q} = \begin{pmatrix} \mathbf{Q}_1 \\ \mathbf{Q}_2 \end{pmatrix}, \qquad (7)$$

where $\mathbf{Q}_1$ is $p \times n$ and $\mathbf{Q}_2$ is $(n - p) \times n$. Then it may be shown that $\mathbf{Q}_1' = \mathbf{X}\mathbf{R}^{-1}$. Thus, if $\mathbf{Q}$ is available, the matrix $\mathbf{X}^* = \mathbf{X}\mathbf{R}^{-1}$ can be extracted as a submatrix.

Orthogonal Polynomials

Low-order **polynomial** functions are frequently used to provide simple curvilinear models for data. If the covariate $\mathbf{x}$ has elements $x_i, i = 1, \ldots, n$, then calculations can in principle be handled as a least squares calculation in which $\mathbf{X}$ has its (i, j)th element equal to $x_i^{j-1}, i = 1, \ldots, n; j = 1, \ldots, p$. This natural representation of the problem produces a matrix $\mathbf{X}$ the columns of which are likely to be strongly **correlated**. This gives coefficients which are strongly correlated, with standard errors which are inflated by amounts which depend on the correlations.

The QR method may be used as discussed in (7) to form the matrix $\mathbf{X}^*$ with orthogonal columns.

The first column of $\mathbf{X}^*$ is a constant, the second is a multiple of $\mathbf{x} - \bar{x}$, the third involves terms up to degree two in $\mathbf{x}$, and so on. Even better is to use recurrence formulas for systems of orthogonal polynomials to generate the columns of $\mathbf{X}^*$ (*see* **Orthogonality**). Such use of orthogonal polynomials gives independent and often more interpretable regression coefficients and avoids numerical instability (*see* **Polynomial Approximation**).

The Deletion and Addition of Columns

Removal of a column of $\mathbf{X}$ is achieved by removing the corresponding column from $\mathbf{R}$ and using a series of Givens rotations to reduce the resulting matrix to upper triangular form. The addition of a further column $\mathbf{x}_{p+1}$ to $\mathbf{X}$ is likewise straightforward, providing $\mathbf{Q}$ is available. A further QR reduction is used to reduce $(\mathbf{R}, \mathbf{Q}\mathbf{x}_{p+1})$ to upper triangular form.

Singular Value Decomposition (SVD)

This decomposition finds application in principal components analysis and in many different related multivariate calculations. It offers yet another approach to least squares calculations [6]. Given an $n \times p$ matrix $\mathbf{X}$, it forms

$$\mathbf{X} = \mathbf{UGV}',$$

where $\mathbf{U}$ is $n \times n$ orthogonal, $\mathbf{V}$ is $p \times p$ orthogonal, and $\mathbf{G}$ is $n \times p$ with its only nonzero elements on the uppermost diagonal, namely the singular values.

One or more singular values that are close to zero indicates that $\mathbf{X}$ is near singular, with the relevant linear relations given by the corresponding columns of $\mathbf{V}$. Note that the singular values of $\mathbf{X}'\mathbf{X}$ are the squares of those of $\mathbf{X}$. The Golub–Kahan algorithm for the singular value decomposition first uses Householder reflections to reduce $\mathbf{X}$ to upper bidiagonal form, i.e. all elements are zero except those on the diagonal or in positions immediately above the diagonal. Repeated planar rotations, (6), then reduce the above diagonal elements to zero [6].

Methods for Singular Matrices

Here we examine several technical issues that arise when matrices are singular or close to singular.

Distance from Singularity

Assume that $\mathbf{X}$ has an initial column of ones and that remaining columns are centered. A statistically motivated measure of the distance of column k of $\mathbf{X}$ from a linear combination of all other columns is the inverse $(s_{kk}s^{kk})^{-1}$ of the *variance inflation factor* $s_{kk}s^{kk}$, where s_{kk} and s^{kk} are the kth diagonal elements of $\mathbf{X}'\mathbf{X}$ and $(\mathbf{X}'\mathbf{X})^{-1}$, respectively. This variance inflation factor is the amount by which the standard error of b_k is multiplied because of correlation between column k of $\mathbf{X}$ and other columns. Note the relationship

$$s_{kk}s^{kk} = \left(1 - R^2_{k|1,\ldots,k-1,k+1,\ldots,p}\right)^{-1}, \quad (8)$$

with the squared multiple correlation $R^2_{k|1,\ldots,k-1,k+1,\ldots,p}$ measuring the dependence of explanatory variable k upon other explanatory variables.

Which are the Linear Dependencies?

Let $\mathbf{r}_k^{(k-1)}$ consist of elements 1 to $k-1$ in column k of $\mathbf{R}$. Let $\mathbf{R}_{11}^{(k-1)}$ be the leading $(k-1) \times (k-1)$ submatrix of $\mathbf{R}$. Then the vector of coefficients in the least squares regression of column k of $\mathbf{X}$ on earlier columns is found by solving for $\mathbf{h}$ in

$$\mathbf{R}_{11}^{(k-1)}\mathbf{h} = \mathbf{r}_k^{(k-1)}.$$

(If $r_{ii} = 0$ for one or more $i < k$, then set $h_i = 0$.)

Suppose that m diagonal elements of $\mathbf{R}$ are zero. Then by determining all such vectors $\mathbf{h}$ we can construct a matrix $\mathbf{H}(p \times m)$ with maximum rank m such that

$$\mathbf{XH} = \mathbf{0}. \quad (9)$$

Columns of $\mathbf{H}$ have the form $(h_1, h_2, \ldots, h_{k-1}, -1, 0, \ldots, 0)'$. The columns of $\mathbf{H}$ are a basis for the orthogonal complement of the row space of $\mathbf{X}$. The general solution to the least squares problem is $\tilde{\mathbf{b}} = \mathbf{b} + \mathbf{Hc}$, where $\mathbf{c}$ is arbitrary. One way to make $\tilde{\mathbf{b}}$ unique is to choose $\mathbf{c}$ so that $\tilde{\mathbf{b}}$ has minimum length, which is itself a least squares problem [8, pp. 106–107, 119]. The easiest choice is $\mathbf{c} = \mathbf{0}$.

A Reflexive g-inverse of R

Let $\mathbf{R}^-$ be obtained from $\mathbf{R}$ by replacing zero diagonal elements r_{ii} with 1, inverting the resulting matrix, and then placing zeros in the rows and columns where $r_{ii} = 0$. Then

$$\mathbf{R}\mathbf{R}^-\mathbf{R} = \mathbf{R}, \mathbf{R}^-\mathbf{R}\mathbf{R}^- = \mathbf{R}^-,$$

which are the conditions for $\mathbf{R}^-$ to be a *reflexive g-inverse* of $\mathbf{R}$. The matrix $\mathbf{R}^-$ may be used in the calculation of variances and covariances of regression coefficients that correspond to the choice $\mathbf{c} = \mathbf{0}$ above.

Applications

We give a few examples where an elegant alternative to matrix inversion reduces computational effort. In part our aim is to move away from an exclusive focus on least squares.

Leverages and Standard Errors of Residuals

In least squares, the matrix $\mathbf{X}(\mathbf{X}'\mathbf{X})^{-1}\mathbf{X}'$ may be calculated as $\mathbf{X}\mathbf{R}^{-1}(\mathbf{X}\mathbf{R}^{-1})'$. If $(\mathbf{X}\mathbf{R}^{-1})'$ is not already available, it may be determined by solving for columns of $\mathbf{Q}_1$ in the lower triangular system of equations $\mathbf{R}'\mathbf{Q}_1 = \mathbf{X}'$ (cf. (7)). The leverage statistic h_i, which is the ith diagonal element of $\mathbf{X}(\mathbf{X}'\mathbf{X})^{-1}\mathbf{X}'$, may be calculated as the sum of squares of elements of the ith column of $\mathbf{Q}_1$. Note also that $\mathbf{I} - \mathbf{X}(\mathbf{X}'\mathbf{X})^{-1}\mathbf{X}' = \mathbf{Q}_2'\mathbf{Q}_2$. Thus $\mathbf{Q}_2$ may be used in calculating the variance–covariance matrix of residuals.

Partial Sums of Squares and Products

We show how to form partial correlations between columns of $\mathbf{Y}$ ($n \times q$), conditional on columns of $\mathbf{X}$ ($n \times p$). Let $\mathbf{Z} = (\mathbf{1}, \mathbf{X}, \mathbf{Y})$, where $\mathbf{1}$ is a column of ones. Now use the QR algorithm to form

$$\mathbf{QZ} = \begin{pmatrix} \sqrt{n} & \mathbf{u}_1' & \mathbf{u}_2' \\ \mathbf{0} & \mathbf{R}_{XX} & \mathbf{R}_{XY} \\ \mathbf{0} & \mathbf{0} & \mathbf{R}_{YY} \end{pmatrix}, \qquad (10)$$

where $\mathbf{u}_1'$ is $1 \times p$, $\mathbf{u}_2'$ is $1 \times q$, $\mathbf{R}_{XX}$ is $p \times p$, $\mathbf{R}_{XY}$ is $p \times q$, and $\mathbf{R}_{YY}$ is $q \times q$.

Then $\mathbf{R}_{YY}'\mathbf{R}_{YY}$ is the matrix of sums of squares and products of the q vectors of residuals from the regressions of columns of $\mathbf{Y}$ on columns of $\mathbf{X}$. The corresponding matrix of partial correlations is $\mathbf{D}^{-1/2}\mathbf{R}_{YY}'\mathbf{R}_{YY}\mathbf{D}^{-1/2}$, where $\mathbf{D}^{-1/2}$ is the diagonal matrix whose elements are the inverses of the square roots of the diagonal elements of $\mathbf{R}_{YY}'\mathbf{R}_{YY}$.

Canonical Correlation

We assume the orthogonal reduction in (10) above. Then computations may be handled by solving the symmetric eigenproblem

$$|\mathbf{R}_{XY}'\mathbf{R}_{XY} - \lambda \mathbf{R}_{YY}'\mathbf{R}_{YY}| = \mathbf{0}. \qquad (11)$$

This may be rewritten as

$$|(\mathbf{R}_{XY}\mathbf{R}_{YY}^{-1})'\mathbf{R}_{XY}\mathbf{R}_{YY}^{-1} - \lambda \mathbf{1}| = \mathbf{0},$$

which can be solved by finding the singular value decomposition of $\mathbf{R}_{XY}\mathbf{R}_{YY}^{-1}$. The **canonical correlations** ϕ_i, where i runs from 1 to min [rank ($\mathbf{R}_{XX}$), rank ($\mathbf{R}_{YY}$)], are given by

$$\phi_i^2 = \frac{\lambda_i}{1 + \lambda_i}$$

([8, pp. 200–202, 206–208]; *see* **Eigenvalue; Eigenvector**).

Canonical Variate Analysis

Canonical variate analysis provides a perspective on **multivariate analysis of variance**. Let $\mathbf{Z} = (\mathbf{X}, \mathbf{Y})$, where now columns of $\mathbf{Z}$ specify the groups to which observations belong. Again the orthogonal reduction of $\mathbf{Z}$ to upper triangular form is an effective starting point for further calculations, leading to an eigenproblem of the same form as for canonical correlation [8, pp. 202–203, 208–210].

Matrix Condition Numbers

A matrix *condition number* κ for a matrix $\mathbf{S}$ provides an indication of the relative sensitivity of $\mathbf{Sd}$ or $\mathbf{S}^{-1}\mathbf{d}$ to small relative changes in the elements of $\mathbf{d}$. One possibility is the *spectral condition number* κ_2, which is the ratio $\lambda_{\max}/\lambda_{\min}$ of the largest to smallest eigenvalue of $\mathbf{S}$.

Let $k = \log_{10} \kappa_2(\mathbf{S})$. In general one can expect to lose k digits of accuracy when solving the linear system

$$\mathbf{Sx} = \mathbf{d}$$

for $\mathbf{x}$, or in computing the inverse of $\mathbf{S}$. Note that $\kappa_2(\mathbf{S}) \geq 1$, which means that relative error can never be expected to decrease in solving a linear system. A matrix whose condition number is no more than

10 or 100 is, from a computational perspective, well-conditioned.

Numerical and Statistical Measures of Conditioning

Let κ_2 be the spectral condition number of the correlation matrix derived from $\mathbf{X'X}$. Then

$$\max_{1 \leq i \leq p} (s_{ii}s^{ii}) \leq \kappa_2 \leq \sum_{i=1}^{p} s_{ii}s^{ii},$$

where s_{ii} and s^{ii} are defined as in (8). This makes a connection between statistical and numerical measures of conditioning [2; 8, p. 211]. The quantity $s_{ii}s^{ii}$ has the benefit that, unlike matrix condition numbers such as κ_2, it is independent of scale.

Note that determination of the minimum value $\min_{\mathbf{b}} \|\mathbf{y} - \mathbf{Xb}\|^2$ is well-conditioned, even if $\mathbf{X}$ is singular.

Components of Larger Computations

The notes on computational methods in [5] demonstrate extensive use of matrix calculations as building blocks for a wide variety of other statistical calculations, analysis of variance with multiple error strata (*see* **Multilevel Models**), **generalized linear models** (GLMs), **generalized additive models** (GAMs), local regression smoothing (loess) (*see* **Graphical Displays**), and **nonparametric regression**; see also [11]. New complications are inevitable as matrix computational methods are used to extend the range of models available to statisticians. In models where a variance–covariance structure must be estimated, the notion of a singularity has subtleties beyond those of ordinary least squares.

Software

Many statistical packages allow the user to specify calculations as a sequence of matrix operations. SAS (in the IML Interactive Matrix Language module), SPSS (MATRIX language), STATA, **S-PLUS**, and Genstat are some of the statistical systems which have extensive matrix computational abilities. Statistical packages have generally stayed with normal equation methods. S-PLUS makes extensive use of modern methods such as QR. Note also the extensive modern matrix abilities in the mathematically oriented languages of MATLAB, Gauss, and Mathematica. MATLAB has been used extensively by numerical analysts [7].

The FORTRAN subroutine package LAPACK [1], and earlier packages LINPACK, and EISPACK from which LAPACK is derived, provide high-quality software to perform calculations referred to in this article. These packages are publicly available from the NETLIB online database, and are also part of the NAG and IMSL subroutine libraries.

References

[1]   Anderson, E., Bai, Z., Bischof, C., Demmel, J., Dongarra, J., Du Croz, J., Greenbaum, A., Hammarling, S., McKenney, A., Ostrouchov, S. & Sorenen, D. (1992). *LAPACK Users' Guide*. SIAM, Philadelphia.

[2]   Berk, K.N. (1977). Tolerance and condition in regression equations, *Journal of the American Statistical Association* **72**, 863–866.

[3]   Björck, A. (1996). *Numerical Methods for Least Squares Problems*. SIAM, Philadelphia.

[4]   Bojanczyk, A.W., Brent, R.P., van Dooren, P. & de Hoog, F.R. (1987). A note on downdating the Cholesky factorization, *SIAM Journal of Scientific and Statistical Computation* **8**, 210–221.

[5]   Chambers, J.M. & Hastie, T.J. (1991). *Statistical Models in S*. Wadsworth and Brooks/Cole, Pacific Grove.

[6]   Golub, G.H. & Van Loan, C.F. (1996). *Matrix Computations*, 3rd Ed. Johns Hopkins University Press, Baltimore.

[7]   Higham, N.J. (1996). *Accuracy and Stability of Numerical Algorithms*. SIAM, Philadelphia.

[8]   Maindonald, J.H. (1984). *Statistical Computation*. Wiley, New York.

[9]   Stewart, G.W. (1982). Linear algebra, computational, in *Encyclopedia of Statistical Sciences*, Vol. 5, S. Kotz, N.L. Johnson & C.B. Read, eds. Wiley, New York, pp. 5–19.

[10]   Stoer, J. & Bulirsch, R. (1992). *Introduction to Numerical Analysis*, 2nd Ed. Springer-Verlag, New York.

[11]   Thisted, R.A. (1988). *Elements of Statistical Computation. Numerical Computation*. Chapman & Hall, New York.

JOHN H. MAINDONALD & GORDON K. SMYTH

Matrix Method to Adjust for Misclassification *see* Misclassification Error

Maximum Concentration *see* Bioequivalence

Maximum Likelihood

The term "maximum likelihood" refers to a general method of **estimation** with important historical and practical significance for biostatistics. Consider a sample $y_1, y_2, \ldots, y_n$ drawn independently from a distribution with density or probability function $f(y; \theta)$ with an unknown vector parameter θ (*see* **Random Variable**). The **likelihood** function is defined as

$$L(\theta) = \prod_{i=1}^{n} f(y_i; \theta).$$

The maximum likelihood estimate (MLE) is the value $\theta = \hat{\theta}$ which maximizes $L(\theta)$ over the set of all possible values for θ. In practice, it is usually more convenient to maximize the logarithm of the likelihood function, $l(\theta) = \ln L(\theta)$. From calculus, it follows that $\hat{\theta}$ satisfies the score equation $\partial l / \partial \theta = 0$.

Early references to the method of maximum likelihood are attributed to **Gauss, Laplace**, and **Edgeworth** [4]. However, the prominent English statistician **R.A. Fisher** is unquestionably responsible for popularizing the technique and for identifying many of its statistical properties [3].

The method has a strong heuristic appeal: choose as your parameter estimate the one which makes the observed data seem most likely. As it turns out, it is often the best estimate possible, particularly in **large samples**. Inference is made easy by the fact that maximum likelihood estimates are **consistent** and asymptotically **normal** under broad regularity assumptions, with a variance that can be estimated from the observed or expected **information matrix**. The MLE is also invariant under one-to-one **transformations** of the parameters, so to obtain the MLE of a transformation of the original parameters, one need only apply the transformation to the original MLE.

Optimal Properties

The following is a list of the most important properties of the MLE in large samples (i.e. $n \to \infty$):

1. *Consistency.* The MLE **converges in probability** to the true value of the parameter.
2. *Asymptotic normality.* The distribution of $n^{1/2}(\hat{\theta} - \theta)$ converges to a normal distribution with zero mean and a covariance matrix which is the inverse of the information matrix $\mathbf{I}$. From a practical point of view it is more convenient to say that $\hat{\theta}$ is approximately distributed as $N(\theta, \mathbf{I}^{-1}/n)$.
3. *Asymptotic efficiency.* The MLE is the best asymptotically normal (**BAN**) estimate in terms of its variance in large samples. Put more precisely, if $\tilde{\theta}$ is another estimate such that $n^{1/2}(\tilde{\theta} - \theta) \xrightarrow{\mathscr{L}} N(\theta, \mathbf{C})$, where $\mathbf{C}$ is a fixed matrix, then $\mathbf{C} \geq \mathbf{I}^{-1}/n$ in the sense that $\mathbf{C} - \mathbf{I}^{-1}/n$ is a positive semidefinite matrix.

Regularity Conditions

It is important to be aware of the general regularity conditions for the optimal properties of the MLE. Most advanced statistics texts have a discussion of these conditions [1, 5], with the classic reference being Cramér [2]. The following three conditions are commonly given:

1. The observed data points $y_1, y_2, \ldots, y_n$ are independently and identically distributed (iid) according to a density or probability function $f(y; \theta)$, where θ has finite dimension m. This condition is less restrictive than it may seem, given that y_i may be a vector. In fact, the method of maximum likelihood is popular and appropriate for many regression problems where the distributions of the data points are not identical, and many texts give less restrictive assumptions.
2. The underlying density or probability function is identifiable, i.e. $f(y; \theta_1) = f(y; \theta_2)$ for all y implies that $\theta_1 = \theta_2$.
3. The density is "smooth" in the sense that f has derivatives up to the third order with finite expectation, and the information matrix

$$\mathbf{I} = E_\theta \left[\frac{\partial^2 \ln f(y; \theta)}{\partial \theta_j \partial \theta_k} \right], \quad j, k = 1, \ldots, m$$

exists and is nonsingular. The latter conditions ensure that the asymptotic covariance matrix exists.

These conditions are satisfied for many models of interest to biostatisticians, such as the **binomial**, normal, and **Poisson** distributions.

Maximum Likelihood Calculations

Maximum likelihood estimation involves finding a global maximum of a function of one or several parameters. For certain models, the solution can be expressed as a simple function of the data. However, more often the solution must be posed as a nonlinear **optimization** problem. Typically, it involves solving a system of nonlinear equations.

The main methods in use today are the Newton–Raphson (NR) or quasi-Newton (QN) methods, and the Fisher scoring (FS) algorithm [6]. The NR algorithm is based on an approximation of the log likelihood by a quadratic function through a Taylor series expansion of the score functions. To implement the NR algorithm, one has to provide second-order derivatives for the log likelihood function – the so-called Hessian matrix. Initial values for the parameters are updated and the process is repeated until convergence is obtained. If the initial value for parameters is close enough to the maximum, the NR algorithm usually converges quickly. However, if the initial value is poorly chosen it may fail. In particular, the Hessian matrix can become non-positive-definite. Upon convergence, at the final iteration, the inverse of the Hessian matrix provides an approximation to the asymptotic covariance of the MLE. In the QN algorithm only first derivatives are used, and the second derivatives are estimated based on results from previous iterations. The QN algorithm involves line search methods, i.e. maximization of the log likelihood along a given ray in the parameter space.

The difference between the NR and FS algorithms is that the latter uses the expectation of the Hessian matrix rather than the Hessian matrix itself as in the NR algorithm. There are two versions of the FS algorithm. In the first version the expectation of the Hessian is approximated as the sum of cross-products of first derivatives. In the second version, the exact calculated information matrix is used. Thus, to use this version of the FS algorithm one has to have a formula for the information matrix as a function of the parameters calculated prior to the maximization procedure.

Other methods are sometimes used for maximum likelihood estimation. One that deserves special mention is the **EM (expectation–maximization) algorithm**. Certain likelihoods may be thought as involving **missing data**, with the most notable example being **random effects** models. The EM method works in this setting by maximizing the expectation of the log-likelihood iteratively for the complete data. This may aid in difficult maximization problems by taking advantage of simple closed-form solutions available for the "M" stage. Other advantages of the EM algorithm include its natural statistical interpretation and its property of producing an increasing sequence of log likelihood values in the specified parameter space. The principal drawback is that it may be relatively slow.

Examples

Estimation of a Proportion

We observe the occurrence of a certain event for n individuals, where y_i is 1 if the event occurs and 0 otherwise. It can be assumed that events are independent among individuals and have the same probability of occurrence θ. The likelihood can be written as

$$L(\theta) = \prod_{i=1}^{n} \theta^{y_i}(1-\theta)^{1-y_i}$$
$$= \theta^m (1-\theta)^{n-m},$$

where m is the number of events observed among the n individuals. The log likelihood is

$$l(\theta) = m\ln(\theta) + (n-m)\ln(1-\theta). \qquad (1)$$

To find the maximum, we consider the following score equation:

$$\frac{\mathrm{d}l}{\mathrm{d}\theta} = m/\theta - (n-m)/(1-\theta) = 0, \qquad (2)$$

which has the unique solution $\hat{\theta} = m/n$.

Logistic Regression

Logistic regression may be viewed as a continuation of the previous example where the probability of the event occurring depends on some other factor. For instance, y could be an indicator of heart disease and x could denote the weight of an individual. We can model the relationship between y and x as the logistic function of the conditional probability of disease,

$$\Pr(y = 1|x) = \frac{\exp(\alpha + \beta x)}{1 + \exp(\alpha + \beta x)}, \quad (3)$$

or, equivalently,

$$\ln[\Pr(y = 1|x)/(1 - \Pr(y = 1|x)] = \alpha + \beta x.$$

Here $\theta = (\alpha, \beta)'$. The assumption is that the log **odds ratio** for the occurrence of disease is linear in the covariate, and β is sometimes referred to as the "log odds" parameter.

Now let $(y_1, x_1), (y_2, x_2), \ldots, (y_n, x_n)$ be values for the disease status and weight of a sample of n individuals. Technically speaking, to write down the likelihood we have to assume that x has a certain distribution which may contain unknown parameters. However, maximum likelihood inference for the logistic regression parameters is not affected by the assumption concerning the distribution of x as long as it does not depend on the parameters α and β. In fact, the values for x_i may be considered as fixed, known constants, and as long as the design matrix (*see* **Experimental Design in Biostatistics**) is of full rank, maximum likelihood estimation is valid. The log likelihood is

$$l(\alpha, \beta) = \sum_{i=1}^{n} y_i \ln \Pr(y = 1|x_i)$$

$$+ \sum_{i=1}^{n} (1 - y_i) \ln[1 - \Pr(y = 1|x_i)]$$

$$= \sum_{i=1}^{n} y_i \ln \frac{\exp(\alpha + \beta x_i)}{1 + \exp(\alpha + \beta x_i)}$$

$$+ \sum_{i=1}^{n} (1 - y_i) \ln \frac{1}{1 + \exp(\alpha + \beta x_i)}$$

$$= \alpha n + \beta \sum_{i=1}^{n} y_i x_i - \sum_{i=1}^{n} \ln[1 + \exp(\alpha + \beta x_i)].$$

A typical graph of the likelihood function is shown in Figure 1. The maximum of the log likelihood is found as the solution to the score equations

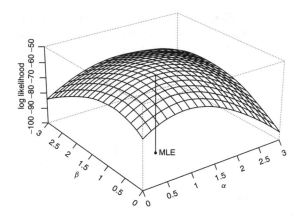

Figure 1 An example of the log likelihood surface and MLE in logistic regression

$$\frac{\partial l}{\partial \alpha} = n - \sum_{i=1}^{n} \frac{1}{1 + \exp(\alpha + \beta x_i)} = 0$$

and

$$\frac{\partial l}{\partial \beta} = \sum_{i=1}^{n} y_i x_i - \sum_{i=1}^{n} \frac{\exp(\alpha + \beta x_i)}{1 + \exp(\alpha + \beta x_i)} x_i = 0.$$

This system of nonlinear equations must be solved iteratively, e.g. by the Newton–Raphson algorithm.

Discussion and Extensions

In theory, the method of maximum likelihood is very simple: determine an appropriate sampling distribution for the data, write down the likelihood as a function of the unknown parameters, and solve for the estimate. Of course, in practice it is not always so easy. Solutions to the likelihood score equations usually must be arrived at by numerical methods, and may be computationally intensive or inaccurate. For some models and data sets it may be difficult to demonstrate that the likelihood has a unique global maximum. Many small-sample MLEs can be shown to be **biased**. The presence of **nuisance parameters** can exacerbate the computational difficulties. Often the MLE is quite non **robust** to **outliers** and, unlike competing general methods such as **least squares** and the **method of moments**, computation of the MLE requires that the distribution of the data be completely parameterized. Uniformly **minimum variance unbiased** (UMVU) **estimation** theory and **Bayesian methods** compete with maximum likelihood estimation with regard to optimal properties, but also require complete specification of the distribution, and may be even harder to implement.

To overcome some of the difficulties of maximum likelihood estimation, modified methods have been proposed such as **restricted maximum likelihood**, conditional likelihood (*see* **Conditionality Principle**), **pseudo-likelihood, quasi-likelihood, partial likelihood**, and M-estimation (*see* **Robustness**). These methods were all inspired by the powerful heuristic appeal and conceptual simplicity of the original formulation of the method of maximum likelihood.

References

[1] Cox, D.R. & Hinckley, D.V. (1974). *Theoretical Statistics*. Chapman & Hall, London.
[2] Cramér, H. (1945). *Mathematical Methods of Statistics*. Princeton University Press, Princeton.
[3] Rao, C.R. (1992). R.A. Fisher: The founder of modern statistics, *Statistical Science* **7**, 34–48.
[4] Stigler, S.M. (1986). *The History of Statistics: The Measurement of Uncertainty Before 1900*. Harvard University Press, Cambridge, Mass.
[5] Stuart, H. & Ord, J.K. (1991). *Kendall's Advanced Theory of Statistics*, Vol. 2. Oxford University Press, New York.
[6] Thisted, R.A. (1988). *Elements of Statistical Computing*. Chapman & Hall, New York.

TOR D. TOSTESON & EUGENE DEMIDENKO

Maximum Tolerated Dose *see* Phase I Trials

Maxwell, Albert Ernest

Born: July 7, 1916, in Rockmount, Co. Cavan, Ireland.
Died: 1996, in Leeds, UK.

Albert Ernest Maxwell was educated at the Royal School, Cavan and at Trinity College, Dublin, where he developed interests in psychology and mathematics. After graduating, 'Max' as he was invariably known to his colleagues, became a mathematics teacher at St Patrick's Cathedral School, Dublin. After only three years, at the age of 25, he was appointed Headmaster. His attempt to understand the behavioral problems of some of his pupils renewed his interest in psychology, a subject he eventually pursued more seriously at the University of Edinburgh where he was awarded a doctorate in 1950.

In 1952 Max left schoolteaching to take up the post of lecturer in statistics at the Institute of Psychiatry, a postgraduate school of the University of London. He was to spend the rest of his working life at the Institute, retiring in 1978 as Professor of Psychological Statistics.

For a number of years Max was a member of the Psychology Department of the Institute, collaborating and advising Professor Hans Eysenck, but he was eventually rewarded with the Headship of his own Biometrics Unit, which had responsibility for helping Institute researchers on all aspects of statistical design and analysis.

Max's main area of expertise was in **multivariate analysis**, particularly **factor analysis**, where his collaboration with Dr D. Lawley resulted in an important account of the mathematical theory behind the technique [1].

Max's teaching skills (no doubt learnt whilst a schoolmaster in Co. Cavan) were legendry and many psychologists obtained a firm grasp of statistical methods from his numerous lecture courses and a number of useful textbooks including [2].

References

[1] Lawley, D.N. & Maxwell, A.E. (1971). *Factor Analysis as a Statistical Method*, 2nd Ed. Butterworths, London.
[2] Maxwell, A.E. (1977). *Multivariate Analysis in Behavioural Research*. Chapman & Hall, London.

BRIAN EVERITT

McKendrick, Anderson Gray

Born: 1876
Died: 1943

McKendrick made important contributions to the mathematical theory of epidemics. He served as a lieutenant-colonel in the Indian Medical Service, and later became Curator of the College of Physicians at Edinburgh. In 1914 [2], he gave the solution of the general homogeneous birth process (*see* **Stochastic Processes**), and this was followed in 1926 by a major paper [3] on stochastic epidemics (*see* **Epidemic Models, Stochastic**). He then turned to deterministic models (*see* **Epidemic Models, Deterministic**), in a series of papers with W.O. Kermack, which included the celebrated Threshold Theorem (*see* **Epidemic Thresholds**). His work is described in some detail in [1].

References

[1]   Irwin, J.O. (1963). The place of mathematics in medical and biological statistics, *Journal of the Royal Statistical Society, Series A* **126**, 1–45.

[2]   McKendrick, A.G. (1914). Studies on the theory of continuous probabilities with special reference to its bearing on natural phenomena of a progressive nature, *Proceedings of the London Mathematical Society* **13**, 401–416.

[3]   McKendrick, A.G. (1926). Applications of mathematics to medical problems, *Proceedings of the Edinburgh Mathematical Society* **44**, 98–130.

McNemar Test

The McNemar test arose in the context of psychology in which two correlated dichotomous responses were to be compared. One example of this test would be an indication of a response or no response under two experimental conditions. The original paper was by McNemar [7]; see also [8].

Armitage and Berry [1] give an example in which we have two culture media and wish to determine if they are equally effective in detecting tubercle bacilli in sputum specimens. The two media, evaluated for the same sample of 50 specimens, give cell counts of positive and negative results, as given in Table 1.

This can be regarded as a single multinomial table in which the cell probabilities, denoted by $\{\pi_{ij}\}$, add to 1. If the two media have the same ability to detect the bacilli, the null hypothesis takes the form $\pi_{i+} = \pi_{+i}$, i.e. that the marginal proportions are the same. This is easily seen to be equivalent to $\pi_{12} = \pi_{21}$. Since only these probabilities are of interest, the hypothesis can be tested referring only

Table 1

		Medium B		
		+	−	Total
Medium A	+	20	12	32
	−	2	16	18
Total		22	28	50

to the counts in these off-diagonal cells. Let the cell counts be denoted by $\{n_{ij}\}$. The (uncorrected) test statistic is given by

$$X^2 = (n_{12} - n_{21})^2 / (n_{12} + n_{21}),$$

which (asymptotically) has a **chi-square distribution** with 1 **degree of freedom** (df). In this case $X^2 = (12 - 2)^2 / (12 + 2) = 7.14$. The test is equivalent to the binomial test that the proportion is 0.5, given that the observation lies in one of the off-diagonal cells. It has also been suggested that a continuity corrected test be used. This is equivalent to the continuity correction for the binomial test. The corrected form is $X^2 = (|12 - 2| - 1)^2 / (12 + 2) = 5.79$. In this case, both statistics are significant at the $\alpha = 0.05$ level.

Examples of this procedure also arise in diagnostic imaging studies when the investigator wishes to determine if a new method provides better diagnostic **sensitivity** and **specificity** than a standard method. In this situation, there are several options: one may compare only the sensitivity (diagnostic performance when the patients have the condition), or the specificity (diagnostic performance when the patients do not have the condition); it is sometimes suggested that the accuracy (proportion correct) be compared, but this comparison is quite sensitive to the proportion of positive and negative subjects, and is not recommended. For the comparison of sensitivity or specificity, a McNemar test can be formed, and the 1 df test can be made. This provides two tests, which may be contradictory in the sense that one test may have higher sensitivity while the other has higher specificity. The two tests may be combined by adding the χ^2 to get a 2 df test. This gives an overall test of common performance [3].

In diagnostic test comparisons, it is important to note that the investigators may be artificially imposing a two-category result on the data. For example, in diagnosing recurrent cancer, the outcomes might be "negative", "resectable", or "not resectable", and the implications of imposing two categories are unclear. In such a case, it seems relevant to examine the 3×3 matrix of categorizations, and use a procedure which formally tests for marginal symmetry. In addition, some misclassifications are more serious than others. This would imply that a weighted procedure might be used. Tests for this are referenced in [6].

The McNemar test can be generalized to equivalence testing [5]. Conditional logistic regression (*see* **Logistic Regression, Conditional**) can be used to adjust for covariates.

Sample size computations are based on comparing a binomial proportion to 0.5. These calculations give the number of discordant pairs (those not represented on the main diagonal). It is then required to determine what fraction of discordant pairs is likely to arise. Various methods have been proposed recently for this (e.g. [4] and [2]).

References

[1]   Armitage, P. & Berry, G. (1994). *Statistical Methods in Medical Research*, 3rd Ed. Blackwell Science, Oxford pp. 127–128.

[2]   Connor, R.J. (1987). Sample size for testing differences in proportions for the paired sample design, *Biometrics* **47**, 207–211.

[3]   Hamdan, M.A., Pirie, W.R. & Arnold, J.C. (1975). Simultaneous testing of McNemar's problem for several populations, *Psychometrika* **40**, 153–162.

[4]   Lachenbruch, P.A. (1992). On the sample size for studies based on McNemar's test, *Statistics in Medicine* **11**, 1521–1527.

[5]   Lee, M.L. & Lusher, J.M. (1991). The problem of therapeutic equivalence with paired qualitative data: an example from a clinical trial using haemophiliacs with inhibitors to Factor VIII, *Statistics in Medicine* **10**, 443–451.

[6]   Mantel, N. & Fleiss, J.L. (1975). The equivalence of the generalized McNemar's tests for marginal homogeneity in 2^3 and 3^2 tables, *Biometrics* **31**, 727–729.

[7]   McNemar, Q. (1947). Note on the sampling error of the difference between correlated proportions or percentages, *Psychometrika* **12**, 153–157.

[8]   Somes, G. (1985). McNemar test, *Encyclopedia of Statistical Sciences*, Vol. 5, S. Kotz & N. Johnson, eds. Wiley, New York, pp. 361–363.

(*See also* **Correlated Binary Data; Matched Pairs with Categorical Data; Rasch Models; Square Contingency Table**)

PETER A. LACHENBRUCH

Mean

The mean is a central concept in both data analysis and statistical theory. The usual sample mean is an arithmetic average of a set of n numerical observations, $x_1, x_2, x_3, \ldots, x_n$,

$$\bar{x} = \frac{\sum_{i=1}^{n} x_i}{n}.$$

The sample mean is nearly universally denoted by the symbol, $\bar{x}$, and is the most commonly used measure of central tendency of a set of numerical data.

In probability, the population mean, expected value or **expectation** of a **random variable** is the analog of the arithmetic or sample mean, $\bar{x}$. In fact, the **law of large numbers** implies that, for an infinitely large sample of independent random variables drawn from a distribution, the sample mean, $\bar{x}$, is equal to the expected value or mean of the distribution.

In any data analysis the usefulness of a summary statistic, such as the mean, depends on the details of the physical or biological process measured and specific summary information needed from the data. The sample mean can often be modified to provide the appropriate summary information. These modifications and their probability model analogs provide a rich source of both theory and numerical description of data sets.

Often each numerical observation does not have equal weight or importance. For example, the numerical observations themselves may be means of subgroups with different numbers of observations in each subgroup. In this case a *weighted mean* or average is used:

$$\bar{x}_w = \frac{\sum_{i=1}^{n} w_i x_i}{\sum_{i=1}^{n} w_i},$$

where w_i is the weight of the ith numerical observation. In the example where each observation represents a subgroup, the weight should be the number of units in the subgroup. This kind of weighted average is found in **analysis of variance, sample survey** analysis, and other more specialized areas.

Weighting can sometimes correct for sampling bias. A special case is when the probability that a unit is sampled is proportional to the variable of interest – an example of size-biased sampling. In this, weighting each observation by $w_i = 1/x_i$ yields

$$\bar{x}_h = \frac{\sum_{i=1}^{n} \frac{1}{x_i} x_i}{\sum_{i=1}^{n} \frac{1}{x_i}} = \frac{1}{\frac{1}{n} \sum_{i=1}^{n} \frac{1}{x_i}},$$

which is called the *harmonic mean*. The harmonic mean is found by taking the average value of the reciprocal of the data, $1/x_i$, and then taking the reciprocal of the average value. The harmonic mean is well defined only for positive data, i.e. when all possible values of the data are greater than 0. For positive data the harmonic mean is always less than or equal to the arithmetic mean.

The *geometric mean* can be used when measurements from natural processes have a distribution that is not symmetric and is **skewed** to the right. For skewed data the sample mean is not an adequate description of the center of the data. Both the theory of the **lognormal** distribution and practical data analysis justify the use of a log transformation of the original data,

$$y_i = \ln x_i.$$

Often the log transformed data will have a nearly symmetric distribution. In this case

$$\bar{y} = \frac{1}{n} \sum_{i=1}^{n} y_i$$

is a good measure of the center of the log transformed data. Transforming $\bar{y}$ back to the original scale of the data yields the geometric mean of x,

$$GM = \exp \bar{y}.$$

Thus, the geometric mean, GM, is the antilog of the mean of the log transformed data. A mathematically equivalent way of expressing the geometric mean is as the nth root of the product of the n observations,

$$GM = \left(\prod_{i=1}^{n} x_i \right)^{1/n}.$$

The geometric mean is only well defined for positive data. For positive data the following inequality

holds for geometric, harmonic, and sample (arithmetic) means:

$$\bar{x}_h \leq GM \leq \bar{x}.$$

One straightforward way to obtain a measure of central tendency that does not depend on the extremes or tails of the data is to first remove or trim the data in both tails of the distribution and then compute the usual arithmetic mean using the remaining data. The result is referred to as a **trimmed** or Winsorized mean.

W. SMITH

Mean Absolute Deviation from Median *see* Robustness

Mean Deviation

The mean deviation d of a data set $x_1, \ldots, x_n$ is defined as

$$d = \frac{1}{n} \sum_{i=1}^{n} |x_i - m|, \tag{1}$$

where m is a location measure, most often the arithmetic **mean**, $\bar{x}$, most naturally the sample **median**, med (which minimizes d over all values of m), or, if known, a population location measure, such as the **expectation** or the median of the population.

It is also called mean absolute deviation (or average deviation), and the mean deviation from the mean is also called mean absolute error (MAE).

Its probabilistic counterpart for a random variable X is the first absolute **moment** with respect to (usually) the expectation (if it exists),

$$\delta = E(|X - EX|). \tag{2}$$

The mean deviation is thus a measure of scale or dispersion, like the **standard deviation** (sd) or the **range**, or the median (absolute) deviation (MAD) $=$ $\text{med}_i(|x_i - \text{med}_j x_j|)$ (the median, not mean, of the absolute differences from the sample median). In general, they all estimate different quantities; but, for example, for large samples from the normal distribution, one can give conversion factors:

$$d = (2/\pi)^{1/2} \text{ sd} \approx 0.7979 \text{ sd}$$

and

$$\text{MAD} \approx 0.6745 \text{ sd} \approx 0.8453 \, d. \qquad (3)$$

The mean deviation is the **maximum likelihood estimator** of the scale parameter δ (and is therefore asymptotically **efficient**) for the double-exponential distribution with density $f_{\mu,\delta}(x) = (2\delta)^{-1} \exp(-|x - \mu|/\delta)$ (μ arbitrary, $\delta > 0$). (The corresponding estimator for μ is the median.)

Around 1900, mean deviation and standard deviation were the two most commonly used scale estimators. Both were usually converted into the *probable error* (the error that would be surpassed with probability one-half) according to the above Eqs (3), with MAD replaced by probable error. The MAD, although the direct (and **nonparametric**) estimate of the probable error, apparently was never used then as an estimator (perhaps because of its low efficiency near the normal distribution, and without awareness of its good **robustness** properties).

In 1920, Fisher [2] proved and stressed the optimality of the standard deviation under strictly normal data and showed that the mean deviation in this case has an **asymptotic relative efficiency** of only $1/(\pi - 2) \approx 88\%$, causing the mean deviation to fall into oblivion. The astronomer Eddington [1, p. 147; 2, footnote, p. 762] maintained that the mean deviation was the better (more accurate) scale measure according to (astronomical) practical experience. There is no contradiction – both were right; real data are never exactly normal. In 1960, Tukey ([6, inserts], with more details and a correction given by Huber [5, p. 3]) showed that less than 0.2% of a very mild form of contamination of a normal distribution suffice to render d better than sd, while for about 5% contamination (a common frequency of gross errors) of the same mild type, d is twice as efficient as sd.

A key to better understanding of these and other facts about the mean deviation is provided by the concepts of robustness theory (the stability theory of statistical procedures). If we add a single observation (e.g. a gross error) in any point x to a large sample with (estimated) parameters m and d, the standardized change of d in the limit of $n \to \infty$ is given by the influence curve or influence function [3]

$$\text{IF}(x) = |x - m| - d, \qquad (4)$$

which increases only linearly with x, while the IF for sd increases quadratically, implying a much higher sensitivity to "dirt" in the tails of the observed distribution (*see* **Robustness**). However, both functions are unbounded; in fact, a single **outlier** moving to infinity carries both estimates to infinity. Hence neither should be used. We say, that their *breakdown point* [3] is zero. By contrast, the MAD tolerates about 50% gross errors before it gives arbitrarily false values; its breakdown point is 50%. There are other scale estimators with positive breakdown point and generally higher efficiency than the MAD (e.g. **trimmed** variances, or Huber's scale estimators – cf. [5]). Using sd or d after (some functioning form of) rejection of outliers prevents the worst, but this approach is a complex procedure usually not well understood, and is less efficient than other robust scale estimators (cf. [4]); nevertheless, it might often be the simplest practical solution.

References

[1]   Eddington, A.S. (1914). *Stellar Movements and the Structure of the Universe*. Macmillan, London.

[2]   Fisher, R.A. (1920). A mathematical examination of the methods of determining the accuracy of an observation by the mean error, and by the mean square error, *Monthly Notices of the Royal Astronomical Society* **80**, 758-770.

[3]   Hampel, F.R. (1974). The influence curve and its role in robust estimation, *Journal of the American Statistical Association* **69**, 383-393.

[4]   Hampel, F.R. (1985). The breakdown points of the mean combined with some rejection rules, *Technometrics* **27**, 95-107.

[5]   Huber, P.J. (1981). *Robust Statistics*, Wiley, New York.

[6]   Tukey, J.W. (1960). A survey of sampling from contaminated distributions, in *Contributions to Probability and Statistics*, I. Olkin et al., eds. Stanford University Press, Stanford.

FRANK HAMPEL

Mean Parameter *see* Exponential Family

Mean Residual Life *see* Survival Distributions and Their Characteristics

Mean Square Contingency *see* Association, Measures of

Mean Square Error

If $\hat{\theta} = \hat{\theta}(Y_1, \ldots, Y_n)$ is an estimator of a parameter θ based on a **random sample** of size n, then the mean square(d) error (MSE) of the estimator is defined as the expected value of the squared deviation of the estimator from the true value to be estimated:

$$\text{MSE}(\hat{\theta}) = \text{E}[(\hat{\theta} - \theta)^2]$$
$$= \int \cdots \int [\hat{\theta}(Y_1, \ldots, Y_n) - \theta]^2$$
$$\times f(y_1; \theta) \ldots f(y_n; \theta) \partial y_1 \ldots \partial y_n,$$

where $f(y; \theta)$ is the density upon which the sample is based. In general, for any estimator $\hat{\theta}$ of a parameter θ, the MSE can equivalently be defined as $\text{E}[(\hat{\theta} - \theta)^2] = \int (\hat{\theta} - \theta)^2 g(\hat{\theta}; \theta) \partial \hat{\theta}$, where $g(\hat{\theta}; \theta)$ is the **sampling distribution** of the estimator $\hat{\theta}$. The MSE is a measure of the closeness of the estimator to the true value. From the following identity:

$$\text{E}[(\hat{\theta} - \theta)^2] = [\text{E}(\hat{\theta}) - \theta]^2 + \text{E}[\hat{\theta} - \text{E}(\hat{\theta})]^2$$
$$= [\text{bias}(\hat{\theta})]^2 + \text{var}(\hat{\theta}),$$

it is seen that the MSE is the sum of the squared **bias** plus the **variance** of the estimator. Thus, the MSE reflects both the bias of an estimator, i.e. how much its expected value differs systematically from the true value, as well as the precision (variance) of the estimator, which measures how much it varies about its expected value or mean due to sampling variability. A good estimator ideally will have a small MSE, reflecting both small bias and small variance. Choosing an estimator with a small MSE often entails a tradeoff between bias and variance.

Subset Selection in Regression and Prediction

Tradeoffs between bias and variance are illustrated in the problem of choosing the "best" set of predictor variables in multiple linear regression (*see* **Variable Selection**). Let y_i be a response measured on the ith individual in a sample of size n. The objective is to relate y_i to a set of p predictors (**explanatory** or independent variables) and to predict future values of y. The standard model writes $y_i = \beta_0 + \beta_1 x_{i1} + \ldots + \beta_p x_{ip} + e_i$, where $x_{i1}, \ldots, x_{ip}$ are p predictors measured on subject i, $\beta_0, \beta_1, \ldots, \beta_p$ are unknown regression coefficients to be estimated, and $e_i, i = 1, \ldots, n$, are independent, identically distributed, residual errors having mean zero and variance σ^2. This model is expressed in matrix notation as $\mathbf{Y} = \mathbf{X}\boldsymbol{\beta} + \mathbf{e}$, where $\mathbf{Y}$ is the $n \times 1$ vector of responses, $\mathbf{X}$ is the $n \times (p + 1)$ design matrix of rank $(p + 1)$ whose ith row is $(1, x_{i1}, \ldots, x_{ip})$, $\boldsymbol{\beta} = (\beta_0, \beta_1, \ldots, \beta_p)'$, and $\mathbf{e}$ is the $n \times 1$ vector of errors. The **least squares** estimate of $\boldsymbol{\beta}$ is $\hat{\boldsymbol{\beta}} = (\mathbf{X}'\mathbf{X})^{-1}\mathbf{X}'\mathbf{y}$, and for a given set of predictors $\mathbf{x} = (1, x_1, \ldots, x_p)'$, the usual predictor of y is $\hat{y} = \mathbf{x}'\hat{\boldsymbol{\beta}}$. This is an **unbiased** predictor, and the *mean squared error of prediction* (MSEP), is defined as $\text{E}(\hat{y} - y)^2 = \sigma^2[1 + \mathbf{x}'(\mathbf{X}'\mathbf{X})^{-1}\mathbf{x}]$. The *mean squared error of the regression coefficients* is defined as $\text{MSE}(\hat{\boldsymbol{\beta}}) = \text{E}(\hat{\boldsymbol{\beta}} - \boldsymbol{\beta})(\hat{\boldsymbol{\beta}} - \boldsymbol{\beta})'$, which equals $\text{var}(\hat{\boldsymbol{\beta}}) = \sigma^2(\mathbf{X}'\mathbf{X})^{-1}$. At times, an objective is to select the "best" subset for predicting y out of a potentially large number p of available predictor variables. Walls & Weeks [5] show that it is possible for the prediction based on a subset of variables to have a smaller MSEP. Partition $\mathbf{X} = (\mathbf{X}_1, \mathbf{X}_2)$, where $\mathbf{X}_1$ is the set of variables included in the regression and $\mathbf{X}_2$ are excluded. Similarly, partition $\boldsymbol{\beta}' = (\boldsymbol{\beta}_1', \boldsymbol{\beta}_2')$ and $\mathbf{x}' = (\mathbf{x}_1', \mathbf{x}_2')$. The least squares estimate of $\boldsymbol{\beta}_1$ based on the subset $\mathbf{X}_1$ is $\tilde{\boldsymbol{\beta}}_1 = (\mathbf{X}_1'\mathbf{X}_1)^{-1}\mathbf{X}_1'\mathbf{y}$, with bias $\text{E}(\tilde{\boldsymbol{\beta}}_1 - \boldsymbol{\beta}_1) = (\mathbf{X}_1'\mathbf{X}_1)^{-1}\mathbf{X}_1'\mathbf{X}_2\boldsymbol{\beta}_2$ and $\text{MSE}(\tilde{\boldsymbol{\beta}}_1) = \sigma^2(\mathbf{X}_1'\mathbf{X}_1)^{-1} + (\mathbf{X}_1'\mathbf{X}_1)^{-1}\mathbf{X}_1'\mathbf{X}_2\boldsymbol{\beta}_2\boldsymbol{\beta}_2'\mathbf{X}_2'\mathbf{X}_1(\mathbf{X}_1'\mathbf{X}_1)^{-1}$. The predicted value of y based on $\mathbf{X}_1$, $\tilde{y} = \mathbf{x}_1'\tilde{\boldsymbol{\beta}}_1$, will generally be biased (the bias is nonzero unless $\mathbf{X}_1'\mathbf{X}_2\boldsymbol{\beta}_2 = \mathbf{0}$), and $\text{MSEP}(\tilde{y}) = \sigma^2[1 + \mathbf{x}_1'(\mathbf{X}_1'\mathbf{X}_1)^{-1}\mathbf{x}_1] + \{[\mathbf{x}_2' - \mathbf{x}_1'(\mathbf{X}_1'\mathbf{X}_1)^{-1}\mathbf{X}_1'\mathbf{X}_2]\boldsymbol{\beta}_2\}^2$, which may be less than $\text{MSEP}(\hat{y})$ based on the full model. In particular, Hocking [2] shows that if $\text{var}(\hat{\boldsymbol{\beta}}_2) - \boldsymbol{\beta}_2\boldsymbol{\beta}_2'$ is positive definite, then (i) $\text{MSE}(\hat{\boldsymbol{\beta}}_1) - \text{MSE}(\tilde{\boldsymbol{\beta}}_1)$ is positive definite, and (ii) $\text{MSEP}(\hat{y}) \geq \text{MSEP}(\tilde{y})$, implying that the reduced model using the subset of variables in $\mathbf{X}_1$ is better in terms of mean squared error both for estimating the regression coefficients $\boldsymbol{\beta}_1$ as well as for predicting y. For example, excluding a single variable X_2 will result in a better estimate of $\boldsymbol{\beta}_1$ and a lower MSEP if $\text{var}(\hat{\beta}_2) > (\beta_2)^2$, i.e. if the variance of the regression coefficient of β_2 estimated in the full model exceeds the square of the true value of β_2. Hocking [2] also proposes considering as a criterion the average decrease in predictive mean squared error over the n points in the sample:

$$\frac{1}{n}\sum_{i=1}^{n}[\text{MSEP}(\hat{y}_i) - \text{MSEP}(\tilde{y}_i)]$$

and discusses how selecting a subset to maximize this criterion is closely related to the use of **Mallows' C_p** and the adjusted R^2 as criteria for subset selection in multiple regression.

The concept that a biased estimator may be preferable in terms of MSE to an unbiased estimator with a large variance also underlies the concept of **ridge regression** [3]. In situations where the p predictor variables are highly intercorrelated (i.e. the problem of **multicollinearity**), they suggest the biased "ridge regression" estimate $\hat{\beta}_k = (\mathbf{X}'\mathbf{X} + k\mathbf{I})^{-1}\mathbf{X}'\mathbf{y}$, where the predictor variables in X have been standardized by subtracting their sample means and dividing by their standard deviations, and the constant k is determined by inspecting the "ridge trace" or plot of $\hat{\beta}_k$ vs. k. For some choice of k, the ridge regression estimate will have smaller MSE than the least squares estimator. **Shrinkage estimators** derived from an **empirical Bayes** approach [1] also typically have a smaller MSE than the usual unbiased estimators. *See also* **James–Stein estimator** [4].

References

[1]   Carlin, B.P. & Louis, T.A. (1996). *Bayes and Empirical Bayes Methods for Data Analysis*. Chapman & Hall, New York.

[2]   Hocking, R.R. (1974). Misspecification in regression, *American Statistician* **28**, 39–40.

[3]   Hoerl, A.E. & Kennard, R.W. (1970). Ridge regression: biased estimation for non-orthogonal problems, *Technometrics* **12**, 55–67.

[4]   James, W. & Stein, C. (1961). Estimation with quadratic loss, in *Proceedings of the Fourth Berkeley Symposium on Mathematical Statistics and Probability*. University of California Press, Berkeley, pp. 361–379.

[5]   Walls, R.C & Weeks, D.L. (1969). A note on the variance of a predicted response in regression, *American Statistician* **23**, 24–26.

MARK D. SCHLUCHTER

Mean Square Successive Difference *see* Randomness, Tests of

Mean Squares *see* Analysis of Variance

Measure Theory *see* Probability Theory

Measurement Error in Epidemiologic Studies

This article is concerned with relating a response or outcome to an exposure and **confounders** in the presence of measurement error in one or more of the variables. We focus almost entirely on measurement error in a continuous or measured variable. When categorical variables (exposed or not exposed, case or control, quintiles of fat) are measured with error, they are said to be misclassified (*see* **Misclassification Error**). There are also many links in this topic with methods for handling missing data and with validation studies (*see* **Missing Data in Epidemiologic Studies; Validation Study**). For further details and a general overview of the topic, see [20]; [30] should be consulted for the linear model.

Before describing the problem, it is useful first to consider a number of specific examples that have had an impact on the development of the field:

1.   Measurement error has long been a concern in relating error-prone predictors such as systolic blood pressure (SBP) to the development of coronary heart disease (CHD). That SBP is measured with error is well known, and estimates

[23] suggest that approximately one-third of its observed variability is due to measurement error. The **Framingham Heart Study** is perhaps the best known **cohort study** in which the role of measurement error in SBP has been a concern for many years. MacMahon et al. [44] describe the important public health implications of properly accounting for the measurement error inherent in SBP. In an (as yet) unpublished paper, David Yanez, Richard Kronmal & Lynn Shemanski have discovered an example also in the CHD context where the failure to account properly for measurement error leads to misleading conclusions based on falsely detected statistical significance.

2.   In measuring nutrient intake, measurement error has been a long-term concern, as has the impact of this error on the ability to detect nutritional factors leading to cancer, especially breast and colon cancer. Typical cohort studies measure diet by means of food frequency questionnaires which, while related to long-term diet, are known to have biases and measurement errors. Other instruments are in use in this field, including food records (essentially diaries), 24 h recalls and (for a limited number of variables such as total caloric intake) biomarkers. Measurement error in nutrient instruments can be very large, for example because of the daily and seasonal variability of an individual's diet, and the **biases** in and loss of **power** to detect nutrient–cancer relationships can be profound. There is still considerable controversy in this field (see [37], [54], and [41]). Because of the cost of cohort studies in nutrition, **case–control studies** are of considerable interest. However, nutrient intakes in case–control studies are measured after the development of disease in cases, and this might cause differential measurement error, a topic we discuss in some detail below (*see* **Nutritional Exposure Measures**).

3.   There are a number of ongoing prospective and case–control studies of disease and serum hormone levels, and this is an area of considerable potential. Measurement error is a major concern here, due to within-individual variation of hormones, as well as various laboratory errors.

4.   In measuring environmental risk factors (*see* **Environmental Epidemiology**), measurement error is a common problem. For example,

measuring household lead levels is an error-prone process, not only because of laboratory and device error, but also because lead levels are inhomogeneous in both space and time, while measurement methods tend to be in fixed locations at fixed times. Because lead exposure has many possible media (air, dust, soil) with possibly correlated errors, the effects of measurement error can be large and complex.

Outline

This article consists of a series of major Sections, as follows:

1.   We first outline the basic concepts of measurement error modeling, making particular distinction between **differential** and **nondifferential measurement error**. We also describe the ideas of functional and structural modeling, as well as indicating how the measurement error problem can be treated as a **missing data** problem.

2.   Following the introductory concepts, we discuss the problem of measurement error as it pertains to the **linear regression** model. Here we introduce the idea of attenuation of regression coefficients, and the biases in parameter estimates caused by measurement error. We also discuss **hypothesis testing**. In the simplest cases, measurement error causes an often large decrease in the power to detect significant effects, while, as indicated above, and as exhibited through the **analysis of covariance**, in an **observational study**, measurement error in a confounder can cause misleading **inferences** about exposure effects.

3.   Having described the effects of measurement error on **estimation** and hypothesis testing, we turn to correcting for the effects due to measurement error. We first describe the two most common methods, known as regression calibration and SIMEX, and also a group of techniques called corrected score methods. We also describe the use of instrumental variables.

4.   **Maximum likelihood** and **Bayesian** estimation form an important component of the measurement error problem, and are described in some detail. We define the **likelihood** function, and show the crucial difference in the likelihood function between the nondifferential and differential measurement error cases; see (13) and (14).

5. While most of the article is based on measurement error in predictors, there is an important literature on response error, which we also review.
6. Case–control studies are important in epidemiology. A distinguishing feature of case–control studies is that the measurement error may be differential. In the differential measurement error case, we indicate that a specific type of data is required, the validation data sets, in which the true predictor can be observed for a subset of the study participants. If the measurement error is nondifferential, then matters are much easier, and the famous result of Prentice & Pyke [55] on the analysis of case–control studies is shown to have an analogue in the measurement error context.
7. There is a significant and developing literature on measurement error in **survival analysis**, and we indicate two possible approaches to the problem.

Measurement error models have a common structure; we illustrate the terms using a breast cancer and nutrition example:

1. An underlying model for a response in terms of predictors, e.g. linear **regression, logistic regression, nonlinear regression**; see Carrell & Ruppert [14]. This is the model we would fit if all variables were observed without error. In what follows, we call Y the response. For example, in the breast cancer and nutrition example, Y is breast cancer incidence fit to covariables using logistic regression
2. A variable which is measured subject to error. This could be an exposure or a confounder. We call this variable X. It is often called the *error-prone* predictor or the *latent predictor*. In the breast cancer example, X is long-term nutrient intake
3. The observed value of the mismeasured variable. We call this W, e.g. nutrient intake measured from a food frequency questionnaire
4. Those predictors which for all practical purposes are measured without error, which we call Z, e.g. age, body mass index
5. We are interested in relating the response Y to the true predictors (Z, X). One method, often called the *naive* method, simply replaces the error-prone predictor X with its measured version

W. This substitution typically leads to biases in parameter estimates and can lead to misleading inferences
6. The goal of measurement error modeling is to obtain nearly **unbiased** estimates of exposure effects and valid inferences. Attainment of this goal requires careful analysis. Substituting W for X, but making no adjustments in the usual fitting methods for this substitution, leads to estimates that are biased, sometimes seriously. In assessing measurement error, careful attention needs to be given to the type and nature of the error, and the sources of data which allow modeling of this error.

It should be obvious that one should design studies and instruments in such a way as best to lessen or to eliminate measurement error. In this article, we demonstrate some of the impacts of ignoring measurement error, ranging from bias in parameter estimates (Figure 1), to loss of power, requiring therefore much larger sample sizes to detect effects (Figure 2) to cases where the type I errors (*see* **Hypothesis Testing**) occur at higher rates than the usual 5% (Figure 3).

Computer Programs

S-PLUS and SAS (*see* **Software, Biostatistical**) computer programs (on Solaris SPARC architecture and for Windows on PCs) which implement many of the methods described in this article (for major **generalized linear models** such as linear, logistic, probit, Poisson and gamma regression) are available at no cost on the World Wide Web at http://stat.tamu.edu/qvf/qvf./html. **Bootstrap standard errors** are available. They have been developed by Raymond Carroll, Henrik Schmiedieche, and H. Joseph Newton.

A set of programs for **logistic regression** (in SAS and FORTRAN) is available from Professor Donna Spiegelman (e-mail stdls@gauss.bwh.harvard. edu). Interested readers should contact her for information concerning extension of these programs to **proportional hazards** and linear regression.

Iowa State University (Department of Statistics, Iowa State University, Ames IA 50011) distributes programs called EV-CARP for linear measurement error models at a cost of $300.

Models for Measurement Error

A fundamental prerequisite for analyzing a measurement error problem is specification of a model for the measurement error process. The *classical error model*, in its simplest form, is appropriate when an attempt is made to determine X directly, but one is unable to do so because of various errors in measurement. For example, consider systolic blood pressure (SBP), which is known to have strong daily and seasonal variations. In trying to measure SBP, the various sources of error include simple machine recording error, administration error, time of day, and season of the year. In such a circumstance, it sometimes makes sense to hypothesize an unbiased **additive error model**, which we write as

$$\text{(the classic model)} \quad W = X + U, \quad (1)$$

where U, the error, is assumed to be independent of X. An alternative model, the *controlled variable or Berkson model* [6], is especially applicable to laboratory studies. As an example, consider the herbicide study of Rudemo et al. [61]. In that study, a nominal measured amount W of herbicide was applied to a plant. However, the actual amount X absorbed by the plant differed from W, e.g. because of potential errors in application. In this case,

$$\text{(the Berkson model)} \quad X = W + U, \quad (2)$$

where U, the error, is assumed to be independent of W.

Determining an appropriate error model to use in the data analysis depends upon the circumstances and the available data. For example, in the herbicide study, the measured concentration W is fixed by design and the true concentration X varies due to error, so that model (2) is appropriate. On the other hand, in the measurement of long-term systolic blood pressure, it is the true long-term blood pressure which is fixed for an individual, and the measured value which is perturbed by error, so model (1) should be used. Estimation and inference procedures have been developed both for error and controlled-variable models.

This hardly exhausts the possible error models. See [20] and [29] for more details and further examples with more complex structure.

Sources of Data

To perform a measurement error analysis, one needs information about the error structure. These data sources can be broken up into two main categories:

1. *internal* subsets of the primary data
2. *external* or independent studies.

Within each of these broad categories, there are three types of data, all of which might be available only in a random subsample of the data set in question:

1. *validation* data, in which X is observable directly
2. *replication* data, in which replicates of W are available
3. *instrumental* data, in which another variable T is observable in addition to W.

An internal validation data set is the ideal, because it can be used with all known analytical techniques, permits direct examination of the error structure and tests of critical error model assumptions, typically leads to much greater precision of estimation and inference, and has strong links to the well-developed theory of missing data analysis (see below). We cannot express too forcefully that, if at all possible, one should obtain an internal validation data set.

With external validation data, one must assume that the error structure in those data also applies to the primary data (see below).

Replication data are used when it is impossible to measure X exactly, as, for example, when X represents long-term systolic average blood pressure or long-term average nutrient intake. Usually, one would make replicate measurements if there were good reason to believe that the replicated mean is a better estimate of X than a single observation, i.e. the classical error model is the target. In the classical error model (1), replication data can be used to estimate the **variance** of the measurement error, U.

Internal instrumental data sets containing a second measure T are useful for **instrumental variable** analysis, discussed briefly later in this article.

Transportability of Models and Parameters

In some studies, the measurement error process is not assessed directly, but instead is estimated from external data sets. We say that parameters of a model can be transported from one study to another if the model holds with the same parameter values in both studies. Typically, in applications only a subset of the model parameters need be transportable.

In many instances, approximately the same classical error model holds across different populations. For example, consider systolic blood pressure at two different clinical centers. Assuming similar levels of training for technicians making the measurements and a similar measurement protocol, it is reasonable to expect that the distribution of the error in the recorded measure is independent of the clinical center one enters, the technician making the measurement, and the value of X being measured. Thus, in classical error models it is often reasonable to assume that the error distribution is the same across different populations, i.e. transportable.

A common mistake is to transport a correction for measurement error from one study to the next. Such transportation is almost never appropriate. For instance, while the properties of errors of measurement may be reasonably transportable, the distribution of the true (or latent) predictor X is rarely transportable, since it depends so heavily on the population being sampled. Problems arise because corrections for measurement error involve not only the measurement error process but also the distribution of X. For example, systolic blood pressure measurements in the MRFIT study and the Framingham Heart Study may well have the same measurement error variance, but the distribution of true blood pressure X appears to differ substantially in the two studies, and the "correction for attenuation" described below cannot be transported from Framingham to MRFIT (see [17] for further details).

Is there an "Exact" Predictor?

We have based our discussion on the existence of an exact predictor X and measurement error models that provide information about this predictor. However, in practice, it is often the case that the definition of "exact" needs to be carefully considered prior to discussion of error models. In the measurement error literature the term "**gold standard**" is often used for the operationally defined exact predictor, though sometimes this term is used for an exact predictor that cannot be operationally defined. Using an operational definition for an "exact" predictor is often reasonable and justifiable on the grounds

that it is the best one could ever possibly hope to accomplish. However, such definitions may be controversial. For example, consider the problem of relating breast cancer risk to the dietary intake of fat. One way to determine whether decreasing one's fat intake lowers the risk of developing breast cancer is to conduct a **clinical trial** in which members of the treatment group are encouraged to reduce fat intakes. If instead one uses observational prospective data, along with an operational definition of long-term intake, one should be aware that the results of a measurement error analysis could be invalid if true long-term intake and operational long-term intake differ in subtle ways.

Differential and Nondifferential Error

It is important to make a distinction between *differential* and *nondifferential* measurement error. Nondifferential measurement error occurs in a broad sense when one would not even bother with W if X were available, i.e. W has no information about the response other than what is available in X. Nondifferential measurement error typically holds in **cohort studies**, but is often a suspect assumption in **case–control studies**.

Technically, measurement error is nondifferential if the distribution of Y given (X, Z, W) depends only on (X, Z). In this case W is said to be a *surrogate*. Measurement error is *differential* otherwise.

For instance, consider the Framingham example. The predictor of major interest is long-term systolic blood pressure, X, but we can only observe blood pressure on a single day, W. It seems plausible that a single day's blood pressure contributes essentially no information over and above that given by true long-term blood pressure, and hence that measurement error is nondifferential. The same remarks apply to the nutrition examples: measuring diet on a single day should not contribute information not already available in long-term diet.

Many problems can be analyzed plausibly assuming nondifferential measurement error, especially when the **covariate** measurements occur at a fixed point in time, and the response is measured at a later time, as is typical in cohort studies.

There are two exceptions that need to be kept in mind. First, in case–control studies, the disease response is obtained first, and then one measures antecedent exposures and other covariates.

In nutrition studies, this ordering of measurement may well cause differential measurement error. For instance, here the true predictor would be long-term dietary intake before diagnosis, but the dietary interview data are obtained only after diagnosis. A woman who develops breast cancer may exaggerate her estimated fat intake, thus introducing **recall bias** (*see* **Bias in Case–Control Studies**). In such circumstances, estimated fat intake will be associated with disease status even after conditioning on true long-term diet before diagnosis.

When measurement error is nondifferential, one can estimate parameters in models for responses given true covariates even when the true covariates are not observable. This is not true when measurement error is differential, except for the linear model. With differential error, one must obtain a validation subsample in which both true covariate measurements and surrogate measurements are available. Most of this article focuses on nondifferential measurement error models. Differential models with a **validation study** are typically best analyzed by techniques for handling missing data (*see* **Missing Data in Epidemiologic Studies; Missing Data; Multiple Imputation Methods**).

Prediction

Prediction of a response is different from estimation and inference for parameters. If a predictor X is measured with error, and one wants to predict a response *based on the error-prone version W of X*, then, except for an important case discussed below, it makes little sense to worry about measurement error. The reason for this is quite simple. If one has an original set of data (Y, W) then one can fit a convenient model to Y as a function of W. Predicting Y from W is merely a matter of using this model for prediction. There is no need then for measurement error to play a role in the problem.

The one situation requiring that we model the measurement error occurs when we develop a **prediction** model using data from one population but we wish to predict in another population. A naive prediction model that ignores measurement error may not be transportable. This context often becomes quite complex, requiring a combination of missing data and measurement error techniques, and to the best of our knowledge has not been investigated in detail in the literature, an exception being [31].

Is Bias Always Towards the Null?

It is commonly thought that the effect of measurement error is to bias estimates of exposure effects "towards the null" (*see* **Bias Toward the Null**). Hence, one could ignore measurement error when testing the **null hypothesis** of no exposure effect, and one could assume that non-null estimates, if anything, underestimate the effect of exposure. This lovely and appealing folklore is sometimes true but, unfortunately, often wrong. We discuss this point in detail below. A numerical example has recently been provided to us by David Yanez, Richard Kronmal & Lynn Shemanski in a heart disease context with seven covariates and a baseline variable. They found that, while an analysis ignoring measurement error showed highly statistically significant effects in all variables, none of the effects was even close to being statistically significant when the analysis took measurement error into account.

Functional and Structural Models

The words *functional* and *structural* have important places in the area of measurement error models. They act as a shorthand terminology for the basic approach one uses to solve the problem. In *functional modeling* nothing is assumed about the Xs; they could be fixed constants (the usual definition) or random variables. In *structural modeling*, X is assumed to be random, and a parametric distribution (usually the **normal**) is assumed. There has traditionally been considerable concern in the measurement error literature about the **robustness** of estimation and inferences based upon structural models for unobservable variates. Fuller [30, p. 263] discusses this issue briefly in the classical **nonlinear regression** problem, and basically concludes that the results of structural modeling "may depend heavily on the (assumed) form of the X distribution". In probit regression, Carroll et al. [23] report that, if one assumes that X is normally distributed, and it really follows a **chi-square distribution** with one **degree of freedom**, then the effect on the likelihood estimate is "markedly negative"; see also [63]. Essentially all research workers in the measurement error field come to a common conclusion: likelihood methods can be of considerable value, but the possible nonrobustness of inference due to model **misspecification** is a vexing and difficult problem.

The issue of model robustness is hardly limited to measurement error modeling. Indeed, it pervades statistics, and has led to the rise of a variety of **semiparametric** and **nonparametric** techniques. From this general point of view, *functional modeling* may be thought of as a group of semiparametric techniques. Functional modeling uses parametric models for the response, but makes no assumptions about the distribution of the unobserved covariate.

There is no agreement in the statistical literature as to whether functional or structural modeling is more appropriate. Many researchers believe that one should make as few model assumptions as possible and favor functional modeling. The argument is that any extra efficiency gained by structural modeling is more than offset by the need to perform careful and often time-consuming **sensitivity analyses**. Other researchers believe that appropriate statistical analysis requires one to do one's best to model every feature of the data, and thus favor structural modeling.

We take a somewhat more relaxed view of these issues. There are many problems, e.g. linear and logistic regression with additive measurement error, where functional techniques are easily computed and fairly efficient, and we have a strong bias in such circumstances towards functional modeling. In other problems – for example, the segmented regression problem [38] – structural modeling clearly has an important role to play, and should not be neglected.

Measurement Error as a Missing Data Problem

From one perspective, measurement error models are special kinds of missing data problems, because the Xs, being mostly and often entirely unobservable, are obviously missing as well. Readers who are already familiar with linear measurement error models and functional modeling will be struck by the fact that most of the recent missing data literature has pursued likelihood and Bayesian methods, i.e. structural modeling approaches. Readers familiar with missing data analysis will also be interested to know that, in large part, the measurement error model literature has pursued functional modeling approaches. We feel that both functional and structural modeling approaches are useful in the measurement error context, and this article pursues both strategies.

The usual interpretation of the classical missing data problem [42] is that the values of some of the variables of interest may not be observable for all study participants. For example, a variable may be observed for 80% of the study participants, but unobserved for the other 20%. The techniques for analyzing missing data are continually evolving, but it is fair to say that most of the recent advances (**multiple imputation,** data augmentation, etc.) have been based on likelihood (and Bayesian) methods.

The classical measurement error problem discussed to this point is one in which one set of variables, which we call X, is *never* observable, i.e. always missing. As such, the classical measurement error model is an extreme form of a missing data problem, but with *supplemental information* about X in the form of a surrogate, which we call W. Part of the art in measurement error modeling concerns how the supplemental information is related to the unobservable covariate.

Because there is a formal connection between the two fields, and because missing data analysis has become increasingly parametric, it is important to consider likelihood and Bayesian analysis of measurement error models – topics taken up later in this article.

Linear Regression and the Effects of Measurement Error

A comprehensive account of linear measurement error models can be found in Fuller [30].

Many textbooks contain a brief description of measurement error in linear regression, usually focusing on **simple linear regression** and arriving at the conclusion that the effect of measurement error is to bias the slope estimate in the direction of 0. Bias of this nature is commonly referred to as *attenuation* or *attenuation to the null*.

In fact, though, even this simple conclusion has to be qualified, because it depends on the relationship between the measurement, W, and the true predictor, X, and possibly other variables in the regression model as well. In particular, the effect of measurement error depends upon the model under consideration and on the joint distribution of the measurement error and the other variables. In **multiple linear regression**, the effects of measurement error vary, depending on: (i) the regression model, be it additive or multiple regression; (ii) whether or not the predictor measured with error is univariate or **multivariate**; and (iii) the presence of bias in the measurement.

The effects can range from the simple attenuation described above to situations where: (i) real effects are hidden; (ii) observed data exhibit relationships that are not present in the error-free data; and (iii) even the signs of estimated coefficients are reversed relative to the case with no measurement error.

The key point is that the measurement error distribution determines the effects of measurement error, and thus appropriate methods for correcting for the effects of measurement error depend on the measurement error distribution.

Simple Linear Regression with Additive Error: Regression to the Mean

We start with the simple linear regression model $Y = \beta_0 + \beta_x X + \varepsilon$, where the scalar X has mean μ_x and variance σ_x^2, and the error in the equation ε is independent of X, has mean zero, and variance σ_ε^2. The error model is additive as in (1). In this classical additive measurement error model, it is well known that an ordinary **least squares** regression ignoring measurement error produces an estimate not of β_x, but instead of $\beta_{x*} = \lambda \beta_x$, where

$$\lambda = \frac{\sigma_x^2}{\sigma_x^2 + \sigma_u^2} < 1. \qquad (3)$$

Thus ordinary least squares regression of Y on W produces an estimator that is attenuated to 0. The attenuating factor, λ, is called the *reliability ratio*.

One would expect that, because W is an error-prone predictor, it has a weaker relationship with the response than does X. This can be seen both by the attenuation and also by the fact that the residual variance of this regression is increased, being not σ_ε^2 but instead

$$\mathrm{var}(Y|W) = \text{residual variance of observed data}$$
$$= \sigma_\varepsilon^2 + \lambda \beta_x^2 \sigma_u^2.$$

This facet of the problem is often ignored, but it is important. *Measurement error causes a double-whammy*: not only is the slope attenuated, but the data are more noisy, with an increased error about the line.

To illustrate the attenuation associated with the classical additive measurement error, the results of a small simulation are displayed in Figure 1.

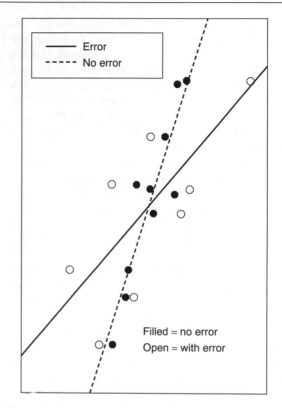

Figure 1 Illustration of additive measurement error model. The filled circles are the true (Y, X) data and the dashed (steeper) line is the least squares fit to these data. The open circles and solid (attenuated) line are the observed (Y, W) data and the associated least squares regression line. For these data $\sigma_x^2 = \delta_u^2 = 1$, $(\beta_0, \beta_x) = (0, 1)$ and $\sigma_\varepsilon^2 = 0.25$

Ten observations were generated with $\sigma_x^2 = \sigma_u^2 = 1$, $(\beta_0, \beta_x) = (0, 1)$, and $\sigma_\varepsilon^2 = 0.25$. The filled circles and steeper line depict the true but unobservable data (Y,X) and the regression line of Y on X. The empty circles and attenuated line depict the observed (Y,W) data and the linear regression of Y on W.

Figure 1 is indicative of a phenomenon called **regression to the mean**. Intuitively, what this means is that the extremes in the observed (W) data are *too* extreme, and that the true X is closer to the mean of the data. In fact, in normally distributed data, if X has a population mean μ_x, then having observed the fallible instrument, the best prediction of X is $\mu_x(1 - \lambda) + \lambda W$, where $\lambda < 1$ is defined in (3). The net effect is that the best (linear) predictor of X is always closer to the overall mean than any observed W.

The foregoing is one facet of regression to the mean. A more common definition is complementary. In a study participant with an unusually large observed W, if one repeats the measurement and obtains a second (replicated) measure, then this replicate is generally less (and often much less) than the original extreme value.

For instance, in a study of true long-term fat intake (X) using a 24 h recall instrument (W), if one focuses on the person with the highest reported fat intake, then (i) that person's true fat intake is most likely less than the observed intake, and (ii) if one repeats the 24 h recall instrument, then the new reported fat intake is likely to be less than the original reported fat intake.

The second part of the "double-whammy" is a loss of **power**. The following example is meant to illustrate this loss of power, and it is easiest to do this illustration in the special case that all variances are known. Suppose that one wants to test the null hypothesis H_0: $\beta_x = 0$ of zero slope against the one-sided alternative H_1: $\beta_x > 0$, using a test with a 5% level (type I error) which has power 80% to detect that the slope $\beta_x = 0.75$. With known variances, in the absence of measurement error, the required sample size is

$$n = \frac{(z_{0.95} + z_{0.80})^2 \sigma_\varepsilon^2}{\sigma_x^2 \beta_x^2},$$

where z_α is the usual α percentile of the normal distribution. With measurement error, the same formula applies, except that, with $\beta_x = 0.75$, one replaces σ_ε^2 by $\sigma_\varepsilon^2 + \lambda \beta_x^2 \sigma_u^2$, σ_x^2 by $\sigma_x^2 + \sigma_u^2$, and β_x by $\lambda \beta_x$. In Figure 2, we plot the sample sizes as a function of the measurement error variance in the case that X has variance $\sigma_x^2 = 1$ and the error about the line has variance $\sigma_\varepsilon^2 = 1$. In the absence of measurement error, approximately 10 observations are required to obtain the desired power. However, if the measurement error variance $\sigma_u^2 = 1$ and thus the reliability = 1/2, then approximately 30 observations are required. Thus, measurement error causes a loss of power. In planning a study with a large measurement error in a covariate, one will typically require a much larger sample size to meet power goals than if there were no measurement error.

It is a common belief that the effect of measurement error is always to attenuate the slope of the regression line, but in fact attenuation depends critically on the assumed classical additive measurement

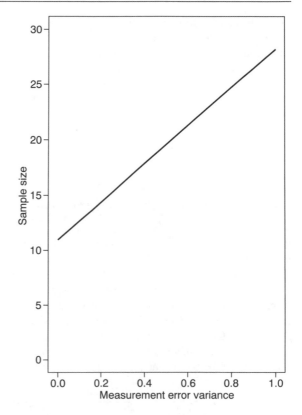

Figure 2 Sample size for 80% power in a one-sided test of level 5% in linear regression, as a function of the measurement error variance. Here the true slope = 0.75, the true variance of X is 1.0, and the true variance about the line is 1.0

error model. Very different results are obtained if measurement errors are differential. One example where this problem may arise is in dietary calibration studies. In a typical dietary calibration study, one is interested in the relationship between a self-administered food frequency questionnaire (FFQ, the value of Y) and usual (or long-term) dietary intake (the value of X) as measures of, for example, the percentage of calories from fat in a person's diet. FFQs are thought to be biased for usual intake, and in a calibration study researchers will obtain a second measure (the value of W), typically from a food diary, a 24h recall, or a short-term biomarker. In this context, it is often assumed that the diary, recall, or biomarker is unbiased for usual intake. If, as sometimes occurs, the FFQ and the diary/recall are given very nearly contemporaneously, it is unreasonable to assume that the error in the relationship between the

FFQ and usual intake is uncorrelated with the error in the relationship between a diary–recall–biomarker and usual intake. This correlation has been demonstrated [29], and gives rise to differential error. It can be shown [20] that, if there is significant **correlation** between the measurement error and the error about the true line, then the regression of Y on W can have a slope biased away from the null. Thus, correction for bias induced by measurement error clearly depends on the nature, as well as the extent, of the measurement error.

Multiple Regression: Single Covariate Measured with Error

In multiple linear regression the effects of measurement error are more complicated, even for the classical additive error model.

We now consider the case where X is scalar, but there are additional covariates Z measured without error. In the linear model the mean is $\beta_0 + \beta_x X + \beta_z Z$. Under the usual conditions of independence of errors, the least squares regression estimator of the coefficient of W consistently estimates $\lambda_1 \beta_x$, where

$$\lambda_1 = \frac{\sigma_{x|z}^2}{\sigma_{w|z}^2} = \frac{\sigma_{x|z}^2}{\sigma_{x|z}^2 + \sigma_u^2}, \qquad (4)$$

and $\sigma_{w|z}^2$ and $\sigma_{x|z}^2$ are the (residual) variances of the regressions of W on Z and X on Z, respectively. Note that λ_1 is equal to the simple linear regression attenuation $\lambda = \sigma_x^2 / (\sigma_x^2 + \sigma_u^2)$ only when X and Z are uncorrelated. *The basic point is that the attenuation depends on the relationships among the covariates.*

The problem of measurement-error-induced bias is not restricted to the regression coefficient of X. The coefficient of Z is also biased in general, unless Z is independent of X [19]. In fact, naive ordinary least squares estimates not β_z but rather

$$\beta_{z*} = \beta_z + \beta_x (1 - \lambda_1) \gamma_z, \qquad (5)$$

where γ_z is the coefficient of Z in the regression of X on Z.

This result has important consequences in epidemiology when interest centers on the effects of covariates measured without error. For example, consider the case that Z is a **binary** exposure variable (exposed or not) which is classified correctly, and X is an important confounder measured with significant error. Then Carroll et al. [19] show that ignoring measurement error produces a **consistent** estimate of

the exposure effect only if the design is balanced, i.e. X has the same mean in both groups and is independent of treatment. With considerable imbalance, the naive analysis may lead to the conclusion that: (i) there is a treatment effect when none actually exists; and (ii) the effects are negative when they are actually positive, and vice versa. In most observational studies the confounder and the exposure are correlated (see [34] and [35]). Errors in measuring the confounders can produce very misleading results.

Multiple Covariates Measured with Error

If multiple covariates are measured with error, then the direction of the bias induced by this error does not follow any simple pattern. One may have attenuation, reverse-attenuation, changes of sign, or an observed positive effect even at a true null model. This is especially the case when the predictors measured with error are correlated or their errors are correlated. In such a problem, there really seems to be no substitute for a careful measurement error analysis.

Correcting for Bias

As we have just seen, the ordinary least squares estimator is typically biased under measurement error, and the direction and magnitude of the bias depends on the regression model and the measurement error distribution. We next describe two commonly used methods for eliminating bias.

In simple linear regression with the classical additive error model, we have seen in (3) that ordinary least squares is an estimate of $\lambda \beta_x$; recall that λ is called the reliability ratio. If the reliability ratio were known, then one could obtain a proper estimate of β_x simply by dividing the ordinary least squares slope by the reliability ratio.

Of course, the reliability ratio is rarely known in practice, and one has to estimate it. If $\hat{\sigma}_u^2$ is an estimate of the measurement error variance (this is discussed below), and if $\hat{\sigma}_w^2$ is the sample variance of the Ws, then a consistent estimate of the reliability ratio is $\hat{\lambda} = (\hat{\sigma}_w^2 - \hat{\sigma}_u^2)/\hat{\sigma}_w^2$. The resulting estimate is $\beta_{x*}/\hat{\lambda}$. In small samples the sampling distribution of this estimate is highly skewed, and in such cases a modified version of the **method of moments** estimator is recommended [30].

The **algorithm** described above is called the *method-of-moments* estimator. The terminology is apt, because ordinary least squares and the reliability ratio depend only on moments of the observed data.

The method-of-moments estimator can be constructed for the **general linear model**, as well as for simple linear regression. Consult the book by Fuller [30], especially Chapter 2.

Another well publicized method for linear regression in the presence of measurement error is *orthogonal regression*. It is fairly rare in epidemiologic situations that the model underlying orthogonal regression holds [15], and we will not discuss the method any further.

Bias vs. Variance

Estimates that do not account for measurement error are typically biased. Unfortunately, correcting for this bias often has a price. In particular, the resulting corrected estimator will be more variable than the biased estimator, and wider **confidence intervals** result. For example, Rosner et al. [60] describe a problem in logistic regression, where the response is the development of breast cancer, and the predictor measured with error is daily saturated fat intake. Ignoring measurement error, they obtained an estimated **odds ratio** for saturated fat of 0.92, with a 95% confidence interval from 0.80 to 1.05. The corrected estimated odds ratio was 0.83 with a confidence interval from 0.61 to 1.12, which is twice as wide as the previous interval.

Attenuation in General Problems

We have already seen that, with multiple covariates, even in linear regression the effects of measurement error are complex, and not easily described. In this Section, we provide a brief overview of what happens in nonlinear models.

Consider a scalar covariate X measured with error, and suppose that there are no other covariates. In the classical error model for simple linear regression we have seen that the bias caused by measurement error is always in the form of attenuation, so that ordinary least squares preserves the sign of the regression coefficient asymptotically, but is biased towards zero. Attenuation is a consequence then of (i) the simple linear regression model and (ii) the classical additive error model. Without (i) and (ii), the effects of measurement error are more complex; we have already seen that attenuation may not hold if (ii) is violated.

In logistic regression, when X is measured with additive error, attenuation does not always occur, but it is typical and generally much like that of linear regression.

Dosemeci et al. [28] give an example of **misclassification error** that shows that trends are not always preserved under nondifferential measurement error. Suppose that 1348 subjects are exposed at no $(X = 0)$, low $(X = 1)$, and high $(X = 2)$ levels to a harmful substance. Suppose that the chance of an adverse outcome is 1/2, 2/3, and 6/7 for no, low, and high exposures, while the chances of the exposures themselves are 0.0059347, 0.8902077, and 0.1038576, respectively. If true exposure could be ascertained, then the expected outcomes would be as in the section of Table 1 labeled "true". If we were to regress Y on the **dummy variables** X_1 indicating low exposure $(X_1 = 1)$, and X_2 indicating high exposure $(X_2 = 1)$, then the true logistic regression parameters for X_1 and X_2 would be $\log 2 = 0.69$ and $\log 6 = 1.79$, respectively, indicating that the two higher exposure levels have response rates higher than the response rate associated with the no-exposure level. The true data clearly indicate a harmful effect due to exposure.

Now suppose, however, that measurement error (in this case misclassification) occurs, so that 40% of those truly at high exposure are misclassified into the no-exposure group, and 40% of those truly at low exposure are misclassified into the high-exposure group. Let W be the resulting variable taking on the three observed levels of exposure, with corresponding dummy variables W_1 and W_2. This is a theoretical example, of course, and one can criticize it for not being particularly realistic, but it is an example of nondifferential measurement error. The observed data we expect to see using the surrogates W_1 and W_2 are also given in Table 1.

The observed logistic regression parameters for W_1 and W_2 are $\log 0.46 = -0.78$ and $\log 0.53 = -0.63$, respectively, indicating that the two higher exposure levels have response rates lower than the response rate associated with the no-exposure level. The observed data suggest a beneficial effect due to exposure, even though the exposure is harmful!

Hypothesis Testing

In this section, we discuss hypothesis tests concerning regression parameters. To keep the exposition simple,

Table 1 A hypothetical logistic regression example with nondifferential measurement error. The entries are the expected counts. The true logistic parameters for dummy variables low and high exposure are $\log 2$ and $\log 6$, respectively, while the observed coefficients for the error prone data are $\log 0.46$ and $\log 0.53$, respectively

Disease status	Exposure = none	Exposure = low	Exposure = high
True			
$Y = 1$	4	800	120
$Y = 0$	4	400	20
Observed			
$Y = 1$	52	480	392
$Y = 0$	12	240	172

we focus on linear regression. However, the results hold in some generality, especially for logistic and **Poisson regression**. We assume nondifferential measurement error and the classical additive error model.

The simplest approach to hypothesis testing calculates the required test statistic from the parameter estimates obtained from a measurement error analysis and their estimated standard errors. Such tests are justified whenever the estimators themselves are justified. However, this approach to testing is only possible when the indicated methods of estimation are possible, and thus requires either knowledge of the measurement error variance, or the presence of validation data, or replicate measurements, or instrumental variables.

There are certain situations in which naive hypothesis tests are justified and thus can be performed without additional data or information of any kind. Here "naive" means that we ignore measurement error and substitute W for X in a test that is valid when X is observed. This Section studies naive tests, describing when they are and are not acceptable.

We use the criterion of asymptotic validity to distinguish between acceptable and nonacceptable tests. We say a test is asymptotically valid if its type I error rate approaches its nominal level as the sample size increases. Asymptotic validity (which we shorten to validity) of a test is a minimal requirement for acceptability.

The main results on the validity of naive tests under nondifferential measurement error are as follows:

1. The naive test of no effects due to X is valid. This means that if one wants to test whether *all*

components of X together have no effect, then it is valid to ignore nondifferential measurement error. Thus, for example, if X is the exposure, then a valid test of the null hypothesis for X is obtained by ignoring measurement error and performing the standard test for the problem at hand.

2. The naive test described above is also fully efficient if X is linearly related to W and Z, but not otherwise [79]. Thus, while in principle one can obtain additional power by a measurement error analysis, many times in practice the naive test of the null hypothesis for X is reasonably efficient.

3. In many problems, more than one covariate is measured with error. For example, suppose that the exposure and one of the confounders are measured with error. Generally, the naive test of the null hypothesis for the exposure is invalid, except under special circumstances, e.g. the exposure and confounder are statistically independent, as are their measurement errors.

4. In general, naive tests for Z are invalid, except possibly if Z is uncorrelated with X. Thus, if X is the exposure and Z is a confounder, then naive tests for significance of the exposure are valid, but they are not valid for testing the significance of the confounder. Somewhat more troubling, though, is the case when X is a confounder related to the exposure Z; here the naive test for the exposure is generally invalid, *even if exposure is measured without error*. We have mentioned this example previously in the case that the exposure is binary (see [19]).

The last point can be demonstrated in the **analysis of covariance**, in which Z is a binary exposure variable and X is a confounder with strong predictive ability. In the analysis of covariance, the model is

$$Y = \beta_0 + \beta_z Z + \beta_x X + \varepsilon,$$

where ε is the error about the line, with variance σ_ε^2. The binary indicator Z takes on the values ± 1, with 50% of the data being unexposed ($Z = -1$) and 50% of the data being exposed ($Z = 1$). Within the unexposed group, X has mean $-\theta/2$ and variance σ_x^2, while, within the exposed group, X has mean $\theta/2$ and variance σ_x^2. The difference between the means for X in the two groups is θ. In a randomized **clinical trial**, one would expect that $\theta = 0$, since

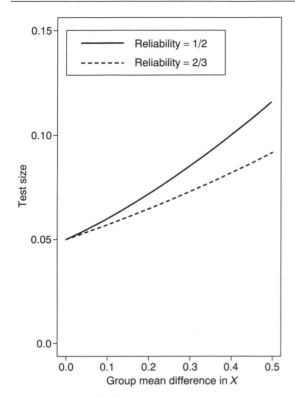

Figure 3 The actual level of a test for exposure effect with a highly predictive covariate measured with error, based on a sample of size $n = 20$. Here the true slope for the covariate $X = 1.0$, the true variance of X is 1.0, the true variance about the line is 1.0, and the reliability is either 2/3 (dashed line) or 1/2 (solid line). The term "Group mean difference in X" is the difference in the mean of X in the exposure group minus the mean of X in the control group

randomization ensures that the population means of X are the same in the exposed and unexposed groups. In nonrandomized studies, one would expect that $\theta \neq 0$. Thus, the larger the value of θ, the more unbalanced is the study. In Figure 3, we plot the level (type I error) of the test for the exposure effect which ignores measurement error as a function of the difference in group means θ. This calculation is done for the case that $n = 20$ (10 exposed and 10 unexposed), $\sigma_\varepsilon^2 = 1$, $\sigma_x^2 = 1$, and $\beta_x = 1$, for reliability ratios $\lambda = 1/2$ and $= 2/3$. The graph shows that if the means of the confounders are sufficiently different, then, instead of a type I error of 5%, the test for exposure effect which ignores measurement error in the *confounder* can have type I error rates higher than 10%, even for such small sample sizes.

Regression Calibration and SIMEX

We now describe two simple, generally applicable approaches to nondifferential measurement error analysis, regression calibration, and simulation extrapolation (SIMEX).

Regression Calibration

The basis of regression calibration is the replacement of X by the regression of X on (Z, W). After this approximation, one performs a standard analysis. This *regression calibration* algorithm was suggested as a general approach by Carroll & Stefanski [16] and Gleser [33]. Prentice [52] pioneered the idea for the **proportional hazard** model, and a modification of it has been suggested for this topic by Clayton [25]; see below. Armstrong [4] suggests regression calibration for **generalized linear models**, and Fuller [30, pp. 261–262] briefly mentions the idea. Rosner et al. [59, 60] have developed the idea for **logistic regression** into a workable and popular methodology, complete with a good computer program. Because of the importance of their contribution to epidemiologic applications, regression calibration is often referred to as "Rosner's Method". Other interesting and important applications and methodology related to regression calibration include work by Whittemore [83], Pierce et al. [51], Liu & Liang [43], and Kuha [39]. In some special cases, regression calibration is equivalent to the classical method of moments bias correction.

The main justifications of the regression calibration approximation are that, for some models, e.g. **loglinear** mean models and **linear regression**, the regression calibration approximation is often exact except for a change in the intercept parameter. For logistic regression, in many cases the approximation is almost exact.

The Regression Calibration Algorithm. The regression calibration algorithm is what Pierce et al. [51] call a "replacement method":

1. Using replication, validation or instrumental data, estimate the regression of X on (Z, W) (see below). This is called the *calibration function*.
2. Replace the unobserved X by its estimate from the regression model, and then run a standard analysis to obtain parameter estimates.

3. Adjust the resulting standard errors to account
    for the estimation at the first step, using either
    the bootstrap or asymptotic methods [20].

The simplest form of regression calibration is the
"correction for attenuation" used in linear regression.
It is easiest to describe in the following situation:

1. X is a scalar.
2. The measurement error is additive, with esti-
    mated error variance $\hat{\sigma}_u^2$.

For estimating the effect of X, the regression calibration estimator is formed by three steps: (i) form
the naive estimator by ignoring measurement error;
(ii) let $\hat{\sigma}_{w|z}^2$ be the regression **mean square error**
from a linear regression of W on Z (this is the sample
variance of the Ws if there are no other covariates Z);
(iii) the regression calibration estimator is defined by
multiplying the naive estimator by $\hat{\sigma}_{w|z}^2/(\hat{\sigma}_{w|z}^2 - \hat{\sigma}_u^2)$.

Estimating the Calibration Function Parameters.
With *internal validation data*, the simplest approach
is to regress X on the other covariates (Z,W) in
the validation data. While linear regression will be
typical, it is not required.

In some problems, an *unbiased second instrument*
T is available for a subset of the study participants.
For instance, one might be interested in $X =$ caloric
intake over a year, but have available only $T =$ the
result of a biomarker experiment using a technique
known as doubly labeled water over a 2 week period,
which does not equal X because it does not take
into account the variability of diet over a year. In
this case one uses the regression of T on (Z,W) as
the calibration function. This is the method used by
Rosner et al. [59] in their analysis of the Nurses'
Health Study.

Finally, in the classical additive error model, one
often has merely a second measurement (a replicate)
for a subset of the study population. One could treat
this replicate as an unbiased second instrument and
apply the method described in the previous paragraph.
If the Ws are not too far from normally distributed,
a more efficient method is to use the so-called best
linear approximation to the calibration function (see
[20, pp. 47–48]). This takes into account that some
of the study participants do have a replicated W
and hence use the data in a reasonably efficient
fashion.

Suppose there are k_i replicate measurements of X_i,
and that $\overline{W}_i$ is their mean. Replication enables us to
estimate the measurement error **covariance matrix**
σ_u^2 by the usual **variance components** analysis, as
follows:

$$\hat{\sigma}_u^2 = \frac{\sum_{i=1}^{n}\sum_{j=1}^{k_i}(W_{ij}-\overline{W}_{i\cdot})^2}{\sum_{i=1}^{n}(k_i-1)}. \tag{6}$$

The calibration function is defined as follows. Sup-
pose the observations are $(Z_i, \overline{W}_{i\cdot})$, where $\overline{W}_{i\cdot}$ is the
mean of k_i replicates. We use **analysis of variance**
formulas. Let

$$\hat{\mu}_x = \hat{\mu}_w = \sum_{i=1}^{n}k_i\overline{W}_{i\cdot}\Big/\sum_{i=1}^{n}k_i, \qquad \hat{\mu}_z = \overline{Z}_{\cdot},$$

$$v = \sum_{i=1}^{n}k_i - \sum_{i=1}^{n}k_i^2\Big/\sum_{i=1}^{n}k_i,$$

$$\hat{\sigma}_z^2 = (n-1)^{-1}\sum_{i=1}^{n}(Z_i-\overline{Z}_{\cdot})^2,$$

$$\hat{\sigma}_{xz} = \sum_{i=1}^{n}k_i(\overline{W}_{i\cdot}-\hat{\mu}_w)(Z_i-\overline{Z}_{\cdot})/v,$$

$$\hat{\sigma}_x^2 = \left\{\left[\sum_{i=1}^{n}k_i(\overline{W}_{i\cdot}-\hat{\mu}_w)^2\right]-(n-1)\hat{\sigma}_u^2\right\}/v.$$

The resulting estimated calibration function which is
used to replace $\mathbf{X}$ in the standard analysis is

$$\hat{\mu}_w + (\hat{\sigma}_x^2, \hat{\sigma}_{xz})\begin{bmatrix}\hat{\sigma}_x^2+\hat{\sigma}_u^2/k_i & \hat{\sigma}_{xz} \\ \hat{\sigma}_{xz} & \hat{\sigma}_z^2\end{bmatrix}^{-1}\begin{pmatrix}\overline{W}_{i\cdot}-\hat{\mu}_w \\ Z_i-\overline{Z}_{\cdot}\end{pmatrix}. \tag{7}$$

Expanded Regression Calibration Models. Rudemo et al. [61], Carroll & Stefanski [16] and Carroll
et al. [20] all describe refinements to the regression
calibration algorithm. Rudemo et al. [61] describe a
bioassay problem (*see* **Biological Assay, Overview**)
with a heteroscedastic Berkson error model. Racine-
Poon et al. [56] describe a similar problem.

There is a long history of approximately consistent
estimates in nonlinear problems, of which regression
calibration and the SIMEX method are the most
recent such methods. Readers should also consult

Stefanski & Carroll [70], Stefanski [67], Amemiya & Fuller [3], and Whittemore & Keller [85] for other approaches.

The SIMEX Method

We now describe a method that shares the simplicity of regression calibration and is well suited to problems with additive or multiplicative measurement error. Simulation extrapolation (SIMEX) is a **simulation**-based method of estimating and reducing bias due to measurement error. SIMEX estimates are obtained by adding additional measurement error to the data in a resampling-like stage, establishing a trend of measurement error-induced bias vs. the variance of the added measurement error, and **extrapolating** this trend back to the case of no measurement error. The technique was proposed by Cook & Stefanski [26], and further developed by Carroll et al. [22] and Stefanski & Cook [73]. See also Stefanski, [68].

An integral component of SIMEX is a self-contained simulation study resulting in **graphical displays** that illustrate the effect of measurement error on parameter estimates and the need for bias correction. The graphical displays are especially useful when it is necessary to motivate or explain a measurement error model analysis.

This Section describes the basic idea of SIMEX, focusing on linear regression with additive measurement error. For this simple model the effect of measurement error on the least squares estimator is easily determined mathematically, as we have shown. *The key idea underlying SIMEX is the fact that the effect of measurement error on an estimator can also be determined experimentally via simulation.* If we regard measurement error as a factor whose influence on an estimator is to be determined, we are naturally led to consider simulation experiments in which the level of the measurement error, i.e. its variance, is varied intentionally.

The SIMEX Algorithm

Suppose that, in addition to the original data used to calculate the naive estimate $\hat{\beta}_{x,\text{naive}}$, there are $M - 1$ additional data sets available, each with successively larger measurement error variances, say $(1 + \zeta_m)\sigma_u^2$, where $0 = \zeta_1 < \zeta_2 < \ldots < \zeta_M$. Of course, the least squares estimate of slope from the mth data set

ignoring measurement error, $\hat{\beta}_{x,m}$, consistently estimates $\beta_x \sigma_x^2 / [\sigma_x^2 + (1 + \zeta_m)\sigma_u^2]$.

We can think of this problem as a nonlinear regression model, with dependent variable $\hat{\beta}_{x,m}$ and independent variable ζ_m, having a mean function of the form

$$\mathcal{G}(\zeta) = \frac{\beta_x \sigma_x^2}{\sigma_x^2 + (1 + \zeta)\sigma_u^2}, \zeta \geq 0.$$

The parameter of interest, β_x, is obtained from $\mathcal{G}(\zeta)$ by extrapolation to $\zeta = -1$. We describe the process schematically in Figure 4.

SIMEX imitates the procedure just described. In the *simulation step*, additional independent measurement errors with variance $\zeta_m \sigma_u^2$ are generated and added to the original data, thereby creating data sets with successively larger measurement error variances. For the mth data set, the total measurement error variance is $\sigma_u^2 + \zeta_m \sigma_u^2 = (1 + \zeta_m)\sigma_u^2$. Next, estimates

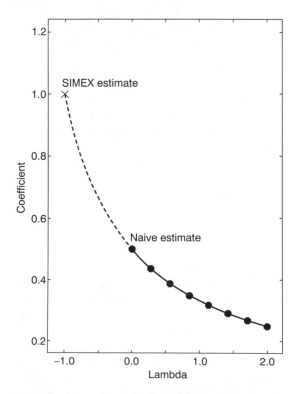

Figure 4 A generic plot of the effect of measurement error of size $(1 + \zeta)\sigma_u^2$ on parameter estimates. The value of ζ is on the x-axis, while the value of the estimated coefficient is on the y-axis. The SIMEX estimate is an extrapolation to $\zeta = -1$. The naive estimate occurs at $\zeta = 0$

are obtained from each of the resulting contaminated data sets. The simulation and reestimation step is repeated a large number of times (to remove simulation variability) and the average value of the estimate for each level of contamination is calculated. These averages are plotted against the ζ values, and regression techniques are used to fit an extrapolant function to the averaged, error-contaminated estimates. Extrapolation back to the ideal case of no measurement error ($\zeta = -1$) yields the SIMEX estimate.

The first part of the algorithm is the simulation step. As described above, this involves using simulation to create additional data sets with increasingly large measurement error $(1 + \zeta)\sigma_u^2$. For any $\zeta \geq 0$, define

$$W_{b,i}(\zeta) = W_i + \zeta^{1/2}U_{b,i},$$
$$i = 1, \ldots, n, b = 1, \ldots, B, \qquad (8)$$

where the computer-generated *pseudo-errors*, $\{U_{b,i}\}_{i=1}^{n}$, are mutually independent, independent of all the observed data, and identically distributed, normal random variables with mean 0 and variance σ_u^2.

Having generated the new predictors, we compute the resulting naive estimates, component by component. For each ζ, do this B times ($B = 100$ usually works fine) and compute their average, $\hat{\beta}(\zeta)$. It is the points $\{\hat{\beta}(\zeta_m), \zeta_m\}_1^M$ that are plotted as filled circles in Figure 4. This is the simulation component of SIMEX.

The extrapolation step of the proposal entails modeling each of the components of $\hat{\beta}(\zeta)$ as functions of ζ for $\zeta \geq 0$, and extrapolating the fitted models back to $\zeta = -1$. In Figure 4 the extrapolation is indicated by the dashed line and the SIMEX estimate is plotted as a cross. Carroll et al. [20] describe practical modifications of the algorithm, and how to estimate variances of parameters. Inference for SIMEX estimators can also be performed via the **bootstrap**. Because of the computational burden of the SIMEX estimator, the bootstrap requires considerably more computing time than do other methods. Without efficient implementation of the estimation scheme at each step, the SIMEX bootstrap may take an inconveniently long time to compute. On my computing system for measurement error models the implementation is efficient, and most bootstrap applications take little time.

We have described the SIMEX algorithm in terms of the additive measurement error model. However, SIMEX applies more generally.

For example, consider multiplicative error. Taking logarithms transforms the **multiplicative model** to the **additive model**. SIMEX works naturally here, in that one performs the simulation step (8) on the logarithms of the Ws and not on the Ws themselves.

With replicates, one can also investigate the appropriateness of different **transformations**. For example, after transformation, the **standard deviation** of the intraindividual replicates should be uncorrelated with their mean, and one can find the transformation (logarithm, square root, etc.) which makes the two uncorrelated.

Example

To illustrate SIMEX, we use data from the Framingham Heart Study, correcting for bias due to measurement error in systolic blood pressure measurements. The Framingham study consists of a series of exams taken two years apart. We use Exam #3 as the baseline. There are 1615 men aged 31–65 in this data set, with the outcome, Y, indicating the occurrence of coronary heart disease (CHD) within an 8-year period following Exam #3; there were 128 such cases of CHD. Predictors employed in this example are the patient's age at Exam #2, smoking status at Exam #1, and serum cholesterol at Exams #2 and #3, in addition to systolic blood pressure (SBP) at Exam #3, the latter being the average of two measurements taken by different examiners during the same visit. In addition to the measurement error in SBP measurements, there is also measurement error in the cholesterol measurements. However, for this example we ignore the latter source of measurement error and illustrate the methods under the assumption that only SBP is measured with error.

The covariates measured without error, Z, are age, smoking status, and serum cholesterol, with $W = \log(\text{SBP} - 50)$. Implicitly, we are defining X as the long-term average of W. We illustrate the analyses for the case where W is the mean of the two transformed SBPs, and σ_u^2 is estimated using (6). The estimated linear model correction for attenuation, or inverse of the reliability ratio, is 1.16; if only one SBP measurement were used, the correction would be 1.33.

Figure 5 contains plots of the logistic regression coefficients $\hat{\Theta}(\zeta)$ for eight equally spaced values of ζ spanning $[0, 2]$ (solid circles). For this example

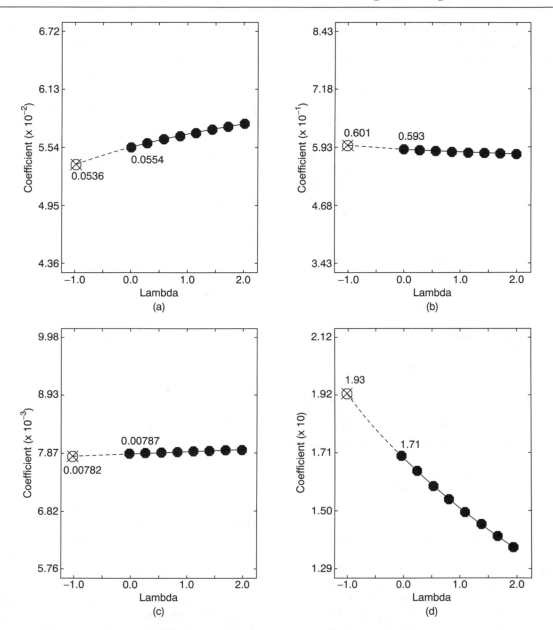

Figure 5 Coefficient extrapolation functions for the Framingham logistic regression modeling. The simulated estimates $\{\hat{\Theta}(\zeta_m), \zeta_m\}_1^8$ are plotted (solid circles) and the fitted rational linear extrapolant (solid line) is extrapolated to $\zeta = -1$ (dashed line), resulting in the SIMEX estimate (cross). Open circles indicate SIMEX estimates obtained with the quadratic extrapolant. (a) Age; (b) Smoking; (c) Cholesterol; (d) log(SBP − 50)

$B = 2000$. The points plotted at $\zeta = 0$ are the naive estimates $\hat{\Theta}_{\text{naive}}$. The nonlinear least-squares fits of $\mathcal{G}_{\text{RL}}(\lambda, \Gamma)$ to the components of $\{\hat{\Theta}(\zeta_m), \zeta_m\}_1^8$ (solid curves) are extrapolated to $\zeta = -1$ (dashed curves), resulting in the SIMEX estimators (crosses). The

open circles are the SIMEX estimators that result from fitting quadratic extrapolants. To preserve clarity the quadratic extrapolants were not plotted. Note that the quadratic-extrapolant estimates are conservative relative to the rational linear-extrapolant estimates in the sense that they fall between the rational linear-extrapolant estimates and the naive estimates.

We have stated previously that the SIMEX plot displays the effect of measurement error on parameter estimates. This is especially noticeable in Figure 5. In each of the four graphs in Figure 5, the range of the ordinate corresponds to a one-standard-error confidence interval for the naive estimate constructed using the information standard errors. Thus Figure 5 illustrates the effect of measurement error relative to the variability in the naive estimate. It is apparent that the effect of measurement error is of practical importance only on the coefficient of $\log(\text{SBP} - 50)$.

Conditional and Corrected Scores for Functional Modeling

Regression calibration and SIMEX are easily applied general methods for nondifferential error. Although the resulting estimators are **consistent** in important special cases such as linear regression and loglinear mean models, they are only approximately consistent in general.

For certain generalized linear models and measurement error distributions there are easily applied functional methods that are fully (and not just approximately) consistent, and make no assumptions about the distribution of X.

We focus on the case of additive normally distributed measurement error with measurement error variance σ_u^2. Although the problem has this parametric error assumption, it also has a nonparametric component: no assumptions are made about the true predictors X.

Suppose for the sake of discussion that the measurement error variance σ_u^2 is known. In the functional model, the unobservable Xs are fixed constants, and hence the unknown parameters include the Xs. With additive normally distributed measurement error, one strategy is to maximize the joint density of the observed data with respect to all of the unknown parameters including the Xs. While this works for linear regression [32], it fails for more complex models such as logistic regression. Indeed, the logistic regression functional maximum likelihood estimator is both inconsistent and difficult to compute [70]. An alternative approach is to change to the structural model and apply likelihood techniques (see below).

In this Section, we consider two functional methods, the conditional-score and corrected-score methods. We start with logistic and gamma–loglinear modeling as important examples for which these techniques apply. The conditional methods exploit special structures in important models such as linear, logistic, Poisson loglinear, and gamma-inverse, and then use a traditional statistical device – conditioning on **sufficient statistics** – to obtain estimators. The corrected-score method effectively estimates the estimator one would use if there were no measurement error.

First consider the **multiple linear regression** model with mean $\beta_0 + \beta_x X + \beta_z Z$, and write the unknown regression parameter as $\Theta = (\beta_0, \beta_x, \beta_z)$. When the measurement error is additive with non-differential measurement error variance Σ_{uu}, the usual **method-of-moments** regression estimator can be derived as the solution to the equation

$$\sum_{i=1}^{n} \psi_* (Y_i, Z_i, W_i, \Theta, \Sigma_{uu}) = 0, \qquad (9)$$

where

$$\psi_* (Y, Z, W, \Theta, \Sigma_{uu}) = (Y - \beta_0 - \beta_x^t X - \beta_z^t Z)$$
$$\times \begin{pmatrix} 1 \\ Z \\ W \end{pmatrix} + \begin{pmatrix} 0 \\ 0 \\ \Sigma_{uu} \beta_x \end{pmatrix}$$

is the *corrected score* for linear regression. If Σ_{uu} is unknown, then one substitutes an estimate of it into (9) and solves for the regression parameters.

The key point to note here is that, in solving (9), we need know nothing about the Xs. This feature is common to all the methods in this Section.

Eq. (9) is an example of an **estimating equation** approach for estimating a set of unknown parameters. The reader can consult the Appendix of [20] for an overview of estimating equations, although this is unnecessary for the purpose of using the methods. Asymptotic standard errors for the estimators can be derived using either the bootstrap or the sandwich formula.

Logistic regression is best handled using the conditional-score method. For example, consider the usual linear-logistic model, where Y is binary and has success probability following the logistic model $H(\beta_0 + \beta_x X + \beta_z Z)$. The conditional score is

$$\psi_*(Y, Z, W, \Theta, \sigma_u^2)$$

$$= \{Y - H[\beta_0 - \beta_x^t \Delta(\cdot) - 0.5\beta_x^t \sigma_u^2 \beta_x$$

$$- \beta_z^t Z]\} \begin{pmatrix} 1 \\ Z \\ \Delta(\cdot) \end{pmatrix}, \qquad (10)$$

where $\Delta(\cdot) = \Delta(Y, W, \beta_x, \sigma_u^2) = W + Y\sigma_u^2 \beta_x$. Eq. (10) is substituted into (9), and the resulting equation is solved numerically.

When Y has a **gamma distribution** with loglinear mean $\exp(\beta_0 + \beta_x X + \beta_z Z)$, it has a variance which is ϕ times the square of the mean. For this important example, the corrected-score estimator is obtained from the corrected score

$$\psi_*(Y, Z, W, \Theta, \sigma_u^2)$$

$$= \begin{pmatrix} 1 \\ Z \\ W \end{pmatrix} - \exp[\Delta(Z, W, \Theta, \sigma_u^2)]$$

$$\times \begin{pmatrix} Y \\ ZY \\ Y(W + 0.5\sigma_u^2 \beta_x) \end{pmatrix}, \qquad (11)$$

where $\Delta(Z, W, \Theta, \sigma_u^2) = -\beta_0 - \beta_x^t W - \beta_z^t Z - 0.5 \beta_x^t \sigma_u^2 \beta_x$.

Unbiased Score Functions via Conditioning

The conditional estimators of Stefanski & Carroll [71] and Nakamura [48] are discussed in detail in Carroll et al. [20, Chapter 6]. They apply to linear, logistic, Poisson loglinear, and gamma inverse regression [the mean is $1/(\beta_0 + \beta_x X + \beta_z Z)$]. Their methods have simple formulas for standard errors, although, of course, as usual, the bootstrap applies.

Exact Corrected Estimating Equations

Suppose that it is possible to find a function of the observed data, say $\psi_*(Y, Z, W, \Theta)$, having the property that

$$E[\psi_*(Y, Z, W, \Theta)|Y, Z, X] = \psi(Y, Z, X, \Theta), \quad (12)$$

for all Y, Z, X, and Θ. Then corrected score function estimators simply replace ψ by ψ_*. Corrected score functions satisfying (12) do not always exist, and finding them when they do is not always easy.

One useful class of models that admits corrected functions contains those models with log likelihoods

of the form

$$\log[f(y|z, x, \Theta)] = \sum_{k=0}^{2} [c_k(y, z, \Theta)(\beta_x^t x)^k]$$

$$+ c_3(y, z, \Theta) \exp(\beta_x^t x);$$

see the examples given below. Then, using normal distribution **moment generating function** identities, the required function is

$$\psi_*(y, z, w, \Theta, \sigma_u^2)$$

$$= \frac{\partial}{\partial \Theta^t} \left[\sum_{k=0}^{2} [c_k(y, z, \Theta)(\beta_x^t w)^k] - c_2(y, z, \Theta) \right.$$

$$\left. \times \beta_x^t \sigma_u^2 \beta_x + c_3(y, z, \Theta) \exp(\beta_x^t w - 0.5\beta_x^t \sigma_u^2 \beta_x) \right].$$

Regression models in this class include:

1. normal linear with mean $= \eta$, variance $= \phi$, $c_0 = -(y - \beta_0 - \beta_z^t z)^2/(2\phi) - \log(\phi^{1/2})$, $c_1 = (y - \beta_0 - \beta_z^t z)/\phi$, $c_2 = -(2\phi)^{-1}$, $c_3 = 0$
2. Poisson with mean $= \exp(\eta)$, variance $= \exp(\eta)$, $c_0 = y(\beta_0 + \beta_z^t z) - \log y!$, $c_1 = y$, $c_2 = 0$, $c_3 = -\exp(\beta_0 + \beta_z^t z)$
3. gamma with mean $= \exp(\eta)$, variance $= \phi \exp(2\eta)$, $c_0 = -\phi^{-1}(\beta_0 + \beta_z^t z) + (\phi^{-1} - 1)\log y + \phi^{-1}\log(\phi^{-1}) - \log[\Gamma(\phi^{-1})]$, $c_1 = \phi^{-1}$, $c_2 = 0$, $c_3 = -\phi^{-1}y \exp(-\beta_0 - \beta_z^t z)$.

Comparison of Methods

The methods are applicable at the same time only in linear regression (where they are identical) and Poisson regression. For Poisson regression the corrected estimating equations are more convenient because they are explicit, whereas the conditional estimator involves numerical summation. For Poisson regression the conditional-score estimator is more efficient than the corrected-score estimator in some practical cases.

Instrumental Variables

We have assumed that it was possible to estimate the measurement error variance, say with replicate measurements or validation data. However, it is not always possible to obtain replicates or validation data, and thus direct estimation of the measurement error variance is sometimes impossible. In the absence of information about the measurement error variance, estimation of the regression model parameters is still possible provided the data contain an *instrumental variable T*, in addition to the unbiased measurement $W = X + U$.

There are three basic requirements that an **instrumental variable** must satisfy: (i) it must be correlated with X; (ii) it must be independent of $W - X$; and (iii) it must be a surrogate, i.e. subject to nondifferential measurement error.

One possible source of an instrumental variable is a second measurement of X obtained by an independent method. This second measurement need not be unbiased for X. Thus the assumption that a variable is an instrument is weaker than the assumption that it follows the classical additive error model.

Instrumental variable estimation in linear models is covered in depth by Fuller [30]. The work described here, outside the linear model, is based on that of Carroll & Stefanski [17] and Stefanski & Buzas [69]. Other pertinent references include [1], [2], and [13].

We have found that instrumental variables require a slightly different notation. For example, $\beta_{Y|1ZX}$ is the coefficient of **1**, i.e. the intercept, in the regression of Y on **1**, Z, and X; $\beta_{Y|1ZX}$ is the coefficient of Z in the regression of Y on **1**, Z, and X. This notation allows representation of subsets of coefficient vectors, e.g. $\beta_{Y|1ZX} = (\beta_{Y|1ZX}, \beta_{Y|1ZX})$ and $\beta_{X|1ZT} = (\beta_{X|1ZT}, \beta_{X|1ZT}, \beta_{X|1ZT})$.

Our analysis is based upon regression calibration in generalized linear models, e.g. linear, logistic, and Poisson regression. It might be useful simply to think of this Section as dealing with a class of important models, whose details of fitting are standard in many computer programs.

The approximate models and estimation algorithms are best described in terms of the composite vectors

$$\mathbf{X} = (\mathbf{1}, Z, X), \qquad \mathbf{W} = (\mathbf{1}, Z, W),$$

$$\mathbf{T} = (\mathbf{1}, Z, T).$$

Define $\beta_{Y|\tilde{\mathbf{X}}} = (\beta_{Y|1ZX}, \beta_{Y|1ZX}, \beta_{Y|1ZX})$.

We note here that, in addition to the assumptions stated previously, we will also assume that the regression of X on (Z, T, W) is approximately linear. This

restricts the applicability of our methods somewhat, but is sufficiently general to encompass many potential applications.

The simplest instrumental variables estimator starts with a (possibly multivariate) regression of $\mathbf{W}$ on $\mathbf{T}$ to obtain $\hat{\beta}_{\mathbf{W}|\mathbf{T}}$. Then Y is regressed on the predicted values $\hat{\beta}_{\mathbf{W}|\mathbf{T}}\mathbf{T}$, which results in an estimator of $\beta_{Y|\mathbf{X}}$.

This estimator is easily computed as it requires only linear regression of the components of $\mathbf{W}$ on $\mathbf{T}$, and then the use of standard regression programs to regress Y on the "predictors" $\hat{\beta}_{\mathbf{W}|\mathbf{T}}\mathbf{T}$.

Carroll et al. [20] describe somewhat more elaborate methods of instrumental variable estimation, which can be more efficient than this simple method, especially if the number of components of T differs from the number of components of W.

Likelihood and Bayesian Structural Methods

This Section describes the use of likelihood methods in measurement error models. There have been a few examples in the literature based on likelihood. See [23], [63], [64], and [78] for probit regression, [84] for a Poisson model, [27], [62] and [81] in logistic regression, and [38] in a **change-point problem**. The relatively small literature belies the importance of the topic and the potential for further applications.

There are a number of important differences between likelihood methods and the methods described in previous Sections:

1. The previous methods are based on additive or multiplicative measurement error models, possibly after a transformation. Typically, few, if any, distributional assumptions are required. Likelihood methods require stronger distributional assumptions, but they can be applied to more general problems, including those with discrete covariates subject to **misclassification error**.

2. The likelihood for a fully specified parametric model can be used to obtain **likelihood ratio** confidence intervals. In methods not based on likelihoods, inference is based on bootstrapping or on normal approximations. In highly nonlinear problems, likelihood-based confidence intervals are generally more reliable than those derived from normal approximations.

3. Likelihood methods are often computationally more demanding, whereas the previous methods require little more than the use of standard statistical packages.

4. **Robustness** to modeling assumptions is a concern for both approaches, but is generally more difficult to understand with likelihood methods.

5. There is a belief that the simpler methods described previously perform just as well as likelihood methods for many statistical models, including the most common generalized linear models. There is little documentation as to whether the folklore is realistic. The only evidence that we know of is given for logistic regression by Stefanski & Carroll [72], who contrast the maximum likelihood estimate and a particular functional estimate. They find that the functional estimate is fairly efficient relative to the maximum likelihood estimate unless the measurement error is "large" or the logistic coefficient is "large". One should be aware, however, that their calculations indicate that there are situations where *properly parameterized* maximum likelihood estimates are considerably more efficient than estimates derived from functional modeling.

Likelihood Specification: Differential and Nondifferential Error

We consider here only the simplest problem in which X is not observable for all subjects, but there are sufficient data, either internal or external, to characterize the distribution of W given (X, Z) (with validation data, we are in the realm of missing data). To perform a likelihood analysis, one must specify a parametric model for every component of the data. Likelihood analysis starts with a model for the distribution of the response given the true predictors. The likelihood (density or mass) function of Y given (Z, X) will be called $f_{Y|Z,X}(y|z, x, \mathcal{B})$ here, and interest lies in estimating $\mathcal{B}$. For example, if Y is normally distributed with mean $\beta_0 + \beta_x X + \beta_z Z$ and variance σ^2, then $\mathcal{B} = (\beta_0, \beta_x, \beta_z, \sigma^2)$ and

$$f_{Y|Z,X}(y|z, x, \mathcal{B}) = \sigma^{-1}\phi[(y - \beta_0 + \beta_x x + \beta_z z)/\sigma],$$

where $\phi(v) = (2\pi)^{-1/2}\exp(-0.5v^2)$ is the standard normal density function. If Y follows a logistic regression model with mean $H(\beta_0 + \beta_x X + \beta_z Z)$,

then $\mathcal{B} = (\beta_0, \beta_x, \beta_z)$ and

$$f_{Y|Z,X}(y|z, x, \mathcal{B}) = H^y(\beta_0 + \beta_x x + \beta_z z)$$
$$\times [1 - H(\beta_0 + \beta_x x + \beta_z z)]^{1-y}.$$

A likelihood analysis starts with determination of the joint distribution of Y and W given Z, as these are the observed variates. There are three components required:

1. A model relating the response to the "true" covariates, see just above.

2. An error model, here called $f_{W|Z,X}(w|z, x, \tilde{\alpha}_1)$. In many applications, the error model does not depend on Z. For example, in the classical additive measurement error model (1) with normally distributed measurement error, σ_u^2 is the only component of $\tilde{\alpha}_1$, and the error model density is $\sigma_u^{-1}\phi[(w - x)/\sigma_u]$, where $\phi(\cdot)$ is the standard normal density function. In the classical error model with independent replicates, W consists of the k replicates, and $f_{W|Z,X}$ is the k-variate normal density function with mean zero, common variance σ_u^2, and zero correlation. A generalization of this error model that allows for correlations among the replicates has been studied [81]. In some application areas, error model structures are studied independently of their role in measurement error modeling, and one can use this research to estimate error models for the problem at hand.

3. A model for the distribution of the latent variable, here called $f_{X|Z}(x|z, \tilde{\alpha}_2)$. Specifying a model for the distribution of the true covariate X given all the other covariates, Z is more difficult. Difficulties arise because: (i) the distribution is usually not transportable, so that different studies yield very different models; and (ii) X is not observed.

Having hypothesized the various models, the likelihood of the observed data under nondifferential measurement error is

$$f_{Y,W|Z}(y, w|z, \mathcal{B}, \tilde{\alpha}_1, \tilde{\alpha}_2)$$
$$= \int f_{Y|Z,X}(y|z, x, \mathcal{B})f_{W|Z,X}(w|z, x, \tilde{\alpha}_1)$$
$$\times f_{X|Z}(x|z, \tilde{\alpha}_2)\mathrm{d}\mu(x). \quad (13)$$

The notation $\mathrm{d}\mu(x)$ indicates that the integrals are sums if X is discrete and integrals if X is continuous.

The likelihood for the problem is just the product over the sample of these terms.

There is a significant difference between the likelihood function in the differential and nondifferential cases. This can be expressed in various ways, but the simplest is as follows. In general, and dropping parameters, the likelihood of the observed data is

$$f_{Y,W|Z}(y, w|z) = \int f_{Y,W,X|Z}(y, w, x|z) \mathrm{d}\mu(x).$$

Using standard conditioning arguments, this becomes

$$f_{Y,W|Z}(y, w|z) = \int f_{W|Y,Z,X}(w|y, z, x) f_{Y|Z,X}(y|z, x)$$
$$\times f_{X|Z}(x|z) \mathrm{d}\mu(x)$$
$$= \int f_{Y|Z,X}(y|z, x) f_{W|Y,Z,X}(w|y, z, x)$$
$$\times f_{X|Z}(x|z) \mathrm{d}\mu(x). \quad (14)$$

Note that the only difference between (13) and (14) is in the error term. In the former, under nondifferential measurement error, W and Y are independent, so that $f_{W|Y,Z,X}(w|y, z, x) = f_{W|Z,X}(w|z, x)$.

What makes differential error so difficult is that, under differential measurement error, we must ascertain the distribution of W given the other covariates *and the response Y*. This is essentially impossible to do in practice unless one has a subset of the data in which all of (Y, Z, X, W) are observed, i.e. a *validation* data set (*see* **Validation Study**).

Numerical Computation of Likelihoods

Typically one maximizes the logarithm of the overall likelihood in the unknown parameters. There are two ways one can maximize the likelihood function. The most direct is to compute the likelihood function itself, and then use numerical optimization techniques to maximize the likelihood. Below we provide a few details about computing the likelihood function. The second general approach is to view the problem as a missing data problem, and then use missing data techniques (*see* **Missing Data**); see, for example, [42] and [75].

Computing the likelihood analytically is easy if X is discrete, as the conditional expectations are simply sums of terms. Likelihoods in which X has some continuous components can be computed using a number of different approaches. In some problems the log likelihood can be computed or very well approximated analytically. In most problems that we have encountered, X is a scalar or a 2×1 vector. In these cases, standard numerical methods such as Gaussian quadrature can be applied, although they are not always very good. When sufficient computing resources are available, the likelihood can be computed using **Monte Carlo** techniques.

Bayesian Methods

Bayesian estimation and inference in the measurement error problem is a promising approach under active development (*see* **Bayesian Methods**). Examples of this approach are given by Schmid & Rosner [65], Richardson & Gilks [57], Stephens & Dellaportas [74], Müller & Roeder [47], Mallick & Gelfand [45], and Kuha [40].

Bayesian analysis of parametric models requires specifying a likelihood (as described above) and a **prior distribution** for the parameters, the latter representing knowledge about the parameters prior to data collection. The product of the prior and likelihood is the joint density of the data and the parameters. Using **Bayes' Theorem**, one can in principle obtain the posterior density, i.e. the conditional density of the parameters given the data. The posterior summarizes all of the information about the values of the parameters and is the basis for all Bayesian inference. For example, the mean, median, or mode of the posterior density are all suitable point estimators. A region with probability $1 - \alpha$ under the posterior is called a "credible set," and is a Bayesian analog to a confidence region.

Computing the posterior distribution is often a nontrivial problem, because it usually requires high-dimensional numerical integration. This computational problem is the subject of much recent research, with many major advances. The method currently receiving the most attention in the literature is the Gibbs sampler (see [66] and [24]; *see* **Markov Chain Monte Carlo**). Also, see Tanner [75] for a book-length introduction to modern methods for computing posterior distributions.

In the Bayesian approach with Gibbs sampling, the Xs are treated as "missing data" (they just happen to be missing for all study subjects unless there is a validation study!). The approach for the classical additive error model is:

1. Assuming nondifferential error, write the likelihood of Y given (X, Z), the likelihood of W given (X, Z), and the likelihood of X given Z depending on parameters, just as in a regular likelihood problem.
2. If X were observable, then the likelihood would be the product of the three terms given above.
3. Select a starting value for the parameters, e.g. from SIMEX.
4. Use a simulation approach to fill in the "missing" Xs, i.e. from the posterior distribution of X given the observed data and the current values of the parameters. In this step, it is rare that the posterior distribution is known exactly, and so one has to use a device such as the Metropolis–Hastings algorithm.
5. Now one has complete data, with Xs all filled in, and one uses simulation to draw a sample of parameters from the posterior distribution of the parameters given the observed data and the current Xs.
6. Repeat the process of generating X and the parameters. These multiple samples of parameters are used to evaluate features of the posterior distribution.

While the procedure is easy to write down, the computations may be difficult.

More importantly, though, is the need to consider the distribution of X given Z. As we emphasized above, the simplest structural approach assumes that X is normally distributed, but this is often a strong assumption. The popularity of functional methods lies in the fact that such methods require no distributional assumptions about the Xs. There is considerable current effort being made to circumvent the problem of model robustness by specifying a flexible distribution for X.

Mixture Modeling

When there are no covariates measured without error, the nonlinear measurement error problem can be viewed as a special case of what are called mixture problems (see [77]). The idea is to pretend that X has a distribution, but to estimate this distribution nonparametrically. Applications of nonparametric mixture methods to nonlinear measurement error models have only recently been described by Thomas et al. [76] and Roeder et al. [58].

An alternative formulation is to let X have a flexible distribution, which covers a wide range of possibilities including the normal distribution. The simplest such model is the mixture of normals, which has been applied by Wang et al. [81] and by Küchenhoff & Carroll [38].

Response Error

In preceding Sections we have focused exclusively on problems associated with measurement error in predictor variables. Here we consider problems that arise when a true response is measured with error. For example, in a study of factors affecting dietary intake of fat, e.g. sex, race, age, socioeconomic status, etc., true long-term dietary intake is impossible to determine and instead it is necessary to use error-prone measures of long-term dietary intake. Wittes et al. [86] describe another example in which damage to the heart muscle caused by a myocardial infarction can be assessed accurately, but the procedure is expensive and invasive, and instead it is common practice to use the peak cardiac enzyme level in the bloodstream as a proxy for the true response.

For a binary response (case or control), see **Misclassification Error**.

The exclusive attention paid to predictor measurement error earlier in this article is explained by the fact that predictor measurement error is seldom ignorable, by which is meant that the usual method of analysis is statistically valid, whereas response measurement error is often ignorable when the response is continuous. Here, "ignorable" means that the model holding for the true response holds also for the proxy response with parameters unchanged, except that a measurement error variance component is added to the response variance. For example, in linear regression models with simple types of response measurement error, the response measurement error is **confounded** with equation error and the effect is simply to increase the variability of parameter estimates. Thus, response error is ignorable in these cases, although of course power will be lost. However, in more complicated regression models, certain types of response error are not ignorable and it is important to account for the response error explicitly in the regression analysis.

Although the details differ between methods for predictor error and response error, many of the basic ideas are similar. Throughout this section, the response proxy is denoted by S. We consider only the case of measurement error in the response, and not the more complex problem where both the response and some of the predictors are measured with error.

We first consider the analysis of the observed data when the response is subject to independent additive or multiplicative measurement error. Suppose that the proxy response S is unbiased for the true response. Then, in either case, the proxy response has the same mean (as a function of exposure and confounders) as the true response, although the variance structure differs. In models such as linear regression, or more generally for **quasi-likelihood** estimation, this means that the parameter estimates are consistent, but inferences may be affected. For example, in linear regression, additive, unbiased response error does not change the mean and simply increases the variance by a constant, so that there is no effect of measurement error other than loss of power. However, for multiplicative, unbiased response error, while the mean remains unchanged, the variances now are no longer constant, and hence inferences which pretend that the variances are constant would be affected. The usual solution is to use a robust covariance estimator, also known as the sandwich estimator (*see* **Generalized Estimating Equations**).

If the proxy response **S** is not unbiased for the true response, then a validation study is required to understand the nature of the bias and to correct for it. In a series of papers, Buonaccorsi [8, 9, 11] and Buonaccorsi & Tosteson [12] discuss the use of adjustments for a biased response. See Carroll et al. [20] for further details.

We call **S** a *surrogate response* if its distribution depends only on the true response and not otherwise on the covariates, i.e. the information about the surrogate response contained in the true response is the same no matter what the values of the covariates. In symbols, if $f_{S|Y,Z,X}(s|y, z, x, \gamma)$ denotes the density or mass function for S given (Y, Z, X), then $f_{S|Y,Z,X}(s|y, z, x, \gamma) = f_{S|Y}(s|y, \gamma)$. In both the additive and multiplicative error models, S is a surrogate. This definition of a surrogate response is the natural counterpart to a surrogate predictor, because it implies that all the information in the relationship between S and the predictors is explained by the underlying response. See Prentice [53] and Carroll et al. [20] for further details.

In general, i.e. for a possibly nonsurrogate response, the likelihood function for the observed response is

$$f_{S|Z,X}(s|z, x, \mathcal{B}, \gamma)$$
$$= \int f_{Y|Z,X}(y|z, x, \mathcal{B}) f_{S|Y,Z,X}(s|y, z, x, \gamma) \mathrm{d}\mu(y).$$
$$(15)$$

There are a number of implications of this formula:

1. If S is a surrogate, and if there is no relationship between the true response and the predictors, then neither is there one between the observed response and the predictors. Hence, if interest lies in determining whether *any of the predictors* contains any information about the response, then one can use naive hypothesis tests and ignore response error. The resulting tests have an asymptotically correct level, but a decreased power relative to tests derived from true response data. This property of a surrogate is important in clinical trials; see Prentice [53] (*see* **Surrogate Endpoints**).
2. If S is *not* a surrogate, then there may be no relationship between the true response and the covariates, but the observed response may be related to the predictors. Hence, naive tests will not be valid in general if **S** is not a surrogate.

Note that one implication of (15) is that a likelihood analysis with mismeasured responses requires a model for the distribution of response error. Except for additive and multiplicative error, understanding such a model requires a validation study.

Case–Control Studies

A *case–control study* is one in which sampling is conditioned on the disease response; it is useful to think that the response is first observed and only later are the predictors observed. A similar design, *choice-based sampling*, is used in econometrics. We use case–control terminology and concentrate on logistic regression models. A distinguishing feature of case–control studies is that the measurement error may be differential.

Two-phase case–control designs, where X is observed on a subset of the data, have been studied by Breslow & Cain [7], Zhao & Lipsitz [87], Tosteson

& Ware [80], and Carroll et al. [18], among others. These designs are significant because the validation, if done on both cases and controls, frees us from the nondifferential error assumption.

We assume that the data follow a logistic model in the underlying source population, although the results apply equally well to the more general models described by Weinberg & Wacholder [82]. For such models, Prentice & Pyke [55] and Weinberg & Wacholder [82] show that when analyzing a classical case–control study one can ignore the case–control sampling scheme entirely, at least for the purpose of estimating **relative risk**. Furthermore, these authors show that, if one *ignores the case–control sampling scheme and runs an ordinary logistic regression*, then the resulting relative risk estimates are consistent and the standard errors are asymptotically correct.

The effect of measurement error in logistic case–control studies is to bias the estimates. Carroll et al. [21] show that, for many problems, one can ignore the case–control study design and proceed to correct for the bias from measurement error as if one were analyzing a random sample from the source population. With nondifferential measurement error, this result applies to the methods we have described previously for prospective studies. Regression calibration needs a slight modification, namely that the regression calibration function should be estimated using the controls only.

Michalek & Tripathi [46], Armstrong et al. [5], and Buonaccorsi [10] consider the normal **discriminant** model. Satten & Kupper [62] have an interesting example of likelihood analysis for nondifferential error validation studies when the validation sampling is in the controls.

Survival Analysis

One of the earliest applications of the regression calibration method was discussed by Prentice [52] in the context of **survival analysis**. Further results in survival analysis were obtained by Pepe et al. [50], Clayton [25], Nakamura [49], and Hughes [36]. While the details differ in substantive ways, the ideas are the same as put forward in the rest of this article, and here we provide only a very brief overview in the case of covariates which do not depend on time.

Suppose that the instantaneous risk that the time T of an event equals t conditional on no events prior to time t and conditional on the true covariate X is

denoted by

$$\psi(t, X) = \psi_0(t) \exp(\beta_x X), \qquad (16)$$

where $\psi_0(t)$ is the baseline **hazard** function. When the baseline hazard is not specified, (16) is commonly called the **proportional hazards** assumption. When X is observable, it is well known that estimation of β_x is possible without specifying the form of the baseline hazard function.

If X is unobservable and instead we observe a surrogate W, then the induced hazard function is

$$\psi^*(t, W, \beta_x) = \psi_0(t) E[\exp(\beta_x X) | T \geq t, W]. \quad (17)$$

The difficulty is that the expectation in (17) for the observed data depends upon the unknown baseline hazard function ψ_0. Thus, the hazard function does not factor into a product of an arbitrary baseline hazard times a term that depends only on observed data and an unknown parameter, and the technology for proportional hazards regression cannot be applied without modification.

The problem simplifies when the event is rare, so that $T \geq t$ occurs with high probability for all t under consideration. As shown by Prentice [53] and others, under certain circumstances this leads to the regression calibration algorithm. The rare event assumption allows the hazard of the observed data to be approximated by

$$\psi^*(t, W, \beta_x) = \psi_0(t) E[\exp(\beta_x X) | W]. \quad (18)$$

The hazard function (18) requires a regression calibration formulation! If one specifies a model for the distribution of X given W, then (18) is in the form of a proportional hazards model (16), but with $\beta_x X$ replaced by $\log\{E[\exp(\beta_x X)|W]\}$. An important special case leads directly to the standard regression calibration model, namely when X given W is normally distributed.

Clayton [25] proposed a modification of regression calibration which does not require events to be rare. At each time $t_i, i = 1, \ldots, k$, for which an event occurs, define the risk set $R_i \subseteq \{1, \ldots, n\}$ as the case numbers of those members of the study cohort for whom an event has not occurred and who were still under study just prior to t_i. If the Xs were observable, and if X_i is the covariate associated with the ith event, in the absence of ties the usual proportional hazards regression would maximize

$$\prod_{i=1}^{k} \frac{\exp(\beta_x X_i)}{\sum_{j \in R_i} \exp(\beta_x X_j)}.$$

Clayton basically suggests using regression calibration within each risk set. He assumes that the true values X within the ith risk set are normally distributed with mean μ_i and variance σ_x^2, and that within this risk set $W = X + U$, where U is normally distributed with mean zero and variance σ_u^2. Neither σ_x^2 nor σ_u^2 depend upon the risk set in his formulation.

Given an estimate $\hat{\sigma}_u^2$, one applies the usual regression calibration calculations to construct an estimate of $\hat{\sigma}_x^2$.

Clayton modifies regression calibration by using it within each risk set. Within each risk set, he applies the formula (7) for the best unbiased estimate of the Xs. Specifically, in the absence of replication, for any member of the ith risk set, the estimate of the true covariate X from an observed covariate W is

$$\hat{X} = \hat{\mu}_i + \frac{\hat{\sigma}_x^2}{\hat{\sigma}_x^2 + \hat{\sigma}_u^2}(W - \hat{\mu}_i),$$

where $\hat{\mu}_i$ is the sample mean of the Ws in the ith risk set.

As with regression calibration in general, the advantage of Clayton's method is that no new software need be developed, other than to calculate the means within risk sets.

Acknowledgment

This work was supported by a grant from the National Cancer Institute (CA-57030).

References

[1]   Amemiya, Y. (1985). Instrumental variable estimator for the nonlinear errors in variables model, *Journal of Econometrics* **28**, 273–289.

[2]   Amemiya, Y. (1990). Instrumental variable estimation of the nonlinear measurement error model, in *Statistical Analysis of Measurement Error Models and Application*, P.J. Brown & W.A. Fuller, eds. American Mathematics Society, Providence.

[3]   Amemiya, Y. & Fuller, W.A. (1988). Estimation for the nonlinear functional relationship, *Annals of Statistics* **16**, 147–160.

[4]   Armstrong, B. (1985). Measurement error in generalized linear models, *Communications in Statistics, Part B - Simulation and Computation* **14**, 529–544.

[5]   Armstrong, B.G., Whittemore, A.S. & Howe, G.R. (1989). Analysis of case-control data with covariate measurement error: application to diet and colon cancer, *Statistics in Medicine* **8**, 1151–1163.

[6]   Berkson, J. (1950). Are there two regressions?, *Journal of the American Statistical Association* **45**, 164–180.

[7]   Breslow, N.E. & Cain, K.C. (1988). Logistic regression for two-stage case-control data, *Biometrika* **75**, 11–20.

[8]   Buonaccorsi, J.P. (1988). Errors in variables with systematic biases, *Communications in Statistics - Theory and Methods* **18**, 1001–1021.

[9]   Buonaccorsi, J.P. (1990). Double sampling for exact values in some multivariate measurement error problems, *Journal of the American Statistical Association* **85**, 1075–1082.

[10] Buonaccorsi, J.P. (1990). Double sampling for exact values in the normal discriminant model with application to binary regression, *Communications in Statistics - Theory and Methods* **19**, 4569–4586.

[11] Buonaccorsi, J.P. (1991). Measurement error, linear calibration and inferences for means, *Computational Statistics and Data Analysis* **11**, 239–257.

[12] Buonaccorsi, J.P. & Tosterson, T. (1993). Correcting for nonlinear measurement error in the dependent variable in the general linear model, *Communications in Statistics - Theory and Methods* **22**, 2687–2702.

[13] Buzas, J.S. & Stefanski, L.A. (1995). A note on corrected score estimation, *Statistics and Probability Letters* **28**, 1–8.

[14] Carroll, R.J. & Ruppert, D. (1988). *Transformation and Weighting in Regression*. Chapman & Hall, London.

[15] Carroll, R.J. & Ruppert, D. (1996). The use and misuse of orthogonal regression in measurement error models, *American Statistician* **50**, 1–6.

[16] Carroll, R.J. & Stefanski, L.A. (1990). Approximate quasilikelihood estimation in models with surrogate predictors, *Journal of the American Statistical Association* **85**, 652–663.

[17] Carroll, R.J. & Stefanski, L.A. (1994). Measurement error, instrumental variables and corrections for attenuation with applications to meta-analyses, *Statistics in Medicine* **13**, 1265–1282.

[18] Carroll, R.J., Gail, M.H. & Lubin, J.H. (1993). Case-control studies with errors in predictors, *Journal of the American Statistical Association* **88**, 177–191.

[19] Carroll, R.J., Gallo, P.P. & Gleser, L.J. (1985). Comparison of least squares and errors-in-variables regression, with special reference to randomized analysis of covariance, *Journal of the American Statistical Association* **80**, 929–932.

[20] Carroll, R.J., Ruppert, D. & Stefanski, L.A. (1995). *Measurement Error in Nonlinear Models*. Chapman & Hall, London.

[21] Carroll, R.J., Wang, S. & Wang, C.Y. (1995). Asymptotics for prospective analysis of stratified logistic case-control studies, *Journal of the American Statistical Association* **90**, 157–169.

[22] Carroll, R.J., Küchenhoff, H., Lombard, F. & Stefanski, L.A. (1996). Asymptotics for the SIMEX estimator in structural measurement error models, *Journal of the American Statistical Association* **91**, 242–250.

[23] Carroll, R.J., Spiegelman, C., Lan, K.K., Bailey, K.T. & Abbott, R.D. (1984). On errors-in-variables for binary regression models, *Biometrika* **71**, 19–26.

[24] Casella, G. & George, E.I. (1992). Explaining the Gibbs sampler, *American Statistician* **46**, 167–174.

[25] Clayton, D.G. (1991). Models for the analysis of cohort and case-control studies with inaccurately measured exposures, in *Statistical Models for Longitudinal Studies of Health*, J.H. Dwyer, M. Feinleib, P. Lipsert et al., eds. Oxford University Press, New York, pp. 301–331.

[26] Cook, J. & Stefanski, L.A. (1995). A simulation extrapolation method for parametric measurement error models, *Journal of the American Statistical Association* **89**, 1314–1328.

[27] Crouch, E.A. & Spiegelman, D. (1990). The evaluation of integrals of the form $\int_{-\infty}^{\infty} f(t)\exp(-t^2)\mathrm{d}t$: applications to logistic-normal models, *Journal of the American Statistical Association* **85**, 464–467.

[28] Dosemeci, M., Wacholder, S. & Lubin, J.H. (1990). Does non-differential misclassification of exposure always bias a true effect towards the null value?, *American Journal of Epidemiology* **132**, 746–748.

[29] Freedman, L.S., Carroll, R.J. & Wax, Y. (1991). Estimating the relationship between dietary intake obtained from a food frequency questionnaire and true average intake, *American Journal of Epidemiology* **134**, 510–520.

[30] Fuller, W.A. (1987). *Measurement Error Models*. Wiley, New York.

[31] Ganse, R.A., Amemiya, Y. & Fuller, W.A. (1983). Prediction when both variables are subject to error, with application to earthquake magnitude, *Journal of the American Statistical Association* **78**, 761–765.

[32] Gleser, L.J. (1981). Estimation in multivariate errors in variables regression model: large sample results, *Annals of Statistics* **9**, 24–44.

[33] Gleser, L.J. (1990). Improvements of the naive approach to estimation in nonlinear errors-in-variables regression models, in *Statistical Analysis of Measurement Error Models and Application*, P.J. Brown & W.A. Fuller, eds. American Mathematical Society, Providence.

[34] Greenland, S. (1980). The effect of misclassification in the presence of covariates, *American Journal of Epidemiology* **112**, 564–569.

[35] Greenland, S. & Robins, J.M. (1985). Confounding and misclassification, *American Journal of Epidemiology* **122**, 495–506.

[36] Hughes, M.D. (1993). Regression dilution in the proportional hazards model, *Biometrics* **49**, 1056–1066.

[37] Hunter, D.J., Spiegelman, D., Adami, H.-O., Beeson, L., van der Brandt, P.A., Folsom, A.R., Fraser, G.E., Goldbohm, A., Graham, S., Howe, G.R., Kushi, L.H., Marshall, J.R., McDermott, A., Miller, A.B., Speizer, F.E., Wolk, A., Yaun, S.S. & Willett, W. (1996). Cohort studies of fat intake and the risk of breast cancer-a pooled analysis, *New England Journal of Medicine* **334**, 356–361.

[38] Küchenhoff, H. & Carroll, R.J. (1997). Segmented regression with errors in predictors: semiparametric and parametric methods, *Statistics in Medicine* **16**, 169–188.

[39] Kuha, J. (1994). Corrections for exposure measurement error in logistic regression models with an application to nutritional data, *Statistics in Medicine* **13**, 1135–1148.

[40] Kuha, J. (1997). Estimation by data augmentation in regression models with continuous and discrete covariates measured with error, *Statistics in Medicine* **16**, 189–201.

[41] Li, L., Freedman, L., Kipnis, V. & Carroll, R.J. (1997). Effects of bias and correlated measurement errors in the validation of food frequency questionnaires. Preprint.

[42] Little, R.J.A. & Rubin, D.B. (1987). *Statistical Analysis with Missing Data*. Wiley, New York.

[43] Liu, X. & Liang, K.Y. (1992). Efficacy of repeated measures in regression models with measurement error, *Biometrics* **48**, 645–654.

[44] MacMahon, S., Peto, R., Cutler, J., Collins, R., Sorlie, P., Neaton, J., Abbott, R., Godwin, J., Dyer, A. & Stamler, J. (1990). Blood pressure, stroke and coronary heart disease: Part 1, prolonged differences in blood pressure: prospective observational studies corrected for the regression dilution bias, *Lancet* **335**, 765–774.

[45] Mallick, B.K. & Gelfand, A.E. (1996). Semiparametric errors-in-variables models: a Bayesian approach, *Journal of Statistical Planning and Inference* **52**, 307–322.

[46] Michalek, J.E. & Tripathi, R.C. (1980). The effect of errors in diagnosis and measurement on the probability of an event, *Journal of the American Statistical Association* **75**, 713–721.

[47] Müller, P. & Roeder, K. (1997). A Bayesian semiparametric model for case-control studies with errors in variables, *Biometrika* **84**, 523–537.

[48] Nakamura, T. (1990). Corrected score functions for errors-in-variables models: methodology and application to generalized linear models, *Biometrika* **77**, 127–137.

[49] Nakamura, T. (1992). Proportional hazards models with covariates subject to measurement error, *Biometrics* **48**, 829–838.

[50] Pepe, M.S., Self, S.G. & Prentice, R.L. (1989). Further results in covariate measurement errors in cohort studies with time to response data, *Statistics in Medicine* **8**, 1167–1178.

[51] Pierce, D.A., Stram, D.O., Vaeth, M. & Schafer, D. (1992). Some insights into the errors in variables problem provided by consideration of radiation dose-response analyses for the A-bomb survivors,

Journal of the American Statistical Association **87**, 351–359.

[52] Prentice, R.L. (1982). Covariate measurement errors and parameter estimation in a failure time regression model, *Biometrika* **69**, 331–342.

[53] Prentice, R.L. (1989). Surrogate endpoints in clinical trials: definition and operational criteria, *Statistics in Medicine* **8**, 431–440.

[54] Prentice, R.L. (1996). Dietary fat and breast cancer: measurement error and results from analytic epidemiology, *Journal of the National Cancer Institute* **88**, 1738–1747.

[55] Prentice, R.L. & Pyke, R. (1979). Logistic disease incidence models and case-control studies, *Biometrika* **66**, 403–411.

[56] Racine-Poon, A., Weihs, C. & Smith, A.F.M. (1991). Estimation of relative potency with sequential dilution errors in radioimmunoassay, *Biometrics* **47**, 1235–1246.

[57] Richardson, S. & Gilks, W.R. (1993). A Bayesian approach to measurement error problems in epidemiology using conditional independence models, *American Journal of Epidemiology* **138**, 430–442.

[58] Roeder, K., Carroll, R.J. & Lindsay, B.G. (1996). A nonparametric mixture approach to case-control studies with errors in covariables, *Journal of the American Statistical Association* **91**, 722–732.

[59] Rosner, B., Spiegelman, D. & Willett, W.C. (1990). Correction of logistic regression relative risk estimates and confidence intervals for measurement error: the case of multiple covariates measured with error, *American Journal of Epidemiology* **132**, 734–745.

[60] Rosner, B., Willett, W.C. & Spiegelman, D. (1989). Correction of logistic regression relative risk estimates and confidence intervals for systematic within-person measurement error, *Statistics in Medicine* **8**, 1051–1070.

[61] Rudemo, M., Ruppert, D. & Streibig, J.C. (1989). Random effect models in nonlinear regression with applications to bioassay, *Biometrics* **45**, 349–362.

[62] Satten, G.A. & Kupper, L.L. (1993). Inferences about exposure-disease association using probability of exposure information, *Journal of the American Statistical Association* **88**, 200–208.

[63] Schafer, D. (1987). Covariate measurement error in generalized linear models, *Biometrika* **74**, 385–391.

[64] Schafer, D. (1993). Likelihood analysis for probit regression with measurement errors, *Biometrika* **80**, 899–904.

[65] Schmid, C.H. & Rosner, B. (1993). A Bayesian approach to logistic regression models having measurement error following a mixture distribution, *Statistics in Medicine* **12**, 1141–1153.

[66] Smith, A.F.M. & Gelfand, A.E. (1992). Bayesian statistics without tears: a sampling-resampling perspective, *American Statistician* **46**, 84–88.

[67] Stefanski, L.A. (1985). The effects of measurement error on parameter estimation, *Biometrika* **72**, 583–592.

[68] Stefanski, L.A. (1989). Unbiased estimation of a nonlinear function of a normal mean with application

to measurement error models, *Communications in Statistics - Theory and Methods* **18**, 4335–4358.

[69] Stefanski, L.A. & Buzas, J.S. (1995). Instrumental variable estimation in binary regression measurement error models, *Journal of the American Statistical Association* **90**, 541–549.

[70] Stefanski, L.A. & Carroll, R.J. (1985). Covariate measurement error in logistic regression, *Annals of Statistics* **13**, 1335–1351.

[71] Stefanski, L.A. & Carroll, R.J. (1987). Conditional scores and optimal scores in generalized linear measurement error models, *Biometrika* **74**, 703–716.

[72] Stefanski, L.A. & Carroll, R.J. (1990). Structural logistic regression measurement error models, in *Proceedings of the Conference on Measurement Error Models*, P.J. Brown & W.A. Fuller, eds. Wiley, New York.

[73] Stefanski, L.A. & Cook, J. (1995). Simulation extrapolation: the measurement error jackknife, *Journal of the American Statistical Association* **90**, 1247–1256.

[74] Stephens, D.A. & Dellaportas, P. (1992). Bayesian analysis of generalized linear models with covariate measurement error, in *Bayesian Statistics 4*, J.M. Bernado, J.O. Berger, A.P. Dawid & A.F.M. Smith, eds. Oxford University Press, Oxford, pp. 813–820.

[75] Tanner, M.A. (1993). *Tools for Statistical Inference: Methods for the Exploration of Posterior Distributions and Likelihood Functions*, 2nd Ed. Springer-Verlag, New York.

[76] Thomas, D., Stram, D. & Dwyer, J. (1993). Exposure measurement error: influence on exposure-disease relationships and methods of correction, *Annual Review of Public Health* **14**, 69–93.

[77] Titterington, D.M., Smith, A.F.M. & Makov, U.E. (1985). *Statistical Analysis of Finite Mixture Distributions*. Wiley, New York.

[78] Tosteson, T., Stefanski, L.A. & Schafer D.W. (1989). A measurement error model for binary and ordinal regression, *Statistics in Medicine* **8**, 1139–1147.

[79] Tosteson, T. & Tsiatis, A. (1988). The asymptotic relative efficiency of score tests in a generalized linear model with surrogate covariates, *Biometrika* **75**, 507–514.

[80] Tosteson, T.D. & Ware, J.H. (1990). Designing a logistic regression study using surrogate measures of exposure and outcome, *Biometrika* **77**, 11–20.

[81] Wang, N., Carroll, R.J. & Liang, K.Y. (1996). Quasi-likelihood and variance functions in measurement error models with replicates, *Biometrics* **52**, 401–411.

[82] Weinberg, C.R. & Wacholder, S. (1993). Prospective analysis of case-control data under general multiplicative-intercept models, *Biometrika* **80**, 461–465.

[83] Whittemore, A.S. (1989). Errors in variables regression using Stein estimates, *American Statistician* **43**, 226–228.

[84] Whittemore, A.S. & Gong, G. (1991). Poisson regression with misclassified counts: application to cervical cancer mortality rates, *Applied Statistics* **40**, 81–93.

[85] Whittemore, A.S. & Keller, J.B. (1988). Approximations for regression with covariate measurement error, *Journal of the American Statistical Association* **83**, 1057–1066.

[86] Wittes, J., Lakatos, E. & Probstfield, J. (1989). Surrogate endpoints in clinical trials: cardiovascular trials, *Statistics in Medicine* **8**, 415–425.

[87] Zhao, L.P. & Lipsitz, S. (1992). Designs and analysis of two-stage studies, *Statistics in Medicine* **11**, 769–782.

RAYMOND J. CARROLL

Measurement Error in Survival Analysis

Let $T \geq 0$ be a failure time variate (*see* **Survival Analysis, Overview**) and $Z = (Z_1, \ldots, Z_p)'$ be a corresponding vector. Suppose that the hazard function is of the **Cox regression model** form [4] $\lambda(t; Z) = \lambda_0(t) \exp(Z'\beta)$, where λ_0 is an unspecified baseline hazard function and β is a regression vector to be estimated. Suppose also that C is a right-censoring variate (*see* **Censored Data**) that is independent of T given Z, so that one observes (X, δ, Z), where $X = T \wedge C$ and $\delta = I[X = T]$. On the basis of an independent random sample (X_i, δ_i, Z_i), $i = 1, \ldots, n$, the standard estimator $\hat{\beta}$ solves

$$\sum_{i=1}^{n} \delta_i \frac{\partial r_i(t)/\partial \beta}{r_i(t)} - \sum_{i=1}^{n} \delta_i \frac{\sum_{l \in R(X_i)} \partial r_l(t)/\partial \beta}{\sum_{l \in R(X_i)} r_l(t)} = 0 \quad (1)$$

where $R(t) = \{l | X_l \geq t\}$ is the **risk set** at time t, $r_l(t) = r_l(t, \beta) = \exp(Z'\beta)$ is the **relative risk** for subject l. This estimator has been justified on the basis of **partial**, marginal, and full-likelihood arguments, and is known to be semiparametric efficient quite generally. See [1] and [10] for development of the asymptotic distribution theory for $\hat{\beta}$.

In many applications some components of the regression vector Z will be measured with error, in which case a vector $W = (W_1, \ldots, W_p)'$ rather than Z will be routinely available (*see* **Measurement Error in Epidemiologic Studies**). For example, in a **nutritional** epidemiology application, Z may consist of Z_1, an individual's long-term (e.g. 10 or 20 years)

average daily intake of fat, along with dietary and nondietary confounding factors, while T is the time from entry into a cohort study until the diagnosis of a specific disease, such as coronary heart disease or colon cancer. The measured fat intake, say W_1, in this context would typically involve self-reported food intakes over a relatively short period of time (e.g. a few days or months). Hence W_1 may differ from Z_1 because of day-to-day or month-to-month variations in actual fat consumptions, because of errors in dietary recording or recall, because of inaccuracies in the nutrient database used to translate foods into nutrients, or due to systematic self-report biases, the magnitude of which may relate to body mass or other "social desirability" characteristics.

If the variation in $W - Z$ is small compared to that for Z, one may simply be able to replace Z by W in (1) and obtain estimates of β having little bias. More generally, some additional data (or assumptions) will be required to estimate the joint distribution of (T, Z, W) and hence to estimate β. In the best of situations, a validation subsample can be obtained that includes (X, δ, Z, W), while only (X, δ, W) is available on the remainder of the sample. More commonly, only a **reliability** subsample consisting of repeated measures of W can be obtained, so that the data consist of $(X, \delta, W_1, W_2, \ldots)$ on the reliability subsample, and (X, δ, W_1) on the remainder of the study cohort [6]. It is typically assumed that the reliability measurement errors have mean zero and are independent of Z, assumptions that appear to be violated in the above nutritional epidemiology context.

Relative Risk Parameter Estimation with a Validation Subsample

Suppose that a **validation** subsample $V \subset \{1, \ldots, n\}$ is selected at random from the study cohort. A "complete case" analysis would use only validation subsample data to estimate β, using (1). Such an analysis would yield consistent, asymptotically normal estimates of β provided that the validation sample size $\to \infty$ as $n \to \infty$, but it may be very inefficient. Toward a fuller use of the data, Prentice [8] considered a model $\lambda(t; Z, W) = \lambda_0(t) \exp(Z'\beta)$, so that given Z, W is not a risk predictor, and derived the induced hazard function $\lambda(t; W) = \lambda_0(t) E[\exp(Z'\beta)|X \geq t, W]$ for nonvalidation sample members. The estimating equation (1) could again be used provided that the induced relative risk $E[\exp(Z'_l\beta)|X_l \geq t, W_l]$ can be appropriately estimated for the nonvalidation subsample. Hughes [5] considers a "naive" analysis that simply inserts $r_l = \exp(W'_l\beta)$ for nonvalidation samples, and shows that the bias in β estimation can be very large, particularly if β is large, in which case the condition $X \geq t$ becomes important as t increases, and the measurement error variation is large. Zhou & Pepe [15] consider the situation in which W is discrete, whence (1) can be applied with $r_l(t)$ a nonparametric estimate of $E[\exp(Z'_l(\beta)|X \geq t, W]$ formed from validation subsample members at risk at t. Asymptotic distribution theory that acknowledges the random variation in these estimated relative risks was also given. Zhou & Wang [16] consider an extension of this method to continuous regression variables using kernel estimation procedures, and noted that difficulties may arise if the number of mismeasured components of Z is large.

Prentice [8] suggested that when the failure probability is small and (Z, W) is jointly normally distributed, then $E[\exp(Z'\beta)|X \geq t, W]$ will be approximately proportional to $\exp[E(Z|W)'\beta]$, suggesting that (1) can then be applied with $r_l(t)$ set equal to a suitable estimate of $\exp[E(Z_l|W_l)'\beta]$. This approach of using a standard estimation procedure with the unavailable regression variable replaced by an estimate of its conditional expectation given the measured value has been termed "regression **calibration**" and has been presented as a mainstay approach in the measurement error monograph by Carroll et al. [2] (*see* **Measurement Error in Epidemiologic Studies**). Recently, Wang et al. [14] have studied the regression calibration approach in the Cox failure time model setting without making a small failure probability assumption. A validation sample was used to fit appropriate regression models for Z on W, and hence to "estimate" the expectation of Z given W. The method performs surprisingly well given its simplicity, although the bias in β estimation may become substantial as β becomes large, particularly if the variation in $W - Z$ may be large relative to that for Z. The authors are currently examining the extent to which such bias can be reduced by recalibration within each risk set, in which case a new regression line is fitted to approximate $E(Z|X \geq t, W)$ for use in the ith term in (1), with $t = X_i$, for nonvalidation sample members. Clayton [3] proposed a more restricted recalibration in which the regression line slope was held constant across risk sets.

Robins et al. [11] discuss semiparametric efficient estimation of β in the presence of a validation subsample. However, the semiparametric efficient estimating function does not have a closed form, so that a functional equation must be solved.

All of these methods, exclusive of the "complete-case" analysis, may break down if the selection probabilities into the validation subsample depend on the elements of Z that are mismeasured. Methods that appropriately condition on the risk set $R(X_i)$ in the ith term in (1) will generally remain valid if the validation subsample selection probabilities depend on the failure times X or censoring indicators δ.

Relative Risk Estimation with a Reliability Subsample

If a validation subsample is unavailable, one requires stronger assumptions to estimate the relative risk parameter β. A classical approach would suppose that a measured regression W_1 is available on the entire sample, that a repeat measure W_2 is available on a randomly selected subsample, and that Z and the errors $W_1 - Z$ and $W_2 - Z$ are mutually independent and normally distributed. It follows that $E(Z|W_1, W_2)$ is a linear function of W_1 and W_2 with coefficients that can be readily estimated, so that a regression calibration approach is again straightforward, with the possibility of risk set recalibration as necessary. These methods have not yet been examined in the literature.

The principal concern in the use of reliability subsample methodology relates to the impact of the strong measurement error model assumptions that are typically untestable. The assumption of independence of the errors $W_1 - Z$ and $W_2 - Z$ is of particular concern in the nutritional epidemiology setting, as persons who underreport the intake of a nutrient using one self-report instrument may also do so using other self-report instruments, as has been shown for protein and total calorie consumption using objective (biomarker) measures [7, 12]. Lack of acknowledgment of such measurement error correlations can evidently yield very biased results in the nutritional epidemiology setting [9]. Greater attention to the development of objective, even if noisy, measures of regression variables, and to corresponding measurement models and estimation procedures is needed in such contexts.

The methods summarized here can be generalized to allow time-varying regression variables. See [13] for an interesting illustration based on repeat measurements on a **time-dependent covariate**.

Acknowledgment

This work was supported by grant CA-53996 from the US National Institutes of Health.

References

[1]   Andersen, P.K. & Gill, R.D. (1982). Cox's regression model for counting processes: a large sample study, *Annals of Statistics* **10**, 1100–1120.

[2]   Carroll, R.J., Ruppert, D. & Stefanski, L.A. (1995). *Measurement Error in Nonlinear Models*. Chapman & Hall, London.

[3]   Clayton, D.G. (1991). Models for the analysis of cohort and case-control studies with inaccurately measured exposures, in *Statistical Models for Longitudinal Studies of Health*, J.H. Dwyer, M. Feinleib, P. Lipsert, et al., eds. Oxford University Press, New York, pp. 301–333.

[4]   Cox, D.R. (1972). Regression models and life tables (with discussion), *Journal of the Royal Statistical Society, Series B* **34**, 187–220.

[5]   Hughes, M.D. (1993). Regression dilution in the proportional hazards model, *Biometrics* **49**, 1056–1066.

[6]   Pepe, M.S., Self, S.G. & Prentice, R.L. (1989). Further results on covariate measurement errors in cohort studies with time to response data, *Statistics in Medicine* **8**, 1167–1178.

[7]   Plummer, M. & Clayton, D. (1993). Measurement error in dietary assessment: an assessment using covariance structured models, part II, *Statistics in Medicine* **12**, 937–948.

[8]   Prentice, R.L. (1982). Covariate measurement errors and parameter estimation in a failure time regression model, *Biometrika* **69**, 331–342.

[9]   Prentice, R.L. (1996). Measurement error and results from analytic epidemiology: dietary fat and breast cancer, unpublished manuscript.

[10] Prentice, R.L. & Self, S.G. (1983). Asymptotic distribution theory for Cox-type regression models with general relative risk form, *Annals of Statistics* **11**, 804–813.

[11] Robins, J.M., Rotnitzky, A. & Zhao, L. (1994). Estimation of regression coefficients when some regressors are not always observed, *Journal of the American Statistical Association* **89**, 846–866.

[12] Sawaya, A.L., Tucker, K., Tsay, R., Willett, W., Salzman, E., Dallal, G.E. & Roberts, S.B. (1996). Evaluation of four methods for determining energy intake in young and older women: comparison with doubly labeled water measurements of total energy expenditure, *American Journal of Clinical Nutrition* **63**, 491–499.

[13] Tsiatis, A.A., DeGruttola, V. & Wulfsohn, M.S. (1995). Modeling the relationship of survival to longitudinal data measured with error: applications to survival and CD4 count in patients with AIDS, *Journal of the American Statistical Association* **90**, 27–37.

[14] Wang, C.Y., Hsu, L., Feng, Z.D. & Prentice, R.L. (1997). Regression calibration in failure time regression. *Biometrics* **53**, 131–145

[15] Zhou, H. & Pepe, M.S. (1995). Auxiliary covariate data in failure time regression analysis, *Biometrika* **82**, 139–149.

[16] Zhou, H. & Wang, C.Y. (1998). Failure time regression analysis with measurement error in covariates, unpublished manuscript.

Ross L. Prentice, C.Y. Wang & X. Xie

Measurement Scale

Many different types of variables occur in statistical investigations. Some are merely classifications, such as a diagnosis into one of three unrelated diseases. Sometimes the classifications have an order, for example the stages of cancer or the common categorization into mild, moderate, and severe. For other variables the order is everything – "preference" recorded on a visual analog scale is an example. Here there are no categorical groups, and yet one can say that one score corresponds to a greater preference than another. Yet other variables seem to impose more sophisticated mathematical relationships between the possible values. With temperature, for example, we can say not only that one temperature is larger than another, but also that the difference between a given pair of temperatures is larger than the difference between some other pair. And, for other variables, we can go even further: for weight or concentration or height we can say that one is twice the other, or half again as large as the other. And, of course, yet other variables are simply counts – the number of cells on a plate, for example.

In fact, many different classifications of variable types have been proposed, often motivated from the perspective of statistical analysis: the set of techniques needed to analyze one type of variable often differs from that needed to analyze another type. However, one classification in particular has had a major impact on statistics. This is the classification into *nominal, ordinal, interval*, and *ratio* scales proposed by the psychophysicist Stevens [17, 18].

Prior to Stevens' work, the emphasis in understanding measurement had been in the physical sciences. The problems there, at least at that stage and at least superficially, seemed more straightforward. Measurement involved assigning numbers to represent the properties of objects, where the objects satisfied (i) an order relationship and (ii) a physical process of addition. The latter is illustrated by the placing of two objects in one pan of a weighing scales, and balancing them by a third object in the other pan. In terms of weight, this third object corresponds to the "physical addition" of the first two. Such a physical addition process is nowadays called *concatenation*. In such situations the notion of "quantity" seems relatively straightforward. Axiom systems describing (i) and (ii), which the objects must satisfy in order for the relationships between them to be representable by order and addition of numbers, were developed by von Helmholtz [22] and Hölder [7]. Campbell [2], in particular, adopted this approach. Of course, even here things are not completely simple: physical concepts such as density are defined in terms of other concepts. They have thus been called "derived" measurements, with the directly measured ones being called "fundamental measurements". Moreover, and more importantly, densities do not physically add in the same way as weight: combine two samples of gas with different densities and the result is something with an intermediate density, not the sum of the densities.

However, in other scientific areas, notably psychology, things are even less clear. In particular, there is often no "physical addition operation" evident. Because of this, notions of measurement in psychology came under much criticism [3]. Stevens tackled these criticisms by pointing out that the numerical representation preserving the relationships between a set of empirical objects was not unique and that the alternative numerical representations are obviously related since they represent the same empirical system. To get from one legitimate numerical representation to another, some transformation or mapping is involved. Stevens suggested that different such mappings defined different *types* or *scales* of measurement. Thus, if any one-to-one mapping was allowed (that is, any mapping which preserved the unique identity of the classes of objects), then the

measurement was on a *nominal* scale. For example, the appearance of a lesion may be classified into one of three distinct types. If any order-preserving mapping was allowed (that is, if any numerical representation which assigned numbers in the same order to the objects was allowed), then measurement was on an *ordinal* scale. For example, "severity" might be encoded so that any alternative encoding would be equally legitimate, provided it had the same order. If any linear transformation was allowed (that is, if rescaling the numbers by changing the units and then adding some constant resulted in an alternative numerical assignment which still preserved the relationships between objects), then the scale was *interval*. Body temperature is an example: this might be measured in degrees centigrade or degrees Fahrenheit, the two being related by a linear transformation. And, finally, if any change of the units yielded an alternative, equally legitimate numerical assignment, then the scale was *ratio*, for example, changing the units of length from inches to centimetres. The physical measurements with which Campbell was concerned were of this last type; Stevens thus generalized the notions of measurement. In each case the class of transformations which lead to another, equally legitimate, representation of the empirical system being modeled is called the class of *admissible* or *permissible* transformations. Mathematically, this class defines the scale being studied.

The notion of admissible transformations has implications for what statistical statements may sensibly be made using the data. If, for example, any numerical assignment which preserves the order of a set of values is equally legitimate, then comparing the arithmetic means of two groups is of dubious value: it may be possible to invert the relative order of the two means by a suitable choice of transformation. To illustrate, suppose that one numerical representation has the values $\{1, 5\}$ for the two objects in one group and $\{3, 4\}$ for the two objects in the other group. Then the mean, 3, of the first group is smaller than the mean, $3\frac{1}{2}$, of the second group. However, consider the alternative numerical assignment $\{1, 7\}$ for the members of the first group and $\{3, 4\}$ for the members of the second. This preserves the order of the numbers – the object which was previously assigned the smallest number has still been assigned the smallest number, and so on. But this new numerical assignment yields respective means of 4 and $3\frac{1}{2}$. Now the mean of the first group is larger than the mean of the second. In general, one's conclusions will be an artifact of one's choice of numerical assignment, and will not reflect any truth about the empirical reality. Thus it seems that statistical arguments must take account of scale type. However, the assumptions made by inferential statistical arguments are distributional, and not scale-specific. Indeed, given a set of numbers, no matter what their scale type, arbitrary statistical statements may be made about those numbers – one is able to compute a *t* statistic and carry out a *t* test whatever the scale type, and this might even seem a sensible thing to do if suitable distributional assumptions are satisfied. The tension between these two viewpoints has stimulated a major debate, running from the time of Campbell and Stevens right up to the present [5, 6, 14, 20, 21]. Its resolution is subtle and lies in awareness of the fact that the objective of statistical analysis is ultimately to make a statement about the empirical system being studied, and not simply about the numbers being used to represent that system. However, this needs to be tempered by the fact that statistical statements applied to what are apparently impermissible transformations of the data may lead to the detection of hitherto unsuspected structures in those data. It seems that if one wants to test strong theories, described in terms of numbers derived by a well-defined mapping from a well-understood empirical system, then the strictures imposed by the theory of scale types should be adhered to. But if one's theories are less stringently formalized, then the constraints of scale type are less important and, indeed, adhering to them may risk missing important discoveries (see [6] and the ensuing discussion).

The nominal, ordinal, interval, and ratio typology is an old one. Since its formulation a huge amount of work has been carried out, partly philosophical, concerned with relating measurement activities to scientific questions, and partly mathematical, concerned with developing axiom systems which an empirical system must obey if it is to be representable by a given numerical system. For reviews of this work see [8–10, 16, 19]. One conclusion of this work has been to show that, for mappings to the real numbers, only certain types of scales can exist, and that Stevens' ordinal, interval, and ratio classification is closely related to this set. However, an interesting anomaly is that for mappings to rational numbers there is an infinite variety of scale types [1]. Since all data are recorded to only a finite number of digits, scientific

mappings are in fact to only a subset of the rationals. Quite what the implication of this is, if any, remains to be seen.

Clearly, physical addition operations hold a central place in measurement theory. Such operations can be mapped to addition, so that very familiar numerical operations can be used. But they are not the only empirical relationships which can be mapped to addition. A completely different class of relationships arises in *conjoint measurement*. Suppose that the objects in the empirical system can be ordered according to attribute *A*, that each object can be described in terms of a pair of attributes (*B, C*), and that each of *B* and *C* can be ordered. Then, subject to certain conditions, it is possible to find numerical assignments such that the relationships between objects can be represented by addition between the assigned numbers (see, for example, [11] and [13]).

So far we have described the aim of measurement as being to assign numbers according to a numerical system within which the relationships correspond to those between the empirical objects. This approach is termed *representational measurement theory*, and is by far the best developed. However, it is not adequate for all situations in which measurement is used. In particular, in many areas of psychology this approach seems to be inadequate, chiefly because it is not clear precisely what empirical system is being modeled. As a consequence, alternative theories have been developed. Chief amongst these is the *operational* approach. This takes the measurement operation as *defining* the attribute being measured. As a consequence, no notion of permissible transformations, and consequently of scale types, can arise. Yet a third theory, termed by Michell [12] the *classical* approach, takes as its starting point that numerical quantities of attributes exist, with the objective of measurement being the determination of the magnitude of these quantities. A key driving force for both the representational and classical approaches is the desire to characterize the relationship between the empirical system and the numerical system. In the operational approach, however, with the assumption of an underlying empirical reality not being necessary, the emphasis is on internal consistency and reproducibility. One might describe the aims of the representational, operational, and classical approaches as being, respectively, to assign, define, and discover numerical representations.

As will be apparent from the above and from the reference list at the end of this article, much of the debate about the fundamental concepts of measurement has occurred in the psychological literature. This is not surprising: in psychology of all disciplines, measurement is difficult. Rarely can the attributes being studied be directly observed, so that subtle indirect measurement procedures have to be devised. Naturally this stimulates debate about the precise nature of the measurement activity and what the resulting numbers actually mean. Earlier manifestations of measurement theory in physics, most notably in *dimensional analysis* [15], although useful, stimulated little debate about underlying principles. Measurement procedures in psychology involve constructing complex instruments which often require collecting many scores or numbers which need to be combined using sophisticated statistical techniques to yield a final measurement. Examples of such methods include **paired comparisons**, Guttman, Likert, and Thurstone scaling factor analysis, and item response theory [4] (*see* **Psychometrics, Overview**). Measurement procedures in medicine can be equally complex: a prime example being attempts to formulate **quality of life** scales.

References

[1]   Cameron, P. (1989). Groups of all order-preserving homeomorphisms of the reals that satisfy finite uniqueness, *Journal of Mathematical Psychology* **31**, 135–154.
[2]   Campbell, N.R. (1920). *Physics: The Elements*. Cambridge University Press, Cambridge.
[3]   Ferguson, A., Meyers, C.S., Bartlett, R.J., Banister, H., Bartlett, F.C., Brown, W., Campbell, N.R., Craik, K.J.W., Drever, J., Guild, J., Houston, R.A., Irwin, J.O., Kaye, G.W.C., Philpott, S.J.F., Richardson, L.F., Shaxby, J.H., Smith, T., Thouless, R.H. & Tucker W.S. (1940). Quantitative estimates of sensory events, *Report of the British Association for the Advancement of Science* **2**, 331–349.
[4]   Hambleton, R.K., Swaminathan, H. & Rogers H.J. (1991). *Fundamentals of Item Response Theory*. Sage, Newbury Park.
[5]   Hand, D.J. (1993). Comment on "Nominal, ordinal, and ratio scales typologies are misleading", *American Statistician* **47**, 314–315.
[6]   Hand, D.J. (1996). Statistics and the theory of measurement (with discussion), *Journal of the Royal Statistical Society, Series A* **159**, 445–492.
[7]   Hölder O. (1901). Die Axiome der Quantitat und die Lehre vom Mass, *Berichte über die Verhandlungen der königlich Sächsischen Gesellschaft der Wissenschaften zu Leipzig, Mathematische-Physiche Klasse* **53**, 1–64.
[8]   Krantz, D.H., Luce, R.D., Suppes, P. & Tversky P. (1971). *Foundations of Measurement*, Vol. 1: *Additive and Polynomial Representations*. Academic Press, New York.
[9]   Luce, R.D. (1996). The ongoing dialog between empirical science and measurement theory, *Journal of Mathematical Psychology* **40**, 78–98.
[10] Luce, R.D., Krantz, D.H., Suppes, P. & Tversky A. (1990). *Foundations of Measurement*, Vol. 3: *Representation, Axiomatization, and Invariance*. Academic Press, San Diego.
[11] Luce, R.D. & Tukey, J.W. (1964). Simultaneous conjoint measurement: a new type of fundamental measurement, *Journal of Mathematical Psychology* **1**, 1–27.
[12] Michell, J. (1986). Measurement scales and statistics: a clash of paradigms, *Psychological Bulletin* **100**, 398–407.
[13] Michell, J. (1990). *An Introduction to the Logic of Psychological Measurement*. Lawrence Erlbaum, Hillsdale.
[14] Niederée, R. (1994). There is more to measurement than just measurement: measurement theory, symmetry, and substantive theorizing, *Journal of Mathematical Psychology* **38**, 527–594.
[15] Porter, A.W. (1933). *The Method of Dimensions*. Methuen, London.
[16] Roberts, F.S. (1979). *Measurement Theory*. Addison-Wesley, Reading.
[17] Stevens, S.S. (1946). On the theory of scales of measurement, *Science* **103**, 677–680.
[18] Stevens, S.S. (1951). Mathematics, measurement, and psychophysics, in *Handbook of Experimental Psychology*, S.S. Stevens, ed. Wiley, New York.
[19] Suppes, P., Krantz, D.H., Luce, R.D. & Tversky, A. (1989). *Foundations of Measurement*, Vol. 2: *Geometrical, Threshold, and Probabilistic Representations*. Academic Press, San Diego.
[20] Velleman, P.F. & Wilkinson, L. (1993). Nominal, ordinal, interval, and ratio scales typologies are misleading, *American Statistician* **47**, 65–72.
[21] Velleman, P.F. & Wilkinson, L. (1993). Reply to comments on Velleman and Wilkinson (1993), *American Statistician* **47**, 315–316.
[22] von Helmholtz, H. (1887). Zählen und Messen erkenntnis-theoretisch betrachet, *Philosophische Aufsätze Eduard Zeller gewidmet*. Leipzig. English translation by C.L. Bryan, *Counting and Measuring*. van Nostrand, Princeton, 1930.

(*See also* **Nominal Data; Ordered Categorical Data**)

DAVID J. HAND